Essentials of Maternal and Neonatal Nursing

Essentials of Maternal and Neonatal Nursing

Carole Ann Kenner, RN,C, DNS
Professor and Interim Department Chairperson
Parent-Child Nursing
College of Nursing and Health
University of Cincinnati

Aileen MacLaren, RN, MSN, CNM
Assistant Professor of Clinical Nursing
University of Miami

SPRINGHOUSE CORPORATION
Springhouse, Pennsylvania

STAFF

Executive Director, Editorial
Stanley Loeb

Director of Trade and Textbooks
Minnie B. Rose, RN, BSN, MEd

Art Director
John Hubbard

Drug Information Editor
George Blake, RPh, MS

Clinical Consultant
Maryann Foley, RN, BSN

Editors
Keith de Pinho, Nancy Priff

Copy Editors
Mary Hardy, Pamela Wingrod

Designers
Stephanie Peters (associate art director), Lesley Weissman-Cook (book designer), Maria Errico, Jacalyn Facciolo, Darcy Feralio

Typographers
David Kosten (director), Diane Paluba (manager), Elizabeth Bergman, Joy Rossi Biletz, Phyllis Marron, Robin Mayer, Valerie L. Rosenberger

Manufacturing
Deborah Meiris (manager), T. A. Landis, Anna Brindisi

Production Coordinator
Caroline Lemoine

Photograph Credits
Lennart Nilsson, from *A Child Is Born,* for fetal development; Harriette Hartigan, Artemis, for birth sequence.

Library of Congress Cataloging-in-Publication Data
Essentials of maternal and neonatal nursing [edited by] Carole Ann Kenner, Aileen MacLaren
    p.   cm.
    Includes bibliographical references and index.
    1. Maternity nursing.   2. Infants (Newborn) — Care.   I. Kenner, Carole.   II. MacLaren, Aileen.
    [DNLM: 1. Maternal-Child Nursing.   WY 157.3 E78]
RG951.E88   1993
610.73'62 — dc20
DNLM/DLC
for Library of Congress   92-49357
ISBN 0-87434-471-9   CIP

CONTENTS IN BRIEF

CONTENTS IN DETAIL

CHAPTER 3 Reproductive Anatomy and Physiology   38

Constance A. Bobik, RN, MSN

UNIT II   THE ANTEPARTAL PERIOD   48

CHAPTER 4 Conception and Fetal Development   49

Leonard V. Crowley, MD; Susan M. Cohen, RN, DSN

Bernadine Adams, RN, BSN, MN

Constance Sinclair, RN, MSN, CNM

Bonnie Mauger Graff, RN,C, MSN, CRNP; Christabel A. Kaitell, RN, BN, MPH, SCM; Joan Engebretson, RN, DrPH; Harriett Linenberger, RN,C, MSN, ACCE

CHAPTER 8 Nutrition and Diet Counseling 107

Ann Brodsky, MS, RD

CHAPTER 9 Antepartal Complications   119

Patricia Ann Mynaugh, RN, PhD; Catherine Dearman, RN, PhD

UNIT III   THE INTRAPARTAL PERIOD

CHAPTER 10   Physiology of Labor and Childbirth

Lynne Hutnik Conrad, RN,C, MSN

CHAPTER 11 Fetal Assessment — 196

Connie Marshall, RN, MSN, Perinatal Clinical Specialist

CHAPTER 14 The Second Stage of Labor

Donna J. van Lier, RN, PhD, CNM

Carole Ann Kenner, RN,C, DNS; Jan Weingrad Smith, CNM, MS, MPH

Aileen MacLaren, RN, MSN, CNM; JoNell Enfantis, RN, MSN, ARNP; Peggy J. Drapo, RN, PhD; Charlotte R. Patrick, RN, MS, MEd; Andrea O. Hollingsworth, RN, PhD

UNIT IV   THE NEONATE

CHAPTER 17   Neonatal Adaptation

Judy Wright Lott, RN, MSN, NNP

CHAPTER 18 Neonatal Assessment   350

Darlene Nebel Cantu, RN,C, MSN; Laura Rodriguez Vaello, RN,C, MSN, NNP; Carole Ann Kenner, RN,C, DNS

CHAPTER 19 Care of the Normal Neonate   381

Carole Ann Kenner, RN,C, DNS; Brook Gumm, RN, MSN; Mary E. Lynch, RN, MS

CHAPTER 20 Infant Nutrition

400

Gail Blair Storr, RN, MN, MEd

CHAPTER 21 Care of High-Risk Neonates and Their Families 422

Laurie Porter Gunderson, RN, PhD; Darlene Nebel Cantu, RN,C, MSN; Laura Rodriguez Vaello, RN,C, MSN, NNP; Ann E. Brueggemeyer, RN, MBA, MSN

CHAPTER 22 Discharge Planning and Care at Home   488

Brook Gumm, RN, MSN; Mary E. Lynch, RN, MS

UNIT V   THE POSTPARTAL PERIOD   511

CHAPTER 23   Physiology of the Postpartal Period   512

Deborah S. Davison, MSN, CRNP

Harriett W. Ferguson, RN,C, EdD; Sarah Elizabeth Whitaker, RN,C, MSN

Paula Maisano Herndon, RN, MS

Annette Gupton, RN, MN

ADVISORY BOARD

CONTRIBUTORS

Bernadine Adams, RN, BSN, MN
Associate Professor, School of Nursing, Northeast
Louisiana University, Monroe

Cynthia L. Armstrong, RN, MSN
Lecturer, Perinatal Graduate Program, School of
Nursing, University of Pennsylvania, Philadelphia

Constance A. Bobik, RN, MSN
Assistant Professor, Brevard Community College, Cocoa,
Fla.

Ann Brodsky, MS, RD
Former Nutritionist, Women's Health Practice,
Champaign, Ill.

Ann E. Brueggemeyer, RN, MBA, MSN
Manager of Education Services, Middletown Regional
Hospital of Nursing, Good Samaritan Hospital,
Cincinnati

Darlene Nebel Cantu, RN,C, MSN
Nursing Faculty, School of Professional Nursing, Baptist
Memorial Hospital System, San Antonio, Tex.

Susan M. Cohen, RN, DSN
Associate Professor and Director of Women's Health
Graduate Program, School of Nursing, University of Texas
Health Science Center at Houston

Lynne Hutnik Conrad, RN,C, MSN
Perinatal Clinical Nurse Specialist, Albert Einstein
Medical Center, Philadelphia

Leonard V. Crowley, MD
Pathologist, Riverside Medical Center; Visiting Professor,
College of St. Catherine, St. Mary's Campus; Clinical
Assistant Professor, University of Minnesota Medical
School, Minneapolis

Debra C. Davis, RN, DSN
Associate Dean and Director of Graduate Studies,
University of South Alabama, Mobile

Deborah S. Davison, MSN, CRNP
Certified Registered Nurse Practitioner, Western
Pennsylvania Cancer Institute, Pittsburgh

Catherine Dearman, RN, PhD
Associate Professor, School of Nursing, Troy State
University, Montgomery, Ala.

Peggy J. Drapo, RN, PhD
Professor and Director of Nurse-Managed Health Center,
College of Nursing, Texas Woman's University, Denton

Joan Engebretson, RN, DrPH
Assistant Professor, School of Nursing, University of Texas
Health Science Center at Houston

Harriett W. Ferguson, RN,C, EdD
Associate Professor, Department of Nursing, Temple
University, Philadelphia

Bonnie Mauger Graff, RN,C, MSN, CRNP
Clinical Faculty, School of Nursing, University of
Pennsylvania, Philadelphia

Christine A. Grant, RN,C, PhD
Assistant Professor, School of Nursing, University of
Pennsylvania, Philadelphia

Brook Gumm, RN, MSN
Clinical Nurse Specialist, Children's Hospital Medical
Center, Cincinnati

Laurie Porter Gunderson, RN, PhD
Associate Professor, College of Nursing and Health,
University of Cincinnati

Annette Gupton, RN, MN
Associate Professor, School of Nursing, and Director of
Manitoba Nursing Research Institute, University of
Manitoba, Winnepeg, Canada

Kathleen Convery Hanold, RN, MS
Director of Women and Infant Services, Barnes Hospital,
Washington University Medical Center, St. Louis

Paula Maisano Herndon, RN, MS
Nursing Education Coordinator, Saint Francis Hospital,
Tulsa, Okla.

Andrea O. Hollingsworth, RN, PhD
Associate Professor and Undergraduate Program Director,
College of Nursing, Villanova (Pa.) University

Christabel A. Kaitell, RN, BN, MPH, SCM
Assistant Professor, School of Nursing, Faculty of Health
Sciences, University of Ottawa, Ontario, Canada

Virginia H. Kemp, RN, PhD
Associate Professor and Director of Center for Nursing
Research, School of Nursing, Medical College of Georgia,
Augusta

Carole Ann Kenner, RN,C, DNS
Professor and Interim Department Chairperson, Parent-Child Nursing, College of Nursing and Health, University of Cincinnati

Harriett Linenberger, RN,C, MSN, ACCE
Student Education Coordinator, Hermann Hospital, Houston

Judy Wright Lott, RN, MSN, NNP
Director of NNP Program, Children's Hospital, Cincinnati

Mary E. Lynch, RN, MS
Assistant Clinical Professor, Department of Family Health Care Nursing, University of California, San Francisco

Aileen MacLaren, RN, MSN, CNM
Assistant Professor of Clinical Nursing, University of Miami

Sylvia A. McSkimming, RN, PhD
Associate Director of Nursing—Research and Education, St. Vincent Hospital and Medical Center, Portland, Ore.

Connie Marshall, RN, MSN, Perinatal Clinical Specialist
Vice President, Conmar Publishing, Inc., Fair Oaks, Calif.

Patricia Anne Mynaugh, RN, PhD
Assistant Professor, College of Nursing, Villanova (Pa.) University

Tommie P. Nelms, RN, PhD
Assistant Professor, School of Nursing, Georgia State University, Atlanta

Charlotte R. Patrick, RN, MS, MEd
Lecturer, College of Nursing, Texas Woman's University, Denton

JoNell Efantis Potter, RN, MSN, ARNP
Adjunct Instructor, School of Medicine, University of Miami

Constance Sinclair, RN, MSN, CNM
Nurse-Midwife, Valley Medical Center, Fresno, Calif.

Gale Robinson Smith, RN, PhD, CS
Assistant Professor, College of Nursing, Rutgers–The State University of New Jersey, Newark

Jan Weingrad Smith, MS, MPH, CNM
Nurse-Midwife, Metropolitan Hospital, New York Medical College, New York

Gail Blair Storr, RN, MN, MEd
Assistant Professor, Faculty of Nursing, University of New Brunswick, Fredericton, Canada

Laura Rodriguez Vaello, RN,C, MSN, NNP
Neonatal Nurse Practitioner–Clinical Nurse Specialist, Baptist Medical Center, San Antonio, Tex.

Donna J. van Lier, RN, PhD, CNM
Nurse-Midwife, Atlanta OB/GYN Associates

Linda Wheeler, MN, EdD, CNM
Associate Professor, School of Nursing, Oregon Health Sciences University, Portland

Sarah Elizabeth Whitaker, RN,C, MSN
Lecturer, College of Nursing and Applied Health, University of Texas at El Paso

Janet K. Williams, RN, PhD, CPNP
Assistant Professor, College of Nursing, University of Iowa, Iowa City

FOREWORD

Courses in maternal and neonatal nursing have changed over the last few years. Those that lasted 8 to 10 weeks—and sometimes 16 weeks—gave the student numerous opportunities and divergent experiences; but these are gone now. Today's typical courses are consolidated into 3, 4, 5, or 6 weeks. The course is intensive, attempting to provide all the necessary information in this shorter time while focusing on the key areas of assessment, normal growth and development, health maintenance, and health teaching.

Also, the semester in which the course is offered varies widely from institution to institution. Some offer this course at the end of the student's schooling, reasoning that the student can use the knowledge gained from medical-surgical courses and apply it here. Others offer this course at the very beginning of the student's schooling, using a developmental approach, focusing on maternal and neonatal events as part of normal growth and development.

No matter which combination of circumstances confronts the student or the instructor, *Essentials of Maternal and Neonatal Nursing* offers the flexibility to meet the needs. First, its organization into self-contained units (described below) enable its user to select elements for a shorter or longer course or to read selectively and intensively on a selected topic. The instructor also can easily use these self-contained units to reorder the information to meet a beginner's needs or a more experienced student's.

Second, this text intentionally provides practical health care knowledge to today's nurse who has to advise women and their families on such topics as family planning, the physiology of conception and fetal development, normal events of the antepartal period, nutritional needs of the pregnant client, the physiology of labor and childbirth, and care of the normal neonate. Additionally, the text meets the nurse's more technical needs by discussing fetal monitoring; neonatal, antepartal and postpartal assessments; the teaching of parents and families; discharge planning—and many other topics. *Essentials of Maternal and Neonatal Nursing* orients the nurse to performing procedures, identifying normal assessment findings, recognizing abnormal assessment findings, anticipating problems, identifying complications, responding to emergencies, and reviewing laboratory studies—all within the framework of the nursing process.

The text is divided into five units. Unit One, The Childbearing Family, focuses on a holistic, family-centered approach to care. It presents a framework for analyzing family structure and function, and describes the nursing process as it is used with the childbearing family. Then it discusses specific nursing care related to family planning, preconception health of the fertile couple, assessment and management of the infertile couple, and genetic screening and counseling. The unit concludes with a detailed discussion of the female and male reproductive systems.

Unit Two, The Antepartal Period, investigates the prenatal factors that enhance maternal health, promote a healthy intrauterine environment, and increase the odds for a healthy neonate. It helps the nurse promote maternal and fetal health by examining the events of pregnancy—from conception through the ninth month—and by delineating the prenatal care required by the pregnant client and her family. It discusses fetal growth and development, surveys the physiologic and psychosocial changes of normal pregnancy, discusses the effects of nutrition on fetal outcome, and details the nurse's role in maintaining high-quality antepartal care. To ensure a comprehensive presentation, this unit also discusses antepartal complications.

Unit Three, The Intrapartal Period, helps the nurse anticipate the needs of the childbearing family and promotes holistic care by emphasizing childbirth as a family-centered event. After describing the physiology of labor and childbirth, the unit explores nursing care related to fetal assessment, comfort promotion, and all stages of normal labor. Stressing health promotion as a nursing goal, it highlights various independent nursing roles, such as teaching, counseling, supporting, and advocating. Again, for comprehensiveness, this unit covers high-risk labor and delivery situations and special procedures.

Unit Four, The Neonate, prepares the nurse to care for the normal neonate, but addresses high-risk neonates and their families, as well. To do this, it investigates the characteristics of neonatal adaptation and relates them to the nurse's physical and gestational-age assessments of the neonate. Then, based on assessment findings, the unit describes nursing care of normal and high-risk neonates and their families. In addition, it discusses neonatal care in the home, where the nurse can gain valuable insights into the functioning, interrelationships, and resources of the family.

Unit Five, The Postpartal Period, begins by describing the anatomic and physiologic changes that restore the body to a nonpregnant state. Based on this information, it discusses nursing care to promote full postpartal recovery. Taking a family-centered approach, the unit also describes psychosocial adaptation to the neonate and explains how the nurse can promote adaptation to the new family structure for all members of the family. The unit also covers home nursing care for the postpartal client.

Eight appendices provide information that the reader will use frequently: the North American Nursing Diagnosis Association (NANDA) Taxonomy of Nursing Diagnoses; NAACOG (the organization for obstetric, gynecologic, and neonatal nurses) Standards for the Nursing Care of Women and Newborns; a Neonatal Weight Conversion Table; a Temperature Conversion Table; 1990 Nutritional Guidelines; Guidelines to Prevent HIV Transmission; Selected Resources for the Disabled Pregnant Client; and Support Resources for Families with Special-Needs Neonates.

A master glossary of more than 500 terms is followed by a thorough index that allows easy access to all information.

Because of reduced course length in many programs, students will have to rely on their textbook partly as a reference. *Essentials of Maternal and Neonatal Nursing* meets this need, too. Its presentation is structured around four recurring key areas: assessment, health maintenance, health promotion, and client teaching. Within this structure, it offers handy, helpful charts, boxed text pieces, and illustrations to assist with student learning.

Its unit organization reflects major instructional concepts; its application of the nursing process illustrates the dynamic connection between nurse and client; its end-of-chapter summaries and study questions encourage readers to test their mastery of essential information; and its chapter bibliographies group references by topic for further study. These features produce a resource that en-

courages critical thinking and fosters professional and attentive care. Written by nurses with outstanding credentials and experience, *Essentials of Maternal and Neonatal Nursing* puts clear, practical, and richly detailed information in the hands of those who need it most—students and practicing nurses who embrace maternal, neonatal, and family care.

Patricia D. Irons, RN, MA
Professor and Chairperson
Department of Nursing
Queensborough Community College
Bayside, New York

PREFACE

To be appropriate and effective, maternal-neonatal nursing care must encompass the three universal standards specified by NAACOG, the organization for obstetric, gynecologic, and neonatal nurses:

1. Care must focus on achieving optimum health potential within the framework of the nursing process
2. Health education must encourage participation in and shared responsibility for health promotion, maintenance, and restoration
3. Policies, procedures, and protocols must clarify the scope of nursing practice and delineate the qualifications of those who administer care.

Essentials of Maternal and Neonatal Nursing helps today's nursing students meet these challenges and standards. The textbook is intended for use in nursing courses that cover physiology, clinical obstetrics, family-centered care, and neonatal care. It provides a balance of these content elements and accurately reflects the nursing model of care, highlighting its holistic nature and focus on health promotion. Although the text was written especially for nursing students, it also will be useful to practicing nurses as a reference or refresher resource.

This succinct, yet comprehensive, textbook is practical, up-to-date, and easy to use. Fully in step with today's nursing curricula, *Essentials of Maternal and Neonatal Nursing* is designed for those who need a broad-based, fundamental understanding of the information and skills required to provide high-quality maternal and neonatal care.

The text consistently uses the nursing process as a format for each nursing care chapter, showing how to apply the nursing process to clinical practice. Each nursing care chapter includes assessment, nursing diagnosis, planning and implementation, and evaluation of care for the client and family. It concludes with documentation of the nursing process, reinforcing the need to assess and intervene accurately and thoughtfully.

The text also distinguishes itself by integrating the latest nursing diagnoses throughout. Each nursing care chapter contains an alphabetized list of representative diagnoses (including problem and etiology statements) ap-propriate for the types of clients the chapter addresses. In each of these chapters, nursing diagnoses also appear in italic type in the "Planning and implementation" section, explicitly linking nursing diagnoses and appropriate interventions. The Appendix includes the complete list of nursing diagnostic categories by functional pattern, as approved by the North American Nursing Diagnosis Association (NANDA).

As recommended by the Maternal-Infant Core Competency Project Regional Conferences, the text provides information in the three domains of learning—cognitive, psychomotor, and affective. It presents cognitive information clearly and logically with an emphasis on critical thinking. To address the psychomotor domain, it provides step-by-step instructions and illustrations for many clinical skills. For the affective domain, it includes a balanced presentation of various sensitive issues related to cultural considerations.

Essentials of Maternal and Neonatal Nursing is organized in five units—The Childbearing Family, The Antepartal Period, The Intrapartal Period, The Neonate, and The Postpartal Period. This organization encourages study of comprehensive and closely focused information, which also can be reviewed later with ease.

The first unit develops the relationship between the nurse and the childbearing family, highlighting family-centered care and use of the nursing process. All subsequent units begin with chapters that present basic information about anatomy, physiology, and, when appropriate, psychosocial concerns. This sets the stage for subsequent chapters in the unit, which move from nursing care for clients with normal findings to those with abnormal findings. The neonatal and postpartal units end with chapters on nursing care at home, a topic of increasing importance to nurses. The instructor who must teach a condensed maternal-neonatal class may choose to focus on chapters that present nursing care related to normal antepartal, intrapartal, postpartal, and neonatal findings.

Useful pedagogical devices assist the reader throughout. See the box on *Pedagogical features* for details. Throughout the text, sidebars and graphic materials hold

PEDAGOGICAL FEATURES

Essentials of Maternal and Neonatal Nursing uses recurring features and set-off material to highlight important themes and types of information. This treatment promotes access to and use of the information. Here are the features and their purposes.

FEATURES	PURPOSES
Learning objectives	• Focus the reader's attention on forthcoming information • Assist in review and recall
Psychomotor skills	• Provide illustrations and step-by-step instructions for detailed assessment techniques, treatments, or other procedures
Emergency alert	• Assists in rapidly identifying serious maternal or fetal problems, assessing their severity, and intervening appropriately
Family considerations	• Suggest appropriate nursing interventions for the client's family • Demonstrate holistic, family-centered care
Fetal status, Maternal status	• Assists the nurse in providing care for two clients at once through assessment reminders, special considerations, and nursing interventions
Cultural considerations	• Provide a short list of assessment tips and special considerations or interventions during care of a client from a culture other than the nurse's own
Client teaching	• Speaks directly to the client and provides useful instructions for self-care • Can be photocopied for the client to take home
Nursing diagnoses	• Present an alphabetized list of appropriate nursing diagnoses based on the chapter's content and the NANDA taxonomy.
Study questions	• Test the reader's understanding of concepts presented • Challenge the reader to recall and apply data
Chapter summary	• Restates major points from the chapter
Bibliography	• Guides the reader to additional resources on specific topics

the reader's attention, promote deeper understanding, and summarize data for easy recall. Vital nursing procedures and descriptions of anatomy and physiology are vividly illustrated. Bulleted lists and tables provide rapid review, and charts efficiently organize larger units of information.

Photographs illustrate noteworthy aspects of childbearing. These include award-winning photographs of fetal development by Lennart Nilsson and of a dramatic birthing sequence by Harriette Hartigan, a nurse-midwife.

Supplementary materials support teaching and learning with this text. For each text chapter, the *Instructor's Manual* includes a chapter overview, suggested lecture topics, suggested critical thinking activities, answers to study questions that appear in the text, and a test bank with answers and rationales. The *Manual* also provides separate pages of test and quiz questions suitable for photocopying plus overhead transparency masters on anatomy, physiology, assessment techniques, and clinical procedures. Test questions also are available on computer disk for the instructor who wants to add, delete, or modify them.

The *Manual* also includes an alternative Table of Contents for those instructors who need an abbreviated course. This alternative recommends 12 chapters instead of 26 and reduces the assigned pages from 610 to 330. Other chapters can be used for reference, or the instructor may elect to include some of them in a revised table of contents.

The text and its supplements reflect years of nursing expertise through its contributors and consultants from the United States and Canada. All contributors are at least master's degree-prepared practicing clinicians, academicians, or researchers. Furthermore, a panel of experts in maternal and neonatal health has reviewed each chapter, and a distinguished advisory board has overseen the total effect of the book. The contributions of all these experts give the student a comprehensive view of this nursing specialty – and a well-illustrated, clinically applicable, and up-to-date text that its readers can continue to use through their years of clinical practice.

UNIT I
THE CHILDBEARING FAMILY

FAMILY CARE

OBJECTIVES

After reading and studying this chapter, the reader should be able to:

1. Describe family care.

2. Discuss the functions of the family.

3. Discuss the various family types.

4. List functions fulfilled by the family.

5. Describe roles typically adopted by family members.

6. Describe the recent social, economic, and family nursing care trends that have affected women and the childbearing family.

7. Describe the important assessment areas for the childbearing family.

8. State examples of nursing diagnoses commonly used for the childbearing family.

9. Discuss approaches to evaluating nursing care and the information necessary for adequate documentation.

INTRODUCTION

Family care involves the delivery of professional, quality health care to all family members based on their needs. To understand those needs, the nurse must apply various family theories, consider the family's culture and religion, and have a working knowledge of family types, functions, roles and dynamics. A full understanding of family care also requires knowledge of the economic, social and political influences on the family.

Families always have needed nursing care to fulfill their health care needs. During the past fifty years, changes have radically altered family structure and function because of today's family variations, family nursing care must address multiple needs and be open and nonjudgmental. Also, the nurse must be aware of family functions and help the client who provides and seeks health care for the family.

Because a family of any type involves close personal relationships, alterations in the health of one member commonly affects other members. Typically, the family plays a critical role in maintaining and promoting the health of its members; and one family member controls the interactions with health care professionals. The nurse, therefore, should take a family-centered approach, drawing on the resources of family members while caring for one of them.

The nurse uses the nursing process to promote the health of the childbearing family by providing family-centered nursing care. This approach includes assessing each family member's health needs, identifying health deficiencies and strengths, and intervening with education and counseling to improve family health. The nurse also involves the client and her partner in health care decision making during pregnancy and after childbirth, such as where the delivery will take place—at home, in a hospital, or in a birth center—and how to participate in the delivery.

Chapter 1 discusses the family and nursing care. The chapter begins by describing some of the classic theories used to study and describe the family. It then discusses the various types of families and the functions of all families, then looks within the family to examine the typical roles of its members and the relationship among them. Finally, the chapter discusses recent trends affecting family nursing care, then describes each step of the nursing process plus documentation of care as it should be used by the nurse caring for the childbearing family.

When providing family nursing care to the client or her neonate, the nurse also cares for the client's family. For example, when providing postpartal home care, the nurse assesses how the client and her family function with the addition of a new member. Therefore, the nurse needs a working knowledge of family functions and dynamics.

THE FAMILY

Until recently, the family was defined as a unit with married parents and dependent children—the nuclear family. Today, however, that definition does not describe increasing numbers of family units. Many different combinations of people who live together may be a family.

FAMILY THEORIES

Many theories have been developed to describe family structure and function. These provide reference points from which to study and understand the family. Typically, sociologists view the family as an open social system in relation to other social systems, such as the church and school. Psychologists examine family interactions and relationships between selected individuals and as a whole. Anthropologists study the family in relation to its environment. Researchers from each of these disciplines use theories to consider the essential elements that define a family and provide a framework for organizing data on the family. The most important family theories include systems, structural-functional, developmental, interactional, and social exchange. (For more information, see *Family theories,* pages 4 and 5.)

FAMILY TYPES

The family is the basic unit of society. It is composed of two or more people who share emotional involvement and live in close geographical proximity (Friedman, 1986).

In the United States, the nuclear family has represented the traditional family structure. Its assignments of responsibilities has been linked to traditional sex-based roles. This family type, however, no longer adequately describes the American family. Contemporary families are changing dramatically in structure and function, adopting various arrangements that defy simple categorizing.

Various family types, ranging from the traditional nuclear and extended families to single parent and alternative life-style families, have evolved in recent decades. The most common family types include nuclear, extended, communal, single parent, blended, cohabiting, and homosexual. (For more information, see *Family types,* page 6.)

FAMILY FUNCTIONS

Nathan Ackerman (1972), well known for his family theory, believes that the family has two basic functions: to ensure the physical survival of the young, which requires providing food, clothing, and shelter; and to help family members grow and develop psychologically and socially. The basic functions—including physical safety, sustenance, personal nurturing, education, and socialization—apply to families everywhere, regardless of their composition, and are essential for maintaining societies (Friedman, 1986).

Physical safety. Young children are helpless and vulnerable; they depend on adult family members to manage and maintain a safe environment. In some cultures, ensuring physical safety may require weapons and physical barriers to protect family members from hostile forces. Although modern families do not face these overt threats, they may face the more subtle but no less hostile threats of drug abuse, interpersonal violence, and such health problems as contagious diseases.

Sustenance. The family provides sustenance to its members in the form of food, water, and shelter. Generations ago, most families provided that sustenance directly; they grew their own food, located and maintained their own water supplies, and built their own homes. With industrialization, however, many families shifted from an agrarian to an urban life-style and became consumers rather than producers. Currently, most families provide sustenance for members by purchasing goods and services. In fact, economic prosperity has become the focal point from which to define part of a family's success.

Personal nurturing. The family is responsible for providing affection, acceptance, and companionship to its members (Friedman, 1986); it is the primary source for personal acceptance, companionship, expression, self-esteem, and the fulfillment of individual goals. The need for love and belonging in a changing world is the foundation from which this family function emerges. Although the mother has traditionally assumed the primary role in providing attention and emotional support for the children, fathers increasingly are involved in this role. Family members demonstrate caring for one another by meeting individual needs for growth and personal fulfillment. The family also provides its members with psychological support, teaches younger members necessary social skills, and develops coping skills that benefit family functioning (Parsons and Bales, 1955; Hill, 1965).

(Text continues on page 6.)

FAMILY THEORIES

Many theories have been developed to describe family structure and function. The chart below describes the five most important family theories and how each applies in the case of a young couple after the birth of their first child.

DEFINITION	MAJOR CONCEPTS	APPLICATION TO NURSING
Systems theory		
• The study of individuals and families as entities rather than as parts of a whole; people are more than the sum of their parts and different from that sum also (von Bertalanaffy, 1969)	• Systems are organized complexities that reflect the influence of variables; family behaviors are determined by relationships among the members • Systems interactions are dynamic and unique • Changes that occur within persons, families, and environments proceed from the simple to complex • Regular changes occur in the evolution of all systems in predictable—but not static—patterns of growth and development • People are open, living systems, and families are always evolving • Every family system has boundaries (physical, emotional, or interpersonal spaces that separate family members), structure, and functions • Every living system has boundaries that maintain individual identity, regulate emotional intimacy, and define rules for relating, which provide the system's structure • Each family member must be allowed to function within personal boundaries, but at the same time remain related to one another • Family boundaries must be clear and flexible • Within the family structure, members carry out role-related functions	• The nurse would define the birth of the child as a creation of a new subsystem, which changes the original system • Open family boundaries facilitate adjustment and adaptation to new roles
Structural-functional theory		
Focus is on social order and how it persists in society	• Society is a system made up of many subsystems called institutions • Each part of society affects every other part; therefore, a change in one part may affect another part • Because society exists in a dynamic equilibrium, the system can function through most types of changes (Schulz, 1982) • Family, religion, and education are all part of the same social system, known as a society • An equal exchange of resources and services exists between the family and society establishing equilibrium (Brown 1931; Parsons and Bales, 1955; Malinowski, 1960; Winch, 1971) • Society persists through marriage, integration of new members, and the actions of members to preserve or alter the established system • The family protects group survival (Brown, 1931) and meets the basic needs of individuals (Malinowski, 1960) • Most children are reared to accept society's values and goals and to pass these to their children	• The nurse would identify the family as nuclear and would assess the couple's role relationships; new roles may be needed to fulfill additional family functions • The functions needed to be assessed include: —provision of a safe environment for the child —provision of sustenance and any needed economic adjustments —socialization of the child, including the couple's preparation for child rearing —affective needs of family members

FAMILY THEORIES *(continued)*

DEFINITION	MAJOR CONCEPTS	APPLICATION TO NURSING
Developmental theory		
Family defined as beginning with marriage, increasing when children are born, diminishing when children leave home, and ceasing when the married couple dies	• Each family member performs various roles and functions throughout the family life-cycle • Family life-cycle and associated tasks are categorized into stages reflecting major developmental steps in a family's life (Duvall, 1984) • Developmental stages are based on patterns of interaction that change with the size of the family, age of the oldest child, school placement of the oldest child, and the function and status of the family before and after the parents bear children	• The nurse would identify the family's developmental level and establish tasks to be completed • Assessment should focus on the family's developmental changes and should address: —adjustment of the new family unit —fulfillment of parental roles —identification and ability to meet the child's needs —adjustment to extended family relationships and role changes
Interactional theory		
Family viewed as an internal network of relationships (Friedman, 1986)	• Individual family roles develop from interaction between family members over specific situations • Those roles persist as long as family expectations remain constant in similar situations • Members are expected to live up to certain social expectations; they may define and redefine their own roles • Roles are not static but change to some degree as family members interact • A married couple's relationship influences each individual in the family, in turn influencing the marital relationship • Change in one partner affects the other, as does change in interactions with the rest of the family	• The nurse would explore the couple's perception of the child and the birth experience • The nurse should establish how the couple expects family roles to change
Social exchange theory		
Reciprocal relationship between partners and the interplay of individual motives, perceptions, and behaviors	• A reciprocal, mutually dependent relationship can exist in which something of value is given by both partners • Rewarding certain behavior will encourage repetition of that behavior • Profit (the reward of a relationship minus its cost) is influential in maintaining a relationship • Exchange of rewards and costs may accommodate and maintain the relationship (Hollander, 1978) • The individual weighs the outcome of an interaction, considers the consequences, and chooses a behavior that will minimize costs and maximize rewards • It emphasizes the individual at the expense of the family	• The nurse examines the interactions between family members and includes an investigation of perceived outcomes • The nurse asks the family members to consider the rewards, costs, and other effects of changes in their family structure and relationship

FAMILY TYPES

The chart below describes the most common family types in today's society.

TYPE	DESCRIPTION

Nuclear	• Is the most readily recognized family type
	• Consists of married couple and their dependent children
	• Lives in a relatively independent household removed from grandparents and other relatives
	• Includes variations:
	  —nuclear dyad
	  —middle-aged or elderly couple
	  —kin-network
	  —second-career family

Extended	• Includes the nuclear family and some or all of the members' relatives • Shares household responsibilities • Provides an overall support system for family members
Single parent	• Typically originates from divorce, death, adoption, unwed motherhood, or a personal choice to forego marriage • Has 90% of children living with the mother • Must perform the functions typically shared by two
Blended	• Is also known as a reconstituted family • Arises when one or both partners lives with children from a previous partner (one or both partners becomes a stepparent) • May have difficulties in establishing roles
Cohabiting	• Is also called a social contract family • Involves an unmarried couple living together in the same household (Cherlin, 1981) • Desire long-term intimacy without legal involvement
Homosexual	• Involves gay or lesbian partners who make an emotional and economic commitment to each other • Has no legal status in most states

Education. The family's educational function is multifaceted, incorporating classroom education, psychomotor skills, social functioning, and emotional and perceptual health. Although parents are not personally responsible for edu-

cating a child, they are responsible for ensuring that the child receives a formal education. In addition to formal education, families must prepare children to function in personal relationships and in society by teaching moral values, instilling a sense of purpose, and providing the direction and motivation needed to attain personal potential. The family's responsiveness to achievements is critical for a child and for building each member's desire to pursue new experiences throughout life.

Socialization. Families assume primary responsibility for teaching children how to be productive members of society. Schools, churches, and other institutions may assume some of this responsibility as well. Children receive their first and most intense socialization within the family, where they learn about values, culture, roles, and beliefs. This function perpetuates the family and prepares for the replacement of society's members. Participation in traditions and ceremonies helps families maintain their place in society and relationships within the family structure (Kertzer, 1989). Rituals may be linked to the family's changing developmental stage—such as graduations, marriage ceremonies, and funerals—and may serve to reinforce such family relationships as holiday celebrations. They may help maintain an ethnic consciousness, such as Bar Mitzvahs. Certain meetings and activities, such as the Girl Scouts, may help family members develop self-concept and personal identification.

FAMILY ROLES

Family members typically carry out their family functions by adopting recurrent patterns of behavior, called roles. These maintain family stability by providing predictability in family functioning. Adoption of roles may be conscious or subconscious; at times, roles may overlap among family members, or they may be unique.

A family's culture, religion, socioeconomic status, and developmental stage influence how roles are assigned and how members function in their roles. According to Beavers (1982), families that function well—mature families—tend to balance roles and functions, communicate openly, respect each member's individuality, and use coping mechanisms that encourage constructive adaptation to everyday problems and periodic crises. (See *Family maturity* for more information.)

Typically, roles correspond to a family's developmental stage, evolving as the family passes from one stage to the next. In the beginning family stage, for example, spouses typically collaborate on all roles. Working together, they provide all the family's needs, sometimes assigning pri-

FAMILY MATURITY

The way family members carry out their roles and relationships indicates the family's level of maturity.

Members of mature families:
• view individuality as an asset, a trait to be encouraged
• express their thoughts and feelings openly and take responsibility for the actions that stem from these thoughts and feelings
• consider the opinions of other family members, respecting each person's perceptions.

Members of immature families:
• are intolerant of divergent ideas
• tend to communicate in a rigid, automatic manner both verbally and nonverbally.

Family maturity tends to develop over successive generations; however, no family reaches complete maturity, and specific circumstances may affect maturity in successive generations. For example, a family member who suffered serious, chronic illness as a child may as an adult expect an inordinate amount of attention and aid from other family members.

mary responsibility for certain functions to one spouse. When children are born, the mother may assume most of the household and nurturing roles, and the father may control family finances. When children enter school, the mother may resume her career and the father may assume more household duties. As the children age, they typically take on roles that include increasing responsibility.

Family roles commonly reflect those the partners experienced in their families. For example, a man will tend to take control of family finances if his father had this responsibility. Role expectations for children also are guided, at least in part, by practices in the parents' families.

A successful family constantly monitors and responds to variables that affect its roles. The family assesses individual and group needs and acts to satisfy those needs through cooperation and healthy functional patterns. Members endeavor to fulfill role responsibilities, give and receive feedback, solve conflicts, and adjust roles as needed to allow each member to grow and develop in a safe, encouraging environment.

Types of roles

Roles may be classified as formal or informal. Formal roles usually are associated with position, such as marital or parental roles. Informal roles may correspond to the family's emotional needs or help to maintain family stability, such as a family scapegoat role.

Although some roles may change and adapt throughout the life of any family, others usually remain consistent, such as that of provider, nurturer, decision maker, problem solver, tradition setter, value setter, and health supervisor (Friedman, 1986). (For more information, see *Family roles,* page 8.)

TRENDS INFLUENCING THE FAMILY

In the late twentieth century, social, economic, and family nursing trends greatly affected families and their nursing care. Key socials trends include a decrease in family size, an increase in the number of women in the work force and of two-career families, and more active participation in health care. Economic trends include growing competition among health care facilities, a rise in consumerism, and the use of such cost-containment policies as prospective payment, alternative delivery systems, direct reimbursement, and regionalization of care, which have significantly changed health care delivery, client reimbursement, and facility operations.

For the childbearing family, nursing care and health care delivery have changed in the past few decades. Before obstetric nursing was a specialty, nurses who worked in obstetrics usually took care of mothers during delivery as labor room nurses or after delivery as postpartal nurses. They were supported by nurses who took care of neonates in the nursery. Each of these nurses took care of their part of the process.

Rubin (1961) was the first to separate maternity and obstetric nursing. She saw the obstetric nurse's role as limited to assisting the obstetrician in the delivery of neonates. The maternity nurse's role, on the other hand, was to help the client fulfill the maternal role. As more parents wanted to take part in deliveries and have their neonate remain with the mother, nursing had to change to provide the care the consumer wanted.

Today's maternity nurse is more of a generalist, taking care of the pregnant client from labor to delivery and then caring for the client and neonate until discharge. Because many facilities have replaced labor and delivery units and nurses with labor-delivery-recovery-postpartal (LDRP) units and maternity nurses, the maternity nurse typically works in an LDRP unit. This nurse plays an independent and interdependent generalist role (Gay, Templeton, Edgil, and Douglas, 1988).

On the other hand, the nursery nurse has become more of a specialist. The new technologies have required the development of neonatal intensive care units (NICUs) and nurses skilled in neonatal critical care. Although the healthy neonate usually receives care from the maternity

FAMILY ROLES

The chart below describes the most common family roles and the functions carried out in each of these roles.

ROLES	FUNCTIONS
Provider	• Ensures that family has food, clothing, shelter, and money • May be split by adult partners
Nurturer	• Offers love, support, care, and reassurance • Maintains or increases the other members' personal development • Usually assumed by one person
Decision maker	• Assumes responsibility for accountability • Assigns family tasks, delegates responsibilities, obtains information, and follows through on outcomes of decisions • Reinforces joint family decisions • Strives to make goals and dreams a reality
Problem solver	• Assumes job of family maintenance • Sets standards of behavior • Assists in modifying behavior when standards aren't met by family members • Includes tasks of disciplinary actions, labeling of behavior as acceptable or unacceptable, identifying deviations in behavior, and monitoring daily family interactions
Tradition setter	• Monitors and responds to anniversaries, birthdays, holidays, and family customs • Maintains family genealogy • Strives to enhance the family's understanding of its place in history and society • May create bridges to the past, with present, and beyond • Cares deeply about family origins and encourages other members to participate
Value setter	• Explores and clarifies the family's belief system • May try to control behavior based on personal beliefs • Establishes standards, allows latitude, and enforces acceptable behavior • Judges behavior on the specific circumstances involved, with judgments changing as the value setter's personal beliefs evolve
Health supervisor	• Examines well-being of family members • Suggests or dictates standards for bathing, eating, dressing, and exercise • Establishes responses to illness and health • Controls the family interaction with health care professionals

nurse, the sick neonate needs care from a neonatal nurse specialist.

NURSING PROCESS AND THE CHILDBEARING FAMILY

Nursing is involved in many of the concerns the family seeks care for today, such as birth options, contraception, maternity care, neonatal care, women's health care, and infertility studies. Today's nurse may assume many roles in family maternity care: direct caregiver, role model, client advocate, change agent, consultant, educator, manager, researcher, liaison, and innovator (Hamric and Spross, 1989; Ryan-Merritt, Mitchell, and Pagel, 1988).

The maternity nurse may decide to be a generalist or specialist in one of many nursing careers for the childbearing family. These career alternatives require different experience, education, and credentials.

The nurse's caring relationship with the client can be mapped out by using the nursing process—a system for making nursing decisions that includes assessment, nursing diagnosis, planning, implementation, and evaluation. The nursing process guides the nurse in providing quality care to the childbearing family in any setting. By following this process and supporting it with thorough documentation, the nurse can develop effective strategies to respond to current and potential needs and problems while promoting family health.

The nurse promotes the health of the childbearing family by providing family-centered nursing care. This approach includes assessing each family member's health needs, identifying health deficiencies and strengths, and intervening with education and counseling to improve family health. The nurse also involves the client and her partner in health care decision making throughout pregnancy and childbirth, such as where the delivery will take place—at home, in a hospital, or in a birth center—and how to participate in the delivery.

ASSESSMENT

Assessment, the first step in the nursing process, involves the orderly collection and careful interpretation of information about a client's health status. Information comes from interviews with the client or family members (subjective data) and from physical examination, medical records, diagnostic test results, and other medical or nursing sources (objective data). Together, subjective and objective data give the nurse information essential for developing an effective care plan.

ASSESSING THE PREGNANT CLIENT: AN OVERVIEW

Providing effective nursing care for the pregnant client requires assessment by the nurse throughout the antepartal, intrapartal, and postpartal periods. Each period presents its own nursing challenges and focus.

Antepartal period

Quality nursing care during pregnancy goes far in ensuring a positive outcome for client and neonate. Thorough, accurate assessment, an essential aspect of this care, begins with baseline data that will help guide subsequent assessment throughout pregnancy, labor, delivery, and the postpartal period.

Antepartal (prenatal) assessment focuses on physiologic, emotional, and socioeconomic considerations. Areas of particular importance include:
• nutrient intake, including unusual cravings
• extent of maternal discomfort and morning sickness
• learning needs related to preparation for labor and delivery
• fetal activity and uterine contractions.

The health history interview should explore the client's and family's attitudes toward the pregnancy and consider the physical, cultural, socioeconomic, genetic, and emotional factors affecting the client and family. If possible, antepartal interviews should include the client's partner, whose attitudes and adaptability may directly affect the client's attitudes toward her pregnancy, delivery, and childrearing.

Physical assessment centers on normal physiologic changes that occur during the stages of pregnancy as well as common indicators of problems that can occur at these stages.

Intrapartal period

Assessment during labor and delivery focuses on:
• the client's and fetus's physiologic adaptation to labor
• any abnormal or unexpected findings during labor
• the client's and family's psychological response to labor.

Relevant health history data include the client's preparation for and knowledge of labor and delivery, onset of labor (including

rupture of membranes, bloody show, and other indicators), and frequency and duration of uterine contractions.

Physical assessment typically includes examining the cervix for effacement and dilation and assessing fetal heart rate and other fetal and maternal physiologic data.

Postpartal period

Assessment after delivery focuses on the client's and neonate's physiologic status and the family's adaptation to a new member. Important factors in postpartal assessment include:
• maternal bleeding and uterine involution
• parent-neonate interaction

• the neonate's transition to extrauterine life (including skin color, respiratory effort, cardiac function, and other physiologic parameters)
• feeding and elimination patterns.

Assessment begins during the first meeting with a client and family and continues throughout the nurse-client relationship. Any change in the family—for example, in composition, socioeconomic status, health status, or relationships among members—requires reassessment and possible alteration in the nursing care plan. For a childbearing client, the nurse will find frequent reassessment necessary to identify the client's and family's changing needs during pregnancy, childbirth, and the postpartal period. (For more information, see *Assessing the pregnant client: An overview.*)

Assessment consists of two parts: health history (the major subjective data source) and physical assessment (the objective portion of the complete health assessment).

Health history

Giving insights into actual or potential problems, the health history provides the nurse with pertinent physio-

logic, psychological, cultural, and socioeconomic information in light of such factors as family life-style and relationships. The health history interview enables the nurse to determine client and family concerns, misconceptions, and other details related to bearing children.

During the health history interview, the nurse begins to establish a relationship with the client and family members based on trust and mutual respect. In addition to information specific to the client's childbearing concerns, the health history interview should supply the nurse with information about cultural, ethnic, religious, socioeconomic, and psychological influences on the client and family as well as information about the family's coping patterns.

Throughout the interview, the nurse must remain aware of verbal and nonverbal cues communicated by the client and family members. To interpret these cues accurately, the nurse must consider them in the context of psychosocial, ethnic, and cultural influences on the client's life. These influences may affect the way a client or family responds to pregnancy, labor and delivery, neonatal care, and other aspects of childbearing.

Physical assessment

After gathering the appropriate subjective information and establishing a rapport with the client during the health history, the nurse performs a physical assessment to collect objective data, which may substantiate or refute the nurse's or client's health concerns.

A physical assessment has three major components:
- general survey, including initial observations of the client's appearance and behavior
- vital signs (including temperature, blood pressure, pulse, and respirations) and anthropometric measurements (including height and weight)
- physical examination, including assessment of body systems, organs, and structures. (For more information on physical examination, see Chapter 7, Care during the Normal Antepartal Period.)

Although the extent of physical assessment varies depending on the client's individual needs, the health care setting, the nurse's level of training, and other factors, the nurse must examine every client to obtain basic physiologic data. During any physical assessment, the nurse should pay particular attention to areas associated with current physical complaints and past problems that the client may have identified during the health history interview. Complete physical assessment involves evaluating all physiologic systems in an organized manner, typically from head to toe or from least invasive (general observation) to most invasive (such as pelvic examination) procedures. Diagnostic studies provide additional important assessment information.

NURSING DIAGNOSIS

After completing the assessment step, the nurse analyzes the subjective and objective data obtained to formulate nursing diagnoses, the next step in the nursing process.

A nursing diagnosis is a statement of an actual or potential health problem that nurses are capable of treating and licensed to treat (Gordon, 1987). Of course, appropriate treatments may involve collaboration with other health care professionals. Determining one or more applicable nursing diagnoses for a client provides the basis for formulating an individualized, effective nursing care plan. Each diagnosis must be supported by clinical information obtained during assessment.

Nursing diagnoses provide a common language to convey the nursing management necessary for each client among the many nurses involved in that client's care. To help ensure standardized nursing diagnosis terminology and usage, the North American Nursing Diagnosis Association (NANDA) has formulated and classified a series of nursing diagnosis categories based on nine human response patterns. These patterns include:
- Exchanging (mutual giving and receiving)
- Communicating (sending messages)
- Relating (establishing bonds)
- Valuing (assigning worth)
- Choosing (selection of alterations)
- Moving (activity)
- Perceiving (reception of information)
- Knowing (meaning associated with information)
- Feeling (subjective awareness of information).

Within each pattern are NANDA-approved nursing diagnosis categories specific to that topic. For example, the human response pattern devoted to *relating* includes such diagnostic categories as "sexual dysfunction" and "parental role conflict." The complete list of NANDA diagnostic categories, arranged by human response pattern, is called the nursing diagnosis taxonomy. (For the complete list, see Appendix 2: NANDA Taxonomy of Nursing Diagnoses.)

Assigning specific nursing diagnoses involves several steps, including clustering assessment data, choosing the appropriate category, and adding specific client information.

Clustering assessment data. Designed to identify broad areas of client need, clustering begins with the nurse's review of assessment data for completeness and accuracy. Whenever possible, the nurse collects assessment data from all involved family members before making a diagnosis. Next, the nurse analyzes assessment data from different perspectives using standards of care, established physiologic norms, and information from other disciplines (psychology or social work to assess family relationships, for example, and sociology to assess cultural influences). Finally, the nurse determines how various data groups relate to one another, clustering them in appropriate groups. This step requires broad-based health care knowledge; the nurse should consult current literature or other health care professionals for help with unfamiliar subject areas.

Choosing nursing diagnosis categories. Using clustered assessment data to identify broad areas of client needs, the nurse chooses one or more appropriate nursing diagnosis categories from the NANDA taxonomy. Each category may address an actual or potential client problem.

Assigning specific nursing diagnoses. After choosing a nursing diagnosis category, the nurse appends specific client information to individualize the diagnosis. A complete nursing diagnosis has three segments: a problem, an etiology, and signs and symptoms (Gordon, 1987). The first segment is the nursing diagnosis category; for example, "ineffective breast-feeding." The second segment states the problem's etiology (causal or contributing factor or factors), introduced by the phrase "related to" or "secondary to." A diagnosis of ineffective breast-feeding could be related to insufficient milk production, for example. The third segment identifies any signs or symptoms that help clarify and individualize the nursing diagnosis. Thus, "ineffective breast-feeding related to insufficient milk production secondary to intermittent bottle feedings" is an example of a complete nursing diagnosis. (For more information on nursing diagnoses, see *Selected nursing diagnoses for the childbearing family,* page 12.)

In some cases, the nurse may need to formulate nursing diagnoses not yet included in the NANDA taxonomy. If this occurs, the nurse should attempt to maintain the three-part nursing diagnosis format.

PLANNING

After completing client assessment and formulating appropriate nursing diagnoses, the nurse develops a care plan appropriate for the client and family. Effective planning focuses on the client's specific needs, considers her strengths and weaknesses, incorporates her participation, sets achievable goals, includes feasible interventions, and is within the scope of the nursing practice setting.

Planning involves three basic steps: setting and prioritizing goals, formulating nursing interventions, and developing a care plan.

Setting and prioritizing goals. After establishing nursing diagnoses, the nurse sets one or more goals for each applicable diagnosis. A goal—the desired client outcome after nursing care—states what the nurse and client expect to achieve to minimize or eliminate a problem. Appropriate goals help guide the selection of nursing interventions and also serve as criteria for evaluating the effectiveness of the interventions. Goals should relate directly to the nursing diagnoses and reflect the desires of the client, family, and nurse, who work together to formulate them. Setting goals with the client helps ensure appropriate and realistic care planning, encourages her involvement, gives her a sense of control, and may improve compliance with the care plan.

An effective goal statement, or outcome criterion, is measurable, realistic, and stated so that the client and family understand it completely. It should include the desired client behavior and predicted outcome, measurement criteria, a specified time for attainment or reevaluation, and other conditions, if any, under which the behavior will occur.

As appropriate, the nurse emphasizes that many health problems are interrelated and can be approached simultaneously; one problem need not be resolved before another is addressed.

After goals are formulated, they must be prioritized. As in goal setting, the nurse should establish priorities together with the client and family. This involves ranking the nursing diagnoses and goals in order of importance, based on an accepted order, such as psychologist Abraham Maslow's hierarchy of human needs (the most frequently used order).

Goals may be short term or long term. Short-term goals may take priority over long-term ones. When prioritizing goals, the nurse and client should account for possible effects of the client's ethnic and cultural background, socioeconomic status, and other factors that can influence goal achievement.

Formulating interventions. After selecting and prioritizing goals, the nurse begins the next planning stage: formulating interventions to facilitate achievement of short- and long-term goals. Nursing interventions consist of strategies, actions, or activities intended to help the client reach established goals by diminishing or resolving problems identified in the nursing diagnoses.

The nurse and client should work together to formulate interventions, analyzing possible strategies and choosing those that seem most likely to achieve goals based on the client's particular circumstances. Interventions may be interdisciplinary, possibly including nursing and medical care, physical therapy, nutritional counseling, social services, and others.

Effective nursing interventions must be based on sound nursing practice, which stems from sound research. Such a knowledge base provides the proper rationales for nursing interventions. The body of knowledge addressing nursing interventions and their effectiveness is increasing; important nursing research studies and other current information can be found in nursing journals, textbooks, and other publications. If possible, the nurse also may consult maternal and neonatal health experts to obtain the latest information on aspects of practice.

Developing a nursing care plan. The nurse develops a nursing care plan by integrating each step of the nursing process: collecting and analyzing health history and physical as-

SELECTED NURSING DIAGNOSES FOR THE CHILDBEARING FAMILY

Listed below under broad topics are examples of nursing diagnoses adapted to clients in maternal and neonatal health settings. These and other diagnoses appear together with related interventions in the "Planning and implementation" section of selected chapters throughout this text. For ease of recognition, nursing diagnoses appear in italic type in individual chapters.

Sexuality concerns
- Altered role performance related to fear of pregnancy
- Altered sexuality patterns related to pregnancy
- Anxiety related to sexual intercourse during pregnancy
- Anxiety related to sexual misinformation
- Body-image disturbance related to pregnancy
- Pain related to sexual position, secondary to pregnancy

Preconception planning
- Altered family processes related to decision to conceive
- Altered nutrition: less than body requirements, related to impending pregnancy
- Altered role performance related to impending pregnancy
- Anxiety related to the decision to conceive
- Body-image disturbance related to impending pregnancy
- Health-seeking behaviors related to contraception
- Knowledge deficit related to contraception and conception
- Knowledge deficit related to self-care activities before conception
- Personal identity disturbance related to the decision to conceive

Infertility
- Altered family processes related to the stress of infertility
- Anticipatory grieving related to infertility
- Anxiety related to infertility tests
- Body-image disturbance related to infertility
- Impaired adjustment related to childlessness
- Ineffective family coping: compromised, related to infertility
- Knowledge deficit related to factors that promote fertility
- Pain related to endometrial biopsy
- Powerlessness related to inability to control fertility
- Social isolation related to lack of children

Genetic disorders
- Altered parenting related to having a child with a genetic defect
- Anxiety related to unknown future health of offspring
- Health-seeking behaviors related to genetic testing
- Ineffective family coping: compromised, related to fear of abnormality in offspring
- Self-esteem disturbance related to awareness of having produced a child with a genetic defect
- Social isolation related to perceived lack of support during decisions regarding pregnancy termination
- Spiritual distress related to possibility of altering reproductive outcome

Labor
- Altered tissue perfusion: decreased placental, related to maternal position
- Impaired gas exchange related to hyperventilation with increasing contractions
- Impaired physical mobility related to electronic fetal monitoring equipment
- Ineffective individual coping related to lack of family support
- Knowledge deficit related to the labor process
- Self-care deficit related to limited mobility during labor

Normal neonate
- Altered parenting related to the addition of a new family member
- Altered patterns of urinary elimination related to renal immaturity
- High risk for fluid volume deficit related to insensible fluid losses
- High risk for infection related to umbilical cord healing
- High risk for injury related to inability to process vitamin K
- Hypothermia related to cold stress
- Ineffective breathing pattern related to transition to the extrauterine environment

Infant nutrition
- Altered family processes related to infant feeding
- Altered sexuality patterns related to requirements of the breast-feeding infant
- Anxiety related to the ability to properly feed the infant
- Body-image disturbance related to physiologic changes secondary to breast-feeding
- High risk for injury related to improper nipple care
- Ineffective breast-feeding related to improper positioning at the breast
- Interrupted breast-feeding related to maternal infection and use of antibiotics
- Sleep pattern disturbance related to the infant's nutritional needs

Comfort promotion
- Anxiety related to labor pain
- Decreased cardiac output related to epidural anesthesia
- Ineffective airway clearance related to general anesthesia
- Knowledge deficit related to analgesia and anesthesia options
- Self-esteem disturbance related to inability to cope with labor pain or negative perception of behavior
- Urinary retention related to spinal anesthesia

sessment data, selecting nursing diagnoses, setting and prioritizing goals, formulating interventions, and evaluating outcomes. The care plan, which can be revised and updated as needed, acts as a written guide for and documentation of a client's care. Also, it helps ensure continuity of care when the client interacts with many nurses, and it facilitates collaboration by all involved health care providers.

The format of nursing care plans varies among health care facilities and sometimes among units in the same facility. All care plans, however, include written nursing diagnoses, goals, interventions, and evaluation criteria. Standardized care plans recently have evolved as a time-saving and efficient method of ensuring documentation of the nursing process approach to care. A standardized care plan incorporates the major aspects of nursing care required by clients with a similar problem, while allowing alterations to reflect individual differences. Such a care plan may be particularly valuable for a client undergoing a short hospitalization with only minor deviations from previous health status, such as a client who experienced an uncomplicated labor and delivery.

IMPLEMENTATION

The next step in the nursing process, implementation involves working with the client and family to accomplish the designated interventions and move toward the desired outcomes. Effective implementation requires a sound understanding of the care plan and collaboration among the client, family, and other members of the health care team, as needed. The implementation phase begins as soon as the care plan is completed and ends when the established goals are achieved. Before and during implementation of any interventions, the nurse reassesses the client as needed to ensure that planned interventions continue to be appropriate. Periodic reassessment helps ensure a flexible, individualized, and effective care plan.

To implement nursing interventions effectively, the nurse needs four types of skills:
- cognitive skills, based on knowledge of current clinical practice and basic sciences
- affective skills, including verbal and nonverbal communication and empathy
- psychomotor skills, involving both mental and physical activity and encompassing traditional nursing actions (for example, taking vital signs and administering medications) and more complex procedures (for example, fetal monitoring)
- organizational skills, such as counseling, managing, and delegating.

EVALUATION

Through evaluation, the nurse obtains additional subjective and objective assessment data that relate to the goals identified in the nursing diagnoses. The nurse then uses these data to determine whether goals have been met, partially met, or unmet. Although evaluation comprises the final step in the nursing process, it actually occurs throughout, particularly during implementation, where the nurse continually reassesses the effect of interventions. Evaluation is directly linked to and must be based on the goals developed for each nursing diagnosis.

When all goals for a particular nursing diagnosis have been met, the nurse and client may decide that the diagnosis is no longer valid. The nurse then documents which goals were met and how and may delete the diagnosis from the nursing care plan. Alternatively, the nurse and client may judge a goal met but still feel that the nursing diagnosis is valid and decide to retain it in the care plan.

If goals have been unmet or only partially met by the target date for goal achievement, the nurse must reevaluate the care plan. Reevaluation involves deciding whether the initial plan was appropriate, whether the time assigned to the plan was realistic, whether the initial goals were realistic and measurable, and whether other factors interfered. Based on this information, the nurse can clarify or amend the assessment data base, reexamine and correct the nursing diagnoses as necessary, establish new goals reflecting the revised diagnoses, and devise new interventions for achieving these goals. The nurse then adds the revised care plan to the original document and records the rationale for these revisions in the nursing notes.

DOCUMENTATION

Although not usually identified as a nursing process step, documentation of nursing care nevertheless is essential to effective care. Documentation serves several functions: It provides communication among members of the health care team, it functions as a discharge planning and quality assurance tool, and it establishes a legal record of care provided.

The nurse may document various care measures—including verbal communication, care plans, team meetings, and staff reports—in the client record.

The client record also serves as legal documentation of the care provided by the health care team. The nurse is bound by law to document accurately and completely all nursing care provided as well as the client's response to that care. Client records commonly are reviewed in litigation regarding alleged malpractice; in the eyes of the

DOCUMENTATION GUIDELINES

Documentation requirements vary among institutions; however, regardless of the format used, data must be documented according to the guidelines listed below.

- Use the appropriate form and write only in ink.
- Write the client's name and identification number on each page.
- Record the date and time of each entry.
- Use only standard accepted abbreviations.
- Document symptoms in the client's own words.
- Be specific; avoid generalizations and vague expressions.
- Write on every line; leave no blank spaces.
- If a certain space does not apply to the client, write NA (not applicable) in the space.
- Do not backdate or squeeze new writing into a previously documented entry.
- Never document another nurse's work.
- Do not record value judgments and opinions.
- Sign every entry with the initial of your first name, last name, and title.

court, if a care measure is not documented on the patient record, it was not provided. (See *Documentation guidelines* for more information.)

The complete client record must be readily accessible to all health care team members at all times. Each institution also must develop mechanisms for ensuring confidentiality of records (American Nurses' Association, 1976).

Regulations regarding the minimal frequency of documentation relative to client status may differ among states and institutions. In all cases, the nurse must use sound professional judgment and document all care provided to help ensure appropriate communication of information and provision of quality care.

CHAPTER SUMMARY

Chapter 1 provided an overview of families and nursing care. Here are the chapter highlights.

Modern families are diverse; no longer can the traditional nuclear family (married parents and dependent children) be considered the only norm.

Family theories allow researchers and clinicians to understand the family by focusing on selected aspects, such as individual relationships and interaction with the environment.

The family's basic functions are to provide its members with physical safety, sustenance, personal nurturing, education, and socialization.

Family members typically adopt certain roles—recurrent patterns of behavior—to allow families to function with some degree of continuity. Roles adopted by one or more family members include provider, nurturer, decision maker, problem solver, tradition setter, value setter, and health supervisor.

Recent social trends that have affected the family include decreased family size, increased numbers of women working outside the home, increased number of two-career families, and the move toward active participation in health care.

Economic trends include growing competition among health care facilities, a rise in consumerism, and the use of such cost-containment policies as prospective payment, alternative delivery systems, direct reimbursement, and regionalization of care, which have significantly changed health care delivery, client reimbursement, and facility operations.

The nurse uses the nursing process in caring for the childbearing family. The nursing process is dynamic and ongoing, with steps typically occurring simultaneously.

Assessment, the foundation for the other steps, involves collecting subjective and objective data about a client's health status. When assessing the health of the childbearing family, the nurse looks for cultural, religious, and socioeconomic factors that influence the client's perception of health and health care, life-style, and childbearing practices.

The nurse organizes and analyzes assessment data to formulate nursing diagnoses, which form the framework for the nursing care plan.

Together, the nurse and family plan goals and interventions to achieve desired outcomes. Planning and implementation require the cooperation of the client, family, nurse, and other health care team members.

Evaluation, commonly viewed as the last step, continues throughout client care, reviewing the client's status in relation to the established goals.

Documentation of the nursing process must be accurate, thorough, concise, current, and in keeping with institutional policy.

STUDY QUESTIONS

1. Discuss the major concepts of the systems theory as it relates to families.

2. How have nursing care and health care delivery changed for the childbearing family?

3. What assessment information is important for the pregnant client during the antepartal period?

4. When planning the care for the childbearing family, what three steps are important?

5. Explain the four types of skills needed by the nurse to implement nursing interventions effectively.

BIBLIOGRAPHY

Ackerman, N. (1972). *Psychodynamics of family life: Diagnosis and treatment of family relationships.* New York: Basic Books.

American Nurses' Association (1976). *Code for nurses with interpretive statements.* Kansas City, MO: American Nurses' Association.

Beavers, W.R. (1982). Healthy, midrange, and severely dysfunctional families. In F. Walsh (Ed.), *Normal family processes* (pp. 45-66). New York: Guilford Press.

Bowen, M. (1978). *Family therapy in clinical practice.* Northvale, NJ: Aronson.

Brown, R. (1931). The organization of Australian tribes. *Journal of Oceania.*

Doherty, W.J., and Jacobsen, N.S. (1982). Marriage and the family. In B.B. Wolman and G. Stricker (Eds.), *Handbook of developmental psychology.* Englewood Cliffs, NJ: Prentice-Hall.

Erikson, E. (1950). *Childhood and society.* New York: Norton.

Friedman, M. (1986). *Family nursing: Theory and assessment.* New York: Appleton-Century-Crofts.

Gay, J., Templeton, J., Edgil, A., and Douglas, A. (1988). Reva Rubin revisited. *JOGNN,* 17(6), 394-399.

Hamric, A., and Spross, J. (1989). *The clinical nurse specialist in theory and practice* (2nd ed.). Philadelphia: Saunders.

Hoff, L. (1989). *People in crisis: Understanding and helping* (3rd ed.). Redwood City, CA: Addison-Wesley.

Hollander, E. (1978). *Leadership dynamics.* New York: Free Press.

Kerr, M., and Bowen, M. (1988). *Family evaluation: An approach based on Bowen theory.* New York: Norton.

Kertzer, D.I. (1989). Lasting rites. *Networker,* July-August, 21-29.

Logan, B., and Dawkins, C. (1986). *Family centered nursing in the community.* Menlo Park, CA: Addison-Wesley.

Malinowski, B. (1960). *A scientific theory of culture.* New York: Oxford University Press.

North American Nursing Diagnosis Association (1990). *Taxonomy I-Revised, with official diagnostic categories.* St. Louis: NANDA.

Parsons, R., and Bales, R.F. (1955). *Family, socialization, and interaction process.* New York: Free Press.

Paxton, J. (Ed.) (1988). *The statesman's year-book. World gazetteer* (3rd ed.). New York: St. Martin's Press.

Ryan-Merritt, M., Mitchell, C., and Pagel, I. (1988). Clinical nurse specialist role definition and operationalization. *Clinical Nurse Specialist,* 2(3), 132-137.

U.S. Bureau of the Census (1987). *Statistical abstract of the United States: 1988* (108th ed.). Washington, DC: U.S. Government Printing Office.

Family theories

Carter, E., and McGoldrick, M. (1988). The family life cycle and family therapy: An overview. In E. Carter and M.K. McGoldrick (Eds.), *The family life cycle: A framework for family therapy* (2nd ed.; pp. 3-20). New York: Gardner Press.

Chadwick-Jones, J.K. (1976). *Social exchange theory: Its structure and influence in social psychology.* New York: Academic Press.

Duvall, E. (1984). *Marriage and family development* (6th ed.). New York: Harper and Row.

Lidz, T. (1983). *The person: His and her development throughout the life cycle.* New York: Basic Books.

Von Bertalanaffy, L. (1969). *General systems theory.* New York: George Braziller.

Family types

Cherlin, A. (1981). *Marriage, divorce, remarriage.* Cambridge, MA: Harvard University Press.

Hill, R. (1965). Generic features of families under stress. In H. Pared (Ed.), *Crisis intervention: Selected readings* (pp. 32-52). New York: Family Service Association of America.

Schulz, D. (1982). *The changing family: Its functions and future* (3rd ed.). Englewood Cliffs, NJ: Prentice-Hall.

Winch, R.F. (1971). *The modern family.* New York: Holdt, Rinehart and Winston.

Recent trends

Centers for Disease Control (1988). Progress toward achieving the 1990 objectives for pregnancy and infant health. *MMWR,* 37(26), 405-413.

Creasy, R., and Resnik, R. (1989). *Maternal-fetal medicine: Principles and practice* (2nd ed.). Philadelphia: Saunders.

Flanagan, J. (1986). Childbirth in the eighties: What next? When alternatives become mainstream. *Journal of Nurse-Midwifery,* 31(4), 194-199.

Hill, D. (1982). Economic constraints in the health care delivery system. In J. Lancaster and W. Lancaster (Eds.), *Concepts for advanced nursing practice: The nurse as a change agent* (pp. 200-215). St. Louis: Mosby.

National Perinatal Association (1989). *NPA Bulletin,* 4(1), Alexandria, VA: Author.

Rubin, R. (1961). Basic maternal behaviors. *Nursing Outlook,* 9(11), 683-686.

Santi, L. (1987). Change in the structure and size of American households: 1970-1985. *Journal of Marriage and the Family,* 49(4), 833-937.

Nursing process

Alfaro, R. (1990). *Applying nursing diagnosis and nursing process: A step-by-step guide* (2nd ed.). Philadelphia: Lippincott.

Carpenito, L. (1989). *Nursing diagnosis: Application to clinical practice* (3rd ed.). Philadelphia: Lippincott.

Doenges, M., Kenty, J., and Moorhouse, M. (1988). *Maternal-newborn care plans: Guidelines for client care.* Philadelphia: F.A. Davis.

Gordon, M. (1987). *Nursing diagnosis: Process and application* (2nd ed.). New York: McGraw-Hill.

Morton, P. (1989). *Health assessment in nursing.* Springhouse, PA: Springhouse Corporation.

Popkess-Vawter, S., and Pinnell, N. (1987). Should we diagnose strengths? Yes—Accentuate the positive. *AJN,* 87(9), 1211-1216.

Stevens, K. (1988). Nursing diagnosis in wellness childbearing settings. *JOGNN,* 17(5), 329-335.

Stolte, K.M. (1986). Nursing diagnosis and the childbearing woman. *MCN,* 11(1), 13-15.

CHAPTER 2

PRECONCEPTION PLANNING AND CARE

OBJECTIVES

After reading and studying this chapter, the reader should be able to:

1. Describe the nurse's role in preconception planning.

2. Identify the risk factors detected during preconception assessment.

3. Discuss the nursing process steps when caring for the fertile client who desires preconception planning.

4. Explain the diagnostic tests used to identify genetic disorder risk factors.

5. Discuss the nursing process steps when caring for the client who has or is at risk for genetic disorders.

INTRODUCTION

Most women assume that pregnancy and child rearing will be a natural part of their adult lives. Many clients prefer to plan the number and timing of births in their family. When clients feel ready to have a child, they may seek help with preconception planning to pave the way for a normal pregnancy and a healthy child. When a client is considering pregnancy, the nurse can enhance health and well-being by assessing the risk of genetic disorders and providing information and services needed to address the client's problems and concerns.

Chapter 2 discusses the nurse's role in assisting the client with preconception planning. It begins by discussing the essential components of male and female fertility. Next, the chapter presents preconception planning for the fertile couple, highlighting nursing interventions that can promote preconception health and minimize risk factors during pregnancy. Lastly, the chapter discusses the care appropriate for clients concerned about genetic disorders. Throughout, the chapter emphasizes the nursing process.

THE FERTILE COUPLE

Fertility results from complex interactions between the hypothalamus, central nervous system, gonads, and pituitary, thyroid, and adrenal glands.

For conception to occur, several events must take place in an environment conducive to ovum fertilization and embryo implantation and growth. The client's ovaries must produce an ovum, and her body must produce sufficient gonadotropic hormones to allow ovum maturation and release. Her partner's testes must produce sufficient mature, motile spermatozoa (sperm), which must travel through his reproductive system and be ejaculated into her vagina. His reproductive system must produce secretions that permit sperm motility; her vaginal and cervical secretions must allow sperm survival. The ovum must enter a patent fallopian tube at the same time that sperm are present in the tube's distal end. The sperm must penetrate the ovum, and the fertilized ovum then must move through the fallopian tube to the uterus.

The client's endometrium must have had sufficient hormonal stimulation to allow implantation of the embryo. Her body must maintain appropriate hormone levels to create a uterine environment that allows the embryo to develop and the pregnancy to continue. If any of these events is interrupted or abnormal, fertilization will not occur or the pregnancy will not be sustained.

To help ensure a normal pregnancy and healthy fetus, the client should begin planning well before conception. Ideally, she should develop and maintain good health habits as soon as she decides to have a child. This is because the embryo's organs are especially sensitive during early development — when the client may not know she is pregnant. Also, pregnancy-related changes may distract the client from focusing on new health habits.

The nurse should pay close attention to the client's developmental status during the preconception stage for insights into the client's motivation and the likelihood of a successful pregnancy.

Whenever possible, the client's partner should be involved in decision making and in preconception planning. For any couple, the decision to become parents should be based on their desires and developmental status as well as their current demands and resources.

ASSESSMENT

To assess the couple's needs related to preconception planning, the nurse obtains a health history and assists with a physical examination and diagnostic studies, as ordered.

Health history

A thorough health history of the client and her partner can provide data that will aid in planning a healthy pregnancy. It also can identify a client who is at high risk for maternal and fetal complications during pregnancy. Demographic data can help make this identification. For example, a client from a low socioeconomic group is more likely to have inadequate prenatal care, poor nutrition, and a poor overall health status. A neonate born to such a client is at high risk for low birth weight and prematurity. (For more information, see *Preconception risk factor identification.*)

In the past, health care professionals focused only on the client's health history. Now, they also assess the partner because research suggests that the partner's health can affect a developing fetus. Also, his positive health habits can serve as a role model to the client and increase her motivation to maintain a healthful life-style before and during pregnancy.

When obtaining a health history from individuals who need help with preconception planning, ask questions about the following topics:
• biographical data
• menstrual and gynecologic history
• obstetric history (including family history)
• medical history
• health care activities

PRECONCEPTION RISK FACTOR IDENTIFICATION

Certain demographic, obstetric, medical, nutritional, and other factors may place a client and fetus at risk for problems during pregnancy. When obtaining a client's preconception health history, the nurse should be especially alert for these factors to help prevent potential problems.

Demography
• Age 15 or younger
• Age 35 or older
• Nonwhite
• Unmarried
• Low socioeconomic status
• Lack of transportation
• Location in rural or isolated area

Obstetric history
• Previous spontaneous or elective abortion
• Previous premature neonate
• Previous perinatal death
• Previous neonate with a congenital anomaly
• Maternal anatomic difficulty, such as a severely retroflexed uterus or a pelvis too small for a normal delivery
• Previous pregnancy-induced hypertension
• Family genetic disorders

Medical history
• Anemia
• Hypertension
• Cardiac, renal, thyroid, or psychological disorder
• Sexually transmitted disease or pelvic inflammatory disease
• Diabetes
• Epilepsy

Nutrition
• 20% or more overweight
• 10% or more underweight

Other risks
• Cigarette smoking (one or more packs daily)
• Moderate to excessive alcohol consumption (from 2 ounces to more than 5 ounces daily)
• Drug use or abuse
• Exposure to teratogens at work or at home

• nutrition habits
• personal habits
• exercise habits
• environmental health
• roles and relationships.

Biographical data. Begin the history by obtaining biographical data from the client and her partner. Particularly note the client's age. A client over age 35 has an increased risk of giving birth to a child with a genetic defect. She and her partner may require genetic counseling. A client under age 16, who is still growing herself, may be ill-prepared physically and psychologically to handle a pregnancy.

Menstrual and gynecologic history. First, determine the client's age at menarche (first menstruation) to help establish a menstrual pattern. Next, ask about the length, regularity, and duration of her menstrual cycles and inquire about blood flow and the presence of blood clots or cramps during the client's menstrual period.

Ask if the client has had pelvic inflammatory disease (PID) or if she or her partner has had a sexually transmitted disease (STD). PID or an STD may cause reproductive tract adhesions that interfere with fertility. For example, a recurrent STD may scar the fallopian tubes, blocking passage of the ovum.

Next, ask the couple which contraceptive method they currently use, how long they have used it, and what difficulties they may have had with it. (For more information on specific methods of contraception, see *Contraceptive methods,* pages 20 to 26.)

A client should stop using oral contraceptives at least 3 months before conception to allow her hormone levels to return to normal. A client who has an intrauterine device (IUD) should have it removed at least 3 months before conception to let the endometrial lining of her uterus return to normal. During this 3-month period, the client should use another contraceptive method, such as a condom or diaphragm.

A client who has used an oral contraceptive for more than 3 years may take longer to become pregnant than one who has not used an oral contraceptive. A client who has had IUD problems, such as PID or heavy bleeding, may have developed uterine scar tissue that can inhibit implantation of a fertilized ovum. That also can cause difficulty in becoming pregnant.

Obstetric history. Determine if the client has had an abortion or miscarriage. A client with a history of spontaneous abortions may need a complete physical examination and extensive laboratory testing to identify and correct the cause. A client who has had an abortion may have adhesions that could cause problems during pregnancy.

Inquire if the client has given birth. If she has, have her describe it. Before conception, a client's obstetric history requires careful evaluation to identify and address any previous obstetric problems, such as premature delivery, perinatal death, or birth of a child with a congenital anomaly. A history of any of these problems increases their likelihood in subsequent births.

If the client has been pregnant before, ask if she had an anatomic problem or pregnancy-induced hypertension (PIH). An anatomic problem, such as an extremely retroflexed uterus or small pelvis, could prolong labor or cause other delivery problems that would require cesarean birth. PIH may recur.

Follow up by asking if the client or any members of her family have given birth to a neonate with a genetic disorder. A family history of genetic disorders indicates the need for genetic counseling.

Medical history. To conclude this portion of the health history, ask if the client has been diagnosed with diabetes; anemia; hypertension; a heart, lung, thyroid, or kidney disorder; hepatitis; epilepsy; or psychological problems. Such conditions may worsen with the stress of pregnancy. To prevent exacerbation of an existing condition, the client will need to know or learn how to manage it. For example, a diabetic client will need to regulate her insulin levels carefully. Such a client also will need a complete physical examination to help determine if the disorder could interfere with her ability to conceive or carry the pregnancy to term.

Health care activities. Ask the client for the date of her last routine checkup and her last gynecologic examination. Her answers will provide information about her level of self-care and will allow you to plan together for subsequent visits.

Inquire about the date of her last rubella (German measles) inoculation and tuberculosis (TB) test. Rubella and TB can cross the placenta, endangering the fetus. Even if she has had rubella or has been inoculated for it recently, she may be tested for immunity and receive a vaccination if she is not immune. A tuberculin test may be performed, if necessary.

Nutrition habits. Have the client perform a 24-hour dietary recall. Poor nutrition before pregnancy can jeopardize fetal well-being. For optimum health for the client and the fetus, the client's diet should include proper amounts of protein, vitamin C, vitamin B complex, folic acid, calcium, iron, and magnesium.

Personal habits. Ask the client how many ounces of alcohol she consumes daily or weekly. As her daily alcohol intake increases, so does the risk of giving birth to a neonate with congenital anomalies, such as intrauterine growth retardation, developmental delays, and craniofacial or limb defects (Rosen, 1983).

(Text continues on page 26.)

CONTRACEPTIVE METHODS

To help a client select the best contraceptive method, describe the methods available and discuss their advantages, disadvantages, and special considerations, including effectiveness. The following chart provides this information for the most common hormonal, mechanical barrier, chemical barrier, natural, and other methods of contraception. *Note:* The chart presents a range from use effectiveness (which reflects actual, sometimes inconsistent, use) to theoretical effectiveness (which reflects correct use of the method at all times).

HORMONAL METHODS

Oral contraceptive

Description
This method may inhibit ovulation by blocking the action of the hypothalamus and anterior pituitary on the uterus. It consists of a series of pills that contain 50 mcg or less of estrogen and 1 mg or less of progestin; "minipills" contain progestin only.

Oral contraceptives are classified as monophasic, biphasic, or triphasic. Monophasic delivers a fixed amount of estrogen and progestin throughout the 21 days. Biphasic delivers a fixed amount of estrogen throughout the 21 days, but an increased amount of progestin on days 11 to 21. Triphasic delivers a progestin dose that changes every 7 days and an estrogen dose that remains fixed for 21 days or changes every 7 days, like the progestin dose.

Advantages
• Offers the lowest failure rate of non-surgical contraceptive methods.
• Does not interfere with sexual spontaneity.
• Helps regulate menstrual cycle.
• May decrease the risk of endometrial and ovarian cancer, ovarian cysts, and noncancerous breast tumors.
• Decreases the incidence of anemia by decreasing menstrual blood flow.
• May decrease the risk of pelvic inflammatory disease (PID) and dysmenorrhea (painful menstruation).
• May decrease or eliminate premenstrual tension.
• May be used to treat menorrhagia (abnormally heavy or long menstrual periods) and endometriosis (ectopic growth and function of endometrial tissue).

Disadvantages
• May cause the following adverse effects: decreased libido (sexual desire), fluid retention, lethargy, depression, dizziness, nervousness, headache, increased appetite, nausea, vomiting, abdominal cramping, diarrhea or constipation, breast enlargement, breast tenderness, spotting or breakthrough bleeding, decreased or increased menstrual flow, vaginal yeast infection, photosensitization, and oily skin and scalp.
• Requires the client to remember to take the pill daily.
• Increases the risk of thromboembolic disorders, cerebrovascular accidents (strokes), and subarachnoid hemorrhage, especially if the client smokes or has hypertension.
• Increases the risk of myocardial infarction, especially in women over age 35 and in those with hypertension, diabetes, or obesity.
• May increase myopia and astigmatism, requiring contact lens refitting or new glasses.
• Increases risk of monilia vaginitis.
• Increases the risk of hepatic lesions, including hepatic adenomas.

Special considerations
• The effectiveness of oral contraception ranges from 98% to 99.5%.
• Oral contraception costs at least $5 per month.
• The benefits of oral contraception may outweigh the risks for healthy non-smokers over age 40.
• Oral contraception is contraindicated in a client with a thromboembolic disorder, benign or malignant liver tumor, impaired liver function, known or suspected breast cancer or estrogen-dependent cancer, or coronary artery disease.
• Oral contraception must be used cautiously in a client with hypertension, epilepsy, asthma, diabetes, kidney disease, gallbladder disease, fibrocystic breast disease, systemic lupus erythematosus, a mental disorder, migraine headaches, or a family history of breast disease or genital carcinoma.
• Oral contraceptives may raise insulin requirements; enhance the metabolism of acetaminophen, lorazepam, and oxazepam; lower the efficacy of anticonvulsants, oral anticoagulants, antihypertensive agents, and hypoglycemic agents; and impair the metabolism of caffeine, diazepam, chlordiazepoxide, metoprolol, propranolol, corticosteroids, imipramine, phenytoin, and phenylbutazone.
• The following drugs may lower the efficacy of oral contraceptives and increase the incidence of breakthrough bleeding: barbiturates, phenylbutazone, phenytoin, primidone, isoniazid, carbamazepine, neomycin, penicillin V, tetracycline, chloramphenicol, griseofulvin, sulfonamides, nitrofurantoin, ampicillin, antihistamines, antimigraine drugs, tranquilizers, and analgesics.
• To increase safety and decrease adverse effects, the physician may prescribe an oral contraceptive with 35 mcg or less of estrogen.
• To reduce the risk of blood clots, the client should discontinue her oral contraceptive 4 to 8 weeks before surgery or if an arm or leg needs a cast.
• A client who wants to become pregnant should discontinue her oral contraceptive, and use another contraceptive method, for 3 months before attempting to conceive, allowing hormone levels to return to normal.
• The client should avoid ultraviolet light and prolonged exposure to sunlight to reduce chloasma (pigment changes that may accompany pregnancy).
• The client should have a complete physical assessment, including a Pap test and breast examination, after the first three to six cycles of pills and every year thereafter.

CONTRACEPTIVE METHODS *(continued)*

Oral contraceptive *(continued)*

• If a client who has taken all pills in the cycle misses a menstrual period, she should begin the next cycle on time. If a client misses a menstrual period and has not taken all the pills on time, or if she misses two consecutive menstrual periods in spite of taking all the pills, she should stop taking the pills and immediately have a pregnancy test. Estrogen and progestin use early in pregnancy has

been associated with a higher risk of birth defects.
• Oral contraceptives should be kept in their original container and out of the reach of children.
• Many types and dosages of oral contraceptives are available. A client who develops adverse reactions to one type may benefit from switching to another type.

• A client who cannot use estrogen can take the mini-pill, which works by altering endometrial and cervical mucus and affecting sperm motility and survival. The pregnancy rate for mini-pill users is 2% to 3% compared to approximately 1% for users of pills containing estrogen and progestin.

Morning-after contraceptive

Description
This method prevents pregnancy after unprotected, mid-cycle intercourse. Medications include estrogen-progesterone combinations (Ovral) and diethylstilbestrol (DES). These medications work primarily by preventing implantation of the fertilized ovum.

Advantages
• Prevents pregnancy in unexpected occurrences, such as rape, condom breakage, diaphragm or sponge displacement, intrauterine device (IUD) expulsion, or loss or omission of oral contraceptive.

Disadvantages
• May cause mild nausea or vomiting for 1 to 2 days.

Special considerations
• The effectiveness of the morning-after contraceptive is 99%.
• Cost is at least $5 per course of therapy.
• The contraindications and cautions are the same as those for an oral contraceptive.
• Morning-after contraceptive use should begin within the first 3 days after intercourse, and preferably within the first 24 hours.
• Morning-after medication is intended only for emergencies, not for regular use.
• The usual DES dosage is 25 mg P.O. b.i.d. for 5 days, starting within 72 hours after intercourse. The usual Ovral or Lo/Ovral dosage is 2 tablets P.O. 24

to 72 hours after intercourse, and 2 more tablets 12 hours later; the usual d-norgestrel dosage, 0.6 mg P.O. up to 3 hours after intercourse; quingestanol acetate, 1.5 to 2 mg P.O. up to 24 hours after intercourse.
• Because a woman exposed to DES in utero has an increased risk of cervical and vaginal cancer, the client may be advised to terminate a pregnancy that DES has not prevented.

MECHANICAL BARRIER METHODS

Cervical cap

Description
A cup-shaped, flexible rubber device, the cervical cap fits snugly over the cervix and is used with a spermicide. Held in place by suction, the cap acts as a barrier to sperm. It is available in four diameters: 22, 25, 28, and 31 mm.

Advantages
• Does not alter hormones.
• Is more convenient than a diaphragm; can be inserted 8 hours before intercourse and requires no spermicide reapplication before repeated intercourse.

Disadvantages
• May cause toxic shock syndrome (severe *Staphylococcus aureus* infection).

• Increases risk of cervicitis and other cervical changes caused by prolonged exposure to spermicides, secretions, and bacteria in and around the cap.
• Requires client to touch her genitalia during insertion and removal.
• May be difficult to insert or remove.
• May produce an allergic reaction.
• May cause vaginal lacerations and abnormal thickening of the vaginal mucosa.
• May produce a strong odor if left in place for more than 36 hours.

Special considerations
• Effectiveness of the cervical cap ranges from 83% to 93%.
• The cervical cap costs at least $50, in-

cluding visits for examination and fitting.
• The cap is not recommended for use by a client with a history of toxic shock syndrome, anatomic abnormalities of the cervix or vagina, acute cervicitis, or vaginal or pelvic infection or by a client who has undergone a cervical biopsy or cryosurgery. It also should not be used during menstruation and for at least 6 weeks postpartum.
• Because the cap is associated with cervical changes, the FDA recommends that it be used only by clients with normal Pap tests and that these clients have another Pap test after the first 3 months of use.

(continued)

CONTRACEPTIVE METHODS (continued)

Cervical cap (continued)

• Clients who are most likely to use the cervical cap include those who cannot be fitted for a diaphragm because of a severely retroverted uterus or decreased vaginal muscle tone, have previously used the diaphragm, or have developed frequent urinary tract infections when using the diaphragm. They also include clients who can no longer use oral contraceptives and those who are breastfeeding.
• The client must be rechecked for proper fit after a weight loss or gain of 15 pounds (6.75 kg) or more, recent pelvic surgery, recent pregnancy, or difficulty with the cap slipping out of place.
• Because the FDA approved the cervical cap recently—in 1989—clients may be unfamiliar with its use, and health care professionals may be unskilled in fitting it.

Diaphragm

Description
The diaphragm is a dome-shaped, flexible rubber device with a thick rim that contains a spring. When placed over the cervix, it acts as a mechanical barrier to sperm. The diaphragm is used with spermicide to create a chemical barrier as well. It comes in different diameters (ranging from 50 mm to 105 mm with 75 to 85 mm most common) and types (coil spring, flat spring, arcing spring, and bow-bent spring).

Advantages
• Causes few adverse effects.
• Protects against sexually transmitted diseases (STDs) when used with a spermicide.
• Does not alter the body's metabolic or physiologic processes.
• Can be inserted up to 2 hours before sexual intercourse.
• Usually undetectable by either partner during intercourse, if properly fitted and inserted.

Disadvantages
• Requires insertion of additional spermicide in the vagina before each act of intercourse and if more than 2 hours have passed between diaphragm insertion and intercourse.
• Requires client to touch her genitalia during insertion and removal.
• Requires physical dexterity for insertion and removal.
• Increases the risk of toxic shock syndrome and urinary tract infections.
• May lead to vaginal ulceration, pelvic discomfort, cramping, or recurrent cystitis, if poorly fitted.
• May produce an allergic reaction, although this is rare.

Special considerations
• The effectiveness of the diaphragm ranges from 82% to 98%.
• The diaphragm costs at least $50, including the office visit, Pap test, fitting charge, and device.

• A diaphragm is contraindicated in a client with a history of toxic shock syndrome or recurrent urinary tract infections, an allergy to rubber or spermicides, or an anatomic abnormality, such as uterine prolapse, uterine retroversion, cystocele, or rectocele.
• It must be fitted by a health care professional because proper fit is essential for contraceptive effectiveness. A nurse practitioner or nurse-midwife can fit a diaphragm and provide the necessary client education.
• The client must be rechecked for proper fit after a weight loss or gain of 15 pounds (6.75 kg) or more, recent pelvic surgery, recent pregnancy, or difficulty with the diaphragm slipping out of place.
• The client should practice inserting and removing the diaphragm in the physician's office or clinic before its first use.

Condom

Description
The condom is a sheath made of thin rubber, processed collagenous tissue, or animal tissue that is worn over the erect penis during intercourse. It prevents sperm from being deposited in the vagina during intercourse.

Advantages
• Is available over the counter (OTC).
• Comes in an easy-to-carry packet.
• Is available in various textures, colors, and contours. A condom with a reservoir tip is recommended to hold the ejaculate.
• Ranges from 0.04 mm to 0.09 mm in thickness. A thicker condom is stronger; a thinner condom allows increased sensation.
• Helps prevent STD transmission, which can reduce infertility rates.
• May decrease the risk of cervical cancer.
• May help prevent premature ejaculation by decreasing glans sensitivity.
• Can help maintain an erection, especially in an older client, because the rim of the condom slightly constricts the penis.
• Can decrease vaginal friction and irritation, if a lubricated condom is used.

Disadvantages
• Decreases spontaneity during sexual activity.
• May produce an allergic reaction to rubber in either partner.
• May break during use, especially if it is used improperly or is of poor quality.
• May decrease sensation for the male client.
• Cannot be reused.

Special considerations
• The effectiveness of the condom ranges from 86% to 97%, but it can be increased to 98% by using it with a contraceptive foam, cream, or jelly.

CONTRACEPTIVE METHODS *(continued)*

Condom *(continued)*

- Although generally inexpensive, a condom may cost up to several dollars.
- Use of a condom actively involves the male client in contraception.

- A latex or other type of rubber condom prevents STDs—including acquired immunodeficiency syndrome (AIDS)—more effectively than a collagenous or animal tissue condom.

- A client allergic to rubber condoms may be able to use animal tissue condoms without problems.

CHEMICAL BARRIER METHODS

Vaginal spermicide

Description
This method may be a foam, cream, suppository, or jelly that contains a sperm-killing chemical.

Advantages
- Is easy to insert.
- Requires no prescription; is available OTC.
- Prevents STDs, such as gonorrhea, trichomoniasis, herpes genitalis, and chlamydia infection.
- Decreases the risk of PID.
- May be used as a backup method during the first several months of oral contraceptive or IUD use.

- Can be used in an emergency, such as when a condom breaks.
- Enhances vaginal lubrication.

Disadvantages
- Can produce an allergic reaction in either partner.
- May leave an unpleasant taste for couples engaging in oral intercourse.
- Must be inserted before each act of intercourse.
- Requires the client to touch her genitalia for insertion.
- May leak from vagina.
- May be difficult for a physically or mentally disabled client to insert.
- May decrease either partner's sensations.

Special considerations
- The effectiveness of vaginal spermicide ranges from 80% to 98%—highest when spermicide is used with a diaphragm or cervical cap.
- Vaginal spermicide costs at least $2 per container.
- Vaginal spermicide is contraindicated in a client who is allergic to spermicides.
- The client should follow package directions for insertion time, which may vary from 15 minutes to 8 hours before intercourse.

Contraceptive sponge

Description
This method consists of a small, doughnut-shaped device made of a soft, synthetic material. It covers the cervix, creating a barrier to sperm, and contains a spermicide that inactivates them.

Advantages
- Does not require fitting by a health care professional; one size fits all female clients.
- Is available OTC.
- Is easy to remove by its attached loop.
- Maintains spermicidal effects for 24 hours, regardless of the frequency of intercourse.

Disadvantages
- Cannot be reused.
- May come apart during removal.
- Requires access to clean water because it must be inserted wet.
- Requires client to touch her genitalia during insertion and removal.
- May cause toxic shock syndrome, especially if left in place for more than 24 hours or during menstruation.
- May produce vaginal dryness by absorbing normal secretions.
- May produce an allergic reaction, although this is rare.

Special considerations
- The effectiveness of the contraceptive sponge ranges from 82% to 91%.
- A box of three contraceptive sponges costs at least $3.
- The sponge is contraindicated in a client who has had toxic shock syndrome.
- The client should not use the contraceptive sponge after an abortion or delivery until approved by her physician, nurse practitioner, or nurse-midwife.

Vaginal contraceptive film

Description
This barrier method consists of a small 2" x 2" semitransparent square of soluble contraceptive film that contains a spermicide.

Advantages
- Does not require fitting by a health care professional.
- Dissolves in normal vaginal fluids, form-

ing a tenacious gel that renders sperm inactive.
- Washes away with natural body fluids.

(continued)

CONTRACEPTIVE METHODS *(continued)*

Vaginal contraceptive film *(continued)*

Disadvantages
- Cannot be reused.
- Must be inserted 15 minutes to 1½ hours before intercourse.
- Must be inserted before each act of intercourse.

- Requires client to touch her genitalia for insertion.

Special considerations
- The effectiveness of the vaginal contraceptive film ranges from 80% to 90%.

- If vaginal irritation occurs, the client should stop using the contraceptive film for 48 hours. If irritation occurs with later use, she should consult her physician or nurse practitioner.

NATURAL METHODS

Rhythm (calendar) method

Description
This method predicts ovulation by mathematically analyzing the length of the client's eight previous menstrual cycles. By this formula, the fertile period extends from the eightteenth day before the end of the shortest cycle through the eleventh day before the end of the longest cycle. During the fertile period, the client should abstain from intercourse to prevent pregnancy.

Advantages
- Requires no drugs or devices.
- Is inexpensive.

- May be acceptable to members of religious groups that oppose birth control.
- Encourages both partners to learn more about the functioning of the woman's body.
- Encourages communication between partners.
- Can be used to avoid or plan a pregnancy.

Disadvantages
- Requires good record keeping before and during use of method.
- Restricts sexual spontaneity during the client's fertile period.

- Requires extended periods of abstinence from intercourse.
- It puts a client with irregular menstrual cycles at high risk for becoming pregnant.

Special considerations
- The effectiveness of the rhythm method ranges from 70% to 85%.
- The rhythm method costs little or nothing in dollars.
- This method may be unreliable if the client is affected by illness, infection, or other factors, such as stress.
- It requires a willingness and ability to monitor body changes.

Basal body temperature (BBT) method

Description
This method identifies ovulation by monitoring the client's daily basal temperature (the lowest body temperature of a healthy individual during waking hours). A client can determine the timing of ovulation after evaluating her BBT for 3 to 4 successive months. In many clients, the BBT drops slightly (0.2° F [0.1° C]) just before ovulation and rises noticeably (0.4° to 0.8° F [0.2° to 0.4° C]) 24 to 72 hours after ovulation. Because the temperature drop cannot be predicted, the client should avoid unprotected intercourse from the first day of her menses until the third day of temperature elevation.

Advantages
- Are the same as the advantages of the rhythm method.

Disadvantages
- Are the same as the disadvantages of the rhythm method.

Special considerations
- The effectiveness of the BBT method ranges from 70% to 75%.
- The BBT method costs few dollars, requiring only the purchase of a BBT thermometer, which is calibrated in tenths of a degree from 96° to 100° F (35.6° to 37.8° C)
- It may be unreliable if the client is affected by illness, infection, or other factors, such as stress.
- It requires a willingness and ability to monitor body changes.

Cervical mucus (ovulation or Billings) method

Description
With this method, the client can identify fertile and infertile days by her cervical mucus characteristics. During the preovulatory and postovulatory phases of the menstrual cycle, cervical mucus is normally yellow or white, sticky, and inelastic. During the ovulatory phase, the mucus becomes clear, thin, and elastic.

Advantages
- Are the same as the advantages of the rhythm method.

Disadvantages
- Are the same as the disadvantages of the rhythm method.

CONTRACEPTIVE METHODS *(continued)*

Cervical mucus (ovulation or Billings) method *(continued)*

Special considerations
- The effectiveness of the cervical mucus method ranges from 70% to 75%.
- The cervical mucus method costs little or nothing in dollars.
- It requires abstention from intercourse during the entire first cycle so the client can chart her mucus characteristics without confusion from semen or sexual lubrication.
- Mucus characteristics may be altered by semen, douches, lubricants, spermicides, or infections.
- The client should abstain from unprotected intercourse if she has any confusion about her mucus characteristics.

Sympto-thermal method

Description
This method combines several natural contraceptive methods to predict ovulation. The couple monitors BBT information and cervical mucus characteristics and watches for secondary signs of ovulation, such as mittelschmerz (ovarian pain during ovulation), increased libido, pelvic fullness, midcycle spotting, and vulvar swelling.

Advantages
- Are the same as the advantages of the rhythm method.

Disadvantages
- Are the same as the disadvantages of the rhythm method.

Special considerations
- The effectiveness of the sympto-thermal method ranges from 78% to 89%.
- The sympto-thermal method costs few dollars, requiring only the purchase of a BBT thermometer.
- This method usually involves the client and her partner and emphasizes their dual responsibility for contraception or conception. For example, the client may identify the signs and symptoms; her partner may record them.
- Additional special considerations are the same as those of the BBT and cervical mucus methods.

Coitus interruptus (withdrawal) method

Description
One of the oldest contraceptive methods, coitus interruptus requires the male to withdraw his penis from the vagina immediately before ejaculation.

Advantages
- Requires no drugs or devices.

Disadvantages
- Has a high failure rate.
- Requires great control on the part of the male client.
- Can interfere with the sexual experience.

Special considerations
- Coitus interruptus is more effective than no contraception, but is not recommended because pre-ejaculatory fluid, which contains sperm, can be deposited in the vagina before ejaculation. When used with extreme care, this method may be up to 75% effective.
- This method costs nothing in dollars.
- After ejaculation, the man must urinate and wash the penis thoroughly before subsequent acts of intercourse.
- Only about 2% of all couples in the United States use this method; couples from other nations use it more frequently.

OTHER METHODS

Intrauterine device (IUD)

Description
An IUD, a plastic device that contains copper or medication (progesterone), can be inserted into the uterine cavity to prevent pregnancy. The exact mechanism of action of the unmedicated types is unknown, but they may work by creating a local, sterile, inflammatory reaction in the uterus. This reaction increases the number of uterine leukocytes, whose by-products are toxic to sperm and embryonic cells. Even if fertilization occurs, this reaction inhibits implantation.

Because many lawsuits are associated with IUD use, few IUDs are available in the United States. One brand, Progestasert, is a T-shaped device that contains 38 mg of progesterone released at a rate of 65 mcg/day, which acts locally on the endometrium to prevent conception. This device must be replaced annually. Another type is impregnated with copper, which is spermicidal.

(continued)

CONTRACEPTIVE METHODS *(continued)*

Intrauterine device (IUD) *(continued)*

Advantages
- Does not interfere with sexual spontaneity.
- Cannot be felt during intercourse.
- Produces no systemic metabolic effects.
- Does not require the client to touch her genitalia to use.

Disadvantages
- Must be inserted and removed by a physician or nurse practitioner.
- May cause dysmenorrhea and increased menstrual flow after insertion. These symptoms occasionally require IUD removal.
- Increases the risk of PID, especially if the client has frequent intercourse with multiple partners.
- May cause uterine cramping on insertion, especially in a nulliparous client.
- Is spontaneously expelled by about 5% to 20% of clients in the first year of use. These clients may benefit from insertion of another type of IUD.
- Increases the risk of ectopic pregnancy in a client who becomes pregnant with an IUD in place.
- Offers no protection against reproductive tract infections.

- Increases the risk of infertility.
- May cause uterine perforation, necessitating surgery, although this is rare.
- May result in sterility or death from septicemia, although this is rare.

Special considerations
- The effectiveness of an IUD ranges from 95% to 96%.
- An IUD costs at least $150, including the examination, insertion, and follow-up care.
- An IUD is contraindicated in a client with a history of ectopic pregnancy, bleeding disorders, anemia, severe dysmenorrhea, concern for future fertility, anatomic disorders that may interfere with proper insertion, abnormal Pap test results, abnormal uterine bleeding, and pelvic infection.
- An IUD usually is not recommended for a nulliparous client who wants to start a family later.
- An IUD should not be used after childbirth or an abortion until uterine involution is complete.

- Some authorities recommend that the client use an additional contraceptive method for the first 3 months after IUD insertion because of the risk of IUD expulsion.
- If the client becomes pregnant when using an IUD, the device should be removed by the seventh week of gestation to decrease the risk of spontaneous abortion, ectopic pregnancy, septic abortion, or premature labor.
- Infection may occur, especially in the first few weeks after insertion. It typically causes abdominal pain, vaginal discharge or bleeding, fever, and chills.
- The client should wait at least 3 months after IUD removal before trying to conceive to allow the uterine environment to return to normal.
- Researchers are studying the use of copper IUDs as "morning-after" contraceptives. They may prevent fertilized ovum implantation and would work most effectively if inserted 5 to 7 days after unprotected intercourse.

If the client or her partner smokes cigarettes, ask how many per day. A pregnant client who smokes one or more packs of cigarettes daily increases the risk of spontaneous abortion, intrauterine growth retardation, premature birth, congenital abnormalities, and decreased neonatal length and head circumference. Secondhand smoke (smoke inhaled from those using cigarettes nearby) also may harm the developing fetus (Alexander, 1987).

Ask the client if she uses any prescription or over-the-counter (OTC) drugs. If she does, record which ones and how often she takes them. Prescription and OTC drugs may pass through her system to the fetus. Some are harmless, but others are dangerous and contraindicated during pregnancy. As part of preconception planning, the client needs to learn about drug use and its effect on a developing fetus. If she must take any drugs, advise her to ask her pharmacist, physician, or nurse about their safety during pregnancy.

Determine if the client uses illegal drugs, such as cocaine. These may be addictive to the fetus and cause additional stress to the fetus during labor and delivery. If these drugs are in the client's circulation during labor, the fetus may be at risk for toxic reactions if the client receives labor medication or anesthesia. Also, addicted neonates usually are ill at birth because they are experiencing drug withdrawal.

Cocaine may cause additional problems. During the first trimester, a cocaine user has an increased risk of spontaneous abortion; during the third trimester, of premature labor. A cocaine user's neonate is at a 15% greater risk for sudden infant death syndrome (SIDS). If the client uses cocaine shortly before giving birth, the fetus or neonate is at increased risk for perinatal cerebral infarction (Smith, 1988).

Exercise habits. Assess the client's exercise patterns. If she exercises regularly, find out what kind of exercise she does, how often, and for how long. Regular exercise before conception will help improve her circulation and muscle tone, preparing her body for a healthy pregnancy. Unless the client has an obstetric complication, such as placenta previa, she should continue moderate exercise throughout her pregnancy.

Environmental health. Have the client describe her job. Specifically inquire about occupational exposure to chemicals, toxic substances, or other environmental hazards. Substances in the workplace may be teratogens (substances that cause abnormal fetal development). Even past exposure to some substances can increase the risk of congenital birth defects in the child. If a client or her partner has been exposed to hazardous substances, she may need amniocentesis and other tests during the pregnancy to check for abnormalities.

Inquire about hobbies that may expose the client to hazardous substances, such as paint, furniture stripper, cleaning solvents, or glue. Also ask about exposure to other hazardous substances at home or in the community. Many common substances can act as teratogens and should be avoided during preconception and pregnancy.

Roles and relationships. Investigate roles and relationships to help assess the client's or couple's readiness for pregnancy and parenthood. Ask each partner a question such as, "What impact do you think a baby will have on your relationship with your partner?" Even a planned pregnancy can stress a relationship. To reduce this stress, the couple should communicate their feelings openly.

Conclude by asking the couple why they decided to have a child now. Certain motives, such as pressure to produce grandchildren, may place undue stress on the relationship. Through active listening, the nurse can help the couple explore their feelings and concerns and consider their own motives.

Physical assessment

Assist with a physical assessment of the client to obtain baseline data, detect any problems, and provide information that can aid in preconception planning. Measure her height, weight, and vital signs. A nurse practitioner would palpate her thyroid, auscultate her heart and lungs, and examine her breasts. Finally, assist with a complete gynecologic examination.

For a client with a history of a particular disorder, assess additional areas. For example, a nurse practitioner would palpate and percuss the liver of a client with porphyria (a hereditary liver disease that affects porphyrin metabolism), which can worsen during pregnancy.

Diagnostic studies

During the gynecologic examination, obtain or assist with obtaining specimens for a Papanicolaou (Pap) test and STD cultures. Also obtain specimens for a complete blood count (CBC), urinalysis, and Venereal Disease Research Laboratory (VDRL) testing.

If the client has a history of a particular disorder, expect to collect additional screening tests. For example, plan to obtain blood for glucose testing if she has diabetes.

NURSING DIAGNOSIS

After a complete assessment has been performed, review the health history, physical assessment, and laboratory study findings. Then formulate appropriate nursing diagnoses based on these findings. (For a partial list of applicable diagnoses, see Nursing Diagnoses: *Preconception planning–Fertile couple*, page 28.)

PLANNING AND IMPLEMENTATION

Based on assessment data and nursing diagnoses, plan care that meets the needs of the client and her partner. Nursing care consists primarily of preconception health promotion, which may require simple reinforcement of health habits or extensive education. It also includes care that helps family members cope with changing roles and relationships.

The prospect of pregnancy may strongly motivate a client to change poor health habits. However, remember to set realistic goals based on her abilities and motivation.

Preconception health

When the client decides to have a child, preconception health promotion is essential. She and her partner should maintain or enhance their health to help ensure the health of the fetus they hope to conceive. Assist them by teaching self-care activities, teaching about fertility and infertility, providing nutrition information, and discussing exercise, rest, and contraceptive discontinuation.

Teach self-care activities. For a client or couple with a nursing diagnosis of *knowledge deficit related to self-care activities before conception,* provide instruction and counseling on life-style changes that can improve their health and that of their fetus.

If the client smokes, explain the effects of smoking on the fetus. If her partner smokes, describe the dangers of secondhand smoke. Stress the importance of controlling the client's exposure to cigarette smoke, and suggest a smoking cessation program in the community.

Advise the client and her partner to limit their alcohol intake. Many authorities recommend consumption of no more than 1 ounce of alcohol a day; others advise con-

PRECONCEPTION PLANNING: FERTILE COUPLE

The following nursing diagnoses address representative problems and etiologies that a nurse may encounter when caring for a client who is planning to conceive. Specific nursing interventions for many of these diagnoses are provided in the "Planning and implementation" section of this chapter.

- Altered family processes related to decision to conceive
- Altered nutrition: less than body requirements, related to impending pregnancy
- Altered role performance related to impending pregnancy
- Anxiety related to the decision to conceive
- Body image disturbance related to impending pregnancy
- Family coping: potential for growth, related to impending pregnancy
- Health-seeking behaviors related to contraception and conception
- Knowledge deficit related to contraception and conception
- Knowledge deficit related to factors that promote fertility
- Knowledge deficit related to self-care activities before conception
- Personal identity disturbance related to the decision to conceive
- Potential activity intolerance related to poor physical fitness before conception

sumption of no alcohol whatsoever. Explain that alcohol consumption can reduce male fertility and, if the client is pregnant, can cause fetal alcohol syndrome. For these reasons, alcohol bottles now display warning labels for pregnant women. If the client or her partner abuses alcohol and wants to stop, provide information about the local chapter of Alcoholics Anonymous or a similar program.

Instruct the client to avoid illegal or recreational drugs, such as cocaine or marijuana, because they can harm the fetus. Tell her to check with her physician, nurse practitioner, or nurse-midwife before taking any prescription or OTC medications, because some of them may endanger the fetus.

If the health history revealed environmental hazards at work, at home, or in the community, help the couple plan ways to avoid them. For example, suggest consistent use of protective clothing and equipment in the workplace, substitution or discontinuation of dangerous substances at home, or relocation if the community has environmental hazards.

Teach about fertility and infertility. To correct a nursing diagnosis of *knowledge deficit related to factors that promote fertility,* candidly discuss fertility and the factors that can

promote it. (For more information, see Client Teaching: *Actions that promote fertility.*) An understanding of these matters will promote health practices that favor fertility.

Provide nutrition information. For any client who wishes to conceive, explain the importance of nutrition to fetal health. Recommend a nutritionally sound diet that contains appropriate proteins, carbohydrates, fats, vitamins, and minerals.

When the nursing diagnosis is *altered nutrition: less than body requirements, related to impending pregnancy,* teach the client how to achieve a balanced diet. Instruct an adult client to include in her daily intake at least two servings from the milk group, two servings from the meat group, four servings from the fruit-vegetable group (including one good source of vitamin C and one of vitamin A), and four servings from the bread group. If the client is an adolescent, instruct her to follow the same daily diet except for the milk group, which should include at least four servings.

Before conception, the client's weight should be appropriate for her height. If her weight is too high, suggest a well-balanced reducing diet or membership in a weight-loss program. If her weight is too low, refer her to a dietitian for an appropriate diet.

Promote exercise and rest. Encourage the client to begin—or continue—an effective exercise program that will improve her overall fitness. This intervention is especially important for a client with a nursing diagnosis of *potential activity intolerance related to poor physical fitness before conception.* Help her select an enjoyable routine that meets her needs. Advise her to perform it at least three times a week for a minimum of 20 continuous minutes each session. For best results, teach her to maintain an exercise pulse rate of 70% to 85% of its maximum capability for her age.

Tell the client to balance exercise with adequate rest before pregnancy, and encourage her to respond to her body's cues. If she feels tired, she should rest. If her nightly sleep is interrupted, she may benefit from an afternoon nap.

Discuss discontinuation of contraception. This intervention addresses a nursing diagnosis of *knowledge deficit related to contraception and conception.* Depending on the client's current contraceptive method, discuss how to discontinue it. If she uses an oral contraceptive, advise her to stop taking it 3 months before attempting to become pregnant. Tell her to rely on another contraceptive method during

CLIENT TEACHING

ACTIONS THAT PROMOTE FERTILITY

To maximize the chance of conception, take these actions that promote fertility.

For the female client
- Always wipe from front to back after urinating or defecating. This keeps your perineal area clean and reduces the risk of vaginal and cervical infections that can cause infertility.
- Avoid using douches, irritating soaps, perfumed bubble baths, and feminine hygiene sprays to prevent genital irritation, which can lead to infection.
- Avoid tight clothing because it limits air circulation to the peri-

neal area. These actions also prevent pH alteration that can compromise fertility.
- Be aware that your ability to become pregnant may be delayed for 2 to 3 months after you stop taking birth control pills or have an intrauterine device (IUD) removed.
- Remain supine with your hips elevated on a pillow and avoid urinating for 1 hour after intercourse to prevent sperm loss.

For the male client
- Avoid exposure to toxic substances and chemicals, which can alter your ability to make sperm.
- Avoid long, hot baths and tight underwear and pants, which

can cause heat and decrease the sperm count over time. Instead, wear loose-fitting pants and underwear, such as boxer shorts.

For the couple
- Eat a well-balanced diet that includes at least two servings from the milk group, two from the meat group, four from the fruit-vegetable group (including one good source of vitamin C and one of vitamin A), and four from the bread group.
- Exercise at least three times a week for a minimum of 20 continuous minutes each session. During your workout, maintain an exercise pulse rate of 70% to 85% of its maximum capability for your age.
- Limit your alcohol intake to no more than 1 ounce of alcohol a day. In men, alcohol can reduce fertility; in women, it can cause fetal abnormalities.
- Avoid using over-the-counter and illegal drugs, and discuss the use of prescription drugs with your doctor. Drugs may affect fertility.

- Avoid environmental hazards at work, at home, or in the community. To do this, use protective clothing and equipment, substitute less dangerous substances at home, or consider a job transfer, if necessary.
- Be alert for the most fertile period: the middle of the woman's menstrual cycle (day 14 of a 28-day cycle).
- Use the basal body temperature (BBT) recording and cervical mucus characteristics to help identify the fertile period.
- Have sexual intercourse every other day during the fertile period to increase the chance of conception.
- Do not use a lubricant during sexual intercourse because it could kill the sperm.
- Have sexual intercourse with the man on top to maximize penetration.

these months to prevent pregnancy while her body returns to its normal hormone levels.

If she has an IUD, urge her to schedule an appointment to have it removed 3 months before conception is desired. Instruct her to rely on a different contraceptive method during this time so that the endometrial lining of her uterus can return to normal before pregnancy.

Provide family care

When a client and her partner have a nursing diagnosis of *family coping: potential for growth, related to impending pregnancy* or *body image disturbance related to impending pregnancy,* plan to discuss the couple's concerns with them. During the discussion, listen actively and encourage open communication between the client and her partner.

Begin by sensitively exploring the couple's decision to conceive. Ask them how they have planned for this event. Candidly discuss potential changes in their life-style and relationship, helping them begin to see themselves as parents and understand the changes in their roles. Also allow them to express concerns about the body changes that will occur with pregnancy. If the client is worried about her body image, encourage her to talk openly with her partner about her fears. Remind her that many men find pregnant women attractive.

EVALUATION

To complete the nursing process, evaluate the effectiveness of nursing care. Keep in mind that health promotion measures adopted before conception need continual evaluation before, during, and after pregnancy.

The following examples illustrate some appropriate evaluation statements:

- The client described the importance of discontinuing her oral contraceptive and of using a barrier method of contraception for 3 months before attempting to conceive.
- The client and her partner agreed to attend smoking cessation classes before conceiving.
- The client and her partner discussed their well-considered decision to have a child.

DOCUMENTATION

Using the appropriate records, document all steps of the nursing process. When caring for a couple who request help with preconception planning, documentation should include:

- significant health history findings
- significant physical assessment findings
- results of diagnostic studies performed
- the couple's understanding of health habits that will prepare them for conception
- instructions given to the couple
- the couple's understanding of instructions
- the couple's emotional readiness for parenting.

THE CLIENT WITH GENETIC CONCERNS

Whether a client is considering pregnancy, is pregnant, or has delivered a neonate, the nurse can enhance health and well-being by assessing the risk of genetic disorders and providing information and services needed to address the client's problems and concerns. Primary responsibilities include:

- assessing for genetic risk factors
- teaching prospective parents about genetic disorders before conception
- answering questions about genetic defects and disorders appropriately
- demonstrating sensitivity to ethical dilemmas faced by the couple at risk for having a child with a genetic disorder
- collaborating with other health care professionals when referring the family for evaluation and treatment of a genetic disorder
- providing nursing care to the family whose neonate has a genetic disorder.

Successful transfer of genetic information from parents to offspring is a crucial step in normal human development. If a parent's genetic material contains an error or defect, or if an error arises during cell division, off-spring may suffer profound deleterious effects. Because genetic factors are involved in many serious disorders, genetics is an important concern for the childbearing family.

When abnormalities arise in cell division and transmission of genetic information to offspring, genetic disorders may result. Ranging from benign alterations to fatal syndromes, genetic disorders number in the thousands and occur at a significant rate before and after birth.

Genetic disorders may result from monogenic (single gene) factors, such as autosomal dominant, autosomal recessive, and X-linked disorders; chromosomal abnormalities, such as changes in the number or structure of chromosomes; or interactions between genetic alterations and the environment.

ASSESSMENT

Assessment for genetic birth defects can be performed at the preconception, prenatal, or postnatal stage. Ideally, genetic risk should be assessed before conception. Even if conception has occurred, however, nursing assessment should include a detailed health history, physical assessment, and review of diagnostic studies.

Health history

When screening for genetic defects, the nurse obtains an extensive health history from the client and her partner, emphasizing family history, exposure to teratogens, and cultural and ethnic background. Assessment questions also should address economic factors, such as the availability of funds to pay for genetic screening tests. Of even greater concern may be the cost of caring for a genetically impaired child. Assess the effect of these factors on family function and make referrals, as appropriate.

The history can reveal the risk of genetic disorders and may aid in diagnosing genetic disorders. Risk factors include:

- previous birth of an affected child
- family history of genetic defects
- intrauterine exposure to known teratogens
- couples who belong to certain population groups at risk for known genetic disorders
- client over age 35
- client's partner over age 40
- history of three or more spontaneous abortions or stillbirths
- consanguinity
- single or multiple congenital abnormalities in a parent or previous offspring

- delayed or abnormal physical or psychological development in a parent or offspring
- mental retardation
- failure to thrive in infancy or childhood
- blindness
- deafness
- family history of neoplasms with known hereditary component, such as retinoblastoma
- infertility
- early onset of common diseases, such as coronary artery disease
- unexpected drug or anesthesia reaction.

To gather complete and accurate data, allow 30 to 45 minutes for the complete interview. Establish and maintain trust by being nonjudgmental about the family history data. Inform the client that all information will be included in the official health record, but none will be shared with others without the client's written permission.

After explaining the purpose of the family history, begin by constructing a three-generation pedigree—a diagram of relationships among family members that includes pertinent comments on each person's health status.

During the health history, ask questions about biographical data; medical, obstetric, and family history; drug use; health habits; environmental and occupational health; finances; and roles and relationships. These questions screen for any health or familial problems that may increase the risk of birth defects.

Biographical data. Record the client's age. The risk of autosomal chromosome anomalies increases with greater maternal age. Determine the ethnic backgrounds of the client and her partner. Some autosomal recessive disorders are more common in certain ethnic groups; individuals in these groups should be informed about their risks, appropriate screening, prenatal testing, and available counseling.

Medical history. The client's health status and that of her partner can help identify potential genetic disorders. Simple questions, such as "Do you have any health problems?" or "Does your partner have any health problems?" may reveal important information.

Obstetric history. Ask the client how many times she has been pregnant and whether any pregnancies have ended in miscarriage, therapeutic abortion, stillbirth, or a child with birth defects. Ask the client to identify genetic variations in partners by whom she has become pregnant. Previous pregnancy loss may indicate increased risk for

birth defects in offspring. Previous therapeutic abortion may have been related to genetic alterations discovered during prenatal diagnostic testing.

Certain infections contracted during pregnancy are known teratogens (such as rubella, toxoplasmosis, and herpes). Determine if the client has been exposed, infected, or vaccinated.

Family history. To begin drawing the pedigree, find out how many children the client has, the sex and age of each, and whether any have health problems. Asking about each child will elicit more complete health information.

Documentation of relatives in the client's generation and the client's parents constitutes minimal information for constructing a three-generation pedigree. Add more family members to the pedigree if they have pertinent health problems. Ask about the health of each of the client's siblings, nieces, nephews, and parents. Also ask if any family members are adopted, which could introduce genetic defects not otherwise present in family members.

Determine if any family members have had Down's syndrome, chromosomal disorders, neural tube defects (NTDs), birth defects, hemophilia, cystic fibrosis, mental retardation, or other inherited disorders. Record each disease or disorder and the family member's relationship to the client.

Drug use. Determine if the client takes any medications or illicit drugs. Some may influence multifactorial inheritance. Nonjudgmental attitudes are essential to obtain honest answers. Communicate that the client's honesty enhances the chances for a healthy infant.

Health habits. Because cigarettes are associated with intrauterine growth retardation, determine if the client smokes. Ask if she drinks because alcohol in sufficient quantity and at critical times is associated with birth defects. Start by asking about a specific amount consumed, such as one six-pack of beer a day, or a fifth of liquor a day. Suggesting an amount that seems high improves the chances of getting a more realistic estimate. This questioning should begin with nonthreatening topics; encourage and support the client to help her feel comfortable answering questions that could seem more threatening.

Environmental health. The unknown dangers of environmental agents make many pregnant clients fearful. A simple question such as "Do you have any other concerns about things that might be harmful to your baby?" may reveal her feelings. Answer questions with factual information when specific risks are known and refer all other questions to specialists.

Occupational health. To identify occupational hazards or teratogens that could increase the risk of multifactorial inheritance or spontaneous genetic changes in genetic information, find out if the client works with dangerous substances and, if so, which ones. Determine if she has been exposed to toxic chemicals, radiation, or X-rays during pregnancy.

Finances. Economic considerations are an important part of the assessment. The cost of genetic testing and counseling may exceed the family's resources. When clients have a financial need, work with them to help find alternate resources, or refer them to a social service agency or genetic counseling unit to obtain needed services. This may be particularly important at the postnatal stage.

Roles and relationships. Assess the effect on the client of being a carrier or having a child with a genetic defect, and investigate the family's readiness and ability to care for a potentially disabled child.

Ask if the client and her partner are blood relatives. Consanguinity increases the chance that the couple will share abnormal genes.

Cultural values can influence decisions and attitudes toward genetic disorders and birth defects. Knowledge that one carries a genetic defect and may produce an abnormal child can threaten self-image. Individual reactions to and resolution of the internal conflict differ widely, even between partners.

After the health history interview, review the history data with the client and her partner, keeping in mind that most cannot answer all questions during the first interview. They may not know family details or may be reluctant to share sensitive information. However, this information is important and should be reviewed during later meetings.

Physical assessment

Genetic screening also includes a thorough physical assessment to determine if malformations (developmental defects) are present. The physical assessment also can help determine if a malformation is isolated or associated with other anomalies. If other anomalies are present, the pattern of abnormalities may have a common genetic cause.

Observations of physical appearance should be as accurate and objective as possible. Record measurements of any structures that appear abnormal (head circumference, for example). Take photographs whenever possible.

Physical examination of family members may be necessary to determine if they have unusual features and if those features are associated with a genetic disorder.

Diagnostic studies

Various studies can be used during each stage of screening—preconception, prenatal, and postnatal—to help identify risks and differentiate among genetic disorders. Screening tests are performed on healthy clients who show no signs of, but have increased risk for, a disorder. Teach the client about the purpose of selected tests and the meaning of results so that she understands what kind of information the testing will provide.

Screening tests must meet sensitivity and specificity criteria without undue false-negative or false-positive results. Therefore, the client should be informed of the limitations of any specific test, and questionable results should be evaluated further.

Assure the client that test results will be kept confidential. Other persons or groups—such as relatives, employers, and insurance companies—should not have access to test results without her permission. Arrange genetic counseling after the screening, as appropriate.

Preconception detection. Screenings for Tay-Sachs disease and sickle cell disease have been available since the early 1970s. Individuals who wish to be screened receive a blood test and genetic counseling. A client who is a carrier will not necessarily develop the disease. However, if the client who carries the sickle cell gene or the Tay-Sachs gene marries a carrier, they will have a 25% (1:4) chance that each child will be affected by the disease.

Recent developments in DNA technology have made molecular detection of DNA alterations possible for a number of genetic disorders, and the list is enlarging.

Prenatal detection. Many hundreds of disorders can be diagnosed prenatally. Examples include Down's syndrome, NTDs, and Tay-Sachs disease. Some prenatal tests are used for screening and others are diagnostic. They include the following procedures:
- *Maternal serum alpha fetoprotein (MSAFP) test.* This test, designed to screen for fetal NTDs, measures alpha fetoprotein (AFP) levels. A high level is associated with possible NTDs; further diagnostic tests are performed then to determine the reason for the abnormal result.
- *Ultrasonography.* Prenatal ultrasonography, which is fetal imaging with ultrasound waves, may be used to detect gross structural abnormalities. Ultrasonography also is used to guide certain prenatal diagnostic pro-

cedures, such as amniocentesis and chorionic villus sampling.

- *Amniocentesis.* This procedure, usually performed between weeks 16 and 20 (occasionally as early as week 13) of pregnancy, provides a sample of amniotic fluid for chromosomal analysis, amniotic fluid AFP, and acetylcholinesterase levels (which may indicate NTD). One common reason for amniocentesis is to detect chromosomal abnormalities in a fetus of a client age 35 or over.
- *Chorionic villus sampling (CVS).* This test, which may be performed 9 to 12 weeks after the client's last menstrual period, allows testing earlier in fetal development than does amniocentesis. Excluding NTDs, disorders that can be identified by amniocentesis also can be identified by CVS.
- *Fetoscopy.* This procedure allows direct fetal visualization via a fiber-optic scope (fetoscope) inserted through the client's abdominal wall; it may be used to obtain fetal tissue samples, such as a skin biopsy. Fetoscopy can be used only during the second trimester.
- *Radiography.* This procedure allows visualization of fetal skeletal or limb malformations; however, it is rarely used because fetal exposure to ionizing radiation has been linked to abnormalities.
- *Amniography.* This procedure allows X-ray visualization of the fetus after instillation of dye into the amniotic sac; radiation dangers have limited its use.
- *Magnetic resonance imaging.* This procedure eventually may provide detailed studies of fetal, uterine, and placental structures; its safety in pregnancy currently is unknown.
- *Cordocentesis.* In this procedure, which targets fetal circulation, fetal blood samples are taken from the umbilical vein; these samples help in assessing fetal hemolytic disease.

Postnatal detection. Testing programs now can screen for more than 10 genetic and metabolic disorders in neonates, some of which will lead to permanent disability or death if untreated. Postnatal identification of genetic disorders also allows for genetic counseling to the couple who are at an increased risk for conceiving other affected children.

NURSING DIAGNOSIS

The nurse uses the client's health history, physical assessment data, and diagnostic studies to develop appropriate nursing diagnoses, which may involve the client, fetus, partner, and other family members. (For a partial list of applicable diagnoses, see Nursing Diagnoses: *Genetic disorders.*)

NURSING DIAGNOSES

GENETIC DISORDERS

The following are potential nursing diagnoses for problems and etiologies the nurse may encounter in clients concerned about genetic disorders. Specific nursing interventions for many of these diagnoses are provided in the "Planning and implementation" section of this chapter.

- Altered family processes related to a client's or partner's feelings about the presence of a genetic risk factor
- Altered family processes related to a physically or mentally disabled family member
- Altered family processes related to financial strains from genetic testing or treatment of a child with a genetic defect
- Altered parenting related to having a child with a genetic defect
- Altered sexuality patterns related to the risk of conceiving a child with a genetic disorder
- Anxiety related to the outcome of genetic evaluation
- Anxiety related to unknown health of offspring
- Caregiver role strain related to having a child with a genetic defect
- Grieving related to the anticipated or actual death of a child
- Ineffective family coping: compromised, related to fear of abnormality in offspring
- Ineffective individual coping related to fear of abnormality in offspring
- Knowledge deficit related to behaviors that can be harmful to the developing fetus
- Knowledge deficit related to genetic defects and their management
- Knowledge deficit related to genetic evaluation and counseling
- Knowledge deficit related to prenatal testing
- Knowledge deficit related to reproductive options
- Knowledge deficit related to the risk of having a child with a genetic defect
- Noncompliance related to ceasing personal behaviors that can harm a developing fetus
- Personal identity disturbance related to awareness of having produced a child with a genetic defect
- Social isolation related to a perceived lack of support during decisions about continuing a pregnancy
- Spiritual distress related to the possibility of terminating a pregnancy

PLANNING AND IMPLEMENTATION

The extent of the nurse's involvement in interventions for clients at risk for genetic abnormalities depends on acquisition of specialized training, characteristics of the work setting (for example, in a clinic where the couple returns repeatedly, a specially prepared nurse may do much of the counseling), the type of genetic disorder involved, and individual needs of the parents and offspring. Specific genetic counseling may be carried out by the family's physician or a specially prepared practitioner. However, the nurse can and should provide interventions as part of the nursing care plan.

Regardless of the nature of a specific genetic disorder, be prepared to address client concerns and problems with prompt management or referrals. To take an active role in managing these problems, implement a care plan focused on education, support, and counseling.

Provide information. The courts have established that health care professionals are legally responsible for informing clients of their risk of transmitting genetic disorders or birth defects based on family history, ethnicity, or teratogen exposure (Shaw, 1986). By extension, the nurse is bound to give clients complete and accurate information about diagnostic tests and their results.

Beginning before conception if possible, identify the client's risk of fetal genetic defects; provide appropriate information about genetic disorders, diagnostic tests, and reproductive alternatives; give emotional support to the client and involved family members; and—with special preparation—offer follow-up genetic counseling.

The client or partner may have a nursing diagnosis of *knowledge deficit related to genetic evaluation and counseling* or *anxiety related to the outcome of genetic evaluation.* Communicate to each family member that screening is voluntary and that all results are confidential. A nurse-midwife, nurse practitioner, or physician will make appropriate referrals for screening tests for family members who wish to learn their specific risks of being carriers.

Inform any client nearing age 35 of the age-related risk for fetal chromosomal abnormality. Assure the client that this increased risk does not result from any deliberate action on her part. Explain the need for and function of appropriate prenatal diagnostic tests.

Aid decision making. After informing the couple about genetic risks for the client and her fetus, help them make decisions about pregnancy. To help the couple explore their feelings and concerns, be sensitive and open but avoid making judgmental observations.

The couple that understands the risks associated with transmission of a genetic disorder will be better equipped to make knowledgeable reproduction decisions. This understanding also may minimize their anxiety about genetic screening and the possibility of having a child with a genetic disorder. When caring for a family at risk for a genetic disorder, determine family members' understanding of the disorder and the risks of passing it to their children. Additionally, assess which risks may arise for the client during pregnancy. Some genetic disorders—such as Marfan's syndrome and cystic fibrosis—can increase the affected client's risk of health complications during pregnancy.

The client at increased risk for bearing a child with a genetic defect may need assistance in deciding on reproductive alternatives. Before becoming pregnant, she may need to choose among several options, including the following:
• accept the risk and attempt pregnancy
• avoid the risk and refrain from pregnancy
• minimize the risk by considering such alternatives as artificial insemination
• monitor the risk by undergoing prenatal diagnostic tests to identify an affected fetus.

Once pregnant, the client may need to choose among several other options, including the following:
• delivery of an affected fetus
• placement of an affected neonate with an adoptive family
• termination of the pregnancy.

Crisis intervention is useful in assisting families with their decisions (Kus, 1985). This approach includes helping the client to identify the problem, generate and evaluate possible solutions, decide on a solution, and implement the decision. This approach is based on the nurse's ability to assist the client in making decisions.

For prospective parents, the decision to terminate the pregnancy when the fetus has genetic disorder will be difficult.

Few resources are available to the family deciding to terminate a pregnancy. The nurse's support and sensitivity are vital, especially in the unit where the termination occurs. A client terminating her pregnancy for genetic reasons may experience a greater depression than one undergoing termination for another reason; follow-up counseling may be necessary.

Assist with pregnancy management. In certain cases, a fetal genetic disorder may require changes in pregnancy management. For example, galactosemia is an autosomal recessive disorder of galactose metabolism that leads to liver disease, cataracts, mental retardation and, in some cases, death. Prenatal diagnosis can determine if a fetus is affected. If so, the client's diet can be modified to restrict galactose intake, which may minimize harm to the fetus.

Assist with genetic counseling. Genetic counseling provides testing, education specific to a particular disorder, presentation of alternatives specific to a particular disorder, and psychological support to help families adjust to genetic disorders. This process requires special educational preparation.

Clients who risk bearing children with genetic disorders or associated birth defects, or who have such disorders themselves, need counseling. This includes anyone with a history of birth defects, genetic disorders, alterations in growth, behavioral or learning disorders, alterations in sexual development, infertility, multiple spontaneous abortions, or stillbirths. Further, clients possibly exposed to teratogens (including alcohol) and clients age 35 or older should be informed about the availability of genetic counseling services.

Inform the client that genetic counseling is nondirective, meaning that she will not be told which decisions to make or how to apply the information presented. Decisions about genetic testing, having children, or having prenatal diagnosis are personal. The genetic counseling team will help the family understand the information available and provide emotional support as family members consider their options.

Typically, genetic counseling services are provided by a team of specialists in medical genetics. Although genetic counseling requires special preparation, the nurse participates as a member of the clinical team. Besides reviewing family histories and providing information, support, and follow-up services, the nurse may coordinate counseling unit activities.

Genetic disorders or associated birth defects may place severe physical, psychological, and economic strains on the client and family. When a genetic or birth defect is identified, the nurse can assist the family in care management, referrals, and successful adjustment. The nurse's roles can include working with the client and family to:
• identify risk factors. The nurse may be the first person to whom the client voices a concern. Nursing responsibility includes understanding the significance of the client's information.
• identify physical or developmental abnormalities from physical assessment data.
• assess the need for referrals to specialty services for genetic evaluations, genetic counseling, or prenatal diagnostic studies.
• facilitate referrals for additional evaluations. The nurse who is acquainted with contact people in specialty clinics in the community is well equipped to ensure that appropriate services are obtained.

• demonstrate sensitivity to attitudes of the client with a genetic disorder, especially regarding reproduction.
• serve as the case manager, including helping family members find appropriate health services.
• prepare the family for the genetic counseling evaluation. The client's realization that something may be wrong can reduce self-esteem as well as create a fear that her children will not be normal.
• correct misconceptions about genetic counseling and its purposes. Some parents fear that they will be told to have no more children, will be blamed for genetic defects, or will be told to terminate a pregnancy.
• explain the typical outcomes from genetic counseling. Besides knowing what to expect, the family needs to understand that all information will be kept confidential. Tell them that they will receive a letter summarizing the conclusions of the genetic evaluation, and that this information can be sent to any other health care professionals they specify.

EVALUATION

To complete the nursing process, the nurse evaluates the effectiveness of nursing care by reviewing the goals attained and the family's involvement and satisfaction with care received. Evaluate every step of the nursing process. As the client's situation changes, revise the care plan as necessary. The following examples reflect appropriate evaluation statements for a client and family at risk for genetic abnormality.
• The client and her family expressed understanding of the risk of transmitting a genetic disorder to their fetus.
• The client underwent prenatal diagnostic testing appropriate to her needs.
• Diagnostic testing revealed no genetic abnormality in the fetus.
• The client made an informed decision about continuing her pregnancy, based on probable neonatal outcomes specific to her situation.
• The client and her family attended genetic counseling sessions.

DOCUMENTATION

Document all components of the nursing process. Information should include:
• risks for genetic disorders or associated birth defects identified through history, family pedigree, physical examination, and diagnostic tests
• results of diagnostic tests

- information provided to the client and her family regarding specific genetic disorders and their ramifications
- the client's response to information provided
- interventions applied and their outcomes
- decisions made by the client and her family, along with her stated reasons for those decisions
- referrals made for diagnostic tests or genetic counseling.

CHAPTER SUMMARY

Chapter 2 described preconception planning and care for the fertile couple and addressed the nurse's role when caring for the client who has or is at risk for transmitting a genetic disorder. Here are the chapter highlights.

During the preconception assessment of the fertile client, the nurse screens the client and her partner for factors that may place the client—or her fetus—at high risk for complications during pregnancy. The nurse also carefully evaluates the couple's current health habits, motives, and plans for having a child and the stability of their relationship.

The nurse can promote preconception health by teaching self-care activities, providing nutrition information, promoting exercise and rest, and discussing discontinuation of contraception. The nurse also provides care for the family.

Genetic disorders result from monogenic factors, chromosomal abnormalities, or multifactorial inheritance.

The health history of a client at risk for transmitting a genetic disorder should include biographical data, medical and obstetric history, family history, drug use, health habits, environmental and occupational factors, financial considerations, and roles and relationships.

Nursing interventions typically required for a client at risk for transmitting a genetic disorder include providing information, helping with decision making, and assisting with pregnancy management.

STUDY QUESTIONS

1. Which factors identified in a client's obstetric history during preconception planning would place her at risk for maternal and fetal complications during pregnancy?
2. After assessing Mrs. Hall, the nurse identifies a nursing diagnosis of *knowledge deficit related to self-care activities before conception.* What information should the nurse provide?
3. When providing information for the couple seeking help with fertility, what information should the nurse teach to the couple to promote fertility?
4. What factors should the nurse be alert for when assessing a client for possible risk of genetic disorders?

BIBLIOGRAPHY

Aaronson, L., and Macnee, C. (1989). Tobacco, alcohol, and caffeine use during pregnancy. *JOGNN,* 18(4), 279-287.

Ad hoc Committee on Genetic Counselling of the American Society of Human Genetics (1975). Genetic counselling. *American Journal of Human Genetics,* 27, 240-241.

American Academy of Pediatrics, Committee on Genetics (1989). Newborn screening fact sheets. *Pediatrics,* 83(3), 449-464.

Baird, P.A., Anderson, T.W., Newcombe, H.G., and Lowry, R.B. (1988). Genetic disorders in children and young adults: A population study. *American Journal of Human Genetics,* 42(5), 677-693.

Chervenak, F.A., Isaacson, G., and Mahoney, M.J. (1986). Advances in the diagnosis of fetal defects. *The New England Journal of Medicine,* 315(5), 305-307.

Clark, M.H., Frankel, M., and Trowbridge, D. (1989). A pedigree primer. *Journal of Pediatric Nursing,* 4(2), 112-118.

Cunningham, F., McDonald, P., and Gant, N. (1989). *Williams obstetrics* (18th ed.). East Norwalk, CT: Appleton & Lange.

Griffith-Kenney, J. (1986). *Contemporary women's health: A nursing advocacy approach.* Menlo Park, CA: Addison-Wesley.

Hamilton, M., Hossam, I., and Whitefield, C. (1985). Significance of raised maternal serum-fetal protein in singleton pregnancies with normally formed fetuses. *Obstetrics and Gynecology,* 65(4), 465-470.

Harris, R. (1988). Genetic counseling and the new genetics. *Trends in Genetics,* 4(2), 52-56.

Jones, S. (1988). Decision making in clinical genetics: Ethical implications for perinatal nursing practice. *Journal of Perinatal and Neonatal Nursing,* 1(3), 11-23.

Kus, R. (1985). Crisis intervention. In G. Bulechek and J. McCloskey (Eds.), *Nursing interventions: Treatments for nursing diagnoses.* Philadelphia: Saunders.

Lewis, S., and Collier, I. (1987). *Medical surgical nursing assessment and management of clinical problems* (2nd ed.). New York: McGraw-Hill.

Lippman, A., Perry, T., Mandel, S., and Cartier, L. (1985). Chorionic villi sampling: Women's attitudes. *American Journal of Medical Genetics,* 22(2), 395-401.

Mattison, D., and Angtuaco, T. (1988). Magnetic resonance imaging in prenatal diagnosis. *Clinical Obstetrics and Gynecology,* 31(20), 353-389.

Mor-yosef, S., Younis, J., Granat, M., Kedari, A,. Milgalter, A., and Schenker, J. (1988). Marfan's syndrome in pregnancy. *Obstetrical and Gynecological Survey,* 43(7), 382-385.

Myhre, C., Richards, T., and Johnson, J. (1989). Maternal serum alpha-fetoprotein screening: An assessment of fetal well-being. *Journal of Perinatal and Neonatal Nursing,* 2(4), 13-20.

President's Commission for the Study of Ethical Problems in Medicine and Biomedical and Behavioral Research (1983). *Screening and counseling for genetic conditions: A report on the ethical, social, and legal implications of genetic screening, counseling and education programming.* Washington, DC: U.S. Government Printing Office.

Rhoads, G., et al. (1989). The safety and efficacy of chorionic villus sampling for early prenatal diagnosis of cytogenetic abnormalities. *The New England Journal of Medicine,* 320(10), 609-617.

Schulman, J., and Simpson, J. (1981). *Genetic diseases in pregnancy: Maternal effects and fetal outcome.* New York: Academic Press.

Shaw, M. (1986). Editorial comment: Avoiding wrongful birth and wrongful life suits. *American Journal of Medical Genetics,* 25(1), 81-84.

Speroff, L. (1987). *The epidemiology of fertility and infertility.* Presentation at the twentieth postgraduate course. Reno: American Fertility Society.

Thompson, J., and Thompson, M. (1986). *Genetics in Medicine* (4th ed.). Philadelphia: Saunders.

Williamson, R., and Murray, J. (1988). Molecular analysis of genetic disorders. *Clinical Obstetrics and Gynecology,* 31(2), 270-284.

Yen, S., and Jaffe, R. (1986). *Reproductive endocrinology: Physiology, pathophysiology, and clinical management* (2nd ed.). Philadelphia: Saunders.

Preconception planning for the fertile couple

Alexander, L. (1987). The pregnant smoker: Nursing implications. *JOGNN,* 16(3), 163-173.

Cranley, M. (1983). Perinatal risks. *JOGNN,* 12(6), 13s-18s.

Rayburn, W. (1984). OTC drugs and pregnancy. *Perinatology and Neonatology,* 8(5), 21-27.

Rosen, T.S. (1983). Infants of addicted mothers. In A. Fanaroff and R. Martin (Eds.), *Behrman's neonatal-perinatal medicine* (4th ed.; pp. 239-252). St. Louis: Mosby.

Smith, J. (1988). The dangers of prenatal cocaine use. *American Journal of Maternal Child Nursing,* 13(3), 174-179.

CHAPTER 3

REPRODUCTIVE ANATOMY AND PHYSIOLOGY

OBJECTIVES

After reading and studying this chapter, the student should be able to:

1. Identify the structures of the external and internal female genitalia.

2. Discuss hormonal regulation of the female reproductive cycle.

3. List the functions of estrogen and progesterone.

4. Describe the menstrual cycle.

5. Identify the structures of the external and internal male genitalia.

6. Discuss hormonal regulation of the male reproductive system.

7. Describe spermatogenesis.

INTRODUCTION

Whatever the practice setting, every nurse will encounter clients concerned about reproduction and sexuality issues, such as family planning, contraception, fertility and infertility, premenstrual syndrome, sexually transmitted diseases, and sexual violence. The nurse will need indepth knowledge of reproductive system anatomy and physiology to provide effective nursing care for such clients. This chapter reviews the structure, function, and hormonal control of the female and male reproductive systems and provides a framework for nursing assessment, planning, and implementation.

FEMALE REPRODUCTIVE SYSTEM

The female reproductive system includes the external and internal genitalia and the accessory organs, the breasts. (For illustrations of external and internal genitalia, see *Female genitalia,* pages 39 and 40.) The genitalia and their related structures respond to sexual stimulation, facilitate reproduction, and produce several hormones that regulate the development of female secondary sex characteristics, the reproductive cycle, and the physiologic changes associated with pregnancy and childbirth.

External genitalia

The vulva consists of the female external genitalia that are visible on inspection: the mons pubis, labia majora, labia minora, clitoris, ducts from Skene's (paraurethral) glands and Bartholin's (vulvovaginal) glands, vaginal orifice, hymen, fossa navicularis, and fourchette.

Internal genitalia

The female internal genitalia are highly specialized organs with one primary function: reproduction. They include the vagina, uterus, fallopian tubes, ovaries, and related structures. Hormones, especially estrogen and progesterone, regulate their development and function. Their blood supply passes through a network of arteries and veins, and innervation is provided through the autonomic nervous system.

FEMALE GENITALIA

These illustrations show the external and internal genitalia of the mature female.

External genitalia

The vulva contains the external genitalia visible on inspection. The mons pubis is a cushion of adipose and connective tissue covered by skin and coarse hair. The labia majora border the vulva laterally from the mons pubis to the perineum. Two moist mucosal folds—the labia minora—lie within and alongside the labia majora and appear darker pink to red.

The introitus (vaginal orifice) and urethral meatus become visible when the labia are spread. Less easily visible are Skene's gland orifices. Bartholin's glands are located laterally and posteriorly on either side of the inner vaginal orifice. The hymen may partially or completely cover the vaginal opening.

Internal genitalia

The vagina, an elastic muscular tube, lies between the urethra and the rectum. The uterus lies between the bladder and the rectum. The uterine corpus is composed of three tissue layers. The *perimetrium,* part of the peritoneum, is the outermost layer.

The middle layer, the *myometrium,* contains three types of muscle tissue. First are longitudinal fibers that contract to help expel the fetus. Second are fibers that wrap around larger blood vessels and ligate them during placental separation. Third are fibers that encircle the fallopian tube exits and the internal cervical os to prevent regurgitation of menstrual flow.

The inner layer of the uterine corpus, the *endometrium,* contains columnar epithelial glands and stromal cells. The endometrium responds to hormonal stimulation and, from menarche to menopause, undergoes monthly degeneration and renewal except during pregnancy.

Two fallopian tubes attach to the uterus at the upper angle of the fundus. Usually nonpalpable, these slender tubes have distal fingerlike projections, called fimbriae, that partially surround the ovaries. Fertilization of the ovum usually occurs in the outer third of the fallopian tube.

Palpable, almond-shaped organs, the ovaries usually lie near the lateral pelvic walls, a little below the anterosuperior iliac spine.

EXTERNAL GENITALIA

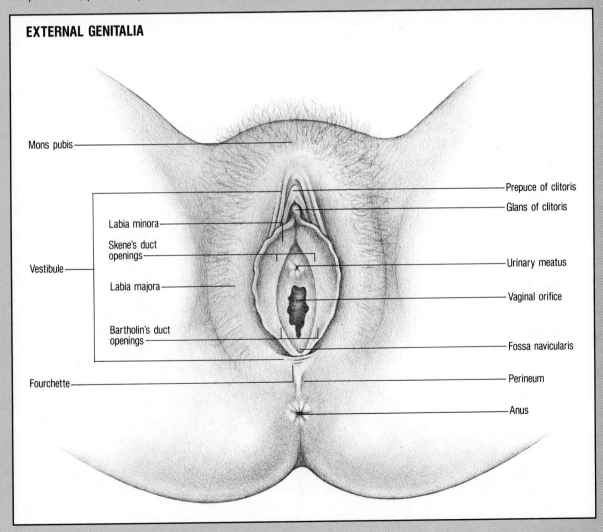

Mons pubis

Prepuce of clitoris

Glans of clitoris

Labia minora

Skene's duct openings

Vestibule

Labia majora

Urinary meatus

Vaginal orifice

Bartholin's duct openings

Fossa navicularis

Fourchette

Perineum

Anus

FEMALE GENITALIA (continued)

INTERNAL GENITALIA—LATERAL VIEW

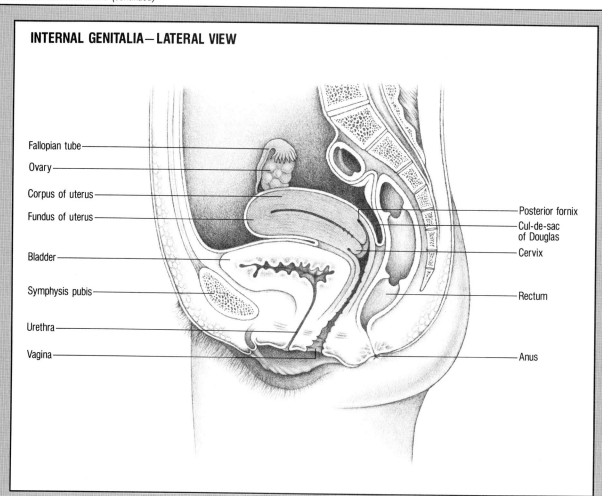

Fallopian tube
Ovary
Corpus of uterus
Fundus of uterus
Bladder
Symphysis pubis
Urethra
Vagina

Posterior fornix
Cul-de-sac of Douglas
Cervix
Rectum
Anus

INTERNAL GENITALIA—ANTERIOR CROSS-SECTIONAL VIEW

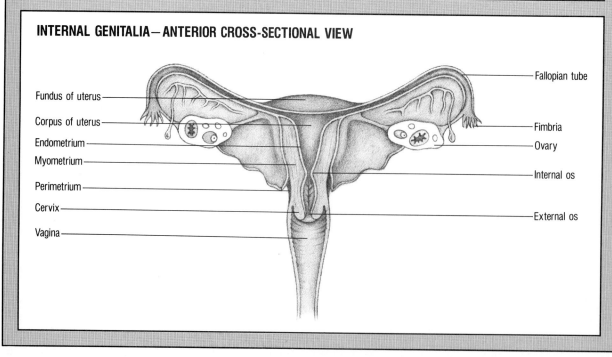

Fundus of uterus
Corpus of uterus
Endometrium
Myometrium
Perimetrium
Cervix
Vagina

Fallopian tube
Fimbria
Ovary
Internal os
External os

Bony pelvis

The female bony pelvis, which resembles a basin, supports the upper torso, protects pelvic structures, and forms the fixed axis of the birth canal. Age, sex, race, and heredity affect pelvic size and shape. The most significant differences between the female and male pelvis are the contours and thickness of the bones. The female pelvic bones are lighter and thinner, and the female pelvis is wider, shallower, and less ovoid. (For more information about pelvic diameters and planes, see Chapter 10, Physiology of Labor and Childbirth.)

Pelvic floor

Muscle pairs and deep fascia in the pelvic floor are accessory structures to the bony pelvis. The pelvic floor contains the upper and lower (urogenital) pelvic diaphragms and muscles of the external genitalia and anus. Pelvic diaphragm ligaments, fascia, and muscles are anchored to the perineal body. Perineal muscles protect pelvic viscera; perform the sphincter action of the urethra, vagina, and rectum; and contract during orgasm.

Related pelvic structures

The pelvis contains urinary and intestinal structures as well as reproductive structures. Urinary structures in-

FEMALE BREAST

The illustrations below show the structure and lymph drainage of the mature female breast. Each breast is composed of glandular (parenchymal), fibrous, and adipose tissue. Glandular tissue in each breast contains 15 to 20 lobes composed of clustered *acini*—tiny, saclike duct terminals that secrete milk. The breasts are supported by fibrous Cooper's ligaments and separated from each other by adipose tissue. The ducts draining the lobules converge to form *lactiferous ducts* and *sinuses* (ampullae), which store milk during lactation. These ducts drain onto the nipple surface through 15 to 20 openings.

The nipple is composed of pigmented erectile tissue that responds to cold, friction, and sexual stimulation. Surrounding the nipple is the areola, a more lightly pigmented circular area. Sebaceous glands known as Montgomery's tubercles dot the areolar surface as small, round papules.

Innervation of the upper breast stems from the third and fourth branches of the cervical plexus. Innervation of the lower breast arises in the thoracic intercostal nerve.

The breasts have an extensive vascular system. Arterial, venous, and lymphatic vessels merge with internal mammary and axillary vessels. Lymphatics deep in the breast drain toward the axilla; other lymphatics drain into the jugular and subclavian veins.

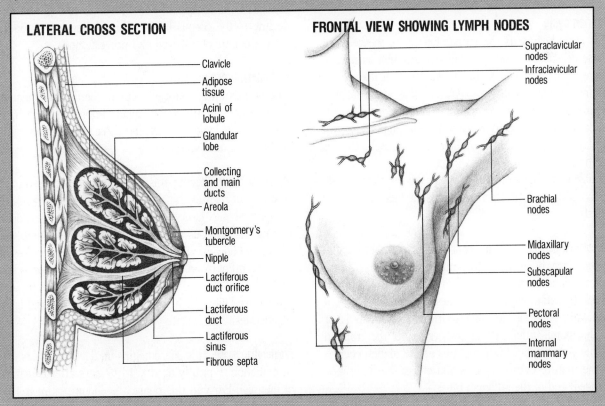

LATERAL CROSS SECTION

- Clavicle
- Adipose tissue
- Acini of lobule
- Glandular lobe
- Collecting and main ducts
- Areola
- Montgomery's tubercle
- Nipple
- Lactiferous duct orifice
- Lactiferous duct
- Lactiferous sinus
- Fibrous septa

FRONTAL VIEW SHOWING LYMPH NODES

- Supraclavicular nodes
- Infraclavicular nodes
- Brachial nodes
- Midaxillary nodes
- Subscapular nodes
- Pectoral nodes
- Internal mammary nodes

clude the ureters, bladder, urethra, and urethral meatus. The pelvis contains four intestinal segments: the rectum, colon, cecum, and ileum. These structures can be affected by changes in the reproductive tract.

Breasts

Highly specialized cutaneous, cone-shaped glands, the breasts are situated on either side of the anterior chest wall over the greater pectoral and the anterior serratus muscles. Vertically, they lie between the third and seventh ribs; horizontally, between the sternal border and the midaxillary line. A nipple is centrally located on each breast. A triangular-shaped portion of breast tissue known as the tail of Spence, or axillary tail, extends into the axilla. (See *Female breast,* page 41, for illustrations of breast structure and lymph drainage.)

FEMALE REPRODUCTIVE CYCLE

The female reproductive cycle, or menstrual cycle, actually involves two simultaneous cycles: the ovarian cycle and the endometrial cycle. (See *Female reproductive cycle* for more information.) A recurring menstrual cycle begins at menarche, continues throughout a woman's reproductive life, and ceases at menopause; it is regulated by hormones produced by endocrine structures.

Ovarian cycle

This cycle begins as the corpus luteum of the previous phase degenerates and hypothalamic stimulation occurs. There are two phases in this cycle. The follicular phase, during which a graafian follicle develops and ruptures, begins on the first day of menstruation and usually lasts 14 days, culminating in ovulation. The luteal phase begins on day 15 and lasts through the end of the cycle. During the first 24 to 48 hours of this phase, the ovum is susceptible to fertilization. Variations in the length of the follicular phase account for variations in menstrual cycle length.

Follicular phase. On the first day of menses, primary follicles in the ovary begin to mature under the influence of pituitary gland hormones. Between days 5 and 7, a single follicle (graafian follicle) dominates and continues to mature while other follicles undergo involution. On day 12 or 13, hormonal influence triggers swelling of the graafian follicle. Around day 14, it ruptures and ovulation occurs, as the mature ovum emerges and enters the fimbriated (fringed) end of the fallopian tube.

Ovulation can produce several clinical signs. Mittelschmerz, abdominal pain in the ovarian region, signals ovulation in many women. Body temperature changes— typically a drop of 0.3° to 0.6° C (0.5° to 1.1° F) and then an increase above basal temperature—may signal ovulation. Evaluation of spinnbarkheit, the elasticity of cervical mucus discharge, can help pinpoint ovulation in many women. This involves aspirating a cervical mucus sample, placing it on a glass slide, pulling upward on the mucus with a forceps, and measuring the length of the resulting mucus threads. Before and after ovulation, cervical mucus threads usually are 1 to 2 cm long. On the day of ovulation, estrogen stimulation causes these threads to lengthen to 12 to 24 cm.

Luteal phase. After ovulation, the ruptured graafian follicle becomes a compact mass of tissue known as the corpus luteum. The corpus luteum produces small amounts of estrogen and progesterone, which stimulate changes in the uterine endometrium that prepare it to receive a fertilized ovum. The corpus luteum continues to secrete hormones for about 8 days. However, if the ovum is not fertilized, the output of estrogen and progesterone decreases as the corpus luteum degenerates. The decreased hormone levels cannot support the endometrium; menstruation then occurs in about 6 days, initiating the next cycle. If fertilization occurs, the gonadotropins produced by the trophoblast (outside layer of the embryonic cell) prevent the decline of the corpus luteum, stimulating it to produce large amounts of estrogen and progesterone.

Endometrial cycle

During this cycle, changes occur in the uterine endometrium that prepare it for implantation of a fertilized ovum. The endometrial cycle has three phases: menstrual, proliferative, and secretory.

Menstrual phase. During this phase, which begins on the first day of menses and lasts approximately 5 days, the compact, spongy layers of the endometrium that developed during the previous cycle are sloughed off and expelled. Menstrual flow is typically dark red from the daily loss of 50 to 60 ml of blood. Approximately 0.5 mg of iron is lost with each ml of blood. While endometrial tissue, cells, and mucus are being discharged, the endometrial basal layer regenerates.

Proliferative phase. This phase begins on day 5 and lasts until ovulation, typically on day 14 (9 days after cessation of menses). Early in this phase, the endometrium is 1 to 2 mm thick and undergoes few changes; cervical mucus

FEMALE REPRODUCTIVE CYCLE

The female reproductive cycle, or menstrual cycle, typically lasts 28 days, although cycles from 22 to 34 days are normal. During the cycle, hormones influence the release of a mature ovum from a graafian follicle in the ovary. Hormones also stimulate changes in the endometrial layer of the uterus that prepare the uterus for ovum implantation. The hormones involved in this cycle are estrogen, progesterone, follicle-stimulating hormone (FSH), and luteinizing hormone (LH). The diagrams illustrate all aspects of the cycle.

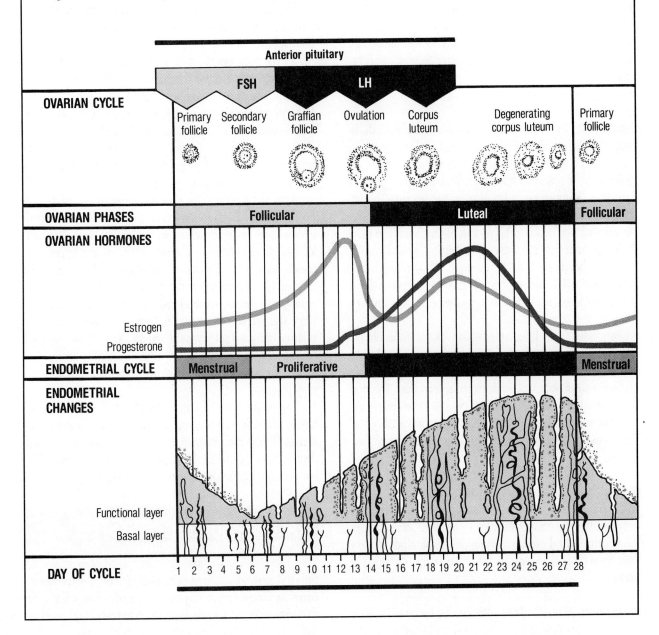

is sparse and viscous. As estrogen secretion increases, the endometrium proliferates and the thickness of the uterine lining increases eight to ten times before ovulation.

Secretory phase. After ovulation, progesterone released by the corpus luteum increases endometrial vascularity and stimulates elongation of the glycogen-producing endome-

trial glands. The secretory phase lasts from day 14 to day 25. At the end of this phase, the endometrium is soft, velvety, edematous, and about 4 to 6 mm thick. Rich with blood and glycogen, it is ready to nourish an implanted fertilized ovum. When fertilization and implantation do not occur, endometrial circulation decreases as blood vessels constrict and then relax and bleed. Tissue necrosis follows ischemia. The subsequent sloughing of the compact and spongy endometrial layers marks the beginning of the next menstrual phase.

Hormonal regulation

Three endocrine structures—the hypothalamus, the pituitary gland, and the ovaries—produce the hormones that regulate the female reproductive cycle. These structures comprise a regulatory loop known as the hypothalamic-pituitary-gonadal axis, which generates physiologic changes through positive and negative feedback mechanisms. Prostaglandins, fatty acid derivatives present in many tissues, also affect the reproductive cycle.

Hypothalamus. The nervous system provides the hypothalamus with sensory data. The hypothalamus then stimulates the pituitary gland to release or suppress appropriate gonadotropic hormones (hormones that regulate gonadal function). Stimulation takes one of two forms. The hypothalamus stimulates or suppresses the release of follicle-stimulating hormone (FSH) or luteinizing hormone (LH) from the anterior pituitary by releasing gonadotropin-releasing hormone (GnRH) or gonadotropin-inhibiting hormone (GnIH). Nerve impulses from the hypothalamus stimulate the release of oxytocin by the posterior pituitary.

Pituitary gland. The anterior pituitary gland (adenohypophysis) produces the gonadotropic hormones FSH, LH, and prolactin. FSH and LH regulate ovarian hormone secretion, and prolactin stimulates milk secretion. The posterior pituitary gland (neurohypophysis) stores oxytocin, a hormone that regulates uterine muscle contractility and the release of milk into the mammary glands during lactation.

Ovaries. The ovaries produce estrogen, progesterone, and a small amount of testosterone. Estrogen and progesterone help regulate the reproductive cycle, testosterone increases the sex drive, and estrogen stimulates pubic and axillary hair growth and sebaceous gland secretion during puberty.

Prostaglandins. All cells in the body produce prostaglandins, but they are especially plentiful in the endometrium of females and the prostate gland of males. In females, prostaglandins affect ovulation, fertility, and uterine motility and contractility. During ovulation, prostaglandins and LH stimulate ovum release and corpus luteum regression. During labor and delivery, they help stimulate uterine motility and cervical dilation.

Hypothalamic-pituitary-gonadal axis function. On the first day of the reproductive cycle, low levels of estrogen and progesterone in the bloodstream stimulate the release of GnRH by the hypothalamus. GnRH stimulates the release of FSH and LH by the pituitary gland. During the first 5 or 6 days of the reproductive cycle, these hormones stimulate follicle development in the ovaries. The maturing graafian follicle releases a potent form of estrogen into the bloodstream, which stimulates the proliferation of uterine endometrium.

As the cycle approaches ovulation on day 14, the level of estrogen in the blood is maintained in a pulsatile manner, and the hypothalamus signals the pituitary to slow FSH secretion and increase LH secretion. A day or so before ovulation, LH production peaks and the follicle reduces estrogen secretion and begins secreting progesterone. LH and progesterone cause follicle swelling and then rupture during ovulation.

After ovulation, LH and prostaglandins stimulate corpus luteum regression. However, the corpus luteum continues to produce progesterone for several days. The high level of progesterone in the blood signals the hypothalamus to stimulate a reduction in FSH and LH secretion by the pituitary gland. Progesterone also stimulates secretory changes in the uterine endometrium that reduce contractility and prepare the uterus for ovum implantation, stimulates changes that prepare the fallopian tube mucosal lining to nourish the ovum, and stimulates lobule and acini development in the breasts and initiates their secretory phase.

The corpus luteum degenerates 8 to 12 days after ovulation, reducing the amount of progesterone in the blood. Unless fertilization occurs, the progesterone level quickly drops below that needed to sustain a fully developed uterine endometrium, and menstruation occurs.

MALE REPRODUCTIVE SYSTEM

The male reproductive system is composed of external and internal genitalia. These organs and their related structures facilitate spermatogenesis, introduce mature spermatozoa into the female reproductive tract, and produce the hormones that regulate male sexual response, development of male secondary sex characteristics, and spermatogenesis. (For an illustration of the organs and structures, see *Male reproductive system*.)

External genitalia

The male external genitalia include the penis and the scrotum. Sexual stimulation causes the normally flaccid penis

MALE REPRODUCTIVE SYSTEM

As shown in these illustrations, the male reproductive system consists of the penis, scrotum and its contents, the prostate gland, and the inguinal structures.

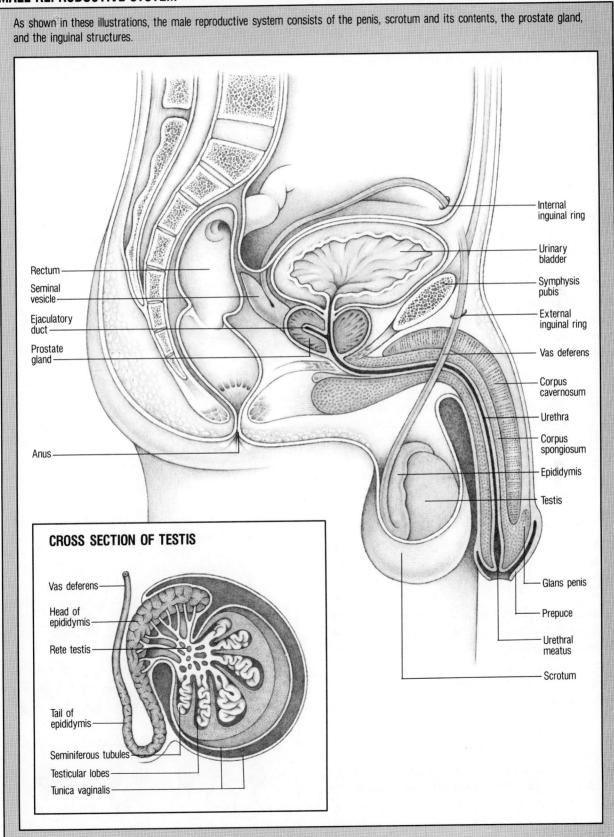

Rectum

Seminal vesicle

Ejaculatory duct

Prostate gland

Anus

Internal inguinal ring

Urinary bladder

Symphysis pubis

External inguinal ring

Vas deferens

Corpus cavernosum

Urethra

Corpus spongiosum

Epididymis

Testis

Glans penis

Prepuce

Urethral meatus

Scrotum

CROSS SECTION OF TESTIS

Vas deferens

Head of epididymis

Rete testis

Tail of epididymis

Seminiferous tubules

Testicular lobes

Tunica vaginalis

to become erect, enabling it to penetrate the vagina and ejaculate semen during coitus. The scrotum contains and protects the testes, the male gonads.

Internal genitalia

The male internal genitalia and related structures include the testes; a duct system composed of seminiferous tubules, epididymis, vas deferens, ejaculatory duct, and urethra; and accessory structures, including seminal vesicles, the prostate gland, bulbourethral glands, and urethral glands. The testes, the male gonads, produce hormones (primarily testosterone) and mature spermatozoa. The duct system transports spermatozoa and other semen constituents through the male reproductive tract. The male reproductive system accessory structures generate the medium that facilitates spermatozoa transport and survival after ejaculation.

Male reproductive development and regulation

Hormones produced by the hypothalamus, pituitary, and testes control male sexual development and regulate spermatogenesis. The hypothalamic-pituitary-gonadal axis responds to positive and negative feedback to maintain hormonal balance.

The male hormone testosterone stimulates sexual development and regulates most aspects of reproductive ability. Testosterone stimulates development of the penis, scrotum, seminal vesicles, prostate gland, genital ductal system, and descent of the testes through the inguinal canal. Shortly after the neonate's birth, testosterone production decreases. It remains low during childhood and increases during puberty, typically between ages 11 and 13. Influenced by testosterone, the penis, scrotum, and testes enlarge, and secondary sex characteristics—including hair growth on the genitalia, face, and chest and voice deepening—develop. Also, testosterone increases sebaceous gland secretion, which influences anabolism (cell-building) and results in increased male musculature, skeletal growth, and metabolism. In the adult male, testosterone affects sexuality and regulates the reproductive function.

Testosterone production continues throughout life, but decreases with age. Because of this decrease as a male ages, his sexual ability declines, muscle mass and hair growth decrease, skin loses elasticity, body fat distribution changes, and bones lose calcium.

Spermatogenesis, the process of spermatozoa formation, occurs in the lobules of the testes and seminiferous tubules. (See *Spermatogenesis* for more information.)

SPERMATOGENESIS

Spermatogenesis, the formation of mature spermatozoa within the seminiferous tubules, occurs in four stages:

- Spermatogonia (primary germinal epithelial cells) grow and develop into primary spermatocytes. Both spermatogonia and primary spermatocytes contain 46 chromosomes, consisting of 44 autosomes and the two sex chromosomes X and Y.
- Primary spermatocytes divide to form secondary spermatocytes. No new chromosomes are formed at this stage; existing pairs divide. Each secondary spermatocyte contains half the number of autosomes (22). One secondary spermatocyte contains an X chromosome; the other, a Y chromosome.
- Secondary spermatocytes divide to form spermatids.
- Spermatids undergo several structural changes to become mature spermatozoa or sperm. Each spermatozoan is composed of a head, neck, body, and tail. The head contains the nucleus; the tail, a large amount of adenosine triphosphate, which provides energy for spermatozoa motility.

Spermatogonia (44 autosomes plus X and Y)

Primary spermatocytes (44 autosomes plus X and Y)

Secondary spermatocytes (22 autosomes plus X or Y)

Spermatids (22 autosomes plus X or Y)

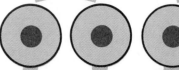 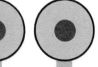

Spermatozoa (22 autosomes plus X or Y)

Hormonal regulation

Sexual development and spermatogenesis are initiated and regulated by the hypothalamic-pituitary-gonadal axis. Early in life, hormone production is inhibited. During puberty, inhibition ceases and the hypothalamus secretes GnRH, which stimulates the anterior pituitary to release LH and FSH. FSH stimulates the production of primary spermatocytes by germinal epithelial cells in the seminiferous tubules and influence the transformation of primary spermatocytes to secondary spermatocytes. At the same time, LH stimulates testosterone production by Leydig's cells in the testes. Testosterone stimulates the maturation of secondary spermatocytes and regulates the development of male secondary sex characteristics. (For additional information, see Chapter 4, Conception and Fetal Development.)

Spermatogenesis continues throughout life. The hypothalamus regulates testosterone production by monitoring blood testosterone levels. When levels fall, the hypothalamus signals the pituitary to increase LH production, which stimulates increased testosterone production in the testes. When levels rise too high, regulatory feedback mechanisms suppress further gonadotropin secretion, causing decreased testosterone production.

CHAPTER SUMMARY

Chapter 3 described the structures and functions of the female and male reproductive systems. Key concepts are as follows.

The organs and structures of female and male reproductive systems facilitate reproduction and provide sexual gratification.

They also produce hormones that regulate the development of secondary sex characteristics and sexual response. In females, hormones also regulate the reproductive cycle; in males, spermatogenesis.

External female reproductive structures include the mons pubis, labia majora, labia minora, clitoris, vaginal orifice, and perineum; internal ones include the vagina, uterus (corpus and cervix), fallopian tubes, and ovaries.

External male reproductive structures include the penis (shaft and glans) and scrotum; internal ones include the testes, seminiferous tubules, epididymis, vas deferens, prostate gland, urethra, seminal vesicles, bulbourethral glands, and urethral glands.

Hormonal stimulation in the hypothalamic-pituitary-gonadal axis initiates and regulates development of the reproductive system and secondary sex characteristics in both sexes.

Menarche, the onset of cyclical menstrual periods, typically begins between ages 11 and 16. Menopause, the period when hormone production and menstruation cease, typically occurs between ages 45 and 60. During the climacteric, the period preceding menopause, hormonal stimulation decreases and menses become irregular.

The ovarian hormones estrogen and progesterone are the primary female hormones that regulate physiologic changes in the ovaries, uterus, and vagina during the female reproductive cycle.

The male hormone testosterone, produced in the testes, stimulates spermatogenesis and the development of male secondary sex characteristics.

Spermatogenesis, the formation and maturation of spermatozoa, occurs in the lobules and seminiferous tubules of the testes. Spermatogenesis begins during puberty and continues throughout life.

STUDY QUESTIONS

1. Discuss the role of the myometrium and endometrium as part of the female reproductive system.
2. What information should the nurse include in a discussion about ovulation?
3. Describe the events occurring during the three phases of the endometrial cycle.
4. What are the functions of the male hormone testosterone?

BIBLIOGRAPHY

Ames, S., and Kneisl, C. (1988). *Essentials of adult health nursing.* Menlo Park, CA: Addison-Wesley.

Auvenshine, M., and Enriquez, M. (1985). *Maternity nursing: Dimensions of change.* Monterey, CA: Wadsworth.

Cunningham, F., MacDonald, P., and Gant, N. (1989). *Williams obstetrics* (18th ed.). Norwalk, CT: Appleton & Lange.

Fogel, C. I., and Woods, N. F. (1981). *Health care of women: A nursing perspective.* St. Louis: Mosby.

Guyton, A. (1986). *Textbook of medical physiology* (7th ed.). Philadelphia: Saunders.

Morton, P.G. (1989). *Health assessment in nursing.* Springhouse, PA: Springhouse Corporation.

Sloane, E. (1985). *Biology of women* (2nd ed.). New York: Wiley.

Spence, A., and Mason, E. (1987). *Human anatomy and physiology* (3rd ed.). Menlo Park, CA: Benjamin/Cummings.

Speroff, L., and Glass, R. (1988). *Clinical gynecology, endocrinology and infertility.* Baltimore: Williams & Wilkins.

Webster, D., and Huges, T. (Eds.). (1986). *Nursing clinics of North America: Women's health.* Philadelphia: Saunders.

UNIT II
THE ANTEPARTAL PERIOD

C H A P T E R 4

CONCEPTION AND FETAL DEVELOPMENT

OBJECTIVES

After reading and studying this chapter, the student should be able to:

1. Describe fertilization.

2. Discuss the events that occur between fertilization and implantation of an ovum.

3. List structures present in the pre-embryo 3 weeks after fertilization.

4. Describe the major developmental events of the embryonic period.

5. Describe the major developmental events of the fetal period.

6. Discuss the hormones produced by the placenta and the function of each hormone.

7. Describe the special characteristics of fetal circulation.

INTRODUCTION

Development of a functioning human being from a fertilized ovum involves a complex process of cell division, differentiation, and organization. Development begins with the union of spermatozoon and ovum to form a composite cell containing chromosomes from both parents. This composite cell divides repeatedly; individual cells increase in size. Beginning approximately 4 weeks after fertilization, daughter cells differentiate—that is, develop specialized properties not possessed by the parent cells, such as the ability to conduct nerve impulses or contract rhythmically. Finally, groups of differentiated cells organize into complex structures, such as the brain and spinal cord, liver, kidneys, and other organs that function as integrated units.

A precise timetable governs each developmental step concurrently with other related phases. During this time, the fetus and mother form a relationship via the placenta that provides an environment conducive to fetal growth and well-being.

The time from fertilization to birth is the period of gestation. Its length can be calculated by two methods. One calculates from the last ovulation (called ovulation age): gestation length from last ovulation approximates 38 weeks. Because few clients know when ovulation occurs, the method using menstrual flow (called menstrual age) is used more commonly. In this method, gestation is calculated from the beginning of the last normal menstrual period: gestation length approximates 40 weeks.

This chapter begins at ovulation—when fertilization can occur—and describes fertilization and factors that can influence it. Three main periods of prenatal development are explained: pre-embryonic, embryonic, and fetal. Additionally, the chapter discusses the environment necessary for normal development throughout the three developmental periods. This discussion includes the decidua, fetal membranes, placenta, and fetal circulatory system.

PRE-EMBRYONIC PERIOD

Beginning with fertilization, the pre-embryonic period lasts for 3 weeks. During this crucial developmental stage, implantation occurs, cells divide rapidly and begin to differentiate, and the placenta and embryo begin to form.

Penetration of a female gamete (ovum) by a male gamete (spermatozoon) marks the beginning of conception. Called fertilization, this event requires coordination of a complex array of physical and chemical factors, some of which begin long before the spermatozoon and ovum join to form a zygote (the single cell resulting from the union of male and female gametes).

The first step needed for fertilization is gametogenesis, where gonadotropic hormones stimulate testicular and ovarian precursor cells to develop into mature gametes.

The second step necessary for fertilization is introduction of spermatozoa into the vagina, either through ejaculation or artificial means. In normal ejaculate, spermatozoa are suspended in seminal fluid, composed of viscous secretions from the seminal vesicles and from the prostate and bulbourethral (Cowper) glands. Ejaculate typically contains about 3 ml of seminal fluid and up to 100 million spermatozoa per ml. Many of the spermatozoa aggregate in the portion of fluid ejaculated first rather than in a uniform distribution throughout the fluid. Ejaculate volume may vary from less than 2 ml to more than 5 ml, depending primarily on the interval between ejaculations.

Only spermatozoa (not seminal fluid) migrate through the cervix and into the uterus. Passage through the cervix is accomplished primarily by active transport. The middle section of each spermatozoon's tail contains enzymes that catalyze energy needed for propulsion, resulting in a lashing motion that propels the spermatozoon forward. Rhythmic uterine contractions move spermatozoa passively through the uterus and toward the fallopian tubes. The spermatozoa spread diffusely over the endometrium and enter both fallopian tubes, where they retain their fertilizing capability for at least 48 hours after intercourse (Cunningham, MacDonald, and Gant, 1989).

Meanwhile, under the influence of follicle-stimulating hormone (FSH) and luteinizing hormone (LH), several ovarian follicles begin to mature during the female reproductive cycle. Granulosa cells surrounding the follicles proliferate, and a layer of acellular material called the zona pellucida forms on the surface of the developing follicle. Fluid accumulates within the layer of granulosa cells, eventually forming a central, fluid-filled cavity within the follicle known as a graafian follicle. At ovulation, the graafian follicle discharges its ovum, which is surrounded by the zona pellucida and several layers of adherent granulosa cells called the corona radiata. The ovum is swept into the adjacent fallopian tube by beating cilia that cover the tubal epithelium; peristaltic contractions of smooth muscles in the fallopian tube wall propel the ovum toward the uterus.

Fertilization is possible only when a descending ovum meets an ascending spermatozoon that has spent several hours in the female reproductive tract.

Several conditions must be met before fertilization may occur, including the following.

- Seminal fluid, which is composed primarily of slightly alkaline secretions of the prostate and seminal vesicles, must protect spermatozoa from destructively acid vaginal secretions.
- Cervical mucus must be thin and conducive to spermatozoa passage. This occurs only during the midportion of the menstrual cycle. Later, cervical mucus thickens in response to progesterone stimulation.
- Spermatozoa count typically must exceed 20 million per ml of seminal fluid.
- Contact must occur between a spermatozoon and an ovum. Spermatozoa have no "guidance system" to direct them toward the ovum. Further, complex mucosal folds inside the fallopian tubes tend to impede and deflect spermatozoa.

When a spermatozoon penetrates an ovum, the spermatozoon's tail degenerates and the head enlarges and fuses with the nucleus of the ovum. This restores the cell's genetic component to 46 chromosomes—23 from the spermatozoon and 23 from the ovum. The fertilized ovum, known as a zygote at the one-cell stage, undergoes a series of mitotic divisions as it continues to travel down the fallopian tube toward the uterus. By the end of the first week after fertilization, the morula (small mass of cells) has begun to implant in the uterine wall.

During the second week of development, known as the *period of twos,* implantation progresses, the inner cell mass forms two germ layers, the blastocyst cavity develops into two cavities, and the trophoblast differentiates into two cell layers.

During the third week of development, known as the *period of threes,* the embryonic disk evolves into three layers, and three new structures are formed: the primitive streak, the notochord, and the allantois. The chorionic villi acquire central cores of mesoderm and now also consist of three layers.

EMBRYONIC PERIOD

Early in the fourth week, the flat, pre-embryonic structure becomes a cylindrical embryo that, over the following 4 weeks, nearly triples in size. Embryonic cells undergo

SYSTEM DEVELOPMENT: WEEKS 2 TO 8

The following chart highlights significant events during pre-embryonic and embryonic development and the times they occur.

SYSTEM	WEEKS	CHARACTERISTIC
Nervous	4 weeks	Well-marked midbrain flexure; neural groove closed; spinal cord extends the entire length of spine
	8 weeks	Differentiation of cerebral cortex, meninges, ventricular foramina, and cerebrospinal fluid circulation
Musculoskeletal	4 weeks	Limb buds appear
	8 weeks	First identification of ossification (mandible, humerus, occiput)
Cardiovascular	2 to 4 weeks	Heart begins to form; blood circulation begins; primitive red blood cells circulate; tubular heartbeat by 24 days
	5 to 7 weeks	Atrial division; heart chambers present; fetal heartbeat present; groups of blood cells identifiable
	8 weeks	Development of heart complete; fetal circulation follows two circuits (two intraembryonic and four extraembryonic)
Reproductive	6 to 8 weeks	Sex glands appear; differentiation of sex glands into ovaries or testes begins; external genitalia appear similar
Endocrine	4 weeks	Thyroid can synthesize thyroxine
Gastrointestinal	4 weeks	Oral cavity and primitive jaw present; stomach, ducts of pancreas, and liver form
Hepatic	4 weeks	Liver function begins
	6 weeks	Hematopoiesis by liver begins
Genitourinary	4 to 7 weeks	Rudimentary ureteral buds present
Respiratory	4 to 7 weeks	Primary lung, tracheal, and bronchial buds appear; nasal pits form; abdominal and thoracic cavities separated by the diaphragm

complex differentiation and develop into primitive organ systems.

Two major events occur during this period.
• Cell differentiation begins.
• Cell organization begins.

Especially during this period, drugs ingested by the mother, some viral infections, radiation, and other environmental factors can seriously disturb embryonic development, possibly leading to congenital abnormalities. (See *System development: Weeks 2 to 8*, and *Embryonic development: Weeks 4 to 8 (days 22 to 56)*, pages 52 and 53, for information about these developmental periods.)

In addition, specialized structures that protect and nurture the embryo—including the maternal decidua and fetal membranes—become fully functional during this period.

Each of the germ layers derived from the inner cell mass will form specific tissues and organs within the embryo. In general, the ectoderm forms the embryo's external covering and the organs that come into contact with the environment. The endoderm forms the embryo's internal lining: the epithelium of the pharynx, the respiratory and gastrointestinal tracts, related organs, and parts of the urogenital tract.

(Text continues on page 54.)

EMBRYONIC DEVELOPMENT: WEEKS 4 TO 8 (DAYS 22 to 56)

During this period, the embryo undergoes rapid growth and differentiation, as illustrated at right. The embryo develops organ systems, limbs, eyes, and ears; the amnion, yolk sac, and connecting stalk unite to form an umbilical cord with two arteries and one vein.

During the fourth week, the center of the embryonic disk grows more rapidly than the periphery as the nervous system begins to form. As a result, the embryonic disk flexes and bulges into the amniotic cavity. The amniotic sac, attached to the lateral margins of the embryonic disk, follows the changing contour of the embryo and bends around it. Part of the yolk sac also becomes enfolded within the embryo, and later will form the intestinal tract, among other important structures.

The lateral margins of the embryonic disk fuse in the midline to form the ventral (anterior) body wall. Fusion is incomplete in the middle of the body wall where the umbilical cord is attached. The portion of yolk sac not enfolded with the embryo protrudes, still connected to the embryo by a narrow duct. It persists for a time but eventually degenerates. The embryo begins to bend into a C-shape. The eyes are pigmented and the auditory pit enclosed.

During the fifth week, the head and heart grow rapidly. The amnion, yolk sac, and connecting stalk unite to form the umbilical cord, containing two arteries and one vein. At this time, the embryo's four limb buds are most vulnerable to injury by teratogens (such as drugs or radiation).

During the sixth week, the head grows larger than the trunk and appears to be bent over the heart area. The eyes, nose, and mouth are more evident. The upper limbs have elbows and wrists. The hand plates develop ridges called finger rays.

During the seventh week, the head continues to enlarge and cerebral hemispheres appear. The face elongates, placing the eyes in a more frontal position. The areas over the heart and liver are prominent because these organs form earlier than others. Limbs continue to develop, especially the fingers.

During the eighth week, the head makes up half of the total embryonic mass. A face occupies its lower half, with a flat nose and recognizable mouth. Eyelid folds have developed and the eyes are far apart. The external ears look similar to their final shape. Arms, legs, fingers, and toes are distinct. Sexual differences may be observed. (For photographs of embryonic development, see pages 58 to 61.)

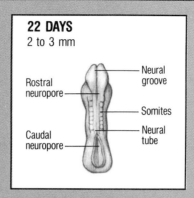

22 DAYS
2 to 3 mm

Rostral neuropore — Neural groove — Somites — Neural tube — Caudal neuropore

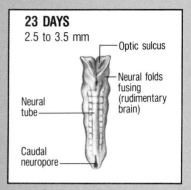

23 DAYS
2.5 to 3.5 mm

Optic sulcus — Neural folds fusing (rudimentary brain) — Neural tube — Caudal neuropore

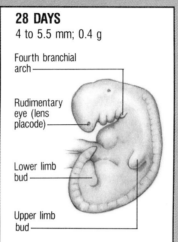

28 DAYS
4 to 5.5 mm; 0.4 g

Fourth branchial arch — Rudimentary eye (lens placode) — Lower limb bud — Upper limb bud

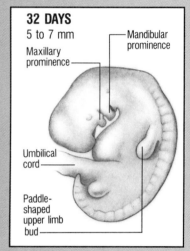

32 DAYS
5 to 7 mm

Maxillary prominence — Mandibular prominence — Umbilical cord — Paddle-shaped upper limb bud

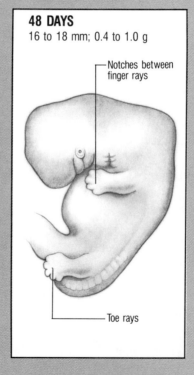

48 DAYS
16 to 18 mm; 0.4 to 1.0 g

Notches between finger rays — Toe rays

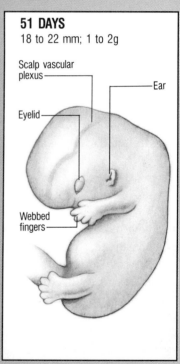

51 DAYS
18 to 22 mm; 1 to 2g

Scalp vascular plexus — Ear — Eyelid — Webbed fingers

24 DAYS
3 to 4 mm

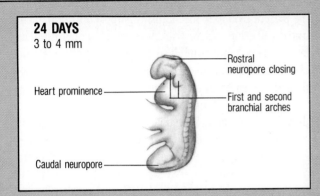

Heart prominence

Rostral neuropore closing

First and second branchial arches

Caudal neuropore

26 DAYS
3.5 to 4.5 mm

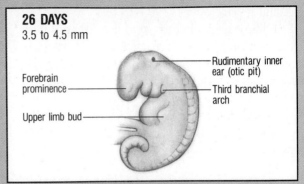

Forebrain prominence

Upper limb bud

Rudimentary inner ear (otic pit)

Third branchial arch

36 DAYS
8 to 9 mm; 0.5 g

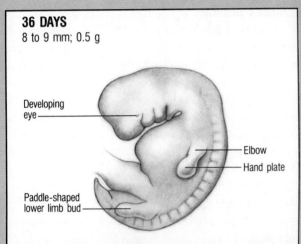

Developing eye

Paddle-shaped lower limb bud

Elbow

Hand plate

41 DAYS
11 to 14 mm

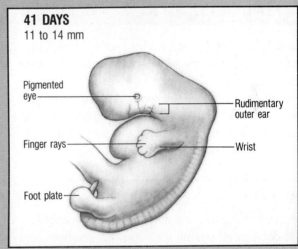

Pigmented eye

Finger rays

Foot plate

Rudimentary outer ear

Wrist

53 DAYS
22 to 24 mm; 1.5 to 2.5 g

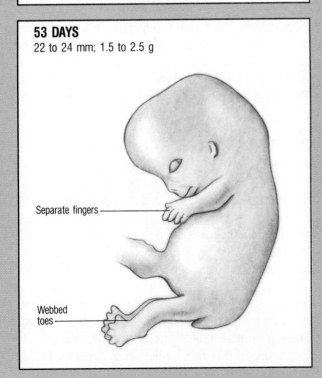

Separate fingers

Webbed toes

56 DAYS
27 to 31 mm; 2 to 3 g

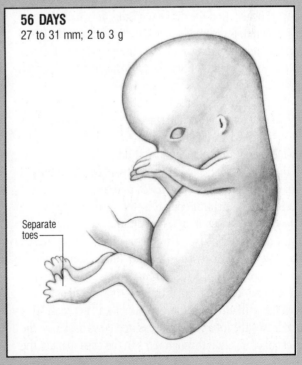

Separate toes

The mesoderm, which is sandwiched between the other two cell layers, forms various supporting tissues, muscles, the circulatory system, and major portions of the urogenital system.

Cell differentiation in each germ layer depends more on location than on inherent characteristics. For example, ectoderm cells transplanted during early development into locations normally occupied by endoderm will differentiate as endoderm cells. The converse is true, too. These transplantations suggest that embryonic cells, which may develop in various ways, are induced into specific development.

FETAL PERIOD

Lasting from weeks 8 to 40, the fetal period involves further growth and development of organ systems established in the embryonic period. When fully developed, fetal organs begin to function and supply part of the fetus's metabolic needs. (See *Fetal development*, page 55 to 61, for illustrations and characteristics of this period.) In addition, the placenta continues to develop.

PLACENTA

A flattened, disk-shaped structure that weighs about 500 g, the placenta is derived from the trophoblast and from maternal tissues. The chorion and the villi are formed from the trophoblast, and the decidua basalis, in which the villi are anchored, is derived from the endometrium. The fused amnion and chorion extend from the margins of the placenta to form the fluid-filled sac enclosing the fetus, which ruptures at birth.

The placenta circulates blood between the mother and fetus so that oxygen and nutrients may be exchanged. This is accomplished through a specialized circulation system in which fetal and maternal blood do not mix.

The fetus is connected to the placenta by the umbilical cord, which contains two arteries and a single vein. The arteries follow a spiral course in the cord, divide on the surface of the placenta, and branch to the chorionic villi. Oxygenated arterial blood from the mother is delivered into large spaces between the villi (intervillous spaces) and delivered to the fetus through the single umbilical vein. Oxygen-depleted blood travels from the fetus to the chorionic villi through the two umbilical arteries. This blood leaves the intervillous spaces and flows back into the maternal circulation through veins in the basal part of the placenta.

Substances (such as oxygen, water, antibodies, and some drugs from the mother and carbon dioxide, urea, and waste products from the fetus) are transferred across the placenta via four mechanisms: simple diffusion, facilitated diffusion, active transport, and pinocytosis. The fetal-placental unit (umbilical cord, placental layers, and chorionic villi) must have developed properly and be functioning for placental transfer to occur.

Maternal protein hormones are not transferred through the placenta, with the exception of small amounts of thyroxine and triiodothyronine. Steroid hormones traverse the placenta freely. Viruses may cross the placenta and infect the fetus, as may some bacteria and protozoa.

Endocrine functions

In addition to providing the means by which the mother nourishes the developing fetus, the placenta also functions as an endocrine organ, producing various peptide, neuropeptide, and steroid hormones. The two major peptide hormones are human chorionic gonadotropin (hCG) and human placental lactogen (hPL). The neuropeptides include gonadotropin-releasing hormone (GnRH), thyrotropin-releasing factor (TRF), and adrenocorticotropic hormone (ACTH). Synthesized by the cytotrophoblast (outer layer of the trophoblast), they may regulate the synthesis and release of peptide hormones from the syncytial trophoblast. The two major steroid hormones are estrogen and progesterone.

Human chorionic gonadotropin. This hormone is a glycoprotein composed of two subunits designated alpha and beta. The alpha subunit also is present in three other glycoprotein hormones: FHS, LH, and thyroid-stimulating hormone. The beta subunit is unique to hCG. Produced by the syncytiotrophoblast (peripheral layer of the trophoblast), hCG can be detected in the mother's serum as early as 8 days after conception, which corresponds to the time the blastocyst is burrowing into the endometrium.

Levels of hCG rise rapidly to about 100 IU/ml at about the tenth week of gestation, and then gradually decline, reaching a low of about 10 IU/ml by the twentieth week and remaining at low levels for the remainder of gestation. For the first 8 weeks of pregnancy, hCG maintains the corpus luteum, which provides the progesterone essential to the pregnancy until the placenta takes over hormone production. This hormone also may regulate maternal and fetal synthesis of steroid hormones, and it stimulates testosterone production by the testes of a male fetus.

The detection of hCG in the blood and urine by immunologic tests specific for the beta subunit of hCG is the

(Text continues on page 62.)

FETAL DEVELOPMENT

The following chart highlights significant events during fetal development and the times they occur.

SYSTEM DEVELOPMENT: WEEKS 8 TO 40

System	Weeks	Characteristic
Nervous	12 to 16 weeks	Structural configuration of brain roughly completed; cerebral lobes delineated; cerebellum assumes prominence
	20 to 24 weeks	Brain grossly formed; myelination of spinal cord begins; spinal cords ends at S-1
	28 to 36 weeks	Cerebral fissures appear; convolutions appear; spinal cord ends at L-3
	40 weeks	Myelination of brain begins
Musculoskeletal	12 weeks	Some bones well outlined; ossification continues
	16 weeks	Joint cavities present; muscular movements detectable
	20 weeks	Ossification of sternum; mother can detect fetal movements (quickening)
	28 to 32 weeks	Ossification continues; fetus can turn head to side
	36 weeks	Muscle tone developed; fetus can turn and elevate head
Cardiovascular	16 to 20 weeks	Fetal heart tone audible with fetoscope
Gastrointestinal	8 to 11 weeks	Intestinal villi form; small intestine coils in umbilical cord
	12 to 16 weeks	Bile is secreted; intestine withdraws from umbilical cord to normal position; meconium present in bowel; anus open
	20 weeks	Enamel and dentin are deposited; ascending colon appears; fetus can suck and swallow; peristaltic movements begin
Genitourinary	8 to 12 weeks	Bladder and urethra separate from rectum; bladder expands as a sac; kidneys secrete urine
	13 to 20 weeks	Kidneys in proper position with definitive shape
	36 weeks	Formation of new nephrons ceases
Respiratory	8 to 12 weeks	Bronchioles branch; pleural and pericardial cavities appear; lungs assume definitive shape
	13 to 20 weeks	Terminal and respiratory bronchioles appear
	21 to 28 weeks	Nostrils open; surfactant production begins; respiratory movements possible; alveolar ducts and sacs appear
	38 to 40 weeks	Pulmonary branching two-thirds complete; lecithin-sphingomyelin (L-S) ratio 2:1
Reproductive	12 to 24 weeks	Testes descend into the inguinal canal; external genitalia distinguishable
Endocrine	10 weeks	Islets of Langerhans differentiated
	12 weeks	Thyroid secretes hormones; insulin present in pancreas

(continued)

FETAL DEVELOPMENT *(continued)*

PHYSICAL DEVELOPMENT: WEEKS 9 TO 40

In the ninth week, the eyelids fuse together, remaining so until the seventh month. The head remains disproportionately large. Limbs are disproportionately small at week 9, but by week 12 the arms have reached normal proportions. Legs and thighs remain small. The liver begins to produce red blood cells, a function taken over by the spleen at about 12 weeks. At 12 weeks, the placenta is complete and fetal circulation has developed. The skin is pink and delicate. Lacrimal ducts are developing.

By the end of week 16, the head makes up one-third of the total size of the fetus, and the brain is roughly delineated. The forehead is prominent, with lanugo (fine hair) growing on it. The chin is apparent, and the ears are placed higher on the head than previously. Fingernails begin to form. The kidneys function, secreting urine, and the fetus begins to swallow amniotic fluid. Sweat glands form. The lower limbs lengthen and the skeleton ossifies. The intestines withdraw from the umbilical cord to their normal position in the abdomen.

By week 17, the fetus's body is covered with lanugo, and sebaceous glands secrete sebum. This forms the vernix caseosa, a cheeselike material that covers the skin, protecting it from the drying action of the amniotic fluid. Many women feel movement, or quickening, between 16 and 20 weeks. Heart tones may be heard with a fetoscope placed over the symphysis pubis. By 20 weeks, the lower limbs are fully formed.

Although gaining weight steadily, the fetus between weeks 21 and 24 appears lean in comparison with a fetus at term. The wrinkled skin is covered with vernix caseosa. The lungs produce surfactant (a respiratory by-product); meconium (fetal excrement) is present in the rectum. The eyes are structurally complete.

The face matures between 25 and 28 weeks; eyelashes and eyebrows form. Eyelids open and close. Skin is red. Most fetuses are considered viable by week 27 if given expert care.

Between 28 and 32 weeks, subcutaneous fat causes the fetus to grow more rounded. Vernix caseosa forms a thick coat over pink skin. Cerebral fissures and convolutions appear. Born at the end of this period, the neonate has a good chance of survival if adequate care is provided.

Subcutaneous fat increases further during weeks 33 through 38. The fetus has hair and fully formed limbs with fingernails and toenails. Earlobes are soft with little cartilage, but stiffen by week 40. Lanugo disappears from the face but remains on the head. Skin on the fetus's face and body becomes smooth. Amniotic fluid volume declines. The skull continues to be the largest body part. All organ systems are developed and can support extrauterine life. In males, the left testicle descends into the scrotum between 37 and 39 weeks. Both testicles are fully descended by 38 weeks. At week 40, lanugo appears on the upper body.

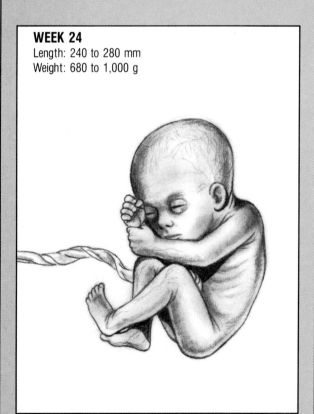

WEEK 24
Length: 240 to 280 mm
Weight: 680 to 1,000 g

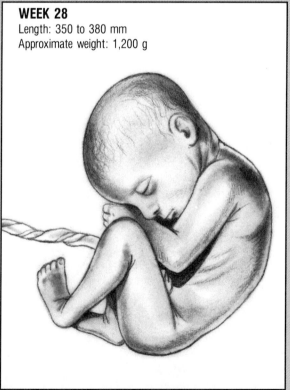

WEEK 28
Length: 350 to 380 mm
Approximate weight: 1,200 g

WEEK 12
Approximate length: 70 mm
Approximate weight: 28 g

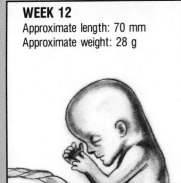

WEEK 16
Length: 100 to 170 mm
Weight: 55 to 120 g

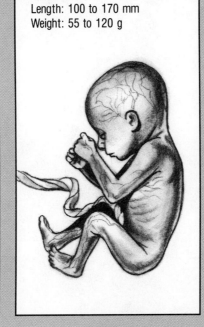

WEEK 20
Length: 160 to 250 mm
Weight: 223 to 310 g

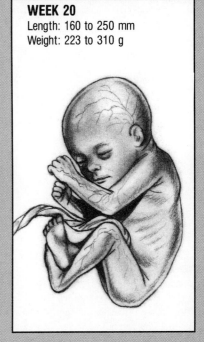

WEEK 32
Length: 380 to 430 mm
Weight: 1,700 to 2,400 g

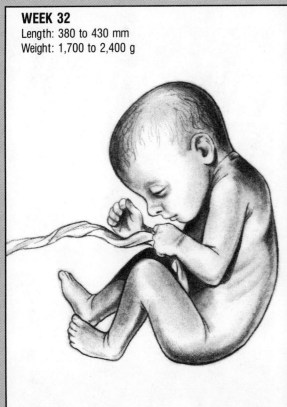

WEEK 38
Length: 480 to 520 mm
Weight: 2,800 to 3,200 g

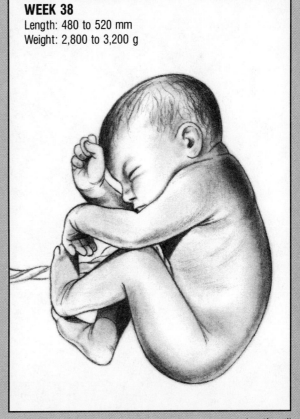

(continued)

FETAL DEVELOPMENT *(continued)*

PHOTOGRAPHIC ESSAY OF EMBRYONIC AND FETAL DEVELOPMENT

Before the client knows for certain that she is pregnant, the embryo is growing rapidly in a cavity beneath the surface of the uterine wall. There, the embryo begins a development that the following classic photographs illuminate.

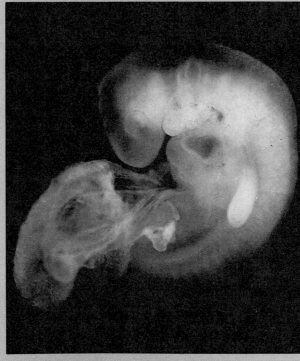

Week 4
Approximate length: 5 cm (0.2")
The embryo has no facial characteristics; the head and neck comprise half the body length.

Week 6
Approximate length: 1.5 cm (0.6")
The embryo floats freely in the fluid-filled amnion. The yolk sac and its stem are still attached but have ceased growing because the liver has begun producing blood cells.

Week 7
Approximate length: 2 cm (0.8")
The umbilical cord has formed, and the heart is beating.

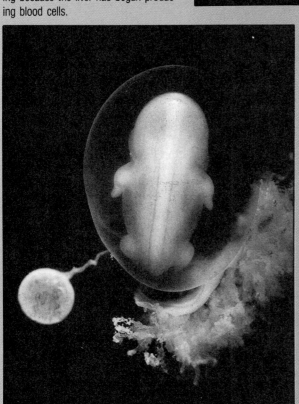

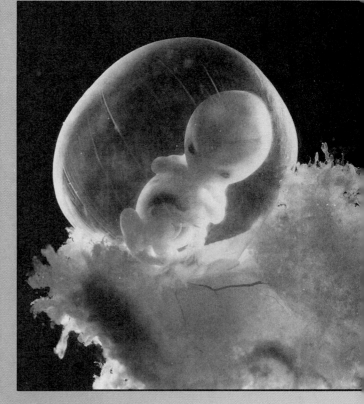

Photographs courtesy of Lennart Nilsson, from *A Child Is Born* (Revised Edition). New York: Dell Publishing, 1986.

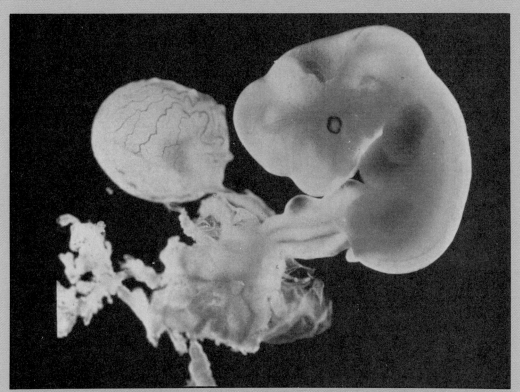

Week 5½
Approximate length: 1 cm (0.4")
Because no bone marrow exists at this stage, the yolk sac is the principal supplier of blood cells. Blood circulation is mostly outside the embryo.

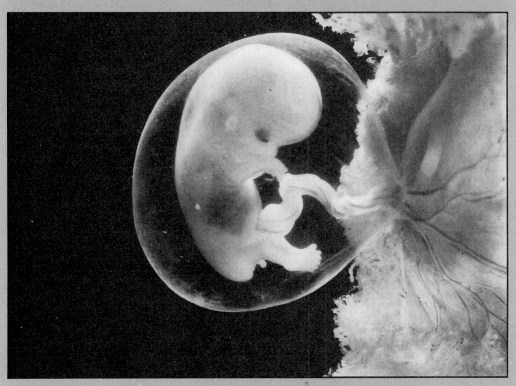

Week 9
Approximate length: 4.5 cm (2")
The placenta has grown where the blastocyst implanted itself in the uterine wall. The fetus receives nourishment through the umbilical cord.

(continued)

FETAL DEVELOPMENT *(continued)*

PHOTOGRAPHIC ESSAY OF EMBRYONIC AND FETAL DEVELOPMENT *(continued)*

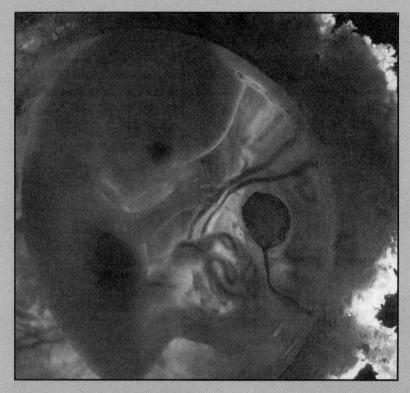

Week 11
Approximate length: 6 cm (2.4")
Blood cells are now produced in the liver and spleen, and the heart is functioning. The face has assumed a baby's profile, and the lips open and close. Although the mother cannot feel the weak legs and arms, they are in constant motion.

Week 18
Approximate length: 25 cm (10")
During constant movement, the fetus may pass a thumb across the mouth. The lips and tongue will respond with a suckling action.

Week 18
Approximate length: 25 cm (10")
Lanugo that follows the whorled skin pattern will be mostly shed before birth. The eyebrows are faintly apparent.

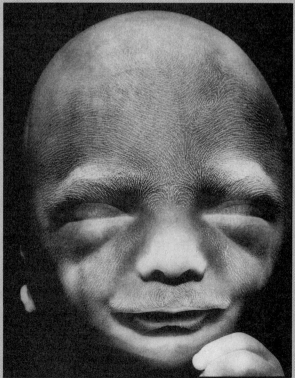

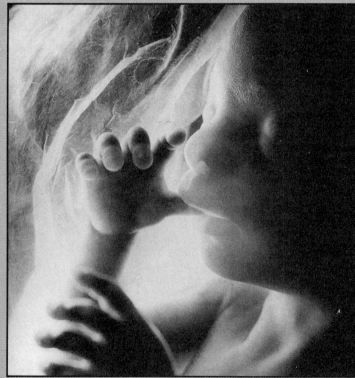

Photographs courtesy of Lennart Nilsson, from *A Child Is Born* (Revised Edition). New York: Dell Publishing, 1986.

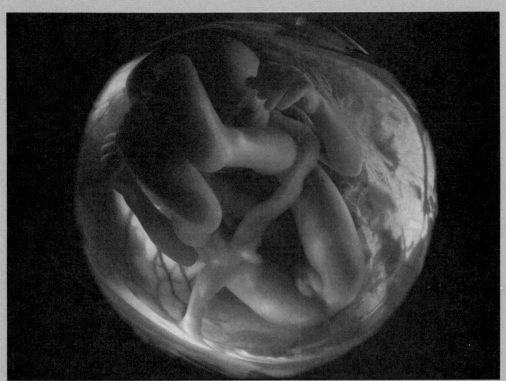

Week 16
Approximate length: 18 cm (7")
One-half the length of a neonate, the fetus has ears that function. Although the eyes have grown shut, they will re-open later. The mother may now feel faint kicks as the fetus moves around.

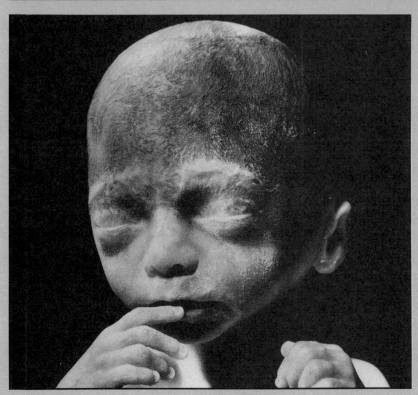

Week 20
Approximate length: 30 cm (12")
Vernix, a protective skin ointment that covers all body surfaces, is especially thick on the upper lip, eyebrows, and scalp.

basis of widely used pregnancy tests. Highly sensitive and specific pregnancy tests can detect hCG in blood and urine even before the first missed menstrual period, and sensitive tests almost invariably are positive if pregnancy causes a missed menstrual period.

Human placental lactogen. Also known as human chorionic somatomammotropin, hPL is a single-chain polypeptide hormone that is produced by the syncytiotrophoblast and has properties similar to pituitary growth hormone. HPL stimulates the maternal metabolism of protein and fat to ensure adequate amino and fatty acids for the mother and fetus. It may antagonize the action of insulin in the mother, decreasing maternal glucose use and making it available to the fetus. The hormone also stimulates the growth of the breasts in preparation for lactation. HPL levels rise progressively throughout pregnancy.

Other peptide hormones. The placenta also produces human chorionic thyrotropin, which has thyroid-stimulating properties, and human chorionic adrenocorticotropin, which has ACTH properties. The physiologic role of these placental hormones is not known. Another placental glycoprotein hormone called inhibin inhibits FSH secretion during pregnancy.

Estrogen and progesterone. Three types of estrogen are produced by the placenta, differing chiefly in the number of hydroxyl groups attached to the steroid nucleus: estrone (E_1), estradiol (E_2), and estriol (E_3). Estrogen production (primarily estriol) and estrogen urinary output increase throughout pregnancy. Progesterone production also increases; progesterone is excreted in the urine as the metabolite pregnanediol.

In contrast to the ovary, which has all the enzyme systems needed for synthesis of both estrogen and progesterone from simple compounds, the placenta lacks important enzymes and is unable to synthesize these hormones completely. To synthesize estrogen, the placenta must be provided with compounds from the fetal and maternal adrenal glands. Most of the steroids produced by the placenta are secreted into the maternal blood.

Because estrogen production depends on an adequate supply of precursor steroids from the fetal adrenal gland, a reduced estrogen output in pregnancy can indicate insufficient fetal adrenal gland development. Anencephaly, a congenital abnormality in which the brain fails to develop, commonly is associated with failure of the adrenal glands to develop normally. In other instances, the fetal adrenal glands may undergo hyperplasia or excessive development. As would be expected, the estrogen output in the urine of

a woman carrying an affected fetus is much increased because of the greater amount of precursor steroids provided to the placenta by the enlarged fetal adrenal glands.

Progesterone is synthesized by the placenta through hydroxylation of maternal cholesterol. Cholesterol is carried to the placenta in low-density lipoprotein particles that become attached to receptors on the surface of the trophoblasts. The particles are carried into the cytoplasm of the cell, where the lipoprotein is converted first to pregnenolone and then to progesterone. Because the fetus plays no part in progesterone biosynthesis, progesterone levels are unaffected by fetal distress or fetal abnormalities.

FETAL CIRCULATION

Because lungs do not function in a fetus, blood is oxygenated by the placenta. Fetal circulation differs from neonatal circulation in that three shunts bypass the liver and lungs and separate the systemic and pulmonary circulations. Because of the shunts, the umbilical vein carries oxygenated blood and the umbilical arteries carry unoxygenated blood. The shunts are:
* the ductus venosus (circulatory pathway that allows blood to bypass the liver)
* the foramen ovale (opening in the interstitial septum that directs blood from the right atium to the left one)
* the ductus arteriosus (tubular connection that shunts blood away from the pulmonary ciculation).

Oxygenated blood returns from the placenta through the umbilical vein. A small amount of this blood passes through the sinusoids of the liver; most is shunted through the ductus venosus into the inferior vena cava. Most of the blood flowing into the right atrium passes through the foramen ovale into the left atrium, bypassing the lungs. Thus, oxygenated blood from the placenta enters the left side of the heart; it is then pumped by the left ventricle into the aorta and then mainly into the vessels of the head and forelimbs.

Unoxygenated blood returns to the right atrium through the superior vena cava and flows downward through the tricuspid valve into the right ventricle. It then is pumped into the pulmonary arteries. Because the lungs are deflated, the blood encounters resistance. Consequently, most of the blood entering the main pulmonary artery bypasses the lungs and flows directly into the aorta through the ductus arteriosis and into the descending aorta. From there, it passes through the two umbilical arteries into the placenta, where the unoxygenated blood can become oxygenated. (See *Fetal circulation* for an illustration and description of this specialized system.)

FETAL CIRCULATION

This schematic representation of blood flow from the placenta through the fetus and back to the placenta shows oxygen exchange during fetal circulation.

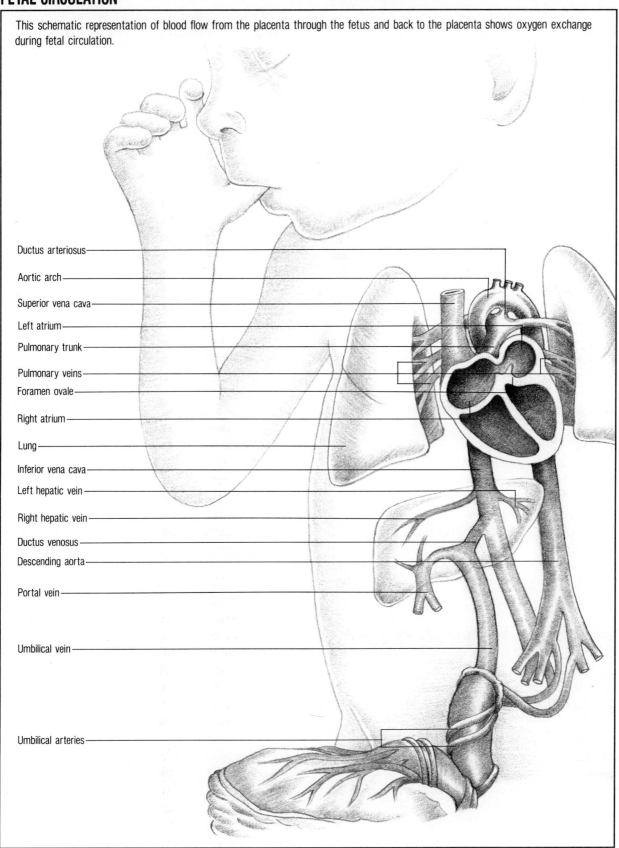

Ductus arteriosus

Aortic arch

Superior vena cava

Left atrium

Pulmonary trunk

Pulmonary veins

Foramen ovale

Right atrium

Lung

Inferior vena cava

Left hepatic vein

Right hepatic vein

Ductus venosus

Descending aorta

Portal vein

Umbilical vein

Umbilical arteries

CHAPTER SUMMARY

Chapter 4 described fetal development during normal gestation. Here are the chapter highlights.

In vivo fertilization can take place only when a mature spermatozoon ascends through a fallopian tube, encounters a mature, descending ovum, and enters and fertilizes it.

Implantation follows fertilization by about 1 week.

Human development from fertilization to birth includes three distinct periods: pre-embryonic, embryonic, and fetal.

All human organ systems are derived from three germ cell layers: ectoderm, endoderm, and mesoderm.

The placenta arises from the trophoblastic tissue layer and supports the fetus by providing the mechanisms for nutrition, respiration, and waste removal.

Placental transfer of substances is accomplished by simple diffusion, facilitated diffusion, active transport, and pinocytosis.

Fetal circulation includes three shunts that bypass the lungs and liver: the ductus venosus, foramen ovale, and ductus arteriosus.

STUDY QUESTIONS

1. Which conditions must be met before fertilization can occur?
2. Describe the events that occur during the period of twos and the period of threes.
3. What two major events occur during the embryonic period?
4. How does blood circulate between the mother and the fetus?
5. Describe the process of fetal circulation.

BIBLIOGRAPHY

Battaglia, F., and Meschia, G. (1986). *An introduction to fetal physiology.* Orlando, FL: Academic Press.

Briggs, G.G., Freeman, R.K., and Yaffe, S.J. (1986). *Drugs in pregnancy and lactation* (2nd ed.). Baltimore: Williams & Wilkins.

Chapman, M.C., Chard, T., and Grudzinskas, G. (Eds.) (1989). *Implantation.* New York: Springer-Verlag.

Crowley, L.V. (1974). *An introduction to clinical embryology.* Chicago: Year Book Medical Publishers.

Crowley, L.V. (1988). *Introduction to human disease* (2nd ed.). Boston: Jones and Bartlet.

Cunningham, F.G., MacDonald, P.C., and Gant, N.F. (Eds.) (1989). *Williams obstetrics* (18th ed.). East Norwalk, CT: Appleton & Lange.

Danforth, D.N., and Scott, J.R. (Eds.) (1986). *Obstetrics and gynecology* (5th ed.). Philadelphia: Lippincott.

Faber, J., and Thornburg, K. (1983). *Placental physiology: Structure and function of fetomaternal exchange.* New York: Raven Press.

Guyton, A. (1986). *Textbook of medical physiology* (7th ed.). Philadelphia: Saunders.

Hacker, N.F., and Moore, J.G. (Eds.) (1986). *Essentials of obstetrics and gynecology.* Philadelphia: Saunders.

Isaacson, G. (1986). *Atlas of fetal sectional physiology.* New York: Springer-Verlag.

Jones, C.T., and Nathaniels, P.W. (1985). *The physiological development of the fetus and newborn.* Orlando, FL: Academic Press.

Moore, K.L. (1983). *Before we were born: Basic embryology and birth defects* (2nd ed.). Philadelphia: Saunders.

Moore, K.L. (1988). *The developing human: Clinically oriented embryology* (4th ed.). Philadelphia: Saunders.

O'Rahilly, R., and Muller, F. (1987). *Developmental stages in human embryos.* Washington, DC: Carnegie Institute of Washington.

Rana, M.W. (1984). *Key facts in embryology.* New York: Churchill Livingstone.

Roberts, D.F. (Ed.) (1976). *The biology of human fetal growth.* Symposia of the Society for the Study of Human Biology Series, vol. 15. New York: Taylor & Francis.

Rolfe, P. (Ed.) (1987). *Fetal physiological measurements.* Woburn, MA: Butterworth.

Sadler, T.W. (1985). *Langman's medical embryology* (5th ed.). Baltimore: Williams & Wilkins.

Speroff, L., Glass, R.H., and Kase, N.G. (1988). *Clinical gynecologic endocrinology and infertility* (4th ed.). Baltimore: Williams & Wilkins.

CHAPTER 5

PHYSIOLOGIC CHANGES DURING NORMAL PREGNANCY

OBJECTIVES

After reading and studying this chapter, the student should be able to:

1. Distinguish among presumptive, probable, and positive signs of pregnancy.

2. Describe the major signs and symptoms used to diagnose pregnancy.

3. Discuss physiologic changes that occur in the maternal reproductive, endocrine, respiratory, cardiovascular, urinary, gastrointestinal, musculoskeletal, integumentary, immune, and neurologic systems during pregnancy.

4. Relate the underlying causes for maternal physiologic changes.

INTRODUCTION

Physiologic changes that occur during pregnancy are among the most dramatic that the human body can undergo. They help the client adapt to pregnancy, maintain health throughout pregnancy, and prepare for childbirth. They also create a safe and nurturing environment for the fetus. Some begin even before the client becomes aware that she is pregnant.

Physiologic changes associated with pregnancy may range from subtle to overwhelming. Although these changes are normal and necessary, they may be uncomfortable and—especially for the primigravid client—even frightening. To care for pregnant clients properly, the nurse must understand the physiologic changes of normal pregnancy, when they occur, and how they are likely to affect the client.

This chapter begins by outlining the presumptive, probable, and positive signs of pregnancy. It then describes the physiologic changes that occur in each maternal body system, the role various hormones play in initiating and regulating body functions during pregnancy, and the signs and symptoms commonly caused by these changes. (For information on nursing care of the antepartal client, see Chapter 7, Care during the Normal Antepartal Period.)

DIAGNOSING PREGNANCY

Early pregnancy produces a constellation of physiologic changes (signs and symptoms) that the health care provider must evaluate as a group before reaching a tentative diagnosis of pregnancy. Some of these changes may be presumptive signs of pregnancy (those that allow an assumption of pregnancy until more concrete signs occur), such as amenorrhea; some may be probable signs of pregnancy, such as abdominal enlargement. Neither presumptive nor probable signs confirm pregnancy because both may be caused by medical conditions. They may suggest pregnancy, however, especially when several are present at once. Probable signs suggest pregnancy somewhat more strongly than presumptive signs. Positive signs, such as fetal heartbeat and palpable fetal movement, prove pregnancy because they cannot be caused by any condition. (For more details, see *Presumptive, probable, and positive signs of pregnancy,* pages 66 and 67.)

(Text continues on page 68.)

PRESUMPTIVE, PROBABLE, AND POSITIVE SIGNS OF PREGNANCY

The following chart lists and describes typical presumptive and probable signs of pregnancy and explains their pregnancy-related and possible other causes. The chart then describes positive signs of pregnancy.

SIGN	DESCRIPTION	PREGNANCY-RELATED CAUSES	POSSIBLE OTHER CAUSES
Presumptive			
Amenorrhea	Absence of menses. Usually the first indication of pregnancy in client with regular menstrual periods.	• Rising levels of human chorionic gonadotropin (hCG) hormone	• Anovulation, blocked endometrial cavity, endocrine changes, medications (phenothiazines), metabolic changes
Nausea and vomiting	Onset typically at 4 to 6 weeks, continuing through first trimester or occasionally longer.	• Rising levels of hCG • Emotional stress • Reduced gastric motility, reflux • Altered metabolism	• Gastric disorders, infections, psychological disorders (pseudocyesis, anorexia nervosa)
Urinary frequency	Begins during first trimester as uterus enlarges; resolves during second trimester when uterus rises out of pelvis; resumes during third trimester when fetus descends into pelvis.	• Enlarging uterus exerts pressure on urinary bladder	• Emotional stress, pelvic tumor, renal disease, urinary tract infection
Breast changes	Enlargement begins early in first trimester. Breasts become tender and may tingle or throb. As pregnancy progresses, nipples enlarge, become more erectile, and may darken. The areolae widen. Veins become more visible.	• Hormonal changes • Growth of secretory ductal system • Increase in glandular tissue	• Hyperprolactinemia induced by tranquilizers, infection, prolactin-secreting pituitary tumor, pseudocyesis, premenstrual syndrome
Fatigue	Malaise, general discomfort, lethargy with no apparent cause.	• Unexplained, although progesterone may play a role	• Anemia, chronic illness
Quickening	Client's first awareness of fluttering movements in lower abdomen, usually at 16 to 20 weeks.	• Movement of fetus	• Excessive flatus, increased peristalsis
Skin changes	May include linea nigra, chloasma, vascular markings, and striae. Because pigment changes may persist, they are not a reliable sign in multigravid clients.	• Increase in melanocyte-stimulating hormone • Increased estrogen • Stretching and atrophy of connective tissue	• Cardiopulmonary disorders, estrogen-progestin oral contraceptives, obesity, pelvic tumor
Probable			
Braun von Fernwald's sign (also called Piskacek's sign)	Fullness and irregular softness of fundus near area of implantation. Can be felt at 5 to 6 weeks of pregnancy.	• Local reaction to implantation; increased blood flow to pelvic organs	• Uterine tumor
Hegar's sign	Softening of uterine isthmus may be felt at 6 to 8 weeks via vaginal or rectovaginal examination.	• Increased blood flow to pelvic organs	• Excessively soft uterine walls

PRESUMPTIVE, PROBABLE, AND POSITIVE SIGNS OF PREGNANCY *(continued)*

SIGN	DESCRIPTION	PREGNANCY-RELATED CAUSES	POSSIBLE OTHER CAUSES
Goodell's sign	Softening of cervix at 6 to 8 weeks.	• Increased blood flow to pelvic organs	• Estrogen-progestin oral contraceptives
Chadwick's sign	Bluish coloration of mucous membranes of cervix, vagina, and vulva at 6 to 8 weeks.	• Engorgement caused by increased blood flow to pelvic organs	• Hyperemia of cervix, vagina, vulva
McDonald's sign	Easy flexion of fundus into cervix at 6 to 8 weeks.	• Increased blood flow to pelvic organs	• Oral contraceptives, uterine tumor
Ladin's sign	Soft, palpable area on anterior middle portion of uterus near junction of uterus and cervix.	• Increased blood flow to pelvic organs	• Oral contraceptives, uterine tumor
Abdominal enlargement	Softening of uterus and fetal growth cause uterus to enlarge and stretch abdominal wall.	• Enlarging uterus	• Ascites, obesity, uterine or pelvic tumor
Braxton Hicks contractions	Uterine contractions beginning early in pregnancy and becoming more frequent after 28 weeks.	• Possibly from enlargement of uterus to accommodate growing fetus	• Hematometra, uterine tumor
Ballottment	Passive movement of fetus. Typically identified at weeks 16 to 18.	• Rebounding of fetus in response to pressure exerted on uterus	• Ascites, uterine tumor or polyps
Uterine souffle	Soft, blowing sound synchronous with maternal pulse.	• Increased vascularity as blood flows through placenta	• Large ovarian tumor, enlarging myoma
Funic souffle	Sharp, blowing sound synchronous with fetal pulse.	• Increased vascularity as blood flows through umbilical cord	• Aneurysm of abdominal aorta, iliac artery, or renal artery
Fetal outline	Fetus may be palpated through uterine wall after 24 weeks.	• Growing fetus	• Subserous uterine myoma
Positive pregnancy test	Based on detection of hCG secreted by chorionic villi. Levels of hCG begin to increase 6 to 8 days after conception, peak at 8 to 12 weeks, and then gradually decline.	• Increased levels of hCG	• Luteinizing hormone is similar to hCG and may cross react in some pregnancy tests.
Positive			
Fetal heartbeat	May be detected as early as week 5 using ultrasound, week 10 using doppler ultrasound, week 12 using fetal electrocardiography, and week 16 using a standard fetoscope.	• Fetal cardiovascular development	• None
Fetal movement on palpation	May be felt as thump or flutter through abdomen after week 18; may be visible after week 20.	• Fetal growth	• None

CHANGES IN BODY SYSTEMS

Physiologic changes that help diagnose pregnancy make up only a small number of the changes that occur in a pregnant client. As the fetus grows and hormones shift, the client's body undergoes physiologic changes, primarily to adapt to the fetus and to prepare for childbirth. Physiologic adjustments occur in each body system.

REPRODUCTIVE SYSTEM

External reproductive structures affected by pregnancy include the labia majora, labia minora, clitoris, and vaginal introitus. These structures enlarge because of increased vascularity; the labia majora and labia minora also enlarge because of fat deposits. Although the structures reduce in size after childbirth, they may not return to their prepregnant state because of loss of muscle tone or perineal injury. For example, the labia majora remain separated and gape after childbirth. In addition, varices may be caused by pressure on vessels in the perineal and perianal areas.

Internal reproductive structures change dramatically to accommodate the developing fetus. Like their external counterparts, these internal structures may not regain their prepregnant states after childbirth.

Ovaries

Once fertilization occurs, ovarian follicles cease to mature and ovulation stops. The chorionic villi, which develop from the fertilized ovum, begin to produce human chorionic gonadotropin (hCG) to maintain the ovarian corpus luteum. The corpus luteum produces estrogen and progesterone until the placenta is formed and functioning. At 8 to 10 weeks of pregnancy, the placenta assumes production of these hormones and the corpus luteum—no longer needed—undergoes involution (reduction in organ size caused by a reduction in the size of its cells).

Uterus

The nonpregnant uterus is smaller than the size of a fist, measuring approximately $7.5 \times 5 \times 2.5$ cm. It weighs approximately 60 to 70 g in the nulliparous client and 100 g in the parous client. In its nonpregnant state, the uterus can hold no more than 10 cc of fluid. Its walls are composed of several overlapping layers of muscle fibers that adapt to the developing fetus and aid in expulsion of the fetus and placenta during labor and childbirth.

The uterus retains the developing fetus for approximately 280 days, or 9 calendar months, and undergoes progressive changes in size, shape, and position in the abdominal cavity.

Enlargement. In the first trimester, the pear-shaped uterus lengthens and enlarges in response to elevated levels of estrogen and progesterone. This hormonal stimulation primarily increases the size of myometrial cells (hypertrophy), although a small increase in cell number (hyperplasia) also occurs. These changes increase the amount of fibrous and elastic tissue to more than 20 times that of the nonpregnant uterus. Uterine walls become stronger and more elastic.

During the first few weeks of pregnancy, the uterine walls remain thick and the fundus rests low in the abdomen. The uterus cannot be palpated through the abdominal wall. After 12 weeks of pregnancy, however, the uterus typically reaches the level of the symphysis pubis and then may be palpated through the abdominal wall.

In the second trimester, the corpus and fundus become globe-shaped, and as pregnancy progresses the uterus lengthens to become oval in shape. The uterine walls become thinner as the muscles stretch; the uterus rises out of the pelvis, shifts to the right, and rests against the anterior abdominal wall. At 20 weeks of pregnancy, the uterus may be palpated just below the umbilicus and reaches the umbilicus at 22 weeks. As uterine muscles stretch, Braxton Hicks contractions may occur, helping to move blood more quickly through the intervillous spaces of the placenta.

In the third trimester, the fundus reaches nearly to the xiphoid process (also called the ensiform process). Between 38 and 40 weeks of pregnancy, the fetus begins to descend in the pelvis (lightening), which causes fundal height to drop gradually. The uterus remains oval in shape. Its muscular walls become progressively thinner as it enlarges, finally reaching a muscle wall thickness of 5 mm or less. At term (40 weeks), the uterus typically weighs approximately 1,100 g, holds 5 to 10 liters of fluid, and has stretched to approximately $28 \times 24 \times 21$ cm.

Progressive abdominal enlargement (accompanied by amenorrhea) is the most observable sign of pregnancy, although posture and previous pregnancies will influence the type and amount of enlargement. Enlargement typically is more pronounced in the multigravid client because the uterus assumes a more forward position after previous pregnancies reduce abdominal muscle tone.

Endometrial development. During the menstrual cycle, progesterone stimulates increased thickening and vascularity of the endometrium, preparing the uterine lining for implantation and nourishment of a fertilized ovum. After implantation, menstruation ceases and the endometrium becomes the decidua, which is divided into three layers: decidua capsularis, decidua basalis, and decidua vera. The decidua capsularis covers the blastocyst (fertilized ovum). The decidua basalis lies directly under the blastocyst and forms part of the placenta. The decidua vera lines the remainder of the uterus.

Vascular growth. As the fetus grows and the placenta develops, uterine blood vessels and lymphatics increase in number and size. Vessels must enlarge to accommodate the increased blood flow to the uterus and placenta. By the end of pregnancy, an average of 500 ml of blood may flow through the maternal side of the placenta each minute (Cunningham, MacDonald, and Gant, 1989). Maternal arterial pressure, uterine contractions, and maternal position affect uterine blood flow throughout pregnancy.

Elongation and softening of the isthmus. After 6 to 8 weeks of pregnancy, the isthmus softens and can be compressed during a vaginal or rectovaginal examination. This compression, known as Hegar's sign, offers one of the most important early signs of pregnancy. As pregnancy advances, the isthmus becomes part of the lower uterine segment. During labor, it expands further.

Cervical changes. In addition to softening, the cervix takes on a bluish color during the second month of pregnancy, becomes edematous, and may bleed easily upon examination or sexual activity.

Hormonal stimulation causes the glandular cervical tissue to increase in cell number and become more hyperactive, secreting a thick, tenacious mucus. This mucus thickens into a mucoid weblike structure, eventually forming a mucus plug that blocks the cervical canal and erects a protective barrier against bacteria and other substances that might enter the uterus.

Perhaps the outstanding characteristic of the cervix is its ability to stretch during childbirth, which is possible because of increased connective tissue, elastic fiber, and enfoldings in the endocervical lining.

Vagina

Estrogen stimulates vascularity, tissue growth, and hypertrophy in the vaginal epithelial tissue. Vaginal secretions—white, thick, odorless, and acidic—increase. The acidity of vaginal secretions helps prevent bacterial infections, but it fosters yeast infections, a common occurrence during pregnancy. This change in pH arises with increased production of lactic acid from glycogen in the vaginal epithelium; increased lactic acid results from the action of *Lactobacillus acidophilus*.

Other vaginal changes include:
• development of the same bluish color as the cervix and vulva due to increased vascularity
• hypertrophy of the smooth muscles and relaxation of connective tissues, which combine to allow the vagina to stretch during childbirth
• lengthening of the vaginal vault
• possible heightened sexual response.

Breasts

During the first trimester, increased levels of estrogen and progesterone enlarge the breasts and cause tenderness. They may tingle or throb. The nipples enlarge, become more erectile, and—along with the areolae—darken in color. Sebaceous glands in the areolae become hypertrophic, producing small elevations known as Montgomery's follicles. Areolae widen from a diameter of less than 3 cm (1½″) to 5 or 6 cm (2″ or 3″) in the primigravid client. Rarely, patches of brownish discoloration may appear on the skin adjacent to the areolae. These patches, known as secondary areolae, may be a sign of pregnancy if the client has never breast-fed an infant.

As blood vessels enlarge, veins beneath the skin of the breasts become more visible and may appear as intertwining patterns over the anterior chest wall. Breasts become fuller and heavier as lactation approaches. They may throb uncomfortably. Increasing hormones cause the secretion of a yellowish, viscous fluid from the nipples known as colostrum. High in protein, antibodies, and minerals but low in fat and sugar as compared with mature human milk, colostrum may be secreted as early as the first several months of pregnancy, but it is most common during the last trimester. It continues for 2 to 4 days after delivery and is followed by mature milk production.

Breast changes are more pronounced in the primigravid than in the multigravid client. In the latter, changes are even less significant if the client has breast-fed an infant within the preceding year because her areola will still be dark and her breasts enlarged.

ENDOCRINE SYSTEM

Together with the nervous system, the endocrine system controls metabolic functions that promote maternal and fetal health throughout pregnancy. Estrogen stimulates and temporarily enlarges the pituitary, thyroid, and parathyroid glands. Other major endocrine changes occur as well.

Pituitary gland

Anterior pituitary hormones help to maintain the corpus luteum in early pregnancy. Two hormones secreted by the anterior pituitary—thyrotropin and adrenocorticotropic hormone (ACTH)—alter maternal metabolism so that pregnancy can progress. Prolactin, another anterior pituitary hormone, increases throughout pregnancy in preparation for lactation.

The posterior pituitary releases two hormones important in pregnancy. Vasopressin (antidiuretic hormone or ADH) helps regulate water balance through its antidiuretic action, and oxytocin stimulates labor and aids in lactation through its effect on breast tissue.

Thyroid gland

As early as the second month of pregnancy, thyroxine (T_4)-binding protein increases and total T_4 rises correspondingly. Because the amount of unbound T_4 does not increase, the client does not develop hyperthyroidism. However, thyroid changes do produce a slight increase in basal metabolic rate (BMR), cardiac output, pulse rate, vasodilation, and heat intolerance. The BMR increases about 15% during the second and third trimesters as the growing fetus places additional demands for energy on the client's system. By term, the client's BMR may have increased 25%. It returns to the prepregnant level within 1 week after childbirth.

In addition, estrogen increases circulating amounts of triiodothyronine (T_3). Because much of this hormone is bound to proteins and is thus nonfunctional (like T_4), its elevation does not lead to a hyperthyroid condition during pregnancy.

Parathyroid gland

As pregnancy progresses, fetal demands for calcium and phosphorus increase. The parathyroid gland responds by increasing hormones during the third trimester to as much as twice the prepregnant level.

Adrenal gland

Increased estrogen raises the levels of cortisol and aldosterone. However, increased cortisol does not significantly increase the metabolism of carbohydrates, fats, and proteins (as it normally would) because much of the cortisol is bound by the cortisol-binding globulin transcortin. Elevated aldosterone minimizes the sodium-wasting effect of progesterone by promoting sodium resorption in the renal tubules.

Pancreas

Although the pancreas itself undergoes no changes during pregnancy, maternal insulin, glucose, and glucagon levels change. As pregnancy advances, fetal growth and development require increased glucose. For example, after ingesting oral glucose, the pregnant client has prolonged hyperglycemia, hyperinsulinism, and reduced glucagon levels. Although the reason for these level shifts is unknown, they probably provide a sustained supply of glucose to the fetus. The placenta secretes a hormone—human placental lactogen (hPL)—that promotes fat breakdown (lipolysis) and provides the client with an alternate source of energy.

However, hPL has a complicating effect. Along with estrogen, progesterone, and cortisol, hPL inhibits the action of insulin, which results in an increased need for insulin throughout pregnancy.

RESPIRATORY SYSTEM

Throughout pregnancy, biochemical and mechanical changes occur in the respiratory system in response to hormonal alterations. As pregnancy advances, these changes facilitate gas exchange, providing the client with increased oxygen.

Anatomic changes

The diaphragm rises by approximately 4 cm during pregnancy, which prevents the lungs from expanding as much as they normally do. The diaphragm compensates by increasing its excursion ability, and the rib cage compensates by flaring from approximately 68 degrees before pregnancy to about 103 degrees in the third trimester. In addition, the anteroposterior and transverse diameters of the rib cage increase by about 2 cm and the circumference increases by 5 to 7 cm. This expansion is possible because increased progesterone relaxes the ligaments that join the rib cage. As the uterus enlarges, thoracic breathing replaces abdominal breathing.

The upper respiratory tract vascularizes in response to increasing levels of estrogen. The client may develop respiratory congestion, voice changes, and epistaxis as capillaries become engorged in the nose, pharynx, larynx, trachea, bronchi, and vocal cords. Increased vascularization also may cause the eustachian tubes to swell, leading to such problems as impaired hearing, earaches, and a sense of fullness in the ears.

Functional changes

Changes in pulmonary function improve gas exchange in the alveoli and facilitate oxygenation of blood flowing through the lungs. The respiratory rate typically remains unaffected in early pregnancy. By the third trimester, however, increased progesterone may increase the rate by approximately two breaths/minute.

Tidal volume and minute volume. Tidal volume (the amount of air inhaled and exhaled) rises throughout pregnancy as a result of increased progesterone and increased diaphragmatic excursion. In fact, the pregnant client will breathe 30% to 40% more air than she does when not pregnant. Minute volume (the amount of air expired per minute) increases by approximately 50% by term. The difference between changes in tidal volume and minute volume creates a slight hyperventilation, which decreases carbon dioxide in alveoli. The resulting lower $PaCO_2$ in maternal blood leads to a greater partial pressure difference of carbon dioxide between fetal and maternal blood, which facilitates diffusion of carbon dioxide from the fetus.

Lung capacity. An elevated diaphragm decreases functional residual capacity (the volume of air remaining in the lungs after exhalation), and decreased functional residual capacity contributes to hyperventilation. Vital capacity (the largest volume of air that can be expelled voluntarily after maximum inspiration) increases slightly during pregnancy. These changes, along with increased cardiac output and blood volume, provide adequate blood flow to the placenta.

Acid-base balance. During the third month of pregnancy, increased progesterone sensitizes respiratory receptors and increases ventilation, leading to a drop in carbon dioxide levels. This increases pH, which might cause mild respiratory alkalosis, except that a decreased bicarbonate level partially or completely compensates for this tendency.

CARDIOVASCULAR SYSTEM

Pregnancy alters the cardiovascular system so profoundly that, outside of pregnancy, the changes would be considered pathological and even life-threatening. During pregnancy, however, these changes are vital to a positive outcome.

Anatomic changes

The heart enlarges slightly during pregnancy, probably because of increased blood volume and cardiac output. This enlargement is not marked and reverses after childbirth.

As pregnancy advances, the uterus moves up and presses on the diaphragm, displacing the heart upward and rotating it on its long axis. The amount of displacement varies depending on the position and size of the uterus, the firmness of the abdominal muscles, the shape of the abdomen, and other factors.

Auscultatory changes

Changes in blood volume, cardiac output, and the size and position of the heart alter heart sounds during pregnancy. These changed heart sounds would be considered abnormal in a client who is not pregnant.

During pregnancy, S_1 tends to exhibit a pronounced splitting, and each component tends to be louder. An occasional S_3 sound may occur after 20 weeks of pregnancy. Definite changes tend not to occur in either the aortic or pulmonic components of S_2. Many pregnant clients exhibit a systolic ejection murmur over the pulmonic area.

Cardiac rhythm disturbances, such as sinus arrhythmia, premature atrial contractions, and premature ventricular systole, may occur. In the pregnant client with no underlying heart disease, these arrhythmias do not require therapy, nor do they indicate development of myocardial disease.

Hemodynamic changes

Pregnancy affects heart rate and cardiac output, venous and arterial blood pressure, circulation and coagulation, and blood volume.

Heart rate and cardiac output. During the second trimester, heart rate increases gradually until it may reach 10 to 15 beats/minute above the prepregnant rate. During the third trimester, heart rate may increase 15 to 20 beats/minute above the prepregnant rate. The client may feel palpitations occasionally throughout pregnancy. In the early months, they result from sympathetic nervous stimulation.

Increased tissue demand for oxygen and increased stroke volume raise cardiac output by up to 50% by the thirty-second week of pregnancy. The increase is highest at rest when the client is lying on her side and lowest when she is lying on her back. The side-lying position reduces pressure on the great vessels, which increases venous return to the heart. Cardiac output peaks during labor, when tissue demands are greatest.

Venous and arterial blood pressure. When the client lies on her back, femoral venous pressure increases threefold from early pregnancy to term. This occurs because the uterus exerts pressure on the inferior vena cava and pelvic veins, retarding venous return from the legs and feet. The client may feel lightheaded if she rises abruptly after lying on her back. Edema in the legs and varicosities in the legs, rectum, and vulva may occur.

Early in pregnancy, increased progesterone levels relax smooth muscles and dilate arterioles, resulting in vasodilation. Systolic and diastolic pressures may decrease 5 to 10 mm Hg. Blood pressure reaches its lowest during the second half of the second trimester and then gradually returns to first trimester levels during the third trimester. By term, arterial blood pressure approaches prepregnant levels.

Brachial artery pressure is highest when the client lies on her back, which causes the enlarged uterus to exert the greatest pressure on the vena cava, and lowest when she lies on her left side, which relieves uterine pressure on the vena cava.

Circulation and coagulation. Venous return decreases slightly during the eighth month of pregnancy and at term increases to normal levels. Blood clots more readily during pregnancy and the postpartal period because of an increase in clotting factors VII, IX, and X.

Blood volume. Total intravascular volume increases during pregnancy, beginning between the tenth and twelfth weeks and peaking at approximately a 40% increase between the thirty-second and thirty-fourth weeks. Volume decreases slightly in the fortieth week and returns to normal several weeks postpartum. The increase consists of two-thirds plasma and one-third red blood cells. The increased blood volume supplies the hypertrophied vascular system of the enlarging uterus, provides nutrition for fetal and maternal tissues, and serves as a reserve for blood loss during childbirth and puerperium.

Hematologic changes
Pregnancy affects red and white blood cells and fibrinogen levels. Bone marrow becomes more active during pregnancy, producing up to a 30% excess in red blood cells if sufficient iron is available. The client may require an iron supplement to increase hemoglobin synthesis.

The increase in plasma volume is disproportionately greater than the increase in erythrocytes, which lowers the client's hematocrit (the percentage of erythrocytes in whole blood) and causes physiologic anemia of pregnancy. The hemoglobin level also decreases. A hematocrit below 35% and a hemoglobin level below 11.5 g/dl indicate pregnancy-related anemia.

Leukocytes increase for unknown reasons during pregnancy, and the white blood cell count rises, ranging from 10,000 to 12,000 mm³. The count may increase to

25,000 mm³ or more during labor, childbirth, and the early postpartal period.

Fibrinogen—a protein in blood plasma—is converted to fibrin by thrombin and is known as coagulation factor I. In the nonpregnant client, levels average 250 mg/dl. In the pregnant client, levels average 450 mg/dl, increasing as much as 50% by term. This increase plays an important role in preventing maternal hemorrhage during childbirth.

URINARY SYSTEM

The kidneys, ureters, and bladder undergo profound changes in structure and function during pregnancy.

Anatomic changes
Significant dilation of the renal pelves, calyces, and ureters begins as early as the tenth week of pregnancy, probably caused by increased estrogen and progesterone. As pregnancy advances and the uterus becomes dextrorotated, the ureters and renal pelves become more dilated above the pelvic brim, particularly on the right side. In addition, the smooth muscle of the ureters undergoes hypertrophy and hyperplasia; muscle tone decreases, primarily because of the muscle-relaxing effects of progesterone.

These changes retard the flow of urine through the ureters and result in hydronephrosis and hydroureter (distention of the renal pelves and ureters with urine), predisposing the pregnant client to urinary tract infection. In addition, because of the delay between urine formation in the kidneys and its arrival in the bladder, inaccuracies may occur during clearance tests.

Hormonal changes cause the bladder to relax during pregnancy, permitting it to distend to hold approximately 1,500 ml of urine. However, hormonal changes and pressure from the growing uterus cause bladder irritation, manifested as urinary frequency and urgency, even if the bladder contains little urine. Bladder vascularity increases and the mucosa bleeds easily. In the second trimester, when the uterus rises out of the pelvis, urinary symptoms abate. As term approaches, however, the presenting part of the fetus engages in the pelvis—exerting pressure once again on the bladder—and symptoms return.

Functional changes
Pregnancy affects renal plasma flow, glomeruler filtration rate, renal tubular resorption, and nutrient and glucose excretion.

Renal plasma flow. Early in pregnancy, renal plasma flow (RPF) increases by an unknown mechanism, rising to 40% to 50% above the prepregnant level by the third trimester. RPF then declines slightly.

Glomerular filtration rate. By the beginning of the second trimester, glomerular filtration rate (GFR) increases as much as 50% by an unknown mechanism; it remains elevated to term. This increase in GFR produces a consequent decrease in some laboratory test values, including blood urea nitrogen and creatinine levels.

Renal tubular resorption. Acting to maintain sodium and fluid balance, renal tubular resorption increases as much as 50% during pregnancy. The sodium requirement increases because the client needs more intravascular and extracellular fluid. Total body water increases also, to a total of about 7 liters more than in the prepregnant state. The amniotic fluid and placenta account for about half of this amount; increased maternal blood volume and enlargement of the breasts and uterus account for the rest.

Late in pregnancy, changes in posture affect sodium and water excretion. The client will excrete less when lying on her back because the enlarged uterus compresses the vena cava and aorta, causing decreased cardiac output. This decreases renal blood flow, which in turn decreases kidney function. The client will excrete more when lying on her left side because, in this position, the uterus does not compress the great vessels. Thus, cardiac output and kidney function remain unchanged.

Nutrient and glucose excretion. The pregnant client loses increased amounts of some nutrients, such as amino acids, water-soluble vitamins, folic acid, and iodine. Glycosuria (glucose in the urine) may occur as GFR increases without a corresponding increase in tubular resorptive capacity. Proteinuria (protein in the urine) is considered abnormal in pregnancy. It may occur occasionally during and after difficult labors.

GASTROINTESTINAL SYSTEM

Changes during pregnancy affect anatomic elements in the gastrointestinal system and alter certain functions. These changes are associated with many of the most discussed discomforts of pregnancy.

Anatomic changes

The mouth and teeth, stomach and intestines, and gallbladder and liver are affected during pregnancy.

Mouth and teeth. The salivary glands become more active, especially in the latter half of pregnancy. The gums become edematous and bleed easily because of increased vascularity. The teeth are unaffected; they lose no minerals to the developing fetus.

Stomach and intestines. As progesterone increases during pregnancy, gastric tone and motility decrease, slowing the stomach's emptying time and possibly causing regurgitation and reflux of stomach contents. The client may complain of heartburn.

The enlarging uterus displaces the stomach upward. In late pregnancy, the uterus displaces the small intestine as well. Hormonal changes and mechanical pressure reduce motility in the small intestine. Reduced motility in the colon leads to greater water absorption, which may predispose the client to constipation. The enlarging uterus displaces the large intestine and puts increased pressure on veins below the uterus, which may predispose the client to hemorrhoids.

Gallbladder and liver. As smooth muscles relax, the gallbladder empties more sluggishly. This prolonged emptying time, along with increased excretion of cholesterol in the bile caused by increased hormone levels, may lead to bile that is supersaturated with cholesterol and predispose the client to cholesterol crystal formation and gallstone development.

The liver does not enlarge or undergo any major changes during pregnancy. However, hepatic blood flow may increase slightly, and the liver's work load increases as the basal metabolic rate increases. Factors within the liver and increased estrogen and progesterone decrease bile flow.

Some liver function studies show drastic changes, possibly caused in part by increased estrogen levels. These changes would suggest hepatic disease in a nonpregnant client.

- Alkaline phosphatase nearly doubles, caused in part by increased alkaline phosphatase isoenzymes from the placenta.
- Serum albumin levels decrease.
- Plasma globulin levels increase causing decreases in albumin globulin ratios.
- Plasma cholinesterase levels decrease.

Functional changes

Nausea and vomiting may affect appetite and food consumption, even while energy demand increases.

Appetite and food consumption. The client's appetite and food consumption fluctuate. Many women experience nausea and vomiting early in pregnancy. Nausea typically is more pronounced in the morning, beginning at 4 to 6 weeks and subsiding by the end of the first trimester. Some women experience this morning sickness at other hours and beyond the first trimester. Severity varies from a slight distaste for food to severe vomiting. Certain odors and the sight of food can trigger an occurrence. Peculiarities in taste and smell also may develop.

Although uncomfortable for the client, morning sickness has no deleterious effects on the fetus. In fact, research suggests that clients who vomit in early pregnancy have a decreased incidence of spontaneous abortion, stillbirth, and premature labor (Klebanoff, Koslowe, and Kaslow, 1985). Morning sickness should be considered abnormal if accompanied by fever, pain, or weight loss.

In addition to the appetite reduction caused by nausea and vomiting, the client's appetite may be reduced by increased hCG levels and changes in carbohydrate metabolism, which are suspected appetite suppressants. Once nausea and vomiting cease, the client's appetite increases along with increasing metabolic needs. However, the old adage of "eating for two" is erroneous. (See Chapter 8, Nutrition and Diet Counseling, for more information.)

Carbohydrate, lipid, and protein metabolism. The client's carbohydrate needs rise to meet increasing energy demands. The client needs more glucose, especially during the second half of pregnancy. Plasma lipid levels increase starting in the first trimester, rising at term to 40% to 50% above the prepregnant level. Cholesterol, triglyceride, and lipoprotein levels increase as well. The total concentration of serum proteins decreases, especially serum albumin and perhaps gamma globulin. The primary immunoglobulin transferred to the fetus-is lowered in the client's serum. (See Chapter 8, Nutrition and Diet Counseling, for a complete discussion of carbohydrate, lipid, and protein metabolism.)

MUSCULOSKELETAL SYSTEM

The client's musculoskeletal system changes in response to hormones, weight gain, and the growing fetus. These changes may affect the client's gait, posture, and comfort.

Skeleton

The enlarging uterus tilts the pelvis forward, shifting the client's center of gravity. The lumbosacral curve increases, accompanied by a compensatory curvature in the cervicodorsal region. The lumbar and dorsal curves become even more pronounced as breasts enlarge and their weight pulls the shoulders forward, producing a stoop-shouldered stance. Increasing sex hormones (and possibly the hormone relaxin) relax the sacroiliac, sacrococcygeal, and pelvic joints. These changes cause marked alterations in posture and gait. Relaxation of the pelvic joints may cause the client's gait to change. Shoe and ring sizes tend to increase because of weight gain, hormonal changes, and dependent edema. Although these changes may persist after childbirth, they more nearly approach their prepregnant states.

Muscles

In the third trimester, the prominent rectus abdominis muscles separate, allowing the abdominal contents to protrude at the midline. The umbilicus may flatten or protrude. After childbirth, abdominal muscles regain tone but typically do not return to their prepregnant state.

INTEGUMENTARY SYSTEM

Skin changes vary greatly among pregnant clients. Of those who experience skin changes, Blacks and brunette Caucasians typically show more marked changes than blondes. Because some skin changes may remain after childbirth, they are not considered an important sign of pregnancy in the multigravid client. The client may need the nurse's help to integrate these skin changes into her self-concept. Skin changes associated with pregnancy include striae gravidarum, pigment changes, and vascular markings.

Striae gravidarum

The client's weight gain and enlarging uterus, combined with the action of adrenocorticosteroids, lead to stretching of the underlying connective tissue of the skin, creating striae gravidarum in the second and third trimesters. Better known as stretch marks, striae on light-skinned clients appear as pink or slightly reddish streaks with slight depressions; on dark-skinned clients, they appear lighter than the surrounding skin tone. They develop most often in skin covering the breasts, abdomen, buttocks, and thighs. After labor, they typically grow lighter until they appear silvery white on light-skinned clients and light brown on dark-skinned clients.

Pigment changes

Pigmentation begins to change at approximately the eighth week of pregnancy, partly from the melanocyte-stimulating hormone and ACTH and partly from estrogen and progesterone. These changes are more pronounced in such hyperpigmented areas as the face, breasts (especially nipples), axillae, abdomen, anal region, inner thighs, and vulva. Specific changes may include linea nigra and chloasma.

Linea nigra refers to a dark line that extends from the umbilicus or above to the mons pubis. In the primigravid client, this line develops at approximately the third month of pregnancy. In the multigravid client, linea nigra typically appears before the third month.

Called the mask of pregnancy, chloasma (or facial melasma) refers to irregular, brownish blotches that appear on the malar prominences (cheek bones) and forehead. Chloasma appears after the sixteenth week of pregnancy and gradually becomes more pronounced until childbirth. Then it typically fades.

Vascular markings

Tiny, bright-red angiomas may appear during pregnancy as a result of estrogen release, which increases subcutaneous blood flow. They are called vascular spiders because of the branching pattern that extends from each spot. Occurring mostly on the chest, neck, arms, face, and legs, they disappear after childbirth.

Palmar erythema, commonly seen along with vascular spiders, are well-delineated, pinkish areas over the palmar surface of the hands. Once pregnancy ends and estrogen levels decrease, these changes reverse.

Epulides, also known as gingival granuloma gravidarum, are raised, red, fleshy areas that appear on the gums as a result of increased estrogen. They may increase in size, cause severe pain, and bleed profusely. An epulis that grows rapidly may require excision.

Other integumentary changes

Nevi (circumscribed, benign proliferation of pigment-producing cells in the skin) may develop on the face, neck, upper chest, or arms during pregnancy. Oily skin and acne from increased estrogen may occur. Hirsutism (excessive hair growth) also may occur, but reverses when pregnancy ends. By the sixth week of pregnancy, fingernails may soften and break easily, a problem that may be exacerbated by nail polish removers.

IMMUNE SYSTEM

Ordinarily, a mature immune system rejects implanted tissue within 2 weeks. During pregnancy, however, the fetus and placenta are protected from the maternal immune system by a mechanism that is not fully understood. The cell layer covering the fetus and placenta may mask antigens, thus preventing detection by sensitized lymphocytes (Cunningham, MacDonald, and Gant, 1989). The placental hormones progesterone and hCG may suppress cellular immunity (Gusdon and Sain, 1981).

NEUROLOGIC SYSTEM

Changes in the neurologic system are poorly defined and incompletely understood. For most clients, neurologic changes are temporary and cease once pregnancy is over. Functional disturbances called entrapment neuropathies occur in the peripheral nervous system from mechanical pressure.

The client may experience meralgia paresthetica—tingling and numbness in the anterolateral portion of the thigh that is caused when the lateral femoral cutaneous nerve becomes entrapped in the area of the inguinal ligaments. This is more pronounced in late pregnancy, as the gravid uterus presses on these nerves and as vascular stasis occurs.

In the third trimester, carpal tunnel syndrome may occur when the median nerve of the carpal tunnel of the wrist is compressed by edematous surrounding tissue. The client may notice tingling and burning in the dominant hand, possibly radiating to the elbow and upper arm. Numbness or tingling in the hands also may result from pregnancy-related postural changes, such as slumped shoulders that pull on the brachial plexus.

Increased metabolism creates the need for greater calcium intake. If the client ingests insufficient calcium, hypocalcemia and muscle cramps may occur.

Lightheadedness, faintness, and syncope may be caused by vasomotor changes, hypoglycemia, and postural hypotension.

CHAPTER SUMMARY

Chapter 5 described the physiologic changes that take place during pregnancy and explained some of their reasons. The chapter includes the following key concepts.

Some of the physiologic changes during pregnancy help in diagnosing it. Signs of pregnancy may be presumptive, probable, or positive. Presumptive and probable signs may be caused by conditions other than pregnancy; positive signs are caused only by pregnancy.

Pregnancy alters every maternal body system, sometimes in ways that would be considered pathological in a nonpregnant client. Although normal, physiologic changes that occur during pregnancy may cause client discomfort and anxiety.

Many pregnancy-induced physiologic changes stem from altered hormone levels, especially estrogen and progesterone.

In the reproductive system, major physiologic changes include enlargement of external reproductive structures; cessation of ovulation and altered ovarian hormone production; uterine enlargement, vascularization, and migration; endometrial development; cervical softening and edema; development of a cervical mucus plug; vaginal vascularization, hypertrophy, and increased secretion; and breast enlargement and milk production.

In the endocrine system, major physiologic changes include increased secretion of the pituitary hormones thyrotropin, ACTH, prolactin, vasopressin, and oxytocin; increased secretion of the thyroid hormones thyroxine and triiodothyronine; increased secretion of parathyroid hormones; increased secretion of the adrenal hormones cortisol and aldosterone; and increased secretion of insulin from the pancreas.

In the respiratory system, major physiologic changes include flaring of the rib cage and a shift from abdominal breathing to thoracic breathing in response to the rising diaphragm, vascularization of the upper respiratory tract, increased tidal volume and minute volume, decreased functional residual capacity, and development of mild respiratory alkalosis.

In the cardiovascular system, major physiologic changes include enlargement and displacement of the heart; changes in heart sounds; increased heart rate and output, venous blood pressure, and blood volume; decreased arterial blood pressure and circulation; enhanced blood clotting; and increased levels of red blood cells, white blood cells, and fibrinogen.

In the urinary system, major physiologic changes include dilation of the renal pelves, calyces, and ureters; elongation and relaxation of the ureters, which results in urinary stasis; relaxation of the bladder walls; bladder irritation, which results in urinary frequency and urgency; and increased renal plasma flow, glomerular filtration rate, and renal tubular resorption.

In the gastrointestinal system, major physiologic changes include increased activity of the salivary glands; edema of the gums; decreased gastric tone and motility; displacement of the large and small intestines; increased gallbladder emptying time; liver function changes, including increased hepatic blood flow, decreased bile flow, and altered results of liver function studies; changes in appetite and food consumption; possible nausea and vomiting; and changes in carbohydrate, lipid, and protein metabolism.

In the musculoskeletal system, major physiologic changes include a shift in the center of gravity, changes in posture and gait, and separation of the abdominal muscles.

In the integumentary system, major physiologic changes include striae gravidarum, linea nigra, chloasma, vascular spiders, palmar erythema, epulides, oily skin, acne, hirsutism, and soft fingernails.

In the immune system, physiologic changes prevent rejection of the fetus and placenta by a poorly understood mechanism.

In the neurologic system, major physiologic changes include entrapment neuropathies; possible muscle cramping caused by insufficient calcium intake; and possible lightheadedness, faintness, and syncope.

STUDY QUESTIONS

1. Mrs. Carr, age 29, comes to the clinic because she thinks that she is pregnant. What signs would confirm that Mrs. Carr is indeed pregnant?
2. What anatomic changes take place in the cardiovascular system during pregnancy?
3. Mrs. Newly, age 32, is a multiparous client, 24 weeks' pregnant, who comes to the physician office for a checkup. Routine laboratory studies show an appreciable drop in her hematocrit. How should the nurse explain this decrease?
4. How does pregnancy affect renal plasma flow and the glomerular filtration rate?
5. Which information should the nurse include when teaching a client about pregnancy-related changes to the skeleton?

BIBLIOGRAPHY

Beischer, N.A., and Mackay, E.V. (1986). *Obstetrics and the newborn: An illustrated textbook* (2nd ed.). Philadelphia: Saunders.

Bobak, I., Jensen, M., and Zalar, M. (1989). *Maternity and gynecologic care* (4th ed.). St. Louis: Mosby.

Cunningham, F., MacDonald, P., and Gant, N. (1989). *Williams obstetrics* (18th ed.). East Norwalk, CT: Appleton & Lange.

Danforth, D.N., and Scott, J.R. (Eds.) (1986). *Obstetrics and gynecology* (5th ed.). Philadelphia: Lippincott.

Guyton, A.C. (1986). *Textbook of medical physiology* (7th ed.). Philadelphia: Saunders.

Neeson, J.D. (1987). *Clinical manual of maternity nursing.* Philadelphia: Lippincott.

Niswander, K.R. (1987). *Manual of obstetrics: Diagnosis and therapy* (3rd ed.). Boston: Little, Brown.

Olds, S., London, M., and Ladewig, P. (1988). *Maternal newborn nursing* (3rd ed.). New York: Addison-Wesley.

Willson, J.R., and Carrington, E.R. (1987). *Obstetrics and gynecology* (8th ed.). St. Louis: Mosby.

Diagnosing pregnancy

Brucker, M.C., and MacMullen, N.J. (1985). What's new in pregnancy tests? *JOGNN,* 14(3), 353-359.

Engstrom, J.L. (1985). Quickening and auscultation of fetal heart tones as estimators of the gestational interval: A review. *Journal of Nurse Midwifery,* 30(1), 25-32.

Gusdon, J.P., and Sain, L.E. (1981). Uterine and peripheral blood concentrations and human chorionic gonadotropin and human placental lactogen. *American Journal of Obstetrics and Gynecology,* 139(6), 705-707.

Munsick, R.A. (1985). Dickinson's sign: Focal uterine softening in early pregnancy and its correlation with placental site. *American Journal of Obstetrics and Gynecology,* 152(7, Pt. 1), 799-802.

Pregnancy-related changes in body systems

Calvin, S., Jones, O.W., Knieriem, K., and Weinstein, L. (1988). Oxygen saturation in the supine hypotensive syndrome. *Obstetrics and Gynecology,* 71(6, Pt. 1), 872-877.

Clapp, J.F. (1985). Maternal heart rate in pregnancy. *American Journal of Obstetrics and Gynecology,* 152(6, Pt. 1), 659-660.

Engstrom, J.L. (1988). Measurement of fundal height. *JOGNN,* 17(3), 172-178.

Hart, M.V., Morton, M.J., Hosenpud, J.D., and Metcalfe, J. (1986). Aortic function during normal human pregnancy. *American Journal of Obstetrics and Gynecology,* 154(4), 887-891.

Klebanoff, M.A., Koslowe, P.A., and Kaslow, R. (1985). Epidemiology of vomiting in early pregnancy. *Obstetrics and Gynecology,* 66(5), 612.

Margulies, M., Voto, L., Fescina, R., Lastra, L., Lapidus, A., and Schwarcz, R. (1987). Arterial blood pressure standards during normal pregnancy and their relation with mother-fetus variables. *American Journal of Obstetrics and Gynecology,* 156(5), 1105-1109.

Tierson, F.D., Olsen, C.L., and Hook, E.B. (1986). Nausea and vomiting of pregnancy and association with pregnancy outcome. *American Journal of Obstetrics and Gynecology,* 155(5), 1017-1022.

CHAPTER 6

PSYCHOSOCIAL CHANGES DURING NORMAL PREGNANCY

OBJECTIVES

After reading and studying this chapter, the student should be able to:

1. List principles that guide the nurse in promoting normal psychosocial adaptation to pregnancy.

2. Identify factors that affect the expectant parents' transition to parenthood.

3. Describe the expectant parents' psychosocial tasks, concerns, fears, dreams and fantasies during each trimester of pregnancy.

4. Discuss the formation of a mother image and a father image during pregnancy.

5. Describe the development of prenatal bonding with the fetus.

6. Describe the effect of pregnancy on the couple's relationship.

7. Identify the primary characteristic of the parents' relationship that favors successful adaptation to pregnancy.

8. Describe the concerns and behaviors of siblings and methods that parents can use to prepare them for the new family member.

9. Describe the grandparents' role and involvement in pregnancy and childbirth.

10. Discuss the cultural variations that may affect the family's psychosocial experience of pregnancy.

INTRODUCTION

Pregnancy and childbirth are psychosocial events that deeply affect the lives of parents and families. Nothing defines the self-concept of most men and women more than the challenge of bearing and raising a child. Pregnancy and childbirth change parents' lives irrevocably, presenting them with a long-term commitment that benefits from intellectual and emotional preparation.

The parents' response to pregnancy and childbirth is affected by psychological, social, economic, and cultural factors and by self-concept and attitudes toward sex-specific and family roles. All of these aspects of childbearing can affect their health and that of their children. Therefore, care of the expectant family presents the nurse with special responsibilities and challenges.

The nurse must promote the family's normal adaptation to and integration of the new family member. To achieve these goals, the nurse should perform these increasingly difficult functions as expertise allows.

• Promote each family member's self-esteem. Listen attentively, elicit questions and concerns, identify preferences and cultural influences, provide anticipatory guidance about emotional and psychological family changes, discuss as fully as needed each family member's necessary roles and tasks, affirm their efforts, inquire about and show concern for each family member's health care needs, and make referrals as needed.

• Involve all family members in prenatal visits, facilitate communication among family members, offer anticipatory guidance about family changes during pregnancy and the postpartal period, help mobilize the family's resources, offer sexual counseling, help the client maximize her family's positive contributions and minimize negative ones, praise the family's efforts, and offer books and other materials that address all family members.

- Promote the family's prenatal bonding (sometimes called attachment) with the fetus. During prenatal visits, share information about fetal development; help the family identify fetal heart tones, position, and movements; and reinforce bonding behaviors—such as patting the abdomen or talking to the fetus—by asking the client or her partner to note and report fetal movements.
- Facilitate resolution of conflicts related to pregnancy and childbirth. Help identify underlying conflicts through reflective communication, validation of feelings, and exploration of dreams and fantasies. Promote conflict resolution by teaching such techniques as personal affirmation and dream interpretation and by suggesting literature that helps identify and resolve conflicts. Refer for counseling any client who cannot resolve conflicts.
- Support adaptive coping patterns through realistic education of the family about pregnancy, childbirth, and the postpartal period. Discuss childbirth and human responses accurately and realistically. Frankly discuss the challenges of parenting.
- Deliver culturally sensitive nursing care. Gather information about the family's customs and beliefs to add to assessment data and to individualize care.
- Identify personal attitudes and feelings about childbearing. Avoid imposing personal values, feelings, and emotional reactions on others. Also, avoid making assumptions about the client and her preferences. Allow her to share her feelings freely.
- Act as an advocate for the expectant family in the health care facility, community, and society. In the facility, suggest more family-centered policies, such as sibling and grandparent visiting hours. In the community, expand childbirth options for expectant families by working to establish a birth center. At the national level, lobby for the health of poor mothers and neonates and for necessary changes in health care by writing to state representatives about laws that fund maternal-neonatal health care and other family services (Thompson, Oakley, Burke, Jay, and Conklin, 1989).

This chapter discusses psychosocial adaptation in expectant parents. For each trimester of pregnancy, it defines the psychosocial tasks and concerns and explores variations that make each pregnancy unique. It explores grandparent and sibling roles and describe how parents can support them. The chapter also investigates cultural influences that can affect psychosocial adjustments.

PREGNANCY: A TIME OF TRANSITION

Pregnancy is a time of profound psychological, social, and biological changes that affect the parents' responsibilities, freedoms, values, priorities, social status, relationships, and self-images. The events of the childbearing year (9 antepartal and 3 postpartal months) also may be unpredictable. Although expectant parents can control some events (for example, by obtaining early prenatal care) and can adopt positive attitudes, they cannot control all that happens during that year.

Many factors can influence the smoothness of this transition:
- support from partner
- support from parents
- support from friends and others
- age
- planned or unplanned pregnancy
- socioeconomic status
- sexuality concerns
- previous childbirth experiences
- previous parenting experiences
- birth stories of family members and friends
- past experiences with health care facilities
- past experiences with health care professionals.

STRESS AND COPING METHODS

The changes and challenges of pregnancy normally produce stress (psychological and physiologic tension that triggers an adaptive change). Ideally, the pregnant woman will cope realistically with the challenges and adapt to the changes, promoting her health. During pregnancy, stress may increase the incidence of neonatal complications by increasing sympathetic nervous system activity and catecholamine release, constricting uterine blood flow, and diminishing fetal oxygenation (Lederman, 1986; Mansfield and Cohn, 1986). During labor, maternal stress may decrease the neonate's Apgar score.

Overcrowding, geographic moves, disturbed personal relationships, concerns about the health of mother and neonate, and economic instability can increase stress during pregnancy, which has been associated with increased incidence of neonatal complications (Lederman, 1986). Expectant fathers commonly find the following concerns stressful: the neonate's health, normality, and condition at birth; the woman's pain during labor; and unexpected events during childbirth (Glazer, 1989).

Reduced anxiety and better adaptation in early pregnancy relate to fewer and less severe pregnancy symptoms. They especially help reduce nausea, backache, dizziness, fatigue, and gastrointestinal distress (Grossman, et al., 1980).

FIRST TRIMESTER

During the first trimester, the family's key psychosocial challenge is resolution of ambivalence. The mother copes with the common discomforts and changes of the first trimester; the father begins to accept the reality of the pregnancy. During pregnancy, both partners may experience vivid dreams about the impending birth. The woman may recall her dreams with greater intensity because she typically is awakened more often at night by heartburn, fetal activity, or a need to urinate. Dreams tend to follow a predictable pattern during pregnancy. By exploring them, expectant parents can better understand themselves and any subconscious conflicts they may have. The couple may use dream examination to help deal with these psychosocial tasks.

Resolution of ambivalence

The first trimester is known as the trimester of ambivalence because parents experience mixed feelings.

Many women have unrealistic ideas about maternal instincts, expecting to feel only loving, happy thoughts about the fetus and motherhood. In fact, most women feel some ambivalence about pregnancy and motherhood. Pregnancy involves stressful changes that force a woman to think and behave differently than she has in the past (Kitzinger, 1984).

Feelings of ambivalence are inevitable and normal, and partners who discuss them usually can resolve their grief and fears and enjoy the gratifications of expecting a child. When partners share feelings, they may find they are experiencing similar conflicts (Shapiro, 1987). Studies of married couples have shown that when the husband receives emotional support during pregnancy, his wife adjusts more easily and enjoys the pregnancy (Parke, 1981).

Coping with common discomforts and changes

In the early weeks of the first trimester, the woman watches for body changes that confirm her pregnancy. Her body image (her mental image of how her body looks, feels, and moves; of her posture, gestures, and physical abilities; and of others' impression of her physical appearance) changes as her breasts enlarge, her menses cease, and she experiences nausea, fatigue, waist thickening, and

general weight gain. Depending on her acceptance of the pregnancy, the woman may enjoy or dread these changes.

Women's sexual responses during pregnancy vary widely. Some women are too uncomfortable during the first trimester to enjoy sexual intercourse; others, especially those who have had a spontaneous abortion, may fear fetal injury. Those who believe sex is for procreation only may feel guilty about sexual activity during pregnancy. Others may feel sexually stimulated by the freedom from contraception, the joy of conception, or the lack of pressure to avoid pregnancy or to have sex on schedule to achieve pregnancy.

A man's sexual response also may change during his partner's pregnancy. He typically will worry about how the pregnancy will change his relationship with his partner. He may feel personally rejected when his partner's fatigue, nausea, and other first trimester discomforts diminish her sexual interest. He may fear causing spontaneous abortion or fetal injury during intercourse.

Because of these fears and concerns, both partners may need extra affection during the first trimester. The nurse should encourage them to communicate and share their feelings and preferences about sexual activities.

Preparation for fatherhood

During the first trimester, the father typically finds the pregnancy unreal and intangible. The idea of the fetus may be abstract to him because he cannot observe physical changes in his partner. Accepting the reality of pregnancy is the father's main psychological task in the first trimester (Miller and Brooten, 1983).

Nonetheless, pregnancy does have an emotional impact on the father, and the child will change his life dramatically. His attachment to the child can be as strong as the mother's, and he can be as competent as the mother in nurturing the child (Cronenwett and Kunst-Wilson, 1981).

Because he is not physically pregnant, the father can choose his degree and type of involvement in the pregnancy. May (1980) studied first-time expectant fathers and identified three fathering styles: the observer, expressive, or instrumental fathering styles. None of these styles is more mature or competent than another. Although each father becomes more involved as the pregnancy advances, his fathering style usually remains consistent (May, 1980).

Regardless of fathering style, the man may experience two psychosocial phenomena during the pregnancy: obsession with his role as provider and couvade symptoms.

Because society values a man's provider role, the expectant father usually ponders the increased financial responsibilities a child will bring. Financial concerns remain a major focus throughout pregnancy, and the man may exert tremendous effort to attain financial security. A disproportionate emphasis on finances may reflect deep doubts about his competence as a father. The more secure he feels about his family's economic status, the more open and nurturing he can be with his partner (Muenchow and Bloom-Feshbach, 1982).

Couvade, french for "to brood" or "to hatch," symptoms refers to the expectant father's experience of up to 39 symptoms of pregnancy, including nausea, weight gain, insomnia, restlessness, headaches, inability to concentrate, fatigue, and irritability (Clinton, 1987). Because these symptoms are not accepted by American society, which expects the father to be strong and supportive, American fathers rarely mention them. However, one study found that 70% of fathers reported one or more couvade symptoms (Strickland, 1987).

Couvade symptoms are not associated with the father's attachment to the fetus and are not limited to first-time fathers (Lemmer, 1987). However, they occur most frequently in fathers who are greatly involved in the pregnancy.

SECOND TRIMESTER

During the second trimester, psychosocial tasks include mother-image development, father-image development, coping with body image and sexuality changes, and development of prenatal attachment. Parents may experience various fears. Feeling dependent and vulnerable, the woman may fear for her partner's safety. In touch with mortality, the man may consider his death and how it would affect his family. He may recall risks he has taken, such as driving recklessly, and make a commitment to be more careful to avoid being taken from his partner and fetus. During the second trimester, the parents' dreams may reflect concerns about the normalcy of the fetus, parental abilities, divided loyalties, and related subjects. To accomplish these tasks, the couple may examine their dreams and fears.

Mother-image development
As the second trimester begins, expectant parents have completed much of the first trimester's grieving. The woman has abandoned old roles and has begun to determine the sort of mother she wants to be (Varney, 1987). Her mother image is a composite of mothering characteristics she has gleaned from role models, readings, and her imagination.

Four aspects of the mother-daughter relationship will influence the woman's mother image:
- her mother's availability in the past and during the pregnancy
- her mother's reaction to the pregnancy, her acceptance of the grandchild, and her acknowledgment of her daughter as a mother
- her mother's respect for the daughter's autonomy and acceptance of her as a mature adult
- her mother's willingness to reminisce about her own childbearing and child-rearing experiences (Lederman, 1984).

Her preoccupation with forming a mother image causes a period of introspection. As a result, she may show less affection, become more passive, or withdraw from her other children, who will react by becoming more demanding. Her partner also may feel neglected during this period.

Father-image development
While the woman develops her mother image, the man begins to form his father image based on his relationship with his father, previous fathering experiences, the fathering styles of friends and family members, and his partner's view of his role in the pregnancy.

As he starts to develop his father image, the man remembers his relationship with his father and sometimes increases contact with his parents. He may have difficulty viewing his father as a grandfather and coming to terms with his position as a father.

Generally, the woman's expectations about her partner's involvement and the quality of their relationship predict the man's role in delivery and child rearing (Reiber, 1976). Some women desire privacy and modesty during childbirth and neither expect nor wish to involve their partners. Others expect their partner's full involvement in tracking fetal movements, attending prenatal visits, and acting as coach, advocate, and primary emotional support during labor.

Coping with body image and sexuality changes
The second trimester often is called a time of radiant health. Physical changes include a heightened sensuality with vasocongestion of the pelvis and increased vaginal lubrication, and 80% of women describe increased sexual gratification, even over prepregnant levels (Colman and Colman, 1977). However, studies show that women become increasingly dissatisfied with their body image as pregnancy progresses, feeling the most dissatisfied during the postpartal period (Strang and Sullivan, 1985).

One study showed that most men feel more positively about the physical changes of pregnancy than do their partners (Moore, 1978).

The way a woman and her partner view her body's changes will affect her sexual responsiveness and self-image.

Development of prenatal bonding

A new phase begins at approximately 17 to 20 weeks, when the woman feels fetal movements for the first time. Because fetal movements are a sign of good health and may dispel the fear of spontaneous abortion, the woman almost always experiences the first flutter of movement positively, even when the pregnancy is unwanted. As a result, she becomes attentive to the type and timing of movements and to fetal responses to environmental factors, such as music, abdominal strokes, and meals.

The woman may demonstrate bonding behaviors, such as stroking and patting her abdomen, talking to the fetus about eating while she eats, reprimanding the fetus for moving too much, engaging her partner in conversations with the fetus, eating a balanced diet, and engaging in other health promotion behaviors (Sherwen, 1987). Bonding is influenced by the woman's health, developmental stage, and culture, but not by obstetric complications, general anxiety, or demographic variables, such as socioeconomic level.

This prenatal bonding requires positive self-esteem, positive role models, and acceptance of the pregnancy. Social support improves this attachment (Cranley, 1981), which in turn increases the woman's feelings of maternal competence and effectiveness (Mercer, Ferketich, De-Joseph, May, and Sollid, 1988). One study demonstrated that women who displayed more bonding behaviors during pregnancy had more positive feelings about the neonate after delivery (Leifer, 1977).

THIRD TRIMESTER

As the third trimester begins, the woman feels a sense of accomplishment because her fetus has reached the age of viability. She may feel sentimental about the approaching end of her pregnancy, when the mother-child relationship will replace the mother-fetus relationship. At the same time, however, she may look forward to giving birth because the last months bring bulkiness, insomnia, childbirth anxieties, and concern about the neonate's normalcy.

During this trimester, psychosocial tasks include adaptation to activity changes, preparation for parenting, partner support and nurture, acceptance of body image and sexuality changes, preparation for labor, and development of birth plans. During the third trimester, a key psychosocial task is to overcome fears the woman may have about the unknown, labor pain, loss of self-esteem, loss of control, and death. The technique of dream and fear examination may help the couple accomplish these tasks.

Adaptation to activity changes

The growing fetus makes daily activities more difficult for the woman and forces her to slow down. This change can affect her emotional state and her family relationships. Decreased social support for the woman on maternity leave can add to anxiety. Further, her increased dependence during pregnancy and decreased activities outside the home may change the family power structure.

Preparation for parenting

As the woman's body grows larger, the man typically catches up with his partner in anticipating and preparing for the neonate. To prepare for parenting, the couple now may focus on concrete tasks, such as preparing the nursery, making decisions about child care, and planning postpartal events.

Partner support and nurture

The couple's ability to support each other through the childbearing cycle is paramount. In a recent study, husbands and wives stated that 80% of their support during pregnancy came from their spouses (Brown, 1987). Other studies found that an egalitarian relationship (one not characterized by the dominance of either member) yields greater satisfaction, greater closeness during the pregnancy, and an easier transition to parenthood (Grossman, et al., 1980; Moore, 1983). Furthermore, relationships that allow flexibility, growth, and risk taking ease role transition.

Acceptance of body image and sexuality changes

Some women are more comfortable with and confident in their bodies during pregnancy, feeling less concerned with each pound of weight gained. Others, however, feel sexually unattractive.

The woman's body image and her partner's feelings affect her sexuality, sometimes diminishing her sexual interest. Some men also experience diminished sexual interest as pregnancy advances. Couples who desire sexual intimacy in the third trimester must be creative, using new positions and techniques. Whether or not the couple remains sexually active, the woman usually desires holding and reassurance.

Preparation for labor

Childbirth education classes can prepare the woman and her partner for labor and delivery. The partner's attendance at prenatal classes and participation in all aspects of pregnancy correlate with his degree of relationship satisfaction (Lederman, 1984). Women who feel supported by their partners during pregnancy and childbirth experience fewer complications and may make an easier postpartal adjustment (May, 1982).

Development of birth plans

A highly dependent woman may allow the health care team to make decisions about the birth plans, assuming that their decisions will be the wisest. A more independent woman may seek health care that is comfortable to her and that fits with her beliefs and knowledge, thus ensuring that her wishes will be honored during labor. A woman who shapes her childbirth experience and who develops realistic expectations of the event has dealt with her fears.

FAMILY AND CULTURAL CONSIDERATIONS

Throughout the pregnancy, the expectant parents may need to prepare siblings for the new family member and involve the grandparents.

The cultural meanings of pregnancy and parenthood influence a woman's psychosocial experience of the childbearing year and her transition to parenthood. Respecting cultural traditions and beliefs maximizes the client's social support and personal integrity and the nurse's effectiveness. (For more information, see Cultural Considerations: *Psychosocial aspects of pregnancy,* page 84.)

Sibling preparation

American parents typically assume that the neonate's birth will make siblings feel displaced and jealous. Siblings may sense this and act as they are expected to act. Rolfe (1985) suggests that parents share the news of an impending birth positively and deal with any feelings that arise.

Awaiting the arrival of a new family member can be confusing or distressing for siblings. To help ease the transition for siblings and parents, the nurse can make the following suggestions to the parents.
• Express positive feelings through such statements as, "We love you so much we wanted another child."

• Deal with the siblings' expressed feelings, accepting these feelings without judgment and affirming the children's lovability.
• Avoid strong statements – positive or negative – about the new family member.
• Discuss which aspects of family life will be changed by the neonate and which will remain unchanged.
• Explain when the neonate is due by creating a calendar that shows the stages of fetal development during the seasons of the birth year. This will help siblings conceptualize the passage of time.
• Explain how the fetus was conceived and answer sex questions simply, truthfully, and individually. Ask for feedback and correct any misunderstandings siblings may have about conception.
• Devise household routines that involve both parents, so that the mother's absence during labor and delivery will not disrupt routines.
• Make bed and room changes early in pregnancy to prevent siblings from feeling displaced by the neonate.
• Involve siblings in preparations for the neonate, such as decorating the nursery or choosing a homecoming outfit.
• Involve siblings in health care. Encourage them to listen to fetal heart sounds, feel fetal movements, and attend childbirth education classes for siblings.
• Instill realistic expectations about the neonate's appearance, behavior, care, and feeding.
• Reminisce with siblings about their births and review baby photographs together.
• Include siblings in health care facility visits. Create a schedule for such visits that includes time for them to rest and be fed. Bring their pictures and toys to the health care facility. Spend time alone with them during visits.
• Plan the neonate's homecoming carefully to minimize sibling distress. Have the mother visit alone with siblings after arriving home, while the father holds the neonate.
• Reward mature behaviors and ignore immature ones.

Grandparent involvement

The grandparent-grandchild bond is second in importance only to the parent-child bond. Grandparents provide a sense of family continuity for their grandchildren, sharing family traditions and religious and moral values. They pass on the family history, provide older role models, and, ideally, affirm the vulnerable new parents' self-esteem.

Because the grandparent role is an imposed one, most grandparents have the right to decide what they will offer to grandchildren. Because the parents are in the central position, they must negotiate intergenerational relation-

PSYCHOSOCIAL ASPECTS OF PREGNANCY

Although each client has personal beliefs and values, her cultural background may influence her psychosocial adaptation during pregnancy as well as her self-care and health promotion measures, health-seeking behaviors, and interactions with health care professionals. When caring for a client from a different culture, the nurse should keep the following considerations in mind.

North American culture

Because the North American culture encompasses various ethnic and cultural backgrounds, no typical view of childbirth exists in America. However, widespread access to medical care and the movement toward family-centered childbirth permit a few generalizations about American attitudes toward pregnancy and childbirth.

In the United States, physicians typically manage a woman's pregnancy. Americans tend to rely heavily on medical intervention to ensure a healthy outcome for the mother and neonate. They usually emphasize technological intervention, including ultrasonography and other tests, to track fetal growth and health.

Americans consider health promotion activities an indication that the woman has accepted her pregnancy. They encourage the woman to get early prenatal care, to monitor her diet carefully, and to eliminate unhealthy practices, such as drinking alcohol and smoking. A pregnant woman who engages in unhealthy practices may meet with disapproval or disdain and may experience guilt and self-doubt.

American men participate in pregnancy and delivery to a greater extent than do men in many other cultures. A large percentage of American men attend childbirth education classes and are present during delivery. Many American men also are taking an increased role in infant care at home.

Asian culture

In the United States, Chinese, Japanese, and Korean clients may practice traditional beliefs or may adopt American customs and practices regarding childbirth.

The Chinese culture values maintaining a balance between the physical and spiritual aspects of life, especially during pregnancy. To help achieve this balance, a pregnant woman may avoid certain foods and drink herbal teas. After delivery, the woman may stay home and rest for 40 days, avoiding strenuous activity. She also may avoid contact with water for 40 days after delivery, believing that a postpartal chill can cause arthritis or body aches.

Japanese-Americans, who have the highest median income and educational level of any American minority group, tend to accept American practices. They view pregnancy as a normal state that requires few changes in the pregnant woman's daily routine. After delivery, the woman controls the neonate's care, although the extended family may participate.

Korean-American women believe that the pregnant woman or a family member experiences a *Tae Mong* (dream that predicts pregnancy). After she becomes pregnant, the Korean woman may read classical literature, view beautiful artworks, and adopt an optimistic and serene attitude to promote health and an easy delivery. Dietary restrictions include balancing hot and cold foods and restricting salty, spicy, or sour foods (Lee, 1989).

Other restrictions include barring men and childless women from the delivery area and keeping the neonate's father away from the mother and neonate for seven days after delivery.

The birth of a first child, especially a son, is an important event in a Korean family, integrating the mother into her partner's family and giving her status and economic security. In traditional Korean families, the mother-in-law is responsible for the pregnant woman's health and care. If she desires a grandson, the Korean mother-in-law will view care of her daughter-in-law as service to Samshin, the goddess of childbirth. Health care professionals should be aware that the Korean client may wish to involve her mother-in-law in decision-making discussions (Sich, 1988).

Southeast Asian culture

Southeast Asian (Vietnamese, Cambodian, and Laotian) women may hold what many Americans consider to be superstitious beliefs, such as the belief that sitting on a step in a doorframe can cause labor and delivery complications, or that a bath after sundown will result in an oversized neonate.

Some Southeast Asian women may see an herbalist or an acupuncturist before seeking Western health care and may refrain from expressing doubts about medications or procedures out of respect for authority. If the health care professional's advice conflicts with traditional beliefs, the Southeast Asian client may deal passively with this conflict, missing appointments or neglecting to fill prescriptions. The health care professional who is alert to such indirect messages can approach the client with an alternate plan (Lee, 1989).

Filipino culture

Filipino women share many traits with Southeast Asian women. They are taught to respect elders, defer to their partners, and avoid confrontation. The nurse who provides care to a Filipino client should be aware that she may wish to deal with issues indirectly and involve the family in planning (Stern, 1985).

Haitian culture

In Haiti, pregnancy is viewed as a matter-of-fact experience that does not need to be discussed. For this reason, Haitian women may not seek prenatal care (Harris, 1987).

Haitian women observe various practices after delivery. They may take a series of three herbal baths, conserve body heat, avoid white foods, and wear abdominal binders (Harris, 1987). The Haitian neonate's name may be chosen by a community leader or an older family member and may commemorate a family member who has died. The name of a deceased family member may signify that the dead person's unfinished business has been passed on to the neonate or that the neonate is expected to carry on a business or profession (Meltzer, 1981).

ships that are comfortable and satisfying for all three generations.

CHAPTER SUMMARY

Chapter 6 described psychosocial needs and tasks of expectant families. Here are the chapter highlights.

Childbearing is vital to most individuals' self-concept and presents unique psychosocial tasks and challenges.

The nurse who cares for the expectant family must promote normal adaptation and integration of the new member by promoting self-esteem, family integrity, prenatal bonding, conflict resolution, and adaptive coping.

To provide appropriate care, the nurse must avoid imposing personal attitudes about childbearing on others.

Various factors can affect an individual's transition to parenthood, such as socioeconomic status and support from the partner, parents, and friends.

In the first trimester of pregnancy, psychosocial tasks for expectant parents include resolving ambivalence; for the mother, coping with discomforts and changes; and for the father, beginning to accept the pregnancy and its implications for his provider role.

In the second trimester, psychosocial tasks include developing a mother image and a father image, coping with changes in body image and sexuality, and developing prenatal bonding.

In the third trimester, tasks include adapting to a slower pace, preparing for parenting, supporting and nurturing the partner, accepting body image and sexuality changes, preparing for labor, and developing birth plans.

The expectant couple may use dream and fear examination to help accomplish psychosocial tasks.

To prepare siblings to accept the neonate, the nurse can suggest ways for parents to involve them in the pregnancy and birth.

Because parents are in the central position, they must negotiate intergenerational relationships that are acceptable to all three generations.

Cultural views of pregnancy and childbirth vary. To provide culturally sensitive care, the nurse must understand the client's cultural background.

STUDY QUESTIONS

1. How might stress affect pregnancy?
2. What aspects of the mother-daughter relationship influence the woman's mother image?
3. What types of behavior would the nurse see when the mother begins to develop parental bonding?
4. John and Mary Gree, expecting their second child in 6 months, ask the nurse how they can best prepare their 4-year-old son for this birth. What suggestions can the nurse make?

BIBLIOGRAPHY

Anderson, S., and DelGiudice, G. (1985). *Siblings, birth, and the newborn*. Seattle, WA: Pennypress.

Boston Women's Health Book Collective. (1985). *The new our bodies, ourselves*. New York: Simon & Schuster.

Friedman, M. (1981). *Family nursing: Theory and assessment* (2nd ed.). East Norwalk, CT: Appleton & Lange.

Grossman, F., Eichler, L., Winickoff, S., Anzalone, M., Gofseyeff, M., and Sargent, S. (1980). *Pregnancy, birth, and parenthood: Adaptations of mothers, fathers, and infants*. San Francisco: Jossey-Bass.

Jones, C. (1987). *Mind over labor*. New York: Viking Penguin.

Kitzinger, S. (1984). *The experience of childbirth* (5th ed.). New York: Penguin.

Mercer, R., Ferketich, S., DeJoseph, J., May, K., and Sollid, D. (1988). Effect of stress on family functioning during pregnancy. *Nursing Research, 37*(5), 268-275.

Miller, M., and Brooten, D. (1983). *The childbearing family: A nursing perspective*. Boston: Little, Brown.

Moore, D. (1978). The body image in pregnancy. *Journal of Nurse-Midwifery, 22*(4), 17-27.

Moore, D. (1983). Prepared childbirth and marital satisfaction during the antepartum and postpartum periods. *Nursing Research, 32*(2), 73-79.

Sherwen, L. (1987). *Psychosocial dimensions of the pregnant family*. New York: Springer Publishing.

Thompson, J., Oakley, D., Burke, M., Jay, S., and Conklin, M. (1989). Theory building in nurse-midwifery: The care process. *Journal of Nurse-Midwifery, 34*(3), 120-130.

Varney, H. (1987). *Nurse-Midwifery* (2nd ed.). Boston: Blackwell-Scientific Publications.

Parents

Bittman, S., and Zalk, S. (1983). *Expectant fathers*. New York: Ballantine Books.

Brown, M.A. (1987). How fathers and mothers perceive prenatal support. *MCN, 12*(6), 414-418.

Clinton, J. (1985). Couvade: Patterns, predictors, and nursing management: A research proposal submitted to the division of nursing. *Western Journal of Nursing Research, 7*(2), 221-243.

Clinton, J. (1987). Physical and emotional responses of expectant fathers throughout pregnancy and the early postpartum period. *International Journal of Nursing Studies, 24*(1), 59-68.

Colman, A., and Colman, L. (1977). *Pregnancy: The psychological experience*. New York: Bantam.

Cranley, M. (1981). *Roots of attachment: The relationship of parents with their unborn*. Birth Defects: Original Article Series, 17(6), 59-83.

Cronenwett, L., and Kunst-Wilson, W. (1981). Stress, social support, and the transition to fatherhood. *Nursing Research,* 30(4), 196-201.

Glazer, G. (1989). Anxiety and stressors of expectant fathers. *Western Journal of Nursing Research,* 11(1), 47-59.

Kornhaber, A. (1987). *Between parents and grandparents.* New York: Berkley Books.

Lederman, R. (1984). *Psychosocial adaptation in pregnancy: Assessment of 7 dimensions of maternal development.* East Norwalk, CT: Appleton & Lange.

Lederman, R. (1986). Maternal anxiety in pregnancy: Relationship to fetal and newborn health status. In H. Werley, J. Fitzpatrick, and R. Taunton (Eds.), *Annual Review of Nursing Research,* Volume 4 (pp. 3-19). New York: Springer Publishing.

Leifer, M. (1977). Psychological changes accompanying pregnancy and motherhood. *Genetic and Psychological Monographs,* 95(1), 55-96.

Lemmer, C. (1987). Becoming a father: A review of nursing research on expectant fatherhood. *MCN,* 16(3), 261-275.

Mansfield, P., and Cohn, M. (1986). Stress and later life childbearing. *Maternal-Child Nursing Journal,* 15(3), 139-151.

May, K. (1980). A typology of detachment/involvement styles adopted during pregnancy by first-time expectant fathers. *Western Journal of Nursing Research,* 2(2), 445-453.

May, K. (1982). Three phases of father involvement in pregnancy. *Nursing Research,* 31(6), 337-324.

May, K. (1987). Men's sexuality during the childbearing year: Implications of recent research findings. *Holistic Nursing Practice,* 1(4), 60-66.

Muenchow, S., and Bloom-Feshbach, J. (1982, February). The new fatherhood. *Parents,* pp. 64-69.

Parke, R. (1981). *Fathers.* Cambridge, MA: Harvard University Press.

Reiber, V. (1976). Is the nurturing role natural to fathers? *MCN,* 1, 336-371.

Rolfe, R. (1985). *You can postpone anything but love: Expanding our potential as parents.* Edgemont, PA: Ambassador Press.

Shapiro, J. (1987). *When men are pregnant: Needs and concerns of expectant fathers.* San Luis Obispo, CA: Impact Publishers.

Strang, V., and Sullivan, P. (1985). Body image attitudes during pregnancy and the postpartum period. *JOGNN,* 14(4), 332-337.

Strickland, O. (1987). The occurrence of symptoms in expectant fathers: The couvade syndrome. *Nursing Research,* 36(3), 184-189.

Cultural references

Harris, K. (1987). Beliefs and practices Among Haitian American women in relation to childbearing. *Journal of Nurse-Midwifery,* 32(3), 149-155.

Lee, R. (1989). Understanding southeast Asian mothers-to-be. *Childbirth Educator,* Spring, 32-39.

Meltzer, D. (Ed.) (1981). *Birth: An anthology of ancient texts, songs, prayers, and stories.* San Francisco: North Point Press.

Sich, D. (1988). Childbearing in Korea. *Social Science Medicine,* 27(5), 497-504.

Stern, P. (1985). A comparison of culturally approved behaviors and beliefs between Filipino immigrant women, U.S.-born dominant culture women, and western female nurses of the San Francisco Bay Area: Religiosity of health care. *Health Care for Women International,* 6(1-3), 123-133.

CHAPTER 7

CARE DURING THE NORMAL ANTEPARTAL PERIOD

OBJECTIVES

After reading and studying this chapter, the student should be able to:
1. Summarize the major components of the antepartal health assessment.
2. Discuss antepartal risk factors that the nurse should assess.
3. Calculate or estimate the expected date of delivery.
4. Explain the importance of previous pregnancies and outcomes to the client's current pregnancy.
5. Describe interventions for common discomforts of pregnancy.
6. List the danger signs of pregnancy.

INTRODUCTION

During the antepartal period, members of the health care team strive to ensure the health of the client and her fetus.

The experienced, specially prepared nurse or the advanced registered nurse practitioner, clinician, or nurse-midwife performs the full physical examination, interprets laboratory data, and takes pelvimetry measurements. The less experienced nurse may conduct the history, take vital signs and weight, gather urine and blood samples, and teach the client and family members.

This chapter begins with client assessment, which is obtained through the health history and physical assessment, occurring during the initial prenatal visit and at scheduled follow-up visits. The assessment section includes instructions for determining the expected date of delivery (EDD). Client assessment is followed by nursing diagnoses

applicable to many antepartal clients, followed by planning and implementing care for the healthy pregnant client. The chapter then presents interventions to help minimize client discomfort during pregnancy and it lists signs of impending danger to the client or fetus. Finally the chapter discusses evaluation and documentation for the antepartal client.

ASSESSMENT

Ideally, antepartal assessment begins when a client seeks health care to confirm a suspected pregnancy and begin prenatal care. During the initial antepartal meeting, the nurse gathers subjective and objective data pertinent to the client's pregnancy and general health.

Assessment should continue regularly throughout the antepartal period. The client may schedule a routine examination every 4 weeks until the twenty-eighth week, every 2 weeks until the thirty-sixth week, and every week until delivery. However, the number of scheduled examinations depends on the client's overall condition.

Repeated contact between nurse and client enables the nurse to monitor the client's well-being, the fetus's development, and the onset of any problems. Also, it provides an opportunity for client teaching.

Besides a health history and physical examination, antepartal assessment includes selected laboratory tests. Follow-up care focuses on maintaining the health and well-being of the client and fetus throughout pregnancy.

HEALTH HISTORY

The health history interview should address all pertinent areas of the client's health—past, present, and potential. The nurse should consider the client's physical appearance and nonverbal communication as well as her verbal responses to questions.

Biographical data. Record the client's name, address, telephone number, birth date, and marital status. Ascertain her reason for requesting care.

The client's age will relate to possible risks she faces during pregnancy. Reproductive risks increase among clients under age 15 and over age 35.

Investigating the client's marital status may give the nurse insight into family support systems, sexual practices, and possible stress factors.

Current pregnancy. After obtaining biographical data, focus on concerns directly related to the pregnancy. Record the client's reasons for believing herself pregnant, including the absence of one or more menstrual periods, nausea, vomiting, urinary frequency, breast tenderness, fatigue, or a positive result on a home pregnancy test.

Ask if the client menstruates regularly, the typical length of her cycle, and the date of her last menstrual period (LMP). Knowing the LMP is useful in predicting gestational age and EDD.

EDD can be calculated using several methods, but Nagele's rule is used most commonly. By Nagele's rule, EDD equals the first day of the last normal menstrual period, minus 3 months, plus 7 days. For example, if the first day of the LMP was September 20, then the EDD will be June 27 of the following calendar year. Nagele's rule is based on a 28-day cycle and must be adjusted if the client has irregular, prolonged, or shortened menstrual cycles.

If the client cannot remember, record her LMP as questionable and rely on other methods—such as the date of quickening, uterine size and growth, and ultrasound—to help predict the EDD.

In addition to requesting the date of the client's LMP, ask her if her last menstrual period differed. Implantation of the fertilized ovum may produce a scant, bloody vaginal discharge at about the time of an expected menstrual period. If the client mistakes this discharge for her monthly flow, she will misinterpret her LMP. In addition, vaginal bleeding or spotting could indicate ectopic pregnancy or a problem with hormonal support of the endometrium.

Ask if the couple planned the pregnancy. If so, they probably desire a child and have primarily positive thoughts about the pregnancy. If not, explore the client's and her partner's desire to maintain the pregnancy and explain options available to them.

Begin assessing the client's educational needs (and her partner's needs, if possible) during the initial visit. Provide the couple with needed information or appropriate referrals. Education helps reduce fears associated with labor and delivery and with postpartal care of both client and neonate. Suggest childbirth education classes when appropriate.

Record the age, health status, and development of other children in the family. It may identify possible areas of family stress and dysfunctional coping behaviors.

After obtaining information on the current pregnancy, investigate possible pregnancy risk factors, as follows.

Previous pregnancies and outcomes. Discussion and documentation of the client's previous pregnancies may help the nurse, the client, and her family anticipate needs and expectations for the current pregnancy. (For more information, see *Documenting previous pregnancies*.)

Make note of birth weights, gestational ages, labor outcomes, and neonatal conditions for each of the client's other children, from the oldest to the youngest. Make special note of any problems or complications she encountered during each pregnancy, labor, and delivery. Such risk factors may warrant special education and guidance. Examples of risk factors include:
• possible cervical incompetence or adhesions resulting from previous abortion
• preterm or postterm labor in a previous pregnancy
• previous cesarean or forceps delivery.

The birth weights of the client's children and their modes of delivery provide information about maternal pelvic size. If any of the client's previous pregnancies ended with a stillbirth or with death during the neonatal period, carefully record factors contributing to the death.

Some risk factors may be linked to ethnic background. Examples include sickle cell disease among Blacks and Tay Sach's disease among Jews. Refer the couple for genetic counseling as needed.

Rh factor may raise the risk of complications for some clients. An Rh-negative client with an Rh-positive partner who previously delivered an Rh-positive neonate and did not receive RhoGAM is sensitized to the Rh factor and will need treatment to prevent complications in subsequent neonates.

DOCUMENTING PREVIOUS PREGNANCIES

One method commonly used to document previous pregnancies is called the TPAL system. The first element, T, stands for the number of term neonates born (after 37 weeks' gestation). The second element, P, stands for the number of preterm neonates born (before 37 weeks' gestation). The third element, A, stands for the number of pregnancies ending in spontaneous or therapeutic abortion. The fourth element, L, stands for the number of children alive.

T P A L

This four-digit system is often confused with the two-digit system (gravida, para). In the two-digit system, *para* refers to the number of pregnancies that resulted in the birth of a viable fetus. It does not address the number of fetuses reaching the point of viability, nor does it address those pregnancies not reaching the point of viability. For example, a woman who was pregnant twice, with one of those pregnancies ending in the birth of viable twins and the other in a full-term live birth, would be gravida 2, para 2. Using the four-digit classification, the woman would be described as gravida 2, para 3003. The four-digit system is a more precise method of describing a woman's pregnancy history.

Be aware that some institutions use T to refer to the number of term pregnancies, not the number of term neonates; refer to institutional policy.

Gynecologic history. The client's gynecologic history may include risk factors for the current pregnancy, independent of whether the client has ever been pregnant.

Ask if the client has had pain or discomfort during menstruation (dysmenorrhea).

Ask if the client has had a vaginal infection or a sexually transmitted disease, either of which could harm the fetus during development or delivery. For example:
- *Candida albicans* can cause thrush.
- Chlamydial infection can cause conjunctivitis and spontaneous abortion.
- Herpes genitalis can cause neonatal death.
- Gonorrhea can cause ophthalmia neonatorum.
- Syphilis and human immunodeficiency virus (HIV) can be transmitted to the fetus in utero.

The following factors increase a woman's risk of contracting HIV infection and acquired immunodeficiency syndrome (AIDS):
- having a bisexual male partner
- using illicit I.V. drugs or having a sexual partner who uses such drugs
- having numerous sexual partners

- having a sexual partner with an unknown drug or sexual history
- receiving, or having a sexual partner who received, blood or blood products (especially before HIV safeguards were established in April, 1985).

After a woman contracts HIV and becomes pregnant, she may pass HIV to her fetus in utero or to her neonate in breast milk.

Determine if the client used a contraceptive before becoming pregnant, and how long she used it. Pregnancy that results from contraceptive failure may raise special risks. For example, an oral contraceptive taken during the first trimester can be teratogenic. A failed IUD can cause spontaneous septic abortion and should be removed by the physician immediately after verification of pregnancy.

Medical history. Collect data about current and previous health factors that may be relevant to the current pregnancy.

Weight. An underweight or overweight client may reflect poor nutrition. An underweight client may deliver a low-birth-weight neonate; an overweight client may be at increased risk for gestational diabetes and pregnancy-induced hypertension (PIH).

Medications and allergies. Determine if the client has taken any prescription or over-the-counter drugs since becoming pregnant. Medications taken in the early weeks of pregnancy may adversely affect fetal development. Ask if the client has any medication allergies.

Viral infections. Determine if the client has had any viral infections since becoming pregnant, such as the TORCH group. The acronym TORCH includes toxoplasmosis, other diseases (chlamydia, group B beta-hemolytic streptococcus, syphilis, and varicella zoster), rubella, cytomegalovirus, and herpesvirus. These infections can harm an embryo or fetus.

Medical treatments or procedures. Inquire whether the client has had any dental treatments, surgery, or X-rays since her last menstrual period. If she had X-rays, was an abdominal shield used? X-rays may be harmful to the fetus, and noxious anesthetics may lead to abortion.

Substance abuse. Attempt to determine whether the client habitually uses substances known to cause or suspected of causing harm to the fetus or to herself.

If the client smokes, ask how many cigarettes per day. Women who smoke deliver, on average, smaller neonates than those who do not smoke. Further, intrauterine growth retardation (IUGR) increases with the number of cigarettes smoked. IUGR was minimal or eliminated when smokers stopped smoking early in the pregnancy (Naeye, 1981). Smoking also may raise the incidence of preterm delivery (Shiono, Klebanoff, and Rhoads, 1986). If the client does not smoke, ask if she is exposed regularly to a smoke-filled environment, which also presents a risk.

If the client drinks alcohol, determine how much and how often. A safe level of alcohol intake during pregnancy has not been determined. However, excessive alcohol intake has serious harmful effects on the fetus. Between weeks 4 and 10 of pregnancy, alcohol intake can affect the fetus's developing facial features, including the jaw, and central nervous system. These effects are more common than full-blown fetal alcohol syndrome. Neonates affected with fetal alcohol syndrome demonstrate microcephaly, growth retardation, short palpebral fissures, and maxillary hypoplasia. Alcohol intake may affect the client's nutrition and may predispose her to complications in early pregnancy, such as abortion. The combined effects of alcohol and cigarettes cause greater fetal anomalies than the sum of their individual effects (Brooten, et al., 1987).

Determine how many cups of caffeinated coffee, tea, and soda the client drinks daily. Although the effects of caffeine are not clearly understood in pregnancy, the client should exercise caution by limiting intake.

Determine if the client has used marijuana, cocaine, heroin, or other illicit drugs before and since becoming pregnant. These drugs pose serious threats to the health of both client and fetus. Marijuana use has been linked to short gestation and high incidence of precipitate labor; it may have effects similar to those of alcohol (Fried, Watkinson, and Willan, 1984). Cocaine use has been linked to increased spontaneous abortions, preterm labor, and abruptio placentae; also, a client who uses cocaine commonly uses other drugs as well. Heroin and cocaine use create neonatal dependency and withdrawal trauma (Landry and Smith, 1987). Additionally, the HIV responsible for AIDS can be transmitted via shared needles used to inject drugs. The virus in a client can pass to the fetus.

Previous medical problems. Elicit information about the client's childhood disease profile, immunizations, past medical conditions and treatments, and surgical procedures.

Some diseases acquired in childhood may confer lifelong immunity. Of those that do not, some may endanger a fetus exposed at certain stages of development. Rubella, for example, may have teratogenic effects on the fetus if the client is exposed during the first trimester. Other problems may occur if the client is exposed during the last trimester. Some immunizations may be recommended during pregnancy because of the client's increased susceptibility. (See *Immunization guidelines during pregnancy* for further information.) Other immunizations, such as rubella, are contraindicated during pregnancy because of the teratogenic effects of the attenuated live virus on the fetus.

Toxoplasmosis can be contracted from organisms in soil or cat feces. Ask if the client gardens or has pets. Toxoplasmosis causes severe congenital anomalies in a fetus infected in the first trimester. During the third trimester, toxoplasmosis attacks the fetus's central nervous system. Infections contracted from bird and dog parasites may put the client and fetus at risk as well.

Certain medical conditions could place a client at high risk or jeopardize the pregnancy. These include bleeding disorders, cancer, cardiac disease, diabetes, epilepsy, gallbladder disease, hepatitis, hypertension, phlebitis, psychiatric problems, renal disease, and urinary tract infection.

Symptoms not associated with possible or probable signs of pregnancy may signal disorders that could have an adverse effect on the pregnancy. Such symptoms warrant investigation.

Ask if the client ever had surgery and, if so, what surgery she had. Previous surgery on the uterus or vagina may have altered their structure, thus increasing the risk of adhesions, which can complicate delivery. Such clients may require a cesarean delivery.

Family health history. Because genetic anomalies and some medical and reproductive conditions are familial, gather family health data. Include the health history of the couple's grandparents, parents, and brothers and sisters.

Ask whether any member of the client's family or her partner's family has had any of the following:
• allergies
• anemias
• bleeding disorders
• cesarean delivery
• children born with congenital diseases or deformities
• diabetes mellitus
• heart disease
• hypertension
• kidney problems
• multiple gestations (such as twins)
• PIH during a past pregnancy.

Psychosocial assessment. Important areas of psychosocial exploration include the client's attitude toward her preg-

IMMUNIZATION GUIDELINES DURING PREGNANCY

The following list gives indications for immunization during pregnancy.

IMMUNIZATION	INDICATIONS
Hepatitis A standard immune globulin	Postexposure prophylaxis
Hepatitis B inactivated virus vaccine	Pre- and postexposure for women at risk of infection
specific immune globulin	Postexposure prophylaxis
Influenza inactivated virus vaccine	Women with serious underlying diseases; public health authorities to be consulted for current recommendation
Measles live virus vaccine	Contraindicated
immune globulin	Postexposure prophylaxis
Mumps live virus vaccine	Contraindicated
Poliomyelitis live virus vaccine	Not routinely recommended for women in U.S., except persons at increased risk of exposure
Rabies inactivated virus vaccine	Indications for prophylaxis not altered by pregnancy; each case considered individually
immune globulin	Postexposure prophylaxis
Rubella live virus vaccine	Contraindicated
Tetanus-diphtheria toxoid	Lack of primary series, or no booster within past 10 years
Varicella immune globulin	Can be considered for healthy pregnant women exposed to varicella to protect against maternal, not congenital, infection

Adapted from American College of Obstetricians and Gynecologists (1991). Immunization during pregnancy. *ACOG Technical Bulletin*, Number 160. Washington, DC: Author.

nancy, her methods of coping with stress, and how cultural and religious beliefs may affect her pregnancy.

Explore any concerns the client or her partner has about the pregnancy. Childbirth education classes may provide the couple with psychosocial support by giving them the opportunity to share concerns with other expectant couples.

Take note of the client's verbal and nonverbal communication patterns, which could reveal problems in adjusting to pregnancy or to impending parenthood. When necessary, refer the client for psychological assistance.

Assess the client's religious and cultural beliefs about pregnancy because they may affect her health practices during pregnancy and predispose her to complications. For example, an Amish woman may refuse recommended vaccinations.

Education and occupation. Educational level may influence the client's attitude toward pregnancy, the quality of her prenatal care and nutritional intake, her knowledge of neonatal care, and the psychosocial changes that accompany childbirth and parenting.

Identifying the client's occupation may help detect environmental hazards or exposure to teratogens, such as dry-cleaning fluids or X-rays. A client who must stand for long periods may develop backache during pregnancy. Her risk of falling increases during the second and third trimesters as her center of gravity changes. Lifting heavy objects may increase the risk of spontaneous abortion.

Ask if the client's employer provides maternity leave and, if so, its duration and financial coverage.

PHYSICAL ASSESSMENT

After collecting complete history data, the nurse assists with or continues the physical assessment. The initial examination provides baseline data against which subsequent changes can be evaluated. (See *Nurse's guide to pregnancy assessment*, page 92, for a list of expected changes.)

Follow-up client visits at regular intervals throughout pregnancy allow the nurse to monitor those changes and detect potential abnormalities.

Conduct all physical examinations in a private and comfortable room, and encourage the client to relax. Work efficiently but without rushing. Drape the client as appropriate to respect her modesty; remain alert for signs of discomfort. Explain pertinent examination steps as they occur.

NURSE'S GUIDE TO PREGNANCY ASSESSMENT

This guide provides an overview of normal changes during pregnancy as seen from weeks 1 through 40.

FIRST TRIMESTER

Weeks 1 to 4
- Amenorrhea occurs.
- Breast changes begin.
- Immunologic pregnancy tests become positive; radioimmuno-assay test is positive a few days after implantation of fertilized ovum; urine hCG test is positive a few days after occurrence of amenorrhea.
- Nausea and vomiting may begin between the fourth and sixth week.

Weeks 5 to 8
- Goodell's sign occurs (softening of cervix).
- Ladin's sign occurs (softening of uterine isthmus).
- Hegar's sign occurs (softening of lower uterine segment).
- Chadwick's sign appears (purple-blue vagina and cervix).

- McDonald's sign appears (easy flexion of the fundus over the cervix).
- Braun von Fernwald's sign (also called Piskacek's sign) occurs (irregular softening and enlargement of the uterine fundus at the site of implantation).
- Cervical mucus plug forms.
- Uterine shape changes from pear to globular.
- Urinary frequency and urgency occurs.

Weeks 9 to 12
- Fetal heartbeat may be detected using ultrasonic stethoscope.
- Nausea, vomiting, and urinary frequency and urgency lessen.
- Uterus becomes palpable just above symphysis pubis by 12 weeks.

SECOND TRIMESTER

Weeks 13 to 17
- Client gains approximately 10 to 12 lb (4.5 to 5.4 kg) during second trimester.
- Placental souffle heard on auscultation.
- Client's heartbeat increases approximately 10 beats between 14 and 30 weeks' gestation. Rate is maintained until 40 weeks' gestation.
- By week 16, the client's thyroid gland enlarges by approximately 25%, and the uterine fundus is palpable halfway between the symphysis pubis and umbilicus.
- Client recognition of fetal movements, or quickening, occurs between 16 and 20 weeks' gestation depending on gravidity and obesity.

Weeks 18 to 22
- Uterine fundus is palpable just below the umbilicus at 18 weeks and is one fingerbreadth above by 22 weeks.
- Fetal heartbeats are heard with fetoscope at 20 weeks' gestation.
- Fetal rebound or ballottement is possible.

Weeks 23 to 27
- Umbilicus appears level with abdominal skin.
- Striae gravidarum usually become apparent.
- Uterine fundus shows evidence of increasing growth.
- Shape of uterus changes from globular to ovoid.
- Braxton Hicks contractions begin.

THIRD TRIMESTER

Weeks 28 to 31
- Client gains approximately 8 to 10 lb (3.6 to 4.5 kg) in third trimester.
- Uterine wall feels soft and yielding.
- Uterine fundus is halfway between the umbilicus and xiphoid process.
- Fetus's outline becomes palpable.
- Fetus is very mobile and may be found in any position.

Weeks 32 to 35
- Client may experience heartburn.
- Striae gravidarum become more evident.
- Fundal height measurement no longer is an accurate indication of gestational age.

- Uterine fundus is palpable just below the xiphoid process at term.
- Braxton Hicks contractions increase in frequency and intensity.
- Client may experience shortness of breath.

Weeks 36 to 40
- Umbilicus protrudes.
- Varicosities, if present, become pronounced.
- Ankle edema becomes evident.
- Urinary frequency recurs.
- Engagement (with or without lightening) occurs.
- Mucus plug is expelled.
- Cervical effacement and dilation begin.

Vital signs. Typically, the assessment begins with vital signs, followed by examination of the head, chest, abdomen, extremities, and pelvic area (when indicated). Alternatively, the examination may follow a body system progression.

At each return visit, ask the client to describe changes that have occurred since the previous visit. Compare these changes with those normally encountered by healthy, pregnant women. Question the client about any symptoms that seem abnormal, such as abdominal pain, vaginal bleeding, headache, or urinary tract pain.

Record the client's temperature, pulse, respirations, and blood pressure. Blood pressure normally remains within the client's prepregnant range. A rise of greater than 30 mm Hg in systolic pressure or 15 mm Hg in diastolic pressure may indicate PIH and should be investigated.

Record the client's height and weight, and compare them against norms for her age and activity level. Weight under 100 lb or over 200 lb may warrant investigation by the client's physician. Failure to gain weight during pregnancy suggests a serious abnormality. Excessive weight gain—more than 2 lb (0.9 kg) weekly—may result from excessive caloric intake, excessive sodium chloride intake, or PIH.

Body systems. When assessing the various body systems, keep the normal physiologic changes of pregnancy in mind. The physical assessment will be modified according to the nurse's educational preparation and clinical expertise.

Musculoskeletal system. Observe the client's posture and gait. These will change later in pregnancy as her center of gravity shifts and hormones relax the pelvic structure.

Endocrine system. On the first visit, palpate the thyroid, which enlarges in about half of all pregnant women because of increased vascularity and hyperplasia.

Respiratory system. On the client's first visit, auscultate the anterior and posterior lung fields. A client in the third trimester may show increased respiratory effort during inspiration.

Cardiovascular system. Expect to hear accentuated heart sounds and, in about 9 out of 10 clients, systolic ejection murmur at 6 to 8 weeks' gestation. The point of maximum impulse may be displaced laterally as the heart moves in response to pressure exerted by the enlarged uterus.

Gastrointestinal system. On the first visit, auscultate bowel sounds. Expect sounds to decrease during pregnancy as a result of reduced peristalsis.

Integumentary system. On the first visit, inspect the client's skin, particularly noting the appearance of pigment changes characteristic of pregnancy: chloasma, linea nigra, and hyperpigmentation of the areolae, nipples, and vulva. Inspect the client's abdomen, noting striae gravidarum as they appear. Progression of these changes should be documented during follow-up care.

Urinary system. On the first visit, palpate and percuss the bladder if uterus placement allows. Obtain a urine sample and test with a dipstick for glucose and protein.

Hematologic system. Observe the client's veins. Pelvic congestion predisposes her to venous varicosities in the legs, vulva, and rectum. Edema in the extremities, although common, may warn of PIH and deserves monitoring.

Neurologic system. On the first visit, check the client's deep tendon reflexes for hyperreflexia, which is seen with PIH.

Reproductive system. Examine the client's breasts and internal pelvic organs only with special preparation and extreme caution.

Maternal status

On the first visit, inspect and palpate the client's breasts, anticipating enlargement and increased nipple size and erectility by about the eighth week. Colostrum may be expressed as early as the twenty-fourth week. Striae on the breasts may become more visible as vascularity and venous engorgement increase throughout pregnancy.

Monitor uterine growth to check the correlation between fetal growth and estimated gestational age. Fundal height is the characteristic used most commonly to monitor uterine growth. (See Psychomotor Skills: *Measuring fundal height,* page 94, for instructions.)

During each visit, palpate the client's uterus for Braxton Hicks contractions, which occur more frequently, last longer, and are more intense later in pregnancy. During the second and third trimesters, palpation of the uterus through the abdominal wall may be affected by abdominal musculature, previous pregnancies, excess or inadequate amounts of amniotic fluid, and IUGR.

Because the pelvic examination is more tolerable with an empty bladder, ask the client to void before beginning the physical examination.

MEASURING FUNDAL HEIGHT

To monitor fetal growth after week 18, the nurse practitioner, nurse-midwife, or physician uses a flexible measuring tape to determine fundal height. The examiner places the client in a supine position and stands at her right side. With one hand, the examiner finds the point on the client's abdomen where soft tissue ends and the firm, round fundal edge begins and measures from that point to the notch at the inferior edge of the sym-physis pubis. The length in centimeters equals approximate gestational age in weeks. For example, a fundal height of 20 cm corresponds with a gestational age of approximately 20 weeks, give or take 2 weeks. After week 32, fundal height measurement does not correlate as well with gestational age because of fetal weight variations, but progressive growth should be evident.

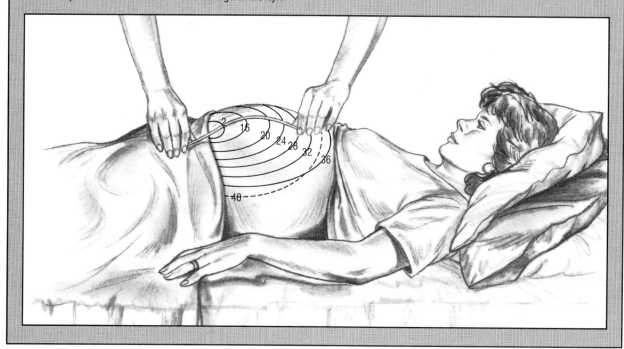

The nurse practitioner uses several measurements to help estimate the capacity of the client's pelvis. If possible, pelvimetry measurements are taken during the first physical examination and again at 36 weeks' gestation; they indicate whether vaginal delivery will be possible.

Typically, a pregnant client undergoes a pelvic examination during the initial assessment and at least once during the final 4 weeks of pregnancy. Late in the pregnancy, the cervix will be soft and cervical dilation may have begun.

Fetal status

Document the client's first report of quickening (fetal movement), which usually occurs between weeks 16 and 20. At each subsequent visit, question the client about the fetus's activity level. If she reports that the fetus is less active, notify the physician immediately.

Assess fetal position using Leopold's maneuvers. (See Chapter 13, The First Stage of Labor, for instructions.) Fe-tal position may vary during pregnancy but, after week 36, it should remain unchanged until delivery.

Assess fetal heart tones, which can be heard with a Doppler device as early as week 10 and with an ordinary fetoscope as early as week 20. In the case of twins or an obese client, detection may be delayed. Early in the pregnancy, listen for fetal heart tones at the midline just above the client's symphysis pubis. Later in pregnancy, they can be heard most clearly through the fetus's back.

If suspected abnormalities arise, the nurse-midwife or physician may prescribe special tests to evaluate fetal well-being. The non-stress test and contraction stress test evaluate the oxygen transfer function of the placenta, predicting possible intrauterine asphyxia in high-risk pregnancies. Other tests of fetal well-being include amniocentesis, chorionic villus sampling, fetoscopy, fetal echocardiography and blood flow studies, percutaneous umbilical blood sampling, alpha-fetoprotein screening, computed tomographic scanning, and magnetic resonance imaging.

COMMON LABORATORY STUDIES

Complete assessment data for a client include the results of various laboratory studies. The chart below lists commonly ordered studies and describes their significance.

BLOOD TESTS

Complete blood count (CBC)
Hemoglobin and hematocrit: Screens for anemia, which may result from a menstrual disorder (such as menorrhagia) or a nutritional deficiency (such as anemia).
White blood cell (WBC) count with differential: Identifies infection, which may be caused by a sexually transmitted disease (STD).

Rubella antibody test
Determines if the client has antibodies to the disease, which is especially important because rubella infection in early pregnancy may cause fetal anomalies.

VDRL test or rapid plasma reagin (RPR) test
Screens for syphilis, which can cause congenital abnormalities if it is transmitted to a fetus.

HIV-III antibody test
Detects antibodies to the AIDS virus. Many health care facilities offer this test for all high-risk clients.

URINE TESTS

Urinalysis
Evaluates the client's urine for glucose, protein, and infection.

Urine culture and sensitivity
Identifies the organism responsible for urinary tract infection and its susceptibility to antibiotics.

OTHER TESTS

Papanicolaou (Pap) test
Identifies preinvasive and invasive cervical cancer.

Wet smear
May detect infection with *Candida albicans*, *Trichomonas vaginalis*, or organisms that cause bacterial vaginosis.

Cervical culture
May detect infection with *Neisseria gonorrhoeae* or *Chlamydia trachomatis*. Confirmation of either of these STDs requires treatment for the client and her partner.

DIAGNOSTIC STUDIES

Diagnostic tests that reflect the client's history and physical findings may include blood type and ABO group, antibody screen, complete blood count, rapid plasma reagent (RPR)

test, sickle cell test, rubella test, urinalysis, cultures for sexually transmitted diseases, Papanicolaou (Pap) test, and others. (Refer to *Common laboratory studies* for more information.)

The nurse practitioner, nurse-midwife, or physician may decide the client will benefit from ultrasonogaphy, which displays a two-dimensional echo image of the fetus and surrounding tissues. Ultrasound examination may be performed to:
• estimate delivery date
• evaluate fetal growth and condition
• investigate the possibility of ectopic pregnancy, hydatidiform mole, and other anomalies of pregnancy
• determine fetal presentation
• estimate fetal weight.

NURSING DIAGNOSIS

After completing the health history and physical assessment, the nurse analyzes the data and formulates appropriate nursing diagnoses. (See Nursing Diagnoses: *Antepartal period,* page 96.)

As much as possible, involve the client in determining appropriate diagnoses, which will increase their usefulness. Also, participation creates a sense of responsibility, retains the client's freedom of choice, and fosters her problem-solving ability.

PLANNING AND IMPLEMENTATION

The planning phase of the nursing process begins after nursing diagnoses are made. Together, the nurse, other members of the health care team, and the client set goals and work out ways to implement the plan of care to meet those goals. During the normal antepartal period, nursing goals typically include comfort promotion for the client, family adaptation to the addition of a new member, promoting maternal and fetal well-being, and relieving discomfort caused by the physiologic changes associated with pregnancy.

ENCOURAGE FAMILY ADAPTATION

Depending on experiences and coping abilities, family relationships may be strengthened or weakened by pregnancy, resulting in a nursing diagnosis of *altered family processes related to inclusion of an additional family member.* Family members may require confirmation that change is healthy or that interventions may be needed to

ANTEPARTAL PERIOD

The following nursing diagnoses are examples of the problems and etiologies that the nurse may encounter when caring for a client in the antepartal period. Specific nursing interventions for many of these diagnoses are provided in the "Planning and implementation" section of this chapter.

- Altered family processes related to inclusion of an additional family member
- Altered nutrition: less than body requirements, related to nausea and vomiting
- Altered urinary elimination related to compression of the urinary bladder
- Altered sexuality patterns related to fear of harming the fetus during intercourse
- Body image disturbance related to the discomforts of pregnancy
- Body image disturbance related to weight gain during pregnancy
- Constipation related to decreased peristalsis
- High risk for injury related to the effect of shifting center of gravity on exercise routine
- Impaired adjustment related to changes in body structure
- Knowledge deficit related to care measures required for optimal pregnancy outcome
- Sleep pattern disturbance related to increased fatigue

maintain a sense of balance in the family. The nurse intervenes to help the family deal with the crises by being supportive and by providing necessary education for childbirth and parenting.

MINIMIZE ANTEPARTAL RISKS

The nurse has the opportunity and responsibility to teach the client and her family about potential risks during the antepartal period and care required to promote maternal and fetal well-being. In addition, without alarming the client, the nurse should urge her to report promptly any signs that could indicate danger to herself or the fetus. (See *Danger signs during pregnancy* for a list of such signs.)

Nutrition. Early in pregnancy, the client may have a nursing diagnosis of *altered nutrition: less than body requirements, related to nausea and vomiting.* Because pregnancy depletes nutrient stores, urge the client to maintain adequate intake of essential nutrients during pregnancy. Insufficient nutrition will not provide adequate nutrients to the fetus for growth and development, and may result in IUGR or other nutrition-related problems. (See Chapter

8, Nutrition and Diet Counseling, for in-depth discussion of this topic.)

Exercise. A client should not start an exercise regimen during pregnancy. However, a client who exercises regularly may continue if she modifies her regimen to prevent a nursing diagnosis of *high risk for injury related to the effect of shifting center of gravity on exercise routine.* Recommend the following guidelines:
- Warm up and stretch to help prepare the joints for activity.
- Exercise for shorter intervals. By exercising for 10 to 15 minutes, resting briefly, and then exercising for another 10 to 15 minutes, the client will decrease the risk of problems associated with shunting blood to the musculoskeletal system and away from the uterus and other vital organs.
- As pregnancy progresses, decrease the intensity of the exercise. This helps compensate for decreased cardiac reserve, increased respiratory effort, and increased weight during pregnancy.
- Avoid prolonged overheating. Strenuous exercise, especially in a humid environment, can raise the core body temperature. Especially in the first trimester, hyperthermia may increase the risk of teratogenesis. The client also should avoid hot tubs and saunas.
- Avoid high-risk activities that require balance and coordination, such as skydiving, mountain climbing, racquetball, and surfing. As pregnancy progresses, the client's changing center of gravity and softened joints may decrease balance and coordination.
- After exercise, cool down with a period of mild activity to help restore circulation and avoid pooling of blood.
- After cooling down, lie on the left side for 10 minutes to improve venous return from the extremities and promote placental perfusion.
- Wear appropriate sports shoes and a support bra.
- Stop exercising and contact the health care practitioner if any of the following occur: dizziness, shortness of breath, tingling, numbness, vaginal bleeding, or abdominal pain.

Substance abuse. Evidence continues to demonstrate that substance abuse represents great risk to the fetus. Encourage the client to stop smoking and avoid alcohol for the duration of pregnancy. Even a reduction in the number of cigarettes smoked daily may improve fetal condition (Naeye, 1981).

Caution the client against indiscriminate use of over-the-counter medications, especially during the first trimester. Inform her about the effect of illicit drugs on

DANGER SIGNS DURING PREGNANCY

The nurse should advise the pregnant client to report immediately any of the following signs and symptoms:
- Fever above 101° F (38.3° C)
- Severe headache
- Dizziness, blurred or double vision, spots before the eyes
- Abdominal pain or cramps
- Epigastric pain
- Repeated vomiting
- Absence of or marked decrease in fetal movement
- Vaginal spotting or bleeding (brown or red)
- Rush or constant leakage of fluid from the vagina
- Painful urination or decreased urine output
- Edema of the extremities and face
- Muscle cramps or convulsions

the developing fetus, and obtain professional counseling for an addicted client or habitual user.

Travel. Most pregnant clients can travel without undue risk to the fetus. However, the risk of accident increases with the amount of traveling. Recommend certain precautions:
- In moving vehicles, wear shoulder and lap belts to reduce injury in case of an accident.
- Do not remain seated for longer than 2 hours. Walk around for approximately 10 minutes to restore circulation.
- Airlines may require a note from a nurse-midwife or physician for customers in later stages of pregnancy. Also, carry a copy of recent medical records in case of emergency.
- As term approaches, determine the availability of medical care at the destination.

Occupation. The client may work throughout pregnancy, provided she faces no environmental hazards, has adequate rest periods, does not engage in hazardous physical activity (such as lifting heavy objects), and feels well.

During the last few weeks, she should avoid standing or sitting for long periods. Recommend that she elevate her legs whenever possible to relieve backache, improve venous return, and reduce edema in her legs. Suggest that she lie on her left side during work breaks, if possible, to enhance placental circulation.

MINIMIZE DISCOMFORTS

Discomforts of pregnancy can cause varying amounts of distress for the client and her family, possibly resulting in

a nursing diagnosis of *body image disturbance related to the discomforts of pregnancy.* These discomforts vary with the stage of pregnancy and the size of the uterus. How women respond to and feel about the changes and discomforts vary greatly.

Discuss the client's comfort level at each antepartal visit and recommend appropriate interventions if she reports problems. (See Client Teaching: *Minimizing discomforts of pregnancy,* pages 98 and 99.)

PROVIDE EDUCATION

The nurse instructs the pregnant client on antepartal care measures in an effort to enhance client and fetal well-being. Although primigravid clients typically need more education, both primigravid and multigravid clients may have a nursing diagnosis of *knowledge deficit related to care measures required for optimal pregnancy outcome.* Education topics should include rest, breast care, childbirth exercises, clothing, personal hygiene, fetal activity monitoring, childbirth and parenting, and sexual activity.

Rest. Adequate rest during pregnancy is important for both physical and emotional health. Women need more sleep when pregnant, especially in the first and third trimesters when they may tire easily. Resilience and resistance to illness depend on adequate rest.

Sleeping becomes more difficult during the third trimester because of the enlarged abdomen, increased urinary frequency, and greater fetal activity. Finding a comfortable position becomes difficult. Encourage the client to try a left lateral position, which reduces uterine pressure on the other organs. Also, teach the client appropriate relaxation techniques to help prepare her for sleep.

Breast care. Teach the importance of proper breast support to promote comfort, retain breast shape, and prevent back strain. This is especially important for the client with large breasts. Recommend that she wear a well-fitting support bra.

Emphasize the importance of cleanliness, especially as the client begins producing colostrum. Recommend that she use warm water to remove colostrum that crusts on the nipples. The client who plans to breast-feed should avoid using soap on her nipples because of its drying effect.

For the client who plans to breast-feed, teach nipple preparation techniques, which reduce soreness by distributing natural lubricants produced by Montgomery's tubercles, stimulating blood flow to the breasts, and developing the protective layer of skin over the nipples. Be-

(Text continues on page 100.)

MINIMIZING DISCOMFORTS OF PREGNANCY

You may find that you suffer from different discomforts as your pregnancy progresses. The following list provides preventive measures that may help relieve these discomforts.

DISCOMFORT	POSSIBLE RELIEF
First trimester	
Nausea and vomiting	• Avoid smelling or eating foods that trigger nausea. • If early morning nausea occurs, eat plain crackers, dry toast, or other dry carbohydrates before getting out of bed. • Keep hard candy at the bedside. • Rise slowly from a lying or sitting position to avoid nausea. • Eat a small meal every 2 to 3 hours. • Avoid fatty or highly seasoned foods. • Eat a bedtime snack high in protein, such as cheese and crackers. • If you arise at night to urinate, drink 8 oz of a sweet beverage, such as apple juice. • Wait for 30 minutes after a meal to drink beverages. • Consult your doctor if vomiting occurs more than once daily or if it continues beyond the sixteenth week.
Urinary frequency and urgency	• Restrict fluids in the evening to reduce having to urinate during the night (daily intake should not go below eight 8-oz glasses). • Void every 2 to 3 hours during the day to reduce urgency and minimize the risk of urine staying in your bladder, which can lead to infection. • Consult your doctor if signs and symptoms of urinary tract infection arise, such as pain, burning, or blood in the urine. • Perform Kegel's exercises (tightening the muscles used to control urine flow) in sets of 10 several times a day to maintain perineal tone and control over urination.
Breast tenderness or tingling	• Wear a well-fitting support bra.
Fatigue	• Rest periodically during the day. • Allow more time for sleep at night.

DISCOMFORT	POSSIBLE RELIEF
First trimester (continued)	
Increased vaginal discharge	• Clean the perineum daily. • Wear cotton-crotch underwear, which allows air circulation. • Use talcum powder to help keep skin dry. Avoid douching, which can lead to infection.
Nasal stuffiness or bleeding	• Use a cool-air vaporizer, especially while sleeping.
Excessive saliva production	• Use an astringent mouthwash regularly.
Second and third trimesters	
Heartburn	• Eat smaller meals at shorter intervals. • Avoid fried or spicy foods. • Avoid lying down immediately after eating. • Maintain adequate fluid intake (six to eight 8-oz glasses daily, 30 minutes after meals). • Avoid citrus juices. • Avoid sodium bicarbonate (baking soda) because it disrupts the sodium-potassium balance. • Use an antacid as recommended.
Ankle edema and varicose veins	• Avoid sitting or standing for long periods. • Avoid garters, knee-highs, or other restrictive bands around your legs. • Avoid crossing your legs. • Wear support or elastic stockings. • Exercise regularly to promote blood flow in your legs. • Elevate your feet and legs whenever possible; support your entire leg rather than simply propping up your feet. • Lie down with your feet elevated several times daily.

MINIMIZING DISCOMFORTS OF PREGNANCY *(continued)*

DISCOMFORT	POSSIBLE RELIEF
Second and third trimesters *(continued)*	
Enlarged veins in the groin	• Support your perineum with two sanitary pads worn inside your underpants. • When elevating your legs, elevate your pelvis as well to avoid pooling of blood in the pelvic area.
Hemorrhoids	• Avoid straining when having a bowel movement. • Use ice packs, warm soaks, and topical ointments and anesthetics. • Eat foods high in fiber to avoid constipation. • Maintain adequate fluid intake (six to eight 8-oz glasses daily, preferably water). • Insert hemorrhoids and lie on one side with your knees drawn up for several minutes. • Consult your doctor if hemorrhoids feel hard, are painful, or if rectal bleeding (more than few spots) develops.
Constipation	• Increase fluid intake to more than eight 8-oz glasses daily, preferably water. • Increase dietary fiber by eating more fruits and vegetables. • Eat prunes, which are a natural laxative. • Exercise daily. • Take time for regular bowel movements. • Take laxatives only as prescribed by your doctor.
Backache	• Use proper body mechanics and good posture. • Perform exercises aimed at restoring body alignment. • Use leg muscles when lifting objects. • Avoid lifting heavy objects. • Recline on a bed or lounge chair to rest back muscles.

DISCOMFORT	POSSIBLE RELIEF
Second and third trimesters *(continued)*	
Leg cramps	• Stretch the calf muscle by standing up, pressing your foot firmly on the ground, and straightening your knee. • While lying face down, ask someone to press down on the back of your knee and flex your foot from the ankle toward your shin. • Use a warm towel or leg massage to relieve discomfort. • Reduce milk intake as suggested by your doctor.
Faintness	• Avoid sudden changes in position (lying to sitting, for example). • Avoid crowds and standing for long periods. • Lie on one side rather than on your back. • When feeling faint, sit down and place your head between your knees.
Shortness of breath	• Use proper posture when standing. • Use pillows to support your back when sitting. • Stretch your abdomen by standing with your hands over your head and deep-breathing.
Insomnia	• Lie on your left side with pillows supporting your back, under your abdomen, and between your legs. • Have a warm, caffeine-free drink or a backrub. • Perform relaxation techniques. • Attempt to alleviate distracting discomforts, such as lower back pain.
Abdominal discomfort, Braxton Hicks contractions	• Lightly massage the abdomen with a slow, circular motion. • Apply cream or lotion for dry skin. • Apply heat to the area.

INCREASING NIPPLE PROTRACTILITY

A client who has inverted nipples can help them protrude by performing Hoffman's exercises or by wearing a special breast shield.

Hoffman's exercises
Teach the client to perform Hoffman's exercises by positioning her thumbs or index fingers on opposite sides of one areola, near the edge. She should then stretch the areola while pressing into the breast to help free any adhesions that could be causing the inversion. Instruct the client to repeat the exercise on the other breast.

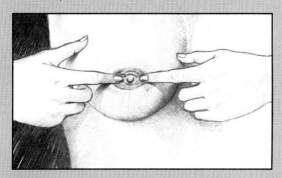

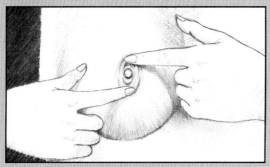

Breast shield
Breast shields, typically more successful than Hoffman's exercises, employ mild suction to draw the nipples out through a hole on the inside of each shield. Used during the third trimester and the postpartal period if necessary, breast shields should not be worn for more than a few hours at a time to minimize their drying effect.

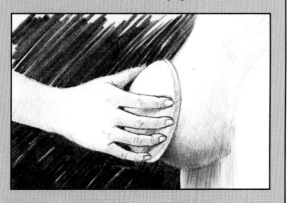

gin teaching the client about nipple preparation in the third trimester. Teach her to grasp the nipple between thumb and forefinger and gently roll and pull it. Because nipple stimulation triggers release of oxytocin, which can cause uterine contractions, do not recommend nipple preparation techniques for clients with a history of preterm labor.

Nipple rolling is more difficult for women with flat or inverted nipples, but it still may be useful. The client with inverted nipples can increase their protractility by performing Hoffman's exercises or wearing special breast shields (such as Woolrich or Eschmann shields) for the last 4 weeks of pregnancy. (See *Increasing nipple protractility* for an explanation of these two techniques.)

Childbirth exercises. Certain exercises help strengthen muscle tone in preparation for delivery and promote more rapid restoration of muscle tone after delivery. Additionally, some physical discomforts of pregnancy can be reduced considerably by faithful performance of body-conditioning exercises. (See Client Teaching: *Prenatal exercises,* pages 101 to 103.)

Clothing. Maternity clothes should be appealing to promote self-esteem and must be loose-fitting to allow for abdominal growth and client comfort. Instruct the client to avoid restrictive clothing, such as garters and tight waistbands, because they can impede venous circulation and encourage or aggravate varicose veins.

A maternity girdle may help a client who exercises during pregnancy or who has a pendulous abdomen that increases spinal curvature and causes backache. Advise against a girdle that has tight leg bands. Underwear should have a cotton lining to allow evaporation and absorption of increased secretions during pregnancy.

Shoes should fit properly, feel comfortable, and have a flat or low wedge heel. Instruct the client to avoid high-heeled shoes because they increase spinal curvature and aggravate backache.

Personal hygiene. The client should bathe daily to remove increased perspiration and vaginal discharge. The client with vaginal bleeding or ruptured membranes must avoid tub baths because of potential bacterial penetration. The client without such problems may shower or bathe, although she may need help getting in and out of the tub.

Remind the client that although her gums may be more tender and bleed during pregnancy, she must maintain good oral hygiene. She should have a dental examination early in pregnancy and any repairs should be done under local anesthesia only. X-rays and repairs that re-
(Text continues on page 103.)

PRENATAL EXERCISES

ABDOMINAL MUSCLES

These exercises will strengthen your abdominal muscles, which support your back, assist with your pushing during childbirth, and promote recovery after childbirth. Before doing any abdominal exercises, however, check with your doctor, nurse-midwife, or nurse practitioner.

Caution: After the fourth month of pregnancy, avoid doing exercises while lying flat on your back. Resume these exercises after your baby's birth.

Resisted knee to chest

Lie flat on your back with your knees bent and your feet flat on the floor. Start with a pelvic tilt and then lift your head toward your chest as your raise one knee toward your abdomen. Grab your leg just below the knee using both hands. Using your leg muscles, try to push the knee toward your feet while your hands pull the knee toward your abdomen. Hold for a count of 5, then release. Repeat on the opposite knee. Do this exercise 5 times at first. Build up to 10 repetitions.

Straight curl up

Lie flat on your back with your knees bent and feet flat on the floor. Bring your chin to your chest as you exhale, continuing forward for about 8". Be sure to curl your back without raising your waist. Then roll back down. Repeat this curl up 5 times at first. Build up to 10 repetitions.

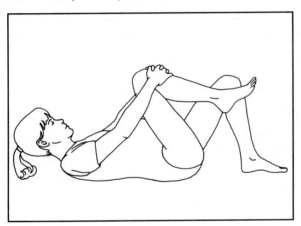

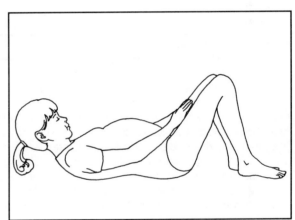

PELVIC MUSCLES

Pelvic exercises can relieve lower back strain and promote good posture. They also will improve abdominal muscle tone, which helps support your growing uterus, deliver your baby, and protect your lower back during pregnancy and throughout life. Pelvic floor muscles support your pelvic organs (the intestines, bladder, and uterus) and help control your urethra, vagina, and anus. During pregnancy, exercise of pelvic floor muscles can increase their strength, giving you greater control and ability to relax during delivery. They can improve healing, strength, and bladder control after childbirth.

Pelvic floor or Kegel exercises

Tighten your pelvic floor muscles by squeezing the urethral and vaginal openings. (You can identify these muscles by trying to stop your urine flow.) You should feel the pelvic floor rise. Hold for a count of 5 and release. Repeat 5 times for a set, and perform a set 8 to 10 times each day.

(continued)

PRENATAL EXERCISES *(continued)*

PELVIC MUSCLES *(continued)*

Pelvic tilt on all fours
Position yourself on your hands and knees with your head and back parallel to the floor. Tighten your stomach muscles and tuck your buttocks under to round the lower back. Hold for a slow count of 5, then release. Do not hold your breath. Repeat this pelvic tilt 5 times at first. Build up to 10 repetitions.

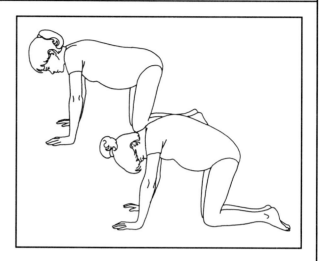

LOWER BACK AND THIGH MUSCLES

Exercises for these muscles will help improve your posture and back stability and increase comfort during childbirth. During these exercises, be careful not to stretch too far because pain may result from separation of the pelvic joints. Because of this potential problem, the tailor stretch and extended leg stretch are optional.

Tailor (Indian style or cross-legged) sit and stretch
Sit on the floor with your knees out and ankles crossed. Hold your back erect to avoid slouching. While in this position, place your hands under your knees. Then press your knees toward the floor while resisting this movement with your hands. Hold for a count of 5, then release. Do this stretch 5 times at first. Build up to 10 repetitions.

Extended leg stretch
Sit on the floor with your legs extended as far apart as comfortable. Gradually stretch your upper body forward without jerking or bouncing. Lead with both hands. Hold for a count of 5, then resume an upright position. Repeat this stretch 5 times at first. Build up to 10 repetitions.

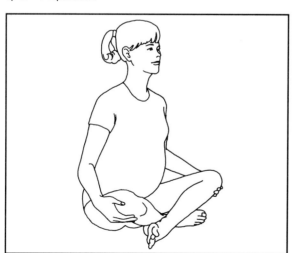

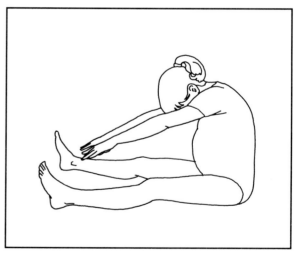

PRENATAL EXERCISES *(continued)*

LOWER LEG MUSCLES

Exercises for your lower leg muscles will promote good circulation, prevent swelling, and increase leg strength.

Calf stretch
Facing a wall, stand with one foot about 12″ in front of the other. Keep your farther leg straight and press your heel to the floor. Bend your nearer knee and lean forward to stretch the calf of your farther leg. Steady yourself with your hands (or arms) against the wall, if desired. Hold for a count of 5, then release. Switch legs and repeat. Do this stretch 5 times at first. Build up to 10 repetitions.

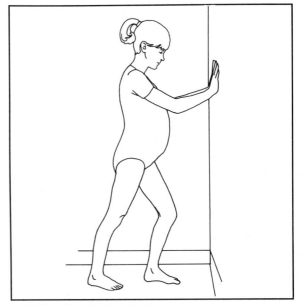

quire systemic anesthesia should wait until after childbirth.

Fetal activity monitoring. Teach the client to assess her fetus's well-being by monitoring movement. Authorities differ on how many movements indicate health in the fetus. Freeman, et al. (1981) suggest that the client should notify her health care practitioner if she feels less than two movements per hour. Other suggestions include six or ten movements per hour; researchers currently are working to determine a reliable standard.

Some clinicians ask clients to use fetal movement records or a fetal activity diary. Keeping a written record of movements at particular times raises the client's awareness of her fetus's activity and her confidence that no problems exist. Further, a drop in fetal activity will be apparent immediately and signal the client to contact her health care practitioner.

Reassure the client that at times she will feel no movement. This may be because the fetus is asleep or because the client cannot feel the movements made. Ultrasound observations have revealed fetuses stretching, rolling, and moving limbs without detection by the mother. Factors that affect fetal activity include drugs, maternal hydration, cigarette smoking, glucose levels, and time of day.

Preparation for childbirth and parenting. Individual and group teaching allows couples to raise questions and seek clarification about any issue related to pregnancy, labor and delivery, the postpartal period, or parenting. Inform every couple of the nearest childbirth education classes. Whether childbirth education occurs in client-teaching sessions with individuals or in classrooms with groups of clients and their partners, it should include the following components:
• physiologic aspects of pregnancy and childbirth
• relaxation techniques
• breathing techniques
• posture and body mechanics
• exercise
• transition to parenthood.

Childbirth education currently emphasizes breathing and relaxation techniques. Various breathing techniques, exercises, and comfort measures during labor are used to promote relaxation. So is information about pregnancy, birth, and parenting, which promotes relaxation by reducing fear of the unknown. Relaxation during labor can help reduce tension, conserve energy, and increase the effectiveness of uterine contractions, resulting in more efficient labor.

Sexual activity. The typical couple has many uncertainties about sexual intercourse during pregnancy. They may worry about harming the client or fetus or about starting labor before term. Additionally, the couple may worry about changes in their desire for each other. An applicable nursing diagnosis may be *altered sexuality patterns related to fear of harming the fetus during intercourse.*

Teach the client and her partner that during normal pregnancy they need not abstain from sexual activity (Reamy and White, 1985). If the client has vaginal bleeding, ruptured membranes, or other complications that could lead to preterm labor, the couple should consult their health care practitioner for advice.

The client's partner may experience changes in sexual desire as well, possibly related to concern over their changing relationship, his own feelings about the pregnancy, discomfort with his partner's changing body and family role, and concern about hurting the fetus. Some men have difficulty seeing their partner as both sexually attractive and a mother. Others find pregnancy arousing (Reamy and White, 1985). The nurse should help the couple communicate openly about these feelings.

EVALUATION

In this step of the nursing process, the nurse evaluates whether nursing diagnoses have been resolved and goals met. Unmet goals may require modification.

Evaluation should take place at each antepartal visit. The nurse observes the client and questions her about problems identified previously. Evaluation statements should reflect actions performed or outcomes achieved for each goal. Examples of evaluation statements for the antepartal period include the following:

- Client accepts her changing body and has confidence in her partner's acceptance of it.
- Client and her partner have enrolled in childbirth education classes.
- Client's weight gain and fundal height are consistent with the calculated EDD.
- Client understands which symptoms could indicate danger to her or her fetus.

DOCUMENTATION

The nurse documents all steps of the nursing process as thoroughly and objectively as possible. This allows more accurate evaluation and better communication between members of the health care team. The nurse must docu-

ment the activities she performs. Therefore, documentation for the normal antepartal initial visit should include minimally:

- the client's vital signs, height, and weight
- age and occupation, social history including smoking, drugs, alcohol
- number of previous pregnancies and complications, if encountered
- danger signs encountered
- fetal activity
- relevant data about the client's other children, family history
- allergies to medications
- psychological profile
- areas of concern
- client teaching accomplished
- date of next visit.

The nurse-midwife or physician may perform and document EDD, LMP, and gestation in weeks; fundal height measurement; fetal heart rate (if gestation exceeds 12 weeks); date of quickening; and pelvic examination findings and collection of vaginal specimens for tests.

Some facilities have charts on which the client can document such data as weight changes, urine test results, and fetal activity during follow-up visits. The nurse should encourage client participation whenever possible.

CHAPTER SUMMARY

Chapter 7 outlined important aspects of nursing care during the antepartal period. Here are the chapter highlights.

Assessment begins with the client's first antepartal visit and continues at regular intervals throughout pregnancy.

The health history should include questions about the current pregnancy, past pregnancies, gynecologic history, medical history (including current symptoms), and family history.

The initial physical assessment should include vital signs, weight, height, and a systematic, progressive assessment of the client's head and chest, abdomen, extremities, and pelvic area (as needed).

Calculation of EDD is commonly performed using Nagele's rule or an obstetric calculator wheel.

Laboratory tests performed routinely on pregnant clients include blood type and ABO group, complete blood count, Pap test, RPR test, sickle cell test, rubella test, urinalysis, and cultures for infectious diseases.

Gestational age may be estimated between weeks 18 and 32 by measuring fundal height in centimeters or by using McDonald's rule. Either method should be augmented by the client's report of quickening and the nurse's auscultation of fetal heart tones.

The nurse follows the nursing process to plan and implement antepartal care.

Interventions typically focus on family preparation for a new family member, promotion of maternal and fetal well-being, and relief of common discomforts of pregnancy.

STUDY QUESTIONS

1. Mrs. Keen, a 24-year-old primigravid client, reports that the first day of her last menstrual period occurred on February 18. What is her EDD using Nagele's rule?
2. During a follow-up visit, the nurse measures Mrs. Keen's fundal height at 22 centimeters. How many weeks pregnant is she?
3. The nurse instructs Mrs. Keen on possible danger signs to report during pregnancy. What information should the nurse include?
4. Mrs. Keen complains of constipation. Which instructions can the nurse give her to help relieve this discomfort?
5. What components should be included in childbirth education?

BIBLIOGRAPHY

Alexander, L.L. (1987). The pregnant smoker: Nursing implications. *JOGNN*, 16(3), 167-173.

American College of Obstetricians and Gynecologists (1985). *Pregnancy exercise program*. Los Angeles: Feeling Fine Programs, Inc.

American College of Obstetricians and Gynecologists (1991). Immunization during pregnancy. *ACOG Technical Bulletin*, Number 160. Washington, DC: Author.

Bush, J.J. (1986). Protocol for tuberculosis screening in pregnancy. *JOGNN*, 15(3), 225-230.

Centers for Disease Control (1989). AIDS and human immunodeficiency virus infection in the United States: 1988 update. *MMWR*, 38(S4), 1-38.

Cnattingius, S., Haglund, B., and Meirik, O. (1988). Cigarette smoking as risk factor for late fetal and early neonatal death. *British Medical Journal*, 297(6643), 258-261.

Cunningham, F., MacDonald, P., and Gant, N. (1989). *Williams obstetrics* (18th ed.). East Norwalk, CT: Appleton & Lange.

Droegemueller, W., Herbst, A., Mishall, D., and Stencheur, M. (1989). *Comprehensive gynecology*. St. Louis: Mosby.

Freeman, R., Garite, R., Mondanlou, H., Dorchester, W., Rommal, C., and Devaney, M. (1981). Postdate pregnancy: Utilization of contraction stress testing for primary fetal surveillance. *American Journal of Obstetrics and Gynecology*, 140(2), 128-135.

Fried, P., Watkinson, B., and Willan, A. (1984). Marijuana use during pregnancy and decreased length of gestation. *American Journal of Obstetrics and Gynecology*, 150(1), 23-27.

Kemp, V.H., and Page, C.K. (1987). Maternal prenatal attachment in normal and high-risk pregnancies. *JOGNN*, 16(3), 179-184.

Klebanoff, M., Nugent, R., and Rhoads, G. (1984). Coitus during pregnancy: Is it safe? *Lancet*, 2(8408), 914-917.

Kleinman, J.C., Pierre, M.B., Madans, J., Land, G.H., and Schramm, W.F. (1988). The effects of maternal smoking on fetal and infant mortality. *American Journal of Epidemiology*, 127(2), 274-282.

Kurth, A., and Hutchison, M. (1989). A context for HIV testing in pregnancy. *Journal of Nurse-Midwifery*, 34(5), 259-266.

Landry, M., and Smith, D.E. (1987). Crack: Anatomy of an addiction, Part 2. *California Nursing Review*, 9(3), 28.

Loveman, A., Colburn, V., and Dobin, A. (1986). AIDS in pregnancy. *JOGNN*, 15(2), 91-93.

Manning, F.A., Morrison, I., Lange, I.R., Harman, R., and Chamberlain, P.F. (1985). Fetal assessment based on fetal biophysical profile scoring: Experience in 12,620 referred high-risk pregnancies. *American Journal of Obstetrics and Gynecology*, 151(3), 343-350.

McKay, S., and Phillips, C. (1984). *Family centered maternity care: Implementation strategies*. Rockville, MD: Aspen Systems.

Naeye, R. (1981). Influence of maternal cigarette smoking during pregnancy on fetal and childhood growth. *Obstetrics and Gynecology*, 57(1), 18-21.

Nichols, F., and Humenick, S. (1988). *Childbirth education: Practice, research, and theory*. Philadelphia: Saunders.

Reamy, K., and White, S. (1985). Sexuality in pregnancy and the puerperium: A review. *Obstetrical and Gynecological Survey*, 40(1), 1-13.

Shepard, M.J., Hellenbrand, K.G., and Bracken, M.B. (1986). Proportional weight gain and complications of pregnancy, labor, and delivery in healthy women of normal prepregnant stature. *American Journal of Obstetrics and Gynecology*, 155(5), 947-54

Shiono, P., Klebanoff, M., and Rhoads, G., (1986). Smoking and drinking during pregnancy: Their effects on preterm birth. *JAMA*, 255(1), 82-84.

Smith, J. (1988). The dangers of prenatal cocaine use. *MCN*, 13(3), 174-179.

Swanson, J. (1980). The marital sexual relationship during pregnancy. *JOGNN*, 9(5), 267-270.

Winslow, W. (1987). First pregnancy after 35: What is the experience? *MCN*, 12(2), 92-96.

Assessment

Engstrom, J.L. (1988). Measurement of fundal height. *JOGNN*, 17(3), 172-178.

Friedrich, E.G. (1988). Current perspectives in candidal vulvovaginitis. *American Journal of Obstetrics and Gynecology*, 158(4), 985-986.

Gilson, G.J., O'Brien, M.E., Vera, R.W., Mays, M.E., Smith, D.R., and Ross, C.Y. (1988). Prolonged pregnancy and the biophysical profile. *Journal of Nurse-Midwifery*, 33(4), 171-177.

Kramer, M.S. (1987). Intrauterine growth and gestational duration determinants. *Pediatrics,* 80(4), 502-511.

Lewis, C., and Mocarski, V. (1987). Obstetric ultrasound: Application in a clinical setting. *JOGNN,* 16(1), 56-60.

Moore, L., Burns, A., Thomas, L., and Skaria, M. (1986). Self-assessment: A personalized approach to nursing during pregnancy. *JOGNN,* 15(4), 311-318.

Nichols, C. (1987). Dating pregnancy: Gathering and using a reliable data base. *Journal of Nurse-Midwifery,* 32(4), 195-204.

Wawrzyniak, M.N. (1986). The painless pelvic. *MCN,* 11(3), 178-179.

Wilson, D. (1988). An overview of sexually transmissible diseases in the perinatal period. *Journal of Nurse-Midwifery,* 33(3), 115-128.

Wise, D., and Engstrom, J.L. (1985). The predictive validity of fundal height curves in the identification of small and large for gestational age infants. *JOGNN,* 14(2), 87-92.

Planning and implementation

Aaronson, L.S., and MacNee, C.L. (1989). Tobacco, alcohol and caffeine use during pregnancy. *JOGNN,* 18(4), 279-87.

Abrams, B.F., and Laros, R.K. (1986). Prepregnancy weight, weight gain and birth weight. *American Journal of Obstetrics and Gynecology,* 154(3), 503-509.

Brooten, D., Peters, M.A., Glatts, M., Gaffney, S.E., Knapp, M., Cohen, S., and Jordan, C. (1987). A survey of nutrition, caffeine, cigarette and alcohol intake in early pregnancy in an urban clinic population. *Journal of Nurse-Midwifery,* 32(2), 85-90.

Brown, J.E. (1988). Weight gain during pregnancy: What is optimal. *Clinical Nutrition,* 7, 181-90.

Brucker, M.C. (1988). Management of common minor discomforts in pregnancy. Part II: Managing minor pain in pregnancy. *Journal of Nurse-Midwifery,* 33(1), 25-30.

Brucker, M.C. (1988). Management of common minor discomforts in pregnancy. Part III: Managing gastrointestinal problems in pregnancy. *Journal of Nurse-Midwifery,* 33(2), 67-73.

Chenger, P., and Kovacik, A. (1987). Dental hygiene during pregnancy: A review. *MCN,* 12(5), 344-343.

Davis, L. (1987). Daily fetal movement counting: A valuable assessment tool. *Journal of Nurse-Midwifery,* 32(1), 11-19.

De Grez, S.A. (1988). Bend and stretch. *MCN,* 13(5), 357-359.

Dohrmann, K.R., and Lederman, S.A. (1986). Weight gain in pregnancy. *JOGNN,* 15(6), 446-453.

Gantes, M., Schy, D.S., Bartasius, V.M., and Roberts, J. (1986). The use of daily fetal movement records in a clinical setting. *JOGNN,* 15(5), 390-393.

Humenick, S.S., and Bugen, L.A. (1987). Parenting roles: Expectation versus reality. *MCN,* 12(1), 36-39.

Poole, C.J. (1986). Fatigue during the first trimester of pregnancy. *JOGNN,* 15(5), 375-379.

Slager-Earnest, S.E., Hoffman, S.J., and Beckmann, C.J. (1987). Effects of a specialized prenatal adolescent program on maternal and infant outcomes. *JOGNN,* 16(6), 422-429.

South-Paul, J., Rajagopal, K., and Tenholder, M. (1988). The effect of participation in a regular exercise program upon aerobic capacity during pregnancy. *Obstetrics and Gynecology,* 71(2), 175-179.

Taubenheim, A.M., and Silbernagel, T. (1988). Meeting the needs of expectant fathers. *MCN,* 13(2), 110-113.

Wallace, A.M., and Engstrom, J.L. (1987). The effects of aerobic exercise on the pregnant woman, fetus and pregnancy outcome. *Journal of Nurse-Midwifery,* 32(5), 277-290.

CHAPTER 8

NUTRITION AND DIET COUNSELING

OBJECTIVES

After reading and studying this chapter, the student should be able to:

1. Explain how physiologic changes during pregnancy affect nutrient needs.

2. List nutritional risk factors affecting antepartal nutrition.

3. Discuss the necessary information to be collected during assessment of the pregnant client's nutritional status.

4. Identify appropriate nutritional goals for the pregnant client.

5. Describe the nursing interventions to maintain adequate nutrition for the pregnant client.

INTRODUCTION

The fetus, like every living organism, needs adequate nutrition to thrive. Encouraging the pregnant client to maintain proper nutrition during pregnancy helps ensure that the nutritional needs of the fetus are met.

Many factors influence the outcome of pregnancy, but few can be controlled as easily by the pregnant client as nutrition. Many pregnant clients want to know how to ensure the health of their fetus through proper nutrition. As a result, antepartal diet and nutrition information has increased dramatically during recent years, providing guidance for the pregnant client.

This chapter investigates how the physiologic changes of pregnancy affect the nutritional needs of the client and her fetus. It discusses the role of specific nutrients in pregnancy as well as factors that may influence nutritional status. It then discusses how the nurse can recognize nutritional risk factors during pregnancy and provide appropriate nursing care using the nursing process. The chapter focuses on assessment, goal-setting for the pregnant client and interventions that help the client meet those goals through healthful food choices.

NUTRITION AND PREGNANCY

Nutrition before conception and during pregnancy is an important factor in the course and outcome of pregnancy.

Before conception, such factors as degree of body fat, body weight, contraceptive method, and alcohol use can influence nutrition and pregnancy outcome.

Antepartal nutrition

Nutritional deprivation during pregnancy, which adversely affects pregnancy outcome and the fetus, can be avoided through nutritional supplementation. Inadequate weight gain, which frequently is used as a measure of nutrition during pregnancy, also may have adverse effects, although a recent study indicates that weight gain and nutritional adequacy are not as strongly related as previously believed (Aaronson and Macnee, 1989).

Nutritional deprivation. Low birth weight is undesirable because it commonly is linked to congenital defects or neonatal mortality. In fact, birth weight may indicate a neonate's overall condition. The lowest rate of neonatal mortality occurs for birth weights between 4,000 and

4,499 g; mortality rates rise for those born under 2,500 g (Brown, 1989).

Prenatal nutritional deprivation may have lasting effects, depending on the stage of development at which it occurs. If malnutrition occurs during the embryonic stage (2 to 8 weeks' gestation) when differentiation of major organs and tissues takes place, irreversible damage may occur. Because organ systems develop at different times during the embryonic stage, malnutrition may cause permanent damage in one organ and not another. If malnutrition occurs when cells primarily are increasing in size (after 8 weeks' gestation), the effects may be reversible (Worthington-Roberts, Vermeersch, and Williams, 1989).

Nutritional supplementation. Improving the pregnant woman's diet by increasing food intake or by adding missing nutritional elements can improve pregnancy outcome. The effects of supplementation depend on the severity of malnutrition. The more undernourished a woman, the greater benefit increased food or added elements will have on her pregnancy outcome.

In the United States, various food programs are available to low-income families who are at high risk for malnutrition. For example, the Special Supplemental Food Program for Women, Infants, and Children (WIC) provides nutrition education as well as coupons for purchasing highly nutritious foods (such as milk, cheese, eggs, iron-fortified cereals, and fruit juices). This national program provides assistance through pregnancy, lactation, and the first 5 years of childhood. Other food programs for eligible families include food stamps obtained from public assistance programs and local food banks when food needs are immediate.

Weight gain during pregnancy. Experts disagree on the amount of weight a woman should gain during pregnancy. However, general recommendations exist for the amount and pattern of weight gain.

Amount of weight gain. Recommendations for weight gain should take the woman's prepregnancy weight into consideration. For a woman entering pregnancy in her ideal weight range, a gain of 24 to 32 lb (11 to 15 kg) is adequate to meet the needs of the mother and fetus. The weight gain is caused by the weight of the fetus and placenta as well as increased adipose tissue, amniotic fluid, blood volume in the uterus, and fat and duct proliferation in the breasts.

Underweight women (less than 90% of ideal body weight) who gain the same amount of weight as ideal-weight women bear neonates at a younger gestational age and of lower birth weight and length. Ideally, an underweight woman should gain the recommended 24 to 32 lb plus the amount that she is underweight, or at least 15 kg (Seidman, Ever-Hadani, and Gale, 1989).

Controversy exists over the amount of gain appropriate for an overweight woman. Although weight gain exceeding the recommended amount is unlikely to harm the fetus, it does place more stress on the woman during delivery. Also, excessive gains may make the previously ideal-weight woman more prone to obesity after delivery.

Recommendations for an overweight woman may range from no gain to a 30-lb gain. However, the most common recommendations for an overweight woman are 16 to 24 lb (7 to 11 kg). Neonatal birth weight increases with maternal weight gain even in overweight women, but the percentage of neonatal gain is not proportional (Seidman, Ever-Hadaini, and Gale, 1989).

Weight gains no greater than 16% to 25% of prepregnant weight are associated with fewer complications during pregnancy, labor, and delivery (Shephard, Hellenbrand, and Bracken, 1986). If weight gain is calculated as a percentage of prepregnancy weight, more individual recommendations can be made. The usual recommended gain is 20% of prepregnant weight.

An adolescent may need additional weight gain, depending on her stage of growth and development. Nonpregnant growth gains must be added to the expected weight gain of pregnancy. Adjustments also are necessary if an adolescent is underweight or obese (American Dietetic Association, 1989).

A woman carrying more than one fetus has higher nutrient needs and therefore should gain more weight. The optimal weight gain for a twin pregnancy is about 44 lb (20 kg) for a woman with an ideal prepregnant weight (Pederson, Worthington-Roberts, and Hickok, 1989).

Pattern of weight gain. During the first trimester of pregnancy, a woman normally should gain 3 to 5 lb (1 to 2 kg). Because of nausea and vomiting, however, she may gain no weight during this time. This does not harm the fetus; the weight gain during the first trimester goes largely to maternal changes, such as the growing uterus and breasts and increased blood volume.

During the second and third trimesters, weight gain is essentially linear, averaging 1 lb (0.5 kg) per week. For a woman with more than one fetus, the pattern of weight gain should parallel that for a single fetus until approximately 20 weeks. During the second half of the pregnancy, weight gain should average 1½ lb (0.7 kg) per week (Pederson, Worthington-Roberts, and Hickok, 1989).

NUTRIENT NEEDS

During pregnancy, a woman's need for many nutrients increases the recommended dietary allowance (RDA)—the daily amount of a nutrient considered adequate for the needs of most healthy people, depending on sex, age, and reproductive status (for example, pregnant or lactating). These nutrients include carbohydrates, fats, and proteins (all energy sources) as well as water, vitamins, and minerals.

RDA STANDARDS

More than 50 nutrients are essential to human life. RDAs have been set by the Food and Nutrition Board of the National Academy of Sciences for 28 nutrients to inform the average, healthy person how much of each to consume daily. RDAs vary for different population groups and are revised periodically to reflect new nutritional knowledge.

Energy. Energy needs increase during pregnancy, and the caloric supply must increase to meet these needs while sparing protein for tissue building. (If calories from sources other than protein are insufficient, the body will burn proteins for energy.) A pregnant woman's energy needs increase 10% to 15%, or about 200 to 300 extra calories/day. (Additional calories may be needed for a woman who is underweight, large-framed, or unusually active). This number is derived by calculating the energy (number of calories) needed for the growth of the fetus and other tissues as well as the energy needed by the mother. The total additional energy needed during a 40-week pregnancy is 60,000 to 75,000 calories (Durnin, 1987).

Although the Food and Nutrition Board states an average increase of 300 calories/day is needed by a pregnant woman, caloric needs are not evenly distributed. During the first trimester, a woman's needs are only slightly higher than for a nonpregnant adult woman. An increase of 150 calories/day for the first trimester and 350 calories/day for the remaining trimesters is recommended (National Research Council [NRC], 1989).

Carbohydrates. The human body primarily uses blood glucose for fuel; because little transformation is required to turn carbohydrates into glucose, carbohydrates are the preferred energy source. Carbohydrates are found in the diet as starches, sugars, and fiber. All carbohydrates, except fiber, provide 4 calories/g.

Despite the general public's impression that starches and sugars are fattening and unhealthy, both are necessary for a balanced diet. Nutrition experts recommend that 55% to 60% of dietary calories come from carbohydrates. This recommendation holds true during pregnancy.

Fats. Fats are a more concentrated source of calories than carbohydrates, providing 9 calories/g. They are provided mostly through the meat and dairy food groups, although grain products also contain a small amount of fat. Fats often are found as a major ingredient in baked foods, such as cakes and cookies, and in candy. They also provide most of the calories in snack chips, salad dressings, butter, margarine, and oils. Although a small amount of fat (providing 30% or less of total daily calories) is needed, this amount usually can be obtained in normal portions of meat, dairy, and grain products. Therefore, no extra fat is necessary during pregnancy.

Protein. This third source of energy supplies 4 calories/g. Protein is the only energy source for which an RDA exists. It is essential for tissue growth and maintenance, formation of essential body compounds (such as hormones and digestive enzymes), water balance regulation, nitrogen balance, antibody formation, and nutrient transport.

The RDA for protein increases from 50 g for a nonpregnant woman to 60 g for a pregnant woman. Although this increase is significant, the average American woman consumes more than 60 g of protein even when not pregnant. Therefore, many women will not need to increase protein intake further during pregnancy.

Although estimates vary, a pregnant woman should consume 30 to 35 calories/kg of body weight (24 calories/kg if overweight) daily for optimal protein use.

Water. Another component essential for human life, water is an important part of the pregnant woman's diet. It is the major component of the fetus, placenta, breasts, and blood.

The human body typically contains 50% to 75% water. Water needs vary according to age, body weight, climate, and activity, but necessary intake is roughly 1 liter of water for each 1,000 calories consumed (NRC, 1989). Beverages provide about two-thirds of water intake; the remaining third comes from solid foods.

Vitamins and minerals. Vitamins are compounds that are needed in small amounts by the body for normal functioning; many serve as coenzymes in cellular reactions.

They can be divided into two groups, fat-soluble and water-soluble.

The fat-soluble vitamins—A, D, E, and K—are stored in body fat and usually are found in fat-containing products. However, water-soluble forms of these vitamins have been developed; therefore, they may be added to low-fat or nonfat foods, such as skim milk. Because fat-soluble vitamins can be stored in the body, toxicity is a greater risk with them than with water-soluble vitamins.

Water-soluble vitamins cannot be stored by the body and must be provided daily by the diet. They include the B vitamins and vitamin C. Folic acid (folacin) intake particularly is critical during pregnancy; the RDA for this B vitamin more than doubles, whereas the RDA for other B vitamins and vitamin C increases only slightly. The RDA for folic acid during pregnancy is 400 mcg, compared with 180 mcg for nonpregnant needs. Because folic acid deficiency during early pregnancy may be associated with birth defects, recommend a supplement containing 400 mcg of folic acid to the client attempting to conceive and advise her to continue this supplementation throughout her pregnancy (NRC, 1989).

Minerals are necessary for normal body functioning; they help maintain acid-base and water balance, act as catalysts in cellular reactions, transmit nerve impulses, and contribute to body structures. Minerals are divided into two categories: Those needed in high amounts (such as calcium, phosphorus, sodium, and magnesium) are called macrominerals; those needed in smaller amounts (such as iron, iodine, zinc, and fluoride) are called microminerals, trace minerals, or trace elements. Calcium needs increase greatly during pregnancy; mineralization of the fetal skeleton requires a large amount of calcium. Although the need for extra calcium is most acute during the last trimester (when the fetal skeleton calcifies), the RDA for calcium throughout pregnancy increases 50%, to a total of 1,200 mg/day, because calcium deposited in maternal bones early in pregnancy is transferred later to the fetus.

The RDA for iron during pregnancy is 30 mg/day, twice that for nonpregnant needs. This increase is caused by several factors. Blood volume increases about 50% during pregnancy, and iron is essential to red blood cells. The placenta also stores a significant amount of iron. The fetus stores a 6-month supply of iron. Between 1,000 and 1,400 extra mg of iron are required over the course of pregnancy—60% going to the maternal plasma, 40% to the placenta and fetus (Winick, 1989).

The need for iron during pregnancy increases gradually; it is sharpest during the last trimester, when the fetus is storing iron.

The body typically absorbs only 5% to 10% of dietary iron. Although this absorption rate doubles during the last half of pregnancy (McGanity, 1987) through unknown mechanisms, dietary intake of iron commonly is insufficient, leading to iron deficiency. Because the fetus draws upon maternal iron reserves, the full-term neonate rarely is iron-deficient.

Because of the high dietary intake of iron needed to maintain iron stores during pregnancy (18 to 21 mg/day), and because most clients do not consume iron-rich foods regularly, the NRC (1989) recommends routine supplementation of iron.

Increasing evidence suggests that multivitamin supplementation before and during the early weeks of pregnancy can reduce the risk of neural tube defect in neonates (Sheppard, et al., 1989). Women who have borne a neonate with neural tube defect should begin supplementation as prescribed by their physician before attempting to conceive again.

With the exception of iron and folic acid, a well-balanced diet, with foods from all four groups, needs no supplementation for a healthy pregnant woman; however, the woman may take vitamins and mineral supplements to ensure adequate intake. Whenever possible, nutrient deficiencies should be corrected by dietary changes. Health care professionals who routinely prescribe vitamin and mineral preparations should caution pregnant clients that the supplement is not a substitute for a balanced diet and that oversupplementation can cause problems. Such preparations contain only some of the approximately 50 recognized essential nutrients, and the nutrients in the supplement may not be well absorbed. Also, vitamin and mineral supplements do not contain the proteins, carbohydrates, fats, or water essential to life.

FACTORS INFLUENCING ANTEPARTAL NUTRITION

A task force from the American College of Obstetricians and Gynecologists and the American Dietetic Association (1978) has identified factors that place a pregnant woman at risk for inadequate nutrition. Some precede conception; others come into play during pregnancy.

Risk factors before conception. These factors can place a woman at nutritional risk if she becomes pregnant: frequent pregnancies, abnormal reproductive history, socioeconomic factors, bizarre food patterns, substance addiction, chronic systemic disorders, prepregnant weight outside the ideal range, and age. Other risk factors identified since the task force include vegetarian diets and breast-feeding.

Risk factors during pregnancy. Various factors can affect nutrition, including anemia, pregnancy-induced hypertension (PIH), multiple gestation (more than one fetus), inadequate or excessive weight gain, pica, gestational diabetes, and lactose intolerance.

NURSING CARE

The nurse can identify a pregnant client's nutritional needs and help her meet them by using the nursing process.

ASSESSMENT

Because nutrition is important throughout pregnancy, the nurse should assess it as early as possible—even before conception, if possible—and reevaluate it frequently. The initial assessment provides baseline information for the nursing care plan.

The initial and subsequent assessments include a health history, physical assessment, and review of laboratory tests.

Health history

To obtain information about nutritional status, gather health history data about the client's age, medical history, contraceptive history, obstetric history, personal habits, socioeconomic status, cultural and religious influences, and nutritional intake.

Age. When collecting biographical data, note the client's age. An adolescent is more likely to be nutritionally at risk than an older client.

Medical history. Assess the client's history for chronic diseases (such as diabetes, cardiac disease, renal disease, and hypertension), and note their dietary implications. Also inquire about any other illnesses or conditions that may affect nutritional status by altering food intake or increasing nutritional needs, such as recent surgery that may increase the body's need for protein.

Ask the client if she has any food allergies or intolerances, such as lactose intolerance. These can affect her food choices and should be addressed during diet counseling.

Contraceptive history. Find out if the client was using contraception recently, and if so, determine which kind. An oral contraceptive or intrauterine device can deplete the body's stores of several nutrients, including vitamin C and pyridoxine. If the client had been using contraception within 3 months of conception, her body may have insufficient stores of some nutrients.

Obstetric history. Record the number of children and their ages. Closely spaced pregnancies can deplete such nutrients as iron and folic acid. If this is the client's first pregnancy, she may require more detailed instructions on nutrition than a multigravid client.

Ask a multigravid client how close to the due dates her children were born and how much they weighed. A history of premature births or low-birth-weight neonates indicates the client may be at risk for poor nutrition; a history of neonates large for their arrival dates indicates she may be at risk for gestational diabetes.

Determine the client's weight gain during each previous pregnancy. Gains of less than 20 pounds or more than 35 pounds in a client in her ideal weight range suggest she needs encouragement to raise her nutrient intake or to control her caloric intake.

Ask the client if she had anemia, gestational diabetes, or other nutritional problems during previous pregnancies. Such problems are likely to recur in subsequent pregnancies. Stress the importance of iron-rich foods in preventing anemia during the current pregnancy.

Find out if the client breast-fed, and if so, her children's ages when she stopped. If she is still breast-feeding, emphasize the importance of increased caloric intake and adequate amounts of protein, calcium, and fluids.

Personal habits. Personal habits that could affect nutritional status include smoking, alcohol consumption, and over-the-counter, prescription, and illicit drug use. Ask about use of nonprescription vitamin and mineral supplements, which may be taken in excess of recommended doses.

Also assess the client's use of caffeine. Some evidence suggests that high caffeine intake is linked to low birth weight (Martin and Bracken, 1987).

Socioeconomic status. The client's occupation, income, educational level, and family may influence her exposure to educational materials, her awareness of community resources, or her knowledge of food and diets. Question the client about her intake of nutritious foods.

Cultural and religious influences. Find out if the client's culture or religion affects her through food restrictions, commonly chosen foods, and cooking methods. Cultural and religious factors may determine which foods the client is likely to include in her diet. Assess whether such factors interfere with proper nutrition.

Nutritional intake. To assess nutritional intake, obtain a diet history from the client using the dietary recall or dietary record methods. Both can be effective; therefore, use the method best suited to the situation and client. Perform a diet analysis after obtaining the information.

Physical assessment

Besides measuring the client's vital signs, record her weight and height and determine the appropriateness of her weight for her height. Remember that height-weight tables apply to nonpregnant clients. However, they may be used as a baseline for evaluating the client's preconception weight and weight gain during pregnancy. If a client is obviously underweight or overweight, her eating patterns may not be optimal for health.

Although the condition of certain tissues, such as the eyes, skin, hair, and teeth, can give information on nutritional status, physical examination is of limited value. Changes in physical state typically do not occur until a particular deficiency is advanced. Dietary assessment and laboratory tests provide a more accurate view of nutritional status.

Laboratory tests

Blood tests exist for almost every nutrient, but the normal levels for many nutrients during pregnancy are unknown. A few nutritionally related blood tests typically are performed during pregnancy, including hemoglobin levels and hematocrit to identify anemia, mean corpuscular volume (MCV) and mean corpuscular hemoglobin concentration (MCHC) to differentiate folic acid and cobalamin (vitamin B_{12}) deficiencies from iron deficiency anemia, a fasting 1-hour glucose tolerance test (GTT) at 24 to 28 weeks' gestation to screen for gestational diabetes, a 3-hour GTT if the 1-hour GTT is elevated, and serum albumin level to detect possible protein deficiency or PIH (Winick, 1989).

NURSING DIAGNOSIS

After reviewing the client's health history data, diet analysis, physical assessment findings, and laboratory test results, the nurse formulates nursing diagnoses for the client. (See Nursing Diagnoses: *Nutrition and diet counseling.*)

NUTRITION AND DIET COUNSELING

The following nursing diagnoses address representative problems and etiologies that a nurse may encounter when caring for a pregnant client. Specific nursing interventions for many of these diagnoses are provided in the "Planning and implementation" section of this chapter.

- Altered nutrition: less than body requirements, related to food aversions
- Altered nutrition: less than body requirements, related to inadequate calcium intake
- Altered nutrition: less than body requirements, related to inadequate finances for food purchases
- Altered nutrition: less than body requirements, related to inadequate nutrient intake
- Altered nutrition: less than body requirements, related to nausea and vomiting
- Altered nutrition: less than body requirements, related to pica
- Altered nutrition: less than body requirements, related to strict vegetarianism
- Altered nutrition: more than body requirements, related to excessive caloric intake
- Anxiety related to effects of food additives on pregnancy
- Anxiety related to weight gain
- Constipation related to insufficient fiber intake
- Knowledge deficit related to antepartal nutrition
- Knowledge deficit related to belief in food myths
- Knowledge deficit related to methods of increasing iron intake and absorption during pregnancy
- Knowledge deficit related to nutritional supplements
- Noncompliance with dietary intake recommendations related to desire to remain thin
- Pain related to heartburn and nausea

PLANNING AND IMPLEMENTATION

Based on the client's assessment findings and nursing diagnoses, the nurse establishes goals and then plans and implements interventions to meet the client's needs.

Basic goals for nutrition throughout pregnancy include:

- adjusting dietary intake to promote appropriate weight gain
- increasing nutrient intake to meet the RDAs for pregnancy
- establishing appropriate food intake patterns for nutrition-related problems, such as anemia and nausea.

Monitor weight gain

Obtain the client's weight at every prenatal visit and compare it to her prepregnancy weight and her previous antepartal weight measurements.

If the client has inadequate weight gain and a nursing diagnosis of *altered nutrition: less than body requirements, related to nausea and vomiting,* suggest ways to reduce discomfort through food choices. (For more information, see Client Teaching: *Altering diet to relieve nausea and vomiting.*)

If a client in her ideal weight range carrying one fetus gains less than 2 pounds per month, encourage her to increase her caloric intake. Conversely, if her gain is more than 6 pounds per month, evaluate her dietary intake to see if she is consuming excessive calories. Follow the same guidelines up to the twentieth week of gestation for a client with twins; after the twentieth week, evaluate her dietary intake if she gains more than 8 pounds per month.

However, verify certain variables recommending increased or decreased caloric intake. Appointments before or after meals may cause a weight difference of 3 to 4 pounds. Seasonal clothing changes also can vary scale weights by several pounds. Clients should schedule visits at approximately the same time of day and wear similar clothing to determine weight gain as accurately as possible.

A sudden large increase in weight after 20 weeks' gestation may be caused by excess fluid retention. Although some fluid retention is normal, it should occur gradually. A sudden shift in fluid balance can be a symptom of PIH, especially if blood pressure elevation and proteinuria are present.

Teach about nutrition

For a client with a nursing diagnosis of *knowledge deficit related to antepartal nutrition,* teach her about basic nutrients and the foods that contain them.

When developing a meal plan with the client, emphasize that the purpose of her diet is to promote fetal health, not to lose weight. Because the term *diet* may be associated with weight loss, use the term *meal plan* instead.

Explain which foods will help the client improve her nutrient intake. Based on the diet analysis, recommend specific foods and portion sizes. For example, instead of saying, "Your diet is low in calcium," explain that her diet is low in the milk group and give examples of foods she could consume, such as low-fat cottage cheese or milk.

Clients who do not consume dairy products may need calcium supplements. However, encourage increased intake of calcium-rich foods, which provide other essential nutrients that calcium supplements lack. The amount pre-

---

CLIENT TEACHING

ALTERING DIET TO RELIEVE NAUSEA AND VOMITING

Two out of every three pregnant women experience some degree of nausea, yet relatively little is known about why nausea occurs or how to relieve it. Many researchers believe nausea is caused by rising estrogen levels early in pregnancy. Nausea typically resolves near the end of the first trimester and does not interfere with nutritional status. However, excessive vomiting can be dangerous, especially if it continues past the first trimester. If excessive vomiting occurs, review your food and fluid intake to ensure adequate nutrition and prevent dehydration.

Although no solution works for everyone, the following recommendations may make you more comfortable.

• Keep crackers or dry toast near you at all times. Eat these when you feel nauseated.
• Eat several small meals instead of three large ones. An overly full or empty stomach may induce nausea.
• Have meals without a beverage. Save liquids for 30 to 60 minutes after the meal to keep your stomach from becoming too full.
• Limit high-fat foods, including oil, margarine, butter, whole-milk dairy products, fatty meats (such as bacon and sausage), salad dressings, and rich desserts. Fat causes higher production of stomach acid, which increases nausea risk.
• Limit spicy foods, particularly pepper-containing foods common in Oriental and Mexican dishes. Such foods also cause your stomach to produce more acid.
• Avoid alcohol, caffeine-containing beverages, and smoking, all of which increase nausea risk.
• Avoid any food that causes stomach discomfort. You may not be able to tolerate certain foods that others can.
• Take time to sit down for meals and chew food well. Eating on the run can lead to stress, which increases nausea risk; chewing your food well decreases the work your stomach must do.

This teaching aid may be reproduced by office copier for distribution to clients. ©1993, Springhouse Corporation.

---

scribed varies according to the client's dairy product intake. If the client consumes no dairy products, the usual recommendation is 1,200 mg. For each cup of milk, yogurt, or equivalent amount of other dairy products that she consumes, subtract 300 mg from the 1,200 mg total.

Absorption of calcium from supplements may be poor. Encourage the client to consume a dairy product when she takes a calcium supplement; the lactose, lactic acid, and vitamin D in dairy products enhances calcium absorption. (Some supplements contain vitamin D.) The sup-

SELECTING FOOD TO INCREASE IRON INTAKE

Iron, an essential mineral, is needed in the blood to carry oxygen throughout the body. Without enough iron, you may look pale, feel tired, or easily become short of breath. However, you may have no obvious symptoms and will not know that you are anemic until after a blood test.

Only 5% to 10% of the iron in food is absorbed by the body. This rate increases to 10% to 20% when needs are high, such as during pregnancy. To cope with this problem, you must increase your intake of iron-rich foods and combine foods for maximum iron absorption.

Iron exists in food in two forms. Heme iron, which is absorbed most readily, is found in meat, fish, and poultry; non-heme iron is found in grains, dried fruits, and vegetables. The type of protein in meats can increase iron absorption from non-heme iron sources. Therefore, eating meat with spinach, an iron-rich vegetable, increases the amount of iron absorbed from the spinach.

Vitamin C has the same effect as meat: Having orange juice along with iron-fortified cereal increases the amount of iron you absorb from the cereal.

To get the maximum iron from your food, take the following steps:
- Eat poultry, fish, and meat often to provide easily absorbable iron and increase iron absorption from other foods.
- Have vitamin C–rich foods with meals. Good sources include oranges, grapefruits, tomatoes, peppers, broccoli, potatoes, watermelon, cantaloupe, and strawberries.
- Choose iron-fortified breads and cereals.
- Eat iron-rich vegetables, such as spinach, broccoli, asparagus, and other dark-green vegetables.
- Cook with iron pots and pans. Using iron cookware can dramatically increase the iron content of your meals. Acidic foods, such as tomato sauce, can leach valuable iron from iron cookware.
- Eat dried fruits or drink prune juice. Fruits usually do not contain iron, but they do pick up the mineral when dried on iron utensils.
- Avoid foods that decrease iron absorption, such as tea and coffee.
- If your doctor has prescribed an iron supplement, be sure to take it with meat or a source of vitamin C. Iron supplements can cause stomach discomfort. They also may darken your stools, which is not harmful. Taking your iron supplement with food should relieve some of the discomfort. Remember to take iron supplements regularly.

Note: Iron can be toxic if taken in large doses; remember to keep your iron supplements out of children's reach.

---

plement should be taken between meals to avoid interfering with calcium absorption.

When developing the client's meal plan, consider the forces that influence her food choices, including food allergies, food preferences, dietary restrictions related to disorders, and cultural, ethnic, and religious factors. Respect her preferences while helping her select appropriate foods to meet her nutritional needs.

Although foods can be chosen to meet nutritional needs for just about every culture or religion, specific nutrients or food groups still may need attention. Even within a given culture or religion, eating patterns vary greatly among individuals.

Discourage pica and encourage a balanced diet. Suggest foods that may offer similar textures or tastes as the nonfood items.

If the client is a vegan, use different food guides to develop the meal plan (Mutch, 1988). These guides may be particularly useful for a client with a nursing diagnosis of *altered nutrition: less than body requirements, related to strict vegetarianism.* One food guide that meets all of the RDAs for most nutrients without including meat is one by the Seventh Day Adventists Dietetic Association (Heath, 1983). This guide calls for:
- four servings of soy milk or soy meat substitutes
- four servings of protein-rich legumes
- six servings of grains
- eight servings of fruits and vegetables.

For an adolescent client, remember that various factors may place her at risk for inadequate nutrition. Whenever possible, include a member of the client's social support structure in the nutrition counseling to ensure outside reinforcement of good eating habits.

Prevent nutrition-related problems

If the client has a nursing diagnosis of *knowledge deficit related to methods of increasing iron intake and absorption during pregnancy,* teach her about iron-rich foods, foods that may increase or decrease iron absorption, cooking techniques to increase iron, and any prescribed iron supplements. Routine iron supplementation has several drawbacks. Iron causes nausea and constipation in one-fifth of women, which contributes to the noncompliance of about one-third of women. Also, iron can reduce the availability of zinc from the diet (Simmer, Iles, James, and Thompson, 1987). Despite these problems, iron-containing multivitamin supplements commonly are prescribed throughout pregnancy and 3 months postpartum. Give the client written instructions to follow at home. (For a sample, see Client Teaching: *Selecting food to increase iron intake.*)

ALTERING DIET TO RELIEVE CONSTIPATION

Constipation is a common complaint during the first and last trimesters of pregnancy. Intestinal movement slows down about 10% during these trimesters, and your growing baby increases pressure on your intestines during the third trimester.

To relieve constipation, make the following dietary changes:
- Increase fruit and vegetable intake to six servings a day. Choose fresh fruit over canned fruit and fruit juices, which contain less fiber. Whenever possible, eat the skins and seeds to increase fiber further.
- Increase grain intake to at least six servings a day. Whenever possible, choose unrefined grains (as in whole wheat bread, brown rice, and bran cereal), which contain more fiber.
- Include legumes (such as beans, peas, and lentils) as meat substitutes. Legumes are good sources of fiber, and they provide calcium and iron as well.
- Include prunes or prune juice, which have a natural laxative effect.
- Increase fluid intake (preferably water) to six to eight 8-oz glasses daily. More fluids help soften the stool.
- Increase exercise. Even a short walk after meals can stimulate intestinal movement.

This teaching aid may be reproduced by office copier for distribution to clients. ©1993, Springhouse Corporation.

If the client has a nursing diagnosis of *constipation related to insufficient-fiber intake,* encourage her to adjust her diet to help correct this problem. (For more information, see Client Teaching: *Altering diet to relieve constipation.*)

Address nutrition-related concerns

If the client has a specific nutritional concern, use active listening to understand her concern fully. She may have a nursing diagnosis of *anxiety related to effects of food additives on pregnancy.* If so, address her concerns. For example, teach her to read labels closely. Encourage her to consume organically grown fresh fruits and vegetables rather than processed foods. If organic produce is not available, encourage her to eat a wide variety of foods to limit the amount of chemicals from any one item.

If the client is concerned about caffeine intake, provide appropriate information. Some studies suggest that a high caffeine intake can cause a neonate to be smaller than average; however, an equal number of studies suggest that caffeine has no effect. To be safe, encourage her to limit caffeine intake to 200 mg/day and list the caffeine content of commonly consumed foods and beverages. For example, a 5-oz cup of automatic drip coffee has 137 mg caffeine, whereas a cola soft drink has 38 mg. If the client intends to breast-feed, recommend that she follow the same limit; caffeine readily crosses into breast milk and can keep her neonate awake.

Teach about weight control

For a client with excessive weight gain and a nursing diagnosis of *altered nutrition: more than body requirements, related to excessive caloric intake,* review her beliefs about antepartal nutrition. She may believe the myth that a pregnant woman must "eat for two." To dispel this myth, remind her that the second person for whom she is eating is very small and requires only 150 extra calories a day during the first trimester and 350 during the second and third trimesters. If the client eats more than that, she may gain more than she needs for her pregnancy and have extra fat to lose after childbirth.

A small amount of food will supply 300 calories, such as two slices of bread with 1 tablespoon of peanut butter and 1 tablespoon of jelly or six crackers and 2 ounces of cheese. Although increases in food intake should be small to limit increases in calories, many of the client's nutrient needs increase substantially during pregnancy. Therefore, she must get the most nutrient value for the calories she consumes. A client who begins her pregnancy at ideal weight should gain between ½ and 1 pound each week. Overweight clients should gain slightly less, underweight clients slightly more.

Remind the client to eat at least four servings of milk, three of meat, four of fruits and vegetables, and four of grains each day. Check portion sizes to ensure she is not over- or underestimating serving sizes. If she gains weight too quickly, review her intake of miscellaneous foods. Foods high in sugar or fats, such as soft drinks, cookies, and snack chips, are considered miscellaneous foods; their intake should be reduced first. The client should limit servings from this group.

The client may limit weight gain by decreasing her use of certain miscellaneous foods in food preparation. For example, an average baked potato has about 150 calories, but 2 tablespoons of margarine raise the total calories to 350. Raw vegetable salads are virtually calorie-free, but salad dressing may contain 50 to 75 calories per tablespoon. Other miscellaneous foods that can drastically increase calories without adding many nutrients include oil, sour cream, cream cheese, mayonnaise, sauces, gravies, and sugar.

Besides eating less of these foods, the client can eat reduced-calorie versions of foods, such as light mayonnaise and diet margarine. Using these items can cut caloric intake from such foods by half.

The client also can check the fat content of required foods, such as dairy products and meat, and choose lower-calorie versions. For example, skim milk has about 7 grams less fat per cup than whole milk, which results in a difference of about 60 calories per cup. The client needs 4 cups of milk per day; therefore, she could decrease her caloric intake by 240 each day or 67,000 calories for the full pregnancy by drinking skim milk. Because approximately 3,500 calories will produce 1 pound of fat, this simple change theoretically could prevent 19 pounds of unnecessary weight gain during pregnancy.

If the client feels hungry after making these dietary changes, tell her to eat more fresh fruits, vegetables, and whole grain products. These high-fiber foods are filling without adding substantial calories.

Warn the client not to reduce her food intake below the minimum recommended number of servings from the four food groups. Maintaining a high-quality diet is important.

Make referrals

Some clients will need more in-depth nutrition education than a nurse can provide. In these cases, refer the client to a registered dietitian. Recognized as the nutrition experts in the health-care field, registered dietitians are found in private practices and hospital settings. Suggest that the client locate one by calling the American Dietetic Association.

If the client has a nursing diagnosis of *altered nutrition: less than body requirements, related to inadequate finances for food purchases,* refer her to appropriate social agencies or programs, such as WIC.

EVALUATION

As with all nursing interventions, an evaluation is necessary to judge the effectiveness of nutritional guidance. State evaluation findings in terms of actions performed or outcomes achieved for each goal. The following examples illustrate some appropriate evaluation statements:
• The client accurately described her antepartal meal plan.
• The client agreed to seek financial assistance through WIC to obtain foods for a balanced diet.
• The client verbalized the basic principles of increasing iron intake and absorption to prevent iron-deficiency anemia.
• The client described ways in which she will decrease foods of low nutritional value to help prevent excessive weight gain.

DOCUMENTATION

When assisting a pregnant client with nutrition and diet planning, documentation should include:
• age
• vital signs
• height, estimated prepregnancy weight, frame
• appropriateness of prepregnancy weight for height and frame
• current weight
• number of weeks pregnant
• appropriateness of weight gain for number of weeks pregnant
• significant attitudes concerning diet and weight
• significant health history findings
• dietary history
• adequacy of diet
• effects of attitudes on nutritional status
• significant physical assessment and laboratory test data
• client teaching performed
• nutrition information given to the client
• assessment of client's comprehension during teaching
• expectations of compliance
• plan for future visits.

CHAPTER SUMMARY

Chapter 8 described how to assist a client with nutrition and diet planning during pregnancy. Here are the chapter highlights.

Nutrition education should begin before conception, if possible, or early in the pregnancy to ensure that the client understands the need for adequate nutrition.

Specific nutrient deficiencies can adversely affect pregnancy outcome; however, nutritional supplements can improve nutritional status.

Commonly used as an indication of nutritional status, optimal weight gain during pregnancy varies according to prepregnancy weight.

To meet nutritional requirements, the client's diet should include adequate amounts of carbohydrates, fats, proteins, water, vitamins, and minerals.

Many factors influence antepartal nutritional needs. Before conception, these factors include frequent pregnancies, abnormal reproductive history, socioeconomic status, bizarre food patterns, vegetarian diets, substance addiction, chronic systemic disorders, breast-feeding, prepregnant weight, and age. During pregnancy, risk factors include anemia, pregnancy-induced hypertension, more than one fetus, inadequate or excessive weight gain, pica, gestational diabetes, and lactose intolerance.

A balanced antepartal diet consists of foods from the four food groups with calories adequate to promote desired weight gain. The client may need vitamin and mineral supplements to meet pregnancy needs in addition to a nutritionally sound diet.

Nutritional assessment, which should be performed as early as possible, includes a health history (including a diet history), physical assessment, and review of laboratory tests.

After establishing nutritional goals for the client, the nurse plans and implements appropriate interventions, which may include teaching about weight control and nutrition, developing a meal plan to prevent nutrition-related problems, discussing client concerns, and making any necessary referrals (such as to a food supplementation program or a dietitian).

STUDY QUESTIONS

1. What is the appropriate amount of weight gain during pregnancy for a woman in her ideal weight range?
2. Which preconception factors place a woman at nutritional risk if she becomes pregnant?
3. How should the nurse intervene for a client with a nursing diagnosis of *knowledge deficit related to antepartal nutrition?*
4. Mrs. Cole, 10 weeks pregnant, complains of nausea and vomiting. What client information should the nurse provide?

BIBLIOGRAPHY

Bender, D. (1987). Estrogens and vitamin B$_6$: Actions and interactions. *World Review of Nutrition and Diet*, 51, 140-188.

Franz, M., Barr, P., Holler, H., Powers, M., Wheeler, M., and Wylie-Rosett, J. (1987). Exchange Lists: Revised 1986. *Journal of the American Dietetic Association*, 87(1), 28-34.

Frisch, R. (1987). Body fat, menarche, fitness, and fertility. *Human Reproduction*, 2(6), 521-533.

Guthrie, H. (1988). *Introductory nutrition* (7th ed.). St. Louis: Mosby.

Heath, P. (Ed.). (1983). *Diet manual including a vegetarian meal plan.* Loma Linda, CA: Seventh Day Adventist Dietetic Association.

Kaufman-Kurzrock, D. (1989). Cultural aspects of nutrition. *Topics in Clinical Nutrition*, 4(2), 1-6.

Mutch, P. (1988). Food guides for the vegetarian. *American Journal of Clinical Nutrition*, 48 (Suppl. 3), 913-919.

National Center for Health Statistics. (1989). Advance report of final natality statistics, 1987. *Monthly Vital Statistics Report*, 38(3).

National Dairy Council. (1989). *Calcium: A summary of current research.* Rosemont, IL: Author.

National Research Council. (1989). *Recommended dietary allowances.* Food and Nutrition Board, Committee on Dietary Allowances. Washington, DC: National Academy Press.

Pennington, J., and Church, H. (1989). *Bowes and Church's food values of portions commonly used* (15th ed.). Philadelphia: Lippincott.

Perri, K., and Franz, K. (1987). Hypocalciuria in preeclampsia. *New England Journal of Medicine*, 317(14), 897-899.

Shephard, M., Hellenbrand, K., and Bracken, M. (1986). Proportional weight gain and complications of pregnancy, labor, and delivery in healthy women of normal prepregnant stature. *American Journal of Obstetrics and Gynecology*, 155(5), 947-954.

Simmer, K., Iles, C., James, C., and Thompson, R. (1987). Are iron-folate supplements harmful? *American Journal of Clinical Nutrition*, 45(1), 122-125.

Winick, M. (1969). Malnutrition and brain development. *Journal of Pediatrics*, 74(5), 667-669.

Worthington-Roberts, B. (1984). Nutrition and maternal health. *Nutrition Today*, November/December, pp. 6-19.

Nutrition and pregnancy

Aaronson, L., and Macnee, C. (1989). The relationship between weight gain and nutrition in pregnancy. *Nursing Research*, 38(4), 223-227.

American College of Obstetricians and Gynecologists. (1987). *Vitamin A supplementation during pregnancy.* American College of Obstetricians and Gynecologists Committee Opinion A, Number 52.

American Dietetic Association. (1989). Nutrition management of adolescent pregnancy: Technical support paper. *Journal of the American Dietetic Association*, 89(1), 105-109.

Brown, J. (1989). Improving pregnancy outcomes in the United States: The importance of preventive nutrition services. *Journal of the American Dietetic Association*, 89(5), 631-633.

Dawson, E., and McGanity, W. (1987). Protection of maternal iron stores in pregnancy. *Journal of Reproductive Medicine*, 32(Suppl. 6), 478-487.

Durnin, J. (1987). Energy requirements of pregnancy: An integration of the longitudinal data from the five-country study. *Lancet*, 2(8568), 1131-1133.

McGanity, W. (1987). Protection of maternal iron stores in pregnancy. *Journal of Reproductive Medicine*, 32(6 suppl.), 475-477.

Mitchell, M., and Lerner, E. (1987). Factors that influence the outcome of pregnancy in middle-class women. *Journal of the American Dietetic Association*, 87(6), 731-735.

Winick, M. (1989). *Nutrition in pregnancy.* Baltimore: Williams & Wilkins.

Worthington-Roberts, B., Vermeersch, J., and Williams, S. (1989). *Nutrition in pregnancy and lactation* (4th ed.). St. Louis, MO: Mosby.

Risk factors and antepartal nutrition

American College of Obstetricians and Gynecologists and American Dietetic Association (1978). *Assessment of maternal nutrition.* Washington, DC: Authors.

Cooper, N. (1988). Nutrition and diabetes: A review of current recommendations. *Diabetes Educator,* 14(5), 428-433.

Gabe, S. (1986). Definition, detection, and management of gestational diabetes. *Obstetrics and Gynecology,* 67(1), 121-125.

Martin, T., and Bracken, M. (1987). The association between low birthweight and caffeine consumption during pregnancy. *American Journal of Epidemiology,* 126(5), 813-821.

Mills, J., and Graubard, B.I. (1987). Is moderate drinking during pregnancy associated with an increased risk for malformation? *Pediatrics,* 80(3), 309-314.

Philpson, E., and Super, D. (1989). Gestational diabetes mellitus: Does it recur in subsequent pregnancy? *American Journal of Obstetrics and Gynecology,* 160(6), 1324-1329.

Raymond, C. (1987). Birth defects linked with specific level of maternal alcohol use, but abstinence still is the best policy. *JAMA,* 258(2), 177-178.

Tallarigo, L., Giampietro, O., Penno, G., Miccoli, R., Gregori, G., and Navalesi, R. (1986). Relation of glucose tolerance to complications of pregnancy in nondiabetic women. *New England Journal of Medicine,* 315(16), 989-992.

Williams, E. (1986). Gestational diabetes mellites and diet control. *Diabetes Educator,* 12(1), 16-17.

Nutrition and fetal development

Overpeck, M., Moss, A., Hoffman, H., and Hendershot, G. (1989). A comparison of the childhood health status of normal birthweight and low birthweight infants. *Public Health Reports,* 104(1), 58-70.

Pederson, A., Worthington-Roberts, B., and Hickok, D. (1989). Weight gain patterns during twin gestation. *Journal of the American Dietetic Association,* 89(5), 642-646.

Seidman, D., Ever-Hadani, P., and Gale, R. (1989). The effect of maternal weight gain in pregnancy on birth weight. *Obstetrics and Gynecology,* 74(2), 240-246.

Sheppard, S., Nevin, N., Seller, M., Wild, J., Smithells, R., Read, A., Harris, R., Fielding, D., and Schorah, C. (1989). Neural tube defect recurrence after "partial" vitamin supplementation. *Journal of Medical Genetics,* 26(5), 326-329.

CHAPTER 9

ANTEPARTAL COMPLICATIONS

OBJECTIVES

After reading and studying this chapter, the student should be able to:

1. Recognize the signs and symptoms of antepartal complications.

2. Discuss the assessment information to be collected for a client with an antepartal complication.

3. Interpret laboratory and diagnostic test data about the client with an antepartal complication and her fetus.

4. Describe the maternal, fetal and neonatal effects for each antepartal complication.

5. Discuss comfort and support measures for the client and her family.

6. Identify common needs of clients experiencing antepartal complications.

INTRODUCTION

A normal pregnancy under ordinary circumstances is accompanied by multiple physiologic and psychological changes. If complications develop, the client can be negatively affected, as can the entire family. Antepartal complications threaten maternal or fetal health and can interfere with normal fetal development, childbirth or transition to parenthood. The discovery of such a complication can change a natural, joyful experience into a time of stress and anxiety. The client and her family may no longer look forward to the birth of a child. Instead, fear may alter their expectations. In addition to worrying about the future, one or more family members, typically the client or her partner, may feel responsible for the problem.

Nursing care must meet physical, psychological, and sociocultural needs. During antepartal complications, the client and her family may need significant emotional support.

Antepartal complications can include medical problems, such as diabetes and anemia; socioeconomic factors, such as poverty and substance abuse; and age-related concerns, such as childbearing during adolescence or maturity. They may exist before conception, as in cardiac disease or infection, or may occur suddenly during pregnancy, as in trauma or an acute condition—like appendicitis—that requires immediate surgery. Other complications of pregnancy, which also can place the mother and fetus at risk, result from pregnancy. These include premature rupture of membranes, preterm labor and delivery, hypertensive disorders of pregnancy, Rh incompatibility, reproductive disorders such as spontaneous abortion, ectopic pregnancy, gestational trophoblastic disease, incompetent cervix and multisystem disorders, such as hyperemesis gravidarum.

This chapter discusses the nursing care for the client experiencing numerous antepartal complications. It begins by addressing the nursing responsibilities common to all clients experiencing antepartal complications. Next, it discusses various antepartal complications, presenting background information about underlying conditions, their causes, treatment, and maternal, fetal and neonatal effects. Each complication is then discussed using the nursing process approach.

NURSING RESPONSIBILITIES

Ideally, all clients should be evaluated for disease and abnormalities before they conceive. Then, nursing care could strive to correct deficiencies and avoid complications. Sometimes, however, the client is first seen after she is pregnant and has a disease that complicates her pregnancy or endangers her fetus. Whether the nurse first sees the client before she is pregnant or during her pregnancy, the nurse can use the nursing process to deliver high-quality care.

ASSESSMENT

To build a useful, current assessment data base, obtain a detailed health history, assist with a thorough physical examination, and collect appropriate diagnostic studies, as ordered. (For more information on fetal diagnostic studies, see *Fetal testing.*)

Health history

Begin by assessing the client's present health status and comparing it with her personal and family health history. This may uncover a previously undetected problem and suggest the need for specific tests. For example, the client with a history of recurring infections (mainly pneumonia and urinary tract infections), bleeding, increased fatigue, poor healing, and general poor health may have undiagnosed anemia. A primigravid client who reports the classic symptoms of diabetes (polyuria, polydipsia, polyphagia, and weight loss) and has a family history of diabetes should receive the 3-hour glucose tolerance test.

Next, ask the client to identify any problems for which she is receiving care, such as a cardiac disease or diabetes. Then investigate signs and symptoms caused by this problem. Note any change in the degree of signs and symptoms, such as increased fatigue, decreased activity tolerance, increased dependent edema, and increased shortness of breath, which may occur during the second and third trimester in a client with cardiac disease. Also, determine if these signs and symptoms resolve with rest. The stress of pregnancy can exacerbate the effects of some disorders, requiring treatment adjustments.

Evaluate the effectiveness of the client's current regimen in managing any previously diagnosed condition. For example, if the client has a congenital heart defect, determine if her treatment has corrected arrhythmias and signs of heart failure. This information may require treatment modifications.

Inquire into the client's past and present obstetric history. Particularly query any obstetric problems, such as spontaneous abortion or stillbirth, that may have been related to an undiagnosed or uncorrected condition. Obstetric problems may recur unless the client is properly tested and treated. For example, a client with a history of hydramnios, unexplained stillbirth, a large-for-gestational-age neonate, or a neonate born with congenital anomalies should receive the 3-hour glucose tolerance test and, if diabetes is confirmed, modify her diet and possibly receive insulin.

Because many infections recur, assess the client's history of infection. Inquire about past treatments and about her and her partner's overall health. Ask about contact with cats, which may expose her to toxoplasmosis. Inquire about childhood diseases and immunizations, which may now protect her from certain infections.

To identify the client's risk of contracting human immunodeficiency virus (HIV) infection and other diseases, question her about drug and substance use, sexual contacts, and blood or blood product transfusions.

If she abuses substances, such as drugs, alcohol, or cigarettes, obtain a complete drug history. If she hesitates to discuss details, assure her that her answers are confidential and are used only to help plan health care for her and her fetus. Combined with the obstetric history, the client's drug history helps determine which drugs the client has taken and if and how they have affected earlier pregnancies and may affect this one. Information about current drug use also guides the health care team toward a treatment plan.

Physical assessment

Obtain the client's vital signs and weight. Document these baseline data and compare them to preconception measurements to detect significant changes. Keep in mind that fever may be associated with anemia or TORCH, HIV, or genitourinary infections. Tachycardia also may be linked to anemia. Hypertension may be related to anemia or diabetes.

Then assist with a head-to-toe physical assessment, including a pelvic examination. Note any abnormalities, which can provide clues to the client's underlying disorder or its progress. For example, pallor, thinness, and poor skin integrity suggest anemia. Renal complications, and other signs of vascular impairment signal advanced diabetes with vascular complications. Skin rash or lesions, enlarged glands or lymph nodes, muscle aches, and joint pain may be associated with a TORCH infection. Urinary frequency or urgency, nausea or vomiting, and vaginal discharge or itching suggest a genitourinary infection. Malaise, weight loss, diarrhea, lymphadenopathy, or evidence of Kaposi's sarcoma (purple or blue lesions) point to HIV infection. Skin abscesses and infections may indicate substance abuse.

Diagnostic studies

Obtain additional assessment data from routine prenatal laboratory tests, including complete blood count (CBC),

(Text continues on page 124.)

FETAL TESTING

The client with an antepartal complication may benefit from antepartal testing, which may be noninvasive (occurring outside the body) or invasive (requiring entry into the body). The chart below describes various antepartal tests, including their purposes, timing, and nursing considerations.

NONINVASIVE TESTS

Ultrasonography

Purpose
- To determine position of the uterus and cervix, size and position of the developing fetus, area of placental formation, and cord insertion site
- To differentiate between a normal and abnormal fetus
- To determine number of fetuses, congenital abnormality, ectopic pregnancy, and amniotic fluid volume
- To diagnose fetal death through absence of fetal heart sounds and fetal movements or by identifying overlapping of fetal skull sutures
- To take fetal measurements (late in pregnancy), including the fetal skull biparietal diameters (BPD), femur length, and crown-rump length (CRL); to verify the presence of fetal organs; to verify cord insertion site and size of placenta; and to determine amniotic fluid volume, which identifies such abnormalities as intrauterine growth retardation and macrosomia

- To estimate gestational age by measuring CRL, BPD, and femur length, calculating the ratios between them, and comparing these measurements and ratios to those expected for various gestational ages
- To provide a baseline that allows meaningful interpretation of fetal growth during the pregnancy

Nursing considerations
- Encourage the client to drink four to six glasses of fluid — but not to void before testing — to increase bladder fullness. Ultrasound waves will not traverse air; the fluid-filled bladder displaces the small bowel and provides a medium that sound waves readily penetrate.
- Be aware that from 24 weeks' gestation to term, estimates of gestational age based on ultrasonography may vary from the actual gestational age. At term, this variation may be 2 to 4 weeks (Kurtz and Needleman, 1988).

Fetal movement count

Purpose
- To provide a rough index of fetal health

Nursing considerations
- Teach the client to record the number of fetal movements during 30 minutes, counted three times daily. Advise her to select times when she can relax and sit down to count these movements, and also when she knows the fetus is active. (Fetal movements normally decrease during fetal sleep periods, when maternal serum glucose levels are low, and during maternal use of tobacco or a central nervous system depressant.)
- Suggest that the client stimulate fetal movements by lying on her left side, eating a light snack, drinking orange juice, touching or moving her abdomen, or making a sudden noise, such as clapping her hands.
- Tell the client to stop counting if she notes five to six movements in each 30-minute period. Advise her to continue count-

ing for an hour or more if she fails to note three movements in 30 minutes (Chez and Sadovsky, 1984).
- Advise the client to contact her health care provider if she notes fewer than 10 movements in two 1-hour periods spaced 12 hours apart, no movements in the morning, fewer than three movements in 8 hours, or if she becomes concerned for any reason. Changes in fetal activity patterns may require additional evaluation.
- Remind the client that wide variations in normal fetal movement exist. However, the pattern of movement should not change greatly during her pregnancy.
- Tell the diabetic client to note fetal movements over 6 to 8 hours and emphasize the importance of becoming familiar with her fetus's activity pattern. Decreased movement occurs with decreased maternal serum glucose levels.

Biophysical profile (BPP)

Purpose
- To predict perinatal asphyxia
- To assess fetal risks
- To detect fetal anomalies

Nursing considerations
- Instruct the client undergoing BPP scoring about its purposes.
- Interpret BPP results for the client and reinforce instructions as the client's care alters.
- Provide psychological support, especially if testing will continue throughout the pregnancy.
- Advise the client that a low score, which may be evidence of fetal compromise, warrants detailed investigation.

(continued)

FETAL TESTING (continued)

Non-stress test (NST)

Purpose
- To assess fetal well-being

Nursing considerations
- Advise the client to eat a snack before the test to help ensure recordable fetal movements.
- Advise the client of the test results. Reactive (favorable) results show two to three fetal heart rate (FHR) increases of 15 or more beats per minute (bpm), lasting for 15 or more seconds over 20 to 30 minutes. These increases occur with fetal movement. Nonreactive (unfavorable) results occur when the FHR response does not rise by 15 or more bpm over the specified time; they may indicate fetal hypoxia. An uninterpretable NST may result from a poor tracing or insufficient fetal activity.
- Instruct the client to touch or rock her abdomen or to drink orange juice if minimal fetal movement occurs during the NST.
- Tell the client with persistent, uninterpretable test results that a nipple stimulation contraction stress test (NSCST) may be needed.

Nipple stimulation contraction stress test (NSCST)

Purpose
- To evaluate the FHR in response to uterine contractions

Nursing considerations
- Be aware that the NSCST is not recommended for clients with a history of premature labor, premature rupture of membranes, abruptio placentae, placenta previa, cesarean delivery with a classical uterine incision, or with current multiple fetuses.
- Advise the client of test results. With negative (favorable) results, late FHR decelerations do not occur with contractions; with positive (unfavorable) results, they do.
- Be aware that the absence of late FHR decelerations indicates proper blood flow, whereas their presence indicates potential impairment in blood flow and possible fetal intolerance of labor. However, a client with a positive NSCST can deliver a healthy neonate.
- Be aware that positive results usually correlate with BPP results.

Fetal acoustical stimulation (FAS)

Purpose
- Same as NST

Nursing considerations
- Describe the test results, which are the same as for the NST.
- Advise the client that the test may be repeated within 24 hours or within a week if no FHR acceleration is detected.

INVASIVE TESTS

Chorionic villus sampling (CVS)

Purpose
- To diagnose fetal karyotype, hemoglobinopathies, (sickle cell anemia, alpha and some beta thalassemias), alpha,-antitrypsin deficiency, phenylketonuria, Down's syndrome, and Duchenne muscular dystrophy (Hogge, Hogge, and Golbus, 1986)

Nursing considerations
- Advise the client that complications of CVS include bleeding, spontaneous abortion, intrauterine infection, membrane rupture, and Rh isoimmunization (Elias, et al., 1985).
- Tell the client that other problems with CVS include inability to obtain a sample, sampling of maternal cells instead of fetal cells, and inaccurate prediction of fetal health.
- Assess the client after the procedure for complications and stabilization. An Rh-negative client should receive Rh$_o$(D) immune globulin to prevent sensitization from CVS.
- Remind the client to return for follow-up studies for continued evaluation of fetal well-being, for laboratory tests for maternal infection, and for amniocentesis, as recommended.
- Assure the client that CVS does not cause neonatal malformations.

Alpha-fetoprotein (AFP) test

Purpose
- To predict open neural tube defects (NTDs), such as spina bifida and anencephaly

Nursing considerations
- Be aware that clients at risk for fetal NTDs are those with a history of having a child with an NTD or with a strong family history of NTDs, those living where NTDs are prevalent (such as England, Ireland, and Wales), and those who are pregnant diabetics (Lemize, 1989).
- Assess the client's understanding of testing procedures and the implications of test results.
- Discuss test results with the client. Elevated MSAFP and AFAFP levels are associated with NTDs; decreased levels, with trisomy 21 (Down's syndrome). However, Schwager and Weiss (1987) found that more than 40% of women studied had elevated AFP levels and delivered normal neonates.
- Provide psychological support throughout the pregnancy. If an abnormal neonate is born, recommend further client evaluation and counseling.

FETAL TESTING *(continued)*

Amniocentesis

Purpose
- To detect genetic disorders
- To diagnose various fetal defects, including chromosomal anomalies, skeletal disorders, infections, central nervous system disorders, blood disorders, inborn errors of metabolism, miscellaneous metabolic disorders, and porphyrias
- To assess fetal lung maturity during the third trimester by evaluating the lecithin/sphingomyelin (L/S) ratio in the amniotic fluid

Nursing considerations
- Be aware that prime candidates for genetic screening by amniocentesis are clients over age 35 and those with a chromosomal or metabolic abnormality in an older child, chromosomal abnormalities in either parent, history of a sex-linked genetic disorder, or a family history of chromosomal or enzymatic abnormality or of NTDs (Willson and Carrington, 1987).
- Advise the client that test results take 2 to 4 weeks because of the complexity of fetal chromosomal diagnosis.
- Advise the client that complications related to amniocentesis include trauma to the client, fetus, umbilical cord, and placenta; premature labor or spontaneous abortion; infection; and maternal isoimmunization with hemolytic disease of the neonate.
- Monitor the client electronically for uterine irritability and alteration in FHR patterns for a few hours after the procedure. Vital signs should remain unchanged.
- Caution the client to observe for decreased fetal movement, persistent uterine contractions, or any abdominal discomfort after the procedure. If these occur, tell her to return immediately for evaluation.

Percutaneous umbilical blood sampling (PUBS)

Purpose
- To diagnose fetal blood disorders, such as coagulopathies, hemoglobinopathies, and hemophilias; congenital infections, such as rubella and toxoplasmosis; and chromosomal abnormalities (Ludomirski and Weiner, 1988)
- To treat Rh isoimmunization through blood transfusions (Dunn, Weiner, and Ludomirski, 1988)

Nursing considerations
- Before the procedure, prepare the client's abdomen by applying a povidone-iodine solution and sterile drapes.
- When assisting with the procedure, maintain sterile technique.
- Teach the client that PUBS can be used to assess, diagnose, and treat fetal anemia. Blood transfusions may be given through direct vascular access. Prompt treatment of the fetus in utero can maintain pregnancy, decreasing prematurity and the risk of death.
- Advise the client that complications of PUBS include chorioamnionitis, premature labor and rupture of amniotic membranes, abruptio placentae, bleeding, laceration or thrombus of an umbilical vessel, and transient fetal arrhythmias (Dunn, Weiner, and Ludomirski, 1988).
- Monitor the fetus with an NST after PUBS. Notify the physician if uterine contractions or FHR decelerations occur. An emergency delivery may be necessary if fetal distress continues.
- Perform a biweekly NST and BPP for fetal assessment until delivery. Inform the client of the importance of these follow-up studies.

Oxytocin contraction test (OCT)

Purpose
- To evaluate the FHR in response to uterine contractions

Nursing considerations
- Be aware that the physician gives standing orders for the nurse to intervene if fetal or maternal problems develop.
- Be aware that the contraindications for this test are the same as those for the NSCST. After three uterine contractions occur, the oxytocin is turned off and the main I.V. line is continued until FHR activity has been evaluated in relation to the contractions.
- Discontinue the infusion if no late FHR decelerations occur.
- If late FHR decelerations occur and do not return to baseline, notify the physician. Turn off the oxytocin, increase the main I.V. line rate, position the client on her left side (to move the gravid uterus away from her inferior vena cava), and administer oxygen. If this positioning does not return the FHR to normal, help the client onto her right side or place her on her hands and knees with her head and chest resting on the bed.
- Be aware that if client repositioning does not return the FHR to baseline, emergency cesarean delivery may be indicated, although this is rare.
- If late FHR decelerations do not occur, or if the decelerations return to baseline immediately after emergency treatment, evaluate fetal well-being further via electronic FHR monitoring for several hours.

coagulation studies, blood glucose levels, electrolyte and cardiac enzyme levels, and urinalysis. Because some infections are asymptomatic, check culture specimen results obtained during the pelvic examination.

Also expect to evaluate the fetus and check the results of any fetal diagnostic studies that were performed.

If the fetus is monitored regularly, compare the results of each test to all others and to the baseline data to identify significant trends.

Perform or assist with other diagnostic studies, depending on the client's condition.

NURSING DIAGNOSIS

After considering all assessment findings, formulate appropriate nursing diagnoses for the client. (For a partial list of applicable diagnoses, see Nursing Diagnoses: *Antepartal complications,* pages 129 and 130.)

PLANNING AND IMPLEMENTATION

After assessing the client with antepartal complications and formulating nursing diagnoses, the nurse develops and implements a plan of care centering on the following common nursing goals:
• promoting the physical well-being of the client and her fetus
• preventing or controlling further complications
• preventing sequelae
• providing emotional support to the client and her family.

Nursing care is holistic and encompasses the client, her fetus, and her family. The nurse monitors client health; teaches about the condition, its management, and effects; promotes adequate rest, exercise, and nutrition; prevents infection; provides support; promotes family well-being; monitors fetal health; and promotes compliance.

EVALUATION

Care of the antepartal client requires a multidisciplinary approach throughout preconception, antepartal, intrapartal, and postpartal periods. The general goals are maintenance of client health and safe delivery of a healthy neonate.

DOCUMENTATION

All steps of the nursing process should be documented as thoroughly and objectively as possible. Thorough documentation allows the nurse to evaluate the effectiveness of the care plan; it also makes this information available to other members of the health care team to ensure consistency of care.

When caring for a client with an antepartal complication, documentation should include:
• baseline and current assessment data for the client, including vital signs, history and physical assessment findings, laboratory and diagnostic test results
• baseline and current assessment data for the fetus, including fetal heart rate – if fetal viability is present
• the client's physical and psychological response to treatment
• medications given and their effectiveness
• pre- and postprocedure care
• the client's physical and psychological response to the limitations caused by her condition
• the family's response to and support of the client.

AGE-RELATED CONCERNS

Most women give birth between ages 20 and 34. Various age-related factors can place an adolescent client (under age 19) or a mature client (over age 34) at risk during pregnancy. (See *Age-related risks during pregnancy.*)

Adolescent client
Pregnancy poses risks to adolescents because of their physical and psychological immaturity, potential for pregnancy complications, lack of prenatal care, and lack of social and economic support systems. The pregnant adolescent may not finish school, which eventually can affect her quality of life, job opportunities and advancements, and economic stability.

Mature client
An older woman who is healthy before pregnancy can reasonably expect a healthy pregnancy, as long as she receives appropriate antepartal care. She also may want genetic counseling and special antepartal testing, such as choronioc villi sampling and amniocentesis for certain physiologic and psychosocial risks.

CARDIAC DISEASE

Pre-existing cardiac disease places about 1% of pregnant women at risk (Gilstrap, 1989). (For more information, see *Functional classifications for cardiac clients,* page 126.)

Common cardiac diseases affecting pregnant clients include rheumatic heart disease, congenital heart defects,

AGE-RELATED RISKS DURING PREGNANCY

The following chart compares the physical and psychosocial risks of pregnancy and their nursing considerations for adolescent and mature clients.

PHYSICAL RISKS	PSYCHOSOCIAL RISKS	NURSING CONSIDERATIONS
Adolescent client		
• Inadequate intake of protein, calories, vitamins, and minerals (especially calcium and iron) for fetal development • Increased risk of maternal, fetal, and neonatal morbidity: pregnancy-induced hypertension (PIH), iron deficiency anemia, cephalopelvic disproportion, sexually transmitted diseases, premature birth, low-birth-weight neonate • Increased maternal, fetal, and neonatal mortality rate	• Arrested psychosocial development or identity confusion • Denial of pregnancy, leading to inability to cope • Avoidance of visits to health care professionals • Late or no prenatal care • Lack of adequate information about pregnancy • Increased desire to sever parent or family ties caused by mistaken beliefs about pregnancy; for example, that pregnancy will punish parents or worsen unstable family relationships or stressful living conditions • Difficulty assuming an adult identity • Failure to complete the tasks of adolescence, such as finishing school • Failure to establish a stable family • Failure to become self-supporting • Failure to bear a healthy neonate • Lack of social, physical, psychological, and financial assistance during and after pregnancy and birth • Lack of parental support • Usurpation of mother role by maternal grandmother, producing role confusion	• Provide prenatal education about pregnancy, fetal development, birth, and infant care, preferably in a setting that makes the client comfortable. (For example, some health centers schedule specific days for adolescent clients, which gives them the comfort of peer support.) • Emphasize the importance of early and continual prenatal care. • Discuss other options, such as adoption and abortion, as the client requests. • Encourage the client to continue formal schooling to help her mature and increase her career opportunities. • Help the client adjust to parenting through individual counseling sessions that identify and plan ways to meet her parenting needs. • Suggest that the client join in peer group discussions to seek help and suggestions from others in similar circumstances. • Help the client obtain financial aid from federal and state programs, such as the Special Supplemental Food Program for Women, Infants, and Children and Aid to Families with Dependent Children. • Promote the client's self-esteem and assist with decision making and problem solving. • Teach the client to recognize and report signs of pregnancy complications. • Teach about tests that should be performed during pregnancy. • Arrange for family counseling to discuss problems and maintain family unity.
Mature client		
• Increased risk of PIH • Increased risk of cesarean delivery • Increased risk of fetal and neonatal mortality • Increased risk of trisomies	• Increased stress level as the pregnancy advances • Difficulty adjusting to work restrictions for a career woman whose identity and self-worth are strongly tied to her work • Isolation from family, friends, and fellow professionals • Encountering ridicule, scorn, rejection, and sympathy instead of congratulations • Loss of support from peers, which may threaten self-esteem and satisfaction with personal and professional decisions	• Encourage the client to maintain her health before and during the pregnancy. • Inform the client and her partner about the availability, benefits, and risks of prenatal tests, such as amniocentesis, chorionic villus sampling, and alpha-fetoprotein testing, and about genetic counseling. • Identify the client's concerns about the antepartal, intrapartal, postpartal, and parenting periods. Reduce her anxiety about these periods by teaching about expected changes. • Counsel the client during pregnancy and prepare her for labor, birth, and parenting. • Teach the client to recognize and report signs of pregnancy complications, such as PIH.

FUNCTIONAL CLASSIFICATIONS FOR CARDIAC CLIENTS

This classification system from the New York Heart Association identifies the client's physical response to her cardiac disease. Before conception, the client's functional capacity should be assessed by a cardiologist to serve as a baseline. After conception, it should be reassessed and compared to the baseline to evaluate the effect of pregnancy on the client's heart.

CLASS	DESCRIPTION
Class I Uncompromised	No limitation of physical activity. A class-I client has no symptoms of cardiac insufficiency or anginal pain.
Class II Slightly compromised	Slight limitation of physical activity. A class-II client is comfortable at rest, but may experience excessive fatigue, palpitations, dyspnea, or anginal pain when engaging in ordinary physical activity.
Class III Markedly compromised	Marked limitation of physical activity. A class-III client is comfortable at rest, but experiences excessive fatigue, palpitations, dyspnea, or anginal pain with slight activity.
Class IV Severely compromised	Inability to perform any physical activity without discomfort. A class-IV client at rest may have symptoms of cardiac insufficiency or anginal syndrome, including choking, spasmodic pain, and shortness of breath. If she performs any physical activity, her discomfort increases.

mitral valve prolapse, and peripartum cardiomyopathy. (For more information, see *Common cardiac diseases*.)

With any cardiac disorder, cardiac decompensation may occur, challenging maternal and fetal health. Rarely, it may lead to maternal or fetal death. Careful medical, obstetric, and nursing care before and during pregnancy can minimize maternal and fetal risks.

ASSESSMENT

If the client's heart maintains adequate output through all the physiologic changes of pregnancy and through delivery, she should be free from cardiac complications. If she maintains her health and prevents complications, her functional classification should not change during pregnancy.

However, physiologic changes of pregnancy may cause cardiac stress, especially during the second trimester. These changes include increased plasma volume and expanded uterine vascular bed, which increase heart rate 10 to 15 beats per minute by the end of pregnancy and boost cardiac output by about 30% between 28 and 32 weeks' gestation. A client who experiences this cardiac stress needs weekly evaluation and may require bed rest, fluid restrictions, or such drugs as digitalis preparations, diuretics, antiarrhythmics, antibiotics, or anticoagulants (usually heparin).

Cardiac stress may intensify in the third trimester and may be severe enough to cause persistent pulmonary effects, such as crackles, tachycardia, tachypnea, dyspnea, or orthopnea. A client who experiences severe cardiac stress should adhere to prescribed treatments and should be monitored weekly for changes in pulmonary effects. To prevent complications, she may need to be placed on bed rest.

Different cardiac conditions affect pregnancy differently. For rheumatic heart disease, maternal mortality increases with active heart disease at the time of pregnancy (Brady and Duff, 1989) and with functional classification. The mortality rate is higher for functional classes IV (6%) and III (5.5%) and decreases significantly with each class, dropping to 0.1% for class I.

Congenital heart defects should pose no problems by themselves during pregnancy. However, pulmonary hypertension associated with a defect, such as Eisenmenger's syndrome (ventricular septal defect with pulmonary hypertension), carries a 30% to 70% maternal mortality rate during pregnancy and the postpartal period. Therefore, the nurse must take steps to prevent circulatory overload (Ramin, Mayberry, and Gilstrap, 1989).

The client with mitral valve prolapse should not have difficulty continuing her pregnancy. However, her obstetrician should monitor her for complications and consult a cardiologist if symptoms worsen.

In the United States, peripartum cardiomyopathy leads to death in 25% to 50% of affected women (Homans, 1985). In others, it may resolve spontaneously, leaving no effects. A client with this disorder should consider future pregnancies carefully because relapses may occur.

For a client with cardiac disease, expect to monitor the results of the CBC, electrolyte levels, and if complications arise, cardiac enzyme levels.

COMMON CARDIAC DISEASES

The chart below lists the clinical findings and treatments for common cardiac diseases that may affect a pregnant client.

DISEASE AND DESCRIPTION	CLINICAL FINDINGS	TREATMENT
Rheumatic heart disease		
Streptococcal infection leading to acute or chronic systemic rheumatic fever and, if untreated, to bacterial invasion of the mitral or tricuspid valve	• Inadequate cardiac functioning (classes I to IV) • Possible signs of right-sided heart failure, such as pitting dependent edema, weight gain, decreased urine output, and jugular vein distention • Possible signs of left-sided heart failure, such as crackles, dyspnea, coughing, tachycardia, tachypnea, and decreased urine output	• If damage is substantial, surgical correction before pregnancy through valvular repair or replacement (preferred) • After surgery, warfarin (Coumadin) or heparin (for the pregnant client) to prevent emboli • Close monitoring of the pregnant client if functional limitations remain after surgery • Daily supplementation with ferrous sulfate and folic acid to maintain hemoglobin at or above 12 g/dl during pregnancy (Brady and Duff, 1989) • Restriction of sodium intake to 2 g daily to prevent excess fluid retention • Depending on the client's functional classification, revision of her medical regimen, which includes digitalis preparations, diuretics, resting in semi-Fowler's position, and proper nutrition
Congenital heart defect		
One of five common defects: **1.** *Atrial septal defect or ventricular septal defect (VSD).* Abnormal opening between right and left atrium or right and left ventricle. **2.** *Tetralogy of Fallot.* Anomaly consisting of four defects, including pulmonic stenosis, VSD, malpositioning of the aorta so that it arises from the septal defect or the right ventricle, and right ventricular hypertrophy. **3.** *Patent ductus arteriosus.* Abnormal communication between the pulmonary artery and aorta. **4.** *Valvular abnormality.* Abnormality of any heart valves, such as narrowing or widening. **5.** *Coarctation of the aorta.* Abnormal narrowing of the aorta, which causes increased aortic pressure and the need for increased ventricular pressure during systole.	• Minor functional limitations after mandatory surgical correction	• Surgical repairs early in life to improve cardiac functioning • If minor functional limitations remain after surgery, close monitoring of the client during pregnancy • Depending on the client's functional classification, revision of her medical regimen, which includes digitalis preparations, diuretics, resting in semi-Fowler's position, and proper nutrition
Mitral valve prolapse		
Lack of support from the chordae tendinae, causing mitral valve leaflets to prolapse into the atrium during ventricular systole	• Typically asymptomatic, but may cause arrhythmias, palpitations, lightheadedness, dizziness, and fatigue	• Life-style adjustments as necessary, such as paced activity and rest periods • Propranolol (Inderal) to treat associated tachyarrhythmias • Close monitoring for signs of complications
Peripartum cardiomyopathy		
Left ventricular dilation and congestive heart failure occurring in the last month of pregnancy or first 6 postpartal months	• Fatigue, weakness, dyspnea, orthopnea, angina, chest pain, palpitations, cough, hemoptysis, and abdominal pain	• Digitalis preparations, diuretics, anticoagulant (heparin), furosemide (Lasix), and bed rest

NURSING DIAGNOSIS

After considering all assessment findings, formulate appropriate nursing diagnoses for the client. (For a partial list of applicable diagnoses, see Nursing Diagnoses: *Antepartal complications.*)

PLANNING AND IMPLEMENTATION

The antepartal client may have a nursing diagnosis of *decreased cardiac output related to valvular dysfunction.* To monitor her status, obtain her vital signs and weight at each prenatal visit. Obtain an ECG periodically, as prescribed. Monitor fluid intake and output. If a client develops pulmonary complications, be aware that a pulmonary artery catheter may be inserted to provide pulmonary pressure measurements.

Teach the client to monitor herself and report significant changes, especially signs and symptoms of potential complications. For example, teach the client with cardiac disease to note increased limitation of activity; presence of or increase in dyspnea, orthopnea, tachypnea, and edema; development of palpitations; significant increase or decrease in heart rate; and chest discomfort.

Inform the client of the need for regular examinations and tests. Advise her of all test results.

Teach about the condition, its management, and effects. The client with cardiac disease may have a nursing diagnosis of *knowledge deficit related to cardiac disease management during pregnancy* or *impaired gas exchange related to decreased cardiac output.* If so, encourage her to assume a semi-Fowler's or a left side-lying position to promote fetal oxygenation by shifting the weight of the pregnant uterus off the major abdominal blood vessels. Suggest ways to arrange pillows for comfort so that her head, neck, and arms are supported in the semi-Fowler's position, and her back, uterus, and legs are supported in the left side-lying position. If the client is hospitalized, administer oxygen, as needed.

Promote adequate rest and exercise. When the client has a nursing diagnosis of *activity intolerance related to altered cardiac function and decreased tissue oxygenation, fatigue related to decreased oxygen-carrying capacity of blood,* or *activity intolerance related to rapid weight gain and fluid retention,* stress the importance of obtaining adequate rest and limiting sodium and fluid intake.

For the client with cardiac disease, identify reasons for limiting activity and benefits of resting before or after activities. Help her find acceptable adjustments to profes-

sional and personal activities and to plan ways to modify her family's schedule to include rest periods. Also, encourage her to sleep at least 10 hours each night and to take morning and afternoon rests, particularly if she has a nursing diagnosis of *sleep pattern disturbance related to cardiac fatigue.*

Prevent infection. The antepartal client may be at increased risk for infection. For example, the client with a cardiac disease has an increased risk for upper respiratory tract infections, which can lead to subacute bacterial endocarditis. Her nursing diagnosis may be *high risk for infection related to altered cardiac status.* To help such a client, discuss the reasons for preventing infection. Encourage her to obtain sufficient rest and recommend that she avoid crowds, drafts, and people with viral infections. Stress the importance of healthful nutrition and adherence to prescribed vitamin and iron supplementation. Arrange for follow-up appointments at mutually agreeable times.

EVALUATION

To evaluate nursing care, determine if specific goals were achieved. The following examples illustrate some appropriate evaluation statements:
- The client accurately described her condition and its limitations on her health.
- The client correctly listed the signs and symptoms of complications in her condition and pregnancy.
- The client endorsed a care regimen that affords her optimum health and functioning.

DIABETES MELLITUS

The most common endocrine disorder in obstetrics, diabetes mellitus occurs in 1 out of approximately every 300 pregnancies (Hibbard, 1988). Although the introduction of insulin therapy for diabetes has reduced fetal mortality from 33% to less than 5% (Swislocki and Kraemer, 1989), the risk of congenital anomalies remains high in clients with insulin-dependent diabetes mellitus (IDDM). However, strict control of maternal serum glucose levels before conception and especially during the first trimester can help reduce this risk. Also, careful medical and nursing care can help the client manage her disorder successfully and deliver a normal, healthy neonate.

Pathophysiology

Diabetes mellitus results from inadequate insulin secretion by the beta cells of the islets of Langerhans in the

ANTEPARTAL COMPLICATIONS

The following nursing diagnoses address representative problems and etiologies that a nurse may encounter when providing care for a high-risk antepartal client. Specific nursing interventions for many of these diagnoses are provided in the "Planning and implementation" section of this chapter.

Cardiac disease

- Activity intolerance related to altered cardiac function and decreased tissue oxygenation
- Activity intolerance related to rapid weight gain and fluid retention
- Altered cardiopulmonary tissue perfusion related to decreased cardiac output
- Altered family processes related to inability to maintain level of functioning within the family
- Decreased cardiac output related to valvular dysfunction
- Fatigue related to decreased oxygen-carrying capacity of blood
- High risk for infection related to altered cardiac status
- Impaired gas exchange related to decreased cardiac output
- Knowledge deficit related to cardiac disease management during pregnancy
- Sleep pattern disturbance related to cardiac fatigue

Diabetes mellitus

- Altered nutrition: less than body requirements, related to altered carbohydrate metabolism
- Altered nutrition: less than body requirements, related to inadequate intake and excessive exercise
- Altered peripheral tissue perfusion related to vascular impairment
- Anxiety related to possible maternal, fetal, and neonatal effects of diabetes
- High risk for infection related to metabolic and vascular abnormalities
- Ineffective management of therapeutic regimen related to hospitalization for poor glucose control
- Knowledge deficit related to the effects of diabetes on pregnancy
- Noncompliance related to specified diet, schedules for serum glucose testing, or insulin administration

Anemias

- Altered nutrition: less than body requirements, related to increased need for intake of iron-rich foods
- Altered peripheral tissue perfusion related to inadequate blood supply
- Anxiety related to maternal and fetal effects of anemia

Anemias (continued)

- Fatigue related to decreased oxygen-carrying capacity of the blood
- High risk for infection related to altered RBC structure and tissue perfusion
- Knowledge deficit related to prenatal care and anemia
- Knowledge deficit related to the effects of anemia on pregnancy
- Pain related to vascular occlusion of sickle cell anemia
- Powerlessness related to frequency of sickle cell crises

Infection

- Altered family processes related to concern over adverse pregnancy outcomes
- Anticipatory grieving related to potential for congenital anomaly or death of fetus or neonate
- Ineffective individual coping related to possibility of delivering a neonate with a congenital anomaly or fatal infection
- Knowledge deficit related to disease transmission and prevention
- Knowledge deficit related to fetal and neonatal effects of maternal infection
- Noncompliance related to incomplete administration of prescribed medication
- Social isolation related to others' fear of disease transmission

Substance abuse

- Altered nutrition: less than body requirements, related to substance abuse
- Altered parenting related to performance of neonatal care while under the influence of a substance
- High risk for infection related to self-administered I.V. drugs
- Impaired tissue integrity related to substance abuse and needle sharing
- Knowledge deficit related to fetal effects of substance abuse
- Noncompliance with drug rehabilitation program related to continued substance abuse
- Self-esteem disturbance related to dependence on a chemical substance

(continued)

ANTEPARTAL COMPLICATIONS (continued)

Trauma or the need for surgery

- Altered family processes related to unexpected change in maternal health status
- Decreased cardiac output related to blood loss from trauma
- Fear related to the effects of trauma or surgery on the fetus
- Impaired gas exchange related to respiratory effects of chest trauma or to surgery and postoperative pain
- Pain related to traumatic injury or surgery

Premature rupture of the membranes

- High risk for infection related to PROM

Premature labor and delivery

- Altered health maintenance related to skipping medication doses
- Knowledge deficit related to at-home uterine monitoring

Spontaneous abortion

- Anticipatory grieving related to loss of pregnancy
- Anticipatory grieving related to potential loss of a fetus through abortion as manifested by expressions of anger
- Denial related to impending loss of pregnancy
- Ineffective family coping: compromised, related to inability to verbalize feelings
- Ineffective family coping: compromised, related to ineffective support as manifested in the partner's expressed frustration with the client
- Situational low self-esteem related to the inability to maintain pregnancy as manifested by crying and by verbalizing guilt

Incompetent cervix

- Anticipatory grieving related to potential loss of a fetus through incompetent cervix
- Caregiver role strain related to prolonged bedrest of the mother
- Impaired physical mobility related to prescribed bedrest
- Ineffective family coping: compromised, related to prolonged bedrest of the mother
- Knowledge deficit related to at-home uterine monitoring

Incompetent cervix (continued)

- Pain from abdominal cramping related to cerclage to repair an incompetent cervix
- Situational low self-esteem related to diagnosis of incompetent cervix

Hypertensive disorders

- Constipation related to bed rest
- Impaired physical mobility related to prescribed bed rest
- Ineffective family coping: compromised, related to prolonged bed rest of the mother
- Knowledge deficit related to hypertensive condition

Ectopic pregnancy

- Anticipatory grieving related to loss of pregnancy
- Anxiety related to the unknown
- Constipation related to bedrest
- Decreased cardiac output related to bleeding at the site of ectopic pregnancy rupture
- Denial related to impending loss of pregnancy
- Denial related to tubal pregnancy as manifested by minimization of symptoms and use of home remedies to relieve symptoms
- High risk for infection related to I.V. therapy
- Potential fluid volume deficit related to intra-abdominal hemorrhage upon rupture of tubal pregnancy

Gestational trophoblastic disease

- Anxiety related to the unknown
- Knowledge deficit related to necessary follow-up care

Rh incompatibility

- Fear related to unknown effect of blood incompatability on the fetus

Hyperemesis gravidarum

- Fluid volume deficit related to persistent vomiting
- Ineffective management of therapeutic regimen, related to hospitalization for persistent vomiting
- Pain related to persistent vomiting
- Situational low self-esteem related to persistent vomiting

pancreas or from ineffective use of insulin at the cellular level. Insulin regulates glucose and its transfer from the blood to body cells, all of which use glucose for energy. It also stimulates protein synthesis and free fatty acid storage in the fat deposits.

Insulin deficiency compromises access to essential nutrients for all body tissues. Without insulin, glucose circulates in the blood stream, unable to enter the cells. The energy-starved cells catabolize fats and proteins for energy, causing ketosis from fat wasting and negative nitrogen balance from protein breakdown and muscle tissue wasting.

The high level of circulating glucose leads to hyperglycemia, which exerts an osmotic force, pulling intracellular fluid into the blood and causing cellular dehydration. When the circulating glucose level exceeds the renal threshold, glucose spills into the urine, causing glycosuria. The urine's high osmotic level prevents reabsorption of water into the renal tubules, causing extracellular dehydration.

These changes produce the four classic signs and symptoms of diabetes:
• polyuria (frequent urination), which develops because the renal tubules do not reabsorb water
• polydipsia (excessive thirst), which is caused by the dehydration of polyuria
• polyphagia (excessive hunger), which results from tissue catabolism and inadequate cellular use of glucose
• weight loss, which occurs when the body burns fat and muscle tissues for energy.

Classifications

The National Diabetes Data Group (1979) classifies diabetes and other types of glucose intolerance as follows.

Diabetes mellitus. This disorder may take three forms: type I, IDDM; type II, non-insulin-dependent diabetes mellitus; and secondary diabetes, or diabetes resulting from another condition, such as a pancreatic, hormonal, or insulin-receptor disorder.

Impaired glucose tolerance (IGT). Formerly called latent or borderline diabetes, this asymptomatic disorder is characterized by normal or slightly elevated fasting levels of plasma glucose but abnormal glucose tolerance test values.

Gestational diabetes mellitus (GDM). This disorder begins or is first diagnosed during pregnancy. A client with GDM may be asymptomatic except for impaired glucose tolerance. GDM has great implications for pregnancy because even mild diabetes increases the risk of fetal or neonatal

morbidity and mortality. GDM may resolve after childbirth or may become IGT or type I or II diabetes mellitus.

ASSESSMENT

All pregnant women experience dramatic changes in carbohydrate, lipid, and protein metabolism. A pregnant diabetic woman is susceptible to hypoglycemia (abnormally low serum glucose level) and hyperglycemia (abnormally high serum glucose level). In some women, however, the growing fetus stresses maternal glucose production and use, disrupting normal carbohydrate metabolism and causing GDM.

In a diabetic client, pregnancy can affect insulin needs. Early in pregnancy, estrogen and progesterone serum levels increase, causing hyperinsulinemia (increased maternal insulin secretion). At the same time, morning sickness may decrease food intake. These changes substantially decrease the need for insulin. Later in pregnancy, human placental lactogen (hPL) levels increase. This hormonal antagonist reduces insulin's effectiveness, stimulates lipolysis, and increases the circulation of free fatty acids. At the same time, the client's food intake usually improves, and maternal and fetal glycogen storage increases. Together, these changes increase the need for insulin (Mestman, 1985). By the third trimester, insulin requirements increase.

Pregnancy also can hasten vascular changes associated with diabetes. Because of this, the diabetic client must be evaluated for hypertension, nephropathy, and retinopathy throughout her pregnancy.

If diabetes is not adequately managed before conception and during pregnancy, it increases fetal and neonatal risks. Preconception diabetic management maintains the client's health and prepares her for pregnancy, allowing fetal development to proceed normally. Blood glucose control throughout pregnancy reduces the risk of congenital anomalies and complications to the same level as that of the general population.

Maternal effects

The severity of the diabetes determines the degree of maternal effects. Uncontrolled diabetes or diabetes associated with vascular damage increases the risk of complications. However, comprehensive health care can control and lessen these risks.

Uncontrolled diabetes causes maternal hyperglycemia, increases the amount of circulating ketones from fatty acid metabolism, and results in ketosis. Decreased gastric motility (a normal change of pregnancy) and hPL's antagonistic effect on insulin further increase circulating glucose, predisposing the client to increased ketosis. Without treatment, she may become comatose, and she or her fetus may die.

Hydramnios (excess amniotic fluid) occurs in about 10% of pregnant diabetic women. Amniotic fluid volume increases to more than 1,500 ml. Although the exact cause of hyramnios is unknown, it may result from increased maternal and fetal circulating blood sugar, which increases fetal urine in the amniotic fluid. The added fluid may increase maternal discomfort later in pregnancy. Also, it occasionally leads to premature rupture of the membranes and premature labor. Although amniocentesis may reduce fluid volume, it is not commonly used for this purpose because it increases the risk of infection, labor stimulation, and placental injury.

The vascular changes of diabetes produce pregnancy-induced hypertension in 20% to 30% of pregnant diabetic clients.

Glycosuria predisposes the pregnant diabetic client to infections, especially monilia vaginitis and urinary tract infections. These non-life-threatening infections usually can be controlled with perineal hygiene, increased fluid intake, and anti-infective agents.

Fetal and neonatal effects
Maternal diabetes may have many adverse effects on the fetus and neonate. It increases the incidence of fetal anomalies and neonatal morbidity and predisposes the neonate to diabetes. Without careful management, it increases the risk of fetal or neonatal death. Neonates born to women with advanced diabetes may display intrauterine growth retardation (IUGR).

Neonates born to mothers with poorly controlled diabetes usually have macrosomia (large body size and birth weight), causing cephalopelvic disproportion and uterine dystocia and requiring cesarean delivery. Macrosomia can affect all fetal organs except the brain. The degree of macrosomia appears to correlate with the degree of maternal hyperglycemia and lack of maternal vascular disease.

Maternal hypoglycemia also leads to life-threatening situations, including lack of fetal nutrition and possible hypotension leading to fetal distress if the mother loses consciousness.

Neonatal hyperbilirubinemia and hypoglycemia also are possible effects of maternal diabetes. Hyperbilirubinemia results when the neonate's immature liver does not metabolize bilirubin. Hypoglycemia may occur after the umbilical cord is severed at delivery because the neonate's pancreas may continue to secrete insulin for a brief time after the maternal glucose supply stops.

Diagnostic studies
Expect to see the following diagnostic tests used to detect diabetes.

Urine glucose testing. Using a urine dipstick (Dextrostix), test the client's urine for glucose at each visit. This test should not be used to determine dietary management or insulin administration. Dextrostix detects glucose in the urine; Ketostix, ketones in the urine.

1-hour (50-gram) diabetes screening test. This oral glucose screening test is recommended for each pregnant client at 24 to 28 weeks' gestation. Advise the client that she does not need to fast before the test. Inform her that a blood sample for glucose testing will be drawn 1 hour after she ingests 50 grams of oral glucose solution. If her plasma glucose level is abnormally high, expect to prepare her for a 3-hour oral glucose tolerance test (Gabbe, 1986).

3-hour oral glucose tolerance test (OGTT). The OGTT may be used to diagnose gestational diabetes. Advise the client to eat a high-carbohydrate diet (more than 200 grams daily) for 2 days before this test. Also tell her to fast from midnight until the test time. When she arrives for her test, explain that a blood sample will be drawn to obtain a fasting plasma glucose level. Then after she ingests 100 grams of oral glucose solution, blood samples for plasma glucose levels will be drawn at 1, 2, and 3 hours. If two or more of the samples show abnormally high glucose levels, the client has gestational diabetes (Gabbe, 1986).

Glycosylated hemoglobin. Used to evaluate diabetic control, this test measures the percentage of glycohemoglobin (hemoglobin with a glucose molecule attached) in the blood, reflecting the blood glucose level during the previous 6 to 8 weeks. When performed monthly, it assists in diabetic management. Elevated glycohemoglobin levels indicate uncontrolled diabetes.

Blood glucose levels. In gestational and insulin-dependent diabetes, this test can be used to manage diabetes. It measures the blood glucose level, which is used to determine dietary changes and insulin dosage (Hollingsworth, 1988; Coustan and Felig, 1988).

Because selective screening may miss previously undiagnosed diabetes, all pregnant clients should be screened for glucose intolerance with a 1-hour (50-gram) diabetes screening test. If screening reveals glucose intolerance, treatment should begin.

NURSING DIAGNOSIS

After considering all assessment findings, formulate appropriate nursing diagnoses for the client. (For a partial list of applicable diagnoses, see Nursing Diagnoses: *Antepartal complications,* pages 129 and 130.)

PLANNING AND IMPLEMENTATION

For a client with diabetes, nursing diagnoses may include *knowledge deficit related to the effects of diabetes on pregnancy.* For such a client, provide information about diabetes, its effects on her and her fetus and neonate, and the treatment. Reassure her that careful management during pregnancy can prevent fetal and neonatal problems. Also, advise her to avoid smoking because of its vasoconstrictive effects on the fetus and herself.

Instruct the client and her partner about diabetes mellitus, home glucose monitoring, and insulin, highlighting the drug's purpose, types, dosage, and administration. Also review the signs and symptoms of hypoglycemia and hyperglycemia.

Reinforce the physician's recommendations for home glucose monitoring, insulin administration, and dietary management. Teach the client about acceptable glucose values, and encourage her to record these levels accurately along with the amount of insulin she self-administers.

If blood glucose cannot be regulated with intermittent insulin administration, a continuous infusion pump may be used or the client may be hospitalized during pregnancy for adjustment of insulin dosages.

Diet. A pregnant client with IDDM should ingest 35 calories/kg of her ideal body weight, or 2,200 to 2,400 calories daily; one with gestational diabetes should ingest 2,000 to 2,200 calories daily. Of these calories, 20% should be from proteins, 50% to 60% from complex carbohydrates, and 25% to 30% from fats (Samuels and Landon, 1986). The client should divide her daily intake into three meals and three snacks, with 25% of calories ingested at breakfast, 30% at lunch, 30% at dinner, and 15% in snacks, especially at bedtime to prevent hypoglycemia during sleep (Gabbe, 1985). The goal of this diet is to regulate blood glucose levels even though protein, carbohydrates, and fats are metabolized at different rates.

Exercise and rest. A diabetic pregnant client should exercise because exercise helps reduce the need for insulin and helps regulate post-meal glucose levels (Schneider and Kitzmiller, 1989). If she exercised before pregnancy, she should continue her usual program. If she did not exercise before pregnancy, she should ease into nonstressful activities under her physician's guidance.

Because muscles use glucose for energy, exercise can decrease blood glucose levels. To correct any glucose deficiencies, the client must report pre- and post-exercise glucose levels to her physician, who can suggest compensatory dietary or insulin dosage changes.

Encourage the diabetic client to obtain adequate rest, including 8 to 10 hours of sleep each night and daily rest periods. Management of the client should include guidelines for effectively incorporating exercise into her daily regimen. The diabetic client may have a nursing diagnosis of *altered nutrition: less than body requirements, related to inadequate intake and excessive exercise.* Suggest that she exercise about 1 hour after meals, when her blood glucose level is elevated, and inform her that she may need the added sugar in hard candy during exercise.

Home glucose monitoring. Home glucose monitoring is an accurate, convenient way to determine the diabetic client's response to treatment. The nurse should provide the client with guidelines for acceptable blood glucose ranges and instruct her to report abnormal values to her physician.

An insulin-dependent diabetic client should monitor her glucose level four times a day, usually after fasting and meals. A client with any other type of diabetes should monitor her blood glucose as prescribed by her physician.

Insulin administration. The goal in diabetes treatment is to keep blood glucose levels within the normal range for pregnancy. If diet management cannot accomplish this goal, insulin therapy should be initiated (Gabbe, 1986). Results of home glucose monitoring enable the physician to prescribe insulin dosages that will meet the client's needs. Insulin therapy for the diabetic pregnant client uses highly purified animal or human insulin preparations, which are less allergenic than synthetic preparations and decrease the risk of maternal allergic reactions. Oral hypoglycemic agents cause prolonged hypoglycemia in the fetus if exposed near term and should not be used during pregnancy.

Insulin is administered subcutaneously. Typically, the client needs a mixture of intermediate-acting (NPH) and short-acting (regular) insulin in the morning and evening. Usually, two-thirds of the total insulin dosage is taken at breakfast, with the remaining third at dinner. Some physicians may prescribe continuous insulin therapy using an insulin pump and regular insulin to maintain blood glucose levels throughout pregnancy.

Monitor fetus. For a diabetic client, regular fetal evaluations are particularly important. Tests for fetal well-being typically include ultrasonography, biophysical profile, fetal movement count, non-stress test, nipple stimulation contraction stress test, and oxytocin contraction test.

During each prenatal visit, monitor fetal status by assessing fetal movement and fetal heart rate. A non-stress test and nipple stimulation contraction stress test may be ordered.

In addition, inform the client and her partner about other diagnostic tests to determine fetal health, including ultrasonography, biophysical profile, oxytocin contraction test, and amniocentesis. Careful examination of the fetus assures the couple that optimum care is being provided and may relieve a client with a nursing diagnosis of *anxiety related to possible maternal, fetal, and neonatal effects of diabetes.* Allow time for questions and discussion of test results.

Prevent infection. The diabetic client is likely to have a nursing diagnosis of *high risk for infection related to metabolic and vascular abnormalities.* Teach such a client to watch for signs of infection, such as redness, warmth, swelling, and fever. Also instruct her to look for broken skin, bleeding, bruises, or slow healing and to report these findings to her physician. Advise her to trim her fingernails and toenails carefully to avoid accidental cuts. Teach her to maintain adequate peripheral circulation by avoiding constricting clothing on her legs. Adequate circulation, especially to the lower extremities, helps decrease the risk of ulceration and infection.

Provide support. The antepartal client may have a nursing diagnosis of *anxiety related to possible maternal, fetal, and neonatal effects of diabetes.* To help such a client, identify her concerns and expect an experienced nurse clinician to provide psychological support and counseling during and after the pregnancy.

Clearly inform the client of the risks for delivering a stillborn or abnormal neonate if anticipated. Maintain honesty and confidentiality through pregnancy testing and discussion of results. Initiate counseling sessions to discuss the client's concerns and fears and provide guidance for future care. If necessary, refer her to a support group or mental health professional.

Promote compliance. To promote compliance with the medical regimen, invite the client to participate in her health care planning. Help her identify her needs throughout the pregnancy, and allow her to become a member of the health care team. Consider the client's educational level

and daily schedule. Respect her judgments and incorporate her prescribed regimen into a workable daily plan.

EVALUATION

To evaluate nursing care, determine if specific goals were achieved. The following examples illustrate some appropriate evaluation statements:
- The client identified changes in her pregnancy caused by the disease.
- The client reported a change in her condition as soon as it occurred.
- The client made an appointment for counseling.
- The client kept all appointments for prenatal care and laboratory tests.
- The client began a regular exercise program.
- The client and her partner made an informed decision about fetal diagnostic testing.
- The client accurately described her condition and its limitations on her health.
- The client planned nutritious meals.

ANEMIAS

Two commons forms of anemia may complicate the antepartal period: iron deficiency anemia and folic acid deficiency anemia.

Iron deficiency anemia results from an inadequate supply of iron for optimal formation of red blood cells (RBCs), producing smaller (microcytic) cells. Insufficient iron stores lead to a depleted RBC mass and, in turn, to a decreased concentration of hemoglobin, which normally transports oxygen throughout the body.

Also known as megaloblastic anemia, pernicious anemia of pregnancy, or macrocytic anemia, *folic acid deficiency anemia* is rare in the United States (Cunningham, MacDonald, and Gant, 1989). Women with multiple gestation and those with hemoglobinopathies or other hemolytic disorders are especially susceptible to developing folic acid deficiency anemia (Cruikshank, 1986b). (For more information, see *Maternal, fetal, and neonatal effects of anemias.*)

Etiology

Pregnancy greatly increases the body's need for iron, and a client may not have adequate iron stores to meet the greater need. Without iron supplementation, the client may develop iron deficiency anemia.

The body uses folic acid to break down and use proteins and to form nucleic acids and heme for hemoglobin.

MATERNAL, FETAL, AND NEONATAL EFFECTS OF ANEMIAS

Iron deficiency anemia, folic acid deficiency anemia, and sickle cell anemia can produce various maternal, fetal, and neonatal effects as described in the chart below.

ANEMIA	MATERNAL EFFECTS	FETAL AND NEONATAL EFFECTS
Iron deficiency anemia	• Poor tissue integrity • Tissue damage at birth • Antepartal or postpartal infection with impaired healing • Excessive bleeding after delivery	• Spontaneous abortion, stillbirth, or small-for-gestational-age (SGA) neonate • Intact fetal iron stores • Fetal distress from hypoxia during later pregnancy and labor, when hemoglobin fails to carry sufficient oxygen to the mother and fetus
Folic acid deficiency anemia	• Urinary tract and other infections • Bleeding complications during delivery • Pancytopenia (reduction of all cellular components of the blood) resulting from immature red blood cell production	• Spontaneous abortion and abruptio placentae complications
Sickle cell anemia	• Pregnancy-induced hypertension • Pulmonary emboli • Pneumonia • Urinary tract infection • Postpartal uterine infection	• Abruptio placentae complications • Intrauterine growth retardation • Prematurity • SGA neonate • Compromised fetal safety that can cause stillbirth and neonatal death when client's crises interfere with general vascular supply

A deficiency may result from inadequate intake of animal protein and uncooked fresh vegetables, malabsorption, or a metabolic abnormality. When deficiency occurs, immature RBCs fail to divide and are released as enlarged cells (megaloblasts). Because they are fragile, many cells are destroyed before they are released into the bloodstream.

During pregnancy, the need for folic acid increases because of tremendous cell multiplication and accelerated erythropoiesis and deoxyribonucleic acid synthesis by the fetus and placenta (Cruikshank, 1986a). This places the pregnant client at risk for folic acid deficiency.

ASSESSMENT

A client with iron deficiency anemia may tire easily and be susceptible to infection and postpartal bleeding. Even minimal blood loss during childbirth may cause an already anemic client to experience difficulty, including decreased blood pressure and dizziness. Other signs and symptoms may include weakness, headache, shortness of breath on exertion, anorexia, pica (craving to eat nonfood substances), irritability, and pallor.

Anemia is diagnosed by blood tests after a thorough health history and physical examination. When iron deficiency anemia is present, the hemoglobin level is below 11 g/liter, and the hematocrit drops below 32%.

For an anemic client, expect to monitor the results of hemoglobin electrophoresis, CBC, folic acid levels, and serum iron measurements.

Folic acid deficiency anemia gradually produces clinical findings, such as decreased hemoglobin levels despite sufficient iron intake, GI distress (including anorexia, nausea, and vomiting), fatigue, weakness, and pallor. In advanced stages, dyspnea and edema may appear.

NURSING DIAGNOSIS

After considering all assessment findings, formulate appropriate nursing diagnoses for the client. (For a partial list of applicable diagnoses, see Nursing Diagnoses: *Antepartal complications*, pages 129 and 130.)

PLANNING AND IMPLEMENTATION

Supplemental iron should be administered to an anemic client before conception to maintain normal hemoglobin concentration. It should be continued during pregnancy. Daily oral doses of 200 mg of elemental iron, supplied in 1 g of ferrous sulfate or 2 g of ferrous gluconate, provide the necessary requirements for a pregnant client with anemia. Divided doses help prevent or decrease adverse gastrointestinal (GI) effects, such as nausea and constipation.

Teach about the condition, its management, and effects. Depending on the client's disorder or problem, provide information about its treatment and care and about the effects they should produce.

Teach the client about her disorder and its effects. This is particularly important for a client with a nursing diagnosis of *knowledge deficit related to the effects of anemia on pregnancy.* Inform her that she should report any evidence of bleeding, especially vaginal bleeding. Identify special needs for the anemic client during pregnancy, such as compliance with iron supplementation.

Promote adequate nutrition. The antepartal client may have a nursing diagnosis of *altered nutrition: less than body requirements, related to increased need for intake of iron-rich foods.* To help such a client, evaluate her food preferences, needs, and restrictions, and estimate the nutritional value of the foods she eats. Incorporate these evaluations into a balanced diet that fulfills nutritional requirements, meets food preferences, and is economical. For any client, outline a pattern of ideal weight gain during pregnancy.

To prevent folic acid deficiency anemia, the client should take 400 mcg of folic acid daily during pregnancy. To treat anemia, she should receive 1 mg of folic acid three times daily. Because iron deficiency anemia almost always coexists with folic acid deficiency anemia, the client also should receive iron supplements.

The nurse should encourage the client to eat foods high in folic acid. The nurse also should teach the client to use little or no water in cooking because folic acid is a water-soluble vitamin that can be removed from foods as they cook.

Depending on the client's underlying disorder, make specific dietary recommendations. To prevent or correct iron deficiency or folic acid deficiency anemia, suggest foods that are rich in these nutrients.

EVALUATION

To evaluate nursing care, determine if specific goals were achieved. The following examples illustrate some appropriate evaluation statements:

- The client accurately described her condition and the potential effects on herself and on the fetus or neonate.
- The client planned nutritious meals.

SICKLE CELL ANEMIA

Sickle cell anemia is characterized by recurring acute, painful, vaso-occlusive attacks known as crises. This disorder can cause organ damage and death. Some pregnant clients with sickle cell anemia can carry to term safely, if they receive careful management. However, nearly one-half the pregnancies of clients with sickle cell anemia end in abortion, stillbirth, or neonatal death. Yet maternal mortality from sickle cell anemia has decreased since 1972 from about 6% to about 1% (Cunningham, MacDonald, and Gant, 1989). (For more information, see *Maternal, fetal, and neonatal effects of anemias*, page 135.)

Etiology

This autosomal recessive disease (inherited from both parents) occurs almost exclusively among individuals of African or Mediterranean descent, especially Blacks. Between 6% and 13% of Black Americans carry the sickle cell trait (heterozygous state of the recessive disorder); 0.2% have sickle cell anemia (Kelton and Cruickshank, 1988).

Sickle cell anemia causes a structural abnormality in hemoglobin molecules (hemoglobin S), causing RBCs to roughen and become sickle- or crescent-shaped. This shape affects the oxygen-carrying capacity and survival of the hemoglobin. It also causes RBC tangling that obstructs blood flow in small blood vessels and organs of high oxygen extraction, such as the spleen, bone marrow, and placenta.

Various factors may precipitate vessel obstruction and subsequent sickle cell crisis. These include infection, stress, dehydration, trauma, fever, fatigue, and strenuous activity. Crisis produces blood stasis, platelet aggregation, local hypoxia, edema, extreme pain, and tissue infarction.

ASSESSMENT

A pregnant client with sickle cell anemia is likely to experience crises during the second half of her pregnancy, although they may occur at any time. Sickle cell crises are characterized by acute, painful, recurring vaso-occlusive attacks that affect the extremities, abdomen, chest, and vertebrae. The client also may experience fever, dehydration, debilitation, hypertension, anemia, pulmonary problems, and osteomyelitis (bone infection).

Sickle cell anemia is diagnosed through laboratory testing with hemoglobin electrophoresis, which can distinguish between sickle cell anemia and sickle cell trait.

NURSING DIAGNOSIS

After considering all assessment findings, formulate appropriate nursing diagnoses for the client. (For a partial list of applicable diagnoses, see Nursing Diagnoses: *Antepartal complications,* pages 129 and 130.)

PLANNING AND IMPLEMENTATION

Teach the client with sickle cell anemia about precipitating factors. Advise her to maintain proper nutrition and hydration. Also instruct her to avoid crowds and individuals with colds or infections to decrease the risk of infection. Stress the importance of noting and reporting signs and symptoms of impending infection to the physician.

During a crisis, the client may need hydration, analgesics, and treatment of infection. Acetaminophen (Tylenol) relieves mild pain; meperidine (Demerol) with a sedative controls severe pain. She also may need a transfusion of RBCs.

During a sickle cell crisis, fetal status should be monitored. Unless the client is in labor or has an arterial oxygen level below 70 mm Hg, antepartal oxygen administration is not necessary.

For a client with sickle cell anemia, emphasize rest and pain-relief measures, such as hot showers or warm baths.

EVALUATION

To evaluate nursing care, determine if specific goals were achieved. The following examples illustrate some appropriate evaluation statements:
• The client correctly listed the signs and symptoms of complications in her condition or pregnancy.
• The client reported a change in her condition as soon as it occurred.

INFECTION

Throughout pregnancy, the client should take measures to avoid infection. If infection occurs despite these measures, the client should be evaluated and treated promptly to prevent maternal and fetal complications. The most common or potentially harmful infections during pregnancy are TORCH, HIV, and genitourinary infections. (For more information, see *Maternal, fetal, and neonatal effects of infections,* pages 138 to 142.)

The acronym TORCH refers to toxoplasmosis, other infections (chlamydia, group B beta hemolytic streptococcus, syphilis, and varicella zoster), rubella, cytomegalovirus, and herpesvirus type 2 infections. These infections can cause major congenital anomalies or death of the embryo or fetus.

HIV infection can cause acquired immunodeficiency syndrome (AIDS), a life-threatening disease that affects the body's immune system, rendering it susceptible to opportunistic infections.

In the first 6 months of 1988, women accounted for more than 10% of reported HIV cases (Cates and Schulz, 1988). The percentage may be higher because many women who carry the virus are asymptomatic.

Genitourinary infections include sexually transmitted diseases (STDs), gynecologic infections, and urinary tract infections. Some of these infections, such as gonorrhea and herpes, can be passed to the fetus as it traverses the birth canal.

ASSESSMENT

For a client with an infection, laboratory data reveal antibody titers and immune status. An abnormally high white blood cell count signals infection. Cultures taken from lesions or drainage samples can be used to identify a specific infecting organism.

NURSING DIAGNOSIS

After considering all assessment findings, formulate appropriate nursing diagnoses for the client. (For a partial list of applicable diagnoses, see Nursing Diagnoses: *Antepartal complications,* pages 129 and 130.)

PLANNING AND IMPLEMENTATION

The client with an infection may have a nursing diagnosis of *knowledge deficit related to disease transmission and prevention.* If so, teach her about the causes of infections, transmission routes, and prevention techniques. Describe the signs and symptoms of common infections, and help her identify predisposing factors. Encourage her to seek medical help if she suspects infection.

Care for the client with an infection involves all family or household members in controlling the infection, assuring satisfactory health for these individuals, and protecting the family caregivers. To accomplish these goals,

(Text continues on page 142.)

MATERNAL, FETAL, AND NEONATAL EFFECTS OF INFECTIONS

The following chart compares the maternal, fetal, and neonatal effects of TORCH, human immunodeficiency virus, and selected genitourinary infections as well as their nursing considerations.

MATERNAL EFFECTS	FETAL AND NEONATAL EFFECTS	NURSING CONSIDERATIONS
TORCH: Toxoplasmosis		
Spontaneous abortion (with widely disseminated infection in early pregnancy) and possibly fatal complications (in an immunosuppressed client)	Stillbirth, premature birth, microcephaly (abnormally small head), hydrocephaly (abnormally large head with accumulation of cerebrospinal fluid in the brain), hypotonia, seizures, coma, mental retardation, blindness, deafness, or chorioretinitis (choroid and retina inflammation)	• Instruct the client to cook meat thoroughly to kill bacteria. • Teach the client to avoid contact with cat box filler, especially if the cats roam outside. Advise the client to wear gloves while gardening. Infected cat box filler or soil may come into contact with hand cuts or contaminate food during preparation.
TORCH: Other — chlamydia		
Pelvic inflammatory disease, dysuria, spontaneous abortion, placental inflammation, and postpartal endometritis 2 to 6 weeks after delivery	Stillbirth, premature birth, neonatal mortality; pneumonia, conjunctivitis (7 to 15 days after birth), or otitis media (Benoit, 1988; CDC, 1989; McElhose, 1988)	• Advise the infected client that her partner also must be examined and treated. • Teach the client that the risk of chlamydia increases with the number of sexual partners and decreases with the use of a barrier method of contraception.
TORCH: Other — group B beta hemolytic streptococcus infection		
Increased risk of septic abortion, chorioamnionitis, postpartal endometritis, arthritis, pyelonephritis, pneumonia, meningitis, and endocarditis	Stillbirth or fetal infection; neonatal infection from delivery (McCracken and Freij, 1987); neonatal susceptibility to pneumonia and septicemia; invasive disease within 7 days of birth, which can lead to death; meningitis within about 24 days, which can lead to death (Simpson, Gaziano, Lupo, and Peterson, 1988)	• Be aware that risk factors include premature labor, premature rupture of membranes, and a prolonged period between membrane rupture and labor. • Remind the client that failure to report signs and symptoms or to appear for prenatal follow-up visits increases the risk of undiagnosed infection. • Be alert for signs of neonatal infection. Be prepared to notify the physician and prepare for blood transfusion and I.V. antibiotic administration.
TORCH: Other — syphilis		
Second trimester spontaneous abortion	Stillbirth, premature labor and birth, congenital infection, and anomalies (if mother is untreated)	• Tell the client that treatment for syphilis typically includes benzathine penicillin G (Bicillin). If she is allergic to penicillin, she may be referred for desensitization before treatment begins. • Be aware that erythromycin is not recommended because of a high failure rate in curing fetal infection. Tetracycline is contraindicated because of effects on fetal teeth and bones, increased incidence of fetal inguinal hernias, and increases in maternal liver toxicity (Sharp, 1986). • Advise the client to return every month to be checked for reinfection. • Advise the client that if she receives adequate antibiotic treatment during pregnancy, the risk to her neonate is low. • Instruct the client to observe for signs and symptoms of premature labor.

MATERNAL, FETAL, AND NEONATAL EFFECTS OF INFECTIONS *(continued)*

MATERNAL EFFECTS	FETAL AND NEONATAL EFFECTS	NURSING CONSIDERATIONS
TORCH: Other — varicella-zoster (herpes zoster, chicken pox) infection		
Possible death from severe varicella pneumonia	Congenital abnormalities, including limb deformity, cortical atrophy, eye abnormalities, skin lesions, and pneumonia (when varicella occurs in the first trimester); neonatal varicella that may lead to pneumonia, encephalitis, and possibly neonatal death (South and Sever, 1986)	• Be aware that maternal infection in the last 4 days of pregnancy and within 48 hours after delivery can cause neonatal varicella. (During its incubation period, the infection is contagious.) • Be aware that vaccines usually are not given during pregnancy. However, varicella-zoster vaccine is under investigation for use in pregnant clients. • Be aware that varicella-zoster immune globulin (VZIG) may be given prophylactically to a pregnant client.
TORCH: Rubella — German measles		
Spontaneous abortion	Congenital anomalies, including cardiac defects (pulmonary artery stenosis and patent ductus arteriosus), intrauterine growth retardation (IUGR), deafness, cataracts, glaucoma, and mental retardation (Pritchard, MacDonald, and Gant, 1985); delayed effects (possibly for decades), such as insulin-dependent diabetes mellitus, sudden hearing loss, glaucoma, and encephalitis (South and Sever, 1986)	• Advise the pregnant client to prevent this disease by avoiding contact with anyone known to have rubella. • Be aware that a negative antibody titer indicates that the client is not immune to rubella. • Advise the client to obtain rubella vaccination after she has delivered. Advise her not to become pregnant for at least 3 months after receiving the vaccine, which contains the live, attenuated virus.
TORCH: Cytomegalovirus infection		
Transplacental transmission of disease to the fetus or transmission to the neonate during vaginal delivery	Severe, permanent damage in about 10% of infected neonates (Cunningham, MacDonald, and Gant, 1989); neonatal hepatosplenomegaly, jaundice, thrombocytopenia, microcephaly, hearing loss, mental retardation, cerebral palsy, epilepsy, blindness, and possibly death	• Be aware that cytomegalovirus can be transmitted by any close contact, including kissing, breast-feeding, and sexual intercourse. • Advise the infected client that she should not breast-feed her neonate because the virus can be transmitted through breast milk. • Be aware that the disease may be fatal to a fetus, although it usually is innocuous in adults and children. • Advise the client that although no treatment exists for cytomegalovirus infection, her physician may prescribe immunotherapy or an antiviral agent. • Expect to isolate the mother and neonate after birth.
TORCH: Herpesvirus type 2 infection		
Discomfort from lesions during the pregnancy, increased incidence of secondary infection, and increased likelihood of cesarean delivery because the virus can be transmitted to the neonate during vaginal delivery	Spontaneous abortion or stillbirth if herpesvirus type 2 becomes active before 20 weeks' gestation (Stagno and Whitley, 1985); premature labor if the virus becomes active later in pregnancy; local infection of the skin, eyes, or mucous membranes (Whitley, et al., 1988); symptoms that develop after birth, such as fever or hypothermia, poor feeding, seizures, and jaundice	• Be aware that the safety of systemic acyclovir (Zovirax) in pregnant clients has not been established. • Expect a vaginal delivery for a client with genital herpes but no lesions. On the day of delivery, obtain a herpesvirus culture from the client and the neonate. • Expect a client with active genital lesions at the time of labor or membrane rupture to have a cesarean delivery to reduce the risk of virus transmission to the neonate. • For a client with genital lesions at or near term but before labor or membrane rupture, collect cultures every 3 to 5 days to monitor viral activity and assess appropriateness of vaginal delivery, as prescribed.

(continued)

MATERNAL, FETAL, AND NEONATAL EFFECTS OF INFECTIONS (continued)

MATERNAL EFFECTS	FETAL AND NEONATAL EFFECTS	NURSING CONSIDERATIONS
TORCH: Herpesvirus type 2 infection (continued)		
		• Be aware that the mother and neonate need not be isolated from each other, although intimacy carries a small risk (about 0.1%) of neonatal infection. • Allow the infected mother to care for her neonate as long as she washes her hands thoroughly before and after touching the neonate. • Reassure the client that she may safely breast-feed her neonate because herpesvirus type 2 is not present in breast milk. • Be aware that the incubation period is 2 to 12 days. A neonate who is symptom-free at birth may display symptoms later.
Human immunodeficiency virus (HIV) infection		
Transplacental transmission of HIV to the fetus or transmission to the neonate through breast-feeding	Possibility of abandonment by parents who leave the neonate in the health care facility permanently, death within a few years (Minkoff, 1988)	• Identify the client at risk for HIV infection and expect serum HIV studies. • Counsel the client about disease transmission to her fetus and partner. • Educate the client and staff about disease transmission to reduce its spread. • Take precautionary measures to prevent contamination from infected body fluids and blood during testing and hospitalization. Alert caregivers to blood and body fluid precautions. • Be aware that diagnosis may be made during pregnancy. Provide support and referrals to counseling for the client faced with the devastating information that she has a terminal illness and her fetus has a 50% probability of contracting the disease transplacentally. • Expect cord blood tests for maternal HIV antibodies at delivery, which indicate maternal infection. Also expect the neonate's blood to be tested for HIV antibodies after delivery and regularly thereafter. If the neonatal titer decreases, the neonate has not been infected. If it increases, the neonate is infected.
Genitourinary infection: Trichomoniasis		
Possible premature rupture of membranes, postpartal endometritis	Neonatal pneumonia	• Advise the client to avoid sexual intercourse or to use condoms. • Reevaluate the couple to assess treatment effectiveness. • Test for gonorrhea and chlamydia, as prescribed, which commonly accompany this infection. • Tell the client to practice thorough perineal hygiene. • Inform the client that unless her partner has been treated effectively, the infection may recur.
Genitourinary infection: Gonorrhea		
Dysuria, urinary frequency and urgency; premature rupture of membranes associated with peripartal fever and chorioamnionitis	IUGR; neonatal sepsis, meningitis, or arthritis; ophthalmia neonatorum (from vaginal delivery); anal, vaginal, and nasopharyngeal infection	• Expect to conduct laboratory tests to rule out other sexually transmitted diseases and to retest late in the third trimester. • Treat the client as prescribed, usually with ceftriaxone I.M., followed by erythromycin for 7 days. Also treat her partner, typically with ceftriaxone and doxycycline. Re-evaluate them to assess treatment effectiveness.

MATERNAL, FETAL, AND NEONATAL EFFECTS OF INFECTIONS *(continued)*

MATERNAL EFFECTS	FETAL AND NEONATAL EFFECTS	NURSING CONSIDERATIONS
Genitourinary infection: Condylomata acuminata		
Increased reproduction of genital warts; possible obstruction of birth canal by warts	Epithelial tumors of mucous membranes on larynx, genital warts, and laryngeal papillomatosis (rare)	• Expect to prepare the client for cryosurgery or laser treatments to remove warts because topical podophyllum resin can be toxic to the fetus. • Expect vaginal delivery except in a client whose warts obstruct the birth canal. • Instruct the client to report recurrence of warts after treatment.
Genitourinary infection: Vaginitis (candidiasis)		
Increased discomforts of pregnancy caused by vaginal itching and discharge	Thrush from delivery if vaginal organisms enter the neonate's mouth	• Be aware that candidiasis commonly occurs in pregnant clients with diabetes mellitus. • Teach the client about candidiasis and support her during occurrences. • Expect to provide local anticandidal preparations for the client and her partner if he has candidal balanitis. • Tell the client to practice thorough perineal hygiene. • Reevaluate the client and her partner to assess treatment effectiveness and to detect recurrence. • Assess the neonate after delivery for signs of thrush, such as creamy, white, slightly elevated plaque inside the mouth, primarily on inner cheeks and tongue.
Genitourinary infection: Vaginitis (bacterial vaginosis)		
Alteration in normal cervical-vaginal environment	Teratogenic effects if the mother is treated with metronidazole (Flagyl) during the first trimester	• Instruct the client to practice thorough perineal hygiene. • Reevaluate the client to assess treatment effectiveness and to detect recurrence. • Be aware that metronidazole should not be administered during the first trimester but may be used in the later trimesters. Evaluate the client for possibility of pregnancy before treatment begins. • Be aware that treatment of the client's partner is not necessary because no counterpart of bacterial vaginosis is recognized in men.
Genitourinary infection: Pelvic inflammatory disease (PID)		
Sterility from tubal infection and scarring; other effects, depending on the infecting organism	Various effects, depending on the infecting organism	• Be aware that PID is rare in pregnancy. However, it may occur in the first weeks of pregnancy. • Instruct the client to receive treatment and take precautions to prevent reinfection. • As prescribed, test the client for chlamydia and herpes, which commonly are associated with PID.
Genitourinary infection: Pyelonephritis		
Increased genitourinary and abdominal discomfort, possibly premature labor	Possible teratogenic effect if the mother is treated with sulfonamides, but evidence is not conclusive.	• Be aware that the incidence of pyelonephritis increases because of the urinary stasis that occurs during pregnancy. • Do not administer sulfonamides to a pregnant client near term.

(continued)

MATERNAL, FETAL, AND NEONATAL EFFECTS OF INFECTIONS *(continued)*

MATERNAL EFFECTS	FETAL AND NEONATAL EFFECTS	NURSING CONSIDERATIONS
Genitourinary infection: Pyelonephritis *(continued)*		
		• Encourage the client to maintain bed rest, drink plenty of fluids, and report worsening of symptoms. • Reevaluate the client to assess the effectiveness of treatment with antibiotics, fluids, and rest and to detect recurrence. • Recommend urologic consultation after delivery to assess for permanent genitourinary changes caused by the infection. • Evaluate for preterm labor and expect treatment with tocolytics, if necessary. • Assess the neonate for elevated bilirubin levels after birth.

educate the family about the infection, its risks, and preventive measures. These measures may include:
• sexual abstinence during the active phases of the disease
• use of a condom during sexual intercourse as recommended by health care professionals
• simultaneous treatment of the client and her partner
• evaluation for reinfection, as indicated by health care professionals
• careful adherence to perineal hygiene measures
• careful attention to proper disposal of body fluids and contaminated needles
• thorough hand-washing after contact with infected areas and before contact with the neonate and others.

For the client with an infection, help the couple identify the neonate's needs as a member of their family. Also, help them identify ways to handle society's fear of disease transmission. Encourage them to obtain information about the disease so that they can prevent transmission.

EVALUATION

To evaluate nursing care, determine if specific goals were achieved. The following examples illustrate some appropriate evaluation statements:
• The client correctly described the potential effects of her condition on herself and on her fetus or neonate.
• The client and family demonstrated correct infection control measures.

SUBSTANCE ABUSE

When a pregnant woman abuses a substance such as illegal drugs or alcohol, it can affect her as well as her child. (For more information, see *Maternal, fetal, and neonatal effects of substance abuse.*)

A pregnant client who abuses substances may suffer physical, psychological, social, and economic consequences. In addition, she may have a spontaneous abortion or premature delivery, or she may develop pregnancy-induced hypertension, hemorrhage, or abruptio placentae.

A pregnant substance abuser is likely to neglect prenatal care because she fears admonishment from health care professionals, lacks the self-esteem to make personal health care a priority, or views prenatal care as unimportant and unnecessary. Yet such a client has a greater need for care because of possible exposure to HIV, STDs, hepatitis, malnutrition, and infection from injection sites—as well as the risk of hypertension, antepartal bleeding, abruptio placentae, spontaneous abortion or stillbirth, and preterm labor (Finnegan and Wapner, 1987; Ronkins, Fitzsimmons, Wapner, and Finnegan, 1988). These factors and risks may arise from poor health, inadequate nutrition, infection, shared needles, multiple sex partners, and drug abuse and its effects.

First-trimester substance abuse has teratogenic effects and increases the risk of spontaneous abortion. Use of cocaine may cause abnormalities in chromosomal structure or numbers and congenital anomalies, such as genitourinary malformations (Chasnoff, Burns, and Burns, 1987; Chasnoff, Griffith, MacGregor, Dirkes, and Burns, 1989). Substance abuse also may cause such problems as IUGR, premature birth, and withdrawal symptoms.

MATERNAL, FETAL, AND NEONATAL EFFECTS OF SUBSTANCE ABUSE

Many abused substances can affect the client and her fetus or neonate, as described in the chart below.

SUBSTANCE	MATERNAL EFFECTS	FETAL AND NEONATAL EFFECTS
Depressants		
Ethanol (alcohol)	Spontaneous abortion	Stillbirth, intrauterine growth retardation (IUGR), short palpebral fissures, microcephaly, mild to moderate mental retardation, irritability, poor coordination, fetal alcohol syndrome (Rodgers and Lee, 1988)
Narcotics heroin, methadone hydrochloride (Dolophine)	Spontaneous abortion, premature rupture of membranes, preterm labor, infections of the placenta, chorion, and amnion	Low birth weight, IUGR, withdrawal symptoms (vomiting, tremors, sneezing, increased muscle tone), seizures, respiratory distress, meconium aspiration with abrupt drug withdrawal, perinatal morbidity and mortality (Finnegan, 1986; Rodgers and Lee, 1988)
Barbiturates phenobarbital (Luminal)	Drowsiness, lethargy, and other reactions such as vertigo, headache, and CNS depression; benefits from use in pregnancy acceptable despite fetal risks if used for serious disorders, such as seizures	Central nervous system depression, seizures, withdrawal symptoms, hyperactivity, decreased sucking reflex, possible teratogenic effects, delayed lung maturity (Wapner and Finnegan, 1982)
Tranquilizers chlordiazepoxide (Librium), diazepam (Valium)	If client overdoses, prolonged hypoxia, malnutrition, poor weight gain, crossdependence on alcohol and barbiturates	Same as for barbiturates, plus tremors, irritability, tachypnea, poor weight gain, sudden infant death syndrome (SIDS), decreased sucking reflex, hypotonia, hypothermia (Wapner and Finnegan, 1982)
Mixed narcotic agonistantagonists pentazocine (Talwin)	Cellulitis, abscesses of arms resulting in infections	Low birth weight, IUGR, addiction (Wapner and Finnegan, 1982)
Stimulants		
Amphetamines amphetamine sulfate (Benzedrine)	Malnutrition, possible ventricular tachycardia and asytole during obstetric anesthesia	Congenital abnormalities, especially cardiac defects and oral clefts (Rodgers and Lee, 1988)
dextroamphetamine sulfate (Dexedrine)	Insufficient nutrition; serious cardiac arrhythmias, ventricular tachycardia, and withdrawal symptoms, including lethargy and profound depression	Withdrawal symptoms, low birth weight, IUGR from poor maternal nutrition, congenital heart defects (Rodgers and Lee, 1988)
Cocaine	Vasoconstriction leading to tachycardia, hypertension, dilated pupils and muscle twitching; myocardial infarction; cardiac and respiratory arrest; increased spontaneous abortion, abruptio placentae, preterm labor	Stillbirth; genitourinary problems, including prune-belly syndrome (congenital absence of abdominal musculature, causing distended, flabby abdomen that is creased like a prune) and hydronephrosis (Chasnoff, Griffith, MacGregor, Dirkes, and Burns, 1989); SIDS (not well documented); depressed interactive behaviors (Rodgers and Lee, 1988)

(continued)

MATERNAL, FETAL, AND NEONATAL EFFECTS OF SUBSTANCE ABUSE (continued)

SUBSTANCE	MATERNAL EFFECTS	FETAL AND NEONATAL EFFECTS
Stimulants (continued)		
Nicotine	Increased risk of neonatal mortality (20 or fewer cigarettes daily); decreased placental perfusion, abruptio placentae, placenta previa, functional anemia, premature rupture of membranes, preterm labor, spontaneous abortion (more than 20 cigarettes daily)	Reduced fetal breathing movements, small for gestational age, low birth weight, increased risk of SIDS, possible death (Rodgers and Lee, 1988)
Psychotropics		
Cannabis sativa (marijuana)	Cross-dependence on nicotine and alcohol	Possible teratogenic effects, prematurity, potential for meconium in amniotic fluid and for meconium aspiration (Wapner and Finnegan, 1982)
Lysergic acid diethylamide (LSD)	Possible spontaneous abortion	Possible prematurity, chromosomal damage or anomalies (Rodgers and Lee, 1988)

ASSESSMENT

Review the results of appropriate laboratory tests for the substance abuser. Urine drug testing provides information about substances abused. Biophysical profile testing assists with fetal health evaluation.

NURSING DIAGNOSIS

After considering all assessment findings, formulate appropriate nursing diagnoses for the client. (For a partial list of applicable diagnoses, see Nursing Diagnoses: *Antepartal complications*, pages 129 and 130.)

PLANNING AND IMPLEMENTATION

If a pregnant substance abuser seeks health care, the nurse should obtain baseline data and determine any health problems. Throughout the client's care, the nurse plays a role in suggesting ways to correct these health problems. For example, the nurse may suggest that the client attempt to control her substance abuse and, if appropriate, refer her to a drug rehabilitation program. On subsequent visits, the nurse could provide nutrition counseling and information about vitamin and iron supplements that may be prescribed. The nurse should help the client to schedule appointments, as necessary, encourage her to keep follow-up appointments, and inform her that she may have to provide a urine specimen for drug screening at each visit to identify the presence, type, and amount of drug abused.

The pregnant substance abuser needs early prenatal care to decrease the risk of congenital anomalies in her neonate. During her early prenatal visits, suggest ways for her to control the type and amount of drugs that she takes. Offer firm support and reassurance during follow-up visits. If she appears for care late in the pregnancy or misses appointments, continue to provide sensitive care at every opportunity during the antepartal, intrapartal, and postpartal periods.

The substance abuser may have a nursing diagnosis of *knowledge deficit related to fetal effects of substance abuse.* If so, teach her about the adverse effects of various substances on her and her fetus and neonate. Help her recognize that substances affect her fetus. Inform her that her neonate will have to undergo withdrawal and will be treated as an addict after birth.

For a client with an opiate or heroin addiction, a controlled substance withdrawal method with methadone administration, although controversial, may be recommended. "Cold turkey" withdrawal is not recommended during pregnancy because of the risk of fetal seizures, hypoxia, and death. A client receiving methadone also should participate in group counseling sessions. A multidisciplinary approach provides comprehensive physical, psychological, social, and economic care to the pregnant substance abuser.

Prevent infection. The client who abuses I.V. drugs risks infection from needles. She may have a nursing diagnosis of *high risk for infection related to self-administered I.V. drugs.* Teach such a client the reasons, causes, signs, and symptoms of infections related to I.V. drug abuse. Explain how such infections can harm her and her fetus.

Good skin integrity decreases the chances of local and systemic infections. Depending on the route of drug administration, the client may have open areas or abscesses on her extremities. Help her maintain skin integrity by evaluating these sites and providing care to prevent systemic infection.

Promote adequate nutrition. A substance abuser may have a nursing diagnosis of *altered nutrition: less than body requirements, related to substance abuse.* When evaluating her dietary habits, also assess her financial status to determine if she has enough money to buy food. Such a client may spend more money on drugs than on basic needs. If necessary, consult a social worker who will determine the client's eligibility for food stamps and Women, Infants, and Children assistance.

Promote family well-being. A client who abuses substances is especially likely to have a nursing diagnosis of *altered parenting related to performance of neonatal care while under the influence of a substance.* This client may benefit from neonatal care instruction during individual counseling sessions or peer group sessions.

EVALUATION

To evaluate nursing care, determine if specific goals were achieved. The following examples illustrate some appropriate evaluation statements:
• The client correctly described the potential effects of her condition on herself and on her fetus or neonate.
• The client planned for neonatal care.
• The client kept all appointments for prenatal care and laboratory tests.

TRAUMA OR NEED FOR SURGERY

A pregnant client suffering from trauma or requiring surgery needs special management. The nurse must be aware of special considerations to provide appropriate client care.

Trauma may result from accidental injury, physical abuse, or other factors. If the injury is major, it can endanger maternal and fetal health. Therefore, a pregnant client who suffers trauma needs immediate, expert health care.

Accidental injury is a major cause of trauma during pregnancy, occurring in 6% to 8% of all pregnancies (Neufeld, Moore, Marx, and Rosen, 1987). For a client who suffers accidental injury, the nurse should focus on maintaining the pregnancy and ensuring maternal and fetal health.

Physical abuse is another common cause of trauma during pregnancy. For an abused client, the nurse should focus on detecting any evidence of damage to the pregnancy, such as vaginal bleeding. (For more information, see *Effects of trauma on pregnancy,* page 146.)

Baden and Brodsky (1985) report that between 25,000 and 50,000 pregnant women undergo surgery each year in the United States for nonobstetric problems. Common surgeries during pregnancy include ovarian cyst removal, acute appendectomy, breast surgery, repairs of incompetent cervix, and surgery for cholecystitis (Rice and Pellegrini, 1985; Willson and Carrington, 1987).

Because of the risks, surgery should be postponed until after delivery, whenever possible, and nonsurgical interventions should be used. Such interventions may include rest, I.V. therapy, antibiotics, and gastric decompression via nasogastric tube. If these measures fail to control the client's condition, they may be used to provide relief until further evaluation is completed and surgery can be performed.

If surgery becomes necessary, the health care team should take a multidisciplinary approach to client preparation. Before surgery, consultants from anesthesiology, perinatology, cardiology, and internal medicine may evaluate maternal and fetal risks to reduce the probability of complications.

ASSESSMENT

Preoperative care begins with chest X-rays and electrocardiography (ECG) which may be required if concerns exist about the client's cardiopulmonary status. During a chest X-ray, the client will wear a shield over her abdomen to protect the fetus from radiation.

Laboratory tests can rule out some potential problems, such as anemia and infection, and provide preoperative baseline data.

NURSING DIAGNOSIS

After considering all assessment findings, formulate appropriate nursing diagnoses for the client. (For a partial

EFFECTS OF TRAUMA ON PREGNANCY

Common causes of trauma during pregnancy include accidental injuries and physical abuse and its psychological stress. The chart below details typical injuries, their effects on pregnancy, and nursing considerations.

COMMON INJURIES	EFFECTS ON PREGNANCY	NURSING CONSIDERATIONS
Accidental injury		
• Falls resulting from too-flexible joints and a displaced center of gravity (Falls may cause fractures of the ankles, legs, or arms, but usually leave the fetus unharmed.) • Blunt abdominal trauma • Crushing injuries from vehicular accidents	• Depending on injury severity and gestational age, maternal and fetal death or fetal death from abruptio placentae • With blunt abdominal trauma during the third trimester, uterine and fetal injury • With fractured pelvis, abruptio placentae, ruptured bladder, retroperitoneal hemorrhage, and shock • With severe head trauma or internal injury hemorrhage, possible maternal death • With severe abdominal trauma sustained during a vehicular accident, uterine rupture and placental separation from the abdominal wall, spontaneous membrane rupture, premature labor, and severely jeopardized fetal health	• Be aware that any trauma may be fatal to the pregnant client and her fetus. Promptly assess and treat the injury as prescribed to decrease the maternal and fetal morbidity and mortality probability. • Ensure an adequate airway and provide oxygen as necessary. • Obtain an accurate clinical and obstetric history to evaluate maternal health. • Assist with a thorough physical assessment and review pertinent diagnostic studies to evaluate maternal health further. • Use electronic fetal monitoring to assess fetal status, as prescribed. • Assess the client's orientation, and inform her of treatment measures and plans for her care. • Position the client on her left side if possible, or insert a wedge under her right hip to decrease aortocaval pressure from the gravid uterus and to increase vascular volume. • Administer I.V. fluids and insert an indwelling urinary catheter, as prescribed. Follow other standard protocols of the health care facility. • Provide continual support throughout the initial period to calm an anxious client. • Perform comfort measures to decrease the amount of pain medication required. Consult with the obstetrician and surgeon about the best pain medications for the client.
Physical abuse		
• Burns • Lacerations • Contusions • Fractures • Head injuries • Dislocations • Penetrating injuries, such as stab or gunshot wounds • Stress-related disorders, such as headaches, insomnia, depression, and suicidal thoughts	• In early pregnancy, possibly no fetal harm because uterus is low in abdominal cavity and protected by amniotic fluid, organs, muscles, and bony pelvis • During late pregnancy, fetal harm because the uterus is protected less by the thinner abdominal wall (Amniotic fluid protects the fetus, unless substantial trauma occurs.) • Compromised fetal development if the client cannot eat or has multiple areas of bleeding • Spontaneous abortion from uterine rupture or placental separation	• Same as for accidental injury. • Remember that late in pregnancy, the gravid uterus is most likely to sustain injury from penetrating abdominal wounds (Slater and Aufses, 1985). • Advise the physically abused client that any physical or psychological abuse is abnormal and harmful to her mental and physical well-being.

list of applicable diagnoses, see Nursing Diagnoses: *Antepartal complications,* pages 129 and 130.)

PLANNING AND IMPLEMENTATION

When surgery is needed, the risk of maternal, fetal, and neonatal morbidity and mortality depends on the stage of the pregnancy and the surgical procedure. Because controversy exists over the fetal risks of various anesthetics in the first trimester, non-emergency surgery should be postponed until the second trimester, which also protects against spontaneous abortion and possible teratogenic effects from medications. Even for abdominal surgery, the second-trimester uterus should not be large enough to interfere with the operative site. Although surgery may induce premature labor, no evidence suggests that a higher incidence of fetal malformations is associated with anesthesia and surgery. (For more information, see *Nursing considerations for the pregnant client requiring surgery.*)

NURSING CONSIDERATIONS FOR THE PREGNANT CLIENT REQUIRING SURGERY

Certain physiologic changes of pregnancy may make surgery difficult. The chart below shows how to overcome these difficulties when caring for the pregnant surgical client.

PHYSIOLOGIC CHANGE	EFFECT ON THE CLIENT	NURSING CONSIDERATIONS
Decreased gastric motility	Increased risk of gastric regurgitation and chemical pneumonitis from pulmonary aspiration of acidic gastric contents	• Expect to administer an antacid to increase gastric pH and decrease the risk of chemical pneumonitis if the client vomits and aspirates during surgery. • Insert a nasogastric tube, as prescribed, for gastric decompression. • Assist with endotracheal intubation, rapid anesthesia induction, or use of regional anesthesia, as prescribed
Weight gain	Difficulty with endotracheal intubation	• Assist with pulmonary assessment during surgical evaluation by anesthesiologist or nurse anesthetist.
Decreased functional pulmonary residual capacity, which can impair oxygenation	Further decrease in functional capacity with general anesthesia and remaining in the supine position	• Oxygenate the client, as prescribed, before anesthesia. • Expect to place a pillow under the client's right hip or tilt the operating room table to the left. • Expect the client to receive regional anesthesia, which reduces hyperventilation, improves maternal oxygenation, and benefits the fetus (preferred in cases where increased cardiac work load is detrimental to the client).
Increased blood volume	Tolerance to blood loss during surgery	• Be aware that the pregnant client may not need blood transfusions as readily as the nonpregnant client.
Aortocaval compression by gravid uterus when the client lies supine	Impaired blood circulation and perfusion	• Expect to place a pillow under the client's right hip or tilt the operating room table to the left to displace the uterus, decreasing vessel compression and maintaining adequate perfusion to the heart, uterus, and placenta. • Use electronic fetal heart rate monitoring during and after surgery to evaluate for fetal distress, as prescribed.
Organ displacement	Difficulty in locating the appendix in a client with appendicitis	• Be aware that after the fifth month of pregnancy the appendix lies at the iliac crest level and continues to rise above it during the last trimester.

EVALUATION

To evaluate nursing care, determine if specific goals were achieved. The following examples illustrate some appropriate evaluation statements:

• The client correctly described the potential effects of her condition on herself and on her fetus and neonate.
• The client's family demonstrated support and concern.
• The client reported a change in her condition as soon as it occurred.

PREMATURE RUPTURE OF MEMBRANES

Premature rupture of the membranes (PROM) is any rupture of the amniotic sac before onset of labor, independent of length of gestation. PROM presents a management challenge because of the divergent opinions surrounding its treatment. It is associated with maternal morbidity and mortality, primarily because of increased incidence of infection. Fetal and neonatal risks include sepsis, preterm delivery, anoxia, respiratory distress syndrome, cord prolapse, and traumatic delivery (Gibbs and Sweet, 1989).

Etiology

Although the etiology of PROM usually is unknown, many conditions predispose a woman to this disorder. Possible factors include incompetent cervix, amnionitis, placenta previa, fetal malpresentation, hydramnios, more than one fetus, and trauma (Gibbs and Sweet, 1989). Besides being a complication of PROM, infection also may be a cause. Some researchers have proposed a link among coitus, inflammation, and PROM. A woman with PROM before term is more likely to have cervical microorganisms than one who does not have PROM (Gibbs and Sweet, 1989).

Incidence

Between 3% and 19% of all deliveries are preceded by PROM (Gibbs and Sweet, 1989). The percentage is significantly higher in preterm pregnancies.

ASSESSMENT

A pelvic examination discloses whether PROM has occurred. Using aseptic technique, a physician, nurse-midwife, or specially prepared nurse uses a sterile speculum to observe the cervix. Direct observation of amniotic fluid seeping from the cervical os confirms PROM. If this fluid is not visible, the practitioner may elect to test with nitrazine paper, which will indicate an alkaline substance by turning blue. (The vaginal area normally is acidic and amniotic fluid is alkaline.)

Nitrazine paper has about a 95% accuracy rate (Gibbs and Sweet, 1989). False-negative results may occur if several hours have elapsed since rupture of the membranes or if the vaginal area has been contaminated with blood, urine, or antiseptic solutions.

Other tests to determine if fluid is amniotic include a smear on a clean slide (amniotic fluid makes a distinctive ferning pattern when it dries), a study of cell structure, and a staining technique to identify fetal fat cells. Because no laboratory or clinical test is foolproof, however, a combination of tests is necessary for an accurate diagnosis.

Ultrasound may be useful in identifying PROM if oligohydramnios (scant amount of amniotic fluid) can be identified on the scan. Once a diagnosis of PROM has been confirmed, the age of the fetus must be determined. If the client cannot remember the exact date of her last menstrual period, ultrasound can be useful in determining fetal age.

NURSING DIAGNOSIS

After considering all assessment findings, formulate appropriate nursing diagnoses for the client. (For a partial list of applicable diagnoses, see Nursing Diagnoses: *Antepartal complications,* pages 129 and 130.)

PLANNING AND IMPLEMENTATION

An inaccurate diagnosis of PROM may lead to unnecessary induction of labor, cesarean delivery, or preterm delivery. Therefore, the physician must make every effort to make an accurate diagnosis of the disorder.

Management of PROM usually involves two distinctly different approaches based on the assessment of risks to both mother and fetus. In active management, labor is induced and, if not effective, a cesarean delivery is performed. In expectant management, no action is taken to speed the onset of labor except in cases of amnionitis or fetal distress.

Because the client may have a nursing diagnosis of *high risk for infection related to PROM,* prophylactic antibiotics may be used. Little agreement exists on their value if labor begins within 24 hours after PROM.

Respiratory distress syndrome (RDS) develops in 10% to 40% of neonates born to clients with PROM. Neonatal sepsis is identified in approximately 10% of neonates, and amnionitis occurs in 4% to 30% (Gibbs and Sweet, 1989). Other neonatal complications include asphyxia, malpresentation, and cord prolapse. Maternal complications include cesarean delivery and endometritis (inflammation of the uterus lining), occurring in 3% to 30% of clients with PROM.

Maternal mortality related to PROM is rare. Neonatal mortality is caused by RDS in 30% to 70% of cases. Anomalies account for 10% to 30% and infection for 3% to 20% (Gibbs and Sweet, 1989).

Infections following PROM are common and potentially severe. A client with oligohydramnios after PROM may have more clinically evident infections than one who did not have oligohydramnios. Amniocentesis for Gram stain and culture of the amniotic fluid sometimes is used to identify infection. Some problems are associated with this diagnostic tool, however. First, amniotic fluid is not always available for testing after PROM. Second, 20% to 30% of clients identified by amniocentesis as having infections do not have clinical signs or symptoms of infection (Gibbs and Sweet, 1989).

Other procedures to identify infection include maternal serum C-reactive protein and fetal movement studies.

EVALUATION

The following examples illustrate some appropriate evaluation statements:
• The client reported a change in her condition as soon as it occurred.
• The client's family demonstrated support and concern.

PRETERM LABOR AND DELIVERY

Defined as any delivery, regardless of the neonate's birth weight, that occurs between 20 and 37 weeks after the client's last menses. Preterm labor and delivery has been a significant cause of perinatal morbidity and mortality for many years (Creasy, 1989). Advances in technology have enhanced medical management of small neonates, but no significant decrease in low-birth-weight, preterm neonates has been documented (Creasy, 1989). The problem of preterm delivery is one of the most significant to be overcome in attempting to improve pregnancy outcome.

Etiology

Many factors can contribute to the onset of preterm labor and delivery, including pneumonia, appendicitis with sepsis, other acute infections, multiple gestation (more than one fetus), poverty, smoking, alcohol abuse, drug addiction, grand multiparity (five or more previous births), teenage pregnancy, and uterine anomalies. Psychological

trauma also may be a contributing factor, as may significant adverse events or chronic stress during the second and third trimesters (Omer and Everly, 1988).

Incidence

Preterm labor and delivery accounts for 5% to 10% of all births in developed countries. Although the percentage is relatively small, this condition accounts for most neonatal deaths. The incidence almost doubles for Black clients (Creasy, 1989).

Maternal age under 19 or over 34 is a significant factor also. A previous preterm labor and delivery is associated with a risk of recurrence of 17% to 30%, with the incidence increasing significantly after two or more preterm labors and deliveries (Creasy, 1989).

Women in lower socioeconomic groups have an increased incidence of preterm labor and delivery. This may be related to nutritional status during pregnancy. A woman who weighs less than 50 kg (112 lb) at the start of her pregnancy is at a higher risk than one who weighs 57 kg (125 lb) or more.

ASSESSMENT

The early symptoms of preterm labor are so subtle that they may be overlooked by the client and the medical and nursing staffs. Because of missed early symptoms, fewer than 25% of clients in preterm labor are candidates for long-term therapy to prevent preterm births (Creasy, 1989). Such therapy is contraindicated by PROM (30% to 40%), advanced cervical dilation (4 cm or more), maternal hemorrhage, and evidence of severe fetal compromise (decelerations in fetal heart rate).

Because the onset of preterm labor is insidious, a primary goal of obstetric care is to prevent it. Many of the factors contributing to preterm labor are reliable indicators and can be used to identify the client at risk. (For more information, see *Identifying the client at risk for preterm labor*, page 150.)

Regardless of the client's problem, assess the fundal height, weight, and vital signs and listen for the fetal heart rate. If the membranes are intact, the physician or nurse-midwife usually will perform a digital pelvic examination of the cervix. Progressive cervical changes may indicate that labor is proceeding; nevertheless, in some cases the physician or nurse-midwife may choose to wait for progressive cervical changes before beginning therapy (Creasy, 1989).

Because urinary tract infections commonly are associated with preterm labor, a urinalysis should be performed to determine whether bacteria are present.

IDENTIFYING THE CLIENT AT RISK FOR PRETERM LABOR

Several factors in the development of preterm labor are of reliable predictive value. Any factor from the high-risk category or any two from the low-risk category call for increased antepartal surveillance.

HIGH-RISK CATEGORY

History factors
- Cone biopsy
- Uterine anomaly
- At least one abortion during the second trimester
- DES exposure
- Preterm delivery
- Preterm labor

Factors in current pregnancy
- Placenta previa
- Hydramnios
- Abdominal surgery
- More than one fetus present
- Cervical dilation
- Effacement greater than 50%
- Uterine irritability

LOW-RISK CATEGORY

Socioeconomic factors
- Low socioeconomic status
- Age: less than age 19 or over age 34
- Single parent
- Work outside the home
- Height: less than 5′ 3″ (160 cm)
- Weight: less than 100 lb (45 kg)
- Cigarettes: more than 10/day

History factors
- Febrile illness
- Pyelonephritis
- First trimester abortion (fewer than 3)
- Less than 1 year since last delivery

Factors in current pregnancy
- Bleeding after 12 weeks' gestation
- Weight gain less than 7 lb (3.2 kg) by 22 weeks
- Albuminuria
- Hypertension
- Bacteriuria
- Weight loss of 5 lb (2.3 kg)
- Febrile illness
- Fetal head engaged at 32 weeks' gestation

NURSING DIAGNOSIS

After considering all assessment findings, formulate appropriate nursing diagnoses for the client. (For a partial list of applicable diagnoses, see Nursing Diagnoses: *Antepartal complications.*)

PLANNING AND IMPLEMENTATION

Management of preterm labor begins with bed rest in the lateral decubitus position and external uterine monitoring of fetal status.

Because the onset of preterm labor is insidious, a primary goal of obstetric care is to prevent its occurrence. Many of the factors contributing to preterm labor are reliable indicators and can be used to identify a client at risk.

Certain hormones—serum estradiol, progesterone, and prostaglandin or its metabolites—have been studied to determine their effect on preterm labor. Serial measurements of these hormones have provided data on their fluctuation, but no relationship has been consistently demonstrated between the levels of any of these hormones and the incidence of preterm labor.

Tocolysis (inhibition of uterine contractions) is a primary tool in caring for a client with preterm labor. Tocolytic drugs are 60% to 88% effective in stopping uterincontractions; however, many of the drugs have adverse effects on both the mother and the fetus. Furthermore, little is known about the cumulative effect of tocolytic drugs used in early gestations and continued over long periods (Givens, 1988). Absolute contraindications to tocolytic drugs include severe pregnancy-induced hypertension, severe bleeding from any cause, chorioamnionitis, fetal death, a fetal anomaly that is incompatible with life, and severe fetal growth retardation. Relative contraindications include mild chronic hypertension, stable placenta previa, uncontrolled diabetes mellitus, fetal distress, and cervical dilation greater than 5 cm (Creasy, 1989).

Tocolytic drugs may be used with success to inhibit labor until term, interrupt labor long enough to transport the mother to a high-risk health care facility, or inhibit labor until prenatal steroids (to increase fetal lung maturity) can become effective. (For an overview of tocolytic agents, see *Drugs used to inhibit labor.*)

Beta-adrenergic agents (isoxsuprine hydrochloride, ritodrine, and terbutaline sulfate) inhibit the contractility of the myometrium. A client taking one of these drugs may have a nursing diagnosis of *altered health mainte-*

DRUGS USED TO INHIBIT LABOR

This chart summarizes the major tocolytic drugs in current clinical use.

MECHANISM OF ACTION	USUAL DOSAGE AND EFFICACY	NURSING IMPLICATIONS
magnesium sulfate		
Acts directly as a calcium antagonist; affects uterine contractility by competing with calcium both inside and outside the cell.	I.V. bolus of 4 grams over 15 to 20 minutes plus 4 to 5 grams I.M. into each buttock, followed by a constant infusion of 2 grams/hour. Stable level is difficult to maintain because of rapid excretion through the kidneys. May work slower than beta-adrenergic agonists. Contractions may not stop immediately.	• Toxicity signaled by a respiratory rate below 15 breaths/minute, hyporeflexia, and urine output below 30 ml/hr. May cause neonatal lethargy, poor sucking reflex, and delayed motility of the gastrointestinal tract. • Monitor respiratory rate, deep tendon reflexes, and urine output every hour. Keep 10% calcium gluconate at bedside as antidote for overdose.
beta-adrenergic agonists (ritodrine and terbutaline sulfate)		
Stimulate beta-adrenergic receptors, which activate an enzyme (adenylate cyclase) that produces cyclic adenosine monophosphate (cAMP). cAMP inhibits the junction of myosin and actin (agents necessary for muscular contractility).	Initially, 50 to 100 mcg of ritodrine/minute by I.V. infusion, increasing by 50 mcg/minute every 10 minutes up to the minimum effective dose. Usual dose is 150 to 350 mcg/minute. Initially, 10 mcg of terbutaline sulfate/minute by I.V. infusion, increasing by 5 mcg/minute every 10 minutes up to 80 mcg/minute. After contractions cease, taper to the least effective dose by decreasing by 5 mcg/minute.	• May cause tachycardia, hypotension, bronchial dilation, increased plasma volume, increased cardiac output, arrhythmias, myocardial ischemia, reduced urine output, restlessness, headache, nausea, and vomiting. • Place the client in a left lateral position to minimize hypotension. • Monitor the maternal and fetal heart rates constantly. • Pulmonary edema is a serious but rare adverse reaction. Monitor weight daily to detect fluid overload.
calcium antagonists (nifedipine)		
Block the flow of calcium through calcium-specific channels in the myometrial cells. Nifedipine appears to target the uterus and has limited cardiac effects.	Initially, 10 mg orally t.i.d.; some patients may require up to 30 mg q.i.d. Maximum daily dosage is 180 mg. Onset of action is within 20 minutes. Use of these medications to inhibit labor remains experimental.	• May cause facial flushing, transiently elevated heart rate, palpitations, headache, dizziness, nausea, and hypotension.
prostaglandin synthetase inhibitors or nonsteroidal anti-inflammatory agents (indomethacin, salicylates, naproxen)		
Inhibit prostaglandin synthetase to decrease the amount of prostaglandins, which interfere with labor.	Dosage varies with drug used. May be used orally or rectally.	• *Fetal effects:* premature closure of ductus arteriosus. *Neonatal effects:* hyperbilirubinemia, altered platelet function, decreased urine output. *Maternal effects:* epigastric pain, rectal intolerance if suppositories are used, interference with platelet function, bleeding. • Monitor client with ruptured membranes carefully. These drugs can mask infection through antipyretic effect.

nance related to skipping medication doses. The client may believe that labor will stop without the drugs.

Magnesium sulfate, used for years to treat hypertensive episodes in pregnancy, is growing in popularity as a tocolytic agent. It has fewer adverse effects than beta-adrenergics and can be used in conjunction with beta-adrenergics or when they are contraindicated. Absolute contraindications to magnesium sulfate include myasthenia gravis, impaired renal function, and recent myocardial infarction.

Oral magnesium, such as magnesium sulfate, also may be used to provide safe, long-term tocolysis although the Food and Drug Administration has not approved it for this use.

Calcium antagonists, agents that regulate the flow of calcium within the cells of the myometrium, are under investigation for use as tocolytic agents. Because calcium is the key element in uterine contractility, calcium antagonists would seem to be the perfect tocolytic agent. However, their use in the inhibition of labor is experimental.

Prostaglandin synthetase inhibitors, such as salicylates, indomethacin, and naproxen, relax the gravid uterus and have been linked to the incidence of postmaturity (overly developed neonate). However, concern about bleeding, prolonged labor, and the potential fetal and neonatal effects has limited their use in preventing preterm labor.

The development in 1985 of a lightweight, highly sensitive tocodynamometer has allowed outpatient monitoring of uterine activity. This in-home monitoring capability is marketed with an intensive perinatal nursing service that incorporates 24-hour nurse availability, daily transmission of recorded uterine activity, weekly physician update, and ongoing client teaching and reinforcement of the treatment plan. An appropriate nursing diagnosis for an outpatient client is *knowledge deficit related to at-home uterine monitoring.* The cost of these programs varies, but many are covered under health insurance plans.

These services were designed exclusively for the high-risk preterm labor group. Monitoring usually is initiated at around 20 weeks' gestation and continues until 36 weeks' gestation.

EVALUATION

To evaluate nursing care, determine if specific goals were achieved. The following examples illustrate some appropriate evaluation statements:
• The client has given a return demonstration of proper use of an at-home uterine monitor.
• The client planned for neonatal care.

HYPERTENSIVE DISORDERS

Hypertension is the third leading cause of maternal mortality in the United States, preceded only by hemorrhage and infection. About 7% of all pregnancies are affected by

PATHOPHYSIOLOGY OF PREGNANCY-INDUCED HYPERTENSION

Pregnancy-induced hypertension (PIH) affects major body systems, including the kidneys, lungs, liver, and uterus. Many of the PIH-induced changes in these systems—such as tissue ischemia and fibrinogen deposits in the vessel walls—can be identified only through postmortem studies.

Effects on kidneys
Low protein levels cause decreased plasma colloidal pressure and allow fluid to shift from intravascular to interstitial spaces, causing edema. Blood flow to the kidneys is decreased by the fluid shift. The decreased blood flow diminishes renal perfusion, which in turn triggers the release of renin that leads to the formation of the potent vasopressor angiotensin. These work to increase the blood pressure to offset the effects of diminished renal perfusion. Renal function becomes inefficient and the glomerular filtration rate decreases. Vascular spasms also decrease glomerular blood flow and constrict glomerular capillaries. Diminished renal function results in albuminuria and increased blood urea nitrogen.

Effects on liver
Vascular spasms result in vessel compression and, in some cases, extravasation (hemorrhage under the liver and in the intra-abdominal cavity). Fibrin clots also may form from elevated plasma fibrinogen levels in gestational hypertension (Ballegeer, et al., 1989).

Effects on lungs
Pulmonary changes resulting from PIH include pulmonary edema and diffuse intrapulmonary bleeding, which could predispose the client to bronchopneumonia.

Effects on placenta
Placental changes from PIH affect the uteroplacental perfusion. These changes include premature aging, degeneration and calcification of tissues, congested intervillous spaces, and arteriolar thromboses. Shanklin and Sibai (1989) have identified extensive endothelial injury in placental biopsy samples of women with PIH. The integrity of uterine vessels and coagulation capabilities also were altered in those women. Rodgers, Taylor, and Roberts (1988) found that serum from preeclampsic women was toxic to endothelial cells maintained in vitro.

hypertension; 6% to 10% of perinatal deaths are associated with hypertensive episodes. According to Hacker and Moore (1986), the hypertensive episode may result directly from the pregnancy itself (pregnancy-induced hypertension, or PIH), or it may predate the pregnancy and result from cardiovascular or renal disease. (For information on how PIH affects major body systems, see *Pathophysiology of pregnancy-induced hypertension.*)

The American College of Obstetricians and Gynecologists accepts the following terms in association with gestational hypertension: preeclampsia and eclampsia, chronic hypertension, PIH, chronic hypertension with superimposed preeclampsia, and transient hypertension (Gilbert and Harmon, 1986). PIH is characterized by hypertension, proteinuria, and edema. It has two basic forms: preeclampsia (a nonconvulsive form marked by the onset of acute hypertension after 24 weeks' gestation) and eclampsia (a convulsive form that occurs between 20 weeks' gestation and the end of the first postpartal week). This syndrome may develop at any point after 20 weeks' gestation or in the early postpartal period. (Hypertension before 20 weeks' gestation usually is associated with gestational trophoblastic disease.) Typically, the syndrome appears in the last trimester and disappears after 42 postpartal days. PIH may be difficult to distinguish from hypertensive states that predate the pregnancy. In addition, a definitive diagnosis of PIH may be impossible unless the client's blood pressure returns to baseline after pregnancy. Severe preeclampsia-eclampsia may be seriously complicated by a syndrome that is given the acronym HELLP. (For more information, see *HELLP syndrome.*)

Chronic hypertension is present and observable before the pregnancy and is diagnosed by week 20 of gestation or extends 42 days after delivery. Chronic hypertensive disease may occur alone or with superimposed PIH.

Other terms used for hypertension associated with pregnancy are toxemia, preeclampsia-eclampsia, and metabolic disease of late pregnancy.

Etiology

The exact cause of PIH is unknown; however, several theories explain aspects of the disorder. Geographic, ethnic, racial, nutritional, immunologic, and familial factors may play a role in its development, as they do in the development of hypertension in other periods of life.

PIH originally was thought to be caused by a circulating toxic substance. That theory, which is responsible for the term "toxemia of pregnancy," has not been proven; therefore, the term is factually incorrect even though it is frequently used (Cunningham, MacDonald, and Gant, 1989).

H.E.L.L.P. SYNDROME

HELLP is a constellation of signs and symptoms which include hemolysis, elevated liver enzymes, and low platelet count (Weinstein, 1982.) This condition is associated with both a high maternal mortality rate (ranges from 0% to 24%) as well as perinatal mortality rate (ranges reported from 17.7% to 60%) (Sibai, 1990). Maternal complications resulting from this syndrome can include disseminated intravascular clotting (DIC), abruptio placentae, acute renal failure, pulmonary edema, and ruptured liver hematoma. Abruptio placentae, intrauterine asphyxia, and extreme prematurity are cited as the primary causes of perinatal death. One third of these infants are severely growth restricted in utero. (Sibai, et al., 1986).

The etiology of this condition is poorly understood. There does not appear to be a precipitating cause. A review of the medical literature indicates professional confusion over terminology, incidence, cause, diagnosis and management of this complex syndrome (Sibai, 1990).

Its precursor, preeclampsia, is usually associated with arteriolar vasospasm, pathologic vascular lesions within multitple organ systems such as the liver, kidneys, cerebrum and placental bed as well as activation of abnormal coagulation. (Barron, 1991). Hypertension and proteinuria do not always occur prior to the onset of HELLP (Sibai, 1990). Accompanying the pathologic changes of preeclampsia, Roberts, et al. (1989) hypothesized that an insult in the maternal system could lead to intravascular platelet activation and agglutination in addition to microvascular endothelial damage. A cycle of vascular endothelial damage leading to platelet agglutination and aggregation with further endothelial injury would then be established. This vascular damage creates the hemolysis (breakdown of red blood cells), referred to as microangiopathic hemolytic anemia, with subsequent ischemia and tissue damage especially within the liver. Although this syndrome usually manifests itself in the third trimester, it has been reported as early as twenty weeks gestation and as late as 48 hours postpartum. (Georgiew, Skortcheva, and Abadjiew, 1990).

The only effective treatment is prompt delivery. These severely compromised clients require tertiary care and aggressive medical management in order to have a successful outcome.

Incidence

The incidence of PIH ranges from 7% to 10% (Rodgers, Taylor, and Roberts, 1988). Factors that predispose a woman to PIH are:

- *Primigravidity.* Most women who develop PIH are pregnant for the first time. The incidence is especially high in those under age 17 or over age 35 (Gavette and Roberts, 1987).
- *Multiple gestation.* The incidence of PIH increases with the number of fetuses.

- *Vascular disease.* Especially associated with PIH are diabetes mellitus, hypertensive renal disease, or essential hypertension.
- *Gestational trophoblastic disease (hydatidiform mole).* The hypertensive syndrome usually appears before 20 weeks' gestation if associated with GTD.
- *Malnutrition or dietary deficiencies.* Deficiencies in proteins and in water-soluble vitamins frequently are associated with the development of PIH (Belizian and Villar, 1980; DeAlvarez, 1978).

As noted, PIH is one of the three major causes of maternal morbidity. Mortality figures in developing countries are 5% to 17% for the mother and 15% to 37% for the fetus. Mortality figures for developed countries are 0.5% to 1% for the mother and 8% to 10% for the fetus when eclampsia, a complication of PIH, occurs (Zuspan and Zuspan, 1986).

ASSESSMENT

Question the client with a hypertensive disorder about the length of her pregnancy because PIH typically occurs after 20 weeks' gestation. Also ascertain if in a previous pregnancy she had elevated blood pressure, proteinuria, or edema in her face, hands, feet, or legs. Ask her if she has vascular spasms, headaches, epigastric pain, visual disturbances, or irritability.

Physical examination will disclose the three classic signs of PIH: elevated blood pressure, proteinuria, and edema—especially of the face (evidenced by puffy eyes, coarse features, and a broad nose). When assessing a client with preeclampsia, weigh her daily, measure urine output every 8 to 12 hours (hourly if necessary), and assess for proteinuria using a reagent strip. Also assess for other indicators of PIH.

Evaluate the client for edema in her legs, hands, and face. To assess for edema, depress the client's skin over a bony prominence, such as the shin bone. In pitting edema, a depression remains in the skin and subcutaneous tissue after the pressure has been removed. The depth of the depression indicates the degree of pitting, which is classified as 1+, 2+, 3+, or 4+. A minor depression that disappears rather quickly indicates 1+ pitting; 4+ indicates a deep depression (approximately 2 cm) that remains for an extended period.

Assessment of deep tendon reflexes (DTRs) may indicate hypo- or hyperreflexia. Elicit the patellar (knee-jerk), biceps, and ankle reflexes. (For additional information, see Psychomotor Skills: *Deep tendon reflexes and ankle clonus.*)

Reflexes should be checked every 4 to 8 hours, depending on the client's condition.

NURSING DIAGNOSIS

After considering all assessment findings, formulate appropriate nursing diagnoses for the client. (For a partial list of applicable diagnoses, see Nursing Diagnoses: *Antepartal complications,* pages 129 and 130.)

PLANNING AND IMPLEMENTATION

Bed rest is prescribed for the client with a hypertensive disorder. Instruct the client to assume a left lateral position to increase renal and uterine perfusion. Increased renal perfusion facilitates diuresis. Other positions may compromise renal and uterine blood flow through compression of the vena cava and aorta. (For more information, see *Drugs used to treat pregnancy-induced hypertension,* page 156.)

Mild preeclampsia

Nursing care is aimed at improving or stabilizing the client. The client may remain at home as long as edema and proteinuria do not increase. A physician, clinical specialist, or nurse practitioner must assess the client at least weekly to determine changes in her condition. As term approaches, data about fetal maturity and cervical status are required in case labor must be induced. For a nursing diagnosis of *knowledge deficit related to hypertensive condition,* teach the client to keep an accurate daily record of weight. She should report a weight gain of more than 1 lb/day. In addition, carefully explain to the client and her family the signs that indicate a deterioration in her condition, such as severe headache, rapid rise in blood pressure, epigastric pain, hyperreflexia (muscle twitching), edema, decreased urine output, or visual disturbances. Instruct her to report such signs to the physician immediately. The client may have a nursing diagnosis of *impaired physical mobility related to prescribed bed rest or constipation related to bed rest.* She must remain on bed rest and maintain a well-balanced, high-protein and high-fiber diet. Protein requirements are 70 to 80 g of protein/day (1 g/kg of body weight/day). The diet must contain adequate fiber and fluids because limited exercise can cause constipation.

The prescribed regimen may become boring and stressful for the client. Family members need to be involved because home management and child care must be assumed by someone else for the remainder of the pregnancy. Diversion is necessary for both the client and young

PSYCHOMOTOR SKILLS

DEEP TENDON REFLEXES AND ANKLE CLONUS

The deep tendon reflexes (DTRs) and ankle clonus provide an important physical sign for the client with pregnancy-induced hypertension. Abnormal DTRs and positive ankle clonus are precursors of seizures and must receive immediate intervention. If reflexes are 4 +, the client will need anticonvulsant therapy; notify the physician immediately. A 3 + reflex indicates that the client is responding to therapy; however, she still will need to be assessed every 4 hours. A 2 + response is normal, indicating that a therapeutic level of medication has been reached. A 1 +

reflex should prompt the nurse to notify the physician of medical treatment changes. Anticipate reduction of anticonvulsant therapy. An absent reflex (0) indicates that a toxic level of anticonvulsant (usually magnesium sulfate) has been reached. Stop the infusion, change the I.V. to "keep vein open" (I.V. rate to maintain patency of I.V. therapy with a solution, such as dextrose 5% in water), notify the physician immediately, and prepare an antidote (50 ml of 10% calcium gluconate) for injection.

Patellar reflex

To elicit the patellar reflex, have the client sit on the bed with one knee flexed and the lower leg dangling over the side. Tap the patellar tendon directly with a reflex hammer. A negative response may indicate depression of reflexes or that the client is not sufficiently relaxed. If she is unable to sit up, place an arm under her knees and raise. She must remain relaxed for an accurate tendon response.

Biceps reflex

To elicit the biceps reflex, flex the client's elbow and place a thumb across the tendon in the antecubital space while supporting her arm with the fingers of the same hand. The reflex hammer will strike the nurse's thumb directly over the tendon. A positive reflex is a slight flexion of the elbow; the nurse will feel a contraction of the tendon under the thumb.

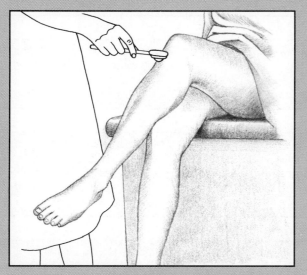

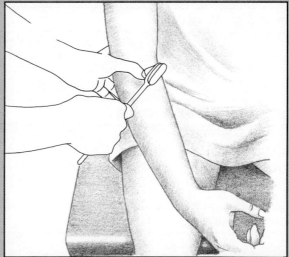

Ankle clonus

To assess ankle clonus, use one hand to support the client's leg with the knee flexed. With the other hand, sharply dorsiflex the foot. Hold in position for a moment, then release. The normal (negative clonus) response is no rhythmic jerking of the foot while it is being dorsiflexed or after release. An abnormal (positive clonus) response is rhythmic jerking of the foot while dorsiflexed as well as when the foot returns to a plantar flexion upon release.

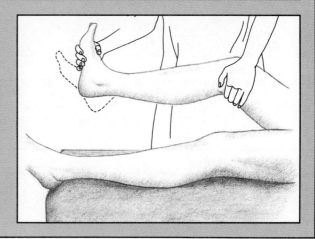

children in the family. Preschoolers cannot understand why their mother stays in bed all day. Ensure that the client and her family understand all aspects of the regimen and why they are necessary. A nursing diagnosis of *ineffective family coping: compromised, related to prolonged bed rest of the mother* may be appropriate in this situation.

Severe preeclampsia

Treatment includes bed rest in a left lateral position. Keep the environment quiet, with minimal stimulation and dim lighting, and follow these procedures.

• Assess vital signs and deep tendon reflexes at least every 4 hours. Record weight daily; measure urine output ev-

ery 1 to 4 hours according to the client's status. The client should maintain a high-carbohydrate, low-fat, 70- to 100-g protein diet with 2 g of sodium/day.

• Perform fundoscopic examinations daily to detect arteriolar spasms, edema, and hemorrhage. Administer sedatives as prescribed. Use a fetal and uterine contraction monitor for signs of labor and fetal well-being.

• If the client's condition improves within 3 to 5 days (for example, if urine output increases or weight decreases by 2 kg or more), further therapy will depend on the gestational age of the fetus. If the fetus is at 38 weeks' gestation or less, the client can be discharged to home care. Instruct her to record the frequency of fetal movement for 1-hour periods, 2 to 3 times daily.

DRUGS USED TO TREAT PREGNANCY-INDUCED HYPERTENSION

This chart summarizes the major drugs used to treat pregnancy-induced hypertension.

MECHANISM OF ACTION	USUAL DOSAGE	NURSING IMPLICATIONS
methyldopa (Aldomet)		
Stimulates central inhibitory alpha-adrenergic receptors; reduces plasma renin activity	Oral: 250 mg t.i.d.; may increase to 500 mg I.V.: initially, three 5 mg boluses 2 minutes apart	• May cause false-positive direct Coombs' test result, sodium retention, constipation, drowsiness
propranolol hydrochloride (Inderal)		
Nonselective beta-adrenergic blocking agent; principally affects myocardial (beta$_1$), bronchial, and vascular smooth muscle (beta$_2$) receptors; may block renin release	Initial I.V.: bolus 0.5 to 3 mg, slow push (do not exceed I mg/minute); may repeat initial dose after 2 minutes Maintenance I.V.: infuse at 2 to 3 mg/hr	• May cause bradycardia, hypotension, short-term memory loss, emotional lability, nausea, vomiting, dry mouth • May potentiate effects of insulin; effects potentiated by furosemide
magnesium sulfate		
Anticonvulsant; prevents and controls seizures in preeclampsia and eclampsia	I.M.: 4 to 5 grams of 50% solution in each buttock I.V.: 4 grams in 250 ml D$_5$W; follow with 1 gram q hr for maintenance	• May cause hypotension, drowsiness, sweating, absent or diminished reflexes, oliguria, respiratory paralysis • Observe deep tendon reflexes every 4 hours. If absent, discontinue medication and notify physician immediately.
labetolol (Trandate, Normodyne)		
Nonselective beta-adrenergic blocking agent	Initial I.V. or oral: 200 mg/day in 2 doses Maintenance: 400 to 800 mg/day in 2 doses	• May cause orthostatic hypotension and dizziness • Check hourly urine output. If below 30 ml/hour, notify physician.
atenolol (Tenormin)		
Selective inhibition of cardiac and lipolytic beta-adrenergic receptors	Oral: 50 mg/day; may increase to 100 mg/day	• May cause bradycardia, hypotension, congestive heart failure • Teach patient to take drug at regular time every day. Monitor blood pressure frequently.

If no improvement is noted, hyperreflexia occurs, the fetus is at 38 weeks' gestation or more, or the lecithin/sphingomyelin (L/S) ratio is appropriate, the physician may elect delivery.

Nursing care for the client with severe preeclampsia is aimed at:
• preventing eclampsia and seizures
• maternal survival with minimal morbidity
• birth of as mature a neonate as possible
• no significant postdelivery complications.

Continue to provide the same monitoring and care that the client received before she was hospitalized. In addition, prepare emergency equipment as soon as the client is admitted in case eclampsia occurs. Emergency equipment should include medications, suctioning apparatus, and in some cases, padded side rails on the client's bed.

Keep emergency anticonvulsant and antihypertensive medications available; these include magnesium sulfate, methyldopa, hydralazine, and propranolol hydrochloride. Be aware of the mechanism of action, usual dosage, and special considerations for each of these medications.

Eclampsia

Hyperreflexia is common just before seizures in the client with preeclampsia. Eclampsia is a complication of PIH. It is preceded by the signs of severe preeclampsia and one or both of the following:
• Tonic (normal tone of muscles) and clonic (alternating between involuntary muscle contraction and relaxation in rapid succession) seizures.
• Hypertensive crisis, in which blood pressure is elevated to such a degree that the client has an increased chance of developing a cerebrovascular accident or shock.

Tonic-clonic seizures are followed by hypotension and collapse and, in many cases, nystagmus, muscle twitching, and coma. Oliguria or anuria also may occur. Disorientation and amnesia delay immediate recovery.

The nurse's first priority during seizures is to ensure a patent airway, then to provide adequate oxygenation.

EVALUATION

To evaluate nursing care, determine if specific goals were achieved. The following examples illustrate some appropriate evaluation statements:
• The client with mild preeclampsia shows a 2-pound weight gain, no proteinuria, and a diastolic blood pressure of 84 mm Hg this visit.
• The client kept all appointments for prenatal care and laboratory tests.

• The client reported a change in her condition as soon as it occurred.
• The client's family demonstrated support and concern.

Rh INCOMPATIBILITY

Hemolytic disease of the newborn, also called erythroblastosis fetalis, is a progressive disorder of the fetal blood and blood-forming organs characterized by hemolytic anemia and hyperbilirubinemia. Erythroblastosis fetalis results from the transfer of red blood cell (RBC)-destroying antibodies from the mother to the fetus. (For more information, see Neonatal Status: *Monitoring when the client and neonate have an Rh incompatibility,* page 158.)

The more severe forms of isoimmune hemolytic disease are associated with $Rh_o(D)$ group incompatibility. Before prophylactic $Rh_o(D)$ human immunoglobulin (RhIg) became available in 1968, this disease occurred in 0.5% to 1% of all term pregnancies in North America. Since immunization with RhIg began, however, the incidence of severe hemolytic disease of the newborn has been reduced drastically (Scott, 1986a).

Etiology

Hemolytic diseases of the newborn, such as erythroblastosis fetalis, hydrops fetalis, and icterus gravis, were found to be linked to the Rh factor. These hemolytic disorders are caused by the hemolysis of fetal RBCs by maternal antibodies. Later research indicated that approximately 90% of clinical cases of hemolytic diseases in neonates followed maternal sensitization (isoimmunization) by Rh antigens (Scott, 1986a). The Rh-negative mother was sensitized by her fetus's Rh-positive RBCs, inherited from the Rh-positive father. (For more information on other hemolytic diseases, see *Other RBC antigen incompatibilities,* page 159.)

Theoretically, maternal isoimmunization also could be caused by a transfusion with Rh-positive or D^u-positive blood. This type of isoimmunization is rare, however, because typing and crossmatching are performed routinely before blood administration. A positive D^u factor would be identified at initial screening and that blood would be labeled as Rh positive (Lloyd, 1987).

Incidence

Almost 65% of the neonates of Rh-incompatible couples are Rh positive. Ten percent to 15% of Caucasian couples will be affected by Rh incompatibility. About 5% of Black couples will be Rh incompatible, and only rarely will an Oriental couple be affected (Scott, 1986a). This difference

NEONATAL STATUS

MONITORING WHEN THE CLIENT AND NEONATE HAVE AN Rh INCOMPATIBILITY

When a client has an Rh incompatibility, neonatal status must be monitored closely through neonatal blood studies and physical assessment, including assessment of the placenta.

Neonatal cord blood studies at delivery
- *Blood type and Rh.* These tests indicate the need, if any, for further assessment of maternal antibody formation.
- *Direct Coombs' test on neonatal cord blood.* This test determines the presence of maternal antibodies attached to the neonate's red blood cells (RBCs). A washed suspension of the neonate's RBCs obtained from the umbilical cord is mixed with Coombs' serum (serum containing antiglobulin). The test is positive—that is, maternal antibodies are present—if the neonate's RBCs agglutinate (clump).
- *Hemoglobin level and hematocrit.* Progressive hemolytic anemia reflects increased production of RBCs (erythropoiesis) as indicated by shifts in hemoglobin level and hematocrit as well as by an increased number of immature RBCs.
- *Blood glucose level.* Increased erythropoiesis increases blood glucose use. Hypoglycemia in the neonate must be recognized and treated early.
- *Indirect or direct serum bilirubin level.* Elevated levels of indirect bilirubin indicate hemolysis of RBCs, which frees bilirubin in the serum.

Postdelivery assessment
- *Yellow-stained vernix (cheeselike covering on the neonate) or umbilical cord.* Evidence of edema (hydrops fetalis), respiratory distress (nasal flaring, intercostal retractions), and alterations in heart rate (bradycardia, tachycardia) or rhythm (arrhythmias) may indicate pleural or pericardial effusions. Pleural or pericardial effusions and ascites indicate cardiac failure.
- *Placental enlargement.* The weight of the placenta is normally one-sixth that of the neonate. In hemolytic disease, the placenta may weigh as much as one-half to three-quarters that of the neonate.
- *Hepatosplenomegaly.* Liver and spleen enlargement indicates increased demands for disposal of bilirubin and increased erythropoiesis.
- *Neonatal pallor with jaundice.* Pallor is caused by RBC hemolysis; jaundice, by increased bilirubin levels. Jaundice typically appears within 24 to 36 hours of birth.
- *Central nervous system manifestations of kernicterus.* These include twitching, irritability, and high-pitched cry.

of incidence among races is related to the proportion of Rh-positive and Rh-negative individuals in each group. For example, Caucasians have a higher proportion of Rh-negative individuals than do Blacks, so they have a greater chance of Rh incompatibility.

The risk of maternal sensitization is less than may be expected. The factors involved include the antigenicity of the antigen, the amount of antigen infused, and the mother's immunologic response to the antigen (Lloyd, 1987). Some clients have a greater antigenic response to the Rh factor. Only about 0.1% of mothers are sensitized during a first Rh-positive pregnancy. The risk of isoimmunization increases with the number of pregnancies if treatment with RhIg is not instituted. About 5% of Rh-incompatible pregnancies produce affected neonates (Scott, 1986a).

Maternal effects from Rh incompatibility have not been identified; however, severe Rh incompatibility results in erythroblastosis fetalis. When fetal blood reacts to the Rh-positive antibodies of the mother, fetal RBCs are destroyed (hemolysis) and fetal hemolytic anemia results. The released blood pigments, or bilirubin, are transported across the placenta, processed by the maternal liver, and excreted in the bile. When the amount of pigments is greater than the maternal liver can process, the neonate will be icteric (jaundiced) at birth. Hyperplasia of the bone marrow and extramedullary (spleen) hematopoiesis occur as fetal compensatory mechanisms to offset fetal anemia, which can lead to cardiac decompensation, cardiomegaly, hepatomegaly, and splenomegaly. A syndrome of generalized edema and ascites known as hydrops fetalis may result. At this point, the fetus will be at serious risk for intrauterine or early neonatal death.

The placenta of the seriously affected fetus is enlarged. The amniotic fluid may be stained a yellowish color from bile pigments. Following delivery, the erythroblastotic neonate becomes icteric because the neonate cannot excrete the bile pigments resulting from RBC hemolysis. Icterus neonatorum (jaundice in the neonate) can occur soon after birth in severe cases.

Generalized pigmentation of brain cells (kernicterus) commonly develops when the serum bilirubin rises to levels that are toxic to the neonate and can lead to death. Serious central nervous system abnormalities, such as choreoathetoid cerebral palsy, may develop and persist if the neonate survives.

Rh hemolytic disease of the neonate occurs once in approximately 150 to 200 full-term pregnancies in the United States (Scott, 1986a). At least 200,000 children are affected each year; 5,000 of these are stillborn. In cases of untreated severe hemolytic disease, about 10% of affected neonates will develop kernicterus. With intra-

OTHER R.B.C. ANTIGEN INCOMPATIBILITIES

Fetal-maternal incompatibility of ABO groups also may cause hemolytic disease. The blood type of a person who has red blood cells (RBCs) with neither the A antigen nor the B antigen is designated as group O. Blood of individuals with group O contains anti-A and anti-B antibodies. Therefore, the group O mother who is pregnant with a fetus whose blood group is A, B, or AB has anti-A and anti-B antibodies that may be stimulated by the pregnancy and may be transferred across the placenta to her fetus. In ABO incompatibility, even the first child can be affected.

The largest percentage of neonates who are affected by ABO incompatibility has blood group A and mothers with blood group O. Black neonates are more likely to develop ABO incompatibility than Caucasian neonates (Cunningham, MacDonald, and Gant, 1989).

The clinical manifestations of fetal-maternal ABO incompatibility typically are mild and short-lasting. However, severe hemolysis with resultant hyperbilirubinemia and kernicterus is possible. No preventive agent is known for use in ABO incompatibility. Treatment of affected neonates is symptomatic, involving phototherapy and increased fluids.

Other, less common RBC antigens also are capable of transplacental isoimmunization. Fortunately, isoimmunization related to these antigens is not common, and serious fetal injury from these factors is unlikely.

uterine (fetal) transfusions, however, that number can be reduced by about 40%. Amniocentesis studies, early delivery of affected fetuses, and exchange or replacement transfusions have decreased the mortality rate.

Complete recovery can be expected in neonates who do not develop kernicterus. If hyperbilirubinemia is treated promptly and effectively, most neonates recover without residual effects or sequelae.

ASSESSMENT

Gather data focusing on previous pregnancies, especially those that ended in abortion. Note any blood replacement therapy the client has received previously.

The physical assessment may not be significant for a client with Rh incompatibility, but diagnostic studies are important. Blood type for ABO and Rh factor is established early in pregnancy to identify a client at risk for isoimmune hemolytic disease. Maternal isoimmunization is probable when antibody screening tests on maternal serum at around 20 weeks' gestation are positive. If the first test is negative, it should be repeated at 32 to 36 weeks. For the indirect Coombs' test, maternal blood serum is mixed with Rh-positive RBCs. In a positive test,

the red cells become coated with Rh antibodies. The dilution of the blood at which this occurs determines the titer or level of maternal antibodies, and the titer indicates the degree of maternal sensitization. If the titer reaches 1:16, an amniocentesis to measure the amount of bilirubin in the amniotic fluid is performed after 36 weeks' gestation.

NURSING DIAGNOSIS

After considering all assessment findings, formulate appropriate nursing diagnoses for the client. (For a partial list of applicable diagnoses, see Nursing Diagnoses: *Antepartal complications,* pages 129 and 130.)

PLANNING AND IMPLEMENTATION

Prophylaxis for Rh isoimmunization requires the use of RhIg. RhIg is not a treatment for isoimmunization because it has no effect against antibodies present in the maternal bloodstream. It provides passive immunity, which is transient and therefore will not affect a subsequent pregnancy. RhIg also prepares RBCs containing the Rh antigen for destruction by phagocytes before the client's immune system is activated to produce antibodies (active immunity). Antibodies formed by an active immune response remain within the individual's bloodstream, presumably for life. RhIg given to an $Rh_o(D)$-negative client who already is sensitized would accomplish nothing. Therefore, RhIg is recommended only for Rh-negative clients at risk for developing Rh isoimmunization. It should not be given to an Rh-positive client because the Rh antibodies could destroy her Rh-positive RBC.

The American College of Obstetricians and Gynecologists (1986) recommendations for RhIg are as follows:
- RhIg is given after delivery or abortion only to a client who is Rh negative and D^u negative, has not already developed isoimmunization, and whose fetus is $Rh_o(D)$ positive or D^u positive. (In a D^u-positive individual, RBCs display a weak positive reaction when tested with standard Rh-typing serums.) RhIg is never given to the neonate or the neonate's father.
- RhIg is not useful for a client who has Rh antibodies.
- RhIg should be administered intramuscularly, not subcutaneously or intravenously.

Assure the Rh-negative client with a nursing diagnosis of *fear related to unknown effect of blood incompatibility on the fetus* that in over 95% of cases, administering RhIg within 72 hours of evacuation of the uterus (by delivery or abortion) prevents isoimmunization to the Rh factor in her fetus.

Rh sensitization also is possible during pregnancy if the cellular layer separating the maternal and fetal circulations is disrupted and fetal blood enters the maternal bloodstream. The cellular layer may be disrupted during amniocentesis or by abruptio placentae.

For the client who is $Rh_o(D)$ negative and RhD^u negative and who has not already formed Rh antibodies, RhIg administered at about 28 weeks' gestation and again within 72 hours after delivery can help prevent Rh isoimmunization.

EVALUATION

To evaluate nursing care, determine if specific goals were achieved. The following examples illustrate some appropriate evaluation statements:

- The client correctly described the potential effects of her condition on herself and on her fetus and neonate.
- The client and her family actively participated in planning care and activities during and after the pregnancy.

SPONTANEOUS ABORTION

Abortion is the termination of a pregnancy at any time before the age of viability. Viability is reached at about 24 weeks' gestation and a weight of over 500 grams, when the fetus is able to survive in an extrauterine environment (Beischer and MacKay, 1986). An abortion may be spontaneous, or the pregnancy may be terminated for medical or therapeutic reasons or for other elective reasons.

The nurse should keep in mind the negative connotations of "abortion" for many people. For this reason, people commonly refer to a spontaneous abortion as a "miscarriage."

An early spontaneous abortion is one that occurs before 12 weeks' gestation; a late abortion, between 12 and 20 weeks' gestation. Births after 20 weeks are considered preterm (Creasy, 1989). Almost 80% of all spontaneous abortions occur before 12 weeks' gestation; of those, the majority occur before 8 weeks (Scott, 1986). Recurrent or habitual abortion is the loss of three of more pregnancies before the age of viability. Such repeated losses can be caused by genetic factors (chromosomal aberrations), anomalies of the reproductive tract (double uterus and its variants), an incompetent cervix, endocrine imbalances (such as hypothyroidism or diabetes mellitus), or systemic disorders (such as lupus erythematosus).

Etiology

A majority of spontaneously aborted fetuses display a problem with implantation or an abnormal genetic or chromosomal makeup that is not compatible with life; the remaining spontaneous abortions result from maternal causes (Beischer and MacKay, 1986). The latter may occur because of an acute infection, such as syphilis, pyelonephritis, or chlamydia trachomatis infection. Abnormalities of the reproductive system are common maternal causes of pregnancy loss during the second and third trimesters. A woman whose mother took diethylstilbestrol (DES) during pregnancy may have spontaneous abortions.

Anything that might interfere with normal ovum implantation and placental development may be related to spontaneous abortion. For example, implantation of the fertilized ovum and placental development can be inhibited by scar tissue on the endometrium, which could result from dilatation and curettage (D&C), previous childbirth, or severe infection. Alterations in hormones, such as progesterone, also may be related to pregnancy loss (Key, 1989).

The risk of early pregnancy loss is increased in women who have a history of first trimester pregnancy loss, uterine defects, chronic infections, or cigarette or alcohol abuse (Deutchman, 1989).

Little can be done to avoid genetic causes of spontaneous abortion. Certain other causes, however, can be prevented. Prepregnancy correction of maternal disorders, immunization against infectious diseases, proper early prenatal care, and prompt treatment of complications of pregnancy can prevent many spontaneous abortions.

Incidence

The exact incidence of spontaneous abortion is difficult to calculate because many early pregnancies are lost for unknown reasons before they are clinically evident. At least 15% of all pregnancies are known to end in spontaneous abortion. However, recent research into the first few days and weeks after conception indicates that the spontaneous abortion rate is far higher than 15%. Researchers postulate that if every woman were continually monitored, the rate might approach 50% (Key, 1989; Scott, 1986).

Classification

According to Key (1989), abortions can be classified according to weight; that is, whether the fetus weighs 500 grams or less. (For a complete classification, see *Assessing different types of abortion.*)

ASSESSING DIFFERENT TYPES OF ABORTION

The nurse must assess the different types of abortion accurately to provide adequate nursing care and emotional support.

DEFINITION	PHYSICAL FINDINGS	MANAGEMENT
Threatened		
Appearance of signs and symptoms of possible loss of embryo	*Bleeding:* slight *Cramping:* mild and intermittent *Expelled tissue:* none *Internal cervical os:* closed *Uterus size:* varies according to length of gestation	Bed rest; sedation; decreased stress; no sexual intercourse, douches, or cathartics. Further treatment depends on specific signs and symptoms. (Blood replacement therapy, I.V. therapy, and antibiotics may be indicated.)
Inevitable (imminent)		
Signs and symptoms indicate certain loss of embryo	*Bleeding:* slight *Cramping:* mild and intermittent *Expelled tissues:* none *Internal cervical os:* open *Uterus size:* varies according to length of gestation	Prompt termination of pregnancy by dilatation and curettage (D&C)
Incomplete		
Part of the products of conception retained in the uterus	*Bleeding:* heavy *Cramping:* severe *Expelled tissues:* some *Internal cervical os:* open *Uterus size:* smaller than expected for length of gestation	Prompt termination of pregnancy by D&C or suction curettage
Complete		
All products of conception expelled from uterus	*Bleeding:* slight to moderate *Cramping:* mild to moderate *Expelled tissues:* all products of conception *Internal cervical os:* closed *Uterus size:* smaller than expected for length of gestation	No intervention needed unless hemorrhage or infection develops
Missed		
Nonviable fetus and other products of conception retained in uterus for 2 months or longer	*Bleeding:* slight *Cramping:* none *Expelled tissues:* none *Internal cervical os:* closed *Uterus size:* smaller than expected for length of gestation	If spontaneous evacuation of the uterus does not occur within 1 month, pregnancy will be terminated. Method of termination will depend on the length of gestation. Client must be monitored for signs of disseminated intravascular coagulation, which may develop if the products of conception remain in the uterus after 5 weeks.
Septic		
Infection of products of conception and endometrial lining of uterus, which may result from attempted interference early in pregnancy	*Bleeding:* varies; malodorous *Cramping:* varies *Expelled tissue:* varies, depending on whether tissue fragments remain *Internal cervical os:* usually open *Uterus size:* varies but will be tender *Other:* fever	Immediate termination of pregnancy by D&C; cervical cultures and sensitivities performed; broad spectrum antibiotic administered; temperature monitored

ASSESSMENT

Signs and symptoms of spontaneous abortion depend on the development of the implantation site, determined by the length of gestation. The three stages of development of the implantation site are:

- *Early (or decidual).* The fertilized ovum, surrounded by decidua, is poorly attached to the uterus. The early stage covers the first 6 weeks of gestation.
- *Intermediate (or attachment).* Chorionic villi in the basal plate of the decidua attach moderately well to the decidua basalis. The intermediate stage extends from 6 to 12 weeks of gestation.
- *Late (or placental).* After 12 weeks of gestation, the placenta is fully formed and firmly attached to the decidua basalis.

During the early stage of placental development, the symptoms of abortion are not severe; bleeding and cramping are minimal. During the intermediate stage, moderate cramping and blood loss are expected because the ovum and its surrounding tissues are larger and more firmly attached to the uterus. Severe pain is associated with a late abortion because the fetus must be expelled. Abdominal cramping, similar to labor, is usual. The amount of bleeding, however, is less than with an intermediate-stage abortion because the placenta remains attached until after the fetus has been delivered. Bleeding is more controlled because of strong uterine contractions.

A client who has a late-stage abortion may experience breast engorgement and lactation. Alterations in hormonal levels subsequent to pregnancy also may be responsible for a labile emotional state (Beischer and MacKay, 1986).

A pregnancy may have been terminated for several days before signs and symptoms become definite. For this reason, the exact date of termination can be difficult to determine. The following laboratory findings are characteristic of abortion.

- *Urine.* A negative or weakly positive urine pregnancy test.
- *Blood.* If blood loss is excessive or prolonged, anemia is probable (hemoglobin level below than 10.5 g/dl or hematocrit less than 32 g/dl). If sepsis occurs following a missed or incomplete abortion (in which portions of the products of conception remain in the uterus), the white blood cell (WBC) count will be greater than 12,000/mm³. (The sedimentation rate will increase with abortion, anemia, or infection and therefore is not useful for diagnostic purposes.)
- *Endocrine.* The hCG, estrogen, and progesterone titers can be minimal in abortions (Cunningham, MacDonald, and Gant, 1989).

A detailed, accurate history focusing on the client's recent health, menstrual, gynecologic, and obstetric history, contraceptive method used, and possible date of conception is necessary for a complete diagnostic evaluation. In addition to obtaining the health history, gather all pertinent information related to the client's physical state. Assess the amount and consistency of blood to determine whether any products of conception have been passed. To help refine the diagnosis, obtain complete pain information, including location, type, and duration.

NURSING DIAGNOSIS

After considering all assessment findings, formulate appropriate nursing diagnoses for the client. (For a partial list of applicable diagnoses, see Nursing Diagnoses: *Antepartal complications,* pages 129 and 130.)

PLANNING AND IMPLEMENTATION

After assessing the client with antepartal complications and formulating nursing diagnoses, the nurse develops and implements a plan of care centering on the following common nursing goals:

- promoting the physical well-being of the client and her fetus
- preventing or controlling further complications
- preventing sequelae
- providing emotional support to the client and her family.

A client with suspected abortion should be referred to a physician immediately because emergency medical intervention may be needed to decrease complications. The client may have a nursing diagnosis of *denial related to impending loss of pregnancy.* To care for this client, save all expelled tissues and clots; maintain a calm, confident, and sympathetic manner; alert the physician to pertinent signs and history (for example, vital signs and amounts of bleeding); and encourage bed rest. Expect to administer sedatives and analgesics. Rest will decrease bleeding, and the medications will ease the client's anxiety. Try to stay with the client, and provide comfort measures usually associated with labor (such as a back rub and a cool cloth for her forehead). The client may be sensitive to any suggestion that she has somehow caused the abortion. The nurse will need to be sensitive to this feeling of vulnerability and be cautious when caring for the family to avoid increasing anxiety. Prepare the client physically and emotionally for D&C, if indicated.

After an abortion, the client may have a nursing diagnosis of *anticipatory grieving related to loss of pregnancy.* To care for this client, provide emotional support, and answer all questions or clarify any information for the client and her family. Question the client and family about family needs and coping mechanisms. Notify clergy to visit and baptize the products of conception, if the client wishes. Religious beliefs directly influence the client's and her family's expectations of care. Accommodating such needs within the facility's constraints enhances care.

Teach the client to wear a comfortable support bra to reduce discomfort from breast engorgement, which may produce anxiety and also will need appropriate intervention (dependent on the physician's orders and the client's preference). Administer RhIg within 72 hours if the client is Rh negative and has not formed Rh antibodies from a previous Rh-positive pregnancy. This medication prevents the formation of maternal anti-Rh antibodies and thereby protects against sensitization from an Rh-positive fetus in future pregnancies. Monitor I.V. infusion and vital signs before, during, and after this procedure. Assess the hemodynamics of the client to maintain her optimal health.

Management of an abortion depends on its type and on the extent of the client's symptoms. An incomplete abortion may be followed by a D&C to remove the remaining tissues. The physician uses dilators to open the cervix and then performs suction curettage. Analgesics or general or local anesthetics may be used. Intravenous oxytocin, in a dextrose 5% in water intravenous solution, may be required to induce uterine contractions. Because retained placental fragments can cause the uterus to remain relaxed following the abortion, the uterine muscles may not constrict uterine vessels, causing hemorrhage during or after the procedure. Additional oxytocin infusion may be required to prevent hemorrhage.

Ergot products, such as methylergonovine, that cause uterine and cervical contractions are contraindicated until the uterus is empty. This reduces the chance of retaining placental fragments. After the procedure, however, the physician may order three or four doses of ergonovine, orally or intramuscularly, if the client's blood pressure is normal. Blood or antibiotics may be ordered in cases of extreme blood loss, anemia, or infection (Beischer and Mackay, 1986; Scott, 1986).

If the cause of the abortion can be determined and eliminated, the chance for a future normal pregnancy is excellent. If no complications (such as infection or hemorrhage) occur, the abortion probably will have no detrimental physical effects on the client.

EVALUATION

To evaluate nursing care, determine if specific goals were achieved. The following examples illustrate some appropriate evaluation statements:
• The client has verbalized understanding of the necessity for having a D&C after a spontaneous abortion.
• The client and family have verbalized feelings of loss appropriately.
• The client's family has demonstrated support and concern.

ECTOPIC PREGNANCY

In ectopic pregnancy, the fertilized ovum is implanted in tissue other than the endometrium (lining of the uterus). More than 95% of ectopic pregnancies occur in the fallopian tubes, usually in the ampullary and isthmic segments. Less than 3% of all ectopic pregnancies are intra-abdominal, and less than 1% of these are implanted in cervical or ovarian tissues (Droegemueller, 1986).

Etiology

The majority of extrauterine pregnancies result from impeded progress of the fertilized ovum through the fallopian tube. The primary causes are tubal obstruction and delayed tubal transport (Osguthorpe and Keating, 1988).

A previous episode of pelvic inflammatory disease with accompanying salpingitis (inflammation of the fallopian tubes) commonly is implicated in cases of tubal obstruction. Salpingitis results in mucosal damage, tubal narrowing, diverticula (sacs or pouches in the tubal wall), and also may impair tubal motility (Osguthorpe and Keating, 1988).

Other conditions that predispose a woman to ectopic pregnancy include:
• previous therapeutic abortion or previous abdominal surgery (presence of scar tissue may affect tubal motility)
• use of an intrauterine device (IUD) for more than 2 years, which can cause a low-grade inflammatory response within the fallopian tubes
• in vivo exposure to DES, which can adversely affect tubal motility
• congenital anomalies that interfere with passage of the fertilized ovum or with implantation
• altered hormonal status that affects tubal motility.

Ectopic pregnancy results from fertilization of the ovum before it migrates to the fallopian tube. This delayed

SIGNS AND SYMPTOMS OF UNRUPTURED AND RUPTURED ECTOPIC PREGNANCY

To act decisively, the nurse must be able to distinguish between the signs and symptoms of unruptured and ruptured ectopic pregnancy.

If unruptured
- Unilateral abdominal cramps and tenderness
- Menstrual changes, such as spotting or a missed period
- Low-grade fever (99° to 100° F [37.2° to 37.7° C])
- Normal pulse
- Nausea and vomiting

If ruptured (additional signs and symptoms)
- Abdominal discomfort from blood accumulation in the peritoneal cavity
- Sudden onset of abdominal pain from blood accumulation in the peritoneal cavity or from tubal rupture
- Shocklike state from ruptured tube or excess blood loss
- Shoulder pain from irritation of the diaphragm from blood accumulation
- Rapid, thready pulse from blood loss and hypovolemia
- Cold extremities from excessive blood loss and decreased blood pressure

transport may leave the zygote in the fallopian tube at the time of implantation.

Incidence

Ectopic pregnancy is the leading cause of maternal death in the first trimester. In the United States, it occurs in 10.8 of every 1,000 pregnancies, and it accounts for 11% of all maternal deaths (CDC, 1990; Lawson, et al., 1988). The majority of ectopic pregnancies occur in women ages 25 to 34 (Loffer, 1986).

The incidence of ectopic pregnancy has increased fourfold over the past 21 years (CDC, 1990). The risk is 1.6 times greater for nonwhite women, and maternal mortality is 3.5 times higher for these women.

Common predisposing factors other than age include infertility and a previous ectopic pregnancy. A woman who has an ectopic pregnancy in one fallopian tube is at increased risk for developing an ectopic pregnancy in the opposite tube. Only 1 in 3 women who experience an ectopic pregnancy will give birth to a live neonate in a subsequent pregnancy (Osguthorpe and Keating, 1988).

Classification

Ectopic pregnancies are classified by the site of implantation, such as tubal or ovarian, because the uterus is the only organ capable of maintaining a term pregnancy. Abdominal pregnancies occur once in approximately 15,000 live births; however, the delivery of a live, term neonate from an abdominal pregnancy occurs only once in approximately 250,000 live births. Intra-abdominal pregnancies also are associated with increased maternal mortality caused by uncontrolled hemorrhage and sepsis.

ASSESSMENT

Gather and record such relevant history as occurrence of abdominal surgery, spontaneous or voluntary abortion, or ectopic pregnancy. Note religious preferences should baptism be requested or administration of blood or blood products be necessary.

Observe for abdominal pain, amenorrhea, and abnormal vaginal bleeding. Abdominal pain is the most consistent finding, occurring in over 90% of cases. The quality of pain varies markedly but usually is described as cramplike. Nausea and vomiting also may occur, along with urinary frequency. Signs of ruptured ectopic pregnancy may occur, including pallor, tachycardia, hypotension, and temperature elevation. Adnexal (lower right or left quadrant near ovary) tenderness occurs unilaterally in about 50% of clients. (For additional details, see *Signs and symptoms of unruptured and ruptured ectopic pregnancy*.)

Complicating ectopic pregnancy diagnosis are the numerous disorders that share many, and possibly all, of the same signs and symptoms. These disorders include appendicitis, salpingitis, abortion, ovarian cysts, and urinary tract infections. Because definitive diagnosis is difficult, the condition may become an obstetric emergency if the ectopic pregnancy is unrecognized until the tube ruptures. Many emergency departments admit clients with a ruptured tubal pregnancy without previous signs or symptoms.

Recently developed tests, like the serum test for beta-subunit human chorionic gonadotropin (beta-hCG), have facilitated the diagnosis of ectopic pregnancy. Beta-hCG, a hormone produced by the trophoblastic cells of the developing placenta, can be detected in minute amounts by radioimmunoassay of the hormone in a blood sample 9 days after ovulation (Romero, 1986). It also can be detected quickly, accurately, and inexpensively by sensitive home urine tests for pregnancy.

Physical signs and laboratory tests other than those for beta-HCG have limited diagnostic value unless tubal rupture occurs. A missed period, adnexal tenderness, or a small adnexal mass, for example, may indicate ectopic pregnancy but also can indicate an ovarian or corpus luteum cyst (Osguthorpe and Keating, 1988).

Once a positive pregnancy test has been obtained, an ultrasound can be performed. If a gestational sac is not visible 5 to 6 weeks after the last menstrual period, an ectopic or abnormal intrauterine pregnancy can be suspected. Although ultrasound can be helpful, it is not a definitive diagnostic tool. First, a pseudogestational sac in the uterus occurs in 10% to 20% of clients with ectopic pregnancy. In addition, intrauterine and ectopic pregnancies can coexist (although rarely) so that the identification of one does not automatically rule out the other. Finally, because of their relatively small size, few ectopic pregnancies can be detected by ultrasound (Osguthorpe and Keating, 1988). Ultrasound has been more effective in ruling out an intrauterine pregnancy than in confirming an ectopic one.

A relatively new assessment development for ectopic pregnancy, endovaginal ultrasound may alter the typical approach (Jain, Hamper, and Sanders, 1988). It is performed by placing a transducer at the external opening of the vagina and directing sound waves into the pelvic cavity. In comparison studies, endovaginal ultrasonography has been more sensitive than traditional transabdominal ultrasound in detecting ectopic pregnancies.

A laparoscopy can be performed to confirm a suspected ectopic pregnancy. Because blood is present in the abdominal cavity in about 65% of clients with unruptured ectopic pregnancies and other conditions not requiring laparotomy, laparoscopy is especially helpful in identifying the bleeding sites.

The most effective diagnosis of an ectopic pregnancy combines these three diagnostic tools. Serum hCG levels in conjunction with ultrasonography and laparoscopy provide accurate information without using an invasive procedure.

Culdocentesis-aspiration or incision through the posterior vaginal fornix-also can be performed to detect intraperitoneal bleeding. Retrieval of nonclotting blood is a positive indication of ectopic pregnancy or other peritoneal bleeding (Romero, 1986). Be aware, however, that a negative (clear fluid) or nondiagnostic (no fluid) result does not ensure the absence of an ectopic pregnancy.

NURSING DIAGNOSIS

After considering all assessment findings, formulate appropriate nursing diagnoses for the client. (For a partial list of applicable diagnoses, see Nursing Diagnoses: *Antepartal complications,* pages 129 and 130.)

PLANNING AND IMPLEMENTATION

A client who exhibits the signs and symptoms of ectopic pregnancy may have a nursing diagnosis of *denial related to tubal pregnancy as manifested by minimization of symptoms and use of home remedies to relieve symptoms.* This client also may have subsequent bleeding and a nursing diagnosis of *decreased cardiac output related to bleeding at the site of ectopic pregnancy rupture.* Contact the physician immediately if signs and symptoms occur, and assess vital signs every 15 minutes or as prescribed. Appropriate laboratory data should be gathered, including blood type, CBC, Rh, crossmatch, and serum hCG. Take the following steps for emergency care:
• Prepare for I.V. fluids with port for medication and a large-bore needle to accommodate blood transfusions if needed.
• Have oxygen at hand to prevent hypoxia related to hypovolemia.
• Gather emergency medications and equipment in case of shock.
• Prepare the client for surgery by explaining the procedure, checking to see if her consent has been obtained, administering prescribed preoperative medication, and completing the surgical checklist.
• Keep the client and her family informed.
• Contact clergy to baptize the fetus if desired by the family, and document their wishes.

After surgery, the client may have a nursing diagnosis of *anticipatory grieving related to loss of pregnancy.* If the client is Rh negative, check to determine if antibodies are present in her blood, and prepare to administer RhIg if she has not formed Rh antibodies from an earlier pregnancy with an Rh-positive fetus. Administer fluids, medications, and treatments as prescribed and based on the client's preference and tolerance. Inform the client and her family if the fetus was baptized. Clarify, if necessary, the physician's explanation of cause, management, and recovery, including chances for future pregnancies.

Effective management of ectopic pregnancy is complex. Hemorrhage is the major problem; bleeding must be controlled quickly and effectively. Because extreme blood loss can lead to shock, ensure that sufficient blood is available for transfusions.

Immediately after an ectopic pregnancy is diagnosed, a laparotomy can be performed to remove the products of conception, control blood loss by evacuating blood and clots, and cauterize bleeding vessels. However, according to Silva (1988), a laparoscopy is preferable to an incision because of lower cost and decreased morbidity.

New developments in laparoscopic surgery allow conservative approaches, including using lasers through the laparoscope to excise the affected area of the fallopian tube. Laser surgery decreases damage to the tube and provides a beneficial hemostatic effect (Huber, Hosmann, and Vytiska-Binstorfer, 1989; Modica and Timor-Tritsch, 1988). In many cases, the affected fallopian tube can be repaired and left in place. Salpingectomy, formerly the treatment of choice, now is reserved for cases in which the tube is significantly damaged or when the client does not wish to maintain fertility.

An interstitial ectopic pregnancy—a pregnancy occurring within a segment of the fallopian tube closest to the uterus—presents a diagnostic and management challenge. This rare form of ectopic pregnancy occurs in about 2.5% of all cases. Because of its location and lack of specific signs and symptoms, interstitial ectopic pregnancy typically is diagnosed through laparoscopy after tubal rupture and hemorrhage. With advances in ultrasonography, however, an eccentric location of the gestational sac can be identified (Weissman, Fishman, and Gal, 1989). Laparoscopic surgery to remove the products of conception can be successful if interstitial pregnancy is identified early, before rupture. If identification occurs concurrently with or after rupture, salpingectomy usually is required. Because the location is adjacent to the uterus, damage may result that will require removal of the uterus.

An ovarian pregnancy requires the removal of the affected ovary. An adherent fallopian tube also may require removal (Cunningham, MacDonald, and Gant, 1989).

An advanced ectopic pregnancy, which typically is abdominal, requires a laparotomy as soon as the client is stable and able to withstand surgery. If the placenta in an abdominal pregnancy is attached to a vital organ such as the liver, no attempt is made to separate or remove the placenta. The umbilical cord is cut flush with the placenta and the placenta is left in situ. Degeneration and absorption of the placenta usually occurs without complications. However, placental degeneration can lead to disseminated intravascular coagulation in some individuals.

EVALUATION

To evaluate nursing care, determine if specific goals were achieved. The following examples illustrate some appropriate evaluation statements:

- The client's vital signs have remained stable.
- The client's ectopic pregnancy rupture site pain has been controlled with an analgesic agent.
- The client has verbalized feelings over the loss of the pregnancy.

GESTATIONAL TROPHOBLASTIC DISEASE

Gestational trophoblastic disease (GTD) may be benign (hydatidiform mole) or malignant (choriocarcinoma). In GTD, trophoblastic cells covering the chorionic villi proliferate, and the villi undergo cystic changes.

In benign GTD, a neoplasm forms on the chorion (outer layer of the membrane containing amniotic fluid) when the chorionic villi degenerate and become transparent vesicles that hang in grapelike clusters (Hilgers and Lewis, 1986). These vesicles contain a clear fluid and may involve all or part of the decidual lining of the uterus. Usually no embryo is present because it has been absorbed.

In malignant GTD—a serious, rapidly developing, but rare carcinoma—neoplastic trophoblasts proliferate without cystic villi and may metastasize.

Etiology

The cause of GTD is unknown. (Several theories relate GTD to a nutritional deficit, specifically an insufficient intake of protein. These theories, however, have not been substantiated.) Because no specific etiology has been determined, prevention techniques are unknown.

Incidence

GTD is reported to occur in about 1 of every 2,000 pregnancies. Recent research indicates, however, that the incidence would be much higher if all cases of the disorder were identified. Some cases are not recognized because the pregnancy is aborted early and the products of conception are not available for analysis.

In most cases, GTD occurs in women who have had ovulation stimulation with clomiphene (Clomid), in women from lower socioeconomic groups, and in older women. The disorder is much more common in the Orient than in the West; for example, it occurs in appproximately 1 of every 200 pregnancies in the Philippines. The reason for the increased incidence among Oriental women is unknown, but nutrition may play a role (Berman and Di-Saia, 1989).

Classification

The classification of GTD depends on whether it is localized or disseminated. A benign neoplasm is well localized in the uterus, whereas a malignant neoplasm may metastasize. The most common site of metastasis is the lungs. However, metastasis to the brain and liver may occur if the disease is allowed to progress (Berman and DiSaia, 1989).

A diagnosis of benign GTD does not denote a benign long-term prognosis, nor does a diagnosis of malignant GTD definitely indicate an unfavorable prognosis. For both diagnoses, close monitoring and thorough follow-up care is vital. (For more information, see "Planning and implementation.")

ASSESSMENT

Question the client about nausea, vomiting, and vaginal discharge (continuous or intermittent). Also ask her about the size of her abdomen. Because GTD typically is accompanied by rapid uterine growth, she may tell you, "I've gotten so big so quickly!"

Assess the client's vaginal discharge, which usually is brownish red. Send a specimen to the laboratory. Measure fundal height; usually the uterus is enlarged out of proportion to the weeks of gestation. A vaginal examination shows thinning and softness of the lower uterine segment. No fetal heart tones are heard nor can any fetal body parts be palpated. Laboratory studies show a reduced hemoglobin level, hematocrit, and RBC count and an increased WBC count and sedimentation rate. Human chorionic gonadotropin titers are extremely elevated. Urinalysis probably will show proteinuria. An ultrasound performed after the third month will show grapelike clusters rather than a fetus.

NURSING DIAGNOSIS

After considering all assessment findings, formulate appropriate nursing diagnoses for the client. (For a partial list of applicable diagnoses, see Nursing Diagnoses: *Antepartal complications,* pages 129 and 130.)

PLANNING AND IMPLEMENTATION

Monitor the client's vital signs, vaginal discharge, and urine for proteinuria. The client may have a nursing diagnosis of *anxiety related to the unknown,* in which she, and probably her partner, will require support when they are given the diagnosis and teaching in the necessary steps of management. If she has to wait for the uterine wall to become firmer before having a D&C, she will be going home knowing that she is not carrying a fetus. Give her time to work this through and verbalize her feelings. Be sensitive to her ability to cope, and assess her family support. After the D&C, routine post-operative care is necessary. The client may have a nursing diagnosis of *knowl-edge deficit related to necessary follow-up care.* GTD can be malignant, making follow-up care extremely important.

Management of GTD involves evacuation of the uterine contents. An induced abortion may be followed by D&C; however, a D&C cannot be performed until the uterine wall becomes firmer and less friable (less easily torn or perforated). Tissue obtained from curettage must be examined by a pathologist for residual trophoblastic cells.

Vacuum suction also may be used to evacuate the uterus. As with a D&C, vacuum suction requires dilatation of the cervix. Whatever the treatment, blood replacement may accompany it (Hilgers and Lewis, 1986).

Because GTD can be malignant, follow-up care must continue for at least 1 year. Recommended care includes:
• hCG levels – once weekly until titers are negative for 3 consecutive weeks; then once monthly for 6 months; then every 2 months for 6 months.
• chest X-ray – once monthly until hCG titers are negative, then every 2 months for 1 year
• no pregnancy – for at least 1 year after all titers and X-rays are negative; an oral contraceptive is indicated to prevent pregnancy.

Continued high or rising hCG titers may indicate recurrent GTD. If the uterus is still intact, a secondary D&C can be performed to evacuate its contents (trophoblastic tissue, which produces the hCG). Curetted tissues are examined to identify signs of progression to choriocarcinoma, which requires a rigorous program of chemotherapy with methotrexate or dactinomycin. If chemotherapy is delayed, the choriocarcinoma has a tendency to rapid and widespread metastasis.

If hCG levels remain within normal limits for 1 year, the couple can anticipate a normal subsequent pregnancy. In this instance, probability of a recurrence of GTD is relatively low, especially if the client is age 40 or younger.

The nurse must be aware of the many options available for dealing with GTD in order to respond to the client's and family's questions about the procedures and probable outcomes.

EVALUATION

To evaluate nursing care, determine if specific goals were achieved. The following examples illustrate some appropriate evaluation statements:
• The client has listed the necessary follow-up for monitoring of GTD.
• The client's family has demonstrated support and concern.

INCOMPETENT CERVIX

Incompetent cervix (or premature dilation of the cervix) is characterized by painless dilation of the cervix without labor or uterine contraction. Depending on the length of gestation, spontaneous abortion or premature delivery may result.

Up to 40% of all perinatal deaths occur in association with pregnancies that terminate between 20 and 28 weeks' gestation. Cervical incompetence is a major contributor to those losses (Beischer and MacKay, 1986).

Etiology
Cervical incompetence may be caused by a previous traumatic delivery or a forceful D&C of the cervix (Scott, 1986). Other etiologic factors may be congenital, such as a short cervix or an anomalous uterus (such as a double uterus or other altered shape).

Incidence
Incompetent cervix occurs in approximately 1 of every 1,000 deliveries, 1 of 100 abortions, and 1 of 5 habitual abortions, where the client has had three or more abortions (Beischer and MacKay, 1986).

ASSESSMENT

The client with this condition does not have uterine contractions or other signs and symptoms of labor. A pelvic examination reveals other signs and symptoms of a dilated cervix possibly accompanied by a congenital problem, such as a short cervix, a double uterus, or a uterus with an altered shape. The client may report a previous traumatic delivery, incompetent cervix, or D&C.

NURSING DIAGNOSIS

After considering all assessment findings, formulate appropriate nursing diagnoses for the client. (For a partial list of applicable diagnoses, see Nursing Diagnoses: *Antepartal complications,* pages 129 and 130.)

PLANNING AND IMPLEMENTATION

Provide basic preoperative and postoperative care for the client undergoing a cerclage of the cervix, paying special attention to vaginal bleeding. Frequently assess for the presence and quality of fetal heart tones. Cervical cerclage may lead to a nursing diagnosis of *pain from abdominal cramping related to cerclage to repair an incompetent cer-*

vix. Decisions about the type of delivery the client will have usually depend on the position of the suture when she begins labor. Many physicians believe that if the suture is maintaining cervical closure, a cesarean delivery should be performed to preserve the suture, thereby maintaining cervical closure in future pregnancies. However, others believe that a cesarean delivery places the client unnecessarily at risk for maternal morbidity when the suture could easily be removed transvaginally (Parisi, 1989). Of course, a suture that has loosened or has become displaced will not maintain cervical closure in subsequent pregnancies. In that case, the suture is clipped and removed when labor begins and vaginal delivery may proceed (Beischer and MacKay, 1986).

Because incompetent cervix usually is not diagnosed until after one or more abortions, this probably is not the first time the client and her partner have had to face delivery complications or the loss of a fetus. Therefore, she and her family will need much support. Applicable nursing diagnoses in this situation include *anticipatory grieving related to potential loss of a fetus through incompetent cervix,* and *situational low self-esteem related to diagnosis of incompetent cervix.* Incompetent cervix can be corrected and the pregnancy maintained by wedge trachelorrhaphy (removal of a wedge from the anterior segment of the cervix with its closure) or by cervical cerclage. The procedure most frequently used is the transvaginal cervical cerclage (McDonald procedure), in which a band of nonabsorbable ribbon (Mersilene) is placed around the cervix beneath the mucosa to constrict the opening. The suture works much like the string on a drawstring bag. The key to the success for the procedure is placing the suture high enough on the cervix so that it will remain in place (Beischer and MacKay, 1986).

The physician typically will wait until 14 to 16 weeks' gestation, if possible, before performing the procedure to avoid having to remove the suture for a spontaneous first trimester abortion.

The pregnancy usually is maintained after cerclage, provided the membranes remain intact and the cervix was not more than 3 cm dilated or more than 50% effaced at the time of the correction. The procedure also may be performed transabdominally if necessary (Parisi, 1989).

EVALUATION

To evaluate nursing care, determine if specific goals were achieved. The following examples illustrate some appropriate evaluation statements:
• The client has verbalized feelings of positive self-esteem.

- The client correctly described the potential effects of her condition on herself and on her fetus and neonate.
- The client and her family actively participated in planning care and activities during pregnancy.

HYPEREMESIS GRAVIDARUM

Sometimes called "pernicious vomiting," this complication of pregnancy involves dehydration and malnutrition. Because hyperemesis begins as simple nausea and vomiting, a definitive diagnosis can be difficult. The client's tolerance for nausea and vomiting, the degree of hydration, her electrolyte balance, and her level of disability all affect the diagnosis. The nurse should realize that every case of nausea and vomiting during pregnancy can be serious.

Mild nausea and vomiting, commonly called "morning sickness," occurs in approximately 50% of all pregnant women during the first trimester. Its physiologic basis is not completely understood. Theories link it to progesterone deficiency, hyperadrenalism, hyperthyroidism, or human chorionic gonadotropin (hCG) in the mother's blood (Key, 1989), but no one theory adequately explains the symptoms. "Morning sickness" is considered a minor, self-limiting nuisance that appears 4 to 6 weeks after a missed menses and disappears after about 14 to 16 weeks of gestation (Key, 1989).

Etiology

The cause of hyperemesis gravidarum is not known. Etiologic theories embrace hormonal alterations, allergic conditions (possibly an autoimmune response to the pregnancy), or a psychosomatic condition (Key, 1989).

Hormonal alterations occur frequently in pregnancy. Progesterone produced by the placenta relaxes the smooth muscle of the uterus to help maintain pregnancy. Progesterone also slows gastric and intestinal motility, which may predispose pregnant clients to emesis. However, hyperemesis has not been directly related to progesterone activity.

Human chorionic gonadotropin levels also may affect emesis during pregnancy. Levels of hCG are elevated in clients with GTD and, according to Berkowitz and Goldstein (1984), many women with GTD develop hyperemesis. (For more information, see "Gestational trophoblastic disease" earlier in this chapter.) Furthermore, hCG levels increase proportionately with placental size and the number of fetuses, and emesis is more probable in clients who are pregnant with more than one fetus. Despite these implied correlations, however, no clear relationship has been established between hCG levels and hyperemesis.

The autoimmune response (allergy) theory has been postulated because hyperemesis terminates with labor.

The psychosomatic theory is based on the fact that nausea unrelated to pregnancy can be psychological. An obnoxious odor, a repulsive sight, or even the recollection of such an odor or sight can cause nausea and vomiting. However, current research findings fall far short of demonstrating a psychosomatic cause of hyperemesis.

Other factors that could be related to hyperemesis are elevated thyroxine (T_4) levels and increased triiodothyronine (T_3) uptake. Another possible explanation is that some clients have a stress reaction pattern that involves gastrointestinal disturbances, such as nausea, vomiting, and diarrhea. Pregnancy could activate that stress pattern.

Incidence

Hyperemesis gravidarum occurs in 7 to 16 of every 1,000 pregnant women (Key, 1989). Its incidence appears to vary with life-style, race, amount of stress, number of gestations, marital status, and age; however, demographic factors are difficult to separate from cultural, sociologic, and environmental ones.

ASSESSMENT

Unremitting nausea and vomiting that persist beyond the first trimester are characteristic of hyperemesis gravidarum. Vomitus ranges from undigested food, mucus, and bile early in the disorder to a "coffee-grounds" appearance in later stages.

Continued vomiting leads to dehydration, ultimately decreasing the circulating blood volume (hypovolemia). Laboratory studies may reveal hemoconcentration and, in severe cases, loss of hydrogen, sodium, potassium, and chloride. Signs of progressive dehydration and impending hypovolemia are weight loss, increased pulse rate, decreased blood pressure, changes in skin turgor, and dry mucous membranes. Dehydration also can lead to confusion and coma as well as to hepatic and renal failure.

The loss of gastric juices from vomiting can lead to metabolic alkalosis. Simultaneously, the client's altered nutritional state can cause metabolic acidosis. The acidosis may partially obscure the alkalosis and result in a mixed acid-base disorder.

Severe malnutrition also may cause hypoproteinemia and hypovitaminosis with resulting hypoprothrombinemia from severe malnutrition and possible hemorrhage.

In severe, long-term cases of hyperemesis gravidarum, the kidneys may cease concentrating urine effectively, causing increased serum levels of urea nitrogen and creatinine.

DRUGS USED TO TREAT HYPEREMESIS GRAVIDARUM

This chart summarizes the major antiemetic agents in current clinical use to treat hyperemesis gravidarum.

MECHANISM OF ACTION	USUAL DOSAGE	NURSING IMPLICATIONS
promethazine (Phenergan)		
Depresses central nervous system and inhibits acetylcholine	I.M.: 12.5 to 25 mg every 4 hours as needed. Also available in oral and rectal forms.	• May cause drowsiness and impair platelet aggregation; observe for bleeding in the fetus. • Safety during pregnancy has not been established.
prochlorperazine (Compazine)		
Blocks dopamine receptors in medullary chemoreceptor trigger zone	Oral: 5 to 10 mg t.i.d. I.M.: 5 to 10 mg every 3 to 4 hours	• May cause glycosuria, dry mouth, nasal congestion, restlessness, insomnia, anorexia, dizziness, postural hypotension, blurred vision. • Safety during pregnancy has not been established.
metoclopramide (Reglan)		
Blocks dopamine receptors in medullary chemoreceptor trigger zone	Oral: 10 mg q.i.d.	• May cause restlessness, anxiety, drowsiness, lassitude, extrapyramidal symptoms. • Safety and efficacy have not been established for therapy that continues longer than 12 weeks. • Safety during pregnancy has not been established.

NURSING DIAGNOSIS

After considering all assessment findings, formulate appropriate nursing diagnoses for the client. (For a partial list of applicable diagnoses, see Nursing Diagnoses: *Antepartal complications,* pages 129 and 130.)

PLANNING AND IMPLEMENTATION

For the client with a nursing diagnosis of *fluid volume deficit related to persistent vomiting and decreased fluid intake,* expect to administer parenteral fluids, electrolytes, vitamins, and proteins as prescribed to counteract dehydration and loss of nutrients. Also be prepared to administer antiemetics as prescribed to decrease vomiting and promote rest. Expect oral intake to be restricted for the first 48 hours followed by cautious resumption of small, dry meals and then by clear liquids. This allows the gastrointestinal system to rest from overstimulation.

For a client with a nursing diagnosis of *pain related to persistent vomiting,* keep the room quiet, pleasant, and well-ventilated to promote rest and relaxation; maintain excellent daily hygiene, especially oral hygiene following vomiting episodes, to promote comfort; and limit visitors to promote client rest.

A client who appears clinically stable may be managed as an outpatient with close follow-up. Hydration with isotonic fluids is essential. In addition, teach the client how to assist with her own treatment—in nutrition, for example. Teach her that small, frequent meals that contain easily digested, high-carbohydrate foods will help to reestablish adequate vitamin and protein levels. Heartburn and reflux esophagitis are common and typically are treated symptomatically.

Antiemetics, a mainstay in treating hyperemesis, also have a mildly sedating effect. (For an overview of antiemetics, see *Drugs used to treat hyperemesis gravidarum.*)

Many clients report episodes of emesis in connection with a particularly stressful incident or aspect of their lives. If possible, a client with hyperemesis should try to avoid or resolve situations that aggravate the condition or increase stress.

An essential aspect of outpatient care is reassurance and support. A debilitated client who is worried about her pregnancy may experience a severe emotional crisis. Make a special effort to give the client emotional support.

For a hospitalized client with severe symptoms, treatment goals are to eliminate vomiting, restore hydration, reestablish electrolyte balance, and supplement vitamin intake. To achieve these goals, restrict oral intake, expect to begin parenteral administration of fluids with electrolytes and supplementary vitamins and minerals, and administer antiemetics. This treatment plan allows rest for the overstimulated gastrointestinal tract while providing necessary nutrients to the body.

Persistent weight loss, acidosis, and malnutrition require total parenteral nutrition to provide adequate protein intake for mother and fetus.

Before, during, and after hospitalization, the client needs a quiet, aesthetically pleasing environment. Maintain a calm, accepting attitude. A perceived lack of tolerance may indicate to the client that the nurse feels the disorder is psychosomatic and that the client does not need hospitalization.

EVALUATION

To evaluate nursing care, determine if specific goals were achieved. The following examples illustrate some appropriate evaluation statements:
- The client has responded to small, frequent feedings by a reduced emesis.
- The client has verbalized decreased pain.
- The client has maintained adequate nutritional status and no weight loss.

CHAPTER SUMMARY

Chapter 9 described antepartal complications and related nursing care for the affected client and her family. The goals for these clients are health maintenance throughout the pregnancy and safe delivery of a healthy neonate. Here are the chapter highlights.

When caring for a client with an antepartal complication, the nurse should obtain a complete health history, perform a thorough physical assessment, and assist with and review diagnostic studies. Depending on the client's needs, the nurse monitors the client's health; teaches about the condition, its management, and effects; promotes adequate rest, exercise, and nutrition; prevents infection; provides support; promotes family well-being; monitors the fetus; and promotes compliance. Evaluation determines if the goals of maintaining client health and safely delivering a healthy neonate were achieved.

A pregnant adolescent is at risk for complications physically and psychosocially because of immaturity, potential for pregnancy complications, lack of prenatal care, and lack of social and economic support systems. Prenatal care and counseling, support groups, and financial assistance can help assure a healthier start for the pregnant adolescent and her fetus.

A mature client who gives birth after age 34 is likely to be prepared for her pregnancy physically, emotionally, and economically. Her needs include sensitive prenatal care and information about genetic testing.

A client with a cardiac disease, such as rheumatic heart disease, a congenital heart defect, mitral valve prolapse, or peripartum cardiomyopathy, can carry to term safely and give birth to a healthy neonate. She must be monitored regularly throughout her pregnancy and may benefit from such treatments as bed rest, fluid restrictions, proper nutrition, and administration of digitalis, diuretics, antiarrhythmics, antibiotics, and anticoagulants.

Care for the client with diabetes mellitus should begin before conception to normalize serum glucose levels and replace oral hypoglycemic agents with insulin. Optimally, the client should achieve normal blood glucose levels before conception and maintain them throughout pregnancy. The nurse should promote diet regulation, insulin therapy, and careful glucose monitoring throughout pregnancy, as prescribed.

Anemia may influence pregnancy and threaten the health of the client and her fetus. Iron deficiency anemia, folic acid deficiency anemia, and sickle cell anemia may worsen with pregnancy. Care for a client with iron or folic acid deficiency anemia includes diet counseling and nutritional supplements. Care for the client with sickle cell anemia includes counseling on crisis prevention, treatment with hydration and analgesics, and infection care.

TORCH infections, including toxoplasmosis, other infections (chlamydia, group B beta hemolytic streptococcus, syphilis, and varicella-zoster), rubella, cytomegalovirus, and herpesvirus, can be devastating to the fetus and neonate. Human immunodeficiency virus—and the risk of AIDS—can be transmitted from the mother to the fetus and neonate, even if the mother is asymptomatic. Genitourinary infections, such as trichomoniasis, gonorrhea, vaginitis, pelvic inflammatory disease, and pyelonephritis, also may influence fetal and neonatal health.

Substance abuse harms the client and her fetus and neonate. It increases the client's risk of other diseases, such as hepatitis B and HIV infection, and commonly is associated with STDs. The nurse should counsel the client and provide information and referrals to educational programs to help her recover from substance abuse.

The client may sustain trauma from accidental injuries or physical abuse during pregnancy. The type and timing of the injury influence pregnancy outcomes. Prompt assessment and treatment of injuries can improve maternal and fetal health. Abused clients need counseling to increase feelings of self-worth and provide support.

Surgery should be avoided during pregnancy, if possible. If surgery cannot be postponed, intervention during the second trimester is preferred. A multidisciplinary approach reduces the risks for the client and her fetus.

PROM, which occurs in 3% to 19% of all pregnancies, has an unknown etiology; however, several factors predispose a client to the condition. These factors include trauma, infection, hydramnios, and fetal malpresentation. Fetal morbidity and mortality rates are high following PROM, and RDS occurs in 30% to 70% of neonates. A key assessment finding includes amniotic fluid leakage. Depending on the risk to the mother and fetus, PROM may be treated with labor induction, cesarean delivery, or antibiotics.

Preterm labor and delivery, which has been a significant cause of perinatal morbidity and mortality for many years, has responded to new technologies with increased survival rates and decreased complications.

PIH, a relatively common antepartal complication, causes increased blood pressure, edema, and proteinuria. PIH is a major cause of maternal and fetal morbidity and mortality. Treatment includes bed rest and prevention of seizures.

Hemolytic disease of the newborn can result from Rh incompatibility or ABO incompatibility. Rh incompatibility results when an Rh-negative client and an Rh-positive partner conceive a fetus with Rh-positive blood. Because of the potential for fetal and maternal blood mixing when the placenta separates after delivery, subsequent pregnancies are at risk for isoimmunization. In most cases, Rh isoimmunization can be prevented with RhIg. ABO incompatibility occurs when a client with blood group O becomes pregnant with a fetus with blood group A, B, or AB.

Spontaneous abortion, also called a miscarriage, can occur at any time before the age of fetal viability (20 to 24 weeks' gestation and a weight of over 500 grams). It typically causes bleeding and pain and is treated with rest, medications, emotional support, and other interventions, as needed.

In ectopic pregnancy, the fertilized ovum is implanted in tissue other than the endometrium. This complication causes bleeding and abdominal pain. If rupture occurs, shock may ensue. The nurse must be prepared to control bleeding, administer transfusions, provide emotional support, and assist with removal of the products of conception.

In GTD, trophoblastic cells covering the chorionic villi proliferate, and the villi undergo cystic changes. GTD may be benign, as in hydatidiform mole, or malignant, as in choriocarcinoma. It is characterized by rapid uterine growth, brownish red vaginal discharge, and a lack of fetal heart tones. Treatment calls for D&C or a similar procedure and at least 1 year of follow-up to detect signs of malignancy.

Incompetent cervix refers to premature cervical dilation. This painless antepartal complication may lead to spontaneous abortion or premature delivery. When caring for a client with an incompetent cervix, the nurse should prepare her for cerclage, provide postoperative care, and offer emotional support.

Hyperemesis gravidarum is a disorder of pregnancy in which excessive nausea and vomiting threaten the continuation of the pregnancy. Dehydration and electrolyte disturbances are common, and hospitalization may be necessary.

STUDY QUESTIONS

1. When Jamie Green, age 16, makes her first visit to the prenatal clinic, she is at 28 weeks' gestation with her first pregnancy. What guidelines will the nurse use in planning Jamie's care?

2. What measures can the nurse use to provide a pregnant client with a history of rheumatic fever the best possible care?

3. Cindy Little, age 22, has had insulin-dependent diabetes mellitus for 6 years. She is 22 weeks pregnant. What information must the nurse review with her about her glucose maintenance?

4. What should the nurse tell a client with sickle cell anemia about the fetal and neonatal effects of the disease?

5. How can the nurse differentiate between rupture of the membranes and urine incontinency?

6. Several hours after receiving an intravenous bolus and intravenous infusion of magnesium sulfate for preterm labor, a client's deep tendon reflexes are 1 + . What actions, if any, are appropriate before the nurse notifies the client's physician?

7. Mrs. Brown, an Rh-negative primigravid 23-year-old client, has reached 28 weeks' gestation. Her partner is Rh positive. Her physician has told her she would receive RhIg at this prenatal visit. She tells the nurse she is afraid of needles and plans to refuse the medication. What are the nurse's responsibilities?

BIBLIOGRAPHY

American College of Obstetricians and Gynecologists (1986). Management of isoimmunization in pregnancy. *ACOG Technical Bulletin,* No. 90.

Beischer, N.A., and MacKay, E.V. (1986). *Obstetrics and the newborn* (2nd ed.). Philadelphia: Saunders.

Beth Israel Hospital Staff (1982). *Obstetrical decision making.* St. Louis: Mosby.

Braunwald, E., Isselbacher, K., Petersdorf, R., Wilson, J., Martin, J., and Fauci, A. (Eds.) (1987). *Harrison's principles of internal medicine* (11th ed.). New York: McGraw-Hill.

Chez, R., and Sadovsky, E. (1984). Teaching patients how to record fetal movements. *Contemporary OB/GYN,* 24(4), 85-86.

Creasy, R.K. (1989). Preterm labor and delivery. In R.K. Creasy and R. Resnick (Eds.), *Maternal-fetal medicine: Principles and practice* (2nd ed.) Philadelphia: Saunders.

Cruikshank, D. (1986a). Medical and surgical complications of pregnancy: Diseases of the alimentary tract. In D. Danforth and J. Scott (Eds.), *Obstetrics and gynecology* (5th ed.; pp. 523-527). Philadelphia: Lippincott.

Cruikshank, D. (1986b). Medical and surgical complications of pregnancy: Neurologic disease. In D. Danforth and J. Scott (Eds.), *Obstetrics and gynecology* (5th ed.; pp. 505-509). Philadelphia: Lippincott.

Cruikshank, D. (1986c). Medical and surgical complications of pregnancy: Urinary tract disease. In D. Danforth and J. Scott (Eds.), *Obstetrics and gynecology* (5th ed.; pp. 505-509). Philadelphia: Lippincott.

Cunningham, F., MacDonald, P., and Gant, N. (1989). *Williams obstetrics* (18th ed.). East Norwalk, CT: Appleton & Lange.

Deutchman, M. (1989). The problematic first-trimester pregnancy. *American Family Physician,* 39(1), 185-198.

Dunn, P., Weiner, S., and Ludomirski, A. (1988). Percutaneous umbilical blood sampling. *JOGNN,* 17(5), 303-313.

Elias S., Simpson, J., Martin., A., Sabbagha, R., Gerbie, A., and Keith, L. (1985). Chorionic villus sampling for first-trimester prenatal diagnosis: Northwestern University Program. American *Journal of Obstetrics and Gynecology,* 152(2), 204-213.

Gibbs, R.S., and Sweet, R.L. (1989). Clinical disorders. In R.K. Creasy and R. Resnick (Eds.), *Maternal-fetal medicine: Principles and practice* (2nd ed.; pp. 656-662). Philadelphia: Saunders.

Gorrie, T.M. (1989). *A guide to the nursing of childbearing families.* Baltimore: Williams & Wilkins.

Hanson, F.W., Zorn, E.M., Tennant, F.R., Marianos, S. & Samuels, S. (1987). Amniocentesis before 15 weeks' gestation: Outcome, risks, and technical problems. *American Journal of Obstetrics and Gynecology,* 156(6), 1524-1531.

Henshaw, S.K., and Silverman, J. (1988). The characteristics and prior contraceptive use of United States abortion patients. *Family Planning Perspectives,* 20(4), 159-168.

Hibbard, B. (1988). *Principles of obstetrics.* Stoneham, MA: Butterworth and Co.

Hogge, J., Hogge, W., and Golbus, M. (1986). Chorionic villus sampling. *JOGNN,* 15(1), 24-28.

Hollingsworth, D., and Resnik, R. (Eds.). (1988). *Medical counseling before pregnancy.* New York: Churchill Livingstone.

Interim report of the Medical Research Council/Royal College of Obstetricians and Gynaecologists Multicentre Randomized Trial of Cervical Cerclage (1988). *British Journal of Obstetrics and Gynecology,* 95(5), 437-445.

Jain, K.A., Hamper, U.M., and Sanders, R.C. (1988). Comparison of transvaginal and transabdominal sonography in the detection of early pregnancy and its complications. *American Journal of Roentgenology,* 151(6), 1139-1143.

Koonin, L., Atrash, H., Rochat, R., and Smith, J. (1988). Maternal mortality surveillance, United States, 1980-1985. CDC Surveillance Summaries, *MMWR,* 37(5), 19-29.

Kurtz, A., and Needleman, L. (1988). Ultrasound assessment of fetal age. In P. Callen (Ed.), *Ultrasonography in obstetrics and gynecology* (2nd ed.; pp. 47-64). Philadelphia: Saunders.

Lemize, R. (1989). Neural tube defects. *JAMA,* 259(4), 558-562.

Lloyd, T. (1987). Rh-factor incompatibility, a primer for prevention. *Journal of Nurse-Midwifery,* 32(5), 297-307.

Ludomirski, A., and Weiner, S. (1988). Percutaneous fetal umbilical sampling. *Clinical Obstetrics and Gynecology,* 31(1), 19-26.

Manning, F., Morrison, I., Lange, I., Harman, C., and Chamberlain, P. (1985). Fetal assessment based on fetal biophysical profile scoring: Experience in 12,620 referred high-risk pregnancies. *American Journal of Obstetrics and Gynecology,* 151(3), 343-350.

Modica, M.M., and Timor-Tritsch, I.E. (1988). Transvaginal sonography provides a sharper view into the pelvis. *JOGNN,* 17(2), 89-95.

Nyberg, D.A., Filly, R.A., Filho, D.L., Laring, F.C., and Mahoney, B.S. (1986). Abnormal pregnancy: Early diagnosis by US and serum chorionic gonodotropin levels. *Radiology,* 158(2), 393-396.

Nyberg, D.A., Mack, L.A., Laing, F.C., and Jeffrey, R.B. (1988). Early pregnancy complications: Endovaginal sonographic findings correlated with human chorionic gonadotropin levels. *Radiology,* 167(3), 619-622.

Parisi, V.M. (1989). Cervical incompetence. In R.K. Creasy and R. Resnick (Eds.), *Maternal-fetal medicine: Principles and practice* (2nd ed.; pp. 447-462). Philadelphia: Saunders.

Pussell, B.A., Peake, P.W., Brown, M.A., Charlesworth, G.A. (1985). Human fibronectin metabolism. *Journal of Clinical Investigation,* 76(1), 143-148.

Rayburn, W.F., and Schad, R.F. (1986). Antiemetics, iron preparations, vitamins and OTC drugs. In W.F. Rayburn and F.D. Zuspan (Eds.), *Drug therapy in obstetrics and gynecology* (2nd ed.; pp. 24-26). East Norwalk, CT: Appleton & Lange.

Sachs, B.P., Brown, D.A.J., Driscoll, S.G., Schulman, E., Acker, D., Ransil, B.J., and Jewett, J.F. (1988). Hemorrhage, infection, toxemia, and cardiac disease 1954-1985: Causes for their declining role in maternal mortality. *American Journal of Public Health,* 78(6), 671-675.

Sadovsky, E. (1985). Fetal movements. In J. Queenan (Ed.), *Management of high-risk pregnancy* (2nd ed.; pp. 183-193). Oradell, NJ: Medical Economics Co.

Schwager, E., and Weiss, B. (1987). Prenatal testing for maternal serum alpha-fetoprotein. *American Family Physician,* 35(4), 169-174.

Scott, J.R. (1986a). Isoimmunization. In D.N. Danforth and J.R. Scott (Eds.), *Obstetrics and gynecology* (5th ed.). St. Louis: Mosby.

U.S. Department of Health and Human Services (1988). *Health, United States, 1987,* Pub. No. (PHS 88-1232). Hyattsville, MD: National Center for Health Statistics.

Willson, J., and Carrington, E. (1987). *Obstetrics and gynecology* (8th ed.). St. Louis: Mosby.

Hypertensive disorders

Abrams, R.S. (1989). *Handbook of medical problems during pregnancy.* Norwalk, CT.: Appleton & Lange.

Ballegeer, V., Spitz, B., Kieckens, L., Moreau, H., Van Assche, A.V., and Collen, D. (1989). Predictive value of increased plasma levels of fibronectin in gestational hypertension. *American Journal of Obstetrics and Gynecology,* 161(2), 432-436.

Barron, W.M. (1991). Hypertension. In W.M. Barron and M.D. Lindheimer (Eds.), *Medical disorders during pregnancy.* St. Louis, MO: Mosby-Year Book.

Belizian, J.M., and Villar, J. (1980). The relationship between calcium intake and edema, proteinuria and hypertension gestosis: A hypothesis. *American Journal of Clinical Nutrition,* 33, 2202.

De Alvarez, R. (1978). Pre-eclampsia, eclampsia, and renal disease in pregnancy. *Clinical Obstetrics and Gynecology,* 21, 881.

Gavette, L., and Roberts, J. (1987). Use of mean arterial pressure (MAP-2) to predict pregnancy-induced hypertension in adolescents. *Journal of Nurse-Midwifery,* 32(6) 357-367.

Georgiew, D.B., Skortcheva, I., and Abadjiew, V. (1990). Early development of HELLP syndrome: A case report. *Gyneologic Obstetric Investigation,* 30(2), 127-128

Gilbert, E.S., and Harmon J.S. (1986). *High-risk pregnancy and delivery.* St. Louis: Mosby.

Hacker, N., and Moore, G. (1986). *Essentials of obstetrics and gynecology.* Philadelphia: Saunders.

Risch, H.A., Weiss, N.S., Clarke, and Roberts, J.M. (1989). Pregnancy-related hypertension. In R.K. Creasy and R. Resnick (Eds.), *Maternal-fetal medicine: Principles and practice* (2nd ed.; pp. 777-823). Philadelphia: Saunders.

Roberts, J.M., Taylor, R.N., Musci, T.J., Rodgers, G.M., Hubel, C.A., and McLaughlin, M.K. (1989). Preeclampsia: An endothelial cell disorder. *American Journal of Obstetrics and Gynecology,* 161(5), 1200-1204.

Rodgers, G.M., Taylor, R.N., and Roberts, J.M. (1988). Preeclampsia is associated with a serum factor cytotoxic to human endothelial cells. *American Journal of Obstetrics and Gynecology,* 159(4), 908-914.

Shanklin, D.R., and Sibai, B.M. (1989). Ultrastructural aspects of preeclampsia: Placental bed and uterine boundary vessels. *American Journal of Obstetrics and Gynecology,* 159(4), 908-914.

Sibai, B.M. (1990). The HELLP syndrome (hemolysis, elevated liver enzymes, and low platelets): Much ado about nothing? *American Journal of Obstetrics and Gynecology,* 162(2), 311-316.

Sibai, B.M., Taslimi, M.M., El/Nazer, A., Amon, E., Mabie, B.C., and Ryan, G.M. (1986). Maternal/perinatal outcome associated with the syndrome of hemolysis, elevated liver enzymes, and low platelet in severe preeclampsia/eclampsia. *American Journal of Obstetrics and Gynecology,* 155(3), 501-509.

Weinstein, L. (1982). Syndrome of hemolysis, elevated liver enzymes, and low platelet count: A severe consequence of hypertension in pregnancy. *American Journal of Obstetrics and Gynecology,* 142(1):159.

Zuspan, F.P., and Zuspan, K.J. (1986). Acute and chronic hypertension during pregnancy. In W.F. Rayburn and F.P. Zuspan (Eds.), *Drug therapy in obstetrics and gynecology* (2nd ed.; pp. 73-92). East Norwalk, CT: Appleton & Lange.

Preterm labor and delivery

Creasy, R.K. (1989). Preterm labor and delivery. In R.K. Creasy and R. Resnick (Eds.), *Maternal-fetal medicine: Principles and practice* (2nd ed.). Philadelphia: Saunders.

Givens, S.R. (1988). Update on tocolytic therapy in the management of preterm labor. *Journal of Perinatal Neonatal Nursing,* 2(1), 21-32.

Gupta, R.C., Foster, S., Romano, P.M., and Thomas, H.M. (1989). Acute pulmonary edema associated with the use of oral ritodrine for premature labor. *Chest,* 95(2), 479-481.

Iams, J.D., Johnson, F.F., and O'Shaughnessy, R.W. (1988). A prospective random trial of home uterine activity monitoring in pregnancies at increased risk of preterm labor, Part II. *American Journal of Obstetrics and Gynecology,* 159(3), 595-603.

Koehl, L., and Wheeler, D. (1989). Monitoring uterine activity at home. *AJN,* 89(2), 200-203.

Omer, H., and Everly, G.S., Jr., (1988). Psychological factors in preterm labor: Critical review and theoretical synthesis. *American Journal of Psychiatry,* 145(12), 1507-1513.

Rayburn, W.F., DeDonato, D.M., and Rand, W.K. (1986). Drugs to inhibit premature labor. In W.F. Rayburn and F.P. Zuspan (Eds.), *Drug therapy in obstetrics and gynecology* (2nd ed.; pp. 172-183). East Norwalk, CT: Appleton & Lange.

Wilkins, I.A., Lynch, L., Mehalek, K.E., Berkowitz, G.S., and Berkowitz, R.L. (1988). Efficacy and side effects of magnesium sulfate and ritodrine as tocolytic agents. *American Journal of Obstetrics and Gynecology,* 159(3), 685-689.

Age-related concerns

Friede, A., Baldwin, W., Rhodes, P., Buehler, J., and Strauss, L. (1988). Older maternal age and infant mortality in the United States. *Obstetrics and Gynecology,* 72(2), 152-157.

Kirz, D., Dorchester, W., and Freeman, R. (1985). Advanced maternal age: The mature gravida. *American Journal of Obstetrics and Gynecology,* 152(1), 7-12.

Robinson, G., Garner, D., Gare, D., and Crawford, B. (1987). Psychological adaptation to pregnancy in childless women more than 35 years of age. *American Journal of Obstetrics and Gynecology,* 156(2), 328-333.

U.S. Department of Health and Human Services (August 15, 1990). *Monthly Vital Statistics Report,* 39(4), Supplement.

Cardiac disease

Brady, K., and Duff, P. (1989). Rheumatic heart disease in pregnancy. *Clinical Obstetrics and Gynecology,* 32(1), 21-40.

Cruikshank, D. (1986d). Medical and surgical complications of pregnancy: Cardiovascular disease. In D. Danforth and J. Scott (Eds.), *Obstetrics and gynecology* (5th ed.; pp. 492-502). Philadelphia: Lippincott.

Gilstrap III, L. (1989). Heart disease during pregnancy. *Clinical Obstetrics and Gynecology,* 32(1), 1.

Homans, D. (1985). Peripartum cardiomyopathy. *New England Journal of Medicine,* 312(22), 1432-1437.

Lee, W., and Cotton, D. (1989). Peripartum cardiomyopathy: Current concepts and clinical management. *Clinical Obstetrics and Gynecology,* 32(1), 54-67.

Ramin, S., Mayberry, M., and Gilstrap, L. (1989). Congestive heart disease. *Clinical Obstetrics and Gynecology,* 32(1), 41-47.

Diabetes mellitus

Coustan, D., and Felig, P. (1988). Diabetes mellitus. In G. Burrow and T. Ferris (Eds.), *Medical complications during pregnancy* (3rd ed.; pp. 34-64). Philadelphia: Saunders

Gabbe, S. (1985). Management of diabetes mellitus in pregnancy. *American Journal of Obstetrics and Gynecology,* 153(8), 824-828.

Gabbe, S. (1986). Definition, detection, and management of gestational diabetes. *Obstetrics and Gynecology,* 67(1), 121-125.

Hollingsworth, D. (1988). Diabetes. In D. Hollingsworth and R. Resnick (Eds.), *Medical counseling before pregnancy* (pp. 271-316). New York: Churchill Livingstone.

Mestman, J. (1985). Medical management of diabetes mellitus. In J. Queenan (Ed.), *Management of high-risk pregnancy* (2nd ed.; pp. 351-360). Oradell, NJ: Medical Economics Co.

National Diabetes Data Group (1979). Classification and diagnosis of diabetes mellitus and other categories of glucose intolerance. *Diabetes,* 28(12), 1039-1057.

Ray, D., Yeast, J., and Freeman, R. (1986). The current role of daily serum estriol monitoring in the insulin-dependent pregnant diabetic woman. *American Journal of Obstetrics and Gynecology,* 154(6), 1257-1263.

Samuels, P., and Landon, M. (1986). Medical complications. In S. Gabbe, J. Niebyl, and J. Simpson (Eds.), *Obstetrics: Normal and problem pregnancies* (pp. 865-977). New York: Churchill Livingstone.

Schneider, J., and Kitzmiller, J. (1989). Medical management of diabetes mellitus during pregnancy. In S. Brody and K. Ueland (Eds.), *Endocrine disorders in pregnancy* (pp. 313-343). East Norwalk, CT: Appleton & Lange.

Spellacy, W. (1987). Diabetes mellitus. In J. Queenan and J. Hobbins (Eds.), *Protocols for high-risk pregnancies* (2nd ed.; pp. 140-143). Oradell, NJ: Medical Economics Co.

Swislocki, A., and Kraemer, F. (1989). Maternal metabolism in diabetes mellitus: Pathophysiology of diabetes in pregnancy. In S. Brody and K. Ueland (Eds.), *Endocrine disorders in pregnancy* (pp. 247-272). East Norwalk, CT: Appleton & Lange.

White, P. (1986). Classification of diabetes complicating pregnancy. The American College of Obstetricians and Gynecologists, *Technical Bulletin* No. 92, May 1986.

Anemias

Cruikshank, D. (1986f). Don't overdo nutritional supplements during pregnancy. *Contemporary OB/GYN,* 27(2), 101-119.

Kelton, J., and Cruickshank, D. (1988). Hematologic disorders of pregnancy. In G. Burrow and T. Ferris (Eds.), *Medical complications during pregnancy* (pp. 65-94). Philadelphia: Saunders.

Martin, J., and Morrison, J. (1984). Managing the parturient with sickle cell crisis. *Clinical Obstetrics and Gynecology,* 27(1), 39-49.

Winick, M. (1989). *Nutrition, pregnancy, and early infancy.* Baltimore: Williams & Wilkins.

Infection

Amstey, M. (1985). Herpes simplex. In J. Queenan (Ed.), *Management of high-risk pregnancy* (pp. 435-437). Oradell, NJ: Medical Economics Co.

Benoit, J. (1988). Sexually transmitted diseases in pregnancy. *Nursing Clinics of North America,* 23(4), 937-945.

Cates, W., and Schulz, S. (1988). Epidemiology of HIV in women. *Contemporary OB/GYN,* 32(3), 94-105.

Centers for Disease Control (1989). 1989 Sexually transmitted diseases treatment guidelines. *MMWR,* 38(S-8), 1-43.

Centers for Disease Control (1989). Update: Acquired immunodeficiency syndrome – United States, 1981-1988. *MMWR,* 38(14), 229-236.

Eschenbach, D. (1988). Infections and sexually transmitted diseases. In D. Hollingsworth and R. Resnik (Eds.), *Medical counseling before pregnancy* (pp. 249-269). New York: Churchill Livingstone.

Gibbs, R., Amstey, M., Sweet, R., Mead, P., and Sever, J. (1988). Management of genital herpes infection in pregnancy. *Obstetrics and Gynecology,* 71(5), 779-780.

Marion, R., Wiznia, A., Hutcheon, R., and Rubinstein, A. (1986). Human T-cell lymphotropic virus type III (HTLV-III) embryopathy. *American Journal of Diseases of Children,* 140(7), 638-640.

McCracken, Jr., G. and Freij, B. (1987). Bacterial and viral infections of the newborn. In G. Avery (Ed.), *Neonatology: Pathophysiology and management of the newborn* (3rd ed.; pp. 917-943). Philadelphia: Lippincott.

McElhose, P. (1988). The "other" STDs: As dangerous as ever. *RN,* 51(6), 52-59.

Minkoff, H. (1988). Managing AIDS in pregnant patients. *Contemporary OB/GYN,* 32(3), 106-114.

Pritchard, J., MacDonald, P., and Gant, N. (1985). *Williams obstetrics* (17th ed.) East Norwalk, CT: Appleton & Lange.

Sharp, H. (1986). Reproductive tract disorders. In D. Danforth and J. Scott (Eds.), *Obstetrics and gynecology* (5th ed.; pp. 551-561). Philadelphia: Lippincott.

Simpson, M., Gaziano, E., Lupo, V., and Peterson, P. (1988). Bacterial infections during pregnancy. In G. Burrow and T. Ferris (Eds.), *Medical complications during pregnancy* (3rd ed.; pp. 345-371). Philadelphia: Saunders.

South, M., and Sever, J. (1986). Viral and protozoal diseases. In D. Danforth and J. Scott (Eds.), *Obstetrics and gynecology* (5th ed.; pp. 551-561). Philadelphia: Lippincott.

Stagno, S., and Whitley, R.J. (1985). Herpes-virus infections of pregnancy, Part II: Herpes simplex virus and varicella-zoster virus infections. *The New England Journal of Medicine,* 313(21), 1327-1330.

Whitley, R., Corey, L., Arvin, A., Lakeman, F., Sumaya, C., Wright, P., Dunkle, L., Steele, R., Soong, S., Nahmias, A., Alford, C., Powell, D., Joaquin, V., and NIAID Collaborative Antiviral Study Group (1988). Changing presentation of herpes simplex virus in neonates. *Journal of Infectious Diseases,* 158(1), 109-116.

Substance abuse

Chasnoff, I., Burns, K., and Burns, W. (1987). Cocaine use in pregnancy: Perinatal morbidity and mortality. *Neurotoxicology and Teratology,* 9(4), 291-293.

Chasnoff, I., Bussey, M., Savich, R., and Stack, C. (1986). Perinatal cerebral infarction and maternal cocaine use. *The Journal of Pediatrics,* 108(3), 456-459.

Chasnoff, I., Griffith, D., MacGregor, S., Dirkes, K., and Burns, K. (1989). Temporal patterns of cocaine use in pregnancy: Perinatal outcome. *JAMA,* 261(12), 1741-1744.

Finnegan, L., and Wapner, R. (1987). Narcotic addiction in pregnancy. In J. Neibyl (Ed.), *Drug use in pregnancy* (pp. 203-222). Philadelphia: Lea & Febiger.

Neerhof, M., MacGregor, S., Retzky, S., and Sullivan, T. (1989). Cocaine abuse during pregnancy: Peripartum prevalence and perinatal outcome. *American Journal of Obstetrics and Gynecology,* 161(3), 633-638.

O'Malley, P., Bachman, J., and Johnston, L. (1988). Period, age, and cohort effects on substance use among young Americans: A decade of change, 1976-1986. *American Journal of Public Health,* 78(10), 1315-1321.

Rodgers, B., and Lee, R. (1988). Drug abuse. In G. Burrow and T. Ferris (Eds.), *Medical complications during pregnancy* (3rd ed.; pp. 570-581). Philadelphia: Saunders.

Ronkin, S., Fitzsimmons, J., Wapner, R., and Finnegan, L. (1988). Protecting mother and fetus from narcotic abuse. *Contemporary OB/GYN,* 31(3), 178-187.

Wapner, R., and Finnegan, L. (1982). Perinatal aspects of psychotropic drug abuse. In R. Bolognese, R. Schwarz, and J. Schneider (Eds.), *Perinatal medicine: Management of the high-risk fetus and neonate* (2nd ed.; pp. 384-417). Baltimore: Williams & Wilkins.

Trauma or need for surgery

Baden, J., and Brodsky, J. (Eds.) (1985). *The pregnant surgical patient.* Mt. Kisco, NY: Futura Publishing.

Franger, A., Buchsbaum, H., and Peaceman, A. (1989). Abdominal gunshot wounds in pregnancy. *American Journal of Obstetrics and Gynecology,* 160(5, Part 1), 1124-1128.

Neufeld, J., Moore, E., Marx, J., and Rosen, P. (1987). Trauma in pregnancy. *Emergency Medicine Clinics of North America,* 5(3), 623-640.

Rice, S., and Pellegrini, M. (1985). Basic principles of teratology. In J. Baden and J. Brodsky (Eds.), *The pregnant surgical patient* (pp. 1-28). Mt. Kisco, NY: Futura Publishing.

Slater, G., and Aufses, A. (1985). Surgical aspects of pregnancy. In S. Cherry, R. Berkowitz, and N. Kase (Eds.), *Rovinsky and Guttmacher's medical, surgical, and gynecologic complications of pregnancy* (pp. 656-663). Baltimore: Williams & Wilkins.

Ectopic pregnancy

Buck, R.H., Joubert, S.M., and Norman, P.J. (1988). Serum progesterone in the diagnosis of ectopic pregnancy: A valuable diagnostic test? *Fertility and Sterility,* 50(5), 752-755.

Centers for Disease Control (June 22, 1990). Ectopic pregnancy—United States, 1987. *MMWR,* 39(24), 401-403.

Droegemueller, W. (1986). Ectopic pregnancy. In D.N. Danforth and J.R. Scott (Eds.), *Obstetrics and gynecology* (5th ed.). St. Louis: Mosby.

Fedele, L., Acaia, B., Parazzini, F., Ricciardiello, O., and Candiani, G.B. (1989). Ectopic pregnancy and recurrent spontaneous abortion: Two associated reproductive failures. *Obstetrics and Gynecology,* 73(2), 206-208.

Huber, J., Hosmann, J., and Vytiska-Binstorfer, E. (1989). Laparoscopic surgery for tubal pregnancy utilizing laser. *International Journal of Gynecology and Obstetrics,* 29(2), 153-157.

Kadar, N., and Romero, R. (1988). Further observations on serial human chorionic gonadotropin patterns in ectopic pregnancies and spontaneous abortions. *Fertility and Sterility,* 50(2), 367-370.

Kuczynski, H.J. (1986). Support for the woman with an ectopic pregnancy. *JOGNN,* 15(4), 306-310.

Lawson, H., Atrash, H., Saftlas, A., Franks, A., Finch, E., and Hughes, J. (1988). Ectopic pregnancy surveillance, United States, 1970-1985. *MMWR,* 37(SSS-5), 9-18.

Lindblom, B., Halin, M., and Sjoblom, P. (1989). Serial human chorionic gonadotropin determinations by fluoroimmunoassay for differentiation between intrauterine pregnancy and ectopic gestation. *American Journal of Obstetrics and Gynecology,* 161(2), 397-400.

Loffer, F.D. (1986). The increasing problem of ectopic pregnancies and its impact on patients and physicians. *The Journal of Reproductive Medicine,* 31(2), 74-77.

Makinen, J.I., Salmi, T.A., Nikkanen, V.P.J., and Juhani-Koskinen, E.Y. (1989). Encouraging rates of fertility after ectopic pregnancy. *International Journal of Fertility,* 34(1), 46-51.

Mecke, H., Semm, K., and Lehman-Willenbrock, E. (1989). Results of operative pelviscopy in 202 cases of ectopic pregnancy. *International Journal of Fertility,* 34(2), 93-100.

Osguthorpe, N.C. (1987). Ectopic pregnancy. *JOGNN,* 16(1), 36-41.

Osguthorpe, N.C., and Keating, K. (1988). Care of the client with ectopic pregnancy. *JOGNN,* 17(1), 32-38.

Pouley, J.L., Mahnes, H., Mage, G., Canis, M., and Bruhat, M.A. (1986). Conservative treatment of ectopic pregnancy. *Fertility and Sterility,* 46(7), 1093.

Romero, R. (1986). The diagnosis of ectopic pregnancy. In A.H. DeCherney (Ed.), *Ectopic pregnancy* (pp. 15-34). Rockville, MD: Aspen Publications.

Schenker, J.G., and Evron, S. (1983). New concepts in the surgical management of tubal pregnancy and the consequent postoperative results. *Fertility and Sterility,* 40(6), 709-723.

Silva, P.D. (1988). A laparoscopic approach can be applied to most cases of ectopic pregnancy. *Obstetrics and Gynecology,* 72(6), 944-947.

Stock, R.J. (1988). The changing spectrum of ectopic pregnancy. *Obstetrics and Gynecology,* 71(6), 885-888.

Timor-Tritsch, I.E., Yeh, M.N., Peisner, D.P., Blesser, K., and Slavik, T.A. (1989). The use of transvaginal ultrasonography in the diagnosis of ectopic pregnancy. *American Journal of Obstetrics and Gynecology,* 161(1), 157-161.

Vermesh, M., Silva, P.D., Sauer, M.V., Vargyas, J.M., and Lobo, R.A. (1988). Persistent tubal ectopic gestation: Patterns of circulating beta-human chorionic gonadotropin and progesterone, and management options. *Fertility and Sterility,* 50(4), 584-588.

Weissman, A., Fishman, A., and Gal, D. (1989). Interstitial pregnancy: A diagnostic challenge. *International Journal of Gynaecology and Obstetrics,* 29(4), 373-375.

Gestational trophoblastic disease

Berman, M.L., and DiSaia, P.J. (1989). Pelvic malignancies, gestational trophoblastic neoplasia, and nonpelvic malignancies. In R.K. Creasy and R. Resnick (Eds.), *Maternal-fetal medicine: Principles and practice* (2nd ed; pp. 1122-1149). Philadelphia: Saunders.

Fine, C., Bundy, A.L., Berkowitz, R.S., Boswell, S.B., Berezin, A.F., and Doubilet, P.M. (1989). Sonographic diagnosis of partial hydatidiform mole. *Obstetrics and Gynecology,* 73(3), 414-418.

Hilgers, R.D., and Lewis, J.L. (1986). Gestational trophoblastic disease. In D.N. Danforth and J.R. Scott (Eds.), *Obstetrics and gynecology* (5th ed.). St. Louis: Mosby.

Khazaeli, M.B., Buchina, E.S., Pattillo, R.A., Soong, S.J., and Hatch, K.D. (1989). Radioimmunoassy of free beta-subunit of human chorionic gonadotropin in diagnosis of high-risk and low-risk gestational trophoblastic disease. *American Journal of Obstetrics and Gynecology,* 160(2), 444-449.

Schlaerth, J.B., Morrow, C.P., Montz, F.J., and d'Ablaing, G. (1988). Initial management of hydatidiform mole. *American Journal of Obstetrics and Gynecology,* 158(6), 1299-1306.

Spontaneous abortion

Berkowitz, R.S., and Goldstein, D.P. (1983). Molar pregnancy: Etiology. In E.S. Hafez (Ed.), *Spontaneous abortion* (pp. 363-372). Hingham, MA: Kluwer Academic Publishers.

Glass, R.H., and Golbus, M.S. (1989). Habitual abortion. In R.K. Creasy and R. Resnick (Eds.), *Maternal-fetal medicine: Principles and practice* (2nd ed.; pp. 437-446). Philadelphia: Saunders.

Hafez, E.S. (1984). Early embryonic loss: Physiology. In E.S. Hafez (Ed.)., *Spontaneous abortion* (pp. 99-114). Hingham, MA: Kluwer Academic Publishers.

Key, T. (1989). Gastrointestinal disturbances. In R.K. Creasy and R. Resnick (Eds.), *Maternal-fetal medicine: Principles and practice* (2nd ed.). Philadelphia: Saunders.

Scott, J.R. (1986). Spontaneous abortion. In D.N. Danforth and J.R. Scott (Eds.), *Obstetrics and gynecology* (5th ed.). St. Louis: Mosby.

UNIT III
THE INTRAPARTAL PERIOD

PHYSIOLOGY OF LABOR AND CHILDBIRTH

OBJECTIVES

After reading and studying this chapter, the student should be able to:

1. Discuss the physiologic changes that commonly signal labor onset.

2. Explain the physiologic changes associated with uterine contractions and cervical effacement and dilation.

3. Explain the cardinal movements of labor.

4. Explain the four stages of labor, discussing what occurs in each stage.

5. Define the five essential factors of labor, and discuss how each affects the physiology of labor and childbirth.

6. Describe maternal physiologic and psychological changes associated with each stage of labor.

7. Explain fetal physiologic responses to labor.

INTRODUCTION

Impending labor and childbirth typically trigger both excitement and apprehension in a pregnant client. Whether about to give birth for the first time (a primiparous client) or experienced from previous childbirth (a multiparous client), she will have many physical and psychological needs. To meet these needs, the nurse must understand the labor process and how it affects the client and fetus.

This chapter begins with a discussion of the physiologic changes that commonly signal labor onset, called premonitory signs and symptoms. Subsequent sections explain the mechanisms of labor, including cervical effacement and dilation and fetal cardinal movements; the four stages of labor; and factors affecting the labor process. The chapter concludes with discussions of physiologic changes that affect the client and the fetus during labor and childbirth.

PREMONITORY SIGNS AND SYMPTOMS OF LABOR

Although several theories of labor onset have been proposed, the exact mechanism has eluded researchers. Instead of a single initiating factor, several maternal, fetal, and placental factors probably interact to initiate labor. These include oxytocin stimulation, progesterone reduction, estrogen stimulation, fetal cortisol production, and the effects of fetal membrane phospholipids, arachidonic acid, and prostaglandins.

Although the exact mechanism that triggers labor remains unclear, certain physiologic signs and symptoms (called premonitory) typically predict the onset of true labor. Some of these signs and symptoms may occur up to 3 weeks before labor onset; others coincide with the beginning of labor.

LIGHTENING

Lightening, subjective sensations experienced by many clients late in pregnancy, occurs as the fetus settles lower in the pelvis, leaving more space in the upper abdomen. In primiparous clients, lightening normally occurs 2 to 3 weeks before labor begins; in multiparous clients, it may not occur until labor actually begins. This downward fetal movement decreases pressure on the diaphragm, easing respiratory effort and allowing the client to breathe more deeply. It also reduces compression of the stomach, allowing the client to eat more at each meal. Accompanying these sensations are a change in abdominal shape and a visible decrease in fundal height, at which time the fetus is commonly said to have "dropped." Lightening also has been associated with a reduction in amniotic fluid volume (Cunningham, MacDonald, and Gant, 1989).

Lightening also may cause discomfort. In some clients, the frequent urge to urinate experienced early in pregnancy returns because the uterus, lower in the pelvis after the fetus has dropped, pushes against the bladder. The client may feel fetal movements much lower in the abdomen, producing a sensation of pressure.

Also, downward pressure on deep leg veins from the enlarged uterus may cause pelvic pressure and edema of the legs. Increased pelvic pressure can lead to or aggravate hemorrhoids or varicose veins; this pressure may cause leg cramps or pain when it impinges on nerves.

BRAXTON HICKS CONTRACTIONS

Throughout pregnancy, the uterus undergoes a series of painless, irregular contractions known as Braxton Hicks contractions. These contractions have been described as pulling or tightening sensations in the uterine fundus. Although Braxton Hicks contractions may occur every 5 to 20 minutes throughout pregnancy, they typically become most noticeable during the last 6 weeks of gestation in primiparous clients and the last 3 to 4 months in multiparous clients (Knuppel and Drukker, 1986). They are the primary cause of false alarms that bring pregnant clients to the hospital thinking that labor has begun. The nurse should assure the client that these contractions are normal, explain that they may become stronger during and following intercourse, and advise rest and relaxation techniques if they produce discomfort.

CERVICAL CHANGES

Late in pregnancy, the cervix begins to change in preparation for dilation and onset of labor. Braxton Hicks contractions move the cervix upward as the lower uterine segment is formed. As a result, the fibrous connective tissue of the cervix loosens, causing the cervix to become softer, thinner, shorter, and more pliable. Prostaglandins also may contribute to cervical softening.

The cervix undergoes its prelabor changes, the mucus plug—which blocks the cervix throughout pregnancy—becomes dislodged. At the same time, some of the cervical capillaries rupture; blood mixes with the mucus, produc-

ing what is known as "bloody show." The client will detect a blood-tinged mucus discharge anytime from several days before labor to the onset of labor. Normally, only a few drops of blood mix with the mucus plug. The nurse should advise the client to notify the physician or nurse-midwife if she passes a larger amount of blood.

RUPTURE OF MEMBRANES

At term, approximately 12% of all pregnant clients experience a spontaneous rupture of membranes (SROM) before labor begins. Within 24 hours, labor will spontaneously begin in about 80% of these clients. The time between SROM and labor initiation depends on the length of gestation. A client who does not deliver within 24 hours after SROM is considered to have prolonged rupture of membranes, a condition that puts her and the fetus at increased risk for infection.

When the rupture occurs, the amniotic fluid may flow profusely or it may dribble. A client may confuse rupture of membranes with urinary incontinence caused by uterine pressure on the bladder. Testing of vaginal discharge with nitrazine paper allows the examiner to distinguish between the two conditions. Normal vaginal discharge and urine are both acidic, but amniotic fluid is alkaline (pH 7.2), which turns yellow nitrazine paper a deep blue upon contact.

Another simple test performs the same function. When allowed to dry on a microscopic slide, amniotic fluid assumes a characteristic fernlike pattern called ferning. Neither urine nor vaginal secretions assume this same pattern.

Another way to identify amniotic fluid is by directly observing pooled fluid within the vagina. The examiner inserts a sterile speculum and then asks the client to cough or bear down. If the membranes have ruptured, the examiner will observe fluid leaking into the vagina.

OTHER SIGNS AND SYMPTOMS

Clients have reported other signs and symptoms shortly before labor onset. A weight loss of 1 to 3 pounds, representing water loss, may result from changes in electrolyte concentrations of body fluids, which are linked to altered estrogen and progesterone levels. The effect of relaxin on pelvic joints may cause or increase sacroiliac discomfort. (Relaxin is a hormone secreted only during pregnancy that seems to soften the sacroiliac, sacrococcygeal, and pubic joints and increase their mobility.) Increased vaginal secretions, resulting from congestion of vaginal mucous membranes, also may occur.

In the last few days before labor onset, the client may experience a burst of energy known as the "nesting instinct." She may feel compelled to clean house and otherwise ensure that everything is ready for the neonate's arrival. The nurse should caution such a client against overexertion and encourage her to rest and build up energy reserves for labor and childbirth.

MECHANISMS OF LABOR

For most clients, labor follows a consistent pattern. As uterine contractions intensify, the cervix effaces and dilates. Propelled by uterine contractions and the client's bearing down efforts, the fetus descends through the birth canal via its cardinal movements.

CERVICAL EFFACEMENT AND DILATION

Myometrial activity at the onset of labor leads to full cervical effacement and dilation. Effacement refers to a progressive shortening of the vaginal portion of the cervix and thinning of its walls as it is stretched by the fetus during labor. Effacement is described as a percentage, ranging from 0% (noneffaced and thick) to 100% (fully effaced and paper thin). With the cervix fully effaced, the constrictive uterine neck is obliterated, and the cervix becomes continuous with the lower uterine segment.

Cervical dilation refers to progressive enlargement of the cervical os from less than 1 cm to about 10 cm (full dilation) to allow passage of the fetus from the uterus into the vagina. Because uterine muscle fibers remain shortened even after a contraction ceases, the uterus elongates and the uterine cavity decreases in size. These actions force the fetus downward toward the cervix. Cervical dilation results from this pressure—referred to as fetal axis pressure—plus the upward pulling of longitudinal muscle fibers over the fetus. Typically, effacement and dilation occur more quickly in multiparous clients than in primiparous clients.

CARDINAL MOVEMENTS

Cardinal movements refer to the typical sequence of positions assumed by the fetus during labor and childbirth. (See *Cardinal movements of labor,* page 182, for illustrations of these positions.)

Descent

Descent refers to the downward movement of the fetus into the pelvic passageway. In a primiparous client, this process may begin several weeks before labor, but further descent usually does not occur until the second stage of labor.

In a multiparous client, descent usually begins with engagement. This downward motion results from one or more forces: contraction of the abdominal muscles, pressure from the amniotic fluid, direct fundal pressure upon the fetus (fetal axis pressure), and the extension and straightening of the fetus. The progression of this downward movement is described as follows:

• *Floating.* The presenting part (the portion of the fetus that enters the pelvic passageway first) moves freely above the pelvic inlet.
• *Fixed.* The presenting part has entered the pelvic inlet and no longer moves but is not yet engaged.
• *Engaged.* The widest part of the presenting part has passed through the pelvic inlet.
• *Midpelvis.* The presenting part has descended halfway to the pelvic floor.
• *On the pelvic floor.* The presenting part has descended to the perineum.

Two other considerations involved in fetal descent are synclitism and asynclitism. These are related to the diameter between the fetal parietal bones and the plane of the maternal pelvic inlet. The measurements and the position of the two can ease or disrupt labor.

Flexion

Resistance from contact with the cervix, pelvic walls, or pelvic floor can flex the head of the fetus. When the head flexes downward so that the chin rests against the chest, the smallest diameter of the head will approach the client's pelvis. In this position, the suboccipitobregmatic diameter (normally about 9.5 cm) will enter the birth canal. If neither flexion nor extension occurs, the occipitofrontal diameter (normally about 11.75 cm) will reach the pelvis first.

Internal rotation

In most cases, internal rotation occurs during the second stage of labor—sometimes during one contraction. During internal rotation, the anteroposterior diameter of the head comes in line with the anteroposterior diameter of the pelvic outlet. When the head meets resistance from the pelvic floor, it rotates approximately 45 degrees left of the midline of the anterior abdominal wall under the symphysis pubis. Internal rotation, caused by twisting of the neck, does not involve movement of the shoulders. The shoulders remain oblique (between a parallel and a perpendicular position).

CARDINAL MOVEMENTS OF LABOR

For a fetus in the vertex (crown or top of head) presentation, labor follows a typical sequence. Inset boxes show the relationship of the fetal skull to the maternal pelvis.

1 Engagement, descent, flexion. The widest diameter of the head passes the level of the pelvic inlet; as the fetus moves downward toward the ischial spines, the head flexes on the chest.

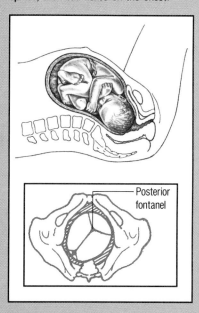

2 Internal rotation. The anteroposterior diameter of the head comes into line with the anteroposterior diameter of the pelvic outlet.

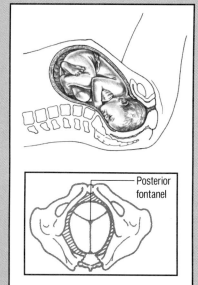

3 Extension. The head extends from the perineum after passing under the symphysis pubis.

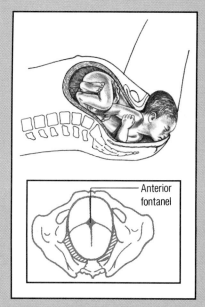

4 External rotation (restitution). The head rotates 45 degrees back to its original position.

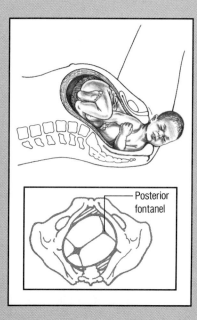

5 External rotation (shoulder rotation). The head rotates an additional 45 degrees to a transverse position; the anterior shoulder passes the perineum.

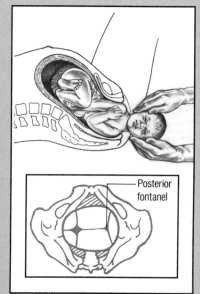

6 Expulsion. The rest of the body is easily delivered by lateral flexion.

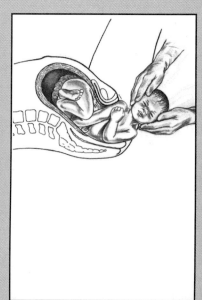

Although most fetuses assume an occiput anterior position following internal rotation, some rotate instead to an occiput posterior or occiput transverse position. These positions occur primarily in clients with abnormal pelvic configurations, such as android or anthropoid pelvises. Approximately 70% of fetuses in either position rotate spontaneously to the anterior position (Scott, 1989). However, failure of the fetus to assume the occiput anterior position can lead to prolonged labor caused by the inability of the fetal occiput to fill the pelvic cavity adequately or to exert equal pressure around the cervical os.

Extension

The head of the fetus remains in a flexed position until it passes under the symphysis pubis and reaches the perineum. The head then extends in response to pressure from uterine contractions, resistance from the pelvic floor, and intra-abdominal pressure from the client's bearing-down efforts.

Extension places the back of the fetus's neck in direct contact with the inferior margin of the symphysis pubis. As the head extends, it passes over the anterior margin of the perineum; then the head drops down, and the chin lies over the client's perineum.

External rotation

Once the head passes the perineum, it rotates 45 degrees, returning to the position it originally assumed during engagement. This is called restitution. Next, the fetus rotates an additional 45 degrees to assume a transverse position as the delivery proceeds. This movement positions the shoulders in line with the anteroposterior diameter of the client's pelvis. The anterior shoulder usually appears first, under the symphysis pubis; the posterior shoulder follows.

Expulsion

Once the shoulders pass the perineum, the remainder of the body is easily pulled upward and away from the perineum, following the natural curve of the pelvic passageway.

STAGES OF LABOR

Labor consists of four distinct stages. Understanding what occurs during each stage will help the nurse anticipate and meet the client's needs in labor.

FIRST STAGE OF LABOR

The first stage of labor is divided into latent, active and transitional phases. Cervical dilation and fetal descent begin during the latent phase, then accelerate during the active and transitional phases. In total, the first stage of labor, including the three phases, lasts 3.3 to 19.7 hours for primiparous clients and 0.1 to 14.3 hours for multiparous clients.

Latent phase

First described by Friedman (1954), the latent phase precedes active labor. In primiparous clients, this phase averages 8.6 hours; in multiparous clients, 5.3 hours. During this time, irregular, short, and mild contractions occur, and the cervix dilates to 3 or 4 cm.

The client may remain at home during the early part of the latent phase. When she enters the hospital, she may complain of abdominal cramping and lower back discomfort. Client behavior typically displays various degrees of excitement and apprehension. If she has not yet passed the mucus plug, she commonly will do so during the latent phase.

Active phase

Transition from the latent to the active phase occurs when the cervix dilates faster than 1.2 cm/hour in primiparous clients and 1.5 cm/hour in multiparous clients. In about 90% of clients, labor has progressed to the active phase by the time cervical dilation reaches 5 cm (Peisner and Rosen, 1986).

During the active phase, the cervix dilates to 7 cm. Contractions occur every 2 to 5 minutes, last 40 to 50 seconds, and are moderately intense. In primiparous clients, the active phase averages 5.8 hours; in multiparous clients, 2.5 hours.

Fetal descent continues throughout the active phase and into the transitional phase. The rate of descent is at least 1 cm/hour in primiparous clients and 2 cm/hour in multiparous clients.

Transitional phase

Occurring when the cervix is dilated between 8 and 10 cm, the transitional phase is the shortest, averaging less than 3 hours for primiparous clients and less than 1 hour for multiparous clients (Friedman, 1978). However, this phase is the most difficult for the client. Intense contractions lasting between 45 and 60 seconds occur every 1½ to 2 minutes. The client may thrash about, lose control of breathing techniques, and experience nausea and vomiting.

SECOND STAGE OF LABOR

The second stage begins with complete cervical dilation and ends with birth. Intense contractions occur every 2 to 3 minutes and last 60 to 90 seconds. For primiparous clients, this stage averages 1 hour; for multiparous clients, 24 minutes. In either case, a second stage longer than 2 hours is considered abnormal.

The beginning of this stage is characterized by an increase in bloody show, rupture of membranes (if this has not already occurred), severe rectal pressure, and a reflex bearing-down with each contraction. As the fetus approaches the perineal floor, the perineum bulges and flattens. As the labia spread, the head appears at the vaginal opening. At this time, the client should assume an active role and push with each contraction. Roberts, Goldstein, Gruener, Maggio, and Mendez-Bauer (1987) report that labor progress and outcome can be enhanced if the nurse discourages the client from sustained breath-holding and encourages pushing, which reinforces the involuntary bearing-down reflex.

Head

To prevent maternal lacerations and damage to the fetus's intracranial area, the nurse or other birth attendant must control the speed at which the head passes the perineum. When necessary, applying pressure over the perineum can maintain flexion of the head.

Once the head emerges, the physician or nurse-midwife must check for the umbilical cord. If the cord is loose around the neck, it should be slipped over the head. If the cord is very tight, fetal hypoxia may occur; therefore, the attendant must clamp and cut the cord while it is still around the neck. The oral and nasal pharynx then are suctioned with a bulb syringe to remove secretions that may be blocking the airway.

Shoulders

Following external rotation of the head, the shoulders pass through the pelvic inlet. After the head emerges, the attendant applies slight downward traction to free the anterior shoulder. After it emerges, gentle upward traction is applied on the head to allow the posterior shoulder to emerge.

Body and extremities

Once the shoulders emerge, the rest of the body, which is narrower than the shoulders, slides out with little or no traction needed.

THIRD STAGE OF LABOR

The third stage begins immediately after birth and ends with the separation and expulsion of the placenta. Strong but usually less painful contractions continue during this stage; their frequency may decrease to every 5 minutes. Normally, the placenta emerges about 5 minutes after the neonate's delivery.

Placental separation

Placental separation usually begins within minutes of birth. As labor nears completion and birth becomes imminent, the uterus begins to contract forcefully. By the time the neonate is delivered, the uterus consists of an almost solid mass of muscle with walls several centimeters thick above the lower segment. This mass differs greatly from the large cavity that previously housed the fetus. The fundal portion lies immediately below the umbilicus.

This decrease in uterine capacity causes the central portion of the placenta to pull away from the uterine wall. Bleeding from blood vessels in the area helps form a retroplacental hematoma. As this hematoma grows, the placenta further separates from the uterine wall. A placenta will not easily separate from a relaxed or boggy uterus because the decreased uterine muscles must first diminish the placental implantation site.

Signs indicating placental separation include lengthening of the umbilical cord, a sudden gush of dark blood from the vagina, and a change in uterine shape from disklike to globular (which the nurse can palpate or see as a visible bulge above the symphysis). The client may have a sensation of vaginal fullness.

Placental delivery

The placenta is expelled through one of two mechanisms. In the Schultze mechanism, the central portion of the placenta separates from the uterine wall before the outside edges do. Then the central portion folds or buckles outward, away from the retroplacental hematoma. When the placenta is expelled, the shiny fetal side (commonly called "shiny Schultze") is visible.

In the Duncan mechanism, the placental edges separate first, followed by the central portion. Then the central portion rolls up and is expelled sideways, so that the rough-surfaced maternal side (commonly called "dirty Duncan") is visible. In the Duncan mechanism, separation may be incomplete, leaving placental fragments that may lead to infection or bleeding. Immediately after delivery, the placenta must be evaluated carefully for completeness, and the client must be assessed for excessive bleeding or a relaxed uterus.

FOURTH STAGE OF LABOR

Beginning with delivery of the placenta and extending through the first 4 hours after childbirth, the fourth stage allows the client's body to adjust to the postpartal stage. She should be assessed carefully for uterine atony, postpartal hemorrhage, and urine retention.

Ideally, the client and her partner should now hold and examine the infant and begin parent-infant bonding.

FACTORS AFFECTING LABOR

Successful labor and childbirth requires coordination of five essential factors, sometimes termed the "five p's":
• passenger (the fetus)
• passageway (the pelvis)
• powers (uterine contractions and bearing-down efforts)
• placental position and function
• psychological response.

For the fetus to move successfully through the pelvis, the contractions and bearing-down efforts must be of adequate intensity and frequency, the placenta must be properly positioned and provide adequate oxygen to the fetus, and the client must be psychologically prepared. Problems involving any of these essential factors may jeopardize safe labor and childbirth and require medical or surgical intervention.

FETUS

Fetal factors affecting labor and childbirth include size and shape of the head, lie, attitude, presentation, position, and station.

Head

The skull is composed of several small, thin, incompletely developed bones, including two frontal bones, two parietal bones, two temporal bones, and one occipital bone in the back, which eventually fuse to form the rigid cranial cavity characteristic of the adult. The largest part of the fetus, the skull also is the least compressible part. However, the skull bones are connected by flexible, membrane-occupied spaces called sutures, which allow alterations in skull shape (called molding). During labor, the skull bones are pressed together and may overlap, reducing the size of the head and facilitating passage through the unyielding pelvis.

Besides allowing for molding, the sutures separating these bones aid in identifying fetal position during labor. The sagittal suture, which runs in an anteroposterior di-

rection, separates the two parietal bones. The frontal suture, an extension of the saggital suture, separates the two frontal bones. The coronal suture separates the parietal bones from the frontal bones. The lambdoidal suture separates the parietal bones from the occipital bone.

Sutures intersect at membranous spaces called fontanels. The anterior fontanel (also called the bregma) is located at the junction of the sagittal, coronal, and frontal sutures. Diamond-shaped, the anterior fontanel measures 3 to 4 cm long and 2 to 3 cm wide. By remaining open until the infant is about 18 months old, this fontanel gives the brain space to grow. The posterior fontanel is located at the junction of the sagittal and lambdoidal sutures. This triangular-shaped fontanel, approximately 2 cm wide, normally closes within 6 to 8 weeks after birth.

During labor, the head goes through movements designed to ensure that its smallest diameter enters the pelvis first. The head can flex or extend about 45 degrees and can rotate about 180 degrees. This ability to flex, extend, and rotate allows its smallest diameters to move down the birth canal and pass through the maternal bony pelvis.

Lie

Fetal lie refers to the position of the fetal spine in relation to the maternal spine. When the two spines are parallel, the fetus is in a longitudinal lie. When the spines are perpendicular, the fetus is in a transverse lie. When the fetal spine is at an angle between the parallel and perpendicular position, the fetus is in an oblique lie. Typically, a fetus in an oblique lie will convert either to a longitudinal or a transverse lie before birth.

Unless the fetus is positioned in a longitudinal lie, a vaginal birth is impossible, and surgical intervention becomes necessary.

Attitude

Fetal attitude refers to overall body flexion or extension, which determines the relationship of fetal parts to one another. The usual fetal attitude in the uterus is vertex, with the head flexed so that the chin rests against the chest, the legs and arms folded in front of the body, and the back curved slightly forward.

The fetus normally exhibits varying degrees of flexion and extension throughout pregnancy, with no ill effects; however, fetal attitude becomes significant during labor and childbirth. With the fetus in a cephalic (head-first) presentation, a fully flexed attitude enables the smallest head diameter to enter the pelvis. As the degree of extension increases, the diameter of the head entering the pelvis also increases, making labor and childbirth more difficult.

Position

Fetal position refers to the relationship of the presenting part to the maternal pelvis. The nurse establishes position by determining three factors: a landmark on the fetal presenting part, whether this landmark faces the right or left side of the maternal pelvis, and whether the landmark faces the front, back, or side of the maternal pelvis. (For more information, see *Determining fetal position.*)

DETERMINING FETAL POSITION

Fetal position is determined by the relationship of a specific presenting part to the front, back, or side of the maternal pelvis. A notation system identifies three features: a landmark on the presenting part (O for occiput, M for mentum, S for sacrum, A for acromion process, and D for dorsal); whether this landmark faces the right (R) or left (L) side of the pelvis; and whether the landmark faces the front (A for anterior), the back (P for posterior), or a side (T for transverse) of the pelvis. Thus, for a fetus with the occiput (O) as the presenting landmark, positioned facing the right side (R) and front (A) of the maternal pelvis, the nurse would identify the position as ROA.

In a vertex presentation (by far the most common), the fetus may assume one of the six positions illustrated below: LOP, LOT, LOA, ROP, ROT, or ROA.

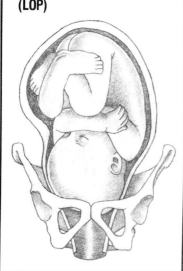

Left occiput posterior (LOP)

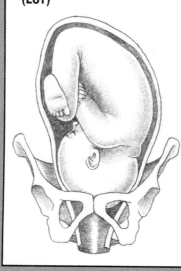

Left occiput transverse (LOT)

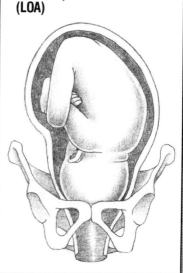

Left occiput anterior (LOA)

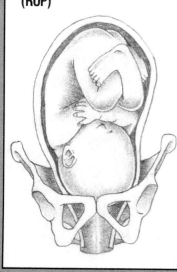

Right occiput posterior (ROP)

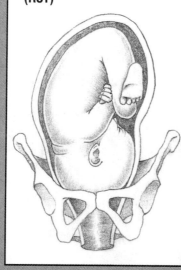

Right occiput transverse (ROT)

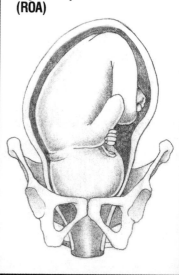

Right occiput anterior (ROA)

Presentation

Fetal presentation refers to the manner in which the fetus enters the pelvic passageway. Presentation is classified according to the presenting part—the portion of the fetus that enters the pelvic passageway first—as:

• cephalic (head-first)

• breech (buttocks-first)

• shoulder

• compound.

(See *Classifying fetal presentation*, pages 188 and 189, for illustrations and descriptions of these presentations.)

Approximately 95% of all births occur with the fetus assuming a cephalic presentation. A shoulder presentation occurs when the fetal spine is perpendicular to the maternal spine. Unless the fetus in this presentation moves to a longitudinal lie, cesarean delivery is necessary. Predisposing factors in a shoulder presentation include placenta previa, neoplasms, fetal anomalies, hydramnios (excess of amniotic fluid), preterm labor, uterine atony, multiple gestation, and premature artificial rupture of membranes.

Before the twenty-eighth week of gestation, approximately 25% of fetuses are in a breech presentation. By the thirty-fourth week of gestation, however, most fetuses move to a cephalic presentation. Nevertheless, 3% to 4% of all term pregnancies involve breech presentation (Oxorn, 1986).

In most cases, the cause of breech presentation cannot be pinpointed; however, numerous maternal, placental, and fetal predisposing factors have been identified. Maternal factors associated with breech presentation include uterine anomalies, uterine relaxation resulting from previous childbirth, myometrial neoplasm, contracted pelvis, oligohydramnios (in which the fetus is restricted to the position it assumed during the second trimester), and hydramnios (in which the fetal position changes easily because of excessive amniotic fluid). Placental factors include the implantation of the placenta in either cornual-fundal region (the horns on either side of the fundus). Also reported to cause a higher incidence of breech presentations is placenta previa, a condition in which the placenta partially or totally covers the cervical os and blocks the fetus from leaving the uterus (Oxorn, 1986). Fetal factors include prematurity, multiple gestation, anencephaly, hydrocephaly (dilation of the cerebral ventricles after obstruction of the flow of cerebrospinal fluid), intrauterine fetal death, and other fetal anomalies.

Station

Fetal station refers to the relationship of the presenting part to the maternal ischial spines. The ischial spines, located at midpelvis, form the narrowest portion of the pelvis through which the fetus must pass. When the largest diameter of the presenting part (usually the biparietal diameter of the head) is level with the ischial spines, the fetus is at station 0. Numbers from 1 to 3 indicate how many centimeters the presenting part is above or below the ischial spines. Thus, a presenting part above the ischial spines is designated as −1, −2, or −3; a presenting part below this point, +1, +2, or +3. When the presenting part is classified as being at greater than station, it is at the pelvic outlet and visible on the perineum.

Successful vaginal birth requires progressive fetal descent from a minus station to 0 and then to a plus station during labor. Lack of this progressive descent with effective uterine contractions may indicate cephalopelvic disproportion or an inappropriately short or tangled umbilical cord. In such cases, cesarean delivery may be necessary.

PELVIS

The passageway through which the fetus must travel during labor consists of the pelvis and soft tissues. Pelvic types and diameters affect labor and childbirth.

The pelvis is partly ligamentous and partly bony. Although Caldwell and Moloy (1933) first categorized four basic pelvic types—gynecoid, android, anthropoid, and platypelloid—a client usually has features of two or more types.

The true pelvis contains three levels, or planes: the pelvic inlet, the midpelvis, and the pelvic outlet. Diameters measured in these three planes indicate the amount of space available for the fetus during birth.

The pelvic inlet has four diameters: the anteroposterior diameter, the transverse diameter, and two oblique diameters. The pelvic inlet's anteroposterior diameter is further divided into the obstetric conjugate, the true conjugate, and the diagonal conjugate diameters. The diagonal conjugate can be measured during a pelvic examination; the other two diameters are estimated from this measurement.

The pelvic diameters can be affected by the client's position during labor, by relaxin (a hormone produced by the placenta) in the system, and by the amount of fat or soft tissue surrounding the pelvis. Assuming a squatting or lateral Sims' position may help increase the pelvic diameters. Relaxin helps to relax the pelvis and increase the pelvic diameters.

(Text continues on page 190.)

CLASSIFYING FETAL PRESENTATION

Fetal presentation may be broadly classified as cephalic, shoulder, compound, or breech. Cephalic presentations comprise almost all deliveries. Of the remaining three, breech deliveries are most common.

CEPHALIC

In the head-down presentation, the position of the fetus may be further classified by the presenting skull landmark, such as vertex, brow, sinciput, or face.

Vertex

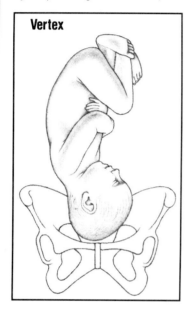

Brow

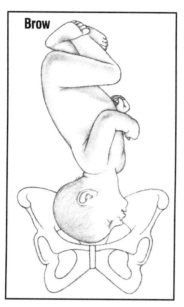

Sinciput

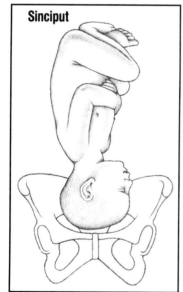

Face

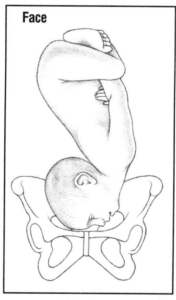

SHOULDER

Although a fetus may adopt one of several shoulder presentations, examination cannot differentiate among them; thus, all transverse lies are called shoulder presentations.

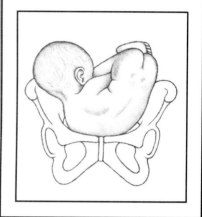

COMPOUND

In this presentation, an extremity prolapses alongside the major presenting part so that two presenting parts appear in the pelvis at the same time.

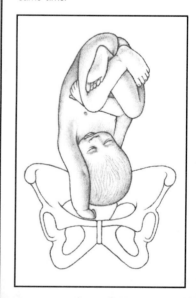

BREECH

In the head-up presentation, the position of the fetus may be further classified as frank, where hips are flexed and knees remain straight; complete, where knees and hips are flexed; footling, where the knees and hips of one or both legs are extended; kneeling, where knees are flexed and hips remain extended; and incomplete, where one or both hips remain extended and one or both feet or knees lie below the breech.

Frank

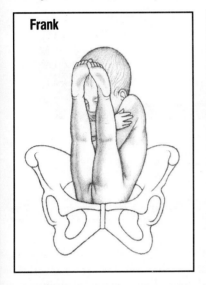

Complete

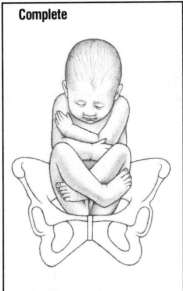

Footling

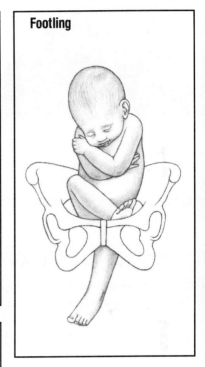

Kneeling

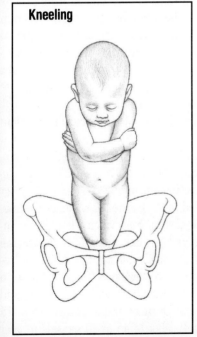

Incomplete

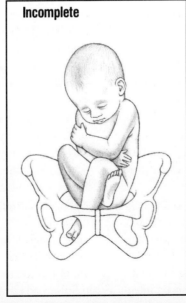

PHASES OF A UTERINE CONTRACTION

As shown in the diagram below, a uterine contraction occurs in three phases: increment (building up), acme (peak), and decrement (letting down). Between contractions is a period of relaxation. The two most important features of contractions are frequency and duration. Frequency refers to the elapsed time from the start of one contraction to the start of the next contraction. Duration is the elapsed time from the start to the end of one contraction.

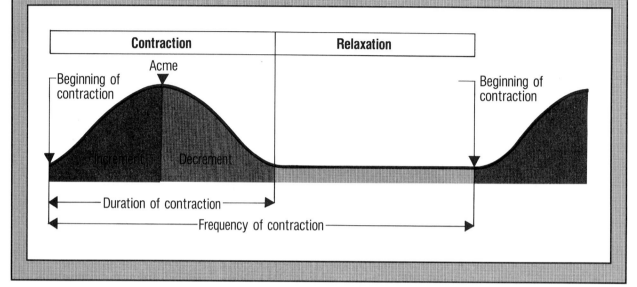

CONTRACTIONS AND BEARING-DOWN EFFORTS

The third of five essential factors in successful labor and childbirth are the powers, also known as uterine contractions and bearing-down efforts. Involuntary uterine contractions and voluntary bearing-down efforts must be adequate in intensity and frequency.

Uterine contractions

Rhythmic tightening of the upper uterine segment musculature, uterine contractions serve several purposes during labor and childbirth. Coordinated and effective uterine contractions promote fetal descent and rotation, cervical effacement and dilation, separation and expulsion of the placenta, and constriction of the uterine vasculature to prevent postpartal hemorrhage.

A uterine contraction begins in response to a change in electrical activity. This change, referred to as a wave of excitation, originates in pacemakers located near the uterotubal junctions. The downward movement of the electrical charge from the upper segment of the uterus to the cervix is known as fundal dominance. Contraction intensity and duration are both greater in the upper uterine segment than in the lower uterine segment.

These three characteristics—fundal dominance, intensity, and duration—help create a coordinated uterine contraction that produces maximum expulsive force. The muscular structure of the uterus (the myometrium) is unique because the fibers remain shortened even after the contraction is over instead of reverting to their precontraction size—that is, the fibers shorten progressively during labor. This is known as retraction or brachystasis. As labor continues, this progressive shortening of fibers results in a thickening of the upper uterine segment and a decrease in uterine size, which impels fetal descent.

For uterine contractions to propel the fetus through the birth canal effectively, several biochemical interactions must occur.

A uterine contraction occurs in three phases: increment, acme, and decrement. (See *Phases of a uterine contraction.*) During the increment and acme phases, waves of excitation, initiated in the pacemakers, induce contractions. As the waves subside, contractions decrease in intensity and duration and conclude in the decrement phase.

During labor, the nurse evaluates the duration, frequency, and intensity of contractions. The duration of a contraction refers to the time between the beginning and end of the contraction. Duration usually ranges from 15 to 30 seconds in early labor to 45 to 90 seconds in later stages. The frequency of contractions is measured from the beginning of one contraction to the beginning of the next. In early labor, frequency ranges from 20 to 30 minutes; in the later stages, it ranges from 2 to 3 minutes.

The duration and frequency of contractions affect both the client and the fetus. Duration greater than 90 seconds and frequency less than 2 minutes increase the risk of uterine rupture and also put the fetus at high risk for hypoxia from uterine vasoconstriction. Excessively long and overly frequent contractions also sap the client's energy and strength during labor, hindering her voluntary bearing-down efforts.

The intensity of a contraction refers to its strength during the acme phase. Intensity can be measured directly with an intrauterine catheter and indirectly by palpation or external monitoring. The normal resting pressure of the uterus between contractions measured via intrauterine catheter is 10 mm Hg; this pressure can increase to 50 mm Hg during acme. When the pressure reaches 15 to 20 mm Hg, blood supply to the uterus and placenta is compromised, and the client begins to feel pain.

Bearing-down efforts

Once uterine contractions have fully effaced and dilated the cervix, the second stage of labor begins and the client's voluntary bearing-down efforts take over. In these efforts, she contracts the diaphragm and abdominal muscles to increase intra-abdominal pressure. This action, which applies pressure to the uterine walls, adds to the pressures from uterine contractions and aids fetal descent and expulsion. The client also experiences a great involuntary urge to push as the head of the fetus descends and pushes against the sacral and obturator nerves.

Positions for labor. Throughout most of the world today, labor and childbirth most often occur with the woman in an upright position. In contrast, the recumbent position remains a Western tradition (Rossi and Lindell, 1986).

Position during labor can affect the frequency and intensity of contractions. For a client in the supine position, contractions may be less intense but more frequent. For one in the lateral position, contractions tend to be more intense but less frequent.

Studies that evaluate the effect of an upright position and walking around during the first stage of labor have yielded inconclusive results (Rossi and Lindell, 1986). However, many women find walking during labor a positive experience. Lupe and Gross (1986) concluded that neither the assumption of various positions nor walking seems to harm the pregnant woman or the fetus or inhibit the progress of labor. Although not conclusive, data suggest that walking, standing, or sitting may shorten labor.

PLACENTAL POSITION AND FUNCTION

Throughout pregnancy and during labor, the fetus depends on the placenta for oxygenated blood and nutrients. Placental malposition or malfunction can hinder labor and childbirth and may compromise the well-being of the fetus. In most cases, the placenta is attached to the upper uterine segment. However, 1 in every 200 to 300 pregnancies involves placenta previa—implantation of the placenta in the lower uterine segment, where it partially or totally covers the cervical os. Besides blocking the os, placenta previa causes the placenta to separate from the uterine wall partially or totally as the cervix dilates, typically causing hemorrhage.

Other conditions can cause placental malfunction. For example, in abruptio placentae, occurring in about 1 in 250 pregnancies, the placenta prematurely separates from the uterine wall. Another condition, uteroplacental insufficiency, impairs the ability of the fetus to withstand the rigors of labor.

PSYCHOLOGICAL RESPONSE

The role that a pregnant woman's mental and emotional state plays in labor and childbirth has received increasing attention over the last several decades. In 1961, Rosengren identified a relationship between a woman's perception of her health state during pregnancy and her behavior during labor. He found that those who adopted a "sick role" during pregnancy had a higher incidence of prolonged, difficult labor. More recent studies point to a relationship between anxiety and the length and difficulty of labor. In particular, researchers have found that high epinephrine levels triggered by maternal anxiety can lead to diminished uterine activity and longer labors (Lederman, et al., 1977). Other researchers have found that women who experienced severe pain or distress-related thoughts may be more likely to experience an inefficient labor (Wuitchik, Bakal, and Lipshitz, 1989).

These and other studies indicate the importance of an appropriate psychological response to the physiologic and emotional demands of labor. Factors that may influence a client's psychological response include preparation for labor, support systems, and coping mechanisms.

MATERNAL SYSTEMIC RESPONSE TO LABOR

Labor produces significant changes in many body systems. Understanding these changes will help the nurse provide better care for the client during labor.

CARDIOVASCULAR SYSTEM

In the first and second stages of labor, cardiovascular system changes primarily affect blood pressure. Cardiac output increases dramatically between contractions as labor progresses, rising 10% to 15% in the first stage of labor and 30% to 50% in the second stage. Contractions during the first stage of labor raise systolic blood pressure readings about 10 mm Hg and diastolic readings from 5 to 10 mm Hg. Because of this fluctuating increase, blood pressure readings between contractions will be the most reliable ones.

Contractions in the second stage raise systolic and diastolic readings an average of 30 mm Hg and 25 mm Hg, respectively. Between contractions, blood pressure may remain elevated by 10 mm Hg systolic and 5 to 10 mm Hg diastolic. This persistent elevation puts a client who already has hypertension at increased risk for complications, such as cerebral hemorrhage (Beischer and Mackay, 1986).

The client's position during labor also can affect blood pressure. The inferior vena cava of a supine client is less compressed as the fetus descends, whereas the aorta remains compressed until delivery, resulting in possible hypertension. Although approximately 90% of clients at term experience supine hypotensive syndrome, only 10% to 15% exhibit signs and symptoms, such as lightheadedness (Albright, Joyce, and Stevenson, 1986). Factors that may increase a client's risk of supine hypotensive syndrome include dehydration, hypovolemia, obesity, multiple gestation, and hydramnios.

A strong contraction reduces blood flow through the uterine artery into the intervillous spaces. Consequently, blood flow is redirected into the peripheral circulation, leading to increased peripheral resistance. This in turn leads to increased blood pressure and decreased pulse rate.

The client's voluntary bearing-down efforts in the second stage of labor greatly alter intrathoracic pressure. As the client performs Valsalva's maneuver (holds her breath and tightens her abdominal muscles), intrathoracic pressure increases, venous return decreases, and venous pressure increases. As blood from the lungs is forced into the left atrium, cardiac output, blood pressure, and pulse pressure all increase, and bradycardia temporarily occurs. These processes reverse when Valsalva's maneuver ceases; however, the nurse must be aware of the long-term effect on the client with a history of cardiac disease. Also, the fetus may experience hypoxia during this time.

Other factors that may alter blood pressure during labor include anxiety, pain, and certain medications. For example, hypotension may result from administration of a narcotic, such as meperidine (Demerol), because of its vasodilating effects or from a regional anesthetic because of its sympathetic blocking effects.

A slow, progressive rise in pulse rate typically occurs during labor. Factors that may exacerbate this rise include pain, anxiety, hemorrhage, infection, certain medications (such as tocolytics), dehydration, increased cardiac output, and decreased plasma volume.

GASTROINTESTINAL SYSTEM

During labor, gastric motility and absorption decrease and gastric emptying time (the time required for the stomach to empty) increases. As a result, a client in labor may vomit food she consumed as long as 24 hours before labor began (Scott, 1989). These normal physiologic responses are enhanced by narcotic administration, which also slows labor.

Solid foods usually are withheld during labor to prevent the risk of aspiration if an emergency arises and general anesthesia is needed. For similar reasons, some physicians advocate giving the client antacids to neutralize gastric acid either during labor or immediately before anesthetic administration. Because gastrointestinal absorption of fluids is not altered, sipping water or chewing ice chips is allowed during labor.

RESPIRATORY SYSTEM

Oxygen consumption increases dramatically during labor, from a normal rate of about 250 ml/minute up to approximately 750 ml/minute during contractions (Knuppel and Drukker, 1986). Both during and between contractions, oxygen consumption increases progressively throughout labor. By the second stage of labor, a client's oxygen consumption may be twice that before onset of labor. This dramatic increase is especially likely in an unmedicated client experiencing extreme anxiety. Resulting hyperventilation can lead to respiratory alkalosis, hypoxia, or hypocapnia. The nurse must monitor the client for signs of such problems and intervene promptly to avoid endangering the fetus.

HEMATOPOIETIC SYSTEM

The normal leukocyte count of 5,000 to 11,000 mm³ may increase to about 25,000 mm³ during labor. This rise occurs particularly during prolonged labor, leading some researchers to link it with strenuous muscle activity or increased stress. Other significant hematologic changes include increased plasma fibrinogen levels and decreased plasma glucose levels and blood coagulation times.

RENAL AND UROLOGIC SYSTEM

During labor, decreased sensory perceptions may impair the client's ability to feel bladder fullness and the urge to void. Also, compression of the ureters by the uterus may impede urine flow. Either of these factors can lead to urinary stasis and, if bladder fullness is profound, possibly impede fetal descent. For this reason, the nurse should encourage the client to empty her bladder every 2 hours during labor.

When engagement occurs and the presenting part of the fetus enters or passes the pelvic inlet, the base of the bladder is pushed upward and forward. Pressure from the presenting part may interfere with blood and lymph drainage from the base of the bladder, leading to tissue edema.

During labor, trace amounts of protein in urine commonly occur because of muscle breakdown. However, levels above trace amounts should alert the nurse to the possibility of pregnancy-induced hypertension.

FLUID AND ELECTROLYTE BALANCE

Labor can have several effects on the client's fluid and electrolyte balance. Increased muscular activity increases body temperature, which in turn causes fluid and electrolyte loss through diaphoresis. Increased respiratory rate and resultant hyperventilation increase fluid loss through evaporation. Vomiting, which may occur during the transitional phase of active labor, also can cause fluid and electrolyte loss. For these reasons, careful monitoring of fluid intake and output is essential during prolonged labor to prevent dehydration and related problems.

FETAL SYSTEMIC RESPONSE TO LABOR

Understanding the normal fetal response to labor helps the nurse quickly identify variations from normal and intervene promptly to prevent further complications.

CARDIOVASCULAR SYSTEM

The normal fetal heart rate ranges from 120 to 160 beats/minute. A rate greater than 160 beats/minute is considered tachycardia; a rate of 120 or less, bradycardia. According to Beischer and Mackay (1986), normal rhythm is fairly constant, with the baseline reflecting a fluctuation of ± 5 to 10 beats over a selected time interval. (See Chapter 11, Fetal Assessment, for a description of the changes.)

Fetal blood pressure is one of several factors responsible for ensuring an adequate exchange of gases and nutrients to and from the fetal capillaries and the intervillous space. Adequate placental and fetal reserve ensures that the fetus can withstand the stresses of anoxia brought on by uterine contractions.

RESPIRATORY SYSTEM

The fetus's breathing activity decreases sharply during labor (Beishcher and Mackay, 1986). Through ultrasonography, an examiner can study these breathing movements and distinguish true preterm labor from false labor.

ACID-BASE STATUS

During pregnancy, the fetus is at risk for both respiratory and metabolic acidosis. Because a major role of the placenta is to function as a fetal lung, any conditions interrupting normal blood flow to or from the placenta will increase fetal $PaCO_2$ and decrease fetal pH (Knuppel and Drukker, 1986).

Since the technique of monitoring fetal capillary blood pH was introduced in the early 1960s, it has gained widespread clinical acceptance because it indicates how adequately tissues are being supplied with oxygen. Measuring PaO_2 indicates the status of the fetus at the time of sampling; however, compared to the pH, PaO_2 may be difficult to measure correctly and may fluctuate rapidly. Because the blood pH is influenced by respiratory and metabolic factors, both rapid (respiratory) and prolonged (metabolic) changes can be detected (Knuppel and Drukker, 1986).

During the first stage of labor, the fetal scalp capillary blood pH is approximately 7.35; during the second stage, approximately 7.25 (Korones, 1986). Values below 7.2 indicate fetal distress. This decrease results from uterine contractions, which inhibit placental exchange, and from decreased maternal pH. Decreased values become more evident during the second stage of labor because the hypoxia associated with pushing leads to metabolic acidosis.

FETAL ACTIVITY

Using ultrasound to study movement during labor, Griffin, Caron, and van Geijn (1985) found that fetal behavioral states present during pregnancy continue during labor. The fetus periodically changes from quiet to active sleep states, in spite of ruptured membranes and uterine contractions that progressively increase in frequency, duration, and intensity.

VITAL SIGNS

During the fetus's quiet sleep state, which normally lasts about 40 minutes, the heart rate variability may decrease. A decrease lasting more than 40 minutes, however, may indicate fetal hypoxia and requires further investigation.

A low maternal temperature has been shown to lead to fetal bradycardia; however, the fetal heart rate returns to normal as maternal temperature rises (Jadhon and Main, 1988). Researchers believe that the temperature of amniotic fluid and the fetus parallel the client's temperature. The fetus responds to lower temperatures with decreased metabolic requirements and a decreased pulse rate.

CHAPTER SUMMARY

Chapter 10 described the physiologic and psychological changes that trigger labor and occur during it. Here are the chapter highlights.

The exact mechanism that triggers labor is unclear.

Premonitory signs and symptoms of labor include lightening, Braxton Hicks contractions, cervical changes, bloody show, rupture of membranes, and a burst of energy.

In most clients, labor follows a consistent pattern. As uterine contractions intensify, the cervix undergoes effacement and dilation to allow passage of the fetus from the uterus into the vagina.

Propelled by uterine contractions, the fetus maneuvers downward through the pelvis via a series of steps known as cardinal movements: descent, flexion, internal rotation, extension, external rotation (restitution and shoulder rotation), and expulsion.

The first stage of labor—comprising latent, active, and transitional phases—extends from the beginning of true labor to complete cervical dilation.

The second stage of labor starts with complete cervical dilation and ends with birth.

The third stage of labor extends from birth to separation and expulsion of the placenta.

The fourth stage of labor encompasses the first 4 hours after childbirth or until the client is stable.

Successful labor and childbirth require coordination of five essential factors, commonly known as the "five p's": the passenger (fetus), passageway (pelvis), powers (uterine contractions and the client's bearing-down efforts), placental position and function, and the client's psychological response.

In about 95% of clients, the fetus assumes the cephalic (head-first) position. Flexibility of the fetal skull bones allows the skull to adapt to the pelvic passageway, a process known as molding.

The client's pelvic type and diameters influence the labor process.

Uterine contractions are involuntary and involve intermittent tightening and relaxing of uterine muscle fibers in response to electrical activity. In the second stage of labor, the client's voluntary bearing-down efforts augment uterine contractions and aid fetal descent and expulsion.

The placenta must be properly positioned to ensure successful childbirth and fetal well-being.

The client's psychological response has a significant effect on labor and childbirth. Factors that may influence this response include preparation for labor, support systems, and coping mechanisms.

Labor causes many physiologic changes in the client's body systems, especially the cardiovascular, gastrointestinal, respiratory, hematopoietic, and renal and urologic systems.

During labor, the fetus experiences significant changes in cardiovascular and respiratory responses, acid-base status, physical activities, and vital signs.

STUDY QUESTIONS

1. Describe the five essential factors affecting labor.
2. Describe how the mother's cardiovascular system responds to labor.
3. Describe what happens to fetal activity during labor.
4. Discuss the three phases of the first stage of labor.
5. Explain the three phases of a uterine contraction and describe what the nurse should evaluate about the contraction.

BIBLIOGRAPHY

Albright, G., Joyce, T., and Stevenson, D. (1986). *Anesthesia in obstetrics: Maternal, fetal, and neonatal aspects* (2nd ed.). Boston: Butterworth.

Burroughs, A. (1986). *Bleier's maternity nursing* (5th ed.). Philadelphia: Saunders.

Cunningham, F.G., MacDonald, P.C., and Gant, N.F. (1989). *Williams obstetrics* (18th ed.). East Norwalk, CT: Appleton & Lange.

Knuppel, R., and Drukker, J. (1986). *High-risk pregnancy.* Philadelphia: Saunders.

Korones, S. (1986). *High-risk newborn infants: The basics for intensive nursing care* (4th ed.). St. Louis: Mosby.

Malinowski, J., Pedigo, C., and Phillips, C. (1989). *Nursing care during the labor process* (3rd ed.). Philadelphia: F. A. Davis.

Morishima, H., Pedersen, H., and Finster, M. (1978). The influence of maternal psychological stress on the fetus. *American Journal of Obstetrics and Gynecology,* 131(3), 286-290.

Peisner, D., and Rosen, M. (1986). Transition from latent to active labor. *Obstetrics and Gynecology,* 68(4), 448-451.

Scott, J.R. (Ed.) (1989). *Danforth's obstetrics and gynecology* (6th ed.). Philadelphia: Lippincott.

Maternal response

Bassell, G., Humayun, S., and Marx, G. (1980). Maternal bearing-down efforts—Another fetal risk? *Obstetrics and Gynecology,* 56(1), 39-41.

Caldwell, W., and Moloy, H. (1933). Anatomical variations in the female pelvis and their effect on labor with a suggested classification. *American Journal of Obstetrics and Gynecology,* 26, 479.

Lederman, R., McCann, D., and Work, B. (1977). Endogenous plasma epinephrine and norepinephrine in last trimester pregnancy and labor. *American Journal of Obstetrics and Gynecology,* 129(1), 5-8.

Lowe, N. (1987). Parity and pain during parturition. *JOGNN,* 16(5), 340-346.

Lupe, P., and Gross, T. (1986). Maternal upright posture and mobility in labor—A review. *Obstetrics and Gynecology,* 67(5), 727-734.

Roberts, J., Goldstein, S., Gruener, J., Maggio, M., and Mendez-Bauer, C. (1987). A descriptive analysis of involuntary bearing-down efforts during the expulsive phase of labor. *JOGNN,* 16(1), 48-55.

Rossi, M., and Lindell, S. (1986). Maternal positions and pushing techniques in a nonprescriptive environment. *JOGNN,* 15(3), 203-208.

Fetal response

Beischer, N., and Mackay, E. (1986). *Obstetrics and the newborn* (2nd ed.). Philadelphia: Saunders.

Griffin, R., Caron, F., and van Geijn, H. (1985). Behavioral states in the human fetus during labor. *American Journal of Obstetrics and Gynecology,* 158(8), 885-886.

Hughey, M. (1985). Fetal position during pregnancy. *American Journal of Obstetrics and Gynecology,* 153(8), 885-886.

Jadhon, M., and Main, E. (1988). Fetal bradycardia associated with maternal hypothermia: 2. *Obstetrics and Gynecology,* 72(3, Pt. 2), 496-497.

Labor: Stages and mechanisms

Friedman, E. (1954). The graphic analysis of labor. *American Journal of Obstetrics and Gynecology,* 68, 1568-1575.

Friedman, E. (1978). *Labor: Clinical evaluation and management* (2nd ed.). East Norwalk, CT: Appleton-Century-Crofts.

Rosegren, W. (1961). Some social psychological aspects of delivery room difficulties. *Journal of Nervous Mental Disorders,* 132, 515.

Oxorn, H. (1986). *Oxorn-Foote human labor and birth* (5th ed.). East Norwalk, CT: Appleton & Lange.

Wuitchik, M., Bakal, D., and Lipshitz, J. (1989). The clinical significance of pain and cognitive activity in latent labor. *Obstetrics and Gynecology,* 73(1), 35-42.

CHAPTER 11

FETAL ASSESSMENT

OBJECTIVES

After reading and studying this chapter, the student should be able to:
1. Identify factors that affect uteroplacental-fetal circulation.
2. Explain the physiology that regulates fetal heart rate.
3. Describe the techniques of electronic fetal monitoring.
4. Identify on a sample monitor strip the baseline fetal heart rate, short- and long-term variability, and any periodic changes present. Explain how uterine activity is monitored.
5. List three alternative methods for fetal monitoring.
6. Explain the importance of proper documentation of monitoring findings, using appropriate terminology.

INTRODUCTION

Early and informed nursing judgments about fetal heart rate (FHR) data can be crucial to performing timely and appropriate nursing interventions. This chapter begins by discussing the intricate physiologic balance between mother and fetus necessary to maintain fetal health and the various conditions that can jeopardize this balance. It continues by describing the principles of and techniques for using electronic fetal monitoring (EFM) to evaluate the FHR, and it discusses the basic guidelines for interpreting FHR patterns. Also discussed are other methods for assessing fetal status, such as fetal scalp blood sampling, fetal acoustic stimulation, and fetal scalp stimulation tests.

The chapter concludes with a section on nursing responsibilities associated with fetal monitoring. Included are discussions of documentation using appropriate terminology, client education and support, and the nurse's legal responsibility for the health of the mother and fetus.

PHYSIOLOGIC BASIS OF FETAL MONITORING

Fetal monitoring provides data about fetal status during the intrapartal period. Hypoxic or nonhypoxic stress on the fetus produces characteristic FHR patterns detectable through electronic monitoring techniques. To detect such patterns accurately, the nurse must understand basic physiologic principles of uteroplacental-fetal circulation and FHR regulation.

UTEROPLACENTAL-FETAL CIRCULATION

During labor, fetal well-being depends on effective oxygen exchange from the maternal circulation through the placenta to the fetus. Any condition or factor that disrupts this circulatory route can compromise fetal well-being.

Factors affecting uteroplacental-fetal circulation

Any condition that decreases maternal cardiac output reduces placental blood flow. During labor, uteroplacental-fetal circulation can be affected by maternal position, uterine contractions, placental surface area and diffusion distance, anesthetics, maternal hypertension or hypotension, and cord compression. The nurse's primary goal is to maintain adequate maternal circulation and perfusion to the placenta so that the fetus can receive the needed oxygen and nutrients.

Maternal position. When a client in labor assumes a supine position, two possible conditions can decrease uterine blood flow. In supine hypotensive syndrome, the gravid uterus compresses the vena cava and hinders blood return to the client's heart. As a result, maternal blood pressure and cardiac output decrease, reducing blood flow to the uterus and decreasing placental perfusion. If the aorta becomes compressed, maternal blood pressure may remain normal but blood flow to the uterus is reduced – a phenomenon known as the Posiero effect. To prevent these problems, the nurse must never allow a client to rest in the supine position, even when her blood pressure remains normal.

The client's position during labor also affects the frequency and strength of uterine contractions, which can influence uterine blood flow (see below). For example, with the client in a lateral recumbent (side-lying) position, contractions typically are less frequent but stronger; in semi-Fowler's position, they are more frequent but less intense.

Uterine contractions. As the uterus contracts, the spiral arterioles delivering blood to the placenta collapse, decreasing or even cutting off blood flow, depending on the strength of the contraction. This decrease results in lower oxygen availability, which can cause stress on the fetus. A healthy fetus with an adequate oxygen reserve usually can tolerate this stress, but a fetus that is compromised because of a low oxygen reserve may cross the fine line from normal stress to distress. Even a healthy fetus has a limited tolerance to prolonged, repeated episodes of hypoxia caused by uterine hypertonus or tetanic contractions, which may result from oxytocin hyperstimulation or abruptio placentae (premature detachment of the placenta from the uterine wall).

Placental surface area and diffusion distance. Any condition that reduces the surface area of the placenta – such as abruptio placentae or placenta previa – also reduces perfusion. Oxygen diffusion through the placental membrane is impaired by conditions that cause a thickened or edematous membrane, such as diabetes mellitus or Rh disease.

Anesthetics. Use of a regional anesthetic – spinal, epidural, or caudal – during labor can impair normal vasoconstriction of peripheral blood vessels. As these vessels dilate and hold more blood, hypotension develops; less blood returns to the heart, decreasing maternal cardiac output and blood flow to the uterus. In response, the fetus may develop a prolonged deceleration of the heart rate.

Maternal hypertension and hypotension. Maternal hypertension decreases blood flow to the uterus directly, through excessive vasoconstriction. It also reduces the total surface area of the placenta by causing placental infarcts and inhibits placental development by producing a prolonged reduction in blood flow.

Maternal hypotension can result from supine positioning, anesthetic administration, and other factors. Regardless of the cause, however, hypotension can decrease the blood return to the heart, reducing maternal cardiac output and blood flow to the uterus.

Cord compression. A common occurrence during contractions, cord compression temporarily decreases oxygen flow to the fetus. When the contraction subsides, oxygen exchange resumes. This event is analogous to the fetus holding its breath and requires further assessment.

FETAL HEART RATE REGULATION

The FHR is regulated by the sympathetic and parasympathetic divisions of the autonomic nervous system and chemoreceptors and baroreceptors. The normal range of the FHR is 120 to 160 beats/minute.

Through the vagal reflex, the parasympathetic nervous system controls the FHR and is responsible for its beat-to-beat (moment-to-moment) changes. When the vagal reflex is stimulated, the FHR decreases. Conversely, stimulation of the sympathetic nervous system increases the FHR.

The autonomic nervous system receives information on blood pressure and oxygen status from chemoreceptors (sensory nerve cells) and baroreceptors (pressure-sensitive nerve endings in the walls of the large systemic arteries), which help the autonomic nervous system stabilize blood pressure.

Chemoreceptors detect even minute changes in tissue oxygen levels and trigger the sympathetic nervous system to increase the FHR so that more blood will circulate to the affected area, increasing tissue oxygenation. As a result, fetal blood pressure increases.

Baroreceptors are extremely sensitive to any elevation in blood pressure. An increase in blood pressure provokes baroreceptors to signal the parasympathetic nervous system to rapidly decrease the FHR. As the FHR decreases, so does fetal cardiac output and blood pressure.

FETAL AND UTERINE MONITORING

Careful monitoring of fetal and uterine functions during labor helps the nurse identify problems before they cause serious complications. Available monitoring methods include manual techniques (fetal heart auscultation and uterine palpation) and internally and externally applied devices for EFM.

FETAL MONITORING

The nurse can monitor the FHR through auscultation, using a fetoscope or an ultrasound stethoscope (Doppler blood flow detector), or through EFM. Each method carries distinct advantages and disadvantages.

Fetoscope and ultrasound stethoscope

Auscultating the FHR during labor traditionally has been considered sufficient monitoring for the low-risk client and fetus (NAACOG, 1988). The fetoscope is a special stethoscope that enhances the nurse's ability to hear the fetal heartbeat. One type is attached to a metal band that fits on the nurse's head and conducts sound. The other type is a stethoscope attached to a 3"-diameter weighted bell that is placed on the client's abdomen.

In contrast, the ultrasound stethoscope uses ultra-high-frequency sound waves to detect fetal heartbeats. Typically, this device consists of a headset, a battery charger, a transducer, and an audio unit. The ultrasound stethoscope can be used as early as the tenth week of gestation.

According to NAACOG (the organization for obstetric, gynecologic, and neonatal nurses) guidelines, the nurse should perform auscultation for the low-risk client every 60 minutes during the latent phase and every 30 minutes during the active phase of the first stage of labor, and every 15 minutes during the second stage; for the high-risk client, every 30 minutes during the latent phase and every 15 minutes during the active phase of the first stage, and every 5 minutes during the second stage (NAACOG, 1990).

A disadvantage of auscultation is that it cannot be used to assess the most important sign of fetal well-being: short-term or beat-to-beat variability of the FHR (Parer, 1984).

Electronic fetal monitoring

Every method for EFM has advantages and disadvantages that the nurse should understand. When the nurse uses this technology accurately and appropriately, EFM is the most reliable means currently available for assessing fetal status in utero.

Electronic fetal monitoring can be used externally (outside the uterus) or internally (in direct contact with the fetus) to establish a continuous record of the FHR and its relationship to uterine contractions. A heart rate pattern that is normal or otherwise within EFM guidelines is a reliable indicator of fetal well-being. At times, abnormal patterns may occur without indicating fetal distress;

however, fetal hypoxia reliably produces changes in the FHR pattern.

External EFM. This technique allows safe, ongoing assessment of the FHR. One widely used method of external EFM is the ultrasound transducer. In this method, a transducer is guided over the client's abdomen to determine the area closest to the fetal heart. After placement, the transducer emits low-energy, high-frequency ultrasound waves and directs them through the abdominal wall toward the fetal heart. These ultrasound waves strike the heart wall and are deflected back through the abdominal wall, where the transducer receives them. The transducer then relays the waves to the fetal monitor, which translates them two ways: into a signal that sounds like a heartbeat and into waveform lines on the monitor strip.

Besides being noninvasive, ultrasound poses no apparent risk for the fetus or mother. This method allows the nurse to monitor baseline FHR, long-term variability, and periodic accelerations and decelerations of the FHR. (See the section on "Fetal heart rate patterns" for more information on these patterns.)

Unfortunately, the monitor can make errors in counting when the FHR falls below 60 beats/minute. It may count both motions of the cardiac cycle (the *lub* and the *dub*), which will falsely double the heart rate, a condition known as doubling. Conversely, with an accelerated FHR of 200 beats/minute or above, the monitor will count only half the beats, a situation known as halving. These problems demonstrate the hazards of relying solely on technology. A nurse who has any question about the accuracy of external EFM should auscultate the FHR to verify the rate.

The phonotransducer and abdominal electrodes are other, less used, types of external EFM devices. The phonotransducer detects the FHR through a microphone placed on the client's abdomen, which amplifies the fetal heartbeat. The abdominal electrodes monitor and record maternal and fetal heartbeats. Both of these methods are less accurate than ultrasound, which has become the most commonly used external monitor.

Internal EFM. Nursing students may wonder why internal EFM is used since external EFM is noninvasive and easier to use. With external EFM, extraneous noises from pulsating maternal vessels and from maternal and fetal movement may interfere with an accurate, clear tracing. The transducer must be repositioned frequently to maintain a clear signal. In contrast, the waveforms produced by internal EFM are not affected by maternal or fetal movement and can produce an accurate tracing of the fetal heartbeat and uterine contractions.

Internal EFM is performed by attaching a small, corkscrew-type spiral electrode to the fetal scalp or buttocks, whichever is the presenting part. The electrode penetrates the presenting part about 1.5 mm and must be attached securely to ensure a good signal. In many health care facilities, nurses with special preparation are allowed to attach these electrodes. A plate is attached to the client's leg to hold the wires from the electrode in place. Most clients consider the leg plate less distracting than the belts used with the ultrasound unit.

The spiral electrode picks up the fetal heartbeat and transmits it to the monitor. The monitor transforms the impulse into a fetal electrocardiogram waveform on an oscilloscope screen and a waveform on the printout. These data are more accurate than those provided by external EFM and allow the nurse to track and calculate beat-to-beat variability in the FHR.

Internal EFM with spiral electrodes can be used only when the client's membranes are ruptured, when the cervix is dilated at least 2 cm, and when the presenting part is at least at the − 1 station.

UTERINE ACTIVITY MONITORING

Like any muscle, the uterus can contract and relax. Its normal resting tone (or baseline tone) is 5 to 15 mm Hg. In the first stage of labor, when the uterus contracts, the tone rises to 50 to 75 mm Hg. During the second stage of labor, when the client does not push, it may rise to 75 to 100 mm Hg with contractions.

Increased uterine activity can result from factors other than normal contractions during labor, including incautious use of oxytocin and abruptio placentae.

Contractions that occur at 3-minute intervals dilate the cervix most effectively and allow sufficient time for the fetus and uterine muscle to reoxygenate. Contractions that occur less than 2 minutes apart or last longer than 90 seconds generally reflect increased uterine activity.

Increased uterine activity can become hyperstimulation, which reduces perfusion to the placenta and can lead to fetal distress. In response to hyperstimulation, the fetus typically displays a prolonged deceleration or late decelerations of the heart rate. Therefore, the nurse must monitor uterine activity as closely as the FHR. Uterine activity can be monitored externally by using palpation or a tocodynamometer or internally with an intrauterine pressure catheter. Telemetry also can be used to monitor the client in labor.

Manual palpation

The manual method of monitoring uterine contractions, palpation requires no special equipment. It does, however, require skill and sensitivity to touch. To palpate uterine contractions, the nurse places the palmar surfaces of the fingers on the top of the uterine fundus where it contracts.

During mild contractions, the fundus indents easily and feels like a chin. In moderate contractions, the fundus indents less easily and feels more rigid, like the tip of the nose. With strong contractions, the fundus is firm, resists indenting, and feels like a forehead. The nurse must remember to palpate a set of at least three contractions to obtain sufficient data to evaluate a uterine contraction pattern.

External tocodynamometer

The tocodynamometer, a pressure-sensitive disk, is attached to an elastic belt strapped on the client's abdomen so that the disk lies directly over the fundus. The pressure exerted by uterine contractions is then amplified and relayed to the FHR monitor, which records the frequency and duration of the contractions. (The tocodynamometer does not record the intensity of contractions.)

If the tocodynamometer is not placed appropriately on the fundus, contractions may not be recorded at all. Also, the tighter the belt is strapped, the stronger the contractions appear on the graph, and vice versa.

Internal intrauterine pressure catheter

When oxytocin is used to stimulate labor, or when labor fails to progress normally, most experts recommend use of an internal intrauterine pressure catheter. This device accurately and continuously records uterine tone and the frequency, duration, and intensity of uterine contractions. It can be used only after the cervix has dilated from 2 to 3 cm and the membranes have ruptured.

In this sterile procedure, the nurse assists the physician or nurse-midwife by filling and irrigating the end of a pliable plastic catheter with sterile water. Then the physician or nurse-midwife inserts the catheter through the vagina and into the cervix, alongside the fetus. The catheter is advanced approximately 18″ until its black mark is visible at the introitus. After insertion is completed, the catheter is irrigated again to clear any bubbles or vernix that may interfere with transmission, and taped to the client's leg; the syringe and catheter are attached to their proper outlets on the strain gauge.

Each uterine contraction compresses the water in the catheter. This pressure is relayed through the plastic tubing to an external pressure-sensitive device, which in turn relays the pressure to an attached monitor that records the pressure as mm Hg on the monitor strip. The contraction is shown on the graph as an inverted "U".

The intrauterine pressure catheter can use various pressure-sensitive devices. One device, the strain gauge, has a plastic dome filled with sterile water that exerts pressure on a membrane within the unit. A more recently developed disposable unit does not require water or a strain gauge. This unit eliminates the time-consuming set-up, irrigation, and calibration required by other types. However, the disposable unit is more expensive and may have to be replaced if the unit is disconnected when the client arises to use the bathroom.

The nurse can speed intrauterine catheter insertion by preparing the equipment in advance—for example, by assembling, irrigating, and calibrating the strain gauge before the catheter is inserted. This gives the nurse time for any necessary troubleshooting.

Telemetry

By using remote monitoring, or telemetry, the nurse can monitor the client in labor as she moves about. External and internal methods are available. For the client with external EFM equipment, a battery-powered, two-way radio transmitter on a shoulder strap allows remote monitoring of the FHR and uterine contractions. The client with internal EFM equipment requires insertion of a transmitter into the vaginal vault after placement of the pressure catheter in the uterus and application of a scalp electrode to the fetal presenting part. Both telemetry methods provide close assessment of the client and allow her to move freely within a specified area and not be confined to bed earlier than she might desire.

A fetus coping well with the stress of labor typically will exhibit a reassuring FHR pattern; a fetus in distress invariably will demonstrate an abnormal pattern. Fetal distress may reveal itself in various combinations of symptoms: an increasing baseline FHR may indicate that the fetus is attempting to compensate for decreased oxygen reserves; late decelerations indicate placental insufficiency and the need for prompt intervention.

FETAL HEART RATE PATTERNS

Labor and delivery put stress on even the healthiest fetus. Accurate interpretation of a monitor strip of fetal heart patterns can help the nurse determine when a fetus has crossed the line from normal stress to distress. (For more information, see *Reading a fetal monitor strip.*)

BASELINE FETAL HEART RATE

The starting point for all fetal assessment is the baseline FHR. Accurate baseline FHR determination serves as a reference for all subsequent FHR readings taken during labor.

The proper time for establishing the baseline FHR is between uterine contractions and when no fetal movement is occurring. Initially, the nurse establishes the baseline FHR by examining approximately 5 to 10 minutes of the FHR on the monitor strip; the baseline FHR is the average rate between contractions during that 5- to 10-minute period. Once a baseline FHR is established, it does not change unless a new rate is present for 15 minutes. In a full-term fetus, baseline FHR normally ranges between 120 and 160 beats/minute. Deviations from the normal baseline FHR include tachycardia, bradycardia, and increased or decreased variability. (For more information, see *Variations on baseline fetal heart rate,* page 202.)

Baseline tachycardia

A baseline FHR exceeding 160 beats/minute indicates baseline tachycardia. Several factors can produce tachycardia in the fetus. The most common cause is maternal fever, which raises the fetal metabolic rate and, consequently, the baseline FHR. Baseline tachycardia also may be the first sign of intrauterine infection with prolonged rupture of membranes. Another possible cause is maternal anxiety, which releases epinephrine that crosses the placenta and increases the baseline FHR. Drugs that can cause fetal baseline tachycardia when used by the mother include parasympathetic blocking agents, such as atropine and scopolamine, and beta sympathomimetics, such as ritodrine and terbutaline. Baseline tachycardia also may be a response to hypoxia.

Baseline bradycardia

A baseline FHR less than 120 beats/minute is termed baseline bradycardia. A baseline FHR below 120 beats/minute without late decelerations, but with normal beat-to-beat variability, can be reassuring. Baseline bradycardia accompanied by late decelerations and little or no variability is an ominous sign of advanced fetal distress from hypoxia and acidosis.

The rare case of congenital heart block produces a baseline bradycardia of 60 to 80 beats/minute. A fetus with heart block must be delivered in a facility where cardiac surgery is available.

READING A FETAL MONITOR STRIP

The monitor strip is divided into two sections. The top section shows the fetal heart rate (FHR), measured in beats/minute (bpm). The nurse reads the strip horizontally and vertically. Reading horizontally, each small square represents 10 seconds. Between each vertical dark line are six squares, representing 1 minute. Reading vertically, each square represents an amplitude of 10 bpm.

The bottom section shows uterine activity (UA), measured in mm Hg. Again, the nurse reads the strip horizontally and vertically. Reading horizontally, each small square represents 10 seconds, with the space between each vertical black line representing 1 minute. Reading vertically, each square represents 5 mm Hg of pressure.

The baseline FHR, the "resting" heart rate, is assessed between uterine contractions and when no fetal movement is occurring. The baseline FHR—normally 120 to 160 bpm—serves as a reference for subsequent heart rate readings taken during contractions.

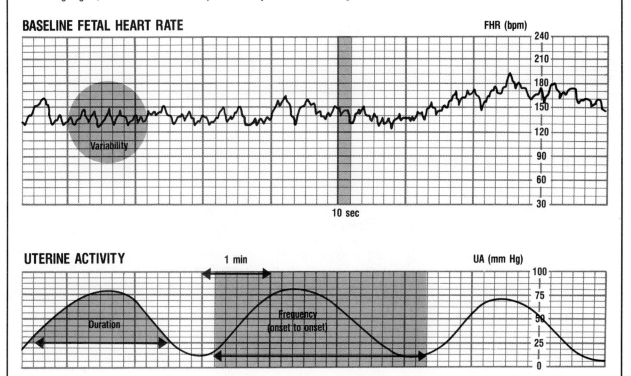

Variability

Variability refers to the beat-to-beat changes in FHR that result from the interaction of the sympathetic nervous system, which speeds up the FHR, and the parasympathetic nervous system, which slows the FHR. It is considered the most important indicator in clinical assessment of fetal well-being.

Variability has two components—long-term and short-term. Long-term variability refers to the larger periodic and rhythmic deviations above and below the baseline FHR. Normal long-term variability ranges from 5 to 20 beats/minute in rhythmic fluctuations, three to five times per minute.

Short-term variability describes the differences in successive heartbeats, as measured by the R-R wave interval of the QRS cardiac cycle. It represents actual beat-to-beat fluctuations in the FHR and the balance between the sym-

pathetic and parasympathetic nervous systems. Short-term variability is considered the most reliable single indicator of fetal well-being; it is classified as absent (0 to 2 beats/minute), minimal (3 to 5 beats/minute), moderate (6 to 25 beats/minute), or marked (more than 25 beats/minute).

Factors increasing variability. In the healthy fetus, movement accelerates the heart rate and increases long-term variability. This concept serves as the basis for assessing fetal well-being with the nonstress test. This test can be performed weekly, usually after week 32 of pregnancy.

The nonstress test indicates fetal well-being if the fetus can accelerate its heart rate two or more times in 15 minutes in response to a stimulus from contractions or fetal movement; if each acceleration increases 15 beats/minute

VARIATIONS ON BASELINE FETAL HEART RATE

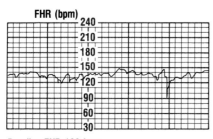

Baseline FHR 130 bpm

By properly interpreting baseline fetal heart rate (FHR), the nurse can determine much about fetal well-being. This chart presents possible causes, clinical significance, and nursing interventions associated with baseline tachycardia (FHR above 160 beats/minute [bpm] persisting for more than 15 minutes) and baseline bradycardia (FHR below 120 bpm persisting for more than 15 minutes). The strip on the left shows representative baseline FHR; variations on baseline are shown in the charts below.

VARIATIONS ON BASELINE	POSSIBLE CAUSES	CLINICAL SIGNIFICANCE	NURSING INTERVENTIONS
Baseline tachycardia **Baseline FHR 170 bpm**	• Early fetal hypoxia • Maternal fever • Parasympathetic agents, such as atropine and scopolamine • Beta-sympathomimetic agents, such as ritodrine and terbutaline • Amnionitis (inflammation of the inner layer of the fetal membrane—the amnion) • Maternal hyperthyroidism • Fetal anemia • Fetal heart failure • Fetal cardiac arrhythmias	Persistent tachycardia without periodic changes usually does not adversely affect fetal well-being—especially when associated with maternal fever. However, tachycardia is an ominous sign when associated with late decelerations, severe variable decelerations, or absence of variability.	Intervene to alleviate the cause of fetal distress and provide supplemental oxygen (7 to 8 liters/minute), as prescribed. Also administer I.V. fluids, as prescribed.
Baseline bradycardia **Baseline FHR 80 bpm**	• Late fetal hypoxia • Beta-adrenergic blocking agents, such as propranolol, and anesthetics • Maternal hypotension • Prolonged umbilical cord compression • Fetal congenital heart block	Bradycardia with good variability and without periodic changes is not a sign of fetal distress if the fetal heart rate remains above 80 beats/minute. However, bradycardia caused by hypoxia is an ominous sign when associated with loss of variability and late decelerations.	Intervene to alleviate the cause of fetal distress. Administer supplemental oxygen (7 to 8 liters/ minute), start an I.V. line, and administer fluids, as prescribed.

above the baseline; and if each acceleration lasts 15 seconds or more.

As the second stage of labor begins (when the cervix becomes fully dilated) and the fetus descends through the birth canal, long-term variability may increase because of mild hypoxia, which results from the increased intensity, duration, and frequency of uterine contractions; this increase is not threatening. However, the nurse should be alert for other changes caused by insufficient fetal oxygenation—such as decreased baseline FHR, prolonged variable decelerations, and decreased short-term variability—and be prepared to intervene appropriately.

When hypoxemia occurs, the fetus responds initially by increasing short- and long-term variability. For example, when uterine contractions occur closer than every 2 minutes or last longer than 90 seconds (a condition known as uterine tachysystole), contractions occur too quickly, preventing complete fetal oxygenation. The fetal stress liberates epinephrine, and variability increases. In this situation, the nurse should notify the physician or nurse-midwife; reduce the frequency of contractions by decreasing the oxytocin and having the client turn to her left side; and administer oxygen by mask and increase I.V. fluids as prescribed.

Factors decreasing variability. Although decreased variability can endanger the fetus, the nurse never should presume fetal distress based solely on a decrease in variability.

Drugs that depress the fetal central nervous system, such as narcotics, or block the action of the fetal parasympathetic nervous system, such as atropine, can decrease variability. When these drugs are administered to the mother, the nurse should expect a decrease in variability and be reassured if no other signs of fetal distress, such as late decelerations, are present.

Fetal dysrhythmias, such as paroxysmal atrial tachycardia and complete heart block, will decrease variability. The sympathetic nervous system becomes dominant and increases the FHR. The nurse should be aware that the higher the FHR, the lower the variability.

Another benign cause of decreased variability is quiet fetal sleep. The fetus normally has sleep-awake cycles lasting 20 to 30 minutes. After a period of normal variability, short- and long-term variability suddenly decrease. This sudden onset, and the absence of such other signs of fetal distress as late decelerations, should reassure the nurse that this is a sleep state, not a sudden catastrophe. When the fetus awakens, the variability reappears just as suddenly.

Two causes of decreased variability that typically do not occur suddenly and are much more dangerous are hypoxia and acidosis. Initially, the fetus may react to hypoxemia with increased heart rate variability. As a continued decrease in oxygen progresses to hypoxia, the heart rate accelerates as the fetus attempts to increase oxygenation. The result is baseline tachycardia and decreased or absent variability. Over time, the lack of oxygen harms the fetal central nervous system. If this cycle of deterioration is allowed to continue, acidosis develops and direct myocardial depression of the FHR occurs. At this stage, the fetus will be near death and may display baseline bradycardia.

PERIODIC CHANGES

Transient accelerations or decelerations from the baseline FHR are called periodic changes and are caused by uterine contractions and fetal movements. They represent the normal rhythmic fluctuations from the fetal resting pulse.

Accelerations

Transient accelerations in the FHR normally are caused by fetal movements and uterine contractions. This type of acceleration typically indicates fetal well-being and adequate oxygen reserve. Accelerations also may be caused by partial umbilical cord compression.

Decelerations

Periodic decelerations from the normal baseline FHR are classified as early, late, or variable, depending on when they occur and their waveform shape. (For more information, see *Common decelerations*, pages 204 and 205.)

Early decelerations. Decelerations that begin early in the contraction are associated with normal FHR variability and are well tolerated by the fetus. They are unaffected by maternal oxygen administration or position changes and require no nursing intervention.

Early decelerations exhibit a uniform waveform shape on the monitor strip, typically mirroring that of the uterine contractions. They arise from pressure on the fontanels produced by uterine contractions when the cervix is dilated 4 to 7 cm. This pressure produces localized hypoxemia that stimulates the chemoreceptors. As the baroreceptors are stimulated, the vagal system decreases the FHR in response. The onset, the lowest point of descent, and the recovery from early decelerations occur exactly in sequence with the contraction.

Late decelerations. These decelerations begin after the beginning of a contraction. The lowest point of a late deceleration occurs after the contraction ends; descent and return are gradual and smooth. The FHR rarely falls more than 30 to 40 beats/minute below the baseline FHR. Late decelerations typically produce U-shaped waveforms.

Usually repetitive, late decelerations occur with each contraction, although in some cases they will occur only with stronger contractions.

Late decelerations are nonreassuring because they indicate uteroplacental insufficiency, which comes from decreased intervillous blood flow. This decreased blood flow leads to inadequate oxygen exchange.

The nurse may counter the underlying cause of uteroplacental insufficiency and may reverse its course by re-

COMMON DECELERATIONS

Decelerations—periodic decreases in fetal heart rate (FHR)—are caused by uterine contractions and fetal movements. This chart illustrates early, late, and variable decelerations, and then lists their possible causes, clinical significance, and appropriate nursing interventions.

EARLY DECELERATION

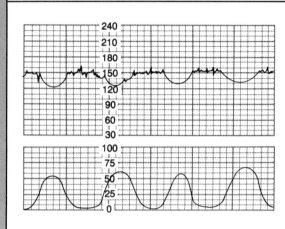

Possible causes
- Compression of the fetus's head

Characteristics
- Descent, peak, and recovery of deceleration waveform mirrors the contraction.

Clinical significance
- Is benign
- Indicates head compression at 4 to 7 cm dilation

Nursing interventions
- Reassure the client that the fetus is not at risk.

LATE DECELERATION

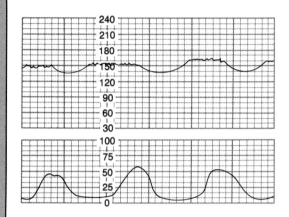

Possible causes
- Uteroplacental circulatory insufficiency (placental hypoperfusion) caused by decreased intervillous blood flow during contractions or structural defect in placenta, such as abruptio placentae
- Uterine hyperactivity caused by excessive oxytocin infusion
- Maternal hypotension or maternal supine hypotension syndrome

Characteristics
- Deceleration waveform begins about 30 seconds after the contraction begins.
- Lowest point of deceleration waveform occurs after the peak of the contraction.
- Recovery occurs after the contraction ends.

moving it. Maternal hypotension usually can be remedied by changing the client's position to her left side and administering I.V. fluids as prescribed. If oxytocin is overstimulating the uterus, it should be discontinued. Then contractions should occur less frequently, giving the fetus more time to reoxygenate, and the late decelerations may disappear.

However, intrinsic causes of uteroplacental insufficiency usually cannot be reversed. Such conditions as diabetes, pregnancy-induced hypertension, and pregnancy of 42 weeks or more may foster a placenta that is structur-

ally incapable of meeting fetal oxygen needs, particularly during labor.

The nurse who recognizes a late deceleration pattern and intervenes appropriately may help prevent fetal hypoxia and asphyxia. If a second late deceleration occurs, the nurse should notify the physician or nurse-midwife and intervene to decrease uterine activity by discontinuing oxytocin, maximize uterine perfusion by turning the client on her left side, administer oxygen by mask, and increase I.V. fluids as prescribed.

If decelerations persist after these interventions and birth is not imminent, the nurse should alert the physician

LATE DECELERATION *(continued)*

Clinical significance
- Indicates uteroplacental insufficiency
- May lead to fetal hypoxia and acidosis, if underlying cause is not corrected

Nursing interventions
- Turn the client on her left side to increase placental perfusion and decrease contraction frequency.
- Increase the I.V. fluid rate to increase intravascular volume and placental perfusion, as prescribed.
- Administer oxygen by mask at 8 to 10 liters/minute to increase fetal oxygenation, as prescribed.
- Notify physician or nurse-midwife.
- Assess for signs of the underlying cause, such as hypotension and uterine tachysystole.
- Take other appropriate measures, such as discontinuing oxytocin, as prescribed.
- Explain the rationales for nursing interventions to the client and her support person.

VARIABLE DECELERATION

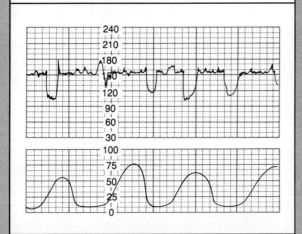

VARIABLE DECELERATION *(continued)*

Possible causes
- Umbilical cord compression causing decreased fetal oxygen perfusion

Characteristics
- Deceleration waveform shows abrupt onset and recovery.
- Waveform shape varies and may resemble the letter U, V, or W.
- FHR commonly decreases to 60 beats/minute.

Clinical significance
- Is most common deceleration pattern in labor because of contractions and fetal movement
- May indicate cord compression
- Is well tolerated if the fetus has sufficient time to recover between contractions and if the deceleration does not last more than 50 seconds

Nursing interventions
- Help the client change positions. No other intervention is necessary, unless fetal distress is present.
- Assure the client that the fetus tolerates cord compression well. Explain that cord compression affects the fetus the same way that breath-holding affects the client.
- Assess the deceleration pattern for reassuring signs: baseline FHR not increasing, short-term variability not decreasing, abrupt beginning and ending of decelerations, and deceleration duration of less than 50 seconds.
- If assessment does not reveal reassuring signs, notify the physician or nurse-midwife; then start I.V. fluids and administer oxygen by mask at 8 to 10 liters/minute, as prescribed.
- Explain the rationales for nursing interventions to the client and her support person.

---

or nurse-midwife again and notify other appropriate personnel. A cesarean delivery may be necessary. The need for cesarean delivery depends on the client's parity and degree of cervical dilation. For example, a primiparous client at 2 cm dilation with uncorrectable late decelerations is not a candidate for a vaginal delivery, but a multiparous client at 9 cm dilation possibly could deliver vaginally without jeopardizing the fetus.

Variable decelerations. When fetal movements or contractions compress the umbilical cord, variable decelerations occur. Dramatic and unpredictable, they vary in shape, duration, depth, and timing. To the client and support person, a variable deceleration may seem to indicate that the fetus's heart has stopped. The nurse should reassure them that these decelerations are the most common patterns during labor and usually are no cause for alarm. The nurse should explain that the decrease in FHR is analogous to the fetus holding its breath during a contraction and then resuming breathing.

Variable decelerations seem dramatic, and at times they can resemble early and late deceleration patterns. Cord compression stimulates the chemoreceptors and baroreceptors, causing the FHR to drop rapidly. A deceleration to 60 beats/minute or below is common.

The deceleration in the FHR produces shapes like the letters V, U, or W on the monitor strip. To tolerate these episodes well, the fetus must have sufficient time between contractions to reoxygenate.

In many cases, variable decelerations are preceded and followed by slight accelerations called shoulders. The FHR accelerates slightly, then decelerates suddenly and sharply; the deceleration ends just as suddenly as it begins. Finally, a small acceleration (the other shoulder) occurs before the baseline FHR is reestablished. These shoulders occur because the contraction occludes only the umbilical vein at first. When the umbilical arteries also are occluded, the deceleration occurs. Shoulders are a reassuring sign.

Variable decelerations can be mild, moderate, or severe. The nurse should know the differences but also should realize that certain fetuses can tolerate severe variable decelerations, while other fetuses have difficulties even with mild ones. Therefore, the nurse must assess the monitor strip according to reassuring and nonreassuring criteria. A reassuring variable pattern has an abrupt onset and end with shoulders; the baseline FHR does not increase, and short-term variability does not decrease.

A nonreassuring pattern includes signs of hypoxemia. At first, variability increases, but the baseline FHR remains within normal limits. Eventually, the FHR accelerates to a baseline tachycardia as the fetus tries to compensate for the growing oxygen deficit. Hypoxia becomes more evident as variability decreases. The shape of the variables may become more rounded, and the onset and end smoother, indicating that the central nervous system is adversely affected.

To help correct variable decelerations, the nurse should try to alleviate cord compression by changing the client's position, using the knee-chest, Trendelenburg, or other positions, as needed. In most cases, maternal repositioning alleviates cord compression, allowing resumption of oxygen flow and fetal reoxygenation.

If maternal positioning is unsuccessful, the nurse should observe for reassuring and nonreassuring signs. If reassuring signs disappear, the nurse should administer oxygen. If variable decelerations persist, other interventions are necessary.

Prolonged decelerations. Although the nurse must notify the physician or nurse-midwife as soon as a prolonged deceleration occurs, it does not automatically indicate cord prolapse or uncorrectable fetal distress.

Also known as a reflex bradycardia, prolonged decelerations occur in response to sudden stimulation of the vagal system by a vaginal examination, electrode application, or similar occurrence. They may persist for several minutes or longer. During deceleration, the FHR exhibits normal or increased variability. The vagal reflex itself may be caused by sudden hypoxemia with or without accompanying carbon dioxide retention and acidosis.

Other common factors also may trigger the vagal reflex that causes prolonged decelerations. When contractions occur closer than every 2 minutes or the uterus develops hypertonus, the sustained pressure on the fetus triggers the vagal reflex and decelerates the FHR. Variability also may increase. While the stimulus is operating, the FHR remains decelerated, commonly at 60 to 90 beats/minute.

In addition, such routine procedures as a vaginal examination and fetal scalp electrode application may trigger a prolonged deceleration. The vaginal examination can cause a temporary uterine tachysystole from prostaglandin release caused by manual manipulation of the cervix. Pressure on the fetal head when the scalp electrode is attached can stimulate the vagal reflex.

Prolonged decelerations also can be caused by such drugs as bupivacaine and lidocaine when used for regional (epidural and caudal) and paracervical blocks. These drugs temporarily increase uterine tone and contraction frequency, which can decrease the FHR. Also, maternal supine hypotension syndrome may cause prolonged decelerations.

Maternal pushing in the second stage of labor puts pressure on the fetus's body. This pressure can trigger a vagal reaction, particularly in the last few minutes before birth. This is one way labor personnel know delivery is imminent.

When prolonged decelerations occur, the nurse first must assess for cord prolapse or imminent delivery. If the client is receiving oxytocin, the nurse should discontinue the drug as prescribed and perform or assist with a vaginal examination. If the examination reveals a pulsating cord, the nurse should intervene using traditional techniques. (See Emergency Alert: *Cord prolapse* in Chapter 16, Intrapartal Complications and Special Procedures.) Katz, et al. (1988) also recommend intervening by rapidly filling the bladder with 500 to 700 ml of normal saline solution to elevate the presenting part and using tocolytics to halt contractions.

If the vaginal examination rules out cord prolapse and imminent delivery, the nurse should assess the client and monitor strip. Uterine hypertonus from oxytocin, anesthetics, or pushing during the second stage of labor can cause prolonged decelerations.

If the deceleration is the result of uterine hypertonus, drugs, or maternal pushing, the nurse should stay with the client and ask another nurse to call the physician, then stop the oxytocin, turn the client on her left side, tell her to stop pushing, administer oxygen by mask, and increase the I.V. fluid rate as prescribed.

In most cases, the deceleration corrects itself in 10 minutes, and the fetus resuscitates itself in 30 to 60 minutes after deceleration ends. During recovery, the FHR shows baseline tachycardia and a few late decelerations. Because tachycardia is a compensatory mechanism that aids fetal reoxygenation, it is a reassuring sign after a prolonged deceleration. The late decelerations verify that the fetus has just experienced hypoxia; they disappear as the fetus recovers.

OTHER FETAL ASSESSMENT TECHNIQUES

Although a normal FHR pattern during labor is a reliable indicator of fetal well-being, an abnormal pattern does not always signal distress. Several tests exist to distinguish the fetus that is in danger from the fetus that exhibits an abnormal pattern requiring no intervention. These tests are performed by the physician or nurse-midwife.

Fetal scalp blood sampling test

At times, fetal hypoxia is suggested by a confusing FHR pattern, such as a sustained flat heart rate without late decelerations. In this case, fetal scalp blood sampling—a process for evaluating the fetus's acid-base status—can be used with fetal monitoring to assess fetal status. When vaginal delivery is anticipated within 30 to 60 minutes but the FHR shows uncorrectable late decelerations with normal variability, fetal scalp sampling can indicate that a cesarean delivery may not be necessary.

Fetal scalp stimulation test

Clark, Gimovsky, and Miller (1984) have suggested that more widespread use of the fetal scalp stimulation test could reduce by half the need for fetal scalp blood sampling. A positive (or reactive) response to stimulating the fetal scalp, either with gentle digital pressure or by applying an Allis clamp, is considered a reliable indicator of fetal well-being. A positive response is marked by an acceleration of the FHR by 15 beats/minute for at least 15 seconds.

Fetal acoustic stimulation test

The fetal acoustic stimulation (FAS) test, also called the vibratory acoustic stimulation test, may be a promising alternative to fetal scalp blood sampling. A positive test for FAS eliminates the need for the more invasive and difficult-to-perform scalp sampling procedure.

In FAS, an electrolarynx vibratory device used at 80 decibels is applied to the client's abdomen for 3 seconds. The sound and vibrations cause an accelerated FHR. A positive result, indicated by an FHR acceleration of at least 15 beats/minute above the baseline FHR for at least 15 seconds occurring two or more times within 10 minutes, indicates fetal well-being. Smith, Nguyen, Phelan, and Paul (1986) found that no fetus with a positive test result had a pH less than 7.25, which is considered within the normal range.

NURSING RESPONSIBILITIES

According to nursing practice standards, the nurse using EFM when caring for a client in labor is held legally responsible for any procedures performed. This means that the nurse is responsible for recognizing abnormal fetal heart patterns and uterine activity, intervening appropriately, and notifying the physician or nurse-midwife whenever necessary. To meet this responsibility, the nurse must have received the special preparation needed to perform EFM procedures and interpret results.

The nurse can be held liable for preparing a client for a procedure to which she did not consent. Therefore, once the physician has explained the procedure and informed consent has been obtained, the nurse must make sure that the client fully understands the procedure that will be performed.

If a nonreassuring pattern occurs, standards of care dictate that the nurse notify the physician or nurse-midwife and then intervene appropriately to prevent further deterioration of fetal status. If the physician does not respond in a timely fashion, the nurse must follow the policy established by the health care facility. In most cases, this means informing the nurse-manager, who can intervene as necessary.

CLIENT TEACHING AND SUPPORT

The nurse should ask the client what she knows about fetal monitoring. The greatest resistance to EFM typically comes from clients who do not understand its purpose. As simply as possible, the nurse should explain how evaluating FHR and uterine contractions can identify possible

DOCUMENTATION CHECKLIST FOR FETAL MONITORING

When assessing the fetal monitor strip and documenting findings, the nurse should ask these questions:
• What is the frequency of contractions?
• How long do the contractions last?
• What is their intensity?
• What is the baseline fetal heart rate (FHR)?
• Is the baseline FHR within the normal range?
• If not, is baseline tachycardia or bradycardia present?
• Are long- and short-term variability present?
• Are accelerations present?
• Are decelerations present? If so, are they early, late, variable, or prolonged?
• Based on the monitor readings, have appropriate nursing interventions been performed and documented?
• What was the outcome of the interventions?

sources of danger to the fetus, emphasizing that a normal FHR is a highly reliable indicator of fetal well-being.

Also, the nurse should describe how EFM can assist the client during labor and delivery by helping her time the frequency and duration of contractions.

The nurse should explain that EFM allows constant tracking of the FHR; even the nurse who is not in the room can view the tracing on the central display at the nursing station and evaluate the data.

Client teaching should include all the possible situations that may cause her undue anxiety. The client should hear the fetal heartbeat and understand that the normal heart rate varies. If the belt moves, the fetal heart tracing may change and the client may think the heart rate is too fast or slow. Therefore, the nurse should demonstrate how moving the belt can cause a false FHR reading. Turning off the microphone on the monitor will eliminate distracting noises.

Applying a fetal scalp electrode and an intrauterine pressure catheter also may cause anxiety about fetal injury. To allay these fears, the nurse should demonstrate the insertion of the scalp electrode so that the client can see that only the tip of the wire slips under the fetal scalp, and explain that the procedure is no more painful than sticking a pin into a thick or calloused area of the finger. The nurse should explain that if the heart rate transmission stops suddenly after the electrode is in place, the electrode has probably fallen off and that this is no cause for alarm.

Before the intrauterine catheter is inserted, the nurse should use an unsterile sample to demonstrate how soft and pliable it is and show the client an illustration of where the catheter is placed in the uterus. The nurse should explain the function of the catheter and the need for data on the strength of contractions, particularly if the client is receiving oxytocin.

Despite the advantages of EFM, the nurse should remember that the client is the focus of the care. She needs to feel that the nurse is monitoring and concerned about her, not a machine.

DOCUMENTATION

The monitor strip is considered a vital part of the medical record. Therefore, the nurse must document all assessments, procedures, and interventions on the monitor strip as well as on the chart. If time is short, the nurse should make the monitor strip the primary place to document because it provides a chronological record of events.

Every health care facility should have a manual of terms and abbreviations for EFM. To avoid legal difficulties, the nurse should use only these terms on the chart and the monitor strip in documenting fetal assessments and interventions. The nurse should call the deceleration or any periodic change by its specific name in charting and in all communication with the physician. (For a list of points to cover when documenting EFM tracings, see *Documentation checklist for fetal monitoring.*)

CHAPTER SUMMARY

Chapter 11 discussed the physiologic basis of fetal monitoring and uterine activity monitoring, explained fetal heart rate patterns and assessment techniques, and discussed nursing responsibilities associated with fetal monitoring, client teaching, and documentation. Here are the chapter highlights:

Uncompromised uteroplacental-fetal circulation is essential to fetal well-being. It is affected by maternal position, uterine contractions, placental surface area and diffusion distance, anesthetics, maternal hypertension and hypotension, and cord compression.

Fetal heart rate is monitored with a fetoscope, ultrasound stethoscope, or external or internal electronic devices.

Uterine activity is monitored with manual palpation, the external tocodyamometer, the internal intrauterine pressure catheter or telemetry.

Important FHR patterns include baseline tachycardia and bradycardia, long- and short-term variability, accelerations, and decelerations (early, late, variable, and prolonged).

Nursing plays a critical role in identifying abnormal FHR patterns that may jeopardize fetal well-being and intervening as necessary.

Other fetal assessment techniques include three tests: fetal scalp blood sampling, fetal scalp stimulation, and fetal acoustic stimulation.

The nurse is responsible for teaching the client about activities and equipment that may be used during fetal assessment.

The nurse must accurately and completely document all nursing activities during the client's care, using nursing diagnoses and terms appropriate to the health care facility.

STUDY QUESTIONS

1. How does maternal position affect uteroplacental circulation?
2. What are the advantages and disadvantages of each method of EFM?
3. Mrs. Thomas, a 29-year-old client at 39 weeks' gestation, is admitted to the labor and delivery area with ruptured membranes. She is attached to a fetal monitor, which shows late decelerations. What are the possible causes of these decelerations?
4. Based on the NAACOG guidelines, how often should the nurse auscultate a client's fetal heart rate?

BIBLIOGRAPHY

ACOG (1989). *Assessment of fetal and newborn acid-base* (Technical Bulletin No. 127.) Washington, DC: Author.

Cunningham, F.G., MacDonald, P., and Gant, N. (1989). *William's obstetrics* (18th ed.). East Norwalk, CT: Appleton & Lange.

NAACOG (1988). Statement: Nursing responsibilities in implementing intrapartum fetal heart rate monitoring. Washington, DC: Author.

NAACOG (1990). OGN nursing practice resource fetal heart rate auscultation. Washington, DC: Author.

Parer, J.T. (1984). Fetal heart rate. In R.K. Creasy and R. Rosnik (Eds.), *Maternal-fetal medicine: Principles and practice*. Philadelphia: Saunders.

Fetal monitoring

Blank, J. (1985). Electronic fetal monitoring: Nursing management defined. *JOGNN,* 14(6), 463-467.

Clark, S. (1989). Do we still need fetal scalp blood sampling? *Contemporary OB/GYN,* 33(3), 75-86.

Clark, S., Gimovsky, M., and Miller, F. (1984). Scalp stimulation test: A clinical alternative to fetal scalp blood sampling. *American Journal of Obstetrics and Gynecology,* 148(3), 274-277.

Freeman, R., and Garite, T. (1981). *Fetal heart rate monitoring.* Baltimore: Williams & Wilkins.

Katz, Z., Shoham, Z., Lancet, M., Blockstein, I., Mogilner, B.M., and Zalel, Y. (1988). Management of labor with umbilical prolapse: A 5-year study. *Obstetrics and Gynecology,* 72(2), 278-281.

Krebs, H.B., Petres, R.E., and Dunn, L.J. (1983). Intrapartum fetal heart rate monitoring: VII. Atypical variable decelerations. *American Journal of Obstetrics and Gynecology,* 145(3), 297-305.

Laeveno, K., Cunningham, F.G., Nelson, S., Roark, M., Williams, M.L., Guzick, D., Dowling, S., Rosenfeld, C., and Buckley, A. (1986). A prospective comparison of selective and universal electronic fetal monitoring in 34,995 pregnancies. *New England Journal of Medicine,* 315(10), 615-619.

Lagrew, D., and Garite, T. (1984). Technology 1985: Reviewing the latest in fetal monitoring equipment. *Contemporary OB/GYN,* 24(special issue), 91-106.

MacDonald, D., et al. (1985). The Dublin randomized controlled trial of intrapartum fetal heart rate monitoring. *American Journal of Obstetrics and Gynecology,* 152(5), 524-539.

Montgomery, J. (1986). Technology 1987: Advantages of the IU catheter and fetal spiral electrode. *Contemporary OB/GYN,* 28 (special issue), 75-84.

Queenan, J., Clark, S., Freeman, R., Johnson, T., and Paul, R. (1988). Symposium: Today's high C/S rate: Can we reduce it? *Contemporary OB/GYN,* 32(1), 154-166.

Rice, P., and Benedetti, T. (1986). Fetal heart rate acceleration with fetal scalp blood sampling. *Obstetrics and Gynecology,* 68(4), 469-472.

Sarno, A., and Phelan, J. (1988). Intrauterine resuscitation of the fetus. *Contemporary OB/GYN,* 32(1), 143-152.

Smith, C., Nguyen, H.N., Phelan, J., and Paul, R. (1986). Intrapartum assessment of fetal well-being: A comparison of fetal acoustic stimulation with acid-base determinations. *American Journal of Obstetrics and Gynecology,* 155(4), 726-728.

Wagner, P., Cabaniss, M., and Johnson, T. (1985). Technology 1986: What's really new in EFM equipment? *Contemporary OB/GYN,* 26(special issue), 91-106.

Yeh, S., Diaz, F., and Paul, R. (1982). Ten-year experience of intrapartum fetal monitoring in Los Angeles County–University of Southern California Medical Center. *American Journal of Obstetrics and Gynecology,* 143(5), 496-500.

CHAPTER 12

COMFORT PROMOTION DURING LABOR AND CHILDBIRTH

OBJECTIVES

After reading and studying this chapter, the student should be able to:
1. Describe the locations and characteristics of pain typically felt during each stage of labor.
2. Identify factors that affect a client's responses to pain during labor.
3. Discuss the types and sources of support for the client in labor.
4. Describe the physical and psychological benefits of support from family and friends to the client in labor.
5. Describe techniques that promote comfort during labor.
6. Discuss nonpharmacologic methods to relieve labor pain.
7. List analgesic and anesthetic agents used to reduce labor pain and discuss their characteristics, administration routes, and adverse effects.

INTRODUCTION

Few women experience painless labor. In fact, many describe it as intolerable, crushing, grueling, and searing. Pain experienced during normal labor follows a predictable cycle of peaks and valleys. Despite its predictable course, however, each client perceives labor pain as a unique, personal experience based on her physical condition, pain tolerance, and psychological background. The nurse must collaborate with other health care providers to assess the client's perception of pain and the degree of comfort achieved through therapy. Because childbirth is a stressful experience for the client, her partner, and other

family members, steadfast support by the nurse can help ease emotional stress and physical discomfort during this time. The nurse plays a key role by helping the client's primary support person function effectively. The nurse also provides direct support, as needed, to the client and to involved family members.

This chapter begins by describing the type and location of pain typically experienced during each stage of labor and the factors influencing labor pain. It then outlines sources of support that may be important to the client, including her partner, parents, children, other family members, and friends. Following the nursing process, it then presents considerations for the client experiencing labor pain, including psychological and physical comfort measures, nonpharmacologic techniques for pain reduction, and pharmacologic options for pain relief.

PAIN DURING LABOR

Even though each client responds to pain uniquely, nursing interventions can help reduce pain perception and alter pain response for most clients. To intervene properly, the nurse should understand the type of pain typically experienced during labor, physical and psychological factors that influence pain perception, and how observation of behavior patterns can clarify a client's response to pain.

During the first stage of labor, pain results primarily from cervical effacement and dilation. At 0 to 3 cm of cervical dilation, the client may describe the pain as an ache or discomfort; at 4 to 7 cm, as moderately sharp; at 7 to 10 cm, as severe, sharp, and cramping.

During the second stage of labor, pain results from friction between the fetus and birth canal and from pressure on the perineum, bladder, bowel, and uterine ligaments.

During the third stage of labor, pain results from ischemia caused by contraction of uterine blood vessels. Impulses are transmitted as in the first stage – through the sympathetic nervous system to thoracic and lumbar vertebrae (T10 to L1).

FACTORS THAT INFLUENCE LABOR PAIN

Many factors affect a client's perception of and ability to cope with pain. These factors may be physiologic, social, or psychological; they include parity, fetal size and position, certain medical procedures, anxiety, fatigue, education level, cultural influence, and coping mechanisms. Knowledge of these influences can help the nurse anticipate, assess, and meet client needs.

Parity

The primiparous client typically experiences longer, more painful labor than the multiparous client, for two reasons. First, the primiparous client's cervix requires greater stretching force because it has never been stretched. This may require contractions of greater intensity during the first stage of labor. Second, the primiparous client may experience increased anxiety and doubt about her ability to tolerate labor pain, feelings that in themselves may focus attention on the pain. Later in labor, the multiparous client typically experiences more intense contractions than the primiparous client (Bonica, 1989); however, experience and previous cervical changes increase the client's ability to cope.

Fetal size and position

A large fetus may disrupt uterine contractions or arrest active labor. Persistent posterior fetal positions also may disrupt contraction efficiency, prolong labor, or cause severe backache by exerting increased pressure on the sacrum.

Medical procedures

Certain procedures, such as augmentation or induction of labor, may affect a client's response to labor pain. Oxytocin – a drug used commonly to augment or induce labor – reportedly creates stronger, more uncomfortable contractions that peak more abruptly than spontaneous contractions. Other actions that increase discomfort include performing a vaginal examination on a supine client, using a tight abdominal belt to secure a fetal monitor, forbidding a client to change positions or walk, and administering an enema, which may produce intestinal and uterine contractions (Jimenez, 1983).

Anxiety

By impeding normal cervical dilation, excessive anxiety may prolong labor and increase pain perception. An anxious client will experience increased cardiac output and blood pressure, and may face increased risk of the following:

• increased levels of epinephrine and norepinephrine (hormones that typically prepare the body for the "fight or flight" response), which may prolong labor, cause hyperventilation, and result in fetal hypoxia. During sustained pain, norepinephrine can decrease blood flow to the uterus by 35% to 70% (Bonica, 1989). Epinephrine increases vasoconstriction and decreases uterine activity.

• increased plasma levels of cortisol (a steroid hormone secreted by the adrenal cortex), which has been associated with longer labor and decreased uterine activity (Lederman, Lederman, Work, and McCann, 1978).

Some anxious clients – particularly those with little childbirth education – may be especially susceptible to escalating anxiety characterized by the fear-tension-pain cycle (Dick-Read, 1970; Jimenez, 1983). Fear and anxiety increase muscle tension, resulting in vasospasm-induced ischemia, which causes pain. This in turn increases anxiety. Education and preparation for labor may reduce fear and anxiety, thus breaking the fear-tension-pain cycle.

Fatigue

Especially if aggravated by sleep deprivation, fatigue may intensify a client's perception of pain during labor and reduce her coping ability. The client may become more tense and anxious if exhaustion prevents her from using learned pain-reduction methods. An exhausted client in a prolonged latent phase may require sedation to relieve anxiety and induce sleep. Anemia worsens feelings of fatigue.

Education

Clients with childbirth education (physical and psychological) experience less fear, tension, and stress during labor; typically, they require less pain medication. After childbirth, these clients tend to have significantly more positive attitudes toward their neonates (Klusman, 1975; Tanzer and Block, 1987). Further, partners educated in childbirth techniques feel a greater sense of control during labor than those not educated.

Culture

A client's cultural background might be expected to influence her behavior during labor, but studies show that culture actually has little effect on how women perceive and react to labor pain; education is the primary factor. Bonica (1989) found that women in Europe, Latin America, Asia, Australia, the Near East, and North America with similar levels of childbirth education exhibited similar verbal, facial, and physical expressions during labor.

The nurse should avoid stereotyping or judging clients by personal standards on such issues as self-control and acceptable modes of expression. Try to view each client's actions according to her own cultural and personal standards.

Coping mechanisms

Normally, people learn to cope with pain through experience, drawing on previously learned coping behaviors when pain recurs. This is one reason why multiparous clients may cope with labor pain more successfully than primparous clients.

Conversely, some painful experiences produce anxiety and fear, possibly affecting the client's self-image and confidence. The nurse should support the client through the pain and remain nonjudgmental.

BEHAVIORAL RESPONSES TO LABOR PAIN

Early in labor, during the latent phase, the client typically can respond to teaching and interventions because contractions have not become intensely painful. The transition to active labor, which may be subtle or obvious, typically marks the point when pain alters the client's behavioral responses. She may lose the ability to focus attention, have difficulty following instructions, and forget proper breathing techniques. She also may withdraw from social interaction, yet fear being abandoned or left alone even for brief periods.

By monitoring for reactions common to women in labor, the nurse can gauge the comfort promotion needs of each client. Such reactions include:
• facial grimacing
• muscle tension and grunting (with bearing-down efforts)
• increased blood pressure, pulse rate, and respirations
• desire for personal contact and touch in early active labor

• withdrawal, irritability, and resistance to touch during the transition to active labor.

SUPPORT DURING LABOR

Support from trusted family members or friends can help an individual gain, regain, and use personal strength during difficult or challenging periods that demand extra energy and resources (Brown, 1986). Several people may be available to assist a client during labor. Her partner, family members, friends, and health care professionals all care about her physical and emotional needs. In addition, nurses, nurse-midwives, and physicians strive to help the family have a positive experience and one that meets each member's wishes and needs. Whatever their cultural, social, economic, or religious background or configuration, most family members who assist the woman in labor will need the nurse's support.

Client benefits and needs

Clients who have a continuous support person during labor can benefit physically and psychologically. Research has found that women with a constant companion during labor had shorter labors, fewer obstetric complications, reduced feelings of pain and anxiety, less use of labor-inducing drugs and anesthesia, more positive feelings about the birth experience, and better coping behaviors than those without a support person.

Although labor and childbirth almost always are associated with pain and anxiety, clients vary in the degree of pain they experience, their tolerance for the pain, and the cultural beliefs that affect their response to the pain. A client who experiences more pain during labor usually will need more support than one who experience less pain.

In addition to differences in pain severity and tolerance, clients differ in their verbal and nonverbal response to pain and in their ability to cope with it. The nurse who assesses a client's pain tolerance and coping skills can use the information to formulate specific strategies for direct client support and for use by the primary support person and others.

Types of support

To maximize effectiveness, support should be tailored to a client's specific needs and personality. One client may prefer quiet hand-holding, for example; another may prefer active coaching. Thus, support may take various forms. The nurse should perform ongoing assessment to ensure that support corresponds to the client's needs and expectations as labor progresses.

The client's belief that support is available should she need it – *perceived support* – may be more important than the actual availability of support (Sarason and Sarason, 1985). She will perceive support if she feels that people care about her feelings and will help her if asked.

Referring to specific steps taken by one person to support another, *received support* may include such actions as touching the client in a caring way, communicating information that she needs, and positioning her to maintain comfort. Received support may be included in one of four categories (House, 1981):

- *Emotional support.* Includes affection, trust, concern, and listening.
- *Appraisal support.* Includes affirmation and feedback.
- *Informational support.* Includes advice, suggestions, directives, and other information.
- *Instrumental support.* Includes money, time, and other such resources.

Sources of support

Mutual confidence, trust, and communication must be present for one person to feel that another is supportive. Although many people may be capable of supporting the client during labor, the typical client prefers to have one trusted person concentrate on her needs, communicate them to others, and provide constant support during labor and delivery.

In North America, the client's partner typically provides support during labor. However, members of some families or cultural groups may prefer a female support person or a family member other than the partner. In some Mexican-American families, for example, a female relative or friend is more likely to act as support person. (For more information, see Cultural Considerations: *Selection of a support person.*)

Regardless of who the client selects as support person, important considerations include the person's ability to provide support and the client's and family's satisfaction with that support. The partner's support can be invaluable to a client in labor.

The partner may assist the client by communicating her needs to health care professionals. The partner also can show concern for the client's needs by being understanding, tolerant, supportive, cooperative, available, communicative, and reliable (Lederman, 1984). These feelings should be accompanied by physical actions, verbal communication, and nonverbal communication. Examples of physical actions include giving the client ice chips, rubbing her back, and bringing her items she may want. Verbal support could include coaching breathing or other pain-coping techniques and praising her for her progress. Non-

CULTURAL CONSIDERATIONS

SELECTION OF A SUPPORT PERSON

The nurse should be sensitive to cultural preferences of each client. Especially when the client and nurse have different cultural backgrounds, the nurse needs to be aware of the client's values, beliefs, and practices that may influence her view of appropriate nursing care. When providing support during the intrapartal period, the nurse should be aware of the following cultural variations:

Many Mexican-Americans choose a female relative or friend as a support person rather than a male partner. In the Mexican-American culture, the extended family is an important part of childbirth. The whole family of female relatives who have experience in childbirth may play a prominent role in the education and support of the pregnant woman (Hahn and Muecke, 1987).

Choi (1986) describes Korean-American beliefs and attitudes toward pregnancy, birth, and postpartal practices. She found that many Korean mothers in the United States continued Korean cultural practices. A woman of middle age who has had many sons and much experience in delivering children customarily attends the pregnant woman during labor and delivery. Men and childless women are not permitted in the labor and delivery area.

The birth culture of the Hmong (refugees from Laos) includes many beliefs important for the nurse to recognize. For example, many Hmong women believe that hospitals are unsafe birthing environments (Nyce and Hollingshead, 1984). According to La Du (1982), Hmong women resented hospital treatment, disliked being forced into a supine position, and had their modesty affronted by being shown their deliveries in mirrors.

verbal support could include holding her hand and stroking her face.

The partner's feelings may greatly affect that person's support of the client. The partner may find labor and delivery progressively more stressful, a feeling that peaks during delivery (Berry, 1988). Expectations on the partner must be realistic and based on the person's ability to cope with personal stress. The nurse should emphasize that health care professionals will be available to help or to assume the primary job if the partner feels overwhelmed.

A first-time support person may feel more anxiety about the role and may need special assistance from the nurse, especially if the person did not attend childbirth education classes. The nurse may have to coach an inexperienced partner in behaviors that will be helpful to the client during labor. An adolescent partner in particular may need appraisal support (support that includes affirmation and feedback) from the nurse, including reassurance that actions are helpful and supportive to the client.

The client's parents (and her partner's parents) usually assume a role different from that of the partner. Typically, they provide more general support and participate for their own pleasure in the birth experience rather than as primary support persons. If the client has no support person, a parent (usually the client's mother) may assume this role. The perceived and received support provided by the client's mother will depend on the quality of their relationship before labor and delivery, on the mother's preparation, and on her ability to cope with her daughter's pain.

In some cultures, female relatives and friends provide support for the client during labor. The partner may take a more passive role or, because of cultural norms, may be forbidden to see the client during labor and delivery. For some families, childbirth represents a culturally recognized event with extended family members in attendance. Although most families gather in a waiting area, some may wish to participate actively. If family participation is not prohibited by facility policy, the nurse should monitor the family's involvement, keep individuals informed of labor progress, and protect the client from unwanted distractions. Avoid making judgments about family preferences or stereotyping a family based on cultural background. Assess and care for each family in appropriate ways.

Occasionally, a client and her partner may wish to have their children witness the birth of a sibling. The couple may feel that group participation will promote family unity. The client may desire the support of older children. At times, a child may ask to view the birth of a new brother or sister. Although many facilities allow children to attend labor and delivery, most require adherence to specific guidelines.

NURSING CARE

To provide care for the client in labor, the nurse must be familiar with various nonpharmacologic and pharmacologic pain-relief methods and provide care for the client and her family. During labor and delivery, the nurse should administer sensitive and appropriate care based on the particular needs of the client and her family. This requires a twofold effort: applying clinical knowledge to assess labor progress and using personal skills to assess the client's and family's needs during this physically and emotionally stressful time.

ASSESSMENT

Assessment of a client experiencing labor pain includes three parts. First is the health history, which investigates any medical factor that could affect the safety or efficacy of pain-reducing pharmacologic agents, ongoing questions about the client's pain perception, and assessment of the client's and family's needs and support. Second is physical assessment, which includes the client, the fetus, and labor progress. Third is follow-up assessment, performed after implementing pain-relief measures to determine their effectiveness.

Health history

Review the client's medical history, asking specifically about medication allergies and any obstetric problems that could affect the choice of pain-relief methods. Determine how much the client knows about childbirth and pain-relief measures, ask about previous experiences with pain and pain-relieving agents, and assess the client's current pain level and psychological reaction to it.

Check carefully for chronic and acute illnesses that could affect labor progress or place the client at risk, including hypertension (chronic or pregnancy-induced), diabetes mellitus, bleeding disorders, complications of pregnancy, chronic respiratory disease, and severe dehydration. A client with one of these conditions may require such special measures as I.V. fluid administration, cardiac and hemodynamic monitoring, or continual nursing assessment when a pain-relief agent is used during labor.

If the client has pregnancy-induced hypertension (PIH), uteroplacental perfusion may be inadequate and gas exchange may be poor. In mild cases of PIH, most analgesic and anesthetic options remain available as long as fetal assessment reveals no signs of compromise.

If the client has diabetes mellitus with no evidence of fetal distress, small doses of narcotic analgesics or an epidural block (discussed in detail later in the chapter) may be used for pain relief. The client will require continuous fetal monitoring, glucose surveillance, and vital sign assessment because of an increased risk of PIH.

The client with placenta previa or abruptio placentae may require caesarean delivery. The anesthesia used depends on the presence or absence of active bleeding and fetal distress. Assess for a history of any chronic respiratory disease, which could cause respiratory depression in the anesthetized client. Also note renal or liver disease, which may affect the metabolism of some agents, possibly resulting in toxicity.

Consider the client's obstetric history when assessing the need for pain-relief measures. Pertinent assessment topics include the length of previous labors, the client's perception of previous labor pain, pain-relief measures used in previous labors, and the client's perception of their effectiveness.

Some obstetric problems may recur in successive pregnancies, resulting in longer, more painful labor or possibly necessitating surgical intervention. These include persistent posterior fetal position and cephalopelvic disproportion.

Assess the client's knowledge of relaxation techniques, positioning, and pharmacologic options for pain relief. Determine client preferences and desires for labor and delivery and identify who will function as the client's main support. Assess the client's reaction to her partner, if he is present. Is he helpful and supportive? Is his anxiety level disturbing to the client?

Assess the client's and family's birth culture for any beliefs and practices that could influence labor and delivery. Birth culture refers to a set of beliefs, values, and norms surrounding the birth process and shared to various degrees by members of a cultural or ethnic group (Hahn and Muecke, 1987). It informs members of the group about the nature of conception, the proper conditions for procreation and childbearing, the mechanism of pregnancy and labor, and the rules and rationales of antepartal and postpartal behavior. The birth culture may influence the client's diet, her response to labor, preferred positions for childbirth, activity restrictions, and family members' roles during childbirth.

Physical assessment

When evaluating possible implementation of comfort promotion or pain-relief measures, consider maternal status, fetal status, and labor progress.

Maternal status. At frequent intervals during labor, ask the client to rate her level of pain using a scale from 1 (lowest) to 10 (highest). Observe her spontaneous verbal and nonverbal expressions to assess discomfort. Keep in mind that excessive anxiety may impede cervical dilation; a small dose of an analgesic agent may relax an anxious client sufficiently to allow cervical dilation and shorten labor.

Fetal status. Carefully consider fetal age and development before administering prescribed pain-relief agents. An immature fetus has a diminished ability to metabolize analgesic or anesthetic agents used to reduce labor pain; the physician or nurse-midwife must carefully consider fetal status before drug administration. (For specific guidelines, see Fetal Status: *Fetal factors that affect drug choice*.)

FETAL STATUS

FETAL FACTORS THAT AFFECT DRUG CHOICE

Certain fetal body systems, such as the renal system, mature less rapidly than others. Rates of development as well as fetal physiology must be evaluated before the physician or nurse-midwife selects pain-relief agents for the client.

- A fetus with an immature blood-brain barrier has increased risk for high drug concentrations in the central nervous system.
- An immature fetus will have less plasma protein available to bind with analgesic and anesthetic agents. As a result, the plasma concentration of free (active) drug is increased.
- A fetus with an immature liver has insufficient enzymes to metabolize such agents.
- A fetus with an immature renal system cannot excrete analgesic and anesthetic agents.

Heart rate offers the primary indicator of fetal well-being. Obtain and document baseline fetal heart rate and pattern before pharmacologic measures are instituted.

Labor progress. Before implementing prescribed pain-relief measures, consider labor progress. Certain factors, such as side-lying positioning or epidural anesthesia, may slow labor. Also consider contraction intensity, frequency, and duration to help determine the need for pain relief.

Assess cervical dilation to ensure that pharmacologic agents are given at the safest times during labor. Systemic narcotics may be given for analgesia during the first stage of labor, but may prolong labor if administered too early in the latent phase. Antianxiety agents also may be used in the latent phase to decrease anxiety and fear. Timing is essential to achieve appropriate pain relief without adversely affecting the fetus.

Follow-up assessment

To determine the effectiveness and safety of comfort promotion and pain-relief measures, continue to assess the client and fetus throughout labor. Observe maternal and fetal vital signs frequently (especially respirations), assess the client's cardiovascular response, and watch for such adverse drug reactions as vomiting, itching, and drowsiness. Also assess the primary support person's feelings and actions to determine their effect on the client.

Pain relief. Assess pain relief continually during nonpharmacologic measures and at 30-minute intervals after analgesic administration. Pain should abate almost immediately after administration of an anesthetic. Assess the duration and degree of pain relief to help anticipate additional pain-relief measures.

Effects on client and fetus. Assess the client's level of consciousness, respiratory rate, blood pressure, and pulse rate. Narcotic analgesics can cause drowsiness that may interfere with effective bearing-down efforts in the second stage of labor. Narcotic analgesics also may produce respiratory depression and hypotension.

To prevent maternal injury, assess for adverse drug reactions (such as nausea and vomiting) and allergic reactions (such as pruritus, urticaria, facial edema, and stridor). Watch for aspiration if a client made drowsy by narcotic analgesics begins to vomit.

After administering pharmacologic agents, assess fetal heart rate according to health care facility protocol. After birth, the neonate's muscle tone, color, and respirations will reflect the effects of pharmacologic agents used on the client.

Support person. Assess the primary support person's goals, expectations, and feelings about labor and delivery. The support person may have a strong desire to photograph the process, which could affect attentiveness to the client's needs. The support person may be nervous about seeing blood or coping with the client's pain. Although discussion of every concern will be impossible, investigate the most critical ones. Discussing feelings and fears may help by itself to allay some of the support person's anxieties.

Although the support person's primary job is to assist the client during labor and delivery, the person also will have individual needs. These needs are complicated further when the client's support person is the expectant father. As labor progresses, the expectant father's attention may shift from the client toward himself and the neonate (Leonard, 1977).

Needs and expectations of expectant fathers have many implications for the nurse. Although they can provide powerful and effective support during labor, they experience great personal stress. They are excited and anxious about the neonate's well-being and about providing adequate support; they may need interventions from the nurse.

NURSING DIAGNOSIS

After assessing the client, fetus, and support persons, review the findings and formulate nursing diagnoses related to comfort promotion and support. (For a partial list of

COMFORT PROMOTION AND SUPPORT

The following list of potential nursing diagnoses are examples of the problems and etiologies that the nurse may encounter when caring for a client in labor as well as the client's support person, family, and friends. Specific nursing interventions for many of these diagnoses are provided in the "Planning and implementation" section of this chapter.

- Anxiety related to labor pain
- Anxiety related to lack of information about labor progress
- Decreased cardiac output related to epidural anesthesia
- Ineffective airway clearance related to general anesthesia
- Knowledge deficit related to analgesia and anesthesia options
- Knowledge deficit related to inadequate preparation for childbirth
- Pain related to the frequency and intensity of uterine contractions
- Self-esteem disturbance related to inability to cope with labor pain or negative perception of behavior
- Self-esteem disturbance related to uncertainty about the effectiveness of support
- Urinary retention related to spinal anesthesia

applicable diagnoses, see Nursing Diagnoses: *Comfort promotion and support.*)

PLANNING AND IMPLEMENTATION

The nurse provides or assists with comfort promotion and pain-reduction measures when caring for a client in labor. The nurse also assists the support persons to ensure adequate and appropriate support for the client and to balance client and family needs.

Comfort measures

Intervene to decrease anxiety, promote hygiene, and help the client find comfortable positions that reduce labor pain and facilitate childbirth. Some clients find these actions adequate to maintain comfort throughout labor.

Decrease anxiety. As contractions grow more frequent and intense, anxiety increases. The client may fear withdrawal of support, abandonment, the unknown, or loss of control. Increased epinephrine and norepinephrine levels raise blood pressure and pulse, diminish myometrial activity, exhaust glucose reserves, and decrease adenosine triphosphate synthesis necessary for uterine contractions.

Anxiety also leads to tension, which may cause additional pain. For a client with a nursing diagnosis of *anxiety related to labor pain,* nursing interventions seek to reduce anxiety, thus decreasing blood pressure and heart rate, allowing greater energy production for effective uterine contractions, and reducing muscle tension and the heightened pain perception caused by tension.

The nurse's presence, confidence, attention, and concern help control the client's anxiety. As labor progresses, keep the client informed, teach and reinforce coping strategies, and assure the client that labor is progressing normally. If assessment reveals that labor is not progressing normally, notify the physician immediately. Reassure, encourage, and praise the client throughout labor. If she becomes discouraged or frustrated, reassure her and help her to choose an alternate method of comfort promotion.

A support person provides comfort, reassurance, and assistance with such pain control techniques as breathing exercises, imagery, and distraction (Copstick, Taylor, Hayes, and Morris, 1986). Helping the client's partner also helps reduce the client's anxiety. Support the partner's efforts to comfort the client. Offer instructions and assistance, as appropriate. Because the client's perception of the partner's efforts may exaggerate the amount of support actually provided, the nurse can most accurately assess the partner's achievements by examining the client's responses to the partner's behavior.

Promote hygiene. Nursing interventions to maintain hygiene can increase the client's comfort level by boosting self-esteem, providing distraction, removing an additional source of discomfort (such as wet sheets), and blocking pain perception. For a client with a nursing diagnosis of *self-esteem disturbance related to inability to cope with labor pain or negative perception of behavior,* the nurse may implement the following hygiene measures.

Showers and bathing. Many labor and delivery areas have showers. A warm water massage (hydrotherapy) directed at the client's back promotes relaxation and counterstimulates pain transmission. Provide a stool in the shower and a supportive bar for the client to grasp or press against during contractions. Assist the client or ask her partner to assist her in the shower, as needed.

Perineal care. Clean the vulva after the client has a vaginal examination, urinates, or defecates. Provide a sanitary pad and belt to help the client feel secure while walking.

Oral hygiene. Provide frequent mouth care, as necessary. For a dry mouth, offer the client ice chips, mouthwash, or a toothbrush or apply a cool, moistened cloth to her lips. For dry lips, suggest petroleum jelly or lip balm.

Linens and clothing. Change soiled or damp linens and gowns frequently. Offer extra pillows for comfort and socks and additional clothing to prevent chilling. If the client grows warm during active labor, help her remove extra clothing.

Position the client for comfort. For a client with a nursing diagnosis of *pain related to the frequency and intensity of uterine contractions,* suggest that she change positions to enhance comfort. During the latent and early active stages, encourage the client to move about. A client in an upright position will have stronger, more regular, and more frequent contractions because gravity helps align the fetus with the pelvic angle as the uterus tilts forward with each contraction. Maintaining this position may shorten labor and reduce pain and medication requirements (Roberts, 1982).

As labor progresses and an upright position becomes uncomfortable, the client might alternate walking with sitting, side-lying, or kneeling to provide rest and vary the intensity and frequency of contractions. If she must remain in bed during labor because of obstetric or fetal conditions, such as premature rupture of membranes with unengaged presenting part or fetal distress, advise her to assume a side-lying position as often as possible to minimize fetal stress and enhance circulation.

Posterior fetal positions typically prolong labor and cause severe sacral pain (known as back labor). To encourage rotation of the presenting part to an anterior position, thus making the client more comfortable, take the following steps:
- Using Leopold's maneuvers, determine the position of the fetus's back. Direct the client to lie on the same side as the fetus's extremities with her upper leg propped on pillows.
- Advise the client to assume an all-fours position and to rock her pelvis to encourage fetal rotation and decrease pain. Kneeling or squatting also may be combined with pelvic rocking, but these positions can be uncomfortable and tiring for a client not accustomed to them.
- Suggest that the client straddle a chair or lean on her partner during contractions. During the second stage of labor, encourage her to use a squatting or side-lying position for pushing. Many birthing beds have squatting bars that allow the client to assume more comfortable, efficient positions for childbirth. After a contraction, the

client can lean back on a supportive wedge or pillow until her next contraction begins. Squatting increases the pelvic angle by approximately 30% and enhances pushing efforts as the vagina widens and shortens. A side-lying position may slow descent in the second stage of labor, but it provides more effective relief for back pain than squatting.

Relaxation techniques

The goal of relaxation techniques is to reduce anxiety and muscle tension, thus quieting or calming the mind and muscles. Relaxation decreases oxygen consumption, heart rate, respiratory rate, arterial blood lactate concentration, and sympathetic nervous system activity (McCaffery and Beebe, 1989).

Typically, relaxation techniques distract the client from pain, increase her sense of control over the pain, and aid sleep and rest. However, not all techniques succeed with all clients; she may have to try several before finding relief. Even when a relaxation method succeeds, relief from fatigue may last only 5 to 20 minutes. Although these methods may reduce distress, they may not relieve pain. Assess whether and when the client needs analgesia or an anesthetic for pain reduction. If and when this becomes necessary, relaxation techniques may increase effectiveness.

Techniques used to promote relaxation include distraction, progressive muscle relaxation, yawning, controlled breathing, imagery, touch, and music therapy. Ensure that the environment is conducive to relaxation. Remove the telephone, dim glaring lights, and maintain the room temperature at 68° to 70° F. Minimize unnecessary interruptions.

Distraction. Distraction can decrease pain perception. Distraction from pain requires that the client focus on stimuli other than the pain sensation. For example, a client in labor may shield herself from contraction pain by focusing on music, rocking, singing to herself, visualizing a scene, or changing positions (McCaffery and Beebe, 1989).

Imagery. Using the imagination to develop sensory images may decrease pain intensity, provide distraction from pain, and increase pain tolerance. Encourage her to imagine being in a peaceful place or being massaged by a gentle flow of water. Use words or phrases that convey pain-relieving images (McCaffery and Beebe, 1989).

Progressive muscle relaxation. This method of alternately tensing and relaxing groups of muscles from head to toe can relax the entire body. Relief of muscle tension reduces pain.

Controlled breathing. Deliberate, controlled breathing decreases anxiety, heart rate, blood pressure, and muscle tension; it also increases oxygenation for the client and the fetus. Concentration on breathing may distract the client from her pain.

Yawning. By stretching the facial muscles, yawning stimulates cardiac activity, increases oxygen in the blood, and expands the lungs. Instruct the client to assume a comfortable position, close her eyes, tense all her muscles, clench her fists, breathe in deeply, and hold it for a few moments. She should yawn as she releases the tension.

Touch. For the typical client, touch conveys a sense of caring and helps aid relaxation. Wiping the client's brow, assisting with effleurage, or massaging her back can reduce tension and increase relaxation. Applying firm pressure may relieve pain. Kneading and stroking muscles improves circulation.

Some clients dislike being touched or massaged, particularly when contractions become more intense or as they enter the transition phase.

Music therapy. Typically, music offers an adjunct to other pain-reducing techniques. It prompts positive associations, aids rhythmic breathing, and distracts the client from environmental noises that might increase anxiety (Hanzer, Lanson, and O'Connell, 1983).

Support person assistance

A support person who helps a client through labor needs assistance from the nurse. A support person with a nursing diagnosis of *knowledge deficit related to inadequate preparation for childbirth* will need even more assistance.

Specific nursing interventions include orienting the support person to the environment, briefly explaining equipment and its use, and informing the support person of the location of restrooms, telephones, and food. Explain that help will be available should the support person need to leave the labor area. With the client's permission, ask the support person to perform such tasks as giving ice chips, performing backrubs, or applying cool cloths. In addition to keeping the support person informed of the client's progress, give brief explanations of potentially disturbing developments during labor, such as bloody show, vomiting, or leg tremors. Avoid using ambiguous or highly technical terms, which may be confusing or frightening.

Remain attentive to the support person's feelings and concerns, keeping in mind the emotional difficulty of watching a loved one in pain. Encourage the support person to focus on the positive aspects of labor rather than on the client's discomfort. Reinforce the importance of support. Emphasize that the support person should avoid asking the client questions during contractions when the client should focus her attention and energy on remaining relaxed. The support person may offer reassuring comments during a contraction but should avoid distracting the client. Demonstrate the gentle and competent care that the client should receive from the support person and health care professionals alike.

In addition to the client and her partner, labor also can affect other family members and support persons, possibly resulting in a nursing diagnosis of *anxiety related to lack of information about labor progress*. Although caring for the client and fetus is the nurse's primary goal and overseeing the primary support person is a secondary goal, the nurse also should try to understand and accept the feelings of family members waiting for the neonate's birth. Waiting is difficult and, during long labors or periods with little word from the nurse or partner, family members and friends may imagine the worst. When appropriate and with the client's permission, allow family members or friends to make brief visits to the labor area for reassurance and to provide support for the client.

Interventions for the unprepared client

A client with no childbirth education presents a special challenge to the nurse, who must provide information and guide the client through comfort promotion and pain reduction.

If the client has no support person, remain with her and assume the support role. Because the client's anxiety and stress level will be high, teach simple relaxation techniques, including controlled breathing. Inform the client of what will happen during labor, why, and how long labor may last.

If the client has a support person, focus on the partner's supporting role. Demonstrate touch, massage, and simple breathing patterns. Describe normal labor stages, expected behaviors, and typical interventions, including comfort measures and pain-relieving agents.

If an unprepared client feels out of control, shifting her focus from pain to relaxation techniques may be difficult. To get the client's attention, try such simple techniques as establishing direct eye contact, calling her by name, asking questions, and whispering in her ear. Coach the client through relaxation techniques (particularly controlled breathing) during a contraction; then have her practice the techniques immediately so that she knows how to use them before the next contraction.

Nonpharmacologic pain control

Comfort measures typically fall short of pain relief, which becomes imperative for most clients as labor progresses. Methods to accomplish this goal without using pharmacologic agents include hypnosis, transcutaneous electric nerve stimulation (TENS), and acupressure or acupuncture.

Hypnosis. In this state of altered consciousness, motor control and perception can be influenced by suggestion. The client attains a state of alertness and heightened concentration through imagery, controlled breathing, and other relaxation techniques. Through intense concentration, the client can diminish pain perception; however, not all clients respond to hypnosis. To assist a client with self-hypnosis, encourage the use of relaxation techniques and provide a tranquil environment free from distraction.

TENS. In TENS, electric currents block pain messages by stimulating large-diameter neural fibers. Impulses travel more quickly along the large fibers than along the small-diameter fibers that transmit pain; thus, electrical counterstimulation blocks or modifies pain perception. TENS stimulation also may release endogenous endorphins, which activate opiate receptors in the brain and spinal cord that decrease the client's response to painful stimuli.

Several European clinical trials have focused on women in labor, showing that TENS provided moderate to good pain relief for about 75% of those studied. Most said that it "modulates" the pain or makes it more tolerable (Perez and Hanold, 1988).

Applied and used properly, TENS appears to have no harmful effects on the client or fetus and can reduce the need for analgesia and anesthesia. However, if the client experiences no pain relief or dislikes the tingling sensation, remove the unit and try other pain-reduction measures.

Acupressure and acupuncture. Based on the Chinese theory that energy travels through the body along 12 major pathways or meridians, acupressure and acupuncture seek to reduce pain and enhance well-being by manipulating key points along those meridians (Lieberman, 1987). In acupuncture, the practitioner stimulates selected trigger points with thin needles. In acupressure, the practitioner uses finger pressure instead of needles.

Pharmacologic pain control

Analgesic and anesthetic agents are the two types of pharmacologic pain relief used during labor. (For a summary, see *Drugs used to relieve labor pain*, pages 220 and 221.)

DRUGS USED TO RELIEVE LABOR PAIN

The following drugs provide analgesia or anesthesia for labor.

DRUG AND INDICATION	POSSIBLE ADVERSE EFFECTS	NURSING CONSIDERATIONS
Narcotic agonists		
meperidine, morphine *Indication:* Alter pain perception	*Maternal:* decreased respirations, orthostatic hypotension, nausea and vomiting, itching, drowsiness *Fetal:* moderate central nervous system (CNS) depression, decreased beat-to-beat variability *Neonatal:* moderate CNS depression, mild behavioral depression	• Review maternal history for drug allergy, substance abuse, chronic respiratory disease, and renal and liver disease. • Frequently assess maternal vital signs, respirations, and level of consciousness. • Assess labor stage and progress. • Use continuous electronic fetal heart rate (FHR) monitoring, if possible. • A degree of neonatal respiratory depression can be anticipated if administered 1 to 2 hours prior to birth. Inject naloxone (0.01 mg/kg) into umbilical cord vein or neonate's thigh, as prescribed.
Narcotic antagonists		
naloxone *Indication:* Reverse respiratory depression caused by narcotic toxicity in client or neonate	*Maternal:* may reverse analgesia if given 5 to 10 minutes before delivery, increasing pain perception *Fetal:* none *Neonatal:* may induce withdrawal symptoms in a narcotic-dependent neonate	• Keep resuscitation equipment nearby during administration. • Do not administer to client with known drug dependency. • Develop a plan for alternate pain relief. • Narcotic antagonists will not reverse respiratory depression caused by sedatives, hypnotics, anesthetics, or nonnarcotic CNS depressants.
Narcotic agonist-antagonists		
butorphanol tartrate, nalbuphine *Indication:* Alter pain perception	*Maternal:* may induce withdrawal symptoms in a narcotic-dependent client; may cause decreased respirations, orthostatic hypotension, nausea and vomiting, itching, drowsiness *Fetal:* moderate CNS depression, decreased beat-to-beat variability *Neonatal:* moderate CNS depression, mild behavioral depression	• Review the client's history for drug allergy, substance abuse, chronic respiratory disease, and renal and liver disease. • Frequently assess maternal vital signs, respirations, and level of consciousness. • Assess labor stage and progress. • Use continuous electronic FHR monitoring, if possible.
Sedative-hypnotics (tranquilizers)		
phenothiazines (promethazine, propiomazine), piperazine (hydroxyzine) *Indication:* Promote rest and sleep; may reduce anxiety and reduce narcotic requirements	*Maternal:* may cause dizziness, lassitude, incoordination, fatigue, euphoria or excitation *Fetal:* decreased beat-to-beat variability; moderate CNS depression, especially with larger doses *Neonatal:* possible hypotonia, decreased feeding, lethargy, and hypothermia	• Review the client's history for drug allergies before administration. • These drugs usually are given only during the early first stage of labor; they may have antiemetic effects.
barbiturates (secobarbital) *Indication:* Decrease anxiety during the prodromal or early latent phase of labor	*Maternal:* possible paradoxically increased pain and excitability *Fetal:* none *Neonatal:* possible CNS depression that can persist for several days	• Barbiturates are administered less commonly than other tranquilizers because of their prolonged depressant effects on the neonate. • Barbiturates should be administered only if delivery is not expected for 12 to 24 hours.

DRUGS USED TO RELIEVE LABOR PAIN *(continued)*

DRUG AND INDICATION	POSSIBLE ADVERSE EFFECTS	NURSING CONSIDERATIONS
Regional anesthetic agents		
bupivacaine, lidocaine, chloroprocaine, mepivacaine *Indication:* Preferred regional method for analgesia and anesthesia during first and second stage of labor; provide anesthesia for vaginal or cesarean delivery; relieve uterine pain (pudendal block relieves perineal pain)	*Maternal:* hypotension (epidural and spinal); delayed analgesia (10 to 20 minutes); one-sided block or ineffective pain relief (spinal); prolonged labor if epidural block given too early; urine retention (epidural and spinal); increased toxicity from vascularity of region (pudendal); hematoma (pudendal); diminished bearing-down efforts (epidural) *Fetal:* transient decreased beat-to-beat variability with lidocaine and mepivacaine; late decelerations; fetal distress secondary to maternal hypotension; about 30% incidence of bradycardia (paracervical) *Neonatal:* CNS depression in presence of severe hypotension; neonatal bradycardia, hypotonia, and decreased responsiveness with accidental fetal intracranial injection (pudendal block)	• Determine baseline maternal vital signs and FHR; assess throughout labor as needed. • Explain procedure and expected feelings as anesthesia is initiated. • *Pudendal:* Assess for diminished bearing-down reflex and fetal symptoms associated with accidental scalp injection. • *Epidural:* Ensure adequate client hydration by administering 500 to 1,000 ml I.V. fluid before injection. Take vital signs every 5 minutes for 30 minutes after injection and report hypotension. Monitor vital signs every 15 minutes throughout continuous epidural infusion. Catheterize if client retains urine. Labor may be augmented with oxytocin if uterine contractions diminish. Assist with positioning and maintain safety (put up side rails). • *Spinal:* Ensure adequate client hydration by administering 500 to 1,000 ml I.V. fluid before injection. Take vital signs every 5 minutes until delivery. Report hypotension, and treat as prescribed. Observe for signs of total spinal block (apnea, unconsciousness, absent blood pressure, absent pulse, pupil dilation). Encourage the client to lie flat for 8 to 10 hours after administration.
General anesthetic agents		
halothane, enflurane, thiopental sodium *Indication:* Anesthesia for cesarean delivery; surgical intervention for obstetric complications, version, extraction, or uterine manipulation	*Maternal:* increased risk of regurgitation and aspiration; increased risk of uterine atony; decreased risk of hypovolemia compared to regional anesthesia *Fetal:* increased risk of fetal CNS depression *Neonatal:* short-term behavioral changes	• Assess for risk of aspiration. Maintain NPO status. • Administer antacid or H₂ blocking agent, as prescribed. • Continuously monitor FHR, especially during induction of anesthesia and in response to anesthesia. • Maintain respiratory support, I.V. fluids, and uterine fundal massage, as necessary, during recovery from anesthesia. • Drowsiness may persist after recovery. Assist with positioning and maintain safety (put up side rails).

Analgesia refers to pain reduction without loss of consciousness. Although the client may continue to perceive pain, an analgesic agent can make it more tolerable by affecting the peripheral nervous system (by relaxing muscles and increasing blood flow) and the central nervous system (CNS).

Anesthesia refers to partial or complete loss of sensation, sometimes with loss of consciousness. Affecting the entire body or only a region of the body, an anesthetic

agent blocks conduction of impulses along pain pathways to the brain.

Regional anesthetic agents are injected into areas surrounding nerves. Types used for labor pain include pudendal block, epidural block, spinal block, saddle block, or paracervical block.

General anesthetic agents render the client unconscious and thus unable to feel pain. These agents may be inhaled or administered I.V. or I.M. Typically, they are used only for emergency cesarean delivery or other surgical interventions because they greatly increase the risk of aspiration, the leading cause of anesthesia-related maternal death.

Ideally, the client should receive information and make choices about pharmacologic options before labor begins. Childbirth education classes typically include such information. The client's obstetrician and anesthesiologist are responsible for describing obstetric analgesia and anesthesia and obtaining written consent to administer these therapies. Provide additional information as needed, including the route of administration, degree and timing of pain relief, impact on labor and the fetus, potential adverse drug reactions, and the effectiveness of the technique selected. In addition, explain how analgesia and anesthesia may interfere with the client's active participation in labor. Describe the immediate and prolonged effects of pharmacologic agents on the neonate. Take steps to ensure that the client's caregivers will support her decision for or against pharmacologic intervention. If a client who planned a "natural" childbirth requires pharmacologic pain relief during labor, help her work through any feelings of guilt or failure and provide reassurance about her decision.

Analgesia. The client may receive an analgesic agent when active labor is established and the cervix begins to dilate. Administration usually takes place via an intravenous or intramuscular injection.

Analgesic agents may cause drowsiness, euphoria, orthostatic hypotension, and dizziness. Use side rails on the bed to ensure client safety if a member of the health care team or a support person cannot be in constant attendance. Caution the client and support person that the client should not get out of bed without a nurse's help.

Categories of systemic analgesic agents used during labor include sedatives, narcotic agonists, mixed narcotic agonist-antagonists, antianxiety agents, and inhalation analgesics.

Sedatives. For the client in the prodromal or latent phase of labor, sedatives allow a few hours of sleep or relaxation before entering active labor. For the client in false labor, sedatives promote rest and stop contractions.

Narcotic agonists. Natural and synthetic opiates, these drugs bind at specific opiate receptor sites in the CNS and alter the client's perception of pain. They depress the CNS, causing drowsiness, euphoria, and reduced respiratory activity. They also stimulate the medullary chemoreceptor trigger zone, producing nausea and vomiting.

Meperidine (Demerol), a synthetic narcotic agonist commonly used during labor, increases pain tolerance and promotes rest between contractions. Administration of meperidine 1 to 3 hours or less before delivery may cause respiratory depression in the neonate. Some researchers also report abnormal reflexes and diminished sucking, alertness, and ability to become and remain quiet for up to 5 days after delivery (Hodgkinson and Hussain, 1982; Cunningham, MacDonald, and Gant, 1989).

Because pain pathways involve transmission via the spinal cord, narcotic agonist administration via epidural catheter is being studied to manage labor pain. Because the drugs act locally on opiate receptors in the spinal cord, this method allows lower doses with greater pain relief and fewer adverse drug reactions than other administration routes. The client still perceives contractions and retains control over the bearing-down efforts.

Adverse reactions to narcotic agonists include nausea, vomiting, pruritus, urine retention, and delayed respiratory depression. After delivery, antiemetics reduce nausea and vomiting, and antipruritics reduce itching. Ambulation improves bladder function.

Regardless of the route of administration, narcotic agonists can cause respiratory depression in the client and neonate. A narcotic antagonist, such as naloxone (Narcan), may be administered to prevent this. For I.V. administration, use the client's I.V. line or the neonate's umbilical vein; for I.M. administration, use the client's gluteal muscle or the neonate's thigh. Administer these agents cautiously in a drug-dependent client because they may induce withdrawal symptoms.

Mixed narcotic agonist-antagonists. These agents produce an analgesic effect unless narcotics already exist in the client's circulation. In this case, they have an antagonist effect and cause withdrawal. Early withdrawal symptoms include yawning, lacrimation, sweating, mydriasis, piloerection, flushing, tachycardia, tremors, and irritability. If withdrawal occurs, notify the physician immediately to prevent fetal adverse reactions. In equianalgesic doses, butorphanol (Stadol) and pentazocine (Talwin) have shown analgesic effects similar to meperidine (Demerol). Both drugs rapidly cross the placenta and can cause CNS depression in the neonate.

Antianxiety agents. These agents increase narcotic effects while they decrease anxiety and relieve nausea. They do not relieve pain directly. Antianxiety agents used commonly during labor include promethazine (Phenergan), hydroxyzine (Vistaril), and promazine (Sparine). Administer antianxiety agents I.M. or I.V.

Regional anesthesia. By blocking pain transmission without altering consciousness, regional anesthesia allows the client to participate in labor and childbirth while decreasing pain perception and the amount of drug that crosses to the fetus. Many physicians advocate regional anesthesia. Its disadvantages include potential CNS toxicity, hypotension, diminished bearing-down efforts, pruritus, urine retention, nausea, and vomiting.

The physician or anesthesiologist administers the anesthetic. Drugs used most commonly include ester-type agents (chloroprocaine hydrochloride, procaine hydrochloride, and tetracaine hydrochloride) and amide-type agents (bupivacaine hydrochloride, etidocaine hydrochloride, lidocaine hydrochloride, and mepivacaine hydrochloride). The choice of agent will differ with the type of anesthetic block used.

Regional anesthesia techniques include local infiltration (including pudendal and paracervical blocks), epidural block, and spinal block. Epidural and spinal blocks carry the risk of hypotension caused by sympathetic blockage. (For descriptions of administration techniques, see *Regional anesthesia administration.*)

Local infiltration. The physician or nurse-midwife may use local infiltration before delivery to perform an episiotomy or after delivery to repair perineal lacerations. This simple method of anesthesia, commonly chosen by prepared clients or clients seeking a more "natural" birth, produces few complications for the client or neonate. The agent is injected directly into perineal tissue. The client may report a brief burning sensation after injection.

Pudendal block. Another form of local infiltration, this block is used during the second stage of labor to numb the perineum and vagina for delivery, episiotomy repair, or forceps delivery. The pudendal block is especially effective for difficult episiotomies or repairing lacerations after delivery. It does not block pain perceived from uterine contractions, but it does decrease bearing-down efforts.

The physician or nurse-midwife injects the drug into the pudendal nerve on each side of the sacrum. Complications include accidental injection into a blood vessel, hematoma, and perforation. If the needle enters the fetus's scalp or cranium, neonatal brachycardia, apnea, and diminished responsiveness may be present after birth.

Paracervical block. Also a type of local infiltration, this technique blocks nerves on either side of the cervix during the active phase of labor, at 4 to 5 cm of dilation. The paracervical block relieves pain stemming from uterine con-

REGIONAL ANESTHESIA ADMINISTRATION

The following chart explains the administration techniques for five types of regional anesthesia.

Local infiltration
Used to numb perineal tissue for episiotomy or laceration repair, this technique involves injection of anesthetic through a 22G needle into the fascia of the perineum. The client may feel a burning sensation.

Pudendal block
Used to block perineal and vaginal pain but not uterine contractions during the second stage of labor, this technique involves injection of 3 to 5 ml of anesthetic into the pudendal nerve on each side of the sacrum. The needle crosses the sacrosciatic notch and passes the tip of the ischial spine.

Paracervical block
Used to anesthetize the uterus and cervix during the first stage of labor, this technique involves insertion of an Iowa trumpet into the lateral fornix of the vagina and injection of 5 to 10 ml of anesthetic. The block provides anesthesia through the second stage of labor.

Epidural block
Used to anesthetize the lower half of the body, this technique involves insertion of an 18G stylet into lumbar interspace 3, 4, or 5. Then the tip of the needle is advanced into the epidural space to administer the anesthetic.

Spinal block
Performed in a similar manner to the epidural block, this technique is used to anesthetize the lower half of the body. However, the needle is advanced somewhat farther, into the subarachnoid space. Thus, the anesthetic is injected directly into spinal fluid. The client loses perception of contractions and ability to bear down. A spinal block to the level of T10 is used for vaginal delivery, to T8 for cesarean delivery.

tractions and cervical dilation. Duration of action is approximately 1 hour.

Use of the paracervical block is rare today. Twenty to thirty percent of fetuses develop bradycardia and subsequently may develop fetal acidosis. Also, a risk exists for inadvertent intracranial injection into the fetus.

Epidural block. The most commonly used method of pain relief during labor, the epidural block provides continuous anesthesia during the first and second stages of labor. This type of anesthesia commonly is used during cesarean deliveries. The anesthesiologist or nurse anesthetist injects a local anesthetic agent into the epidural space, located between the dura mater and the ligamentum flavum, at the lumbar region of the spinal column (third to fifth lumbar inner space). Although the client's pelvis and legs feel heavy, she retains some ability to move and bear down.

Continuous epidural infusion is a variation on the epidural block. The client receives continuous infusion of dilute anesthetic agents through an indwelling epidural catheter, a method that maintains continuous drug levels, reduces the amount of drug needed, and decreases the risk of hypotensive crisis (Morrison and Smedstad, 1985). The same precautions should be exercised with the indwelling epidural catheter as with the standard method.

Contraindications for epidural anesthesia include coagulopathy problems, allergic reactions, placental insufficiency, and infection at the puncture site. If a virus, such as herpes, is present on the skin at the site of epidural injection, further dissemination of the virus may occur (Ravindran, 1982). An epidural block should be used with caution if the client has high or low blood pressure. (For more information, see Emergency Alert: *Hypotensive crisis.*)

Disadvantages of epidural anesthesia include the need to have skilled anesthesia personnel or a physician on hand to monitor the client and fetus. Further, it may prolong labor, cause difficulty in voiding, increase oxygen use, and increase the risk of forceps delivery because of the client's diminished bearing-down efforts.

Administering epidural anesthesia requires much skill; areas of unanesthetized tissue, ineffective anesthesia, or inadvertent spinal anesthesia may result from improper infusion. Maternal hypotension may occur from sympathetic blockade, producing vasodilation, loss of peripheral resistance, and CNS toxicity. The client may feel chilled from peripheral temperature changes and may experience postpartal urine retention, necessitating catheterization.

Spinal block. This technique resembles the epidural block except that the needle penetrates the meninges and enters the subarachnoid space. The anesthesiologist mixes a single injection of anesthesia with a sample of the client's cerebrospinal fluid and injects it into the third, fourth, or fifth lumbar inner space. The client loses feeling and motor ability in the lower portion of her body. Numbness extends from the umbilicus to the toes for vaginal delivery and from the xiphoid process to the toes for cesarean delivery. A low spinal block, or saddle block, may be used during the second stage of labor if placental extraction or instrumental delivery becomes necessary.

As with an epidural, a spinal block may lead to vasodilation that can cause hypotension and fetal hypoxia. The anesthetic agent could spread, causing a total spinal

EMERGENCY ALERT

HYPOTENSIVE CRISIS

Hypotensive crisis may occur after spinal or epidural anesthesia because of the spread of the anesthetic agent through the spinal canal. A sympathetic blockade produces marked hypotension from loss of peripheral resistance, decreased venous return, and decreased cardiac output. Decreased placental perfusion occurs with maternal hypotension, resulting in fetal bradycardia.

Signs and symptoms
- Fetal bradycardia
- Decreased beat-to-beat variability
- Maternal hypotension (20% or greater drop from baseline blood pressure or less than 100 mm Hg systolic)

Treatment and nursing considerations
- Turn the client to the left lateral position to increase uterine perfusion.
- Infuse I.V. fluid rapidly, as prescribed.
- Administer oxygen by mask, as prescribed.
- Elevate the client's legs.
- Notify the anesthesiologist.
- Administer a vasopressor (such as ephedrine) I.V. or I.M., as prescribed.
- Stay with the client and monitor blood pressure and fetal heart rate frequently.

block, apnea, reduced blood pressure and pulse, and unresponsiveness. Contraindications for spinal block are similar to those for epidural block. Adverse reactions include post-spinal headache, shivering, and urine retention.

Epidural and spinal blocks. Because epidural and spinal anesthesia cause hypotension (produced by vasodilation), I.V. fluids (preferably lactated Ringer's solution) are necessary. Expect to infuse 500 to 1,000 ml of fluid before administration of epidural or spinal anesthesia and to maintain an I.V. infusion for fluid and possible emergency drug administration should hypotension occur. Monitor vital signs every 5 minutes for the first 30 minutes after initiation of epidural anesthesia and every 15 minutes throughout epidural infusion. Monitor vital signs every 5 minutes after administration of spinal anesthesia until delivery, and monitor as prescribed for up to 24 hours after delivery.

Administration of epidural or spinal anesthesia requires that the client be placed in a sitting or side-lying position with shoulders parallel and legs slightly flexed to reduce hypotension. Epidural anesthesia does not affect motor pathways but, because the legs are numb, they seem heavy and are difficult to move. A spinal block produces motor paralysis. Ensure the client's safety by using side rails and assisting with position changes.

Signs and symptoms of anesthesia overdose include circumoral numbness, dizziness, and slurred speech. Maternal and fetal hypoxia may result, causing tachycardia. Be alert for these signs and symptoms, and notify the physician or anesthesiologist if they occur. Treatment of toxicity includes administering oxygen and I.V. fluids.

General anesthesia. Because it requires intubation and increases the risk of aspiration, general anesthesia (where the client loses consciousness) usually is used only when the client undergoes emergency cesarean delivery, intrauterine manipulation, or other surgical intervention. General anesthesia may be attained through inhalation or I.V. drug administration. Inhalation involves high concentrations of the same agents used for inhalant analgesia (nitrous oxide, halothane, and enflurane). The intravenous agent thiopental sodium (Pentothal) produces deep anesthesia and may cause depression in the neonate.

Before anesthesia induction, a nurse anesthetist or anesthesiologist may have the nurse apply pressure to the client's cricoid process during intubation. This occludes the esophagus and reduces the risk of aspiration should the client vomit.

To avoid compressing the vena cava once the tube is in place, move the client from the supine position before anesthesia administration begins. Many obstetric operating room tables provide left lateral tilt capability to displace the gravid uterus off the vena cava. If the table cannot be tilted, insert a wedge beneath the client's right hip. After client positioning, administer oxygen and fluids as prescribed just before anesthesia administration.

Administer a clear antacid—such as sodium citrate—a few hours before surgery to reduce the client's risk of aspiration of acidic stomach contents while anesthetized. If the client requires emergency surgery, the antacid may be administered 30 minutes or less before the procedure. Turning the client from side to side enhances antacid effectiveness and promotes mixing of the antacid with gastric contents. In addition, many anesthesiologists now routinely decrease gastric acidity by administering an H_2 antagonist, such as cimetidine (Tagamet), before surgery.

Because of delayed gastric emptying during pregnancy, the client who requires emergency surgery may be at increased risk for regurgitating, which can cause chemical pneumonitis and death. To reduce gastric volume, some obstetricians forbid clients from drinking anything while in labor.

Because inhalation agents may cause cardiac arrhythmias, monitor the maternal electrocardiogram continuously throughout anesthesia administration and during recovery. Uterine atony, also produced by inhalants, may lead to uterine hemorrhage. Fetal and neonatal hypoxia also may occur with deep induction anesthesia, which reaches the fetus in about 2 minutes. If the client received an I.V. anesthetic agent, monitor the neonate closely for depression.

EVALUATION

Evaluation findings should be stated in terms of actions performed or outcomes achieved for each goal. The following examples illustrate appropriate evaluation statements for the client experiencing labor pain.

- The client demonstrated knowledge of such comfort promotion techniques as controlled breathing and progressive muscle relaxation.
- The client expressed understanding of pain-relief measures available to her.
- The client reported relief from pain after administration of regional anesthesia.
- Fetal heart rate remained stable after anesthesia administration.
- The support person actively influenced the client's breathing pattern during contractions.
- The support person massaged the client's back and applied a cool cloth to her forehead.
- The support person maintained composure despite discomfort with the client's level of pain.
- Family members expressed gratitude for regular reports on the client's progress.

DOCUMENTATION

The nurse must document all findings and actions taken using the nursing process. Documentation applicable to the client experiencing labor pain includes:

- comfort measures taken and their effectiveness
- analgesic agents administered and their effectiveness
- anesthetic agents administered and their effectiveness
- vital signs
- changes in uterine contractions after drug administration
- changes in fetal heart rate after drug administration
- client preferences for participation by the primary support person and family members
- statements made by the client and partner about their feelings during labor
- instructions given to the support person

• actions taken by the support person, such as applying a cool cloth to the client's forehead
• client reactions to the support person's assistance.

CHAPTER SUMMARY

Chapter 12 described comfort promotion techniques, client support, and pain-reduction methods for the client in labor. Here are the chapter highlights.

Although labor pain proceeds through a predictable series of peaks and valleys, each client perceives her pain uniquely, based on her physical condition, pain tolerance, and psychological profile.

Factors that influence the intensity of labor pain include parity, fetal size and position, certain medical procedures, anxiety, fatigue, childbirth education level, culture, and coping mechanisms.

Comfort measures, support, and reassurance can reduce the client's emotional tension and discomfort. The nurse helps maintain client comfort by decreasing her anxiety, promoting hygiene, positioning the client comfortably, and helping with relaxation techniques.

Each client and family require various types and amounts of support. The client's perception that support is available to her (perceived support) may be more helpful to her emotional well-being than acts of support (received support).

Types of support include emotional, appraisal, informational, and instrumental. Common sources of support include the client's partner, their parents, other family members, and friends.

Nonpharmacologic techniques used to minimize and control pain perception in labor include hypnosis, TENS, acupressure, and acupuncture.

Pharmacologic pain-relief measures should promote maternal analgesia without risk to client or fetus.

Analgesics may be initiated when active labor begins, via an intravenous, intramuscular, or subcutaneous route. Drug categories used include sedatives, narcotic agonists, mixed narcotic agonist-antagonists, and antianxiety agents.

Regional analgesia and anesthesia techniques require injection of an anesthetic agent into nerve tissue. Techniques include local infiltration, pudendal block, paracervical block, epidural block, and spinal block.

General anesthesia, used for cesarean delivery or other surgical intervention, may be administered by inhalation or injection.

STUDY QUESTIONS

1. Describe how primiparity affects labor pain.
2. Ms. Rose, age 25, is admitted to the labor and delivery area in active labor. She reports that her labor pains are growing in intensity and that she prefers to avoid drug-induced pain relief. She has had no childbirth education and is alone. How can the nurse intervene with this client?
3. For which possible maternal and fetal adverse effects should the nurse assess when a client receives morphine for analgesia?
4. Mrs. Taft is scheduled to receive regional anesthesia. What are the advantages and risks associated with this type of anesthesia?

BIBLIOGRAPHY

Berry, L.M. (1988). Realistic expectations of the labor coach. *JOGNN*, 17(5), 354-355.

Bonica, J.U. (1989). Labour pain. In P. Wall and R. Melzack (Eds.), *Textbook of pain* (2nd ed.). New York: Churchhill Livingstone.

Collins, B.A. (1986). The role of the nurse in labor and delivery as perceived by nurses and patients. *JOGNN*, 15(5), 412-418.

Copstick, S.M., Taylor, K.E., Hayes, R., and Morris, N. (1986). Partner support and the use of coping techniques in labor. *Journal of Psychosomatic Research*, 30(4), 497-503.

Cunningham, R., MacDonald, P., and Gant, N. (1989). *Williams obstetrics* (18th ed.). East Norwalk, CT: Appleton & Lange.

Dick-Read, G. (1970). *Childbirth without fear.* New York: Harper & Row.

Fenwick, L. (1984). Birthing: Techniques for managing the physiologic and psychosocial aspects of childbirth. *Perinatology/Neonatology*, 6, 51.

Gaston-Johansson, F., Fridh, G., and Turner-Norvell, K. (1988). Progression of labor pain in primiparas and multiparas. *Nursing Research*, 37(2), 86-90.

Kintz, D. (1987). Nursing support in labor. *JOGNN*, 16(2), 126-130.

Lederman, R., Lederman, E., Work, B.A., and McCann, D.S. (1978). The relationship of maternal anxiety, plasma catecholamines, and plasma cortisol to progress in labor. *American Journal of Obstetrics and Gynecology*, 132(5), 495-500.

Lederman, R.P. (1984). *Psychosocial adaption in pregnancy.* East Norwalk, CT: Appleton & Lange.

Lieberman, A.B. (1987). *Easing labor pain: The complete guide to achieving a more comfortable and rewarding birth.* New York: Doubleday.

McCaffery, M., and Beebe, A. (1989). *Pain: Clinical manual for nursing practice.* St. Louis: Mosby.

Melzack, R., and Wall, P. (1965). Pain mechanisms: A new theory. *Science*, 150(699), 971-979.

Nettelbladt, P., Fagerstrom, C.F., and Uddenberg, N. (1976). The significance of reported childbirth pain. *Journal of Psychosomatic Research,* 20(3), 215-221.

Nichols, F., and Humenick, S.S. (1988). *Childbirth education: Practice, research, and theory.* Philadelphia: Saunders.

Nicholson, J., Gist, N.F., Klein, R.P., and Standley, K. (1983). Outcomes of father involvement in pregnancy and birth. *Birth,* 10(1), 5-9.

Perez, P., and Hanold, K. (1988). The use of transcutaneous nerve stimulation in the first stage of labor. In M. Rathi (Ed.), *Current perinatology.* New York: Springer-Verlag.

Reading, A.E., and Cox, D.N. (1985). Psychosocial predictors of labor pain. *Pain,* 22(3), 309-315.

Roberts, J. (1982). Which position for the first stage? *Childbirth Educator,* (1), 35.

Sosa, R., Kennell, J., Klaus, M., Robertson, S., and Urrutia, J. (1980). The effect of a supportive companion on perinatal problems, length of labor, and mother-infant interaction. *The New England Journal of Medicine,* 303(11), 597-600.

Wolff, B.B., and Langley, S. (1975). Cultural factors and the response to pain: A review. In M. Weisenberg (Ed.), *Pain: Clinical and experimental perspectives.* St. Louis: Mosby.

Client support

Anderberg, G.J. (1988). Initial acquaintance and attachment behavior of siblings with the newborn. *JOGNN,* 17(1), 49-54.

Barnard, K. (1978). The family and you, Part 1. *MCN,* 3(2), 82-83.

Bennett, A., Hewson, D., Booker, E., and Holliday, S. (1985). Antenatal preparation and labor support in relation to birth outcomes. *Birth,* 12(1), 9-16.

Brown, M.A. (1986). Social support during pregnancy: A unidimensional or multidimensional construct? *Nursing Research,* 35(1), 4-9.

Copstick, S.M., Taylor, K.E., Hayes, R., and Morris, N. (1986). Partner support and the use of coping techniques in labor. *Journal of Psychosomatic Research,* 30(4), 497-503.

Fishbein, E.G. (1984). Expectant father's stress – due to the mother's expectations? *JOGNN,* 13(5), 325-328.

Honig, J.C. (1986). Preparing preschool-aged children to be siblings. *MCN,* 11(1), 37-43.

Horn, M., and Manion, J. (1985). Creative grandparenting: Bonding the generations. *JOGNN,* 14(3), 233-236.

House, J. (1981). *Work, stress, and social support.* Reading, MA: Addison-Wesley.

Hunter, M., Philips, C., and Rachman, S. (1979). Memory for pain. *Pain,* 6(1), 35-46.

Leonard, L. (1977). The father's side: A different perspective on childbirth. *The Canadian Nurse,* 73(2), 16-20.

Maloni, J.A., McIndoe, J.E., and Rubenstein, G. (1987). Expectant grandparents class. *JOGNN,* 16(1), 26-29.

Peddicord, K., Curran, P. and Monshower, C. (1984). An independent labor-support nursing service. *JOGNN,* 13(5), 312-316.

Raphael, D. (1976). *The tender gift: Breastfeeding.* New York: Schocken Books.

Reading, A.E., and Cox, D.N. (1985). Psychosocial predictors of labor pain. *Pain,* 22(3), 309-315.

Sarason, I.G., and Sarason, B.R. (1985). Social support – insights, from assessment and experimentation. In I.G. Sarason and B.R. Sarason (Eds.), *Social support: Theory, research, and applications* (pp. 39-50). Hingham, MA: Kluwer Academia.

Sosa, R., Kennell, J., Klaus, M., Robertson, S., and Urrutia, J. (1980). The effect of a supportive companion on perinatal problems, length of labor, and mother-infant interaction. *The New England Journal of Medicine,* 303(11), 597-600.

Cultural references

Choi, E.C. (1986). Unique aspects of Korean-American mothers. *JOGNN,* 15(5), 394-400.

Hahn, R.A. and Muecke, M.A. (1987). The anthropology of birth in five U.S. ethnic populations: Implications for obstetrical practice. *Current Problems in Obstetrics, Gynecology, and Fertility,* 10(4), 133-171.

La Du, E.B. (1982). A study of the birthing practices of a group of recently immigrated Hmong women. Master's thesis in nursing, School of Nursing, Oregon Health Science University, Portland.

Nyce, J.M., and Hollingshead, W.H. (1984). Southeast Asian refugees of Rhode Island: Reproductive beliefs and practices among the Hmong. *Rhode Island Medical Journal,* 67(8), 361-366.

Nonpharmacologic pain control

DiFranco, J. (1988). Music for childbirth. *Childbirth Educator,* (8), 36-41.

Hanzer, S.B., Lanson, S.C., and O'Connell, A.S. (1983). The effect of music on relaxation of expectant mothers during labor. *Journal of Music Therapy,* 20(2), 50-58.

Hilbers, S., and Gennaro, S. (1986). *Non-pharmaceutical pain relief.* In NAACOG Update Series, Vol. 5. Princeton, NJ: Continuing Professional Education Center.

Jimenez, S. (1983). *Application of the body's natural pain relief mechanisms to reduce discomfort in labor and delivery.* In NAACOG Update Series, Vol. 1. Princeton, NJ: Continuing Professional Education Center.

Klusman, L.E. (1975). Reduction of pain in childbirth by alleviation of anxiety during pregnancy. *Journal of Consulting and Clinical Psychology,* 43(2), 162-165.

Melzack, R. (1984). Acupuncture and related forms of folk medicine. In P. Wall and R. Melzack (Eds.), *Textbook of pain.* New York: Churchhill Livingstone.

Tanzer, D., and Block, J.L. (1987). *Why natural childbirth?* New York: Schocken Books.

Velovsky, I., Platonov, K., Ploticher, U., and Shugom, E. (1960). *Painless childbirth through psychoprophylaxis.* Moscow: Foreign Languages Publishing House.

Wideman, M.V., and Singer, J.E. (1984). The role of psychological mechanisms in preparation for childbirth. *American Psychologist,* 39(12), 1357-1371.

Pharmacologic pain control

Albright, G.A., Joyce, R.H., and Stevenson, D.K. (1986). *Anesthesia in obstetrics* (2nd ed.). Boston: Butterworth.

Bonica, J. (1980). *Obstetric analgesia and anesthesia.* Amsterdam: World Federation of Societies of Anesthesiologists.

Gibbs, C.P. (1985). Anesthetic management of the high risk mother. In V.V. Sciaria, R. Depp, and D.A. Eschenbach (Eds.), *Gynecology and obstetrics.* New York: Harper & Row.

Hodgkinson, M.A., and Hussain, F.J. (1982). The duration of effect of maternity administered meperidine on neonatal neurobehavior. *Anesthesiology,* 56, 51-52.

ICEA (1988, February). ICEA position paper: Epidural anesthesia for labor. *International Journal of Childbirth Education,* 3(1).

Kuhnert, B.R., Linn, P.L., and Kuhnert, P.M. (1984). Effect of maternal epidural anesthesia on neonatal behavior. *Anesthesia and Analgesia,* 63(3), 301-308.

Kuhnert, B.R., Linn, P.L., and Kuhnert, P.M. (1985). Obstetric medication and neonatal behavior: Current controversies. *Clinics in Perinatology,* 12(2), 423.

Morrison, D.H., and Smedstad, K.G. (1985). Continuous epidurals for obstetric analgesia. *Canadian Anesthesiology Society Journal,* 32(2), 101.

Ravindran, R.S. (1982). Epidural analgesia in the presence of herpes simplex virus (type 2) infection. *Anesthesia and Analgesia,* 61(8), 714-715.

CHAPTER 13

THE FIRST STAGE OF LABOR

OBJECTIVES

After reading and studying this chapter, the student should be able to:

1. Differentiate between true labor and false labor.

2. Obtain pertinent health history information during the client's admission to the labor and delivery area.

3. Describe physical assessment techniques used during admission to the labor and delivery area.

4. Interpret laboratory data for the client and fetus.

5. Describe how to assess the client and fetus during the first stage of labor.

6. Implement comfort and support measures for the client and her family.

7. Identify common variations in the first stage of labor and their specific nursing interventions.

8. Describe the impact of cultural background and family support on the childbearing process.

INTRODUCTION

The first stage of labor begins with the onset of regular, rhythmic uterine contractions that cause progressive cervical changes. It ends with complete cervical dilation of approximately 10 cm. Labor, however, is much more than a physiologic process that allows the fetus to enter the world. It is also the dramatic culmination of the gestational period—a significant life event that represents a pivotal point in the lives of the mother, father, neonate, and other family members. It is a psychological and developmental task that demands rigorous adaptation.

During the first stage of labor, nursing care must meet the client's physical, psychosocial, and cultural needs. To provide this kind of care, nursing responsibilities typically include:

• interpreting history, physical, and laboratory findings and evaluating their possible effects on labor

• assessing the progress of labor and adapting nursing care to meet individual needs

• maintaining client safety through ongoing assessments

• promoting client comfort in a supportive environment that encourages active participation

• recognizing variations in labor and intervening promptly

• teaching the client and her family about the childbirth process and discussing the benefits, risks, and alternatives related to any procedures

• enhancing the client's and support person's self-esteem and childbirth experience by encouraging active participation and development of realistic goals

• integrating the psychosocial and cultural needs of the client and her support person and adapting care to meet individual differences.

This chapter describes how to manage all of these responsibilities. It begins with preadmission care, describing how to gather the health history and physical assessment data needed to evaluate maternal and fetal status and how to distinguish between true and false labor. It also describes how to perform a more detailed, postadmission assessment that includes psychosocial and laboratory study data and how to formulate appropriate nursing diagnoses based on this assessment data. Then it discusses how to plan and implement initial care and ongoing care, including activities to monitor the client and provide comfort and support. The chapter describes variations in the first stage of labor and concludes with a brief discussion of documentation.

NURSING CARE BEFORE ADMISSION

Before any client can be admitted for care in the labor and delivery area, she must be in true labor or show signs of a medical complication, such as hypertension, that could affect her or the fetus during labor and delivery. To make this determination, the nurse performs an initial assessment that focuses on the imminence of the birth and on fetal stability. This assessment, which includes a brief history and physical examination, should provide sufficient data to distinguish true labor from other conditions that mimic it, such as false labor, urinary tract infection, "terminal pregnancy blues" (generalized physical discomfort and emotional distress near the end of pregnancy), and abruptio placentae. However, if delivery appears imminent, omit the preadmission assessment and admit the client immediately.

INITIAL ASSESSMENT

Set the tone for the initial assessment by making appropriate introductions. Briefly describe nursing activities during this assessment and maintain the client's privacy and confidentiality to gain her trust and ease anxiety.

During the introductory period, observe the client closely to identify clues to her labor status. Postures, facial expressions, or gestures that connote tension, anxiety, or pain may accurately reflect a client's labor progress. Perspiration, varying breathing patterns, lack of concentration, and frequent position changes can indicate discomfort or stress during and between contractions. Involuntary grunting or breath holding may signal the onset of the second stage of labor. To help form an accurate initial impression, relate the client's behavior to her cultural background. (See Cultural Considerations: *Response to pain.*)

If the client is in active labor, shorten the initial assessment and prioritize the questions. Focus on collecting data about her current labor status. Refer to prenatal records, if available, and use the previously documented information. Engage the client's support person in conversation to reduce anxiety, especially if the client is in active labor.

Perform a brief physical examination to determine labor progress and fetal well-being. Be sure to help the

CULTURAL CONSIDERATIONS

RESPONSE TO PAIN

Although each client has personal beliefs and values, her cultural background may influence her behavior.

Martinelli (1987) found that the response to pain varies among clients and among cultures. One study of 75 Lamaze-trained clients found that, among ethnic groups, response to labor pain differed significantly—even when anxiety was minimal. Clients from some groups, such as Italians and Hispanics, tended to use body language and expressions freely; those from other groups, such as Vietnamese, Irish, and Native Americans, tended to respond passively and did not openly display discomfort.

To help a client from a different cultural background cope with her pain effectively, be aware of your personal and cultural views and take a nonjudgmental approach. During the health history, identify the client's cultural background and determine how it may affect her response to pain.

client find a comfortable position for the assessment, especially if she is in active labor. Calmly conduct the history and physical assessment between contractions.

Health history
During the initial health history, gather biographical data and investigate the client's health status, health promotion and protection behaviors, and roles and relationships as they relate to her pregnancy, labor, and forthcoming delivery.

To help prioritize this information, obtain health history information in this order:
- biographical data
- expected delivery date
- previous pregnancies and outcomes
- previous labors and deliveries
- contractions
- rupture of amniotic membranes
- bloody show (a pink-tinged or blood-tinged mucus discharge) or vaginal bleeding (a bloody discharge without mucus)
- pregnancy-related health problems
- other health problems
- fetal movements
- prenatal care
- roles and relationships.

Also obtain and document any other information required by the health care facility.

Biographical data. Obtain the client's name, address, and other biographical information required by the health care facility. Particularly note her age, because it can affect labor progress and outcome. (For more information about these concerns, see Chapter 16, Intrapartal Complications and Special Procedures.)

Expected delivery date. Ask the client her expected delivery date or "due date." This information will help in assessing for a preterm or postterm neonate, determining gestational age, and evaluating fetal size.

Previous pregnancies and outcomes. Find out the client's gravidity (number of pregnancies) and parity (number of births). Also determine if any of the pregnancies ended in spontaneous or induced abortions and if all of her children are living. If any of her children are dead, ask about the cause.

Gravidity and parity affect the duration of—and potential for complications in—successive labors. Generally, each labor shortens because the cervix and pelvic soft tissues offer less resistance and the uterus becomes more efficient, which promotes more rapid fetal expulsion. After more than five births, however, the uterus may lose its muscle tone, reducing its efficiency.

Information about induced or spontaneous abortions helps in planning the client's care. It also reconciles the number of children with the number of pregnancies.

Previous labors and deliveries. Ask the client the date of her last delivery and the length of her last labor—information that can help predict the progress of the current labor and delivery. If the client's last delivery was within the past 10 years and without complications, labor should progress rapidly and smoothly.

Inquire about the birth weight of the newborns in previous pregnancies. Determine if any were born prematurely or required cesarean delivery. Then ask if the client or any of her previous newborns developed complications.

Contractions. Ask the client to describe the frequency and duration of her present contractions. Find out when they began and determine the frequency and duration of those first contractions. This can help predict the client's labor progress and help distinguish true labor contractions from false labor (Braxton Hicks) contractions. (See *Characteristics of true and false labor.*)

Follow up with questions about the location of pain during the contractions. The location and nature of the pain help differentiate true labor from false labor, urinary tract infections (UTIs), and abruptio placentae.

CHARACTERISTICS OF TRUE AND FALSE LABOR

The information in this chart helps the nurse determine whether the client is in true labor.

CHARACTERISTIC	TRUE LABOR	FALSE LABOR
Contractions	Regular and rhythmic	Irregular
Pain	Discomfort that moves from the back to the front of the abdomen	Mild discomfort or pressure in the abdomen and groin; may be relieved by walking
Fetal movement	Unchanged	May intensify
Fetal descent	Progressing	Unchanged
Show	Pinkish mucus, possibly with the mucus plug from the cervix	None
Cervix	Progressing effacement and dilation	Unchanged after 1 to 2 hours

Rupture of amniotic membranes. Determine the condition of the amniotic membranes and, if possible, the amniotic fluid. If the client is unfamiliar with medical terms, word questions in simple terms, such as, "Has your bag of waters broken?" Find out when the membranes ruptured and if they broke with a gush or in a trickle. If the client's membranes have ruptured, ask her to describe the amniotic fluid color. Also inquire if the fluid had an odor and if it has been leaking continuously since the membranes ruptured.

A client may confuse urinary incontinence, increased vaginal secretions, or the mucus plug with rupture of membranes. Clear or pink-tinged fluid is normal. Green-tinged or yellowish green–tinged fluid signifies passage of meconium, a sign of fetal stress that requires immediate assessment. Port wine–colored fluid may indicate bleeding, as in abruptio placentae. Malodorous fluid suggests infection.

Bloody show or vaginal bleeding. Determine if the client has had any bloody show or vaginal bleeding. Increasing bloody show may signal the onset of the second stage of labor. Vaginal bleeding may signal placenta previa or abruptio placentae and subsequent fetal distress.

Pregnancy-related health problems. Focus on the current pregnancy. Ask if the client had any problems, such as bleeding, anemia, infections, or increased blood pressure. Also inquire if she underwent any special tests. Ultrasonography or amniocentesis can provide information about fetal status or the expected delivery date.

Other health problems. Ask if the client has any medical problems, such as diabetes, heart disease, high blood pressure, or kidney disease. Continue the initial assessment by inquiring about the client's antepartal health promotion and protection behaviors.

Fetal movements. Have the client describe current fetal movements and find out if their frequency has changed from the usual rate over the past several days. A fetus usually moves at least 10 times a day.

Prenatal care. Ask if the client has received regular prenatal care. Lack of prenatal care—or of recent prenatal care—increases the risk of complications and may affect the client's care. If the client has had prenatal care, ask who provided it and where. The client's prenatal records can guide the complete health history and physical assessment.

Roles and relationships. Evaluate the roles and relationships that may affect—or be affected by—the client's labor and delivery. Ask a question such as, "Will someone be with you during labor?" to help identify the client's support person for inclusion in the plan of care. Ask the client which family members and friends have accompanied her to the unit. This information can help facilitate family support and participation in the client's care.

Physical assessment
The initial physical assessment includes evaluation of:
• vital signs
• fetal heart tones
• uterine contractions
• fetal lie (relationship of the fetal long axis to the maternal long axis)
• fetal presentation (fetal part that enters the maternal pelvis first and can be touched through the cervix)
• fetal position (relationship of the leading fetal presenting part to a point on the maternal pelvis)
• engagement (descent of the fetal presenting part into the maternal pelvis)
• estimated fetal weight
• edema and deep tendon reflexes
• amniotic membranes

• cervical changes, fetal descent, and other factors determined by vaginal examination.

Vital signs. For a client in labor, vital signs provide necessary information about maternal and fetal health. They also provide baseline data for future comparisons.

First, check the client's blood pressure, which should range from 90 to 140 mm Hg systolic and from 60 to 90 mm Hg diastolic. A rise of 30 mm Hg systolic and 15 mm Hg diastolic above the client's usual blood pressure may signal anxiety, fear, or pregnancy-induced hypertension (PIH).

The client's temperature should normally range from 98° to 99.6° F (36.2° to 37.6° C). A temperature elevation may signal dehydration; a serious obstetric infection, such as chorioamnionitis (fetal membrane inflammation); or another type of infection, such as a UTI.

Pulse rate should typically range from 60 to 90 beats/minute. An elevated pulse rate may be caused by anxiety, pain, infection, dehydration, or drug use.

Respirations should normally range from 16 to 24 breaths/minute. Increased respirations may indicate hyperventilation, anxiety, pain, or infection. Decreased temperature, pulse, and respirations do not commonly occur during labor.

Fetal heart tones. Assess the fetal heart tones to evaluate fetal well-being. If the health care facility requires, use a fetal heart monitor for this part of the assessment. (See Chapter 11, Fetal Assessment.) Otherwise, assess the heart tones via auscultation. (For an illustrated procedure, see Psychomotor Skills: *Auscultating fetal heart tones.*) A variation from the normal fetal heart rate of 120 to 160 beats/minute may indicate fetal distress.

Uterine contractions. Distinguish true labor from Braxton Hicks contractions by using an external fetal monitor or palpating the client's abdomen. Note the frequency, duration, and intensity of the uterine contractions. Also observe the client during and between contractions to estimate her level of discomfort. (For more information, see Psychomotor Skills: *Palpating uterine contractions,* page 234.) Ask the client's support person to record the contraction pattern, if possible.

Fetal lie, presentation, and position. Perform Leopold's maneuvers to determine the fetal lie, presentation, and position. Leopold's maneuvers help detect potential problems, such as breech presentation or transverse lie, that require physician or nurse-midwife evaluation. Also, they help antic-

AUSCULTATING FETAL HEART TONES

The nurse auscultates fetal heart tones to assess the fetal heart rate, which provides information about fetal viability and stress. To auscultate fetal heart tones, follow these guidelines.

1 Place the earpieces of an ultrasound stethoscope in your ears and press its bell gently on the client's abdomen. Start listening at the midline about midway between the umbilicus and the symphysis pubis. As an alternate auscultation method, listen with a fetoscope on your head with the bell extending from the center of your forehead. Then press the bell about ½″ into the client's abdomen. Remove your hands. With either method, move the bell slightly from side to side, if needed, to the point where the heart tones are loudest.

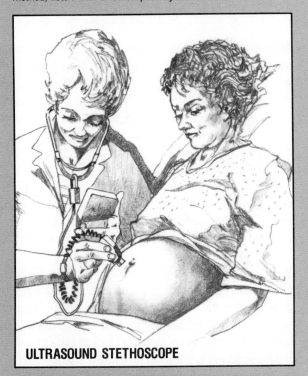

ULTRASOUND STETHOSCOPE

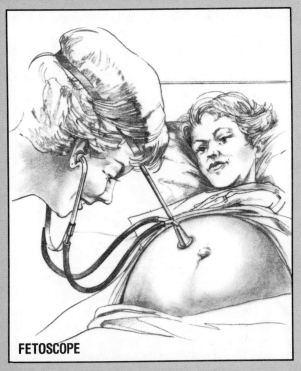

FETOSCOPE

2 Listen throughout several contractions and for at least 60 seconds afterwards to establish the well-being of the fetus. The normal fetal heart rate is 120 to 160 beats/minute. Check the fetal heart rate every 30 to 60 minutes during early labor, every 15 minutes during active labor, and every 5 minutes during the second stage of labor. Remember that heart rate accelerations and decelerations occur periodically during contractions and fetal movements.

3 If fetal heart tones are difficult to hear, perform Leopold's maneuvers to determine the fetal position and find the site where the heart tones are likely to be heard best. Refer to this illustration, which divides the abdomen into quadrants, and start listening at the point indicated by the position. If the fetal heart tones still are not clear, move in the direction indicated by the arrows. The fetus is likely to be in one of the following positions: left sacral anterior (LSA), left occiput anterior (LOA), left occiput posterior (LOP), right sacral anterior (RSA), right occiput anterior (ROA), or right occiput posterior (ROP). For example, with the fetus in a cephalic presentation, fetal heart tones are loudest midway between the client's umbilicus and the anterior superior spine of the ilium; in a breech presentation, tones are loudest at or above the level of the umbilicus.

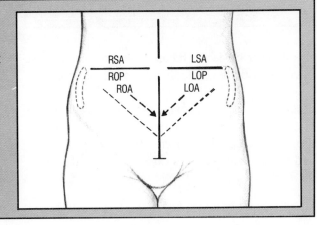

PALPATING UTERINE CONTRACTIONS

Assessment of uterine contractions by palpation requires no special equipment. It does, however, demand nursing skill and sensitivity to touch. To palpate uterine contractions effectively, the nurse follows these steps.

1 Place the palmar surface of the fingers on the client's uterine fundus and palpate lightly. Note the uterine tightening and abdominal lifting that occurs with contractions. Keep in mind that each contraction has three phases: the increment (building up) phase, the acme (peak) phase, and the decrement (letting down) phase.

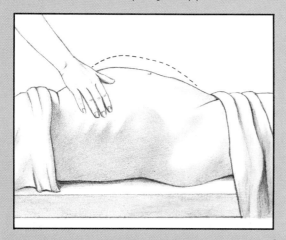

2 Palpate during several contractions, determining their frequency, duration, and intensity. To assess frequency, time the period between the beginning of one contraction and the beginning of the next. To evaluate duration, time the period from the onset of uterine tightening to its relaxation. While the uterus is tightened, determine the intensity of the contraction by pressing the fingertips into the fundus. During mild contractions, the fundus indents easily and feels like a chin. In moderate contractions, the fundus indents less easily and feels more rigid, like the tip of a nose. With strong contractions, the fundus is firm, resists indenting, and feels like a forehead.

ipate the course of labor. (For an illustrated procedure, see Psychomotor Skills: *Performing Leopold's maneuvers*.)

Engagement. Palpate the abdomen to verify engagement. After engagement, labor may progress more quickly. In any client, an unengaged fetus increases the risk of umbilical cord prolapse and warrants close supervision during labor.

Estimated fetal weight. Assess the fetal weight by measuring the fundal height. (See Chapter 7, Care during the Nor-

mal Antepartal Period.) Then correlate the estimated weight with the gestational age to identify a fetus that is large or small for gestational age.

Edema and deep tendon reflexes. Inspect and palpate the client's extremities for edema. Slight localized edema of the feet and ankles is normal late in pregnancy. However, edema of the face (especially in the periorbital area and bridge of the nose), hands, or pretibial area may signal generalized edema and PIH, especially if accompanied by brisk deep tendon reflexes or clonus. If these signs are present, notify the physician immediately.

Amniotic membranes. Whether or not the client reported a sudden gush of fluid during the health history, check the amniotic membranes. Inspect the vaginal opening for obvious fluid leakage. If fluid is present, test it with nitrazine paper. A positive test result (in which the paper turns bright blue) may confirm rupture of the amniotic membranes or may indicate nitrazine paper contamination with sterile lubricant, semen, or bloody show.

If the membrane status is in doubt, expect the physician or nurse-midwife to confirm or rule out ruptured membranes by inspecting the cervical os through a speculum and examining the fluid through a microscope.

Vaginal examination. The vaginal examination determines the client's labor progress by assessing cervical changes, confirming amniotic membrane status, and evaluating fetal position and descent. If specially educated in this skill, the nurse may conduct the vaginal examination. Otherwise, the nurse assists a physician or nurse-midwife.

To prepare for a vaginal examination, gather the appropriate equipment based on the health care facility's procedures and the maternal and fetal status. For example, if the fetus shows signs of distress, obtain electronic fetal monitoring equipment with an internal catheter or electrode for insertion during the examination. Then help the client into a comfortable lithotomy position and drape her to maintain dignity.

During the examination, talk to the client. Help her relax her vaginal muscles by suggesting conscious relaxation techniques. After the examination, clean the client's perineum and change the disposable pad under her buttocks, as needed. Cover the client with her bed sheet, if she desires. Explain the examiner's findings, as appropriate, and answer any questions.

Immediately document vaginal examination findings. Include the date, time, findings, the examiner's name, and any procedures that were performed, such as an amni-

PERFORMING LEOPOLD'S MANEUVERS

Leopold's maneuvers allow the nurse's systematic evaluation of the client's abdomen to determine fetal position. This technique is generally reliable except in clients who are obese or who have hydramnios (excess amniotic fluid).

Before performing Leopold's maneuvers, have the client void and lie supine with her abdomen uncovered. To reduce abdominal muscle tension, place a pillow under her shoulders and ask her to draw her knees up slightly. Warm your hands before touching the client's abdomen to avoid startling her or causing discomfort.

1 Use the first maneuver to determine which part of the fetus lies in the upper uterus. Facing the client, lightly palpate her upper abdomen with both hands. The head feels round and firm. The buttocks feel softer and have bony prominences.

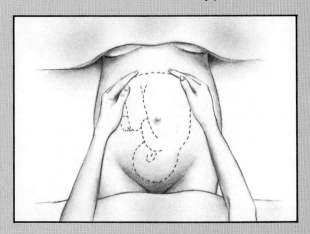

2 Perform the second maneuver to locate the back. Using gentle pressure, palpate the left side of the client's abdomen with the palm of your right hand while steadying the opposite side with your left hand. Repeat the maneuver with your right hand steadying and your left hand palpating. On one side of the client's abdomen, the back of the fetus should feel firm and smooth; on the opposite side, the extremities should feel like small irregularities or protrusions.

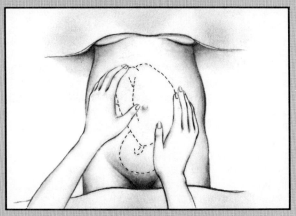

3 Carry out the third maneuver to identify the presenting part (the part of the fetus above the pelvic inlet). Using the thumb and fingers of your dominant hand, grasp the client's abdomen just above her symphysis pubis. The fetal part found here should be the opposite of the one found in the upper abdomen. If the head is palpated and can be moved gently back and forth, it is not yet engaged.

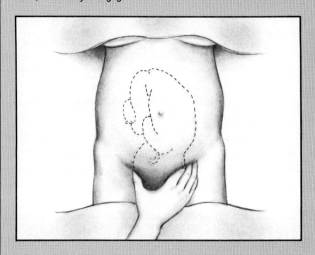

4 Perform the fourth maneuver to determine the descent of the presenting part. Stand facing the client's feet. Then gently move your hands down the sides of the client's abdomen toward her symphysis pubis, noting which side has greater resistance. This resistance is caused by a normal bony prominence of the fetus's head, either the brow (a narrow prominence) or the occiput (a broad prominence). If the head is flexed, the brow will be palpated on the side opposite where the back was identified. If the head is extended, the occiput will be palpated on the same side as the back.

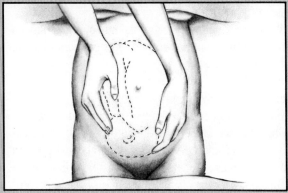

VARIATIONS IN THE FIRST STAGE OF LABOR

In the first stage of labor, variations may occur in the childbirth process, such as premature rupture of membranes (PROM), or may involve the fetus, such as occiput posterior positioning.

Premature rupture of membranes
PROM refers to rupture of the amniotic sac before the onset of labor. It occurs in approximately 10% of clients with term pregnancies. Of these, about 80% will begin labor spontaneously within 24 hours. PROM may occur in clients with normal pregnancies, but it also occurs commonly in those with multiple gestation, hydramnios, or fetal malpresentation.

When a client reports fluid leakage on admission, obtain a thorough history to rule out such conditions as urinary incontinence, vaginal discharge, or loss of the cervical mucus plug. To help confirm or rule out PROM, determine the time of occurrence, the time of last sexual intercourse, and the quantity, color, and odor of the fluid.

Then inspect the perineum for obvious fluid leakage. If no fluid is apparent, assist with or conduct a vaginal examination. In addition to the usual equipment, gather a sterile vaginal speculum, sterile cotton swabs, microscope slides, and nitrazine paper.

If specially prepared to perform this procedure, inspect the cervical os through a speculum, using strict sterile technique. Because PROM increases the risk of chorioamnionitis, be especially careful to prevent any contamination. Amniotic fluid pooling in the vaginal vault or oozing from the cervical os signals PROM.

Using a sterile cotton-tipped applicator, take fluid from the cervical os and spread it on a slide to dry. Microscopic evaluation of this fluid can confirm the presence of amniotic fluid — and PROM — through sodium chloride crystallization, or ferning.

Do not insert nitrazine paper into the vagina, because the paper is not sterile. Instead, touch the paper to the speculum blade after removing the speculum from the vagina. The paper will turn bright blue if the fluid is alkaline with a pH of 7.0 to 7.5. This result can confirm PROM, although it is less reliable than the microscopic evaluation.

When PROM is confirmed, treatment begins. Some experts believe that the fetus must be delivered within 12 to 24 hours. This may require induction of labor with oxytocin or cesarean

birth. Other experts allow labor to progress naturally. When caring for a client with PROM, use the following interventions:
• Monitor fetal heart tones every 30 minutes. Tachycardia may indicate infection; bradycardia indicates hypoxia, which suggests umbilical cord compression.
• Evaluate the client's pulse and temperature at least every 2 hours to detect signs of infection (pulse rate over 90 beats/ minute or temperature over 99.6° F [37.6° C]).
• Postpone vaginal examinations until after the client begins active labor to avoid introducing infectious organisms.
• Provide frequent perineal care.
• Ensure adequate hydration with oral or I.V. fluids, as prescribed.
• Encourage the client to rest until labor begins.
• Stimulate labor by walking, if the client's condition permits.

Occiput posterior positioning
This fetal malposition occurs when the fetal occiput descends the pelvic inlet posteriorly in the oblique diameter instead of in the transverse diameter. It forces the vertex to press against the sacrum. This prolongs the active phase of labor and makes it more painful, especially in the lower back, producing what is called back labor. The position can cause hypotonic uterine dysfunction and, if incomplete rotation occurs, a deep transverse arrest of the fetal head or cephalopelvic disproportion, which may require surgical intervention or forceps delivery.

Occiput posterior positioning affects 15% to 30% of all clients. However, given sufficient time and adequate uterine contractions, most fetuses in this position rotate anteriorly. To care for a client with an occiput posterior fetus, take the following steps:
• Help the client change positions frequently to promote fetal rotation.
• Keep the bladder empty, which provides more room for the fetus to rotate.
• Use sacral massage and counterpressure to relieve lower back pain.
• Administer analgesics to relieve pain, as prescribed.

otomy or placement of fetal scalp electrode or intrauterine pressure catheter.

With additional preparation, the nurse may conduct a vaginal examination to assess cervical position, dilation, effacement, and station.

Before labor begins, the cervix typically lies in the posterior part of the vagina. During labor, it rotates forward to midposition. A tight muscular band in the vagina may be mistaken for cervical dilation when the cervix actually is closed and posterior. To locate cervical position accurately, palpate the entire vagina with the fingertips.

Dilation, effacement, and station vary as labor progresses. The initial assessment findings will provide a

baseline for later evaluations of labor progress and will help in planning the client's care.

If dilation is present without fetal descent, use caution during later vaginal examinations to prevent membrane rupture and umbilical cord prolapse. (See *Variations in the first stage of labor.*)

PREPARATION FOR ADMISSION OR DISCHARGE

Review all of the health history and physical assessment findings to develop a complete clinical picture of the client. Consider the health care facility's policy for admission. If the client is in true labor or meets the standards for admission, continue to prepare her for delivery. If she is in false labor and she and the fetus are in stable condition, call the physician or nurse-midwife for discharge orders and instructions for the client's return.

For a client who must be discharged, suggest comfort measures and explain medical orders. Keep the client's safety in mind when providing instructions. Suggest that a warm tub bath or shower assisted by a family member can ease discomfort. Propose drinking warm milk or herbal tea and reclining semi-upright with pillows under her knees to promote rest. Encourage hydration with clear liquids and nourishment with light meals rich in carbohydrates. Suggest a massage by the client's support person to promote comfort.

Instruct the client to return to the health care facility if her membranes rupture, if she develops bleeding, if her contractions become more intense, or if she shows signs of infection, such as fever. Advise her to return if normal fetal movements change dramatically.

Document the client's discharge. Record the initial assessment findings and recommendations that the client received for follow-up with the health care provider.

The client may linger in the facility because of such factors as her distance from the health care facility, access to transportation, ability to cope with her current status, or her family's concerns and ability to assist her at home.

NURSING CARE AFTER ADMISSION

Clients and their support persons enter the labor and delivery unit in widely varying emotional states and degrees of preparedness. Regardless of the family's emotional state or preparation on admission, the nurse should make every effort to create a calm, welcoming environment. This will help decrease their apprehension and stress and promote a more positive childbirth experience.

ORIENTATION

After the client has been officially admitted, acquaint her and her support person with their physical environment. Introduce yourself as the nurse who will care for them, and ask the client and her support person the names they prefer to be called. Remind the client to give any money, jewelry, or other valuables to her family for safekeeping.

To promote relaxation and comfort during labor, many clients bring special items from home, such as pillows, nightgown, fan, radio or tape player, camera, and pictures or personal objects to use as focal points. Help the client and her support person arrange these items to create a

personal space that does not block access to the client or equipment. Convey respect for their rights by being nonjudgmental about their preferences, as long as they do not interfere with safety codes or institutional policies.

Orient the client and her support person to the call light, bed adjustment control, equipment to be used, and to the location of the bathroom, lounge, and telephone. A thorough orientation will help reduce their anxiety and convey openness to their needs, encouraging them to participate fully.

An informed consent is obtained before any procedure is performed on a client in labor. The physician or nurse-midwife should inform the client of each procedure's benefits, risks, and alternatives and obtain the consent. Then the nurse should allow time to answer the client's questions and discuss her concerns. If medications or the stress of labor compromises the client's ability to make rational decisions, include her support person or a family member in discussions about care and procedures. Document the client's—or her family's—consent in her records.

ONGOING ASSESSMENT

After the client is admitted, complete her health history, perform a detailed physical assessment, and collect laboratory data. The assessment data will serve as the basis for developing a care plan for the client and her family.

Health history

This interview supplements the initial health history, which emphasized the client's current labor status, with questions that review all body systems and assess her psychosocial status. If the client's prenatal record includes this information, do not collect it again. If her record is unavailable or if she does not have frequent contractions or severe pain, assess the following areas in this order:
• family history
• medical and surgical history
• activities of daily living
• psychosocial status.

Vary the length of the ongoing health history based on the client's condition. If the client's labor is progressing rapidly, shorten the interview.

Family history. Begin by asking the client if anyone in her family has a disorder that may affect her labor and delivery, such as diabetes or hypertension. A client with a family history of these disorders may develop complications during the stress of labor.

Medical and surgical history. Determine if the client is allergic to any medications, anesthetics, foods, or other substances. Inquire whether she has ever had a blood transfusion. If so, find out when and determine if it caused any reactions. Particularly note any history of transfusion reactions. Ask what kind of surgery she has had. If she received an anesthetic during surgery, find out which type and how well she tolerated it.

Activities of daily living. Ask the client whether she uses alcohol, cigarettes, or prescription, over-the-counter, or street drugs. If she does, find out how much she consumes daily and when she consumed it last. Use of alcohol or drugs may endanger maternal and fetal health. It also may interfere with labor and the effects of prescribed analgesics or anesthetics, which may require dosage adjustments based on the timing of the last ingestion. Cigarettes reduce fetal weight and produce maternal respiratory congestion, causing difficulty if the client receives a general anesthetic.

Ask when the client had her last food and drink. If general anesthesia is necessary, this information can signal the possibility of vomiting and airway obstruction.

Determine how well the client has been sleeping and resting. The quality and quantity of the client's sleep and rest may determine how much energy she has for labor.

Inquire about her weight before becoming pregnant and ask how much weight she has gained during her pregnancy.

Psychosocial status. A psychosocial assessment is an important part of the total evaluation. Key factors that influence a client's response to labor include her personality, previously established reaction patterns, and other childbirth experiences. Other influential factors include her relationship with her support person, relationship with her mother, general attitude toward conception, and feelings about the timing of this pregnancy. A client also may be affected by her perception and acceptance of herself as a woman, partner, and mother as well as by various social, cultural, and economic adjustments required during childbearing.

The psychosocial assessment provides information that can be used to enhance the client's coping skills and intervene in self-defeating or stressful behaviors. This will help build her self-confidence, which can promote her sense of control over the process, decrease her stress, and ultimately promote a positive childbirth experience, maternal and fetal well-being, and maternal-infant bonding.

Observe the client carefully to obtain a full picture of her current psychosocial status. Note how she presents herself for care by considering her general appearance, facial expression, posture, and body language. Also study her verbal and nonverbal cues to help determine how she is coping. Pose questions that investigate the following areas:

Cultural or ethnic background. Have the client describe her background. Culture and ethnicity can affect expectations and perceptions of childbirth. A culturally sensitive, nonjudgmental nurse can find out what the client expects and try to meet her needs.

Child care considerations. Ask about the client's plans for breast-feeding or bottle-feeding the neonate. If she has not made a decision about feeding, discuss the options with her. If she has made a decision, support it. If the client has other children at home, ask how old they are. Also determine if she feels the need for help with child care or household management when she goes home. A client discharged shortly after delivery may need referral to a social service or home care nurse agency if she has inadequate help.

Knowledge and concerns about labor and delivery. If the client has attended childbirth education classes, find out which type. This information provides an estimate of her knowledge of labor and delivery and allows proper nursing support for her chosen childbirth method.

To assess the client's understanding of—and worries about—her impending labor and delivery, pose such questions as, "What do you know about labor and delivery?" and "Do you have any concerns or fears about childbirth?"

Knowledge and concerns can affect the client's childbirth experience. Lack of knowledge can lead to nonproductive efforts and stress. Encourage the client to share her concerns.

Goals for labor and delivery. To obtain this information, ask such questions as, "What are your goals for labor and birth?" or "How would you like your support person to participate?" The client's answers can help determine whether her goals are realistic and flexible and aid in planning for the support person's participation.

Conclude the assessment by finding out what kind of support the client prefers during labor and delivery. Note the client's preferences, and help her support person and family understand them.

Physical assessment

Focus the physical assessment on findings that could affect labor, delivery, and maternal or fetal well-being. The following health history findings require detailed physical assessment:

- *Skin rash or lesions, especially on the genitals.* These signs may indicate a sexually transmitted disease, such as herpes, that could be transmitted to the fetus.
- *Jaundice.* This sign may signal liver disease, which could reduce the client's ability to clear anesthetics and medications from her body.
- *Visual difficulties.* These symptoms may result from elevated blood pressure, which occurs in PIH.
- *Headaches, dizziness, or syncope.* These symptoms also may be linked to PIH.
- *Signs and symptoms of upper respiratory tract infections, such as congestion or rhinorrhea (nasal discharge).* Such effects may cause problems if the client receives general anesthesia or undergoes intubation. They also may indicate cocaine use.
- *Edema.* A client with generalized or excessive edema may have PIH or a kidney disorder that may cause labor complications.
- *Indigestion, nausea, vomiting, or diarrhea.* These gastrointestinal problems can lead to dehydration, which depletes the energy needed for labor.
- *Signs and symptoms of dehydration, such as thirst or dry mucous membranes.* A dehydrated client will need fluids to maintain her blood volume and prevent further problems.
- *Vaginal itching.* This symptom may signal a vaginal infection that could be transmitted to the fetus.
- *Vulvar varicosities or hemorrhoids.* A client with these swollen, tortuous veins should be monitored for pain or thrombosis during labor.
- *Dysuria (burning or pain on urination).* This symptom suggests a UTI, which could increase the client's discomfort during labor and delivery.
- *Problems with back, pelvis, or abduction of legs that involve stiffness, difficulty in moving, or pain.* Any of these problems may make the client uncomfortable when in the lithotomy position. Back problems may worsen during labor.
- *Varicosities in legs.* A client with this condition may develop thrombosis and reduced blood flow to the legs during contractions.
- *Calf pain.* This symptom may indicate that thrombosis has occurred.

Laboratory studies

Review all of the client's laboratory data. Consider the results of routine antepartal studies, special antepartal tests (if the client has a chronic disease, such as diabetes, or an obstetric concern, such as a genetic disorder), and the rou-

---

NURSING DIAGNOSES

FIRST STAGE OF LABOR

The following potential nursing diagnoses are examples of the problems and etiologies that a nurse may encounter when caring for a client in the first stage of labor. Specific nursing interventions for many of these diagnoses are provided in the "Planning and implementation" sections of this chapter.

- Altered placental tissue perfusion related to maternal position
- Anxiety related to fear of death during childbirth
- Anxiety related to hospital environment
- Impaired gas exchange related to hyperventilation with increasing contractions
- Impaired physical mobility related to electronic fetal monitoring equipment
- Ineffective family coping: compromised, related to client's hospitalization
- Ineffective family coping: compromised, related to client's pain
- Ineffective individual coping related to absence of extended family
- Ineffective individual coping related to lack of family support
- Knowledge deficit related to admission procedures in the labor and delivery area
- Knowledge deficit related to appropriate relaxation techniques
- Knowledge deficit related to labor progress
- Knowledge deficit related to obstetric procedures
- Pain related to uterine contractions
- Potential fluid volume deficit related to restricted oral intake and increased fluid output
- Self-care deficit related to limited mobility during labor

---

tine studies performed on admission to the labor and delivery area. (See *Common laboratory studies*, page 240.)

NURSING DIAGNOSIS

The nurse reviews all health history, physical assessment, and laboratory test findings. Based on these, the nurse formulates nursing diagnoses for the client, fetus, support person, or other family members, as needed. (For a partial list of applicable diagnoses, see Nursing Diagnoses: *First stage of labor.*)

INITIAL PLANNING AND IMPLEMENTATION

After assessing the client and fetus, the nurse plans and implements routine admission procedures, such as intravenous (I.V.) fluid infusion and skin preparation. The

COMMON LABORATORY STUDIES

The chart below lists commonly ordered studies and describes their significance to the pregnant client.

ROUTINE PRENATAL TESTS

ABO blood typing and Rh typing
Identify blood type and Rh factor—vital information if the client needs a blood transfusion. Also point out potential Rh incompatibility with the fetus if the client is Rh-negative.

Antibody screening test (indirect Coombs' test)
Detects anti-Rh$_o$(D) antibodies in the client's blood and evaluates the need for Rh$_o$(D) immune globulin administration.

VDRL test or rapid plasma reagin (RPR) test
Screens for syphilis, which can be transmitted through the placenta to the fetus after the eighteenth week of pregnancy.

Rubella antibodies test
Determines whether the client has antibodies to the disease. If not, she must avoid exposure to rubella during the first trimester to prevent transmittal to the fetus, which could cause anomalies.

Gonorrhea culture
Detects gonorrhea, which typically is asymptomatic in women. During childbirth, gonorrhea in the cervix can cause a neonatal eye infection and a serious puerperal infection for the client.

Complete blood count
Hemoglobin and hematocrit: Screen for anemia, which may reduce the ability of the blood to carry oxygen to the fetus.
White blood cell (WBC) count with differential: Identifies infections and blood dyscrasias, which could lead to complications when labor stresses the client's body systems.
Platelet count: Assesses clotting mechanisms and alerts to potential bleeding problems during delivery.
Red cell indices: Identify specific type of anemia if hemoglobin and hematocrit are low, and guide specific treatments.

Urinalysis
Albumin: Screens for pregnancy-induced hypertension and renal disease, which can worsen during pregnancy.
Microscopic analysis: Screens urine for red blood cells, WBCs, casts, epithelial cells, and microorganisms, which may indicate renal disease or infection.

Papanicolaou (Pap) test
Identifies cervical cancer. Also screens for herpes simplex Type 2, which can be transmitted to the fetus during passage through the birth canal.

SPECIAL PRENATAL TESTS

Alpha-fetoprotein test
May identify fetal anomalies, such as anencephaly, spina bifida, and other neural tube defects. Very high levels may identify omphalocele (herniation of fetal viscera through the abdominal wall), other anomalies, or fetal death.

HIV antibody test
Detects the acquired immunodeficiency syndrome (AIDS) virus, which can be transmitted to the fetus, requiring infection precautions during labor and delivery.

Two-hour postprandial plasma glucose test
Evaluates for gestational diabetes.

Hemoglobin electrophoresis
Identifies hemoglobinopathies, such as sickle cell anemia and thalassemia, which may be passed genetically to the fetus.

Hepatitis B surface antigen test
Screens for hepatitis B, which can infect the fetus, producing low birth weight and acute liver changes.

ROUTINE ADMISSION TESTS

VDRL test or rapid plasma reagin (RPR) test
Detects infection with syphilis.

ABO blood typing and Rh typing
See above. Most health care facilities require these tests on admission of a client who has not had a prenatal workup or whose results are not available.

Hemoglobin and hematocrit
Track levels of these blood components, because many clients develop anemia, especially late in pregnancy.

Urinalysis
Assesses for changes in urine composition, which may occur as pregnancy stresses the kidneys.

---

nurse should prioritize these procedures based on the labor progress, the ease of implementation, and the client's comfort, safety, preference, and need to move about.

I.V. fluid infusion

Because anesthetics delay gastric emptying and relax the swallowing reflex, which may cause subsequent aspiration, the physician is likely to limit the client's intake to minimum oral fluids and ice chips. However, a client in labor may perspire heavily, breathe rapidly, and urinate frequently, creating the potential for a fluid volume deficit. Therefore, the physician or nurse-midwife may order continuous I.V. fluid infusion.

Expect to administer I.V. fluids to a client with a nursing diagnosis of *potential fluid volume deficit related to restricted oral intake and increased fluid output.* Also plan to use this intervention under the following circumstances: maternal exhaustion and dehydration; fetal distress; oxytocin induction or augmentation; grand multiparity (more than five births); history of postpartal hemorrhage; potential for uterine overdistention and atony caused by such factors as multiple gestation, macrosomia, or hydramnios; a life-threatening obstetric or medical condition, such as abruptio placentae, PIH, or diabetes; or potential need for surgery or regional anesthesia.

If an I.V. is ordered, prepare the specified I.V. fluid, such as normal saline or lactated Ringer's solution. Plan to start the I.V. in the client's cephalic vein just above the wrist, if possible. If blood samples have not yet been obtained for laboratory studies, gather the appropriate vials and take samples before starting the I.V. Then infuse the fluid at the prescribed rate.

During the infusion, watch for signs of fluid overload, infiltration, and phlebitis. Also, watch for restlessness or agitation, which can dislodge the catheter.

Skin preparation
In most health care facilities, complete skin preparation, or prep, has been omitted or replaced by removal of hair from the lower third of the labia or from around the part of the perineum where an episiotomy or laceration would be repaired. When any type of prep is ordered, perform the procedure according to the health care facility's policy.

Enema administration
For a client in labor, enema administration is no longer a routine procedure. However, if an enema is ordered, administer it according to the health care facility's policy.

ONGOING PLANNING AND IMPLEMENTATION

During the first stage of labor, continually monitor the status of the client and the fetus as well as the labor progress. Also provide comfort and support to the client, and plan and implement care for her family.

Do not let any activities interfere with the client's ability to work with her body (efforts to coordinate breathing with contractions) or with her support person's assistance during labor. Instead, encourage the support person's active involvement, use gentle touch and calm verbal assur-

ance to show respect for their efforts, and when appropriate, communicate that all is going well. Repeatedly praise the client's efforts and validate her feelings.

Monitor vital signs
To help provide safe care, evaluate the client's vital signs as often as required by health care facility policy.

During the early phase of labor (0 to 3 cm of cervical dilation), assess the client's blood pressure, pulse, and respirations hourly, if no problems are anticipated or discovered. Monitor her temperature every 4 hours throughout labor, unless she has ruptured membranes or a temperature above 99.6° F (37.5° C). In these instances, monitor her temperature every 2 hours while checking her pulse. Be sure to record all findings.

During the active phase of labor (4 to 10 cm of cervical dilation), check blood pressure, pulse, and respirations every hour (if normal). When the client reaches transition, the final part of the active phase of labor, evaluate at least every 30 minutes.

Monitor uterine contractions
The policy of the health care facility – and the physician's or nurse-midwife's orders – will determine exactly how often uterine contractions must be monitored. However, most facilities provide similar guidelines. Unless a deviation occurs, the nurse must assess contractions every hour during the early phase and every 30 minutes during the active phase of the first stage of labor.

The facility's policy and physician's or nurse-midwife's orders also will determine whether uterine contractions are monitored by abdominal palpation or electronic fetal monitoring (EFM). Regardless of the method used, monitor the intensity, frequency, and duration of the contractions. Uterine activity can be affected by maternal exhaustion or dehydration, rupture of membranes, medication, position changes, and increased anxiety. Any of these factors needs closer monitoring than usual.

When monitoring contractions, pay careful attention to the relaxation period between them. Resting uterine tonus can become abnormally elevated, making the intensity of the contractions difficult to assess. If palpation reveals that the uterus is not relaxing adequately between contractions, the client may have abruptio placentae or dysfunctional labor. This uterine hypertonicity can decrease placental perfusion, causing severe fetal hypoxia and distress.

Monitor fetal response to labor
Frequently evaluate the fetus to maintain well-being. (See Fetal Status: *Fetal evaluations during labor,* page 242.)

FETAL EVALUATIONS DURING LABOR

During labor, the nurse must frequently monitor the fetus—as well as the client—to help maintain their health. To assess fetal status accurately, the nurse follows these steps.

- Auscultate the fetal heart rate, rhythm, and response to contractions at least every 30 minutes in the early phase of labor, every 15 minutes during active labor, and every 5 minutes in the second stage of labor. As an alternate technique, evaluate fetal heart rate patterns using an electronic monitor at least every 30 minutes in the early phase of labor, every 15 minutes during active labor, and every 5 minutes in the second stage of labor.
- Note the amniotic fluid color when the membranes rupture.
- Evaluate the results of fetal scalp sampling and pH testing, if prescribed.

Depending on the health care facility's policies, assess the fetus by auscultating fetal heart tones or using EFM.

Monitor labor progress

Perform or assist with vaginal examinations, as needed, to monitor cervical dilation, effacement, station, and other indicators of labor progress.

The frequency of vaginal examinations generally depends on the client's condition and the nurse's ability to observe the contraction pattern, bloody show, client's behavior, level and location of discomfort, and fetal heart tones.

Vaginal examination frequency also depends on the risk of introducing infection. A vaginal examination must be done on admission, before the client receives any medication, when verifying entry into the second stage of labor, when the client develops an increased urge to push, and after spontaneous rupture of membranes.

Monitor urinary function

Evaluate the client's urine output and assess for proteinuria and ketonuria, especially if the client has a nursing diagnosis of *potential fluid volume deficit related to restricted oral intake and increased fluid output.* The client should urinate at least every 2 hours, and her urine should contain no protein or ketones.

During active labor, the client may develop bladder distention with decreased urine output. This increases her discomfort, impedes labor progress by preventing fetal descent, and can lead to postpartal UTIs. To detect bladder distention, check for an irregularity in the lower abdomen or a distinct bulge over the symphysis pubis while monitoring uterine contractions and fetal heart tones. If she cannot urinate and shows signs of increasing distention, inform the physician or nurse-midwife and obtain an order for straight catheterization.

The presence of protein in urine (proteinuria) may signal the onset of PIH, or it may indicate that the urine was contaminated with vaginal secretions, amniotic fluid, or perspiration. To aid diagnosis of PIH, check for other signs, such as elevated blood pressure, edema, and exaggerated deep tendon reflexes. If you detect these signs, notify the physician or nurse-midwife.

Ketonuria may indicate dehydration or maternal exhaustion. If ketonuria is present, notify the physician or nurse-midwife, and monitor the client and fetus more closely.

Provide comfort and support

During childbirth, the client not only needs physical care but also a supportive human presence, pain relief, acceptance, information, and reassurance. By constantly providing for the client's physical comfort and emotional support, the nurse can meet most or all of these needs.

When caring for a client in the first stage of labor, individualize her care by selecting comfort and support measures that are most effective for her. These measures include creating a supportive atmosphere, promoting good positioning and walking, maintaining hygiene, conserving energy, promoting rest and effective breathing, integrating cultural beliefs and practices, educating the client and advocating on her behalf, and relieving pain.

All of these measures help reduce the client's anxiety and prevent stress on the fetus. Furthermore, increased maternal anxiety is associated with uterine dysfunction and intrauterine hypoxia that can lead to physiologic disturbances in neonates (Lederman, Lederman, Work, and McCann, 1985; Sosa, Kennell, Klaus, Robertson, and Vrrutia, 1980).

Tailor all comfort and support measures to the client's condition and phase of labor. In early labor, the client may be excited or apprehensive but usually is talkative and sociable. She can be distracted easily with a diversional activity, such as watching television, reading, taking a walk, or even sleeping.

As active labor begins, the client becomes more serious and preoccupied with her contractions. She may become quiet and withdrawn, or panicked and verbal; she may begin to doubt her ability to cope. Companionship and a relaxed, quiet atmosphere can aid her concentration and coping abilities and can promote rest. Breathing techniques may help her maintain self-control.

During the transition phase, contractions grow rapid and intense. The client becomes self-absorbed, restless, irritable, and hypersensitive and may develop nausea, vomiting, hiccups, belching, or a natural amnesia. Increased perspiration with intermittent chills and hot flashes may sweep quickly over her. She may feel discouraged or panicky. During this phase, do not leave her alone. Provide constant reassurance, firm guidance in using modified breathing techniques, and steadfast physical and emotional support and comfort. Although the transition phase is the most painful, analgesics are used with caution because the amount needed to reduce the pain would depress the fetus and because this phase usually is very brief.

Create a supportive atmosphere. Be sensitive to the family's need to create a supportive environment. Intervene, as needed, to prevent a nursing diagnosis of *ineffective family coping: compromised, related to client's hospitalization; anxiety related to fear of death during childbirth;* or *anxiety related to the hospital environment.* Help the family personalize the environment to enhance the client's comfort, security, and privacy and improve the labor progress by reducing anxiety and pain (Simkin, 1986).

Promote good positioning and walking. During labor, a client may be confined to bed because of concomitant procedures, such as labor induction, epidural anesthesia, or pain relief through analgesia or sedation; convenience in monitoring maternal and fetal well-being; or the policy of the health care facility. Such a client may have a nursing diagnosis of *impaired physical mobility related to electronic fetal monitoring equipment.* For a client who must remain in bed, help her maintain a lateral—rather than supine—position to enhance labor efficiency, comfort, and safety. The lateral (side-lying) position is commonly used to prevent maternal vessel compression and hypotension. This position promotes maternal and fetal circulation, enhances comfort, increases maternal relaxation, reduces muscle tension, and eliminates pressure points.

When allowed freedom of movement, most clients will change positions many times to maximize comfort and enhance labor progress. If the client is not confined to bed, help her find comfortable positions that allow adequate maternal and fetal surveillance. By using alternative positions, such as forward-leaning sitting, squatting, sitting, standing, or hands and knees, she can enhance her labor progress, comfort, and safety. These interventions will help a client with a nursing diagnosis of *altered placental tissue perfusion related to maternal position.*

Also help the client walk around, if possible. Although long walks may tire her, brief walks can decrease pain and improve comfort (Caldeyro-Barcia, 1979). They also can shorten labor by encouraging fetal descent, using gravity to promote application of the presenting part against the cervix, and allowing better alignment of the uterus with the vaginal canal and the presenting part with the cervix (Fenwick and Simkin, 1987).

Contraindications to walking include exhaustion, preterm labor, vaginal bleeding, medication administration, fetal intolerance to labor, an unengaged fetus with cervical dilation or ruptured membranes, fetal malposition, and precipitous labor.

Maintain hygiene. During active labor, the client perspires heavily and produces increased vaginal secretions (with intact membranes) or a constant flow of wet, sticky vaginal drainage (with ruptured membranes). These activities may compromise hygiene, add to general discomfort, and result in a nursing diagnosis of *bathing or hygiene self-care deficit related to limited mobility during labor.*

To maintain hygiene and promote comfort, suggest a warm shower or, if her membranes have not ruptured, a tub bath, to the client who is allowed to walk. As an alternative, perform a sponge or bed bath, providing meticulous perineal care. Change the client's gown and sheets whenever they become saturated. Also change the disposable underpad, especially after a vaginal examination. Frequently wipe the client's face and neck with a cool, clean washcloth, especially during the transition phase. To help her feel fresh, suggest using her own toiletries, if available, and powder her skin or comb her hair.

Provide mouth care during labor. Encouraging the client to brush her teeth or use mouthwash can help freshen her breath, remove any stale taste, and moisten her mouth and throat, which can become dry if oral fluids are restricted. Offer frequent sips of water or allow her to suck on ice pops, hard candy, or a washcloth saturated with ice water. These techniques are especially effective during the transition phase. To soothe dry, cracked lips, suggest applying lip balm or petrolatum and using lemon and glycerin swabs.

Conserve energy and promote rest. Help the client work with her body by using a conscious relaxation technique, especially if she has a nursing diagnosis of *knowledge deficit related to appropriate relaxation techniques.* (See Chapter 12, Comfort Promotion during Labor and Childbirth.) This intervention not only will promote the client's self-esteem and sense of control, but also will conserve her energy and promote comfort. To promote rest between contractions, maintain a calm, quiet atmosphere and organize nursing tasks to minimize disturbances.

Based on the client's preference, use a gentle touch to promote relaxation. (See Chapter 12, Comfort Promotion during Labor and Childbirth.) Some clients find these techniques restful and reassuring and respond well even to simple hand-holding. Others find them offensive or intrusive, especially if they develop hyperesthesia (increased sensitivity, usually in the skin).

Use massage to promote relaxation and help the client remain in control. Teach the support person to perform a counterpressure massage on the lower back, sacrum, and buttocks to help ease labor discomfort. During the transition phase, a back or foot massage can be especially effective. Show the client how to use effleurage (a light, fingertip self-massage) on her lower abdomen to decrease pain. (See Chapter 7, Care during the Normal Antepartal Period.)

The use of visual imagery, quiet speech, eye contact, and appropriately timed analgesia also can promote rest and conserve energy. So may soft music and a cool breeze created by a hand-held fan, especially during the transition phase. (See Chapter 12, Comfort Promotion during Labor and Childbirth).

Promote effective breathing. Effective breathing patterns help the client work with her body efficiently and can break the anxiety-pain-hyperventilation cycle that may occur even in a prepared client. They also can help prevent or correct a nursing diagnosis of *impaired gas exchange related to hyperventilation with increasing contractions.*

If the client has learned certain breathing patterns in childbirth education class, reinforce her learning and support her efforts. If she has not attended classes, briefly teach her how to breathe effectively.

Integrate cultural beliefs and practices. Clients from various cultures may have labor practices and beliefs about childbirth that differ greatly from the nurse's. For example, a client's cultural background may forbid the use of a support person. (See Cultural Considerations: *Using a labor support person.*)

Be sensitive to the client's beliefs and customs. Find out about her cultural background and individual preferences. Then provide care that shows respect for her health attitudes, beliefs, and behaviors during labor. For a client with a nursing diagnosis of *ineffective individual coping related to absence of extended family,* for example, get family members as involved in the labor process as possible rather than having them wait in another area.

CULTURAL CONSIDERATIONS

USING A LABOR SUPPORT PERSON

Although each client has personal beliefs and values, her cultural background may influence her behavior. When caring for a client from a different culture, the nurse should keep the following considerations in mind.

Not every culture encourages the use of a labor support person. Even in the United States, a support person has gained wide acceptance only within the past 20 years. The following two examples illustrate how a client's cultural background can affect her ideas about a labor support person—and her nursing care.

In the Orthodox Jewish faith, certain religious laws require modesty to maintain personal dignity. Even a husband, despite his intimate relationship with his wife, is forbidden to observe her directly when she is immodestly exposed. Therefore, if an Orthodox Jewish couple enter the labor and delivery area, the nurse should be sensitive to their beliefs by draping the client appropriately during vaginal examinations and perineal care, and by giving the husband an opportunity to leave the room during care in which his wife's body is exposed (Lutwak, Ney, and White, 1988).

In Dempsey and Gesse's study (1985) of Cuban refugees, most clients expected the father to be present through labor and birth "so he knows what his wife is going through and what will happen." When caring for a Cuban client, the nurse should provide opportunities for the father's involvement whenever possible.

To integrate a client's cultural beliefs into her care, first identify these beliefs by asking open-ended questions, such as, "Would you like any special people or items with you during labor?" or "Would you like anything else now that I've explained our procedures?" By acknowledging the existence of cultural variations, the nurse can incorporate them in the care plan as long as they do not compromise the safety of the client or fetus.

Educate and advocate. For each client and her family, provide simple, factual information about such things as labor progress, procedures, and medications. This will decrease the client's fear, tension, and pain and increase her and her support person's confidence in their ability to cope. It also will address nursing diagnoses, such as *knowledge deficit related to labor progress* and *knowledge deficit related to obstetric procedures.*

Advocate on the client's behalf, especially when acute care is needed, as with fetal distress. Continue to encourage the client and her support person to participate in the birth as much as possible.

FAMILY CARE

INVOLVEMENT IN LABOR

Traditionally, the focus of childbearing has been on the client's role in pregnancy, labor, delivery, and parenting. Today, the client may share the labor and birth with her partner or support person as well as other family members. To promote the effective involvement of these people, the nurse can use the following interventions.

For the partner or support person
- Promote confidence in the ability to support the client through this demanding period.
- Welcome the support person on admission, using the person's preferred name to encourage relaxation.
- Include the support person in the client's history and physical assessment, if both desire this participation.
- Evaluate goals for the support person's involvement. Keep in mind that involvement may range from being present during labor to active coaching throughout.
- Assess the support person's physical and emotional needs and plan ways to address them during labor.
- Reduce anxiety and feelings of awkwardness by showing concern for the support person's interest and participation in childbirth.
- Make the support person feel important to the client's comfort and support.
- Direct care and support measures if the support person is hesitant or unprepared. Demonstrate or suggest the following comfort activities: hand holding, fanning, wiping the client's face with a cool cloth, offering clear liquids or ice chips, providing a sacral counterpressure massage, and helping her to walk or find a comfortable position.
- Reinforce the prepared support person's knowledge of conscious relaxation and breathing techniques.
- Facilitate the prepared support person's interaction and foster successful sharing. Encourage the support person's participation. Do not try to take over or intervene.
- Suggest appropriate times for the support person to take a break to eat, rest, or attend to personal hygiene. This prevents the person from feeling overwhelmed or trapped. Offer to stand in for the support person during breaks. Time these

breaks to prevent disappointment and frustration if birth occurs while the support person is away.
- Help the support person listen to the fetal heart tones, whenever desired.
- Inform the support person of routine changes in fetal heart rate patterns and their significance.
- Assure the support person that frequent monitoring does not indicate a problem.
- Keep the support person involved if a crisis arises during labor. Help allay feelings of helplessness and fear by remaining calm and confident, sharing information, and providing reassurance that the health care team is doing everything possible.

For the grandparents
- Be sensitive to the impact that unfamiliar and perhaps frightening modern birthing equipment and procedures may have on the grandparents. Explain the equipment and procedures, as needed.
- Regularly inform anxious family members outside the labor and delivery area of the client's progress.
- Advise the family about necessary medical treatments or procedures. Reassure them that the health care team is doing everything possible to provide safe, high-quality care.

For the siblings
- Introduce yourself to the children and the person who will be caring for them and answering their questions.
- Be aware that a child's response to childbirth depends on maturity and interest.
- Maintain a calm, matter-of-fact attitude to reassure the children that everything is proceeding normally. Most children will assimilate the information casually.

Relieve pain. Labor is physically demanding. Some clients experience extreme pain; others experience merely bothersome cramping. For a client with a nursing diagnosis of *pain related to uterine contractions,* try different measures to relieve pain. Use progressive relaxation techniques, biofeedback, acupressure, or visual imagery, along with paced breathing, frequent repositioning, and the emotional and physical assistance of her support person. Or try alleviating her pain through analgesia and anesthesia, depending on safety considerations, labor progress, maternal and fetal well-being, and her preference and coping ability. (See Chapter 12, Comfort Promotion during Labor and Childbirth.)

Care for the family
Throughout labor, provide care not only for the client and fetus, but also for the family. Each family requires individualized interventions based on needs and childbirth goals. For a family with a nursing diagnosis of *ineffective family coping: compromised, related to the client's pain,* for example, suggest ways to provide comfort for the client. (See Family Care: *Involvement in labor.*)

Keep in mind that some people choose not to participate in a family member's childbirth experience. The partner may prefer not to be involved; the client may not want her partner to see her during labor. Respect each person's preferences and avoid imposing personal values.

EVALUATION

Evaluate the effectiveness of nursing care by reviewing the goals attained and the family's involvement and satisfaction with the care. Remember that evaluation stimulates continued reassessment – and improvement – of the effectiveness of nursing care throughout the intrapartal period. The following examples illustrate appropriate evaluation statements for a client in the first stage of labor.

- The client and her family understood admission procedures, equipment, and the expectations of the health care team as evidenced by clear, two-way communication.
- The client used a relaxation method that worked for her during the active phase of labor.
- The support person took effective comfort measures, as evidenced by the client's ability to rest between contractions.
- The support person actively participated in labor by helping the client cope.

DOCUMENTATION

Document assessment findings and nursing activities as thoroughly and objectively as possible. Thorough documentation not only allows evaluation of the effectiveness of the nursing care plan, but also makes data available to other members of the health care team, which helps ensure consistent care. To document as accurately as possible, make sure the entries describe events exactly, completely, and in chronological order.

Although each health care facility may require documentation of slightly different information, most require the nurse to record the following information on the continuing labor record after initial assessment is completed:

- client's vital signs
- fetal heart rate pattern (variability, baseline, periodic changes, and use of external or internal monitor)
- uterine contraction pattern (intensity, frequency, and duration)
- vaginal examination findings (cervical dilation, effacement, station, position, and status of membranes)
- spontaneous or artificial rupture of membranes and description of amniotic fluid
- application of internal fetal scalp electrode or intrauterine pressure catheter
- client's position changes or behaviors, such as crouching or vomiting
- fluid intake and output
- administration of medications, oxygen, I.V. fluids, and epidural anesthesia

- client's response to treatments received
- presence of family members
- physician or nurse-midwife visits with the client.

CHAPTER SUMMARY

Chapter 13 described how to assess and care for the client, fetus, and family during the first stage of labor. Here are the chapter highlights.

A significant life event, labor is a physiologic, psychological, and sociocultural process.

Before a client may be admitted to the labor and delivery area, the nurse performs an initial assessment to differentiate true labor from false labor and to obtain baseline information about the labor status. The health history portion of this assessment focuses primarily on obstetric data. The physical assessment portion includes a vaginal examination and evaluation of vital signs, fetal heart tones, uterine contractions, fetal lie, fetal presentation, fetal position, engagement, fetal weight, edema and deep tendon reflexes, and amniotic membrane status.

The client with true labor contractions is admitted to the labor and delivery area, where the nurse orients her and her support person to the environment and helps them arrange special items from home to create a personalized space.

After the client is admitted, the nurse performs ongoing assessments. As time permits, the nurse obtains more health history information, collecting data about the client's body systems, past, and psychosocial status. The nurse also performs specific physical assessments based on the health history and reviews laboratory data from routine prenatal, special prenatal, and routine admission tests.

Initial and ongoing assessment findings serve as the basis for the remaining nursing process steps during labor and delivery.

Initially, the nurse's planning and implementation may include I.V. fluid administration, as prescribed. Less common procedures include skin preparation and enema administration.

Ongoing planning and implementation should include monitoring of vital signs, uterine contractions, fetal response to labor, labor progress, and urinary function. It also should include provisions for client comfort and support, such as creating a supportive atmosphere, promoting good positioning and walking, maintaining hygiene, conserving energy, providing for rest, promoting effective breathing, integrating cultural beliefs, educating the client, advocating on her behalf, and relieving pain. In addition, the nurse should plan and implement strategies for family care.

Variations in the first stage of labor include premature rupture of membranes and occiput posterior positioning. The nurse must be prepared to intervene appropriately.

The nurse should evaluate all care provided to determine how well it achieves goals and meets the client's needs. The nurse thoroughly documents all assessment findings and care in the format required by the health care facility. In most labor and delivery areas, the nurse must record such things as the client's vital signs, fetal heart rate patterns, uterine contraction patterns, and vaginal examination findings as well as application of an internal fetal scalp electrode or intrauterine pressure catheter, use of medications or oxygen, and presence of family members.

STUDY QUESTIONS

1. Mrs. Jones arrives at the labor and delivery area requesting admission. For which characteristics should the nurse assess to determine if Mrs. Jones is in true labor?
2. Which interventions should the nurse take to ensure the health of the fetus if Mrs. Jones's membranes rupture spontaneously?
3. Describe how the occiput posterior fetal position can affect a client's labor and how the nurse can best intervene in this situation.
4. Identify the necessary steps for assessing fetal status during labor.
5. What characteristics would nursing assessment reveal when Mrs. Jones is in the transition phase of labor?
6. How can the nurse involve Mrs. Jones's children during the labor process?

BIBLIOGRAPHY

Auvenshine, M., and Enriquez, M. (1985). *Maternity nursing: Dimensions of change.* Boston: Jones and Bartlett.

Chagnon, L., and Easterwood, B. (1986). Managing the risks of obstetrical nursing. *MCN,* 11(5), 303-310.

Cunningham, F.G., MacDonald, P.C., and Gant, N.F. (1989). *William's obstetrics* (18th ed.). East Norwalk, CT: Appleton-Century-Croft.

Feldman, E., and Hurst, M. (1987). Outcomes and procedures in low risk birth: A comparison of hospital and birth center settings. *Birth,* 14(1), 18-24.

Fenwick, L., and Simkin, P. (1987). Maternal positioning to prevent or alleviate dystocia in labor. *Clinical Obstetrics and Gynecology,* 30(1), 83-89.

Guidelines for perinatal care (2nd ed.) (1988). Washington, DC: American Academy of Pediatrics and ACOG.

Hoffmaster, J.E. (1983). Labor and intrapartum care. In L.J. Sonstegard, K.M. Kowlaski, and B. Jennings (Eds.), *Women's health, volume II, Childbearing* (pp.109-173). New York: Grune & Stratton.

Horn, M., and Manion, J. (1985). Creative grandparenting: Bonding the generations...participation in the birth experience. *JOGNN,* 14(3), 233-236.

Knuppel, R.A., and Drukker, J. (1986). *High risk pregnancy: Medical management and nursing care.* Philadelphia: Saunders.

Myers, S.T., and Stolte, K. (1987). Nurses' responses to changes in maternity care: Technologic revolution, legal climate and economic changes, part II. *Birth,* 14(2), 87-90.

Pollack, L. (June 1988). Commentary: Reconsidering the risks and benefits of intravenous infusion in labor. *Birth,* 15(2), 80.

Sheen, P.W., and Hayashi, R.H. (1987). Graphic management of labor: Alert/action line. *Clinical Obstetrics and Gynecology,* 30(1), 33-41.

Simkin, P. (1986). Stress, pain, and catecholamines in labor: Part 1, a review. *Birth,* 13(4), 227-233.

Standards for obstetric, gynecologic, and neonatal nursing (3rd ed.) (1986). Washington, DC: NAACOG.

Van Lier, D.J., and Roberts, J.E. (1986). Promoting informed consent of women in labor. *JOGNN,* 15(5), 419-422.

Varney, H. (1987). *Nurse-midwifery* (2nd ed.). Boston: Blackwell Scientific Publications.

Whitley, N. (1985). *A manual of clinical obstetrics.* Philadelphia: Lippincott.

Preparation for childbirth
Dick-Read, G. (1987). *Childbirth without fear* (5th ed.). New York: Harper & Row.

Maloni, J.A., McIndoe, J.E., and Rubenstein, G. (1987). Expectant grandparents class. *JOGNN,* 16(1), 26-29.

Nichols, F.H., and Humenick, S.S. (1988). *Childbirth education: Practice, research and theory.* Philadelphia: Saunders.

Phillips, C., and Anzalone, J. (1982). *Fathering, participation in labor and birth* (2nd ed.). St. Louis: Mosby.

Fetal monitoring
Electronic fetal monitoring: Joint ACOG/NAACOG statement (1988). Washington, DC: NAACOG.

Snydal, S. (1988). Responses of laboring women to fetal heart rate monitoring: A critical review of the literature. *Journal of Nurse-Midwifery,* 33(5), 208-216.

Cultural references
Bates, B., and Turner, A.N. (1985). Imagery and symbolism in the birth practices of traditional cultures. *Birth,* 12(1), 29-35.

Dempsey, P.A., and Gesse, T.C. (1985). The childbearing Cuban refugee: A cultural profile. *Urban Health,* 14(5), 32-37.

Hedstrom, L.W., and Newton, N. (1986). Touch in labor: A comparison of cultures and eras. *Birth,* 13(3), 181-186.

Laderman, C. (1988). Commentary: Cross-cultural perspectives on birth practices. *Birth,* 15(2), 86-87.

Lutwak, R., Ney, A.M., and White, J. (1988). Maternity nursing and Jewish law. *MCN,* 13(1),44-46.

Martinelli, A.M. (1987). Pain and ethnicity: How people of different cultures experience pain. *AORN,* 46(2), 273-281.

Michaelson, K.L. (Ed.) (1988). *Childbirth in America: Anthropological perspectives.* Westport, CT: Bergin & Garvey.

Nursing research

Caldeyro-Barcia, R. (1979). The influence of maternal position on time of spontaneous rupture of the membrane, progress of labor and fetal head compression. *Birth and the Family Journal,* 6(7), 7-15.

Jones, S.P. (1984). First time fathers: A preliminary study. *MCN,* 9(2), 103.

Lederman, R.P. (1984). *Psychosocial adaptation in pregnancy: Assessment of seven dimensions of maternal development.* East Norwalk, CT: Appleton & Lange.

Lederman, R.P., Lederman, E., Work, B.A., and McCann, D.S. (1985). Anxiety and epinephrine in multiparous women in labor: Relationship to duration of labor and fetal heart rate pattern. *American Journal of Obstetrics and Gynecology,* 153, 870-877.

Lowe, N.K. (1987). Parity and pain during parturition. *JOGNN,* 16(5), 340-346.

Sosa, R., Kennell, J., Klaus, M., Robertson, S., and Vrrutia, J. (1980). The effect of a supportive companion on perinatal problems, length of labor, and mother-infant interaction. *New England Journal of Medicine,* 303(11), 597-600.

CHAPTER 14

THE SECOND STAGE OF LABOR

OBJECTIVES

After reading and studying this chapter, the student should be able to:

1. List characteristics of the onset and progression of the second stage of labor and its typical length for primiparous and multiparous clients.

2. Describe assessment of a client in the second stage of labor.

3. Explain how bearing-down efforts should change as the second stage progresses and how bearing-down efforts may differ among clients.

4. Describe how the various position changes can help a client during the second stage of labor.

5. Outline the nurse's responsibilities during delivery and immediately afterward.

INTRODUCTION

The second stage of labor begins with complete cervical dilation and ends with delivery of the neonate. It requires exhaustive maternal efforts coupled with strong, effective uterine contractions. The client will need substantial emotional support and encouragement. During this highly emotional and stressful period, the nurse must meet the needs of the client, family, and fetus as well as monitor the progress of labor, prepare the environment and equipment needed for delivery, and evaluate the neonate's status after delivery.

This chapter covers characteristics of second stage of labor onset, phases, and duration. Following the nursing process steps, the chapter then presents assessment topics, nursing diagnoses, and interventions pertinent to the client in the second stage of labor. Finally, the chapter presents guidelines for nursing care of the neonate immediately after delivery. Overall, the chapter gives guidelines for nursing care that is safe and comforting for the client and family during the expulsive phase of labor.

CHARACTERISTICS OF THE SECOND STAGE

The transition from the first to the second stage of labor signals impending birth. The nurse should be aware of the onset of the second stage, of phases typically experienced during this stage, and of expected duration.

Onset

Several characteristics indicate a transition from the first to the second stage of labor, including some or all of the following:

- an increasing urge to push, possibly accompanied by perineal bulging in a multiparous client
- an increase in bloody show, caused by greater cervical dilation
- grunting
- gaping of the anus
- involuntary defecation
- bulging of the vaginal introitus
- spontaneous rupture of the membranes, if this has not occurred
- abrupt onset of early decelerations (beginning early in the contraction) in fetal heart rate (FHR), possibly

caused by compression of the fetus's head during descent into the pelvic canal. (Such FHR changes, although common, should be reported to the physician or nurse-midwife.)

Phases

Some authorities divide the second stage of labor into two distinct phases. The first phase lasts from complete dilation of the cervix until the presenting part reaches the pelvic floor. The second phase lasts from when the presenting part reaches the pelvic floor until birth.

During the first phase, the client may feel a strong urge to bear down. Typically, these urges are short, manageable, and occur at the peak of each contraction. They may assist in the final retraction of the cervix before fetal descent. During the second phase, the client typically feels an uncontrollable urge to push; during this phase, bearing-down efforts are most effective at expelling the fetus.

Duration

For primiparous clients, the second stage of labor averages 66 minutes, ranging from 48 to 174 minutes. For multiparous clients, the second stage averages 24 minutes, ranging from 6 to 66 minutes (Friedman, 1989). The duration depends on the combined effects of fetal, maternal, psychological, and environmental factors.

Fetal factors that may affect duration include physical condition, size, station, position, molding, rotation, and rate of descent. Maternal factors include parity, labor position, fatigue level, age, degree of expulsive efforts, strength of uterine contractions, size and shape of the bony pelvis, resistance or relaxation of soft tissues, and such obstetric interventions as anesthesia and episiotomy (Cunningham, MacDonald, and Gant, 1989).

Psychological factors that may affect duration include the client's emotional readiness, degree of relaxation, and level of trust in her care providers. The client's preparation for childbirth—from reading, childbirth education classes, information handed down from female relatives, and inner spiritual resources, for example—also affect her reaction to labor, which may influence its duration (Kitzinger, 1984; Peterson, 1984).

Environmental factors, which include bright lights, noise, and hectic activity, may increase the client's anxiety, lengthening labor. A quiet, relaxed environment can shorten labor (McKay and Roberts, 1985; Odent, 1986; van Lier, 1985).

This complex interplay of diverse factors may preclude an accurate prediction of how long the second stage of labor will last, even for a multiparous client. Although the client and her family have little control over such physical factors as the size of the fetus or degree of pelvic resistance, they can influence other factors, such as the positions the client assumes during labor.

Some authorities consider abnormal any second stage of labor that lasts longer than 2 hours. However, authorities do not agree on the effect of a prolonged second stage. Some suggest a correlation between a prolonged second stage and infant mortality, postpartal maternal hemorrhage, neonatal seizures, puerperal febrile morbidity, and changes in neonatal acid-base status (Hellman and Prystowski, 1952; Minchom, et al., 1987; Wood, Ng, Hounslow, and Benning, 1973). Others have found no difference in neonatal deaths, low 1-minute Apgar scores, and postpartal hemorrhage (Cohen, 1977; Reynolds and Yudkin, 1987).

Although a prolonged second stage of labor (over 2.9 hours in a primiparous client or 1.1 hours in a multiparous client) may indicate a disorder and deserves careful monitoring, it does not necessarily give sufficient reason to terminate labor; if labor is progressing and the fetus displays no signs of distress, some authorities recommend allowing labor to continue until vaginal delivery occurs (Friedman, 1989). The client and fetus should undergo continual monitoring and documentation as labor progresses.

NURSING CARE

To provide the best possible care, the nurse should apply the nursing process when caring for a client in the second stage of labor. During this stage, the nursing process addresses the client, fetus, and labor progress.

ASSESSMENT

During the second stage of labor, assessment occurs more frequently than during the first stage. As delivery nears, assessment becomes continuous, and the nurse will care for one client exclusively. Beginning early in the second stage and continuing until delivery, the nurse assesses maternal vital signs, cervical dilation, contractions, bearing-down efforts, FHR, fetal descent, amniotic fluid, and the emotional response of the client and support person.

Vital signs. Take vital signs at least every 15 minutes and more often if the client has continuous epidural anesthesia, is hypertensive, or has other complicating conditions. Bearing-down efforts may increase client blood pressure, pulse, and respirations. Take blood pressure as necessary between contractions, but use discretion if pressure has been stable and birth is imminent. A temperature rise of one degree may occur even in the absence of infection, but a temperature over 100° F should be reported to the physician or nurse-midwife. Dehydration may play a role in temperature elevation.

Cervical dilation. When characteristics of the second stage appear (such as increased bloody show and facial perspiration, decreased restlessness, shaking of the extremities, and involuntary bearing-down efforts), expect a vaginal examination to be performed to confirm dilation and assess the presenting part, fetal station, status of the fetal membranes, and color of the amniotic fluid.

Some clients have a strong urge to bear down before the cervix dilates completely. This can cause edema and tissue damage, and it may impede fetal descent. If examination reveals incomplete dilation and the client has a strong urge, help the client avoid bearing down. Help her onto her forearms and knees, a position that may decrease the urge to bear down by relieving pressure on the rectum. Instruct her to pant or blow through each contraction until examination reveals that the cervix has receded completely. To maintain her comfort as long as possible in this position, raise the head of the bed and place several pillows under her arms. Some facilities use a large bean bag to support clients in this position.

In some clients, incomplete dilation may be felt as an anterior "lip" of the cervix. This condition stems from uneven pressure of the presenting part on the cervix; all of the cervix recedes except for a small anterior portion. The physician or nurse-midwife may reduce an anterior lip of the cervix manually, using two fingers to ease the cervix over the fetus's head by pressing against it during a contraction. The client can aid reduction by bearing down during the pressing. Keeping the fingers in place during the next contraction will help the physician or nurse-midwife determine whether the lip has been effectively reduced.

Fetal bradycardia to 90 beats/minute may occur for 1 to 2 minutes after manual reduction of the lip. This may result from vagal stimulation and typically resolves on its own. If not, notify the physician or nurse-midwife and initiate standard nursing care for fetal bradycardia.

Contractions. Assess the strength, frequency, and duration of uterine contractions every 15 minutes during the second stage. Contractions that have occurred every 2 or 3 minutes may extend to every 5 minutes during this stage, allowing the client to rest between contractions. Some clients have more frequent contractions and report unceasing pain. This pain may relate to increasing pressure

from the presenting part and difficulty relaxing between contractions. When the second stage lasts longer than 2 hours, uterine contractions may decrease in strength and frequency. The physician or nurse-midwife should evaluate the need for oxytocin (to stimulate labor) and assess for cephalopelvic disproportion or other abnormalities.

If the client has had epidural anesthesia, the support person or nurse may need to cue her when a contraction begins so that she can position herself to bear down.

Bearing-down efforts. Assess the effectiveness of the client's bearing-down efforts and her energy resources as the second stage progresses. Remind her to bear down at the peak of each contraction and to continue bearing down to the end of the contraction to facilitate fetal descent. After assessing the progress of the first few contractions in the second stage, notify the physician or nurse-midwife of the client's status. If descent is delayed, or if the client complains of increased pain, fatigue, or frustration, the physician or nurse-midwife will identify the problem and intervene appropriately.

Although epidural anesthesia can be useful in the first stage of labor, it may create problems for a client in the second stage; the amount of sensory and motor block necessary to relieve pain may reduce, delay, or abolish bearing-down efforts. Moreover, epidural anesthesia may lengthen the second stage and increase the need for forceps or vacuum assistance (Chestnut, Vandewalker, Owen, Bates, and Choi, 1987). If the client's bearing-down efforts produce little descent, even with direct coaching, then the anesthetic agent may have to wear off slightly or be administered in reduced amounts before the client can bear down effectively. Reassure the client that, although the pain will increase somewhat, her improved pushing efforts will help deliver the neonate more quickly.

Fetal heart rate. Assess the FHR more frequently during the second stage of labor than during the first, based on the client's risk status, underlying medical conditions, medications and anesthetic agent used, and any alterations in FHR patterns that arose during the first stage. For a low-risk client, auscultate FHR every 5 minutes or use an electronic fetal monitor, depending on the client's wishes, the physician's or nurse-midwife's preference, and facility policy. Although a standard fetoscope may be used for manual auscultation of FHR, a Doppler ultrasound device typically is less obtrusive (Sleep, Roberts, and Chalmers, 1989). If the client finds repeated FHR auscultation disruptive, consider switching to electronic monitoring. A client with complications placing her at risk may require

ASSESSING AND MANAGING FETAL HEART RATE CHANGES

Variability in the fetal heart rate (FHR) during the second stage of labor is an indicator of fetal well-being. Yet variations can be difficult to interpret. The nurse can use the following basic guidelines to help interpret and manage FHR changes.

- Baseline FHR should remain within 20 beats/minute of the rate identified early in labor. A slight decline in this baseline is common, probably resulting from vagal stimulation from increased pressure on the fetus's head during descent into the pelvis.
- The FHR fluctuates more during the second stage of labor than during the first stage. Accelerations typically have no adverse effect on the neonate. In fact, the absence of accelerations should be investigated.
- Decreased FHR variability, especially if accompanied by bradycardia, decelerations, or lack of accelerations, may be cause for concern. Decreased FHR variability has been associated with decreased umbilical cord blood pH, which reflects fetal distress.
- Second-stage FHR decelerations and bradycardia have been reported in 50% to 90% of all FHR tracings and usually produce no lasting adverse effects. In contrast, pronounced or prolonged decelerations require prompt delivery.
- Terminal bradycardia (FHR below baseline immediately before delivery) is common and probably stems from compression of the fetus's head, vagal stimulation, umbilical cord compression, and impaired uteroplacental perfusion (Ohel, 1978; Herbert and Boehm, 1981). It typically lasts only a few minutes and produces no adverse effects.
- Scalp stimulation may help in evaluating fetal condition when bradycardia occurs; FHR acceleration in response to stimuli offers a reliable sign of fetal well-being. If the fetus develops bradycardia, the physician or nurse-midwife may press the fetus's scalp with a finger while performing a vaginal examination. If the FHR rises, the fetus is not seriously acidotic. If delivery is not imminent, try raising the FHR by repositioning the client, offering oxygen by mask, and encouraging her to breath through contractions rather than to push (Roberts, 1989).

electronic monitoring, possibly with an internal scalp electrode to detect fetal distress or beat-to-beat variability.

Changes in the FHR become more difficult to interpret during the second stage because they occur more frequently and with more variation than during the first stage (Roberts, 1989). In fact, 50% to 90% of healthy neonates display some abnormality in heart rate during the expulsive phase of labor (Graziano, Freeman, and Bendel, 1980; Krebs, Petres, and Dunn, 1981). Variations in the

FHR may result from umbilical cord compression, fetal descent, and maternal bearing-down efforts.

Although few studies focus on the outcomes of second stage FHR changes, Hon and Quilligan (1967) found a correlation between a normal FHR pattern and a normal Apgar score. (Apgar scoring is described in detail later in this chapter.) Specific results of FHR alterations may not be obvious. Usually, however, accelerations pose little danger; decelerations and changes in variability should be monitored closely. (See Fetal Status: *Assessing and managing fetal heart rate changes.*)

Descent. The fetus normally begins descent during active labor; if descent has not begun by 7 cm of cervical dilation, an abnormality may exist. Failure to descend occurred in approximately 4% of clients in a large sample (Friedman, 1989). Causes included:

- a large fetus (over 4,000 g)
- cephalopelvic disproportion
- fetal malposition, primarily persistent occiput transverse or occiput posterior positions.

Begin assessing descent when cervical dilation is between 7 and 8 cm (usually during the first stage of labor) by measuring the relationship between the fetus's head and the client's ischial spines. Suspect an abnormality if no descent occurs after a primiparous client bears down for 1 hour or a multiparous client bears down for ½ hour. Be careful to distinguish between actual descent and increased swelling of the fetus's scalp, which may give the illusion of descent.

Amniotic fluid. Note any change in the color of the amniotic fluid during the second stage of labor because it may indicate fetal distress. When tainted with meconium, amniotic fluid becomes green and may range in consistency from thin (1 + or 2 +) to thick (3 + or 4 +). Thick amniotic fluid may contain particulate meconium. An increase in bloody show, which commonly occurs early in the second stage, may cause pink-tinged amniotic fluid. Port wine–colored fluid may indicate abruptio placentae. Notify the physician or nurse-midwife of any change in amniotic fluid color.

Emotional responses. Assessment of the client's emotional status and that of her support person becomes increasingly important as labor continues. Both may experience fatigue and frustration, especially early in the second stage. When told that she can push, the client may feel relief and anticipation that labor will end soon. The support person and health care team may feel a surge of renewed energy as well.

Clients may respond in various ways to the sensation of bearing down. Some respond well because bearing down allows them to give in to the urge they feel and do something positive with the pain (van Lier, 1985). These clients may express satisfaction in working hard, receiving positive feedback, and seeing results from their efforts. Others respond poorly to bearing down, especially if the fetus is in a posterior position or if the client fears spontaneous perineal lacerations.

Immediately after delivery, the client may experience a range of emotions and reactions, including relief that the pain has diminished, a sense of achievement, exhaustion, and pleasure or disappointment in the appearance or sex of the neonate.

NURSING DIAGNOSIS

Based on continuous assessment and monitoring throughout the second stage of labor, the nurse formulates nursing diagnoses specific to the client, fetus, support person, or other family members, as necessary. (For a partial list of applicable diagnoses, see Nursing Diagnoses: *Second stage of labor.*)

PLANNING AND IMPLEMENTATION

During the second stage of labor, the nurse must plan and act almost simultaneously. After detecting the onset of the second stage and assessing maternal and fetal well-being and labor progress, notify the physician or nurse-midwife of the client's status and of any maternal or fetal complications (such as meconium-stained amniotic fluid, fetal distress, or recent narcotic administration).

As the second stage progresses, the nurse should provide the client with emotional support, coordinate her bearing-down efforts, assist with positioning, monitor hydration, facilitate delivery, and care for the neonate immediately after birth.

Provide emotional support. Especially for the primiparous client, the second stage of labor may result in a nursing diagnosis of *anxiety related to duration of labor* or *ineffective individual coping related to exhaustion.* Help resolve these problems by providing emotional support and reassurance. Provide general emotional support to the client by assuring her if labor is progressing normally, that she will not be left alone, and that the physician or nurse-midwife will be summoned. Depending on the support person's participation, the nurse's role can range from reassuring to active coaching during the second stage. If the support person participates actively and re-

---

NURSING DIAGNOSES

SECOND STAGE OF LABOR

The following diagnoses address representative problems and etiologies that the nurse may encounter when caring for a client during the second stage of labor. Specific nursing interventions for many of these diagnoses are provided in the "Planning and implementation" section of this chapter.

- Altered urinary elimination related to epidural or spinal anesthesia
- Anxiety related to duration of labor
- Anxiety related to not meeting labor expectations
- Fatigue related to duration of labor, energy expenditure, and possible lack of sleep
- Fluid volume deficit related to restricted fluid intake and fluid loss during labor efforts
- Hopelessness related to prolonged bearing-down efforts that produce little progress
- Impaired tissue integrity related to perineal and vaginal lacerations or to episiotomy
- Ineffective breathing pattern related to painful uterine contractions and bearing-down efforts
- Ineffective individual coping related to exhaustion
- Knowledge deficit related to typical duration of labor
- Pain related to rapid delivery or fetal malposition
- Pain related to uterine contractions and stretching of vaginal and perineal tissues

---

sponds appropriately to the client's efforts, the nurse will need to supply only positive feedback and encouragement.

Reassure the client that each expulsive effort helps to move her baby down and out. Suggest that the client imagine herself opening and her baby moving down the birth canal and out.

Choose words carefully because clients in labor are highly vulnerable and sensitive to suggestions that they are not succeeding. Even mildly critical remarks intended to make the client try harder may be hurtful.

The client who becomes exhausted and discouraged during this stage of labor will want to know how much longer the effort must continue. Never try to estimate when birth will occur. Instead, suggest concentrating on and working with the contractions, perhaps by changing position or exhaling forcefully (blowing) instead of pushing through the next one. Encourage the client to rest or doze between contractions. Affirm that labor is hard work that can seem to take forever, but that she is making progress and will get through it. Encourage her to draw energy from her supporters.

Especially during this stage, the client's support person may need emotional support, a brief break, or gentle direction. If the client's bearing down does not accomplish quick results, the supporter may need reassurance that the FHR remains normal and that 1 to 2 hours of bearing down is not uncommon. If necessary, suggest such concrete tasks as holding the client's leg, supporting her body in selected positions, massaging her back, offering ice chips, or preparing a cool cloth for her forehead.

Coordinate bearing-down efforts. During painful periods, the client may have a nursing diagnosis of *ineffective breathing pattern related to painful uterine contractions and bearing-down efforts.* Help resolve this problem by coordinating the client's bearing-down efforts.

As the second stage progresses, bearing-down urges become more intense and aid in expelling the neonate. Encourage the client to bear down with each contraction. Although the nurse need not discourage bearing down early in the second stage, it produces the most pronounced result later in the stage. Never chastise a client who cannot resist the urge to bear down. (See *Alternative ways of bearing down.*)

If bearing-down efforts produce inadequate results, give positive suggestions for change between contractions, help the client into an alternative position, and encourage her to push through the pain rather than pull back from it. If she pulls back out of fear that she will hurt herself, try placing warm washcloths on the perineum to decrease any burning sensation.

Assist with positioning. Position changes may be especially helpful for a client with a nursing diagnosis of *pain related to rapid delivery or fetal malposition.* The side-lying position helps slow a rapid delivery and may reduce perineal tension. The forearms-and-knees position can reduce back pain related to labor. When the fetus is in an occiput-posterior position or descends slowly, the client may benefit from a squatting position. If she squats on the toilet, use a flashlight to maintain a steady view of the perineum. Be sure to consider the advantages and disadvantages of a position before suggesting a change to the client.

If the client assumes a lithotomy position for delivery, maximize her participation and bearing-down efforts by placing two pillows, a bean bag, or a backrest behind her shoulders or at the small of her back. Alternatively, the client can lean against her support person to help maintain a more upright position.

For some clients, a birthing chair may help maximize comfort while meeting fetal needs and allowing the health care team to monitor maternal and fetal status. Used for bearing down and for delivery, the birthing chair is particularly suitable for primiparous clients because of the longer pushing phase. A tired client who has tried several positions in bed may benefit from the birthing chair's hand grips and back support. The client may assume a side-lying position in the birthing chair, as well as various degrees of upright and recumbent positions. Drawbacks to the birthing chair include a risk of increased blood loss and perineal edema (Sleep, Roberts, and Chalmers, 1989); also, the forearms-and-knees and squatting positions are not feasible. The chair should not be used by a client who has received an epidural block because she will lack the physical control needed to transfer to the chair.

Monitor hydration. A client who shows decreased bearing-down efforts after a period of effective efforts may have a nursing diagnosis of *fluid volume deficit related to restricted fluid intake and fluid loss during labor efforts.* Continue to offer her juice, water, or tea. If bearing down lasts more than 2 hours, start an I.V. line to deliver fluids, as prescribed.

Facilitate delivery. As delivery approaches, nursing responsibilities include making a judgment about when to transfer the client to the delivery room (or when to summon the physician or nurse-midwife), preparing the delivery area, preparing the client, and assisting with delivery.

Transfer to the delivery room. Judging when to transfer a client to the delivery room and when to summon the physician or nurse-midwife is a learned skill. The goal is to allow sufficient time for the client to reach the delivery room before giving birth, but not to allow so much time that the client and staff have an extended wait. Obviously,

ALTERNATIVE WAYS OF BEARING DOWN

Traditionally, nurses have taught and reinforced the following method of bearing down: the client takes a cleansing breath, exhales, bears down to a count of 10 four times inhaling quickly between counts, and then takes a final cleansing breath. Typically, she assumes a C-shaped position curled around the fetus, holding her knees, with head bent.

Two alternative styles for bearing down include the open-glottis method and the urge-based method. In the former, the client releases air through the glottis while bearing down. Theoretically, this reduces stress on the fetus. In the latter, the client bears down as she feels the urge and in the manner that feels right to her.

Because childbirth educators teach all three bearing-down methods, the nurse should be familiar with each one and work to achieve the most comfortable and effective method for each client.

early arrival is better than delivery of the neonate en route to the delivery room. Always consider the client's labor history, current progress, and rate of descent.

Many health care facilities feature combined labor and delivery rooms, where the client labors, delivers, and recovers in the same room with the same staff.

Prepare the delivery area. Make all necessary physical preparations for the impending birth. This includes gathering and setting up needed equipment (including a radiant heat unit, in some cases) and reviewing the client's and physician's or nurse-midwife's wishes for the delivery.

If the client plans to give birth in the labor bed, place extra pads under her buttocks to absorb the blood and amniotic fluid that emerge after delivery. If she will require transfer to a delivery room, ensure that the route contains no obstacles. If delivery occurs en route, be sure the side rails of the bed are raised and that the client remains draped. Try to plan ahead for emergencies; for example, check needed supplies at the start of each day to ensure that all are present and within reach. Know how to operate all delivery room equipment, including stirrups, infant resuscitation equipment, and the bed.

Set up the instrument pack and delivery pack specified by the facility, gloves for the members of the health care team, and any special supplies or equipment requested by the physician or nurse-midwife. Equipment should include the following: a sterile drape to go under the client's buttocks, clamps and scissors for the umbilical cord, a bulb syringe, a dry sterile towel and warm blanket for the neonate, and (usually) a needle holder and syringes. Many health care facilities use a drape pack that contains an abdominal drape, two leggings, and a drape for under the buttocks.

Additional supplies for the neonate may include a radiant heat unit, suctioning equipment with catheters (sizes 5, 8, and 10), oxygen bag and mask (sizes for premature and full-term neonates), laryngoscope with endotracheal tubes (sizes 2.5, 3.0, and 3.5), extra bulb syringes and neonatal suction (DeLee) catheters, feeding tubes, syringes and needles, and neonatal resuscitation drugs, such as naloxone hydrochloride (neonatal injection, 0.02 mg/ml), sodium bicarbonate, epinephrine, 10% dextrose in water, and reagent strips.

Prepare the client. Do not break the delivery room bed (bend down the lower end so that the client can assume the lithotomy position) until a nurse, physician, or nurse-midwife is in position in case the fetus descends rapidly. Once the client is positioned in the delivery room bed, prepare the perineum by swabbing with an antiseptic solu-

tion and, if necessary, by trimming long pubic hairs. (See Psychomotor Skills: *Preparing the perineum,* page 256.)

A client in the lithotomy position should place her feet in the stirrups or leg holders. Align her knees at equal heights, and check that her legs are abducted at similar angles. Open the drape pack for the physician or nurse-midwife, and assist with draping, as needed. Follow universal blood and body fluid safety precautions throughout delivery.

Prepare the support person for delivery by giving instructions on hand-washing and assisting with gown or scrub suit, boots, cap, and mask according to facility policy.

Assist with delivery. While the physician or nurse-midwife scrubs and dons gown and gloves, adjust lighting as necessary to observe the perineum, which will verify if delivery is imminent. If the client finds bright light distracting, dim the overhead lights but maintain perineal illumination. (For photographs of the steps of childbirth, see *Photographic essay on the second stage of labor,* pages 258 and 259.)

As the fetus's head crosses the perineum, perineal tissue may lacerate spontaneously. Perineal damage extensive enough to require sutures occurs in two-thirds of primiparous clients (Sleep, Roberts, and Chalmers, 1989). This spontaneous trauma can cause discomfort to a degree that dominates the experience of early motherhood; sometimes it results in significant disability during the following months and years (Kitzinger, 1984).

To circumvent this potential problem, the physician or nurse-midwife may perform an episiotomy, either midline or mediolaterally. Possible benefits of episiotomy include prevention of damage to the anal sphincter and rectal mucosa (third- and fourth-degree lacerations), easier repair and better healing than a spontaneous laceration, prevention of trauma to the fetus's head, and prevention of serious damage to pelvic floor muscles (Banta and Thacker, 1982).

The nurse does not assist with the performance or the repair of an episiotomy but should communicate the client's wishes to the physician or nurse-midwife. Further, the nurse should provide care and support during and after an episiotomy.

In theory, prenatal perineal massage by the partner may offer an alternative to episiotomy for reducing perineal damage (Avery and Burket, 1986). In addition, the nurse, physician, or nurse-midwife can "iron out" the perineal tissue firmly with lubricated fingers as the fetus's head moves onto the perineum. Some clients may find touch disruptive, particularly because of edema and the increased vascularity of the perineal tissue (Noble, 1983).

PREPARING THE PERINEUM

After the client assumes the position she will maintain for delivery, the nurse uses an antiseptic solution to clean her perineum of discharge that accumulated during labor. Explain the procedure to the client; assure her that it involves no pain but that the solution may feel cool. Always scrub outward from the vaginal orifice to avoid contaminating it. Always use a fresh sponge when beginning to clean a different area. To clean the perineum, follow these steps.

1 Follow hand-washing protocol. Open a sterile prep tray and either add antiseptic solution to the sterile container or add sterile water to the antiseptic sponges. Expect to use at least six sponges. Don sterile gloves.

2 Use a sponge to scrub gently back and forth from the client's clitoris to her lower abdomen. Apply just enough pressure to remove any discharge.

3 Clean from the outer labia majora up one inner thigh and halfway to the knee. Repeat with another sponge on the opposite leg.

4 Starting at the clitoris, cleanse downward over one labia majora, making one sweep past the anus. Repeat with another sponge on the opposite side.

5 Clean from the top of the vulva downward over the perineum and anus in a single motion.

6 Rinse with sterile water, if desired, by pouring from the vulva downward.

7 Replace the wet pad beneath the client's buttocks with a dry, sterile pad.

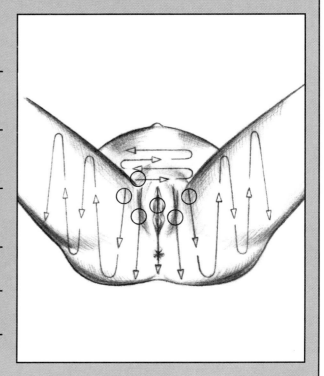

Care for the neonate. Immediately after delivery of the head (before the neonate begins to breathe and before delivery of the body), the physician or nurse-midwife suctions the neonate and ensures an adequate airway and normal breathing. After the neonate's delivery, nursing care shifts from the client (now cared for by the physician or nurse-midwife) to the neonate. Complete the clamping of the umbilical cord, perform an initial assessment, dry and wrap the neonate, continue to suction the upper airway as needed, and initiate bonding between the neonate and parents within the first few minutes after delivery.

Clamping the umbilical cord. The physician or nurse-midwife holds the neonate at or below the level of the client's introitus to facilitate transfer of blood until the umbilical cord is clamped. Before clamping, assist with collection of cord blood for analysis according to facility protocol. Typically, the physician or nurse-midwife draws blood from the umbilical vessels into a purple-top (hep-arinized) tube and stores it in the health care facility refrigerator in case further studies are needed. Blood type and a direct Coombs' test can be obtained from this sample if the client is Rh negative.

To cut the umbilical cord, the physician or nurse-midwife may apply two Kelly clamps (or one Kelly and one plastic clamp) and cut between them. If the physician or nurse-midwife and facility policy permit, ask the client and support person if they would like to cut the cord.

Assessing the neonate. Note the time of birth and the condition of the neonate's airway, amount of mucus, and respiratory efforts. Mucus may be greater following fast descent or cesarean delivery because fetal thorax compression does not force fluid from the respiratory tract. Continue with assessment of the umbilical cord as well as heart rate, color, tone, and neonate's physical condition.

Inspect the umbilical cord for obvious abnormalities and verify that it contains two arteries and one vein. The presence of only one artery and one vein has been associated with congenital kidney and cardiac problems. Notify the pediatric personnel of any abnormalities.

Assign an Apgar score at 1 minute and 5 minutes after delivery, preferably while the neonate lies on the client's abdomen supported by the client, partner, or nurse. (For instructions, see *Assigning an Apgar score.*)

Explain the Apgar score's meaning to the client and her partner. Just after the neonate's delivery, perform a quick physical examination to detect obvious congenital anomalies, birthmarks, or bruises associated with delivery. Make note if the neonate passes meconium or urine in the delivery room.

Initiate parent-infant bonding. As soon as the neonate's breathing has been established and the umbilical cord clamped, lay the neonate on the client's abdomen and cover both with a warm blanket. Urge the client and her partner to dry the neonate if necessary while maintaining skin-to-skin contact.

If the neonate's condition warrants placement in a radiant heat unit, position the unit and deliver care within

ASSIGNING AN APGAR SCORE

A method of indicating neonatal vigor, the Apgar score combines the results of five individual assessments: heart rate, respirations, muscle tone, reflex irritability, and color. Typically assigned by the nurse at 1 minute and 5 minutes after the neonate is delivered, the score may reveal the need for resuscitation, confirm trauma during delivery, and indicate congenital anomaly, among other findings. If heart rate is less than 100 beats/minute or respirations are absent, request help and initiate resuscitation immediately.

ASSESSMENT STEPS

Use the guidelines below to assign a score from 0 to 2 in each assessment category. Be sure to follow the appropriate assessment procedures.

Heart rate
Using a stethoscope, count heartbeats for 30 seconds and multiply by 2. Alternatively, feel for a pulse at the base of the umbilical cord or over the heart. If heart rate exceeds 100 beats/minute, give a score of 2. A heart rate under 100 beats/minute warrants a 1, and no detectable heartbeat should receive a 0.

Respirations
After counting and observing, assign a score of 2 for vigorous crying or regular respirations. Irregular, shallow, or gasping respirations score a 1, and absent respiratory effort gets a 0.

Muscle tone
Normally, the neonate's elbows are flexed and thighs and knees drawn up. If the limbs return to this position quickly after being extended, assign a score of 2. If muscles have some tone but do not respond briskly, give a 1. Assign a 0 for flaccid muscles.

Reflex irritability
Insert a bulb syringe into one of the neonate's nostrils or lightly flick the sole of one foot. If the response is a vigorous cry, assign a score of 2. Some motion and weak crying warrants a 1; no response rates a 0.

Color
Observe the skin or mucous membranes for pallor or cyanosis. If the neonate appears completely pink, assign a score of 2 (few neonates receive this score). Acrocyanosis, which refers to bluish hands and feet and applies to most neonates, receives a score of 1. A completely pale or blue neonate receives a score of 0. (In a dark-skinned neonate, check the palms of the hands and soles of the feet to determine pallor or cyanosis.)

Add the scores assigned in each assessment category to arrive at a total Apgar score. The highest score possible is 10; the lowest is 0. Interventions, if necessary, are based on the score.

INTERVENTIONS

A neonate with a score of 8 to 10 is normal and needs only routine interventions. Aspirate the mouth and nose with a bulb syringe. Dry and wrap the neonate in warm blankets. Perform a brief physical examination.

A score of 5 to 7 indicates mild respiratory, metabolic, or neurologic depression. Stimulate breathing by gently but firmly slapping the soles of the feet or rubbing the spine or sternum. Administer 100% oxygen via bag and face mask. If the neonate shows no improvement and the mother received a narcotic analgesic, expect to administer 0.01 mg/kg of naloxone I.M.

A score of 3 or 4 requires interventions as described above; also, the neonate may require a feeding tube to decompress the stomach. Expect to maintain oxygen administration until the neonate's heart rate exceeds 100 beats/minute and skin is completely pink.

A score of 0 to 2 indicates severe depression and requires immediate intubation and bag ventilation at 40 to 60 breaths/minute with pressures high enough to move the upper chest. Closed chest cardiac massage is performed for bradycardia under 60 beats/minute or cardiac arrest. Resuscitation drugs also are needed.

PHOTOGRAPHIC ESSAY ON THE SECOND STAGE OF LABOR

The second stage of labor begins with complete cervical dilation and ends with birth. Intense contractions occur every 2 to 3 minutes and last 60 to 90 seconds. For primiparous clients, this stage averages 1 hour; for multiparous clients, 15 minutes. To provide appropriate care, the nurse must be familiar with the steps involved, as shown in the following photographs.

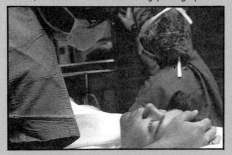

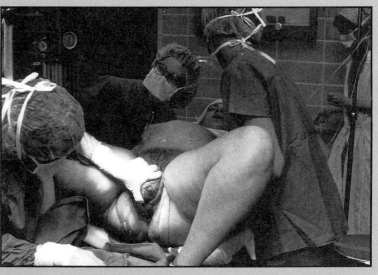

The primary support person and the nurse provide emotional support, coaching, and reassurance to the client entering the second stage of labor. The nurse continuously monitors the client's progress.

As the fetus approaches the perineal floor, the perineum bulges and flattens. As the labia spread, the head appears at the vaginal opening (crowning). At this time, the client should assume an active role and push with each contraction.

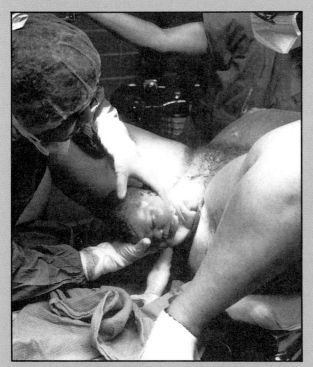

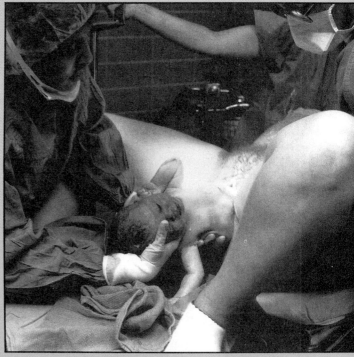

The birth attendant grasps the side of the head and usually applies gentle traction downward to deliver the anterior shoulder, then upward to deliver the posterior shoulder. (In this photograph, the posterior shoulder has emerged first.)

Once the shoulders have emerged, the rest of the body, which is narrower, can slide out with little or no traction needed; but the head and shoulders need support.

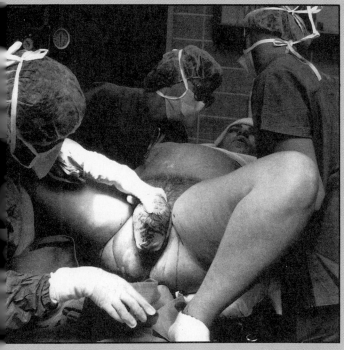

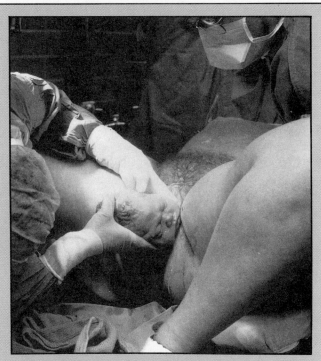

As the fetus's head emerges, it passes over the anterior margin of the perineum; the head then drops down, and the chin lies over the perineum.

To prevent maternal lacerations and damage to the fetus's intracranial area, the birth attendant must control the speed at which the head passes the perineum. When necessary, applying pressure over the perineum can maintain flexion of the head.

External rotation of the head brings the shoulders in line with the anteroposterior diameter of the client's pelvis.

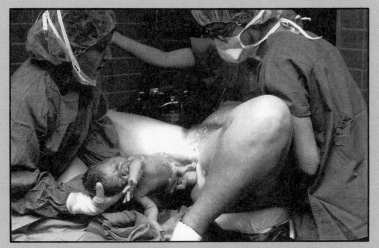

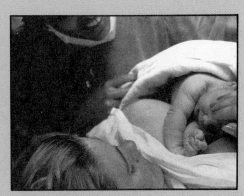

While the birth attendant holds the neonate at or below the level of the client's uterus, the nurse assists with collection of cord blood, if required, and with clamping of the cord before it is cut. The time of the neonate's complete extraction—the time of birth—is recorded.

The nurse initiates bonding between the client and neonate with skin-to-skin contact.

the client's view. Place the dried neonate, unwrapped, on top of a dry blanket. (Radiant heat only warms outer surfaces.) A modified Trendelenburg position will help drain mucus from the airways, if needed.

Assess the client's and partner's response to the neonate. Many new parents feel insecure and will value the nurse's support and instruction. Assist parents if they ask how to hold their infant. Praise them for holding their infant securely and for any other appropriate behavior, such as talking to the infant or observing the infant's responses. Give feedback about the infant's condition, such as, "The toes and hands are bluish right now but this is typical; they should change to pink within a few hours," or "It is normal for your infant's head to be molded after delivery. It will become more rounded over the next few days."

EVALUATION

Evaluate the effectiveness of nursing care by reviewing the goals attained and the outcome of the second stage of labor for the client, support person, and neonate. The following are examples of appropriate evaluation statements.
• After adopting a forearms-and-knees position, the client reported a decrease in the urge to push.
• The client bore down productively during the final phase of the second stage of labor.
• The client and her partner expressed appropriate bonding behavior with the neonate immediately after delivery.
• The client and her partner each held the neonate properly shortly after delivery.

DOCUMENTATION

The nurse documents initial and ongoing assessment findings, pertinent characteristics of the client and support person, and all nursing activities and interventions as completely as possible.

Although documentation records vary among health care facilities, most require the nurse to document at least the following whenever appropriate:
• vital signs (blood pressure, pulse, temperature)
• vaginal examination findings (cervical dilation, station, position, crowning)
• uterine contractions (duration, frequency, intensity)
• bearing-down efforts
• amniotic fluid (color and amount)
• fluid intake and output
• emotional responses (such as crying, screaming, expressions of fatigue or frustration)
• presence of support person or others
• transfer to delivery room or birthing chair
• perineal preparation
• time of birth (full extraction of neonate)
• names of all people in the room at the time of birth
• fetal heart rate (variability, baseline, periodic changes, use of external or internal fetal monitor)
• episiotomy or lacerations and description of repairs
• positioning and behaviors
• Apgar scores
• resuscitation, if necessary
• passage of meconium or urine
• any neonatal abnormalities or umbilical cord variations
• initial parent-infant bonding.

CHAPTER SUMMARY

Chapter 14 described the second stage of labor. This stage requires great effort from the client and strong support from the nurse. In addition, the nurse must monitor labor progress, assess for abnormalities and impending delivery, and assist with delivery and immediate care for the neonate. Here are the chapter highlights.

The second stage of labor, which lasts from complete cervical dilation to delivery, typically takes about 1 hour for primiparous clients and about ½ hour for multiparous clients. Although variations are common, a second stage that takes more than 2 hours may indicate abnormality.

Indications of the transition from first stage to second stage may include an increasing urge to push, increased bloody show, grunting, a gaping anus, involuntary defecation, bulging of the vaginal introitus, spontaneous rupture of membranes, and early decelerations in the FHR.

Assessment during the second stage should include vital signs; degree of cervical dilation; the strength, frequency, and duration of contractions; effectiveness of bearing-down efforts; FHR; rate of descent; and color of the amniotic fluid.

Planning and implementation involves providing emotional support for the client and family, coordinating the client's bearing-down efforts, assisting the client into positions that increase comfort and assist bearing-down efforts, monitoring hydration, preparing for delivery, and caring for the neonate immediately after delivery.

Nursing care required immediately after delivery includes drying and inspecting the neonate for obvious abnormalities, clamping the umbilical cord, assigning an Apgar score at 1 and 5 minutes, and encouraging parent-infant bonding.

STUDY QUESTIONS

1. Which characteristics would nursing assessment reveal when a client moves from the first to the second stage of labor?

2. Mrs. Tuttle, a 27-year-old primaparous client, is in the second stage of labor. Her cervix is fully dilated and the fetus's head is beginning to descend. She is bearing down with each contraction. During each contraction, the fetal heart rate drops to 60 beats per minute, then returns to the baseline. What are the possible causes of this drop?

3. During the delivery, the physician performs a midline episiotomy on Mrs. Tuttle. What are the benefits of this procedure?

4. Mrs. Tuttle delivers a baby boy. At 1 minute after delivery, he has a heart rate of 102 beats per minute, shallow respirations, flaccid limbs, moderate reaction to insertion of bulb syringe in one nostril, and blue hands and feet. What Apgar score should this neonate receive? How should the nurse respond?

BIBLIOGRAPHY

Avery, M.D., and Burket, B.A. (1986). Effect of perineal massage on the incidence of episiotomy and perineal laceration in a nurse-midwifery service. *Journal of Nurse-Midwifery,* 31(3), 128-134.

Banta, D., and Thacker, S.B. (1982). The risks and benefits of episiotomy: A review. *Birth,* 9(Spring), 25-30.

Butani, P., and Hodnett, E. (1980). Mothers' perceptions of the labor experience. *Maternal-Child Nursing Journal,* 9(Summer), 73-82.

Church, L.K. (1989). Water birth: One birthing center's observations. *Journal of Nurse-Midwifery,* 34(4), 165-170.

Cohen, W.R. (1977). Influence of the duration of second stage labor on perinatal outcomes and puerperal morbidity. *Obstetrics and Gynecology,* 49(3), 266-267.

Cohen, W.R. (1984). Steering patients through the second stage of labor. *Contemporary OB/GYN,* 24(1), 122-141.

Cunningham, F.G., MacDonald, P.C., and Gant, N.F. (1989). *Williams obstetrics* (18th ed.). East Norwalk, CT: Appleton & Lange.

Engelmann, G.J. (1882). *Labor among primitive peoples showing the development of the obstetric science of today* (reprint). New York: AMS Press.

Friedman, E. (1989). Normal and dysfunctional labor. In W.R. Cohen, D. Acker, and E. Friedman (Eds.), *Management of labor* (pp. l-18). Rockville, MD: Aspen.

Hellman, L.H., and Prystowski, H. (1952). The duration of the second stage of labor. *American Journal of Obstetrics and Gynecology,* 61, 1223-1233.

Kitzinger, S. (1984). *The experience of childbirth* (5th ed.). New York: Penguin.

McKay, S.R. (1981). Second stage labor—has tradition replaced safety? *AJN,* 81(5), 1016-1019.

McKay, S.R., and Roberts, J.E. (1985). Second stage labor: What is normal? *JOGNN,* 14(2), 101-106.

Minchom, P., Niswander, K., Chalmers, I., Dauncey, M., Newcombe, R., Elbourne, D., Mutch, L., Andrews, J., and Williams, G. (1987). Antecedants and outcomes of very early neonatal seizures in infants born at or after term. *British Journal of Obstetrics and Gynaecology,* 94(5), 431-439.

Noble, E. (1981). Controversies in maternal effort during labor and delivery. *Journal of Nurse-Midwifery,* 26(2), 13-22.

Noble, E. (1983). *Childbirth with insight.* Boston: Houghton-Mifflin.

Odent, M. (1986). *Birth reborn.* New York: Pantheon.

Peterson, G.B. (1984). *A personal growth approach to childbirth* (2nd ed.). Berkeley, CA: Mindbody Press.

Reynolds, J.L., and Yudkin, P.L. (1987). Changes in the management of labour. *Canadian Medical Association Journal,* 136(10), 1041-1045.

Roberts, J., and Mendez-Bauer, C. (1980). A perspective of maternal position during labor. *Journal of Perinatal Medicine,* 8(6), 255-264.

Sleep, J., Roberts, J., and Chalmers, I. (1989). Care during the second stage of labour. In M.W. Enkin, M.J.N.C. Keirse, and I. Chalmers (Eds.), *A guide to effective care in pregnancy and childbirth.* Oxford, England: Oxford University Press.

Turner, M.J., Webb. J.B., and Gordon, H. (1986). Active management of labour in primigravidae. *Journal of Obstetrics and Gynecology,* 7, 79-83.

Whitley, N. (1975). Uterine contractile physiology: Application in nursing care and patient teaching. *JOGNN,* 4(5), 54-58.

Whitley, N. (1985). *A manual of clinical obstetrics.* Philadelphia: Lippincott.

Wood, C., Ng, K. H., Hounslow, D., and Benning, H. (1973). Time—an important variable in normal delivery. *Journal of Obstetrics and Gynaecology of the British Commonwealth,* 80(4), 295-300.

Maternal position

Caldeyro-Barcia, R.Y. (1978). The influence of maternal position during the second stage of labor. In P. Simlein and C. Reinke (Eds.), *Kaleidoscope of childbearing: Preparation, birth, and nurturing* (pp. 31-42). Seattle: Pennypress.

Carr, K.C. (1980). Obstetric practices which protect against neonatal morbidity: Focus on maternal position in labor and birth. *Birth and the Family Journal,* 7(Winter), 249-254.

Drahne, A., Prang, G., and Werner, C. (1983). The various positions for delivery. *Journal of Perinatal Medicine,* 10(Supplement 2), 72-73.

Haukeland, I. (1981). An alternative delivery position: New delivery chair developed and tested at Kongsberg Hospital. *American Journal of Obstetrics and Gynecology,* 141(2), 115-117.

Humphrey, M.D., Chang, A., Wood, E.C., Morgan, S., and Hounslow, D. (1974). A decrease in fetal pH during second stage of labour, when conducted in the dorsal position. *Journal of Obstetrics and Gynecology of the British Commonwealth,* 81(8), 600-602.

Irwin, H.W. (1978). Practical considerations for routine applications of left lateral Sims' position for vaginal delivery. *American Journal of Obstetrics and Gynecology,* 131(2), 129-132.

Kurz, C.S., Schneider, R., and Huch, R. (1982). The influence of the maternal position on the fetal transcutaneous oxygen pressure (tcP0$_2$). *Journal of Perinatal Medicine,* 10 (Supplement 2), 74-75.

Lehrman, E.J. (1985). Birth in the left lateral position: An alternative to the traditional delivery position. *Journal of Nurse-Midwifery,* 30(4), 193-197.

Liu, Y.C. (1989). The effects of the upright position during childbirth. *Image: Journal of Nursing Scholarship,* 21(1), 14-18.

Mendez-Bauer, C., Arroyo, J., Garcia-Ramos, C., Menendez, A., Lavilla, M., Izquierdo, F., Villa Elizaga, I., and Zamarriego, J. (1975). Effects of standing position on spontaneous uterine contractility and other aspects of labor. *Journal of Perinatal Medicine,* 3(2), 89-100.

Roberts, J. (1980). Alternative positions for childbirth, Part II: Second stage of labor. *Journal of Nurse-Midwifery,* 25(5), 13-19.

Schneider-Affeld, F., and Martin, K. (1982). Delivery from a sitting position. *Journal of Perinatal Medicine,* 10(Supplement 2), 70-71.

van Lier, D.J. (1985). Effect of maternal position on second stage of labor. Unpublished doctoral dissertation. University of Illinois at Chicago, Health Science Center, Chicago, IL.

Comfort measures

Bloom, K.C. (1984). Assisting the unprepared woman during labor. *JOGNN,* 13(5), 303-306.

Chestnut, D.H., Vandewalker, G.E., Owen, C.L., Bates, J.N., and Choi, W.W. (1987). The influence of continuous epidural bupivacaine analgesia on the second stage of labor in nulliparous women. *Anesthesiology,* 66(6), 774-780.

Tryon, P. (1966). Use of comfort measures as support during labor. *Nursing Research,* 15(2), 109-118.

Fetal effects

Apgar, V. (1966). The newborn (Apgar) scoring system: Reflections and advice. *Pediatric Clinics of North America,* 13(3), 645-650.

Caldeyro-Barcia, R. (1979). The influence of maternal bearing-down efforts during second stage on fetal well-being. *Birth and the Family Journal,* 6(Spring), 17-21.

Caldeyro-Barcia, R. (1979). The influence of maternal position on time of spontaneous rupture of the membranes, progress of labor, and fetal head compression. *Birth and the Family Journal,* 6(Spring), 7-15.

Caldeyro-Barcia, R., Giussi, G., Storch, E., Poseiro, J., LaFaurie, N., Keffenhuber, K., and Ballejo, G. (1981). The bearing-down efforts and their effects on fetal heart rate, oxygenation and acid base balance. *Journal of Perinatal Medicine,* 9(Supplement 1), 63-67.

Graziano, E., Freeman, W., and Bendel, R. (1980). FHR variability and other heart rate observations during second stage labor. *Obstetrics and Gynecology,* 56(1), 42-47.

Herbert, C. and Boehm, F. (1981). Prolonged end-stage fetal heart rate deceleration: A reanalysis. *Obstetrics and Gynecology,* 57(5), 589-593.

Hon, E.H., and Quilligan, E.J. (1967). The classification of fetal heart rate, Part II: A revised working classification. *Connecticut Medicine,* 31(11), 779-784.

Krebs, H., Petres, R. and Dunn, L. (1981). Intrapartum fetal heart rate monitoring, Part V: Fetal heart rate patterns in the second stage of labor. *American Journal of Obstetrics and Gynecology,* 140(4), 435-439.

Ohel, G. (1978). Fetal heart rate in the second stage of labour and fetal outcome. *South African Medical Journal,* 54, 1130-1131.

Roberts, J. (1989). Managing fetal bradycardia during the second stage of labor. *MCN,* 8(6), 41-47.

CHAPTER 15

THE THIRD AND FOURTH STAGES OF LABOR

OBJECTIVES

After reading and studying this chapter, the student should be able to:

1. Describe physical assessment during the third stage of labor.

2. Describe placental separation and delivery.

3. Discuss nursing interventions for a client with uterine atony.

4. Explain neonatal assessment and care during the third and fourth stages of labor.

5. Discuss normal assessment findings during the fourth stage of labor.

6. Describe abnormal fourth-stage findings and possible nursing interventions.

7. Identify comfort measures to assist the client and her family.

8. Describe measures to promote bonding between the parents and the neonate.

INTRODUCTION

The third stage of labor begins with delivery of the neonate and ends with delivery of the placenta. It may last from a few minutes to 30 minutes. For most clients, this stage occurs without incident and produces a blood loss of less than 500 ml. However, postpartal hemorrhage may occur, signaling an obstetric emergency.

In this stage, the nurse assesses the client for homeostasis, placental status and delivery, and perineal repair. The nurse also evaluates the neonate's adaptation to the extrauterine environment and assesses the family's re-

sponse to the client and neonate. The nurse must respond quickly to changing circumstances, resetting priorities as needed.

The fourth stage of labor begins after delivery of the placenta and lasts about 1 hour. It marks the beginning of the "fourth trimester" (the first 3 postpartal months), during which the client recovers from the stresses of labor and physiologically returns to a nonpregnant state. During this stage, the client, her partner, and the neonate experience heightened awareness and sensitivity as they further their bonding (Rubin, 1984).

During the third and fourth stages of labor, the client's cultural beliefs can influence her self-care and health promotion measures, interactions with health care professionals, and care of and bonding with the neonate. To provide adequate care, the nurse should become acquainted with the client's cultural beliefs and exercise care to avoid stereotyping her.

In most facilities, the client, her partner or support person, and the neonate remain together during the fourth stage of labor. In others, the neonate may be moved to the nursery while the client remains in the labor and recovery area. Therefore, the type of nursing care needed will depend on facility policy.

Nursing goals for the third and fourth stages of labor relate to the physiologic adaptation and changing needs of the client and her neonate. They typically include:

• maintaining homeostasis of the client and neonate
• providing necessary equipment, supplies, and medications
• promoting bonding and family interaction
• initiating breast-feeding, if the client desires.

To meet these goals, nursing responsibilities usually include:
- observing for signs of placental separation
- assisting with placental delivery
- examining the placenta for intactness and number of umbilical cord vessels
- assisting with perineal repair
- observing the neonate's adaptation to extrauterine life, including assessment of respiratory and cardiovascular status
- evaluating the neonate's temperature and keeping the neonate warm
- preparing the neonate for interaction with the parents
- monitoring maternal blood pressure, pulse, and respirations and neonatal heart rate and respirations
- evaluating the amount and character of uterine bleeding
- monitoring uterine location and contractility
- evaluating the suture line if perineal repair was performed
- recognizing abnormal findings and intervening appropriately
- enhancing client and family self-esteem by promoting bonding
- evaluating neonate-parent interaction
- promoting comfort and safety for the client and her neonate
- helping the client meet fluid and nutrient needs
- teaching the family about postpartal recovery and neonatal feeding and care
- addressing the cultural needs of the client and her family, and
- adapting nursing care to meet those needs
- documenting the client's status and care as well as that of her neonate.

This chapter describes the third and fourth stages of labor and discusses how the nurse provides appropriate care based on careful assessment. It begins immediately after the birth of the neonate, discussing information obtained at the birth. Then it discusses common variations of the placenta and explores related nursing interventions. The chapter describes continuing assessments, clearly distinguishing between normal findings and variations and signs of potential problems. It concludes with a discussion of continuing nursing responsibilities, including promotion of bonding and preparation for discharge.

NURSING CARE DURING THE THIRD STAGE OF LABOR

During this stage, the nurse may care for the mother and neonate simultaneously. To provide the best possible care, the nurse should apply the nursing process.

ASSESSMENT

Because the third stage of labor is brief, rapidly assess maternal vital signs and the status of the placenta, perineum, fundus, and neonate. (For more information, see *Placental variations.*)

Maternal vital signs. Assess vital signs frequently, reporting changes or abnormal findings to the physician or nurse-midwife immediately. An increasing pulse rate followed by increased respirations and decreased blood pressure may be the first signs of postpartal hemorrhage and hypovolemic shock, which can occur rapidly. These complications are relatively common and typically result from uterine atony and excessive blood loss during placental separation and delivery or from perineal lacerations.

Changes in the client's level of consciousness and vital signs (rising systolic pressure, decreased pulse, and irregular respirations) may indicate increased intracranial pressure caused by rupture of a cerebral aneurysm, which may be precipitated by the increased cardiac output and stress of bearing down during the second stage of labor. However, this complication is rare.

Restlessness, tachypnea, and tachycardia may signal amniotic fluid embolism, another rare complication that may occur when amniotic fluid enters the maternal circulation during placental separation.

Placenta. After delivery of the neonate, watch for these normal signs of placental separation:
- a sudden gush or trickle of blood from the vagina
- increased umbilical cord length at the vaginal introitus
- change in the shape of the uterus from discoid (disk-shaped) to globular (globe-shaped)
- change in the position of the uterus to a location at or above the client's umbilicus.

These signs indicate normal progress of the third stage of labor. They occur when the size of the uterine cavity decreases while the size of the inelastic placental tissue remains constant. As the placental tissue buckles and begins separating from the uterus, bleeding from open decidual arterioles forms a clot between the placental tissue and the uterine wall. This retroplacental clot further

PLACENTAL VARIATIONS

After delivery of the placenta, the nurse assesses it carefully, documenting any variations from the norm, such as a placenta that is not intact. The nurse also notes umbilical cord variations, such as unusual insertion into the placenta or an abnormal number of umbilical cord vessels. The illustrations below show some common variations and their significance.

NORMAL PLACENTA

Normally, the placenta is delivered intact and no fragments remain in the uterus. It has many lobes with smooth, rounded edges and consistent color throughout, indicating adequate tissue perfusion. The placenta at term is flat, cake-like, round or oval, 15 to 20 cm in diameter, and 2 to 3 cm in breadth at its thickest parts. The maternal side is lobulated and the fetal side is shiny. It has no calcifications, discolorations, malformations, cysts, or other abnormalities.

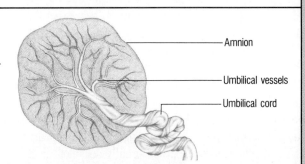

— Amnion

— Umbilical vessels

— Umbilical cord

PLACENTAL VARIATIONS

Battledore placenta
In this placental variation, the umbilical cord inserts in the margin (edge) of the placenta. This normal variation occurs in about 10% of gestations.

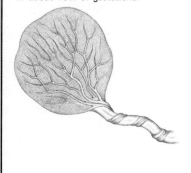

Velamentous insertion
Occurring in about 1% of gestations, a velamentous insertion occurs when the cord vessels branch from the membranes to the placenta. A velamentous insertion poses a danger because, if the membranes rupture, the cord vessels will rupture, leading to fetal hemorrhage. Blood vessels also may rupture, leading to hemorrhage between the amnion and chorion. Compression of the vessels during labor could explain fetal heart rate changes, indicating anoxia.

If velamentous insertion is detected when inspecting the delivered placenta, the danger to the fetus has passed.

Succenturiate lobe
A succenturiate lobe is an aberrant lobe or entire cotyledon (subdivision of the uterine surface of the placenta) that is separate from the placenta but connected to its main body by blood vessels. Occurring rarely, a succenturiate lobe may tear away from the main portion of the placenta during separation and expulsion. If left in the uterus, a succenturiate lobe can cause postpartal hemorrhage or infection. It also may cause vasa previa (presentation of the cord's blood vessels in front of the fetus's head during labor and delivery). Vasa previa, which also may occur with velamentous insertion, endangers the fetus because the fetus's head can compress the unprotected vessels, reducing fetal oxygen supply. Also, the unprotected vessels may be ruptured easily, leading to life-threatening hemorrhage.

shears the placenta from the uterine wall and maintains hemostasis by controlling arteriolar blood flow.

When these signs occur, expect placental delivery shortly. After the placenta separates completely, it descends to the lower uterine segment. Myometrial contractions, which may have subsided temporarily, return at 4- to 5-minute intervals and propel the placenta into the vagina. At this point, the client may push to help expel the placenta. The mechanism for pushing is similar to, but less intense than, that used during the second stage of labor.

Note the mechanism of placental expulsion. The Duncan mechanism (sometimes called the "dirty Duncan") occurs when the dark, rough, maternal side of the placenta appears first. The Schultze mechanism (or "shiny Schultze") occurs when the glistening fetal side appears first. The mechanism of expulsion usually does not affect the client's outcome.

As the placenta is delivered, examine its intactness, number of lobes, texture, and color. Examination of the placenta determines whether fragments remain in the uterus and provides additional information about the neonate's status. Calcifications, discolorations, malformations, cysts, or other abnormalities may indicate poor placental function, explain fetal distress in labor and low birth weight, and indicate the need to evaluate the neonate more thoroughly.

Assess the umbilical cord and its insertion into the placenta. Some cord variations pose potential hazards to the neonate. For example, the normal umbilical cord contains three vessels: two arteries and one vein. Fewer than three vessels correlates with various congenital anomalies. Other cord variations are benign.

Perineum. If the client underwent an episiotomy or sustained lacerations, assist with surgical repair of the tissue by providing adequate light, suture material, a local anesthesia kit (if necessary), and client support. The perineum is stitched in layers to maintain its visual integrity. Assess for an intact suture line, and note the degree of swelling, oozing, or discoloration caused by bruising or hematoma formation.

If the physician or nurse-midwife did not perform an episiotomy, assist with inspection of the perineum for lacerations or edema. Also assist with inspection of the vagina and cervix for lacerations or retained placental fragments.

Fundus. Palpate the fundus to determine its location and consistency. After the placenta is delivered, the fundus normally is midline, 1 to 2 cm below the umbilicus, and firmly contracted. A boggy (soft and poorly contracted) fundus is a sign of uterine atony (lack of muscle tone).

The following factors commonly are associated with uterine atony and the potential for postpartal hemorrhage:
• history of postpartal hemorrhage with previous delivery
• delivery of a large-for-gestational-age neonate
• hydramnios
• multiple fetuses
• extended stimulation of labor with oxytocin (Pitocin)
• bladder distention
• traumatic delivery
• grand multiparous client (more than 5 childbirths)
• anesthesia or excessive analgesia.

If uterine atony is not identified and corrected, postpartal hemorrhage can occur. (For more information, see Psychomotor Skills: *Uterine palpation and massage.*)

Neonate. Depending on facility policy, the physician, nurse-midwife, or nurse assesses the neonate immediately after delivery by assigning an Apgar score. (For more information, see Chapter 14, The Second Stage of Labor.)

Continue to assess the neonate throughout the third stage of labor, focusing on evaluation of respiratory and cardiovascular status.

NURSING DIAGNOSIS

Based on assessment findings, formulate nursing diagnoses for the client. (For a partial list of applicable diagnoses, see Nursing Diagnoses: *Third and fourth stages of labor,* page 274.) Then use the assessment findings and diagnoses to define care priorities during the postpartal period.

PLANNING AND IMPLEMENTATION

Routine care includes hygienic care, repositioning and transferring the client to the recovery area (or assisting recovery in the labor-delivery-recovery area), providing neonatal care, and promoting bonding.

Provide hygienic care. At this stage, the client may have a nursing diagnosis of *high risk for infection related to perineal laceration* or *high risk for infection related to episiotomy.* Immediately after the physician or nurse-midwife has finished inspecting or repairing the perineum, help prevent infection by cleaning the client's vulva with sterile water. Using a wet towel or gauze, wipe from the urethral area to the rectal area. Discard used gauze after each pass. Dislodge and remove dried blood or fecal material, leaving the perineal area free of bacterial contamination.

PSYCHOMOTOR SKILLS

UTERINE PALPATION AND MASSAGE

Through uterine palpation, the nurse can assess the location and firmness of the fundus. Uterine massage can help stimulate uterine contractions, which promote involution and prevent hem- orrhage. Also, blood clots may be expelled during uterine massage. To perform uterine palpation and massage, expose the lower abdomen and follow these steps.

1 Place one hand at the level of the symphysis pubis, cupping it against the abdomen to support the fundus and prevent downward displacement. Keep in mind that the elasticity of the ligaments supporting the uterus and the stretching experienced at term place the postpartal uterus at risk for inversion if it is not fixed in place during palpation and massage.

2 Place the other hand at the top of the fundus, cupping it against the abdomen.

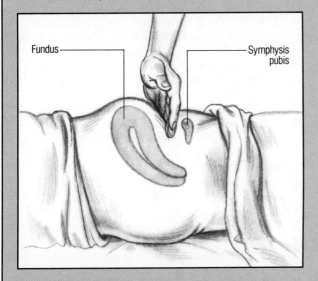

Fundus — Symphysis pubis

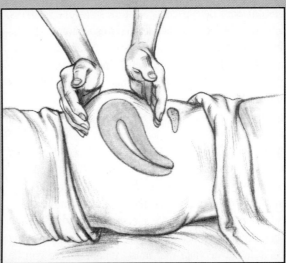

3 Gently compress the uterus between both hands. Note the level of the fundus above or below the umbilicus in finger- breadths or centimeters. (One fingerbreadth measures about 1 cm.) Also note the firmness of the fundus.

4 To massage the fundus, use the side of the hand above the fundus. Without digging into the abdomen, gently compress and release, always supporting the lower uterine segment with the other hand. Observe for lochia flow during massage.

5 Massage long enough to produce firmness. Because the fundus is tender, use only enough pressure to produce desired results without causing discomfort.

Using a downward movement, apply a clean perineal pad. Remove all delivery drapes and immediately place them in a linen hamper.

To prevent a nursing diagnosis of *potential altered body temperature related to evaporation of perspiration and muscle fatigue,* help the client change from her soiled delivery gown into a clean gown, and cover her with a clean, warm bath blanket. Change her gown even if it is not obviously soiled, because dampness from perspiration can cause chilling.

Reposition and transfer the client. To prevent hip joint disloca- tion and a nursing diagnosis of *potential for injury related to maternal positioning* or *altered tissue perfusion related to sudden change in pelvic or abdominal blood volume,* pay close attention to body dynamics and homeostasis when repositioning the client. When helping her lower her legs from stirrups or from the flexed position, advise her to bring her legs together and lower them simultaneously.

A client who has had a local anesthetic and must transfer from the delivery table to a recovery bed will need assistance in moving. Ask another member of the health care team to help stabilize the bed and keep the client's perineal pad in place as you help her move.

If spinal or epidural anesthesia was used during delivery and the client cannot control her legs, use a draw sheet or roller for the transfer and have other team members assist to ensure client safety.

After the client has been repositioned, transfer her to the recovery area or allow her to remain in the labor and delivery area, depending on facility policy.

Care for the neonate. While the neonate remains with the mother or parents, provide appropriate care. (For specific nursing care, see Neonatal Status: *Third and fourth stages of labor.*) Be especially alert for signs of cold stress, which may include an accelerated respiratory rate; labored respirations; and an increased metabolic rate accompanied by hypoglycemia, which indicates greater use of glucose stores. (For more information about cold stress and heat loss in the neonate, see Chapter 17, Neonatal Adaptation, and Chapter 19, Care of the Normal Neonate.)

Promote bonding. During the third stage of labor, the family may have a nursing diagnosis of *family coping: potential for growth, related to neonate's birth.* For this reason, the neonate's introduction to the parents is paramount. The physician or nurse-midwife places the neonate in the mother's arms even before the cord has stopped pulsating or been cut. A neonate that must remain supine can lie on the mother's abdomen. While assessments and procedures are performed, keep the mother and neonate together.

Encourage both parents to touch and talk to the neonate immediately. If the parents are afraid to touch the neonate, reassure them. Upon hearing the parents' voices, the neonate should gaze in their direction and may open the eyes fully if they are shaded from the light.

While the client is being repositioned or transferred to another bed, encourage the father or support person to hold the neonate. If the client plans to breast-feed, allow the father to place the neonate in her arms.

When the neonate is transferred to a crib, warmer, or the nursery, encourage the father or support person to remain with the neonate and report weight and activity to the mother. This helps parents and neonate maintain contact and continue bonding.

EVALUATION

Before the fourth stage of labor begins, evaluate nursing care provided during the third stage. In many facilities, the delivery nurse continues to care for the mother; in oth-

---

NEONATAL STATUS

THIRD AND FOURTH STAGES OF LABOR

When caring for the mother during the third and fourth stages of labor, the nurse also must assess and provide care for the neonate.

Assessment

To assess the neonate's respiratory status, count respirations and note skin color. Respirations should range from 40 to 60 breaths/minute. Except for the hands and feet, which may have a blue tinge, the neonate's skin color should be similar to that of the parents.

To assess cardiovascular status, palpate the heart rate or auscultate it through a stethoscope at the point of maximum impulse. The rate should range from 120 to 160 beats/minute, increasing with crying and activity. Palpate the femoral pulse for presence and quality. Lack of a femoral pulse may indicate coarctation of the aorta, a congenital cardiovascular condition.

Assess respiratory and cardiovascular status at 1 and 5 minutes, then at 5-minute intervals unless the situation warrants more frequent assessment. Evaluate the neonate each time the mother is assessed routinely.

Nursing care

An important aspect of care during this time is maintenance of the neonate's temperature. Temperature regulation depends on metabolism of brown fat, which accumulates during the last 3 months of gestation. If hypothermia occurs, the metabolic rate increases to produce heat; this can cause respiratory distress, a condition that can progress to metabolic acidosis and require aggressive intervention. To prevent this, keep the neonate warm.

Dry the neonate thoroughly immediately after delivery. Skin-to-skin contact with the mother provides the warmest environment for the neonate because heat from her body conducts to the neonate. If the mother holds the neonate, cover both with a warm blanket. If she does not, keep the neonate wrapped in warm blankets under a radiant warmer.

The neonate's largest surface area and area of greatest potential heat loss is the head. After drying the scalp, cover it with a stockinet cap or, if facility practice dictates, a plastic bunting head covering.

Other routine neonatal care includes applying identification bands and footprinting, as facility practice dictates. Place a numbered identification bracelet on the neonate's wrist and opposite ankle and on the mother's wrist. Take two sets of neonate footprints, one for the chart and one for the parents. Encourage the support person to participate in footprinting and explain the need for this identification to the mother.

In most facilities, the neonate is weighed and measured in the nursery and receives vitamin K and eye prophylaxis (ophthalmic anti-infective treatment) there as well. Encourage the support person to accompany the neonate and to return to the client and inform her of the neonate's vital statistics. However, if these procedures occur in the delivery area, be prepared to perform them.

ers, another nurse assumes care for the mother after transfer to the recovery area. In either case, evaluate maternal status by reviewing and comparing assessment data and considering the effectiveness of nursing interventions.

The following examples illustrate appropriate evaluation statements:
• The client's placenta was delivered intact.
• The client's fundus was firm.
• The client's blood loss was within normal limits.
• The neonate adapted appropriately to the extrauterine environment, as shown by stable temperature, heart rate of 120 to 160 beats/minute, and respirations between 40 and 60 with no nasal flaring or grunting.
• The client held and gazed at the neonate immediately after delivery.
• The father touched and talked to the neonate.

DOCUMENTATION

The nurse usually documents assessments and activities of the third stage on the delivery record. The nurse also may be required to complete special forms, such as neonate footprint papers.

Although each health care facility may require documentation of slightly different information, most expect the nurse to record the following on the delivery record:
• episiotomy or laceration repair
• drugs or fluids administered
• time, method, and completeness of delivery of the placenta
• maternal and neonatal vital signs
• interaction between parents and neonate
• maternal status at the time of transfer to the recovery area
• neonatal status at the time of transfer to the recovery area or nursery.

NURSING CARE DURING THE FOURTH STAGE OF LABOR

The nurse uses the nursing process to care for a client during the fourth stage of labor. To interpret assessment data properly and make decisions about care, the nurse must understand the physiology of the recovery period, including shifts in internal pressures and changes in the cardiovascular, respiratory, urinary, reproductive, gastrointestinal, and musculoskeletal systems.

ASSESSMENT

Maternal status can change rapidly during the fourth stage of labor, and such life-threatening complications as postpartal hemorrhage can occur. Therefore, frequent assessments are necessary. Begin the assessment by reviewing subjective and objective data obtained during the previous stages of labor. (This review has special importance for the nurse providing care in a recovery room separate from the labor and delivery area.) Continue the assessment by collecting current data.

If the neonate stays with the mother during this period, continue to maintain the neonate's warmth and monitor cardiovascular and respiratory status.

Health history
First, review all data obtained on admission and throughout labor and delivery. The following elements of the client's history help interpret fourth stage assessment findings.

Vital signs. Postpartal deviations from the client's baseline can indicate hemorrhage, pregnancy-induced hypertension (PIH), dehydration, or infection.

Obstetric history. The client's gravidity and parity help predict her uterine contractility and response to oxytocic medication. For example, a multiparous client may have inadequate muscle contractility because childbirth commonly causes a loss in uterine muscle tone.

The client's obstetric history can provide other clues about her probable postpartal recovery. For example, a client who experienced postpartal hemorrhage after a previous childbirth has greater risk for hemorrhage after this one (Varney, 1987).

Labor duration and progress. Prolonged labor can lead to uterine atony, particularly if accompanied by many hours of oxytocic stimulation. It also may cause dehydration and exhaustion, which may result in circulatory and musculoskeletal problems. Precipitous labor and delivery can cause uterine atony, predispose the client to hemorrhage, and produce lacerations or cervical tears that may increase blood loss.

Physical assessment
Begin client assessment after the neonate is stabilized and during or immediately after perineal repair. Assess the client's vital signs and level of consciousness.

After any perineal repair is complete and the client has been helped into a more comfortable position, assess postpartal parameters and evaluate her discomfort, recovery from analgesia and anesthesia, and fatigue, hunger, and thirst. Also observe the family's response to the neonate's birth.

Postpartal parameters. During this assessment, evaluate vital signs, fundus, lochia (blood, tissue, and cells shed from the uterus immediately after delivery and continuing for several weeks), perineum, leg pain, and tremors. (For more information, see *Parameters of postpartal assessment.*)

Assess these parameters at least every 15 minutes during the fourth stage. In situations that deviate from the norm, such as a sudden drop in blood pressure or a large increase in bright red lochia, alert the physician or nurse-midwife.

Discomfort. With each assessment during the fourth stage, determine the client's discomfort. Determine the character, intensity, and source of discomfort, such as uterine contractions, laceration repair, or perineal hematoma. Sources of discomfort during the fourth stage of labor directly relate to the length and intensity of labor, the conduct of the delivery, the presence of perineal trauma, and uterine muscle contractility (which affects hemorrhage control). A report of discomfort coupled with physical assessment findings may indicate a problem, such as hematoma formation.

Uterine contractions. Once the placenta has been delivered, the myometrial fibers contract to control blood flow from open vessels at the placental site. Sometimes called afterpains, these contractions are experienced differently by each client. For example, the multiparous client tends to need stronger and longer contractions to firm the uterus than the primiparous client, and those stronger contractions produce more intense afterpains. Postpartal contraction pain also may intensify if oxytocic drugs (Pitocin, Methergine) have been administered to control uterine bleeding.

Episiotomy, laceration repair, or perineal hematoma. A client who has undergone an episiotomy or laceration repair may experience a dull aching or burning sensation from edema and disruption of muscle and nerve tissue. Although some pain is inevitable, severe, throbbing, or increasing pain may signal a serious problem.

An episiotomy, performed during the second stage of labor, can cause great discomfort during the fourth stage. During the second stage, perineal sensitivity is dulled by continuous pressure from the fetal head and by a local anesthetic, which may be injected before the episiotomy.

When fetal head pressure is released and normal circulation resumes in the area, the perineum can become extremely tender.

If the client also incurred minor sublabial tears that required no surgical repair, she may experience a burning sensation during voiding, when acidic urine passes over open wounds. Fear of this burning may cause her to postpone voiding, leading to urine retention, bladder distention, and uterine displacement and atony.

Dull aching or burning constitute normal episiotomy pain. Pain that throbs, increases, or does not respond to comfort measures may indicate an abnormality, such as perineal, vulvar, or vaginal hematoma.

A hematoma can form when blood seeps into the tissue because open blood vessels are not closed adequately during episiotomy repair. Characteristically, it swells gradually and reddens or becomes purple. Symptoms may include increasing and throbbing perineal pain, tachycardia, restlessness, and, in severe cases, hypotension.

Cervical and vaginal hematomas pose potential problems during the fourth stage. They produce various discomforts, from a vague inability to achieve comfort to a throbbing sensation in the vagina that cannot be relieved by comfort measures. A hematoma may not be readily apparent on perineal inspection.

Other discomforts. During the fourth stage, the client may experience other discomforts related to second-stage occurrences, such as the exertion and method of pushing, use of regional anesthesia, or positioning during delivery.

The client may experience a dull ache in the sacral area caused by pressure from the fetus's head. If she pushed for an extended time, she may experience discomfort in her abdomen, arms (from holding her legs or a side rail), or upper shoulders and ribs (from curling up and bearing down). If she pushed from her upper chest while contracting her face and neck muscles, she may experience aching behind her eyes and a red or blotchy facial discoloration.

A client who maintained an extended lithotomy position or braced herself with her legs may experience constant leg pain or aches. This pain must be differentiated from that caused by a thrombus or hypertension through assessment for Homan's sign (sharp calf pain with dorsiflexion of the foot), which is not found with muscular aches.

Recovery from anesthesia and analgesia. If the client received an anesthetic or other medications during labor and delivery, evaluate her recovery with each assessment during the fourth stage. As the effects of the drugs begin to dissipate,

PARAMETERS OF POSTPARTAL ASSESSMENT

For each postpartal assessment parameter, this chart describes assessment techniques, normal and abnormal findings, and related nursing interventions. During the fourth stage of labor, the nurse must assess these parameters at least every 15 minutes.

ASSESSMENT TECHNIQUE	FINDINGS	NURSING INTERVENTIONS
Vital signs		
Palpation of the pulse for a full minute, observation of respiratory rate and rhythm, and blood pressure auscultation; temperature usually taken 1 hour after birth	**Normal findings** • Pulse within 4 to 17 beats/minute of predelivery rate • Respiratory rate within 2 to 4 breaths of predelivery rate • Systolic and diastolic blood pressure within 10 mm Hg of predelivery pressure	**For a client with normal findings** • Repeat assessments every 15 minutes until stable; then repeat according to facility policy or as prescribed. • Assess for orthostatic changes in blood pressure and increase in pulse if the client reports lightheadedness when rising or walking.
	Abnormal findings • Rapid pulse rate, characteristic of hemorrhage • Pulse rate more than 17 beats/minute slower than predelivery rate, which may indicate heart block or other postpartal cardiac anomaly • Depressed respiratory rate, which can result from medications or anesthesia • Tachypnea, which indicates oxygen need from hemorrhage or shock • Hypotension (less than 10 mm Hg between systolic and diastolic measurements), which may suggest extensive blood loss and impending shock • Hypertension (15 mm Hg increase in diastolic, 30 mm Hg systolic), which may occur with pregnancy-induced hypertension (PIH) • Elevated temperature, which may be caused by dehydration, fatigue, or infection	**For a client with abnormal findings** • Notify the physician or nurse-midwife. • Repeat vital sign assessments at least every 5 minutes along with other assessments. • Maintain fluid balance, as needed. • Be prepared to administer oxygen and medications, as prescribed. • If hypertension is present, check the client's reflexes. A client with PIH who develops symptoms will show brisk reflexes with ankle clonus.
Fundus		
Palpation	**Normal findings** • Fundal height between the umbilicus and 1 to 2 cm below the umbilicus • Fundus at midline, firm, and about the size of an average cantaloupe	**For a client with normal findings** • Repeat fundal palpation every 15 minutes with other assessments. • Teach the client the significance of a well-contracted uterus. Teach her to palpate her fundus and practice fundal massage.
	Abnormal findings • Boggy (soft, poorly contracted) uterus, deviated from midline and above the umbilicus, which suggests atony, clot retention, or a full bladder	**For a client with abnormal findings** • Massage the fundus until it becomes firm and clots are expressed. • Reassess the fundus at least every 5 minutes. • Encourage the client to void. • Encourage the client who has chosen to breast-feed to begin because nipple stimulation causes the pituitary gland to release oxytocin. • Administer oxytocic medications, if prescribed.

(continued)

PARAMETERS OF POSTPARTAL ASSESSMENT *(continued)*

ASSESSMENT TECHNIQUE	FINDINGS	NURSING INTERVENTIONS
Lochia		
Inspection of lochia flow and observation for clots at the perineum while assessing the fundus. Check to ensure that blood is not pooling under the client.	**Normal findings** • Bloody fluid with no clots • Scant (1″ stain on perineal pad), light (1″ to 4″ stain), or moderate (4″ to 6″ stain) flow within 15 minutes	**For a client with normal findings** • Repeat the assessment in 15 minutes.
	Abnormal findings • Heavy flow (saturation of one or more perineal pads) in 15 minutes or less, which indicates excessive bleeding and possible uterine atony • A steady trickle of bleeding in a client with a well-contracted uterus, which may indicate cervical, vaginal, or perineal laceration	**For a client with abnormal findings** • Evaluate for uterine atony. • Massage the fundus. • Notify the physician or nurse-midwife, who may need to evaluate the client's condition further.
Perineum		
Inspection. Remove the perineal pad, position the legs so that the perineum can be observed, and use an adequate light source. Alternatively, position the client in the left or right lateral position with the upper leg flexed. Raise the upper buttock slightly to observe the perineum. Ask the client to contract and relax the perineal muscles to assess muscle function. Place a clean pad on the perineum and help the client into a comfortable position.	**Normal findings** • Intact perineum, possibly with slight edema (depending on the duration of the second stage of labor), and painless contraction of perineal muscles (if no episiotomy was performed) • Incision with approximated edges (straight edges meeting without separations), minimal swelling, no discoloration or bleeding from the incision, no discomfort on contraction of perineal muscles, and possible burning sensation in the incision area when voiding (if episiotomy was performed)	**For a client with normal findings** • Maintain cleanliness and comfort if the perineum is intact. • Assess the perineum every 15 minutes in a client with an episiotomy. Place an ice pack on the perineum to increase comfort and decrease edema. Initiate perineal care after assessing the area.
	Abnormal findings • Swelling and discoloration, which may indicate hematoma development • Bleeding, which may indicate unligated blood vessels • Dehiscence (separation of the suture line)	**For a client with abnormal findings** • Report edema, discoloration, or dehiscence immediately. • If signs of hematoma exist, monitor for signs of impending shock, such as restlessness and changes in respirations, pulse, and blood pressure.
Leg pain and tremors		
Dorsiflexion of the foot. Support the client's thigh with one hand and her foot with the other. Then bend her leg slightly at the knee, and firmly and abruptly dorsiflex the foot.	**Normal findings** • No discomfort in the calf or popliteal space • No ankle clonus	**For a client with normal findings** • Encourage client activity. • Repeat this assessment every 15 minutes.
	Abnormal findings • Pain in the calf or popliteal space, which may result from a thrombus • Ankle clonus, which may result from PIH	**For a client with abnormal findings** • Report findings. • Obtain elastic stockings and advise the client to wear them as prescribed. • Instruct the client not to massage her legs. • Monitor for signs of embolism, such as shortness of breath, rapid drop in blood pressure, elevated heart rate, ashen coloring, and sweating.

evaluate the client's condition and response to pain. As numbness from regional or local anesthesia diminishes, she may experience sudden and intense pain in the perineum and at the episiotomy site. Assess the character, intensity, and location of pain, and monitor response to measures such as repositioning and applying ice. These assessments will help distinguish between normal discomfort and pain that signals a problem.

If the client had continuous regional anesthesia, assess the return of motor function to her legs. During each postpartal assessment, note the color and temperature of her legs and toes and her ability to move them.

When the physician or nurse-midwife removes the epidural catheter after discontinuing regional anesthesia, observe and document catheter removal.

If regional anesthesia was employed, observe the lumbar-area puncture site for drainage or bleeding.

If spinal anesthesia was administered, instruct the client to remain supine until motor function returns.

Fatigue, hunger, and thirst. Depending on the duration of labor and the second stage, the client may experience extreme fatigue or exhaustion immediately after delivery. Shaking or tremors may indicate muscle exhaustion or PIH. To differentiate normal postpartal tremors from those caused by PIH, evaluate the client's blood pressure, assess for ankle clonus by dorsiflexing the foot, and assess deep tendon reflexes.

After the neonate is born, the client may feel extremely hungry and thirsty, especially if she was restricted to ice chips or clear fluids during labor and if her labor was long. Keep in mind that labor and delivery consume a great amount of energy and, when preceded by a period of restricted food and fluid intake, may leave a client with a caloric and fluid deficit.

Assess nutritional status by testing the first urine with a reagent strip to identify ketones, a sign of fat metabolism caused by insufficient available carbohydrates.

If the client's labor was uncomplicated, honor her requests for food and fluids after delivery. Begin by administering sips of water or clear juice to assess for normal swallowing and for nausea.

Response to birth. Assess the parents' response to the neonate's birth at least once during the fourth stage of labor. Sensitive postpartal assessment of family interaction can provide valuable information that predicts future family interactions.

Bear in mind that responses to birth vary greatly, ranging from joy to relief and from pleasure to withdrawal. Childbirth is a profound physical and emotional experience. Parents may need to reconcile the pain of labor and delivery with the happiness that a child can bring.

The parents' first response to the neonate may be colored by their expectations for a perfect child, experience of pregnancy, culture, the consistency of the actual birth with expectations about it, and the child's normalcy.

Their response to the labor and birth may vary according to their culture, family expectations (including sex and appearance of the neonate), past birth experiences, and overall perspective (Avant, 1988; Choi, 1986; Mercer, 1981; Wadd, 1983; Lee, 1982).

Observe the new family as they experience one another. If they rely on another member, such as a grandmother or aunt, as the primary caregiver, include that member in the bonding experience.

Mother's response. Rubin (1963) describes the progress a mother makes in touching her child. She begins by touching the neonate with her fingertips and proceeds to use her entire hand. The en face position (in which the neonate's face turns toward the mother and they look directly at each other) indicates positive bonding.

The mother may want to count the neonate's fingers and toes to assure herself of her child's normalcy. She may express concern about the neonate's color, breathing, crying, or lack of crying. These concerns reflect the mother's attempt to establish her child's reality and health.

Father's response. Greenberg and Morris (1976) describe the relationship of a father's early contact with his child to his subsequent involvement with the child. The term "engrossment" defines positive bonding between father and child, characterized by tactile, visual, and verbal activities by the father that are directed to the neonate. Touching the neonate's skin, looking closely at the neonate, and expressing feelings of elation all indicate the father's engrossment.

NURSING DIAGNOSIS

Carefully review assessment findings and use them to develop appropriate nursing diagnoses. (For a partial list of applicable diagnoses, see Nursing Diagnoses: *Third and fourth stages of labor,* page 274.)

PLANNING AND IMPLEMENTATION

Although the fourth stage of labor is brief and focuses on assessment, planning is necessary and may occur during assessment. During this stage, interventions may include maintaining appropriate maternal positioning and activ-

THIRD AND FOURTH STAGES OF LABOR

The following nursing diagnoses address representative problems and etiologies that a nurse may encounter when caring for a client during the third and fourth stages of labor. Specific nursing interventions for many of these diagnoses are provided in the "Planning and implementation" sections of this chapter.

Third stage of labor
- Altered cerebral tissue perfusion related to sudden change in pelvic or abdominal blood volume
- Caregiver role strain related to prolonged labor and delivery
- Decreased cardiac output related to postpartal hemorrhage
- Family coping: potential for growth, related to neonate's birth
- High risk for altered body temperature related to evaporation of perspiration and muscle fatigue
- High risk for infection related to episiotomy
- High risk for infection related to perineal laceration
- High risk for injury related to maternal positioning
- High risk for injury related to neonatal birth trauma
- Impaired gas exchange related to excess secretions in the neonate
- Ineffective breathing pattern related to excess secretions in the neonate
- Ineffective individual coping related to the birth experience
- Pain related to perineal trauma

Fourth stage of labor
- Altered nutrition: less than body requirements, related to food restriction and energy expenditure during labor and delivery
- Altered parenting related to unmet expectations about childbirth
- Altered parenting related to unmet expectations about the neonate's capabilities
- Decreased cardiac output related to postpartal hemorrhage
- Fluid volume deficit related to fluid loss from perspiration during labor and delivery
- Fluid volume deficit related to fluid restriction during labor and delivery
- High risk for infection related to perineal trauma
- Pain related to difficult labor and delivery
- Pain related to episiotomy
- Pain related to maternal positioning
- Pain related to severe uterine contractions

ity, preventing hemorrhage, maintaining hygiene and comfort, maintaining fluid balance, meeting nutritional needs, and promoting bonding.

Maintain appropriate maternal positioning and activity. To prevent a nursing diagnosis of *pain related to maternal positioning,* position the client for maximum comfort during her recovery. Adjust her position based on such considerations as the need to prevent postspinal anesthesia headache.

For fundal and perineal assessments, help the client into the supine position. Between assessments, suggest that she assume a semi-Fowler's, high Fowler's, or lateral position, which may be more comfortable and give her a better position from which to view or breast-feed the neonate.

The events of labor and delivery determine the client's activity during the fourth stage. If she experienced an uncomplicated labor and delivery, received little or no analgesia, delivered the neonate with her perineum intact, or delivered with a local anesthetic agent for an episiotomy, she may be able to walk and may appreciate the opportunity.

Before helping the client out of bed for the first time, check her blood pressure. Some clients experience orthostatic hypotension after delivery and may require assistance. For this reason, help her rise slowly to prevent dizziness and weakness, and accompany her on her first walk to prevent a fall.

Expect a client who experienced a long or difficult labor and delivery, received a regional anesthetic, or was heavily medicated during or after delivery to remain in bed and be less active.

Advise a client who experienced postpartal hemorrhage to remain in bed until she stabilizes completely, which may take hours. Take special care to assist her when she first rises from bed.

Prevent hemorrhage. To help prevent a nursing diagnosis of *decreased cardiac output related to postpartal hemorrhage,* monitor the client closely and take measures to prevent uterine atony and hemorrhage. Massage her uterus gently during each assessment, and teach her to do so at regular intervals. If the fundus is boggy, continue massaging until it becomes firm and all clots are expressed.

To prevent uterine atony, administer oxytocin, as prescribed. (For more information, see Selected Major Drugs: *Fourth stage of labor.*) Encourage breast-feeding, which helps contract the uterus by stimulating the release of endogenous oxytocin.

Encourage voiding to prevent bladder distention, which displaces the uterus and can cause atony. Depending on

SELECTED MAJOR DRUGS

FOURTH STAGE OF LABOR

This chart summarizes the drugs commonly used during the fourth stage of labor.

MAJOR INDICATIONS	USUAL ADULT DOSAGES	NURSING IMPLICATIONS
oxytocin (Pitocin)		
Ineffective uterine contractions after delivery of the placenta; heavy amount of lochia	1 to 4 ml (10 to 40 units) in 1,000 ml D_5W or normal saline solution I.V., infused at a rate to control bleeding, usually 20 to 40 milliunits/minute; many clinicians follow with ergonovine maleate or methyl-ergonovine maleate I.M.	• Administer drug I.M. or by I.V. infusion, never by bolus injection. If possible, use an infusion pump or a drip regulator to ensure accurate delivery. • Monitor the client's heart rate, central nervous system (CNS) status, blood pressure, uterine contractions, and blood loss every 15 minutes. • Watch for signs of hypersensitivity, such as blood pressure elevation. In a client who had a long labor accompanied by infusion of oxytocin and large volumes of parenteral fluid, watch for signs of water intoxication, such as edema; oxytocin has an antidiuretic effect. • Use appropriate comfort measures to control pain caused by uterine contractions.
ergonovine maleate (Ergotrate) and methylergonovine maleate (Methergine)		
Prevent or control postpartal hemorrhage	For both drugs, 0.2 mg I.M. every 2 to 4 hours to a maximum of five doses	• Be aware that these drugs may be given if oxytocin does not control postpartal bleeding. • Assess the client's vital signs (especially blood pressure) before administration. • Do not administer this drug before delivery of the neonate because it can cause tetanic contractions. • Do not administer this drug if the client is hypertensive. • Watch for adverse reactions, which may include severe hypertension and signs of cerebral hemorrhage (such as loss of consciousness), myocardial infarction (such as chest pain), and retinal detachment (such as blurred vision). • Monitor the client's blood pressure, pulse rate, uterine contractions, and vaginal bleeding. Report sudden changes in vital signs, frequent periods of uterine relaxation, and any change in lochia character or amount. • Use appropriate comfort measures to control pain caused by uterine contractions.
acetaminophen (Tylenol)		
Relief of mild to moderate pain caused by episiotomy or uterine contractions	325 to 650 mg P.O. every 3 to 4 hours as needed	• Assess the client's need for analgesia. Her discomfort may increase with oxytocin administration and development of vaginal or perineal hematoma. • Monitor the client's response to the drug; hypersensitivity (very rare) may cause general malaise, rash, and sweating. *(continued)*

SELECTED MAJOR DRUGS

FOURTH STAGE OF LABOR *(continued)*

MAJOR INDICATIONS	USUAL ADULT DOSAGES	NURSING IMPLICATIONS
meperidine hydrochloride (Demerol)		
Relief of moderate to severe pain caused by uterine contractions	25 to 100 mg I.M., depending on the client's weight and degree of pain	• Drug should be used only for short-term management of pain. • Assess the client's need for analgesia. Evaluate the drug's appropriateness in relation to the client's vital signs, history of drug sensitivity, and degree of discomfort. • Obtain the client's baseline blood pressure and pulse and respiratory rates before administering this drug. Assess vital signs regularly to determine the client's response to the drug. • Observe for adverse reactions, such as dry mouth, dizziness, and respiratory depression. • Keep naloxone hydrochloride (Narcan) readily available to reverse respiratory depression.
promethazine hydrochloride (Phenergan)		
Adjunct to narcotic administration to sedate client and control nausea related to narcotic administration	12.5 to 25 mg P.O., I.M., or rectally every 4 to 6 hours	• Use with caution in a client with hypersensitivity to this drug or with CNS depression. • Assess the client's need for analgesia and nausea control. Evaluate the drug's appropriateness in relation to the client's vital signs, history of drug sensitivity, and degree of discomfort. • Monitor the client's vital signs and CNS status regularly. • Observe for adverse effects, such as transient hypotension, drowsiness, tinnitus, nervousness, hysteria, blurred vision, and seizures. • Advise the client to rise slowly, and assist with ambulation.

the client's condition, use the following interventions to prevent bladder distention—and postpartal hemorrhage.
• Provide a bedpan.
• Help the client walk to a bathroom.
• Apply warm water over the perineum to encourage muscle relaxation.
• Use the sound of running water as a psychic stimulant.
• Catheterize the client, if prescribed.
• Encourage fluid intake.
• Maintain hygiene and comfort.

Maintain hygiene and comfort. The client may have a nursing diagnosis of *pain related to severe uterine contractions, pain related to episiotomy, pain related to difficult labor and delivery,* or *high risk for infection related to perineal trauma.* For such a client, take measures that increase comfort and promote hygiene, which not only help prevent

infection but also enhance comfort. Use the following general interventions to maintain client comfort and hygiene.
• Remove collected secretions, such as lochia and perspiration.
• Teach the client self-care activities that ensure continued cleanliness.
• Provide clean, warm clothing and blankets.
• Change perineal pads and underpads after each assessment or more frequently, if appropriate.
• Clean the perineum at least once during the fourth stage with warm, clear water.
• Teach the client perineal care techniques, including wiping from front to back after urinating or defecating and rinsing the perineal area regularly with warm, clear water.

To help relieve discomfort caused by uterine contractions, use the following interventions.

- Administer analgesic agents, as prescribed.
- Reduce the rate of continuous oxytocin infusion, as prescribed.
- Teach abdominal effleurage (light, fingertip massage over the abdomen) to ease the pain of contractions.
- Place a pillow over the client's lower abdomen and help her assume a prone position, if her condition allows. The uterus should contract strongly several times and the pain should subside for a while. When the pain subsides, help the client assume a comfortable position.
- Offer a modified bed bath to remove perspiration and relax sore muscles.
- Offer a back and neck massage to relieve tension and stiffness caused by labor, pushing, or positioning.

Use the following interventions to help relieve perineal pain.

- Apply an ice pack to the area.
- Apply witch hazel compresses to the area.
- Encourage the client to contract and relax the perineal muscles (Kegel exercises).
- Administer analgesic agents, as prescribed.

The following interventions may help relieve discomfort caused by tremors, such as those from chills (unrelated to PIH).

- Wrap warm blankets around the client's feet or head.
- Provide warm oral fluids if the client's condition warrants.
- Adjust the room temperature.

Maintain fluid balance and meet nutritional needs. During the fourth stage of labor, nursing diagnoses may include *fluid volume deficit related to fluid restriction during labor and delivery, fluid volume deficit related to fluid loss from perspiration during labor and delivery,* or *altered nutrition: less than body requirements, related to food restriction and energy expenditure during labor and delivery.* If the client has one of these nursing diagnoses, employ the following interventions.

- Monitor temperature, pulse rate, and blood pressure and compare them to baseline measurements to estimate the extent of the deficit.
- Provide oral fluids.
- Regulate I.V. fluids as directed by the physician or nurse-midwife.
- Provide nourishment according to the client's preference, if not contraindicated by complications. Assess the appropriateness of her food choices and recommend easily digestible alternatives, if necessary.

Promote bonding. According to Rubin (1984) and other experts, the postpartal client experiences at least 1 hour of heightened awareness and sensitivity to her surroundings, especially to the neonate, unless she received depressant medications. Bonding commonly begins at this time, unless the client is distracted by pain or her environment.

Once the neonate is stabilized, the client may become increasingly concerned about herself. She may wonder why she still looks pregnant, why uterine contractions continue, and why she feels perineal discomfort. These personal concerns may delay bonding.

Rubin (1984) describes the first 1 or 2 days after childbirth as a time of "taking in," when the client exhibits dependent behavior and requires some "mothering" herself. Her needs relate to comfort, nutrition, and sleep, and she may focus on one or all of these during the first hour after delivery. Nursing interventions can help prevent a nursing diagnosis of *altered parenting related to unmet expectations about childbirth* or *altered parenting related to unmet expectations about the neonate's capabilities.*

Paukert (1982) suggests the following ways to promote family involvement and parent-infant bonding:

- immediate, continuous mother-infant contact
- anticipatory guidance regarding the neonate's needs and abilities
- establishment of an emotionally warm and sensitive environment.

Bonding typically begins during pregnancy as the client relates to the reality of the fetus. Bonding intensifies for both parents when they first see their infant. Typically, the neonate is quiet and alert during the first hour after delivery, and the mother experiences a surge of energy and heightened sensitivity at this time. Afterwards, the neonate and mother may sleep or rest.

Some child development experts place great importance on initial bonding and its role on the future of the parent-neonate relationship (Klaus and Kennell, 1982). However, if the immediate postpartal situation does not permit extended contact, assist the family when bonding becomes practical.

Consider the family structure when assisting with bonding. If the client is an adolescent, for example, encourage her mother or other primary caregiver to become involved during bonding.

Immediately after delivery, try promoting mother-infant bonding by encouraging the breast-feeding client to hold the neonate to her breast. During breast-feeding, the mother and infant face each other, have skin-to-skin contact, and interact as the mother responds to the feel, smell, and movement of her infant.

Help the client breast-feed as long as the neonate desires because breast-feeding positively influences bonding, and unrestricted breast-feeding does not cause or increase nipple discomfort (Carvalho, Robertson, and Klaus, 1984). Also, colostrum (yellow fluid secreted by the mammary glands during pregnancy and after childbirth until milk is produced) transmits immunoglobulins, fat-soluble vitamins, calories, and fluid to the neonate.

EVALUATION

At the end of the fourth stage of labor, evaluate the effectiveness of nursing care while making a final assessment of the client's stability. The following examples illustrate some appropriate evaluation statements.
• The client's fundus is firm and located 1 cm below the umbilicus.
• The client's perineum is intact.
• The father and other family members held the neonate.
• The neonate opened both eyes fully and responded to the parents' voices.
• The client used effleurage to reduce postpartal discomfort.
• The client began breast-feeding her neonate.

After the fourth stage of labor, a facility with birth areas or units may transfer the client from the birthing room to a room with an adjacent nursery where the neonate will be placed. A more traditional facility may transfer the neonate to a central nursery and move the client to a postpartal room. Finally, if the family wishes to go home, the client and neonate may be discharged a few hours after birth.

Before the transfer occurs, assess the client's ability to leave the delivery area via stretcher or wheelchair and the neonate's stability for transfer in the client's arms or by nursery personnel. Also check the client's and neonate's name bracelets before they are moved. A client who is drowsy from medication should not carry her neonate and may need to be transferred via stretcher with the side rails up.

DOCUMENTATION

As part of the nursing plan of care, document all nursing care provided as well as the client's response to the care. In addition to a verbal report, a written record will help the postpartal nurse meet the client's individual needs.

Although each health care facility may require documentation of slightly different information, most require the nurse to record the following information:
• client's vital signs
• location and consistency of the uterus
• amount and quality of lochia

• condition of perineum
• presence or absence of ankle clonus and calf pain upon dorsiflexion of the client's foot
• parents' response to the neonate's birth
• client discomfort
• reports of fatigue, hunger, or thirst
• urinary status (whether patient has voided)
• drugs, fluids, and food given to the client.

CHAPTER SUMMARY

Chapter 15 described the third and fourth stages of labor. Although relatively brief, these stages are critical periods of physical and psychological adjustment. Nursing care during this time is based on an understanding of the physiologic responses to birth and a complete assessment of the beginning of involution. Nursing interventions are directed toward recognizing deviations that place the client at risk, maintaining comfort and hygiene, and promoting bonding. Here are the chapter highlights.

The third stage of labor begins with delivery of the neonate and ends with delivery of the placenta. The fourth stage of labor begins after delivery of the placenta and lasts for about 1 hour.

During the third stage of labor, the nurse assesses maternal vital signs, which may indicate postpartal hemorrhage or other complications; the placenta for intactness, number of blood vessels, and presence of variations; the perineum, which may have been altered by an episiotomy or lacerations; and the fundus, which may indicate uterine atony or postpartal hemorrhage.

The nurse also assesses the neonate during the third stage of labor, focusing on respiratory, cardiovascular, and temperature status.

Nursing interventions during the third stage of labor focus on maternal hygiene, repositioning, and possible transfer to the recovery area; neonatal warmth and identification; and bonding for the new family.

Involution (return to the prepregnant state) begins in the fourth stage of labor. Physiologic changes occur in the respiratory, cardiovascular, renal, gastrointestinal, and musculoskeletal systems and within the uterus and perineum.

Assessment during the fourth stage of labor begins with a review of data obtained during previous stages. The nurse performs a physical assessment every 15 minutes, evaluating vital signs, fundus, lochia, perineum, leg pain, and tremors. The nurse also assesses the client's discomfort; recovery from analgesia and anesthesia; fatigue, hunger, and thirst; and response to the neonate.

Nursing interventions during the fourth stage focus on preventing uterine atony and postpartal hemorrhage through fundal massage, oxytocin administration, initiation of breast-feeding, and prevention of bladder distention.

If postpartal hemorrhage occurs, nursing interventions include immediately notifying the physician or nurse-midwife, performing continuous fundal massage, increasing oxytocin administration, elevating the client's legs, and administering oxygen.

The nurse can promote bonding by encouraging the parents to hold the neonate and helping the client breast-feed.

Other interventions during the fourth stage include maintaining appropriate positioning, activity, hygiene, comfort, fluid balance, and nutrition.

The nurse must evaluate and document all assessments and care before the client and neonate are prepared for discharge or transferred to another area for continuing care.

STUDY QUESTIONS

1. Mrs. Dougherty, a 30-year-old primiparous client, has delivered an 7-lb, 12-oz girl without complications. Which findings indicate that Mrs. Dougherty's placenta has separated?

2. After placental delivery, the nurse palpates the fundus. Which findings would be considered normal?

3. How frequently should the nurse assess Mrs. Dougherty during the fourth stage of labor? Which parameters should the nurse assess?

4. After assessing Mrs. Dougherty, the nurse finds that she has saturated her perineal pad completely in 10 minutes. What does this indicate? How should the nurse intervene?

5. Mrs. Dougherty complains of perineal pain. Which nursing interventions are appropriate?

BIBLIOGRAPHY

Cunningham, F.G., MacDonald, P., and Gant, N.F. (1989). *Williams obstetrics* (18th ed.). East Norwalk, CT: Appleton & Lange.

Hangsleben, K. (1983). Transition to fatherhood: An exploratory study. *JOGNN*, 12(4), 264-270.

NAACOG (1986). *Standards for obstetric, gynecologic, and neonatal nursing* (3rd ed.). Washington, DC: Author.

Varney, H. (1987). *Nurse-midwifery* (2nd ed.). St. Louis: Mosby.

Bonding

Anderson, G. (1977). The mother and her newborn: Mutual caregivers. *JOGNN*, 6(5), 50-57.

Dean, P., Morgan, P., and Towle, J. (1982). Making baby's acquaintance: A unique attachment strategy. *MCN*, 7(1), 37-41.

Greenberg, M., and Morris, N. (1976). Engrossment: The newborn's impact upon the father. *Nursing Digest*, 4(1), 19-22.

Klaus, M., and Kennell, K. (1982). *Parent-infant bonding* (2nd ed.). St. Louis: Mosby.

Paukert, S. (1982). Maternal-infant attachment in a traditional hospital setting. *JOGNN*, 11(1), 23-26.

Reiser, S. (1981). A tool to facilitate mother-infant attachment. *JOGNN*, 10(4), 294-297.

Taubenheim, A. (1981). Paternal-infant bonding in the first-time father. *JOGNN*, 10(4), 261-264.

Virden, S. (1988). The relationship between infant feeding method and maternal role adjustment. *Journal of Nurse-Midwifery*, 33(1), 31-35.

Physiologic research

Carvalho, M., Robertson, S., and Klaus, M. (1984). Does the duration and frequency of early breast-feeding affect nipple pain? *Birth*, 11(2), 81.

Gabbe, S. (1988). Current practices of intravenous fluid administration may cause more harm than good. *Birth*, 15(2), 73-74.

Maternal adaptation

Avant, K. (1988). Stressors on the childbearing family. *JOGNN*, 17(3), 179-185.

Carlson, S. (1976). The irreality of postpartum: Observations on the subjective experience. *JOGNN*, 5(5), 28-30.

Gruis, M. (1977). Beyond maternity: Postpartum concerns of mothers. *MCN*, 2(3), 182-188.

Lee, G. (1982). Relationship of self-concept during late pregnancy to neonatal perception and parenting profile. *JOGNN*, 11(3), 186-190.

Martell, L., and Mitchell, S. (1983). Rubin's "puerperal change" reconsidered. *JOGNN*, 13(3), 145-149.

Mercer, R. (1981). The nurse and maternal tasks of early postpartum. *MCN*, 6(5), 341-345.

Rubin, R. (1961). Puerperal change. *Nursing Outlook*, 9(12), 753-755.

Rubin, R. (1963). Maternal touch. *Nursing Outlook*, 11(11), 828-831.

Rubin, R. (1984). *Maternal identity and the maternal experience*. New York: Springer Publishing.

Sheehan, F. (1981). Assessing postpartum adjustment: A pilot study. *JOGNN*, 10(1), 19-23.

Nursing process

Harr, B., and Hastings, J. (1981). Parturition care planning. *JOGNN*, 10(1), 54-57.

Honan, S., Krsnak, G., Petersen, D., and Torkelson, R. (1988). The nurse as patient educator: Perceived responsibilities and factors enhancing role development. *Journal of Continuing Education in Nursing*, 19(1), 33-37.

Sherwen, L. (1987). MICC: The maternal-infant core competency project: Report of phase I. *Journal of Professional Nursing,* 3(4), 230-241.

Tepas, K. (1988). Thermoregulation in newborns. March of Dimes Series 1: The first six hours after birth, Module 1. March of Dimes Birth Defect Foundation.

Cultural references

Choi, E. (1986). Unique aspects of Korean-American mothers. *JOGNN,* 15(5), 394-400.

Newton, N. (1970). Childbirth and culture. *Psychology Today,* 4(6), 74-75.

Thomas, R., and Tumminia, P. (1982). Maternity care for Vietnamese in America. *Birth,* 9(3), 187-190.

Wadd, L. (1983). Vietnamese postpartum practices: Implications for nursing in the hospital setting. *JOGNN,* 12(4), 252-258.

CHAPTER 16

INTRAPARTAL COMPLICATIONS AND SPECIAL PROCEDURES

OBJECTIVES

After reading and studying this chapter, the student should be able to:

1. Identify factors or conditions that place a client, fetus, or neonate at risk for complications during delivery.
2. Assess for signs and symptoms that indicate the potential for or presence of an intrapartal complication.
3. Describe the emotional and psychological needs of a client and her family during an intrapartal complication.
4. Identify the priority needs of a client and fetus during a potentially life-threatening intrapartal complication.
5. Describe the nursing assessment of a client experiencing an intrapartal complication.
6. Discuss specific nursing interventions for a client experiencing an intrapartal complication and her fetus or neonate, based on her condition.
7. Identify emergencies that may arise when caring for a client with an intrapartal complication and describe appropriate nursing interventions.
8. List the indications and contraindications for selected obstetric procedures.
9. Discuss the nursing process when caring for a client and family undergoing a special obstetric procedure.

INTRODUCTION

Childbirth can be a time of change and stress, but the emotional and physical demands of labor usually can be managed by the healthy childbearing family. For most healthy clients, labor and delivery proceed normally. However, complications do occur, placing the intrapartal client at risk, raising the client's fear, and threatening the health and well-being of the client and fetus.

Conditions associated with the intrapartal client and complications include age-related concerns; chronic disorders, such as cardiac disease, diabetes mellitus, infection, and substance abuse; pregnancy-related conditions, such as pregnancy-induced hypertension (PIH) and Rh isoimmunization; reproductive system disorders related to uterine, membrane and amniotic fluid, umbilical cord, placental, and pelvic factors; systemic disorders of the pregnant client; and fetal complications. (See Chapter 9, Antepartal Complications, for more information.)

The intrapartal client at risk may be less well equipped to handle the emotional and physical demands of labor because of her struggle with the uncertainties of the pregnancy outcome. She probably was monitored closely during pregnancy and begins labor keenly aware of the risks for herself, her fetus, or her neonate. Indeed, she may be anxious or frightened about the effects of labor and delivery on her medical or obstetric condition.

The client may be unprepared for a positive childbirth experience, believing that cesarean delivery is inevitable or that she or her neonate will die during delivery.

Because the intrapartal client with a complication may believe she is not healthy or normal, her anxieties about pain and the lack of control over labor and delivery may be exaggerated. This anxiety can compound her intrapartal problems because increased maternal anxiety is associated with labor dysfunction, delivery complications, fetal distress, and altered maternal-infant bonding (Gabbe and Main, 1988).

In contrast to clients at risk who invested extra time, expense, and care to produce a healthy pregnancy are those who are at risk because they received late – or no – prenatal care. In the United States in 1985, 5% of all neonates were born to women who did not receive prenatal care. Such women and their neonates are at risk because of their socioeconomic status, poor health, or both. Lack of prenatal care increases the risk of perinatal morbidity and mortality (Brown, 1988).

A pregnancy with complications has a much higher chance of perinatal complications (problems for the mother and her fetus or neonate). Many conditions create an unfavorable intrauterine environment that does not support normal fetal growth or oxygenation. The fetus is especially sensitive to hypoxia, stress, and trauma. Signs of fetal distress, such as fetal heart rate (FHR) abnormalities and meconium-stained amniotic fluid, may develop more quickly during labor.

For a neonate of a client with complications, perinatal concerns involve the significant increase in the morbidity and mortality associated with prematurity, postmaturity, or low birth weight (Knupple and Drukker, 1986). These conditions predispose the neonate to birth trauma, perinatal asphyxia, meconium aspiration, hypoglycemia, heat loss, polycythemia, and death (Korones, 1986).

Although the goal of care is a safe, satisfying delivery that produces a normal, healthy neonate, this goal may not be achieved. If a neonate is born seriously ill, disabled, or without hope for survival, the parents' worst fears are confirmed. If perinatal death or disability occurs, the family will need assistance with coping and grieving. The nurse plays a vital role in detecting intrapartal complications, assisting in their resolution, and providing the client with appropriate care.

Occasionally, a client may require special assistance to ensure a normal delivery. This assistance could be aimed at changing the fetus's orientation in the uterus, initiating or enhancing uterine contractions, aiding the client in moving the fetus through the birth canal, or delivering the neonate surgically. To provide the best possible care, the nurse should understand the special obstetric procedures a client may undergo, be able to explain these procedures to the client and her family, and be able to assist as needed.

The chapter begins by discussing the nursing care relevant to any client at risk for or experiencing intrapartal complications. Then, using the nursing process, the chapter describes appropriate nursing care for each of the conditions associated with intrapartal complications. Throughout the chapter, where appropriate, special non-surgical and surgical obstetric procedures, their indications, contraindications, and risks are discussed.

NURSING RESPONSIBILITIES

For the client at risk and her family, the nurse must provide basic intrapartal care. (See Chapters 13, 14, and 15, on the four stages of labor.) In addition, the experienced nurse must understand the complexities of labor and delivery for a client at risk for or experiencing an intrapartal complication and provide specialized care at a critical-care level of specialized practice. These responsibilities should not be undertaken by the beginning nurse.

To manage the nursing care of the intrapartal client at risk, the nurse must perform specialized maternal and fetal monitoring (which demands advanced knowledge and skills), be familiar with the technology used to improve perinatal outcomes, and be ready to provide nursing care as an important part of a specialized perinatal team.

Every pregnant client should have been evaluated for medical and obstetric complications before the intrapartal period because early findings can assist health care professionals in correcting deficiencies and avoiding intrapartal complications. Sometimes, however, a client at risk is first encountered during the intrapartal period or a problem develops late in the pregnancy that goes undetected until admission to the labor and delivery area. In either situation, however, the nurse can use the nursing process to deliver high-quality care.

ASSESSMENT

As with any client who seeks admission for labor and delivery, the nurse obtains the intrapartal client's health history, conducts an abbreviated physical assessment, and assists in collecting specimens for appropriate laboratory tests. (For basic assessment information and procedures, see Chapters 13, 14, and 15, on the four stages of labor.) With an intrapartal client with or at risk for complications, however, the nurse must make additional assessments, be aware of maternal and fetal risks, and be prepared to notify the physician of significant findings, as described below. (For more information, see *Selected intrapartal conditions and risks.*)

Health history

When taking a history, keep in mind that a client may perceive a common, normal variation as a problem. Depending on the intrapartal client's condition, adjust the

SELECTED INTRAPARTAL CONDITIONS AND RISKS

During the intrapartal period, the nurse should be alert to certain conditions that may pose risks for the client and her fetus or neonate, as shown in the chart below.

CONDITION	MATERNAL RISKS	FETAL OR NEONATAL RISKS
Age (adolescent client)	• Psychosocial problems • Panic related to lack of control • Uterine dysfunction, which may cause prolonged labor or precipitous birth • Labor arrest • Abruptio placentae • Cesarean delivery related to cephalopelvic disproportion (CPD) or insufficient cervical dilation	• Low birth weight (LBW) or intrauterine growth retardation (IUGR) • Prematurity • Fetal distress caused by reduced perfusion of the fetal-placental unit and insufficient oxygenation • Meconium aspiration • Perinatal asphyxia • Hypoglycemia • Neonatal respiratory or central nervous system (CNS) depression • Neonatal infection, especially with a sexually transmitted disease
Age (mature client)	• Increased anxiety for neonate • Multiple gestation (more than one fetus) • Placenta previa in a multiparous client • Preterm labor • Premature rupture of membranes (PROM) • Labor dysfunction and postpartal hemorrhage, especially in a client with uterine leiomyoma • Prolonged or arrested labor, which can require oxytocin (Pitocin) administration or cesarean delivery • Malpositioning • CPD	• Chromosomal abnormalities, open neural tube defects, or cardiac defects • LBW or IUGR • Breech presentation • Small for gestational age (SGA) or large for gestational age (LGA) • Fetal distress • Meconium aspiration • Perinatal asphyxia • Neonatal respiratory or CNS depression • Stillbirth
Cardiac disease	• Cardiac decompensation • Pulmonary edema • Congestive heart failure • Maternal death • Preterm labor, if certain cardiac drugs were used	• Increased risk of congenital heart defects • IUGR • Fetal hypoxia or asphyxia
Diabetes mellitus	• Hypoglycemia • Hydramnios • Hyperglycemia • Diabetic ketoacidosis • Preterm labor • Excessive postpartal bleeding from uterine atony or birth trauma	• Hydramnios • Congenital malformations • Fetal distress • Fetal death, especially in a client with diabetic ketoacidosis • Macrosomia, which can lead to birth trauma • Neonatal hyperinsulinism leading to hypoglycemia • Respiratory distress syndrome • Polycythemia • Hyperbilirubinemia • Hypocalcemia

(continued)

SELECTED INTRAPARTAL CONDITIONS AND RISKS *(continued)*

CONDITION	MATERNAL RISKS	FETAL OR NEONATAL RISKS
Infection	• PROM • Premature labor • Fever	• Premature neonate • Neonatal infection or sepsis • Respiratory distress syndrome • Fetal death
Substance abuse	• Preterm labor • Precipitous birth • Abruptio placentae • Maternal infection • Psychosocial problems, such as isolation • Interactions between abused substance and drugs administered during delivery	• LBW or SGA neonate caused by IUGR • Premature neonate • Neonatal infection • Congenital malformations • Neonatal withdrawal symptoms
Pregnancy-induced hypertension	• Insufficient perfusion of vital organs, including fetal-placental unit • Seizures, hypertonic uterine activity, and abruptio placentae, if the client develops eclampsia • Preterm labor	• Premature neonate • Toxicity in neonate, if magnesium sulfate was administered to client • IUGR
Rh isoimmunization	• Placental hypertrophy with uteroplacental insufficiency • Chorioamnionitis • Abruptio placentae • Hydramnios, which may cause inefficient contractions • Preterm labor and delivery	• Fetal hypoxia and distress • Anemia • Jaundice • Liver, spleen, and heart enlargement • Anasarca (severe, generalized edema) • Myocardial failure

approach to the health history, augmenting the basic interview with appropriate questions. These questions depend on the client's age, disorder, and labor status.

Physical assessment

During the physical assessment, modify the standard examination to meet the intrapartal client's needs, and note significant findings that are related to her condition.

Laboratory tests

Unless otherwise ordered, expect to collect all standard admission laboratory tests. (For details, see Chapter 13, The First Stage of Labor.) Consider the client's condition when reviewing the results.

NURSING DIAGNOSIS

The nurse reviews all health history, physical assessment, and laboratory test findings and then formulates nursing diagnoses appropriate for the intrapartal client. (For a partial list of applicable diagnoses, see Nursing Diagnoses: *Intrapartal complications.*)

PLANNING AND IMPLEMENTATION

Some nursing interventions for the intrapartal client at risk for or with an intrapartal complication are the same as those for any other intrapartal client. For example, the nurse must assess the client and fetus, assist in labor management, promote comfort, assist with delivery, provide emotional support, promote bonding, perform client teaching, and care for the client's family. However, when caring for this type of client, the nurse must be prepared to respond to intrapartal emergencies and may need to approach the usual labor and delivery tasks differently and modify normal intrapartal care.

Nursing care in this situation requires advanced nursing knowledge and skills. The nurse must be prepared to participate as an integral member of the perinatal team and work closely with the physician to achieve

NURSING DIAGNOSES

INTRAPARTAL COMPLICATIONS

The following nursing diagnoses address problems and etiologies the nurse may encounter when caring for the client with intrapartal complications. Specific nursing interventions for many of these diagnoses are provided in the "Planning and implementation" section of this chapter.

Intrapartal complications and special procedures
- Altered family processes related to mother's prolonged hospitalization and bed rest
- Anxiety related to fear of death during childbirth
- Anxiety related to uncertain maternal or perinatal outcome
- Caregiver role strain related to complications and required treatments
- Impaired gas exchange related to required obstetric or special procedure
- Ineffective family coping: compromised, related to unexpected need for obstetric procedure
- Knowledge deficit about obstetric procedure or condition
- Potential fluid volume deficit related to restricted oral intake
- Powerlessness related to complications that threaten pregnancy
- Situational low self-esteem related to the inability to have a normal pregnancy

Age-related concerns
- Body image disturbance related to labor and delivery
- Decisional conflict related to offering the neonate for adoption
- Fear related to labor and delivery
- Knowledge deficit related to labor and delivery

Cardiac disease
- Altered cardiopulmonary tissue perfusion related to stress of labor on an abnormal heart
- Altered renal tissue perfusion related to intrapartal blood loss
- Decreased cardiac output related to intrapartal blood loss
- Pain related to labor and delivery

Diabetes mellitus
- Altered nutrition: less than body requirements, related to increased glucose needs
- Fear related to possible congenital malformations from uncontrolled diabetes
- Powerlessness related to condition that threatens maternal and fetal health

Infection
- Anxiety related to unexpected fetal outcome
- Ineffective denial related to socially unacceptable infection
- Ineffective individual coping related to disruption of bonding
- Social isolation related to isolation precautions

Substance abuse
- Altered nutrition: less than body requirements, related to substance abuse
- Fear related to removal and loss of neonate by statute
- Ineffective individual coping related to lack of family support
- Ineffective individual coping related to prospect of prosecution

- Knowledge deficit related to infant care
- Social isolation related to substance abuse

Pregnancy-induced hypertension (PIH)
- Altered cardiopulmonary tissue perfusion related to elevated blood pressure
- Altered renal tissue perfusion related to elevated blood pressure
- Decreased cardiac output related to vasospasm of PIH
- High risk for injury related to seizures
- Knowledge deficit related to PIH treatments

Rh isoimmunization
- Altered parenting related to the neonate's transfer to the neonatal intensive care unit
- Ineffective family coping: compromised, related to lack of opportunity for bonding

Reproductive system disorders
- Anxiety related to abnormally prolonged labor
- Anxiety related to uncertain maternal or perinatal outcome
- Fatigue related to prolonged labor
- Fear related to real or potential threat to fetus or self
- High risk for alteration in maternal hemodynamic status caused by hemorrhage
- High risk for fetal compromise related to alteration in the fetal-placental unit
- High risk for fetal compromise related to premature delivery and inadequate placental perfusion
- High risk for fetal injury secondary to fetal hypoxia and traumatic delivery
- High risk for infection related to amniotomy
- Ineffective individual coping related to exhaustion and anxiety
- Pain related to abnormally prolonged labor

Systemic disorders
- Anxiety related to uncertain perinatal outcome
- Decreased cardiac output related to hemorrhage
- High risk for alteration in maternal hemodynamic status caused by hemorrhage

Fetal complications
- Anticipatory grieving related to death of the fetus
- Anxiety related to uncertain perinatal outcome
- Dysfunctional grieving related to the death of the fetus
- High risk for fetal injury secondary to fetal hypoxia and traumatic delivery
- Pain related to abnormally prolonged labor
- Powerlessness related to having to carry a dead fetus
- Situational low self-esteem related to the inability to have a normal pregnancy

optimal outcomes. For example, nursing care for the intrapartal client with cardiac disease may require a one-to-one nurse-client ratio. Care for the intrapartal diabetic client focuses on maintenance of euglycemia (normal blood glucose levels) and prevention and identification of fetal distress. For an infected client, intrapartal care calls for prompt, aggressive medical treatment of the infection and planning for immediate care of the neonate to help prevent illness. For a client with PIH, care demands skills and expertise that seek to detect preeclampsia, prevent eclampsia, and deliver a healthy neonate.

The family of the intrapartal client at risk is likely to be very concerned about the client and her fetus or neonate. The nurse must provide sensitive nursing care adapted to the family's needs. (For more information, see Family Care: *Intrapartal clients at risk.*)

EVALUATION

During the final step of the nursing process, the nurse evaluates the effectiveness of nursing care. The nurse should state all evaluations in terms of actions performed or outcomes achieved for each goal.

DOCUMENTATION

The nurse documents assessment findings and nursing activities as thoroughly and objectively as possible. Thorough documentation not only allows evaluation of the effectiveness of the care but also makes data available to other members of the health care team, which helps to ensure consistent care. To document as accurately as possible, ensure that the entries describe events exactly, completely, and in chronological order.

Record physician management decisions and how nursing care was accomplished. Make sure to record all information required by the health care facility. Examples of appropriate documentation topics include:
• maternal vital signs
• labor progress and outcome
• FHR
• medications given, time of administration, and effectiveness
• laboratory studies and their values
• interactions among client and family.

ADOLESCENT CLIENT

Various age-related factors can place an adolescent client (under age 19) at risk during labor and delivery. If an adolescent has maintained a healthy, uncomplicated preg-

---

FAMILY CARE

INTRAPARTAL CLIENTS AT RISK

The family of an intrapartal client at risk is likely to experience extreme anxiety for her and her fetus. Family members may feel left out, isolated from the client, and intimidated by the setting, equipment, and staff. If they focus on the gravity of the client's condition, they may lose sight of the impending celebration of birth.

To help reduce anxiety for the client's family (which may help reduce her anxiety as well), the nurse should be sensitive to their concerns and include a family member in her care if the client chooses. When providing family-centered care, the nurse might use the following interventions.

• Encourage the family member's presence at the client's bedside for reassurance.
• Encourage the family member to use touch or massage to reduce the client's discomfort and anxiety.
• Teach the family member to help the client with relaxation and breathing techniques.
• Instruct the family member to promote comfort by applying a cool cloth to the client's brow or by providing mouth care.
• Allow the family member to fan the client, as needed.
• Keep other family members informed of the client's progress and provide reassurance to them.
• Explain unfamiliar equipment and procedures and the reasons for their use.
• Discuss choices about positioning, analgesia, and anesthesia with the client and family member.
• Clarify and interpret the prescribed treatment for the family, as needed.
• Discuss impending vaginal or cesarean delivery with the client and family member.
• Encourage the family member to take frequent breaks to prevent fatigue.
• Incorporate the family's cultural preferences into the care plan whenever possible.
• Attempt to establish realistic childbirth goals with the client and her family. Support their decisions about care.

---

nancy, is over age 15, is in good general health, and has had early and consistent prenatal care, adequate nutrition, and family support, she may progress through labor and delivery normally. Her risk for intrapartal complications may be no greater than that for the general population (Hollingsworth, Kotchen, and Felice, 1985).

Even if she has maintained a healthy pregnancy, however, she is likely to be at risk for psychosocial problems during labor and delivery. These are especially common because of unfamiliar surroundings, a sense of isolation, heightened fears and fantasies about labor and delivery, and the forthcoming responsibilities of motherhood.

She also may be at risk for physical problems. A client under age 15 or a multigravid adolescent client over age 15 is at considerably higher risk for poor maternal, fetal, or neonatal outcomes related to birth (Moore, 1989). About 14.5% of neonates born to adolescents under age 15 weigh 2,500 g or less as compared to about 6.9% of neonates born to women in their twenties (Slap and Schwartz, 1989). Low-birth-weight (LBW) neonates of adolescent mothers have higher morbidity and mortality rates. In adolescents, generally smaller stature, lower preconception weight, and insufficient antepartal weight gain contribute to LBW neonates.

Of the approximately 5% of pregnant women in the United States who have received little or no prenatal care, about 14% are under age 18 (Brown, 1988). Insufficient prenatal care and other factors may produce an LBW neonate who displays respiratory or central nervous system depression at birth, has a low Apgar score, and is at increased risk for developing sudden infant death syndrome, or SIDS (Institute of Medicine, 1985).

ASSESSMENT

When caring for an adolescent intrapartal client, the nurse obtains a health history, assists with a physical assessment, and collects laboratory test results as for any client who seeks admission for labor and delivery. In addition, the nurse must make specific assessments and be prepared to notify the physician of significant findings.

Health history

When assessing an adolescent client, be aware that this may be her first experience in a health care facility. If she is in active labor, she may panic because she is unprepared and feels out of control. She may perceive history questions as unimportant and may be unwilling or unable to answer them because of fear or ignorance. To calm her and obtain the necessary information, include her support person in the interview and attempt to gain her trust and cooperation. If birth seems imminent, concentrate on the most important history questions and gather data quickly.

After determining her age, parity, and labor status, ask her about length of pregnancy, prenatal care received, and the presence of any complications. This information can direct the physical assessment. Be aware, however, that the adolescent may not know her last menstrual period (LMP), making gestational age assessment and subsequent prediction of intrauterine growth retardation (IUGR) or prematurity inaccurate.

When investigating her obstetric history, particularly note complications that may recur, such as PIH, abruptio placentae, and postpartal hemorrhage. Typically, a young multiparous client has closely spaced pregnancies, rapid labors, and small neonates, all of which predispose her to precipitous (extremely rapid) delivery.

Determine the client's preconception weight and antepartal weight gain. Smaller maternal body size and poor gestational weight gain have been associated with LBW infants, who may not tolerate the stresses of labor well because of poor placental perfusion (Mercer, 1987; Winick, 1989).

Discuss her use of tobacco, alcohol, or drugs—substances that are used by many adolescents. (For more information, see "Substance abuse" later in this chapter.) These substances compromise fetal and neonatal health.

When evaluating the adolescent client's psychosocial status, be sure to assess her coping methods and support systems. Her ability to cope depends on her developmental stage, preparation for childbirth, family support, and flexibility of the health care team (Corbett and Meyer, 1987). She may need constant support during the intrapartal period.

Physical assessment

An adolescent may feel embarrassed or shy about being examined by a "stranger." Her lack of control over her labor may make her feel vulnerable, restricted, and confused. To gain a sense of control over something, she may rebel against the physical assessment and other facility procedures. Provide reassurance, remain calm but firm, and explain each step of the assessment before performing it.

Measure the client's vital signs as accurately as possible. Keep in mind that her anxiety may distort her initial vital signs. Nevertheless, her baseline blood pressure measurement will help detect PIH, and temperature and pulse rate will help detect infection or severe anemia.

Note fundal height, estimate fetal weight, and determine fetal presentation. These assessments can identify LBW, prematurity, malposition, and malpresentation. Alert the physician to any suspicious findings for further evaluation.

Assist with a pelvic examination to determine labor progress, pelvic adequacy, the imminence of delivery, and the possibility of cephalopelvic disproportion (CPD). Gaining the client's trust is important for this examination. If the client resists this evaluation, expect it to be delayed until she is more settled. Remember that she may perceive a forced pelvic examination as an assault and that she has the right to refuse any procedure.

Laboratory tests

During the pelvic examination, specimens to detect sexually transmitted diseases (STDs) and chorioamnionitis, which can cause neonatal complications, may be collected. Expect to collect specimens for all routine laboratory tests if test results are not available on the client's prenatal chart. Expect to obtain blood and urine specimens to test for anemia, STDs, hepatitis, rubella, Rh type and antibody screening, and urinary tract infections, especially if the client has not received prenatal care. Because needles and blood can be frightening to an adolescent client, provide reassurance and support when collecting specimens.

NURSING DIAGNOSIS

The nurse reviews all health history, physical assessment, and laboratory test findings and then formulates nursing diagnoses appropriate for the client. (For a partial list of applicable diagnoses, see Nursing Diagnoses: *Intrapartal complications,* page 285.)

PLANNING AND IMPLEMENTATION

Closely observe the adolescent client for development of PIH, which can be sudden. Pay careful attention to her blood pressure, urine protein levels, degree of edema, and deep tendon reflexes. (For more information, see "Pregnancy-induced hypertension" later in this chapter.)

Assess fetal status with intermittent external monitoring so that the adolescent client can get out of bed and be unrestricted, if all parameters are normal. If the client feels threatened by electronic fetal monitoring (EFM), explain that it helps determine her fetus's tolerance of labor. If the fetus shows signs of distress or IUGR, anticipate continuous EFM by internal fetal scalp electrode.

Labor management

During labor, an adolescent client can become demanding if she fears abandonment and isolation. She may want and need constant support. She may bite, pinch, or cling to the nurse, especially during pelvic examinations. These actions are common in a client with a nursing diagnosis of *fear related to labor and delivery.*

To help the client regain her composure, set limits and maintain a calm, confident approach. Also provide clear directions and descriptions. Elicit the help of her partner or a family member to provide support. Keep in mind, however, that an adolescent client may act out expected roles to gain her family's attention and become more hyperactive and helpless when they are present.

To enhance her coping ability, remain nonjudgmental and provide constant, positive encouragement about her progress and behavior. Direct her primary support person to provide comfort measures and labor coaching to help her through childbirth so that she may recall this event as an accomplishment.

For an adolescent client, carefully assess labor progress and screen for such problems as uterine dysfunction or labor arrest. The adolescent's immature uterus may have an uncoordinated contraction pattern, and her labor may not progress without augmentation. Because her pelvis may not be fully developed, she may have CPD and a difficult labor.

Assist with delivery

To promote a positive childbirth experience for the adolescent client, emphasize the normality of her experience and promote bonding, which ultimately may enhance the mother-infant relationship.

Throughout labor and delivery, provide supportive coaching and encouragement. Make every effort to decrease the drama and enhance the intimacy and joy of the experience. A client who fears trauma and mutilation from giving birth may have a nursing diagnosis of *knowledge deficit related to labor and delivery.* Such a client may benefit from encouragement to "push the baby out so you can hold the baby in your arms." If the client expresses concern that her body will never be the same and has a nursing diagnosis of *body image disturbance related to labor and delivery,* provide reassurance by explaining what she can expect as she goes through the postpartal period.

Promote bonding

The adolescent's experience of labor and delivery affects her bonding with her neonate. To promote bonding, express acceptance of, provide support to, and convey respect for the adolescent client.

Adolescents seldom relinquish their neonates for adoption (Brucker and Muellner, 1985). However, if the client chooses to do so, be sure to give her time with her neonate immediately after birth. This brief transition period helps the client begin grieving and allows her to say goodbye to her neonate. It may help her resolve a nursing diagnosis of *decisional conflict related to offering the neonate for adoption.* It also may help her understand her accomplishment as a woman, her ability to manage labor, and her success. This fosters maternal bonding with the neonate and may affect her enjoyment of relationships with future children (Mercer, 1987).

EVALUATION

During the final step of the nursing process, the nurse evaluates the effectiveness of nursing care. The nurse should state all evaluations in terms of actions performed or outcomes achieved for each goal. The following examples illustrate appropriate evaluation statements:

- The client had an uneventful labor and delivery free of complications.
- The client expressed satisfaction with her decision to keep her neonate or to give up her neonate for adoption.
- The client reported positive feelings and a sense of accomplishment related to her childbirth experience.

DOCUMENTATION

Documentation should include the following:

- maternal vital signs
- continuous labor progress
- coping responses during labor
- interactions among the client and support person during labor
- FHR patterns.

MATURE CLIENT

Typically, mature primigravid clients are in better health, are better educated and better nourished, and have a higher standard of living than adolescent clients (Jennings, 1987). Although they are at increased risk for some medical and obstetric complications, they usually proceed well through pregnancy and delivery (Acker, 1987), possibly because they tend to seek early prenatal care, are highly motivated and compliant, and receive monitoring throughout pregnancy and delivery (Queenan, Freeman, Niebyl, Resnik, and Simpson, 1987).

Typically, the mature intrapartal client has been screened prenatally for fetal chromosomal abnormalities, multiple gestation (more than one fetus), gestational diabetes, PIH, appropriate fetal growth, placenta previa, and a tendency for premature labor. A healthy mature client has the same intrapartal nursing needs as a younger client. Her greatest nursing needs will be psychosocial.

For mature clients, aging or obesity are responsible for many intrapartal risks, including diabetes mellitus, gestational diabetes, PIH, chronic hypertension, thrombophlebitis, chronic renal disease, collagen disease, and uterine leiomyoma (benign neoplasm of the uterine smooth muscle), which can affect labor and delivery (Oats, Abell, Andersen, and Beischer, 1983; Calandra, Abell, and

Beischer, 1981). Mature clients also are at higher risk for premature rupture of the membranes (PROM) and preterm labor (Naeye, 1983).

The neonate of a mature client is at increased risk for chromosomal abnormalities (including Down's syndrome), open neural tube defects, and cardiac defects. This is especially significant to nursing care if the client declined prenatal genetic screening or ultrasonography, because she may not be prepared for the birth of a neonate with a disorder.

If the mature client has hypertension or PIH, her neonate is at risk for LBW or IUGR caused by uteroplacental insufficiency. Intrapartal risks for an LBW neonate include increased fetal distress, meconium aspiration, and neonatal depression.

If the client is obese, her neonate may be born with macrosomia from her nutritionally unbalanced diet or from gestational diabetes. Intrapartal concerns for a macrosomic fetus include stillbirth or birth trauma from shoulder dystocia.

ASSESSMENT

When caring for a mature intrapartal client, the nurse obtains a health history, assists with physical assessment, and collects laboratory tests as for any client who seeks admission for labor and delivery. In addition, the nurse must make specific assessments and be prepared to notify the physician of significant findings.

Health history

When taking a history, keep in mind that a client may perceive a common, normal variation as a problem. Depending on the intrapartal client's condition, adjust the approach to the health history, augmenting the basic interview with appropriate questions. These questions depend on the client's age, disorder, and labor status.

Early in the interview, obtain the mature client's LMP and estimated delivery date, and calculate gestational age because of her increased risk for preterm labor. Also ask about any vaginal fluid leakage, which signifies rupture of amniotic membranes, because the mature client has an increased risk for PROM.

Inquire about any medical or obstetric problems because this information can help guide the plan of care. For example, a client with a chronic medical problem, such as diabetes mellitus or cardiac disease, will need additional specialized intrapartal care.

Determine if the client has a history of infertility. If so, ask how it was treated. Treatment with drugs that stimulate ovulation can predispose her to multiple gestation and accompanying risks, such as premature labor, malpresentation, and dystocia.

Also inquire if she has had any previous spontaneous abortions, has been trying to conceive for a long time, or conceived via artificial insemination. If so, she may be more anxious about this pregnancy outcome and may need close maternal and fetal monitoring during labor, if only to reassure her of normal progress.

Ask if she has had prenatal and genetic screening. For a client who has not been screened, be prepared for the possibility of a neonate with serious chromosomal abnormalities, and plan to alert the neonatal team to the client's history when delivery is imminent. Keep in mind, however, that genetic screening cannot detect all abnormalities; a client who was screened may give birth to a neonate who needs intensive care.

Perform a psychosocial assessment to identify any needs that must be addressed in the plan of care. Determine if the client is anxious about this birth or about other children at home. Find out if she has been managing a high-stress career. Anxiety and stress can affect fetal growth and can increase the risk of complications during labor and delivery (Resnik, 1988).

Assess the client's understanding of her condition and care. A mature primigravid client is likely to have planned her pregnancy and may be knowledgeable about her prenatal health. She may use various community resources, be well-read, and be highly motivated to have a controlled and successful labor and delivery (Winslow, 1987a).

Also evaluate the client's coping skills. They may be well developed, and she may be better able to express her concerns or fears about labor and delivery than a younger client. However, she may have a strong need to be in control (Winslow, 1987b). Such a client may respond well to a nurse who encourages her participation in the plan of care, is sensitive to her needs for adaptation to labor, and supports her role transition.

Physical assessment

For a mature client, establish a baseline blood pressure and assess for signs and symptoms of PIH. Evaluate fundal height for evidence of a fetus that is small for gestational age (SGA) or large for gestational age (LGA), hydramnios (if she has gestational diabetes or her fetus has an anomaly), or multiple gestation, which are more common in mature multiparous clients.

Ascertain fetal position to detect breech presentation, which occurs more frequently in mature clients (Kirz, Dorchester, and Freeman, 1985).

Laboratory tests

Unless otherwise noted, expect to collect all standard admission laboratory tests. (For details, see Chapter 13, The First Stage of Labor.) Consider the client's condition when reviewing the results.

NURSING DIAGNOSIS

The nurse reviews all health history, physical assessment, and laboratory test findings and then formulates nursing diagnoses appropriate for the client. (For a partial list of applicable diagnoses, see Nursing Diagnoses: *Intrapartal complications*, page 285.)

PLANNING AND IMPLEMENTATION

Although every intrapartal client and fetus should be assessed continuously, the mature intrapartal client at risk for or with a complication and fetus may require more frequent or additional types of surveillance, depending on the condition.

Assess vital signs and symptoms to detect impending PIH. Identify evidence of fetal stress by initiating EFM and obtaining a baseline monitor strip. Early detection of fetal distress allows prompt intrapartal treatment.

Labor management

Labor dysfunctions are relatively common in mature clients. Researchers have demonstrated a relationship between advancing maternal age and increasing frequency of labor dysfunctions (Halfar, 1985), labor protraction, and labor arrest (Queenan, Freeman, Niebyl, Resnik, and Simpson, 1987). These dysfunctions may result from decreased efficiency of the aging myometrium or from increased incidence of CPD, uterine leiomyoma, and fetal malposition, such as occiput posterior and occiput transverse (Acker, 1987).

Because of the increased risk of labor dysfunctions for the mature client, carefully monitor her contraction pattern, which can affect the efficiency of contractions. Also assess fetal position, which can help determine the duration of labor.

If contractions cease and cervical dilation or fetal descent are arrested, anticipate assisting with I.V. fluids, oxytocin (Pitocin) augmentation, and continuous EFM, unless signs of fetal distress or CPD exist.

Assist with delivery

For a healthy mature client with no detectable intrapartal risks, expect a vaginal delivery. If labor dysfunction occurs or CPD is identified, prepare for a cesarean delivery, as prescribed.

Research has found that mature clients are more likely to need cesarean delivery, although the reasons for them remain unclear. They also found an increased tendency to use epidural anesthesia, which could account for some labor dysfunction (Kirz, Dorchester, and Freeman, 1985). This research also documented an increased incidence of vacuum extractor and forceps deliveries among mature clients. This could result from decreased efficiency of the aging myometrium, decreased maternal stamina, and increased use of epidural anesthesia.

Anticipate the complications that may arise in the labor and delivery area. If the client has had oxytocin augmentation after a difficult labor, postpartal hemorrhage related to uterine atony may occur. Alert the neonatal team to attend an imminent delivery if assessments suggest neonatal abnormality.

EVALUATION

The following examples illustrate appropriate evaluation statements:
• The client had an uneventful labor and delivery without complications.
• The client and her partner and family regularly received information about labor progress and fetal status.
• The client began bonding with her neonate immediately after delivery.

DOCUMENTATION

Documentation should include the following:
• maternal vital signs
• continuous labor progress
• coping responses during labor
• interactions between the client and support person during labor
• FHR patterns.

CARDIAC DISEASE

Maternal cardiac disease complicates nearly 1% of all pregnancies and is a major cause of maternal death in the United States (Greenspoon, 1988). The intrapartal period poses the greatest risk for the client with cardiac disease because the hemodynamic changes of pregnancy peak at this time.

Labor can produce sudden, profound changes in the cardiovascular system. During each contraction, pain and increased venous blood return from the uterus raise cardiac output 20%. Mean arterial pressure rises and is followed by a reflex bradycardia. Uterine contractions can compress the aorta and iliac arteries, forcing more blood to the upper torso and head (Samuels and Landon, 1986).

Intrapartal management of the client with a cardiac disease requires the expertise of an obstetrician, cardiologist, anesthesiologist, and obstetric nurse with critical-care skills. The client needs intensive obstetric and cardiac monitoring. Interventions are based on the client's degree of cardiac decompensation (inability of the heart to compensate for impaired functioning). Even a client with minimal activity limitation during pregnancy can experience sudden worsening of the disease during labor. The nurse should be familiar with the normal changes of pregnancy and with the maternal and fetal consequences of cardiac disease. (For more information, see Chapter 9, Antepartal Complications.)

ASSESSMENT

When caring for an intrapartal client with cardiac disease, the nurse obtains a health history, assists with physical assessment, and collects laboratory tests as for any client who seeks admission for labor and delivery. In addition, the nurse must make specific assessments and be prepared to notify the physician of significant findings.

Health history

A client with cardiac disease requires careful assessment of cardiovascular status. Inquire if she has recently had difficulty breathing, experienced chest pains or dizzy spells, or has felt increased fatigue. Severe dyspnea, chest pain on exertion, increasing fatigue, or syncope suggest significant cardiac disease or decompensation and should be reported promptly to the physician.

Obtain a complete medication history. Any delay in medication administration during labor and delivery may affect the client's cardiovascular status and general well-being.

Drugs used to treat cardiac disease potentially can harm the fetus and affect the perinatal outcome. Some cardiac medications may have teratogenic effects; others may precipitate preterm labor. Oral anticoagulants are potential teratogens when taken during the first trimester. After the first trimester, they increase the risk of intrauterine bleeding (Hall, Pauli, and Wilson, 1980).

Propranolol, a beta blocker used to treat hypertension and tachyarrhythmias, can cause a constantly high uterine tone (uterine muscle contraction without relaxation) and result in preterm labor (Ueland, 1989). The drug may produce neonatal respiratory depression, sustained bradycardia, and hypoglycemia when taken late in pregnancy or immediately before delivery (Rubin, et al., 1984).

Thiazide diuretics can harm the fetus, especially when used in the third trimester or for extended periods. They may cause severe neonatal electrolyte imbalance, jaundice, thrombocytopenia, and liver damage (Anderson, 1970). However, drugs such as quinidine and the cardiac glycosides are not known to have teratogenic effects or cause problems with use during the third trimester of pregnancy.

Physical assessment

When assessing the client with cardiac disease, be especially alert for dependent edema, crackles in the lower lung fields, jugular vein distention, cyanosis, clubbing, diastolic murmurs, cardiac arrhythmias, and loud, hard systolic murmurs. Depending on their severity, these findings may indicate cardiac decompensation and must be reported immediately to the physician.

Laboratory tests

Unless otherwise noted, expect to collect all standard admission laboratory test. (For details, see Chapter 13, The First Stage of Labor.) Consider the client's condition when reviewing the results.

NURSING DIAGNOSIS

The nurse reviews all health history, physical assessment, and laboratory test findings and then formulates nursing diagnoses appropriate for the client. (For a partial list of applicable diagnoses, see Nursing Diagnoses: *Intrapartal complications,* page 285.)

PLANNING AND IMPLEMENTATION

Frequently check the maternal pulse, respirations, and blood pressure, and maintain strict fluid intake and output records, as prescribed. Expect continuous EFM as well as continuous maternal electrocardiogram monitoring; hemodynamic monitoring with an arterial line, central venous pressure, or indwelling pulmonary artery catheter may be ordered as well. Keep resuscitation equipment near the client at all times.

Labor management

For the client with cardiac disease, keep in mind that maternal position, contractions, and anesthesia can affect cardiovascular status during labor and delivery.

Close observation is particularly important for a client with cardiac disease because she is likely to have a nursing diagnosis of *altered cardiopulmonary tissue perfusion related to stress of labor on an abnormal heart* or *altered renal tissue perfusion related to intrapartal blood loss.*

Promote proper positioning for the client with cardiac disease, especially if she has a nursing diagnosis of *altered cardiopulmonary tissue perfusion related to stress of labor on an abnormal heart.* She must avoid the supine position because it can increase venous return, stroke volume, and cardiac output and can decrease the heart rate. During labor, encourage use of the lateral recumbent position, which improves cardiac emptying and promotes oxygenation. During delivery, do not elevate the client's legs fully in the lithotomy position because this increases venous return and may overload the heart (Greenspoon, 1988).

Promote comfort

For a client with a nursing diagnosis of *pain related to labor and delivery,* keep in mind that labor pains can cause maternal tachycardia and elevate blood pressure, increasing the stress on the heart. Effective analgesia should minimize this effect.

Expect the client to receive regional anesthesia, such as epidural anesthesia, to relieve pain during labor and delivery. Regional anesthesia is particularly useful in a client with cardiac disease because it decreases cardiac output and heart rate and acts as a peripheral vasodilator that reduces venous return to the heart. However, it can cause hypotension, requiring close blood pressure monitoring (Sullivan and Ramanathan, 1985).

Assist with delivery

During the second stage of labor, bearing down can reduce venous blood flow to the heart by increasing intrathoracic pressure. When the client stops bearing down, cardiac output and blood pressure increase rapidly. Therefore, instruct the client to avoid bearing down in the second stage or expect the physician to use epidural anesthesia, which eliminates the bearing-down reflex. After the cervix is dilated fully, labor should progress naturally through the second stage. Uterine contractions usually produce fetal descent; the physician allows it to proceed unless labor continuation would jeopardize the client or her fetus. Keep in mind that some physicians prefer to shorten the second stage by using low forceps or vacuum extraction (Greenspoon, 1988).

If the client with cardiac disease delivers vaginally, expect her blood volume to be redirected to central circulation and cardiac output to increase dramatically. Monitor her closely and observe for abrupt changes in cardiac status.

For a client who undergoes a planned cesarean delivery, expect a blood loss of about 1,000 ml, causing a temporary decrease in cardiac output and blood pressure (Greenspoon, 1988). This client has a nursing diagnosis of *decreased cardiac output related to intrapartal blood loss.*

Prepare for acute neonatal problems because the neonate of a client with cardiac disease has an increased risk of morbidity and mortality. A client with congenital heart disease has an increased risk of giving birth to a neonate with congenital heart disease. Antepartal maternal cyanosis is associated with preterm labor, resulting in LBW or a premature neonate. Maternal cyanosis and tachycardia also may cause hypoxia and fetal death. Keep the neonatal team advised and alert them when birth is imminent so that they can be present in the delivery room (Ueland, 1989).

Plan to assess the client continuously for at least 24 hours after delivery. Cardiac output increases immediately after delivery, when blood that had been diverted to the uterus reenters the central circulation. A client with cardiac disease who cannot tolerate these postpartal changes may develop decompensation and congestive heart failure. Prompt medical intervention may be required for such a client. Therefore, the nurse must be able to recognize any change and report it immediately to the physician.

EVALUATION

The following examples illustrate appropriate evaluation statements:
• The client assumed labor positions that supported cardiac function.
• The client and her partner and family regularly received information about maternal and fetal status.
• The client delivered successfully without further maternal or neonatal complications.

DOCUMENTATION

Documentation should include the following:
• maternal vital signs
• fluid intake and output
• cardiac and pulmonary assessment findings
• FHR patterns
• equipment and medications used.

DIABETES MELLITUS

During pregnancy, a client with diabetes mellitus requires close monitoring and management to prevent intrapartal problems. Prevention of hyperglycemia before conception and during pregnancy improves perinatal outcomes but does not remove all risks (Mills, et al., 1988). Uncontrolled diabetes is associated with increased maternal, fetal, and neonatal morbidity and mortality. (For more information about the maternal, fetal, and neonatal effects of diabetes, see Chapter 9, Antepartal Complications.)

Uncontrolled diabetes can cause hydramnios (excessive amniotic fluid). It also is associated with hypertensive disorders, such as chronic hypertension and PIH, which affect 15% to 30% of all pregnant clients with diabetes (Cousins, 1987). Women with diabetes also are at risk for preterm labor and, if associated with vascular changes, placental abnormalities.

Neonates of diabetic mothers whose diabetes has not been well controlled have a higher morbidity and mortality rate than those born to nondiabetic mothers. They also are at risk for neonatal hypoglycemia at birth and for macrosomia, which can lead to birth trauma. A neonate of a pregestational diabetic client is at increased risk for congenital malformations, especially if the client's glucose levels were uncontrolled during fetal organ development (Mills, et al., 1988).

ASSESSMENT

When caring for diabetic intrapartal client, the nurse obtains a health history, assists with physical assessment, and collects laboratory tests as for any client who seeks admission for labor and delivery. In addition, the nurse must make specific assessments and be prepared to notify the physician of significant findings.

Health history
When assessing a diabetic client, determine when she last ate and took insulin. An omitted or reduced insulin dose can cause a surge in blood glucose levels. Insulin deficiency can lead to diabetic ketoacidosis (DKA)—an acute complication of diabetes characterized by hyperglycemia, metabolic acidosis, electrolyte imbalance, coma, and possibly maternal and fetal death.

Physical assessment
When assessing the diabetic client, be especially alert for signs of hyperglycemia, such as unusual thirst; increased

urine output; and continuous, deep, rapid breathing. Also watch for signs of hypoglycemia, such as faintness, trembling, impaired vision, and changes in level of consciousness.

Laboratory tests

For a diabetic client, carefully check blood glucose levels, as prescribed. The insulin-dependent diabetic client is at risk for DKA when blood glucose levels approach 300 mg/dl (Hollingsworth and Moore, 1989).

If an elective induction or repeat cesarean delivery is planned, the physician may perform an amniocentesis to determine the lecithin/sphingomyelin (L/S) ratio and phosphatidylglycerol (PG) level. These test results provide information about fetal lung maturity, which helps determine whether a vaginal delivery is possible or cesarean delivery is necessary as well as the timing of delivery.

NURSING DIAGNOSIS

The nurse reviews all health history, physical assessment, and laboratory test findings and then formulates nursing diagnoses appropriate for the client. (For a partial list of applicable diagnoses, see Nursing Diagnoses: *Intrapartal complications,* page 285.)

PLANNING AND IMPLEMENTATION

For an intrapartal client with diabetes, expect to observe and report on her fetus, renal and cardiovascular functions, glucose levels, and insulin and glucose infusions.

Assess the fetus. To detect fetal distress, assess the fetus continuously through EFM and evaluate maternal blood glucose levels hourly. Glucose levels should range from 60 to 100 mg/dl (3.3 to 5.6 mmol/liter). Even short periods of maternal hyperglycemia during labor can lead to neonatal hypoglycemia (Ryan, O'Sullivan, Skylar, and Mintz, 1982).

Assess renal and cardiovascular functions. If the client has diabetes-related renal disease, anticipate strict recording of her fluid intake and output during labor and delivery. When administering I.V. fluids, expect to use an infusion pump to regulate the exact dosage. Because chronic hypertension usually accompanies renal disease, closely monitor her blood pressure also.

Frequently assess for edema, proteinuria, and hyperactive deep tendon reflexes. Keep in mind that chronic hypertension and PIH are common among diabetics.

Carefully evaluate and document these findings. Report abnormal findings promptly to the physician.

A client with a history of cardiovascular complications caused by diabetes requires close cardiac monitoring. Such a client is at high risk for complications and may need followup by the critical care team.

Assess glucose levels and infusions. Expect to check the diabetic client's blood glucose levels carefully during and immediately after the intrapartal period. The physician will attempt to maintain her glucose levels within the target range using a continuous I.V. insulin and glucose regimen. Regimens vary from minimal glucose and no insulin to 5 g of glucose/hour and 1 to 2 units of insulin/hour, adjusted according to hourly glucose levels (Knuppel and Drukker, 1986). Regardless of the insulin regimen used, glucose is necessary to compensate for the energy expenditure of labor (Jovanovic and Peterson, 1982). Insulin infusion may be needed until delivery of the placenta; glucose, until the client consumes food.

The client who is to have a planned cesarean delivery or induced labor the following morning should be instructed to take nothing by mouth after midnight and to skip her morning dose of insulin.

Check the client's blood glucose levels immediately after delivery and at least every 4 hours thereafter. After the client begins eating, the physician may reinstitute insulin administration when hyperglycemia recurs. The client's antepartal insulin dose serves as a guide to her postpartal dose. Be aware, however, that a lower dose may be prescribed after delivery because of the rapid decline in placental hormones and cortisol, which reduces opposition to insulin.

Labor management. In a client with hydramnios, anticipate a large gush of fluid when the diabetic client's membranes rupture, which can cause umbilical cord prolapse. Be prepared to intervene appropriately. (For more information, see "Umbilical cord prolapse" later in this chapter.)

Assist with emergencies. In a client with insulin-dependent diabetes mellitus, poorly controlled blood glucose levels and insulin deficiency can lead to DKA, which can cause intrauterine fetal death (Knuppel and Drukker, 1986). DKA produces maternal acidosis, which causes fetal acidosis and fetal distress. Until prompt treatment restores maternal homeostasis, the client and her fetus will remain in jeopardy. (For more information, see Emergency Alert: *Diabetic ketoacidosis.*)

EMERGENCY ALERT

DIABETIC KETOACIDOSIS

For a client with diabetes, the stress of labor can trigger ketoacidosis. This form of acidosis is accompanied by ketone accumulation in the blood and can lead to coma and death if not treated promptly. It also can compromise the fetus.

The following chart will help the nurse identify the signs and symptoms of diabetic ketoacidosis (DKA) and prepare to intervene or assist appropriately. Keep in mind that correction of maternal DKA should reverse fetal compromise.

Signs and symptoms
- Hyperglycemia and ketonuria
- Signs of dehydration, such as poor skin turgor, flushed dry skin, oliguria, and confusion
- Hypotension
- Deep, rapid respirations
- Decreased level of consciousness, possibly leading to coma
- Fruity or acetone-like breath odor
- Nausea and vomiting

Nursing considerations
- Confirm DKA by obtaining arterial blood gas (ABG) levels, as prescribed; using a reagent strip to evaluate the client's urine for ketones; using a reflectometer to monitor blood for a glucose test; and sending for baseline laboratory studies, such as electrolyte and serum blood glucose levels.
- Summon health care team members, including the obstetrician, diabetologist, and internist.
- Record hourly fluid intake and output on a flowsheet.
- Document blood glucose and urine acetone levels, laboratory test results for ABG levels and electrolyte studies, maternal vital signs, and fetal heart rate (FHR)
- Start an I.V. line with an isotonic solution, such as normal saline solution, as prescribed.
- Monitor the client's cardiac status with a bedside ECG monitor, if possible. On an ECG strip, hyperkalemia may produce small P waves, a prolonged PR interval, widened QRS complex, and tall peaked T waves. It can precipitate cardiac arrhythmias and typically occurs in DKA when potassium is pulled from cells into the blood. Attempt to maintain serum potassium in the 4 to 5 mEq/liter range. Expect to draw blood to check serum potassium levels every hour.
- Administer short-acting regular insulin, as prescribed. Before administering insulin, however, ensure that fluid replacement has been initiated.
- Monitor blood glucose levels every hour.
- Administer I.V. glucose only after the client's blood glucose level falls below 250 mg/dl.
- Assess the FHR and variability continuously.

Assist with delivery. If the diabetic client has controlled blood glucose levels during pregnancy and shows no signs of placental insufficiency, anticipate a vaginal delivery after the onset of spontaneous labor. Vaginal delivery at term is preferred with a normal L/S ratio and PG level, indicating fetal lung maturity, and if the fetus shows no evidence of macrosomia or compromise.

Anticipate a difficult delivery if the fetus has macrosomia because it can cause shoulder dystocia and lead to maternal and neonatal birth trauma. If the client experienced a difficult delivery, she may have vaginal and perineal lacerations and excessive postpartal bleeding.

If fetal distress or maternal problems occur, assist with a cesarean delivery if needed. The delivery should be planned carefully to minimize maternal and neonatal morbidity and mortality; the neonatal team should be present at the delivery. (For more information, see *Indications for planned delivery for the diabetic client,* page 296.)

A heel stick of the neonate to obtain a blood sample for glucose testing may be performed in the delivery area. During the intrapartal period, maternal hyperglycemia may lead to neonatal hyperinsulinism and hypoglycemia, causing a rapid drop in the blood glucose level in the first 30 to 60 minutes after birth. Neonatal hypoglycemia may be asymptomatic or produce such signs as twitching, jitteriness, hypotonia, apnea, and seizures. If hypoglycemia is detected, keep the neonate warm until treatment (such as dextrose and water feeding or I.V. glucose therapy) can begin, probably in the neonatal intensive care unit.

EVALUATION

The following examples illustrate appropriate evaluation statements:
- The client's blood glucose levels remained within acceptable limits.
- The client displayed no signs of hypoglycemia or hyperglycemia.
- The client delivered a stable neonate.
- The client experienced spontaneous labor at term.
- The client and her family regularly received information about maternal, fetal, and neonatal status.

DOCUMENTATION

Documentation should include the following:
- maternal and fetal vital signs
- fluid intake and output
- blood glucose levels
- insulin and glucose administration.

INDICATIONS FOR PLANNED DELIVERY FOR THE DIABETIC CLIENT

For a diabetic client, the following assessment findings may uncover the need for a planned delivery. Depending on the severity of these findings and the client's condition, planned delivery may include an induced vaginal delivery or a cesarean delivery.

- Fetal distress
- Signs of intrauterine growth retardation, such as inadequate fundal height and abnormal findings on ultrasonography
- Estimated gestation duration greater than 42 weeks
- Pregnancy-induced hypertension
- Signs of markedly failing renal function, such as decreasing urine output
- Macrosomia with a fetus greater than 4,000 g

INFECTION

Infections are a major cause of maternal, fetal, and neonatal death. During the intrapartal period, they are more common in clients with premature labor, PROM (especially before 36 weeks' gestation), fever, or fetal death.

The primary perinatal infections are bacterial or viral and are caused by such organisms as group B beta-hemolytic streptococcus, herpes simplex virus (HSV), or hepatitis B virus. They may be transmitted to the fetus through an infected uterus or birth canal and can lead to morbidity or mortality because the fetus's immature immune system cannot fight off these life-threatening organisms. Fungal (candidiasis) or protozoal (trichomoniasis) infections are not potentially fatal (Benoit, 1988).

Many factors can predispose a client to intrapartal infection, including obesity, severe anemia, poor hygiene, uncontrolled diabetes, chronic renal or respiratory disease, and a depressed immune response (Balgobin, 1987). Clients at increased risk for STDs, which are the most common intrapartal infections (Cates and Holmes, 1987), constitute a large and varied population, including but not limited to:
- unmarried women
- women under age 24
- women with multiple sex partners, especially with a history of treatment for STDs
- women treated for recurrent vaginitis or a previous STD (Wilson, 1988; Spence, 1989).

During labor, predisposing factors to infection (especially chlamydia) may include preterm labor, prolonged labor, prolonged PROM (rupture that occurs more than 24 hours before labor), use of such invasive equipment as internal fetal scalp electrodes or intrauterine pressure catheters, and multiple vaginal examinations.

ASSESSMENT

When caring for an intrapartal client with infection, the nurse obtains a health history, assists with physical assessment, and collects laboratory tests as for any client who seeks admission for labor and delivery. In addition, the nurse must make specific assessments and be prepared to notify the physician of significant findings.

Health history

Because any woman may contract an infectious disease and because it may have grave consequences, assess all intrapartal clients for infection, noting symptoms of, and risk factors for, infection. Early recognition of intrapartal infection allows prompt treatment and helps prevent its spread.

During the admission interview, review the client's history of antepartal illness, possible exposure to STDs, and any treatments received. This information may point to a serious infection, such as an STD, which may be asymptomatic when the disease is most virulent (Krieger, 1984).

Ask the client about recent exposure to colds or viruses or whether she has a persistent cough or fever. Inquire about past or current urinary tract infections, which typically recur during pregnancy. These questions also may uncover evidence of infection.

Also inquire about general signs and symptoms of infection, such as fever, chills, fatigue, and anorexia as well as specific signs and symptoms of upper respiratory, genitourinary, and other infections.

During the client's obstetric history, rule out prolonged PROM, which can lead to chorioamnionitis. Note the onset of labor to rule out prolonged labor, which can predispose the client to infection.

Physical assessment

When assisting with the physical assessment, be alert for signs of dehydration, maternal or fetal tachycardia, fever, chest congestion, uterine or other abdominal tenderness, costovertebral angle tenderness, perineal lesions, and purulent, malodorous vaginal secretions. These signs suggest infection.

Even if the client displays no obvious signs of infection, be vigilant about following infection control guidelines (Centers for Disease Control, 1987). Assume that any client may be infected with the human immunodeficiency virus (HIV) or hepatitis B virus, and observe universal precautions with every client.

Laboratory tests

Anticipate the laboratory tests ordered for the client with an infection, which may include a complete blood count with differential; erythrocyte sedimentation rate; blood culture; urinalysis; urine culture and sensitivity test; cervical, vaginal, and lesion cultures; chest X-rays; and culture and microscopic evaluation of amniotic fluid. These tests help pinpoint the type and degree of infection.

NURSING DIAGNOSIS

The nurse reviews all health history, physical assessment, and laboratory test findings and then formulates nursing diagnoses appropriate for the client. (For a partial list of applicable diagnoses, see Nursing Diagnoses: *Intrapartal complications,* page 285.)

PLANNING AND IMPLEMENTATION

Expect to administer I.V. fluids immediately to improve hydration, reduce fever, and prevent maternal exhaustion (Balgobin, 1987). Use external EFM to avoid further contamination of the fetus. After collecting blood or vaginal cultures to identify the infecting organism, administer I.V. antibiotics, as prescribed. For example, unless contraindicated by the client's allergies, expect to give a broad-spectrum antibiotic combination. Carefully assess maternal and fetal responses to infection treatments during the intrapartal period.

Assist with delivery

Once an intrapartal bacterial infection is identified, labor induction or augmentation with oxytocin may be prescribed to shorten the diagnosis-to-delivery time to less than 12 hours (Balgobin, 1987). The number of vaginal examinations should be limited and amniotomy should be avoided. Provide meticulous perineal care. Anticipate spontaneous vaginal delivery, depending on the severity of the infection and the maternal and fetal tolerance to labor.

Expect to avoid cesarean delivery in the infected client because it increases the risk of maternal morbidity and postpartal endometritis five- to ten-fold (Balgobin, 1987). However, if the client has active lesions from herpes simplex virus (HSV) infection or has had an HSV genital infection up to 2 weeks before delivery, anticipate a cesarean delivery (if her amniotic membranes have not ruptured). If PROM occurs less than 4 to 6 hours before the client is admitted, anticipate a cesarean delivery to prevent the fetus from coming into contact with lesions in an infected birth canal.

When anticipating delivery for an infected client, summon the neonatal team so that they are ready for the potentially ill neonate. The neonate may be premature and at increased risk for sepsis; lung maturity problems, such as respiratory distress syndrome, also are likely. If the client received adequate antibiotics for sepsis during labor, the neonate is less likely to have respiratory depression at birth; if not, the neonate may require resuscitation.

Coordinate family care and communicate all pertinent information to the nursery and postpartal teams. After delivery, collect specimens for culture from the mother, neonate, and possibly the placenta, and send them to the laboratory, as prescribed. These cultures may reveal previously undetected infection in the mother and infection transmission to the neonate.

Provide emotional support

An intrapartal client with an infection will need emotional support because of anxiety for herself and her neonate. If her infection requires isolation precautions, she also may feel isolated or dehumanized because the health care team must wear gowns, gloves, and masks. She may have a nursing diagnosis of *anxiety related to unexpected fetal outcome or social isolation related to isolation precautions.* For such a client, provide emotional support and reassurance.

If she has an active HSV infection, she and her partner may be concerned about cesarean delivery and the chance of having a neonate with a potentially fatal infection. While preparing the client for cesarean delivery, provide reassurance and teach her and her partner about the virus and the rationale for surgery.

Also be aware that the client and her partner may harbor guilt, resentment, or embarrassment because of the stigma of this STD. Reassure the client that only the staff responsible for her care will be aware of her diagnosis. The client may invent another, less emotionally charged, reason for cesarean delivery, such as persistent breech or slow labor progress, so that others are not aware of the HSV infection. Such a client may have a nursing diagnosis of *ineffective denial related to socially unacceptable infection.* If so, maintain her confidentiality and respect her preferences.

For any client with an infection, explain the disorder and its ramifications, which may include separating her from her neonate at birth. If so, encourage her to express her frustration and sadness at this prospect (Knupple and Drukker, 1986). This may help prevent a nursing diagnosis of *ineffective individual coping related to disruption of bonding.*

EVALUATION

The following examples illustrate appropriate evaluation statements:
- The client verbalized an understanding of the need for infection control techniques.
- The client's family expressed support and concern for the client.
- The client safely delivered a stable neonate.

DOCUMENTATION

Documentation should include the following:
- maternal vital signs, especially temperature
- fluid intake and output
- character of vaginal secretions, especially color and odor
- fetal heart rate
- client's physiologic response to necessary treatments
- family's response to, and support of, the client.

SUBSTANCE ABUSE

During pregnancy, substance abuse can lead to serious perinatal risks. Substance abusers tend to have unplanned pregnancies or may be uncertain when the pregnancy began. They may have suboptimal nutrition, smoke heavily, abuse multiple drugs, and seek prenatal care late, if at all (Frank, et al., 1988).

These actions put the substance abuser and her fetus at risk during the intrapartal period. For example, cocaine use during pregnancy causes maternal and fetal vasoconstriction, tachycardia, and elevated blood pressure. These effects reduce blood flow to the fetus and can induce uterine contractions. Cocaine use also increases the risk of preterm labor, delivery of an LBW or SGA neonate (MacGregor, et al., 1987), and abruptio placentae (Burkett, Banstra, Cohn, Steele, and Palow, 1990).

Substance abuse also can cause problems that may affect the antepartal period and lead to intrapartal problems. For example, severe nutritional deficiencies and STDs, which are common among women who abuse drugs, compromise fetal health (Lynch and McKeon, 1990). Substance abuse can produce social isolation, which can affect the client's ability to cope with labor. Use of nonsterile needles can cause maternal infection or embolization, which can affect maternal and fetal health.

Some states have strict laws regarding substance abuse and child protection. For example, if the client used or tested positive for drugs during the antepartal or intrapartal periods, Florida law mandates home environment evaluation and referral of the client for drug treatment before the neonate can be discharged (Florida Statute, 1987).

ASSESSMENT

When caring for a substance abusing intrapartal client, the nurse obtains a health history, assists with physical assessment, and collects laboratory tests as for any client who seeks admission for labor and delivery. In addition, the nurse must make specific assessments and be prepared to notify the physician of significant findings.

Health history

The admission interview is the ideal time to assess the client for substance use, abuse, or withdrawal. With careful questioning, probe sufficiently to discover if substance abuse is a problem and, if it is, determine the client's current status. This is especially important because the substance abuser may enter the health care facility without revealing her problem (Miller, 1989).

Explore past and present substance use in a nonjudgmental manner. Remember that the substance abuser is likely to be anxious or depressed and to display abrupt behavior changes. She may lack self-confidence and have low self-esteem. If she is afraid, she may be hostile and aggressive.

Begin the history by determining the client's first use of cigarettes, alcohol, and drugs, and then lead to a current substance abuse history. To evoke honest responses, ask nonthreatening questions, such as, "When was the last time you had a drink?"

Review the client's medical history for clues to prior substance abuse, such as serum hepatitis, venous thrombosis, thrombophlebitis, cellulitis, abscess, hypertension, STDs, and human immunodeficiency virus (HIV) infection. Such complications are associated with substance abuse and use of drug equipment.

Pay close attention to the client's complete obstetric history. Substance abuse may have complicated previous pregnancies and may cause problems in this one. Illicit drug use during pregnancy can affect the client and her fetus or neonate.

The client who abuses substances may experience menstrual irregularities or amenorrhea. As a result, she may be unaware of her pregnancy until she begins to look pregnant or feel fetal movement. Because of this, determination of gestational age may be difficult, especially if she has not had prenatal care. Maternal nutritional deficiencies and drug exposure in utero can cause IUGR, further complicating gestational age determination (Frank, et al., 1988).

During the history, evaluate the client's feelings about her pregnancy. The substance abuser may have ambivalent feelings about pregnancy. Carefully document her responses and bonding behaviors, such as talking about the fetus and touching her abdomen. This information can help health care professionals make decisions about the neonate's safety.

Physical assessment

Observe the client's physical appearance for signs of substance abuse. Note drowsiness, lethargy, or a malnourished, gaunt, or untidy appearance. Also note extremely dilated or constricted pupils; track marks, abscesses, or edema in the arms or legs; and inflamed or indurated nasal mucosa.

Laboratory tests

Because of the client's life-style, she may have multiple infections and diseases. Expect to perform all routine intrapartal tests as well as tests for hepatitis, tuberculosis, STDs, and HIV infection, as prescribed. If the client admits to substance abuse or shows its clinical indications, expect a urine toxicology screen to be performed for confirmation, as prescribed.

NURSING DIAGNOSIS

The nurse reviews all health history, physical assessment, and laboratory test findings and then formulates nursing diagnoses appropriate for the client. (For a partial list of applicable diagnoses, see Nursing Diagnoses: *Intrapartal complications*, page 285.)

PLANNING AND IMPLEMENTATION

For a substance abuser, closely assess vital signs for maternal or fetal tachycardia, depressed maternal respirations, and elevated blood pressure.

Labor management

Carefully monitor the client's labor progress. Because the substance abuser is at increased risk for precipitous birth, evaluate her labor progress quickly and be prepared for a rapid delivery.

After labor begins, the substance abuser may delay coming to the facility because of fear or may use drugs to ease her labor pains and not realize that delivery is imminent. For these reasons, she is at risk for giving birth outside the facility or en route.

Keep in mind that labor management for a substance abuser is the same as for any other client. Medical management may include early artificial rupture of the membranes. Illicit drug use shortly before delivery increases the risk of fetal distress. Therefore, amniotic fluid must be evaluated for color, such as meconium staining and blood, and quantity. Anticipate continuous external EFM to assess fetal well-being.

Promote comfort

Analgesia for the substance abuser's labor pain will not contribute to her drug problem. However, observe her for interactions between analgesics and illicit drugs. Because the substance abuser commonly is not accompanied by friends or family, provide nonpharmacologic comfort measures and coach her through labor to reduce her feelings of isolation.

Assist with delivery

Work closely with the neonatal team to ensure continuity of care. The neonate of a substance abuser is at increased risk for congenital malformations, prematurity, and IUGR. About two-thirds of neonates born to heroin or methadone users are born with withdrawal symptoms; cocaine-dependent neonates commonly experience painful abstinence symptoms that may last up to 3 weeks (Landry and Smith, 1987). Anticipate the need for a neonatologist or pediatrician at delivery because the neonate may require resuscitation and intubation.

Provide emotional support

The substance abuser who is aware of child protection laws may fear prosecution or worry that her neonate will be taken from her. She may have a nursing diagnosis of *ineffective individual coping related to prospect of prosecution* or *fear related to removal and loss of neonate by statute.* If so, try to understand her fears and the difficulty of her decision to seek intrapartal care at the health care facility. Express acceptance of and patience with the client.

The substance abuser who gives birth without the support of her family or friends may have a nursing diagnosis of *social isolation related to substance abuse* or *ineffective individual coping related to lack of family support.* If so, stay with her as much as possible, coach her through labor, and provide reassurance and support.

Promote bonding

State laws and social service representatives may determine if the substance abuser can take her neonate home. While her home environment is being evaluated, promote bonding and offer information about the neonate's needs. To help foster early bonding, follow these guidelines:

• Accept the client's condition in a nonjudgmental manner.
• Offer information about the neonate's condition.
• Explain facility policies briefly and directly.
• Encourage contact, such as holding the neonate after birth and planning for nursery visits.

EVALUATION

The following examples illustrate appropriate evaluation statements:

• The client received analgesia to relieve labor pain.
• The client expressed an understanding of her labor progress.
• The client demonstrated signs of bonding with her neonate by holding him and gazing at him after birth.

DOCUMENTATION

Documentation should include the following:

• FHR
• maternal vital signs
• maternal contractions and labor progress
• maternal response to analgesia
• interactions between analgesia and illicit drugs
• signs of mother-infant bonding.

PREGNANCY-INDUCED HYPERTENSION

A hypertensive syndrome that occurs during pregnancy, pregnancy-induced hypertension (PIH) has two forms: preeclampsia (causing hypertension, proteinuria, and edema and possibly causing oliguria, headache, blurred vision, and increased deep tendon reflexes) and eclampsia (causing convulsions along with the signs of preeclampsia). Affecting about 5% of all pregnancies (Knupple and Drukker, 1986), preeclampsia may progress to eclampsia suddenly or gradually. The client with PIH may be very ill. Failure to recognize and appropriately manage PIH accounts for about 1% of maternal deaths in the United States (Roberts, 1989).

PIH is characterized by insufficient perfusion of many vital organs, including the fetal-placental unit (all fetal and maternal systems that work together to exchange nutrients, excrete toxins, and perform other functions); it is completely reversible with pregnancy termination, but symptoms may remain for 24 to 48 hours after delivery. The client may report sudden weight gain, varying degrees of edema, numbness in her hands or feet, headache, or vision problems; small warning signs of increasing preeclampsia.

The major goal of preeclampsia management is prevention of eclampsia. To achieve this goal, the nurse must understand the pathophysiology, progression, and prognosis of the disorder, and must recognize and immediately report to the physician the classic signs of preeclampsia. (For more information on PIH, see Chapter 9, Antepartal Complications.)

ASSESSMENT

When caring for an intrapartal client with PIH, the nurse obtains a health history, assists with physical assessment, and collects laboratory tests as for any client who seeks admission for labor and delivery. In addition, the nurse must make specific assessments and be prepared to notify the physician of significant findings.

Health history

Assess the client for signs and symptoms of PIH, especially those of increasing severity. Expect her to complain of symptoms in various body systems because PIH reduces perfusion to nearly all tissues.

Inquire about the client's pattern of weight gain during pregnancy. A gain of 5 pounds in one week is a warning sign of preeclampsia. Ask about edema of the hands, feet, or face—a common, early sign of preeclampsia. If edema is severe, the client will require further evaluation for other signs of preeclampsia.

Also ask about other signs and symptoms that may suggest PIH. Complaints of tightness and intermittent numbness in her hands and feet indicate ulnar nerve compression from edema. Complaints of epigastric pain or stomach upset may signal hepatic distention, a warning sign of impending preeclampsia. Headache and mental confusion indicate poor cerebral perfusion and may precede seizures. Visual disturbances, such as scotomata, indicate retinal arterial spasm and edema (Roberts, 1989).

Physical assessment

The client's prenatal blood pressure should be compared to her current readings. In preeclampsia, blood pressure increases by at least 30 mm Hg systolic or 15 mm Hg diastolic. If the prenatal blood pressure is unknown, a blood pressure of 140/90 mm Hg after 20 weeks' gestation suggests PIH. Severe preeclampsia exists when blood pressure is 160 mm Hg or more systolic or 110 mm Hg or more diastolic and significant edema and proteinuria are present. However, eclampsia can occur with much lower blood pressure.

Laboratory tests

For all intrapartal clients, test a random urine specimen with a protein-sensitive reagent strip to screen for proteinuria, one of the three classic signs of PIH. Be aware that urine contamination with blood or amniotic fluid will cause a false-positive result because these fluids contain protein.

If results indicate proteinuria, expect to collect a 24-hour urine specimen for quantitative analysis, as prescribed. Severe preeclampsia exists when urine protein measures 3+ or 4+ on a reagent strip or 5 g or more (or 300 mg/liter) on a quantitative analysis.

NURSING DIAGNOSIS

The nurse reviews all health history, physical assessment, and laboratory test findings and then formulates nursing diagnoses appropriate for the client. (For a partial list of applicable diagnoses, see Nursing Diagnoses: *Intrapartal complications,* page 285.)

PLANNING AND IMPLEMENTATION

Before delivery, the client must be stabilized and the fetal-placental unit closely monitored. Cardiovascular monitoring with an indwelling pulmonary artery or central venous pressure catheter for the client with severe PIH may be prescribed, especially if she is oliguric. This allows closer monitoring of blood pressure and intravascular volume, which is particularly important with a nursing diagnosis of *altered renal tissue perfusion related to elevated blood pressure.*

Determine the client's level of consciousness. As a result of drugs used to treat PIH, she may show depressed vital signs and may sleep between contractions. As long as her respiratory rate is normal, do not be alarmed, but continue to monitor her closely.

The client will require continuous EFM to detect signs of placental insufficiency and evaluate fetal well-being. Keep in mind that the seizures of eclampsia cause maternal hypoxia and can produce fetal bradycardia. After seizures stop, FHR should return to baseline.

Labor management

Because a client with eclampsia is likely to be lethargic or semicomatose, she may have a reduced response to uterine contractions. Therefore, expect to monitor her uterine contractions closely, palpating the abdomen frequently.

She may display hypertonic uterine activity and develop vasospasm, which increases the risk of abruptio placentae. A sustained rigid abdomen with severe pain (which the semicomatose client may not notice or report) indicates possible abruptio placentae and must be reported to the physician immediately.

Assist with emergencies

A client with PIH always is at risk for eclampsia; prepare to carry out the physician's orders for management. About 5% of clients with preeclampsia develop eclampsia, which is characterized by seizures (Sibai, Lipshitz, and Anderson, 1981). Most seizures occur during the intrapartal period and the first 48 hours of the postpartal period, suggesting that these are the periods in which preeclampsia is most likely to develop into eclampsia (Roberts, 1989). The number of seizures a client experiences can vary from 1 to 20.

Clients most at risk for seizures are those who have not received adequate prenatal care and those with unrecognized PIH of increasing severity. However, no specific signs and symptoms can be used to predict the development of seizures (Sibai, Lipshitz, and Anderson, 1981). Therefore, treatment of all clients with preeclampsia is based on concerns for the few who may develop eclampsia.

For any client with PIH, nursing care includes taking seizure precautions, assisting with prevention or treating of seizures, assessing maternal and fetal response to treatment and related disorders.

Taking seizure precautions. To avoid general injury to the client, pad the side rails of her bed. This precaution is particularly important for a client with a nursing diagnosis of *high risk for injury related to seizures.* (Never use a padded tongue depressor to keep the client from biting her tongue during a seizure—it is ineffective and may cause further injuries.)

If necessary, establish an airway and administer oxygen. To prevent aspiration of secretions, position the client on her side. If she is oliguric, position her on her left side to increase urine excretion and uterine perfusion.

To reduce the nervous system irritability that usually precipitates seizures, dim the lights and reduce unnecessary noise. Organize care to avoid frequent disturbances. Keep the number of people at her bedside to a minimum, but allow a family member to remain with her. This may help reduce her anxiety and help keep the family informed and involved in her care.

Assist with prevention or treatment of seizures. Magnesium sulfate ($MgSO_4$) is the treatment of choice for seizures because it is effective and relatively safe, although it can be toxic for the client and fetus. It depresses neuromuscular transmission, which diminishes hyperactive reflexes and prevents seizures. It also reduces cerebral edema and intracranial pressure, which cause mild vasodilation.

Expect to administer $MgSO_4$ I.V. or I.M. For I.V. use, initially give 4 g in a 20% solution slowly over 20 minutes. (To treat seizures, expect to administer 4 g of $MgSO_4$ I.V. over 20 minutes [Knupple and Drukker, 1986].) Follow this I.V. bolus infusion with continuous I.V. infusion of 1 to 2 g/hour, as prescribed.

Although rarely prescribed, $MgSO_4$ may be given I.M. using a deep, Z-track injection in the upper outer quadrant of the buttocks with a 3″, 20G needle. Administer the I.M. loading dose of 5 g injected into each buttock, followed by 5 g every 4 hours in alternating gluteal muscles. If more than 6 hours elapse between doses, expect to give the loading dose again.

Assess maternal and fetal response to treatment. The therapeutic blood level of $MgSO_4$ is 2.5 to 7.5 mEq/liter; signs of toxicity may appear when the level exceeds 7 mEq/liter (Hayashi, 1986). Monitor the client closely to detect signs of $MgSO_4$ toxicity, such as hypotension, respiratory paralysis, and reduced reflexes. Assess the patellar reflex or, if the client has received epidural anesthesia, the biceps reflex. (Epidural anesthesia may depress the patellar reflex.) Alert the physician if the reflex is absent. Loss of the patellar or other deep tendon reflex may indicate that $MgSO_4$ is approaching toxic levels. However, because this can occur with concentrations lower than the therapeutic level, $MgSO_4$ therapy is not based solely on this observation. At best, the patellar reflex is a gross measure of plasma concentration. Monitor and document deep tendon reflexes every hour for the client receiving $MgSO_4$.

Monitor and document the client's respiratory rate every 15 minutes, and inform the physician if the respiratory rate is depressed. Also note a urine output of less than 25 ml/hour. $MgSO_4$ is excreted by the kidneys, and any renal impairment may lead to magnesium retention and toxicity. Monitor the client's fluid intake and output every hour. Carefully measure and document urine output each hour and before administering a dose of $MgSO_4$. Expect to insert an indwelling urinary catheter for accurate monitoring.

Because $MgSO_4$ is not an antihypertensive drug, expect to continue to monitor the client's blood pressure closely, and record these measurements every 15 minutes. If the blood pressure remains significantly elevated, expect

to give a drug such as hydralazine (Apresoline) to control hypertension.

Several drugs may be used in combination to lower blood pressure, induce or augment uterine contractions, and relieve pain. Monitor the client's response to this multiple drug therapy to assess its effectiveness and detect any adverse reactions.

Keep calcium gluconate at the client's bedside in case of $MgSO_4$ overdose. As prescribed, administer 1 g of calcium gluconate in 10 ml of a 10% solution I.V. over 3 minutes.

Expect to continue administering $MgSO_4$ throughout labor and delivery and for at least 24 hours afterward. Document the infusion dosage so that the recovery nurse can continue therapy properly.

Fetal levels of $MgSO_4$ correlate with maternal blood levels. Anticipate continuous fetal monitoring during the intrapartal period. Be aware that $MgSO_4$ therapy may cause a transient loss in beat-to-beat variability with internal fetal monitoring.

Assess for related complications. A small percentage of clients with eclampsia develop pulmonary edema with a nursing diagnosis of *altered cardiopulmonary tissue perfusion related to elevated blood pressure*. To detect this complication, auscultate the client's lungs at least every half hour and monitor her fluid intake and output at least every hour.

According to Roberts (1989), about 20% of clients with PIH are at increased risk for disseminated intravascular coagulation (DIC). Therefore, expect to obtain specimens for clotting studies, and carefully observe all orifices and puncture sites for increased serosanguinous drainage. Report any abnormal findings immediately. If the client shows signs of DIC and spontaneous hemorrhage, prepare for expeditious vaginal or cesarean delivery.

Assist with delivery

Although PIH resolves shortly after delivery, delivery usually is not desirable until the fetus reaches sufficient maturity. However, delivery will be mandatory in a client whose blood pressure cannot be controlled, whose weight gain (from edema) continues despite bed rest, and whose proteinuria increases. In such a client, delivery is justified even when the estimated gestational age falls below 30 weeks (Knupple and Drukker, 1986).

In an unstable client, cesarean delivery is undesirable because it could contribute to maternal stress and complications. Ideally, the fetal-placental unit is monitored closely, the client is stabilized and monitored closely, and she delivers vaginally.

After the client is stabilized, prepare for vaginal or cesarean delivery, depending on her condition and physician management. Ideally, she would deliver vaginally to avoid the complications of surgery. If the cervix is likely to respond to oxytocin—that is, if it is soft, open, and not posterior in position—and the client and fetus are stable, induced vaginal delivery is preferred. If assessments reveal fetal distress or an estimated fetal weight of less than 1,500 g, cesarean delivery is preferred.

As a result of the stress of PIH, the client may have a shorter labor and a precipitous delivery. Prepare to intervene quickly for such a client.

Alert the neonatal team to be present for delivery, especially if the neonate is premature, which is common in clients with severe preeclampsia. Work with the neonatal team and prepare for care of the neonate.

If the client received $MgSO_4$ during labor, prepare for potential neonatal effects. $MgSO_4$ toxicity may occur in the neonate, producing respiratory depression, hypotonia, and hypotension (Knupple and Drukker, 1986).

EVALUATION

The following examples illustrate appropriate evaluation statements:
• The client's blood pressure was stabilized.
• The client's fluid intake and output were balanced.
• The client delivered a stable neonate.
• The client did not develop seizures.
• The client and her neonate remained free of further complications.

DOCUMENTATION

Documentation should include the following:
• maternal vital signs, especially blood pressure measurements
• central venous pressure readings
• respiratory assessment findings
• urine reagent strip results
• deep tendon reflexes
• FHR
• fluid intake and output
• signs of bleeding
• drugs administered and their effects
• $MgSO_4$ levels, if administered.

Rh ISOIMMUNIZATION

Rh isoimmunization refers to sensitization and immune response of maternal blood antibodies to fetal blood antigens, which can create a serious blood incompatibility between the two during pregnancy. This can lead to erythroblastosis fetalis (hydrops fetalis or hemolytic disease of the newborn).

Erythroblastosis fetalis is a serious hemolytic disease of the fetus and neonate that produces anemia; jaundice; liver, spleen, and heart enlargement; and anasarca (severe generalized edema) and may lead to myocardial failure. It also may cause placental hypertrophy, which can contribute to fetal hypoxia and death (Knupple and Drukker, 1986) and accounts for a significant percentage of fetal morbidity and mortality (Queenan, 1985).

Rh isoimmunization results when a client has Rh-negative blood and her fetus has Rh-positive blood. However, this is becoming more rare because most Rh-negative women now receive $Rh_o(D)$ immune globulin (RhoGAM) during antepartal and postpartal care, which provides passive immunization against the Rh antigen.

Today, hemolytic disease of the newborn occurs more commonly when the client develops a sensitivity to other foreign blood antigens. This sensitization is known as nonimmune hydrops fetalis. Maternal factors that contribute to development of nonimmune hydrops include multiple gestation; perinatal infections, especially syphilis or cytomegalovirus infection; previous transfusion of blood that contained foreign antigens; diabetes mellitus; thalassemia; or PIH (Sachs, 1987). (For more information about isoimmunization, see Chapter 9, Antepartal Complications.)

Unlike other high-risk intrapartal clients, the client with Rh isoimmunization does not feel ill. However, if she knows the consequences of isoimmunization, she may experience extreme guilt and anxiety because of her body's actions against her fetus. She may have endured frequent invasive tests and close fetal monitoring to prevent fetal death. She may view the intrapartal period as the culmination of a trying time.

ASSESSMENT

When caring for a client with Rh isoimmunization, the nurse obtains a health history, assists with physical assessment, and collects laboratory tests as for any client who seeks admission for labor and delivery. In addition, the nurse must make specific assessments and be prepared to notify the physician of significant findings.

Health history

When collecting history data from an isoimmunized client, ask about the antepartal progression of the disorder. She may be extremely knowledgeable about the frequent surveillance of her fetus.

Inquire about her obstetric history, which may provide information about Rh problems. For example, her fetus may be at increased risk for developing erythroblastosis fetalis if she did not receive $Rh_o(D)$ immune globulin during her previous pregnancy.

Also, determine the client's expectations for and concerns about her pregnancy. This information may help guide the nursing care plan.

Physical assessment

During the physical assessment, observe for signs of chorioamnionitis, such as maternal or fetal tachycardia, fever, uterine or other abdominal tenderness, and purulent vaginal secretions with rupture of the membranes. An isoimmunized client may develop chorioamnionitis if her amniotic fluid becomes contaminated during intrauterine blood transfusions or amniocentesis, which commonly is performed in pregnant clients with Rh problems.

Also note signs of abruptio placentae, such as a painful, taut abdomen, or hydramnios, such as excessive abdominal distention and dyspnea. These obstetric conditions are associated with isoimmunization.

Laboratory tests

Lung maturity studies, such as L/S ratio and PG level, may guide plans for an isoimmunized client to have a premature delivery.

NURSING DIAGNOSIS

The nurse reviews all health history, physical assessment, and laboratory test findings and then formulates nursing diagnoses appropriate for the client. (For a partial list of applicable diagnoses, see Nursing Diagnoses: *Intrapartal complications,* page 285.)

PLANNING AND IMPLEMENTATION

Because abruptio placentae is more common in isoimmunized clients, observe carefully for signs of vaginal bleeding or uterine tetany, such as continuous uterine contractions without relaxation.

During labor, continuous internal EFM with a fetal scalp electrode to monitor FHR and with an intrauterine pressure catheter to monitor uterine contractions may be employed, depending on gestational age and delivery op-

tions. Closely observe the FHR for signs of fetal distress or hypoxia. Fetal distress in Rh isoimmunized premature fetuses, especially in the absence of labor, indicates the need for cesarean delivery. Hypoxia may result from placentomegaly, which causes insufficient fetal perfusion. Severe fetal hemolysis may lead to congestive heart failure in the fetus. If an abnormal FHR emerges, expect to assist the physician with fetal scalp sampling to estimate fetal tolerance of labor and to determine if cesarean delivery is required.

Labor management

If the client has hydramnios, her uterine contractions may be inefficient, producing uncoordinated labor patterns with coupling (doubling of inefficient contractions) or hypotonic contractions. For such a client, the physician may rupture the membranes by needling them slowly and carefully. This helps prevent a sudden gush of amniotic fluid, which can cause cord prolapse or vertex malpositioning of the fetus on descent.

Promote comfort

Know that analgesia and anesthesia may be restricted during labor because of fetal immaturity and instability. Be prepared to use nonpharmacologic pain relief measures and to offer labor coaching to the client.

EVALUATION

The following examples illustrate appropriate evaluation statements:
• The client expressed an accurate understanding of her condition and that of her fetus.
• The client delivered a stable neonate.

DOCUMENTATION

Documentation should include the following:
• FHR
• signs of maternal bleeding
• maternal vital signs, especially temperature measurements
• maternal labor pattern.

UTERINE DISORDERS

Many uterine factors can affect the progress of labor. Uterine contractions, the primary power of labor, play a critical role in determining whether labor is normal or dysfunctional. (For more information, see *Dysfunctional labor,* page 306.)

Other intrapartal complications related to the uterus include postterm labor, precipitate labor, uterine rupture, uterine inversion, and structural abnormalities.

Dysfunction

Uterine dysfunction may be classified as hypotonic or hypertonic. In hypotonic dysfunction, the more common of the two, contractions grow less frequent and less powerful as labor continues. Eventually, they become too weak to produce adequate cervical dilation. Hypotonic dysfunction typically occurs during the active phase of labor.

Hypertonic dysfunction, which typically occurs during the latent phase of labor, is characterized by intense, painful contractions unaccompanied by normal cervical dilation.

Postterm labor

When pregnancy lasts 42 weeks or longer, labor is considered postterm and may be impeded if the fetus is LGA – a condition that could result in CPD.

Precipitate labor

Characterized by rapid progression, precipitate labor typically lasts less than 3 hours. It may result from decreased resistance of soft tissue in the birth canal or by abnormally strong uterine contractions (Cunningham, MacDonald, and Gant, 1989). Although research suggests that precipitate labor poses no greater risk to the client and fetus than does normal labor (Oxorn, 1986), some experts believe that precipitate labor increases the risk of maternal lacerations and fetal intracranial hemorrhage and asphyxia. Additional risks include unattended delivery, fetal hypoxia from intense uterine contractions, and decreased uterine tone after delivery.

Uterine rupture

A serious medical emergency, rupture of the uterus may occur before or during labor. A complete rupture tears all layers of the uterus, establishing direct communication between the uterine and abdominal cavities. In an incomplete rupture, the myometrium tears, but the peritoneal covering of the uterus remains intact (Oxorn, 1986).

Uterine rupture occurs more frequently after previous cesarean delivery and during prolonged labor, difficult forceps delivery, and oxytocin administration. Although signs and symptoms of uterine rupture vary widely with location and severity, they typically include abdominal pain, vaginal bleeding, hypovolemic shock, and fetal dis-

tress. If rupture occurs during labor, contractions may cease.

Uterine inversion

In this rare, potentially life-threatening emergency, the uterus turns inside out so that its internal surface protrudes into or beyond the vagina. Uterine inversion may occur before or after delivery of the placenta. Although the cause may not be apparent, excessive traction on the umbilical cord and attempts to deliver the placenta manually while the uterus is relaxed may be contributing factors. The client may experience significant blood loss and shock. The clearest sign of uterine inversion is the craterlike depression that forms in the abdomen during the third or fourth stage of labor.

Structural abnormalities

Although uncommon, abnormalities of the uterus, cervix, and vagina may block normal labor and delivery. Improper development may produce duplications of all or part of the reproductive structures (Jackson, 1990). The most common abnormality is a septate uterus.

ASSESSMENT

Nursing assessment of the client with hypotonic or hypertonic dysfunctional labor patterns requires continuous, careful monitoring of labor progress and fetal status. To distinguish hypotonic uterine dysfunction from problems caused by CPD, the nurse-midwife or physician may perform an amniotomy and initiate internal fetal and uterine monitoring.

When assessing contractions, keep in mind that hypertonic uterine dysfunction typically is seen during the latent phase of labor and is characterized by painful contractions of increased intensity. Though painful, the contractions are not able to produce normal cervical dilation.

Critical assessment criteria for possible postterm labor include accurate determination of gestational age and fetus's size. Gestational age can be determined from the client's history (date of last menstrual period and day of quickening), physical assessment, and ultrasonography. The ultrasound examination also will reveal the fetus's size.

Evidence suggests that fetal distress and meconium release occur twice as frequently and meconium aspiration syndrome occurs eight times as frequently in postterm pregnancies as in normal pregnancies (Usher, Boyd, McLean, and Kramer, 1988). Therefore, postterm pregnancies require careful assessment of fetal well-being, including fetal monitoring according to facility policy.

DYSFUNCTIONAL LABOR

When a fetus fails to move out of the uterus and through the birth canal, or when this progression takes an abnormally long time, the client is in dysfunctional labor. (Other terms used to describe dysfunctional labor include dystocia, prolonged labor, and failure to progress.) Experts estimate that dysfunctional labor has a 1% to 7% incidence (Oxorn, 1986). Depending on the circumstances involved, it may threaten the health or life of the client and fetus.

Dysfunctional labor has several causes. Altered uterine muscle contractility can prevent cervical dilation and effacement, thus blocking fetal descent. Altered muscle contractility may result from abnormalities of the uterus or bony pelvis or fetal position and presentation. Administration of narcotic or anesthesic agents, primiparity, and maternal exhaustion are other causes (Oxorn, 1986). In many cases, the cause cannot be identified with certainty.

According to Friedman (1989), the latent phase can be considered prolonged if it exceeds 14 hours for a multiparous client or 20 hours for a nulliparous client.

The most important factors in assessing labor progress are cervical dilation and fetal descent. Without cervical dilation, descent cannot occur. Most nulliparous clients show cervical dilation of at least 1.2 cm per hour during active labor; most multiparous clients dilate by at least 1.5 cm per hour during active labor. Dilation of less than these rates constitutes a prolonged active phase. The active phase is divided into three phases. The acceleration phase occurs when the rate of cervical dilation begins to increase; the phase of maximum slope, when cervical dilation is almost complete; and the deceleration phase, when the rate of cervical dilation slows.

Progression of labor can be depicted by plotting cervical dilation in centimeters against elapsed time. In normal labor, the resulting graph will form an S-shaped curve, as shown below (Friedman, 1989). In dysfunctional labor, the dilation curve will become flattened or strung out.

Effects of prolonged labor on the fetus may include hypoxia, asphyxia, and physical injuries during descent. In many cases, dysfunctional labor is an indication for cesarean delivery.

COMPARISON OF NORMAL AND DYSFUNCTIONAL LABOR PROGRESSION

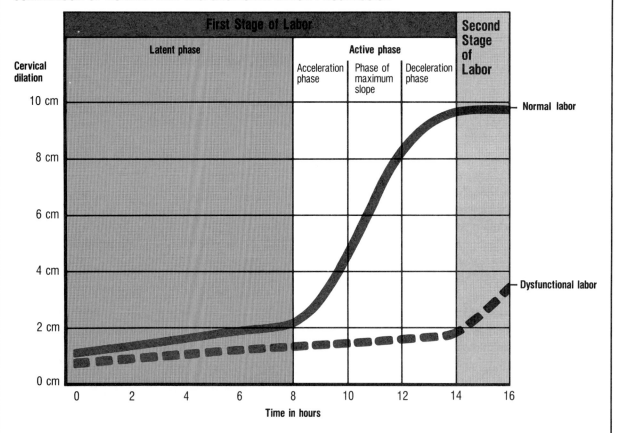

Adapted from Figure 1-1 of *Management of Labor,* 2nd edition, by W.R. Cohen, D.B. Acker, and E.A. Friedman (Eds.), page 5, with permission of Aspen Publishers, Inc., ©1989.

A client with a history of precipitous labors may not progress through the stages of labor in a normal manner; monitor this client closely.

Assessment of uterine rupture requires careful monitoring of bleeding, fetal status, and the client's vital signs and laboratory test results.

When assesing a client with uterine inversion, carefully monitor blood loss and vital signs to detect shock – an emergency situation. Be prepared to assist other members of the health care team in the attempt to reverse the uterus.

Structural abnormalities are assessed by the nurse-midwife or physician.

NURSING DIAGNOSIS

The nurse reviews all health history, physical assessment, and laboratory test findings and then formulates nursing diagnoses appropriate for the client. (For a partial list of applicable diagnoses, see Nursing Diagnoses: *Intrapartal complications,* page 285.)

PLANNING AND IMPLEMENTATION

The fetus of a client with a hypertonic uterine dysfunction may have a nursing diagnosis of *high risk for fetal injury secondary to fetal hypoxia and traumatic delivery.* Continuous, careful monitoring of labor progress and fetal status is essential because fetal hypoxia may occur. Be aware of any signs of fetal distress and be prepared to intervene appropriately.

A client with hypertonic uterine dysfunction may have a nursing diagnosis of *ineffective individual coping related to exhaustion and anxiety.* She may be given narcotic analgesia to produce sleep for several hours. Upon awakening, she may have a normal, progressive labor pattern. This intervention is used only if the membranes are intact and no evidence of fetal distress is detected because this treatment delays delivery (Cunningham, MacDonald, and Gant, 1989).

The client with a dysfunctional labor pattern may have a nursing diagnosis of *pain related to abnormally prolonged labor.* The client and her support person will need updates on labor progress and the results of all assessments. They may grow physically or emotionally exhausted, discouraged, and anxious. To prevent excessive fatigue, suggest rest periods for the support person during times when someone else can attend the client; tell the support person that the client will not be left alone. Provide information and support, as needed, especially if cesarean delivery becomes necessary.

A client with hypotonic uterine dysfunction may have a nursing diagnosis of *anxiety related to abnormally prolonged labor.* Such a client may receive an amniotomy followed by oxytocin to augment her contractions. Although labor augmentation differs from labor induction with oxytocin, take similar precautions and care for the client as if labor were being induced.

A client with postterm labor may undergo labor induction and, if induction fails, cesarean delivery. (See "Cesarean delivery" later in this chapter.)

A client with a history of a precipitous labor will need careful and constant monitoring of fetal and maternal status. Prolonged periods of uterine contractions with decreased periods of uterine relaxation may lead to periods of fetal hypoxia.

If a client experiences uterine rupture, surgical intervention must take place immediately to save the fetus's life and, at times, the client's life. After cesarean delivery, the surgeon will repair the ruptured uterus if it can sustain a future pregnancy or remove it if it cannot. If uterine inversion occurs, immediate interventions must be taken to save the client's life, including blood transfusions and surgical reinversion of the uterus. This emergency situation requires the nurse's assistance.

Some vaginal and cervical anomalies may be repaired surgically; some may not interfere with labor and delivery. Uterine anomalies may contribute to spontaneous abortion, preterm birth, and malpresentation.

Induction of labor

Uterine contractions may be induced through hormone injection or through amniotomy. Induction may be necessitated by an emergency when medical or obstetric problems threaten the health of the client or fetus. The physician also can use labor induction methods to strengthen natural contractions. Occasionally, labor may be induced by choice if the client has a term pregnancy and is free of complications.

The two most common induction methods are amniotomy and intravenous synthetic oxytocin (Pitocin or Syntocinon) infusion. An experimental procedure involves administration of prostaglandin (PGE_2) gel. (For more information, see *Labor induction with PGE_2 gel,* page 308.)

Amniotomy. To accomplish an amniotomy, a physician or nurse-midwife artificially ruptures the amniotic membranes to augment or induce labor. Some call the procedure artificial rupture of the membranes, or AROM. (For an illustration, see *Amniotomy,* page 308.)

The physician or nurse-midwife performs the procedure under sterile conditions with the client in the lithot-

LABOR INDUCTION WITH P.G.E.₂ GEL

Although still experimental, administration of prostaglandin (PGE₂) as a gel into the cervix, vagina, or extra-amniotic space may induce cervical changes and uterine contractions.

To administer PGE₂ gel extra-amniotically, the physician inserts a catheter through the cervical canal and instills 0.3 to 0.4 mg of the drug. The client remains recumbent for at least 1 hour after administration, and the obstetric team continuously monitors the fetal heart rate and uterine activity. The client's vital signs should be checked every hour for the first 4 hours. Most clients will experience mild uterine contractions.

PGE₂ gel causes few adverse effects; vomiting, fever, or diarrhea occur in only about 0.2% of cases. The drug almost never hyperstimulates uterine contractions, and fetal effects are minimal (Rayburn, 1989; Cunningham, MacDonald, and Gant, 1989).

omy position. During and immediately after the procedure, the obstetric team monitors the fetus to ensure that the umbilical cord has not prolapsed.

Amniotomy improves the efficiency of uterine contractions because prostaglandins are released with the rupture of membranes, initiating uterine activity; once this has begun, the release of endogenous oxytocin further stimulates labor (Petrie and Williams, 1986). Amniotomy is most effective when the client's cervix is soft, dilated, anteriorly positioned, and effaced to some degree and the fetal presenting part has contacted the cervix.

AMNIOTOMY

The physician or nurse-midwife dons a sterile glove, guides a sterile amniohook into the cervix, and punctures the amniotic sac to augment or induce labor.

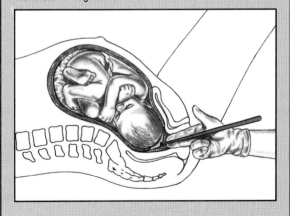

If amniotomy fails to induce labor, the physician may initiate oxytocin infusion. If this fails, cesarean delivery may be required.

Intravenous oxytocin. During natural labor, the posterior lobe of the pituitary gland releases the hormone oxytocin. This hormone stimulates strong, rhythmic contractions of the uterine muscle. Estrogen production increases during pregnancy, which in turn increases the sensitivity of the uterus to minute amounts of oxytocin. Because oxytocin stimulates such a powerful response, the physician can induce labor by infusing minute amounts of it.

Oxytocin infusion may cause excessive or tetanic uterine contractions that last longer than 70 seconds each, occur more often than once every 3 minutes, and increase intrauterine pressure to more than 75 mm Hg. These excessive contractions may rupture the uterus or rush labor and delivery, resulting in cervical and perineal lacerations. They also may reduce oxygen to the fetus, reducing or disrupting heartbeat.

Excessive contractions or reduced FHR warrants an immediate halt to oxytocin infusion. The oxytocin level will drop by half within about 3 minutes, and the tetanic contractions usually will return to a normal level (Cunningham, MacDonald, and Gant, 1989; Hacker and Moore, 1986).

Oxytocin has a potent antidiuretic action. An infusion of 20 mU/min or more markedly decreases the free water clearance of the kidneys, in turn reducing urine production. Avoid giving the client large amounts of fluid, particularly dextrose 5% in water, during oxytocin infusion to avoid possible water intoxication (Cunningham, MacDonald, and Gant, 1989).

EVALUATION

The following examples illustrate appropriate evaluation statements:
- Five hours after initial oxytocin infusion, the client gave birth vaginally.
- The client exhibited no signs of infection after amniotomy.
- The client and her fetus completed labor and delivery safely with little or no additional complications.
- The client and her support person and family received regular updates about her condition and the status of the fetus, as the situation allowed.
- The client remained as comfortable as possible during dysfunctional labor.

• The client and her support person received support and encouragement from the nursing staff during complications.

DOCUMENTATION

Documentation should include the following:
• maternal vital signs
• maternal contraction rate and intensity
• medications given, time of administration, and effectiveness
• oxytocin dosage, time of initiation, and duration of infusion
• fetal heart tones, variability, and any abnormal patterns
• induction methods used, if any
• time of amniotic sac rupture and amount and color of amniotic fluid.

MEMBRANE AND AMNIOTIC FLUID DISORDERS

Several complications may arise during labor that are linked to the membranes and amniotic fluid. They include hydramnios, oligohydramnios, and amniotic fluid embolism.

Hydramnios

Normally, amniotic fluid volume equals approximately 1,000 ml at term. In hydramnios, volume reaches or exceeds 2,000 ml and is associated with fetal anomalies, the most common being congenital anomalies of the central nervous and gastrointestinal systems.

Hydramnios occurs in about 0.9% of all pregnant clients; the risk increases in clients with diabetes. In 90% of mild cases, the cause of hydramnios cannot be determined (Hill, Breckle, Thomas, and Fries, 1987). Ultrasonography and physical assessment are used to diagnose this condition.

Oligohydramnios

The counterpart of hydramnios, oligohydramnios refers to an abnormally small amount of amniotic fluid. Its cause is unknown, but a normal reduction in amniotic fluid after week 36 may create or aggravate the condition in postterm pregnancies. Reduced amniotic fluid is associated with maternal hypertension, fetal congenital anomalies, IUGR, and risk to the fetus's life. Experts are unsure about the degree to which fluid may be reduced before such adverse responses occur.

Amniotic fluid embolism

A rare obstetric disorder, amniotic fluid embolism has a maternal mortality rate approaching 80% (Clark, 1987). The fetal mortality rate also is high. In this syndrome, amniotic fluid enters the maternal circulation and causes respiratory distress and shock (Oxorn, 1986). Classic symptoms include sudden onset of dyspnea and hypotension, possibly followed by cardiopulmonary arrest. Other significant signs include chest pain; cyanosis; frothy, pink-tinged sputum; tachycardia; and hemorrhage. Coagulopathy affects approximately 40% of clients with this syndrome and may be the cause of death in those who survive the initial hemodynamic insult.

Although it occurs primarily during labor, amniotic fluid embolism has occurred during first and second trimester abortions and even during the postpartal period (Clark, 1987). Most clients who die from this disorder do so within 30 minutes after its onset. Diagnosis is confirmed by cytologic detection of fetal squamous cells and lanugo in a blood sample aspirated through the central line used for hemodynamic monitoring.

ASSESSMENT

The client with hydramnios may experience dyspnea during labor and may be comfortable only with the head of the bed elevated. The enlarged uterus also may place additional pressure on the vena cava. Assess the client frequently for supine hypotensive syndrome. The fetus of a client with ogliohydramnios may experience fetal distress from umbilical cord compression and requires close monitoring during labor.

Assess vital signs closely in a client with amniotic fluid embolism, particularly respiration and heart rate. Also monitor blood test results, particularly coagulation studies.

NURSING DIAGNOSIS

The nurse reviews all health history, physical assessment, and laboratory test findings and then formulates nursing diagnoses appropriate for the client. (For a partial list of applicable diagnoses, see Nursing Diagnoses: *Intrapartal complications,* page 285.)

PLANNING AND IMPLEMENTATION

The management of hydramnios depends on the severity of the client's symptoms, which may include dyspnea and increased edema of the legs and vulva from increased uterine pressure on the venous system. The client may experience discomfort severe enough to require hospitalization. Amniocentesis may be able to alleviate the discomfort; however, because fluid production continues, relief is temporary.

When oligohydramnios has been diagnosed before delivery through ultrasonography, prepare the client for possible abnormal fetal appearance, including dry, leathery skin and urinary tract or musculoskeletal anomalies.

The treatment of a client with amniotic fluid embolism includes maintaining oxygenation and cardiac output as well as managing any coagulation problems, recognizing the symptoms of respiratory distress and shock, and knowing emergency procedures for respiratory and cardiac arrest.

EVALUATION

The following examples illustrate appropriate evaluation statements:
• The client and her fetus completed labor and delivery safely with little or no additional complications.
• The client and her support person and family received regular updates about her condition and the status of the fetus, as the situation allowed.
• The client and her support person received support and encouragement from the nursing staff during complications.

DOCUMENTATION

Documentation should include the following:
• maternal vital signs
• maternal contraction rate and intensity
• maternal fluid intake and output
• medications given, time of administration, and effectiveness
• vaginal examinations and results
• vaginal discharge, type, and amount
• laboratory studies and their values
• fetal heart tones, variability, and any abnormal patterns.

UMBILICAL CORD DISORDERS

Anomalies involving the umbilical cord typically are not detected until delivery. Some may threaten the fetus's life. Complications that may arise during labor include abnormal cord implantation, abnormal cord length, and cord prolapse.

Abnormal cord implantation

Normally, the umbilical cord inserts in the center of the placenta. In a velamentous (membranous) insertion, the cord vessels separate into branches before reaching the placenta and the cord inserts into the membranes rather than the placental disk (Oxorn, 1986). Occasionally with a velamentous insertion, fetal vessels in the membranes cross the internal os and take up a position ahead of the fetal presenting part. This potentially serious condition, known as vasa previa, may be discovered during a pelvic examination when the examiner feels vessels through the cervical os (Cunningham, MacDonald, and Gant, 1989).

Abnormal cord length

On average, an umbilical cord measures 55 cm (22″). An excessively long cord raises the risk of knots and prolapse or a nuchal cord. A short cord may contribute to abruptio placentae.

Cord prolapse

Displacement of the umbilical cord to a position at or below the fetus's presenting part most commonly occurs when amniotic membranes rupture before fetal descent. The sudden gush of fluid carries the long, loose cord ahead of the fetus toward and possibly through the client's cervix and into the vagina. Serious damage may occur when the fetus compresses the cord, interrupting blood flow from the placenta. Factors that increase the risk of cord prolapse include hydramnios, more than one fetus, ruptured membranes, a transverse or breech lie, a small fetus, a long umbilical cord, a low-lying placenta, premature delivery, and an unengaged fetal presenting part.

Umbilical cord prolapse incurs a high infant mortality rate if not detected and treated immediately. Diagnosis of cord prolapse is based on observation of the cord outside the vulva, feeling the cord during a vaginal examination, or observation of fetal distress. (For more information, see Emergency Alert: *Umbilical cord prolapse.*)

ASSESSMENT

In a client with possible cord prolapse, auscultate fetal heart tones to assess well-being. If the fetus shows any signs of distress, expect to assist with a vaginal examination.

In a client with vasa previa, the nurse-midwife or physician may feel the cord vessels through the cervical os. Abnormal cord length, however, cannot be assessed before delivery.

UMBILICAL CORD PROLAPSE

If not corrected within 5 minutes, umbilical cord prolapse may cause fetal hypoxia, central nervous system damage, and possible death. Fortunately, rapid assessment and intervention by the health care team can help the client and fetus survive this traumatic event. Discussed below are the signs and symptoms of cord prolapse and appropriate interventions until emergency cesarean or forceps delivery can take place.

Signs and symptoms
• Client reports feeling the cord "slither" down after membrane rupture
• Visible or palpable umbilical cord in the birth canal
• Violent fetal activity
• Fetal bradycardia with variable deceleration during contractions

Nursing considerations
• Immediately summon another member of the health care team who can notify the physician and prepare the team for a prompt delivery or emergency surgery.
• Place the client in a Trendelenburg or knee-chest position with her hips elevated. Either position will shift the fetus's weight off the cord. (Two gloved fingers also can assist in pushing the fetus's presenting part off the cord while the operating room is being prepared.)
• Do not attempt to press or push the cord back into the uterus. This may traumatize the cord, stop blood flow to the fetus, or start an intrauterine infection.
• Expect to assist in giving the client supplemental oxygen by face mask at 10 to 12 liters/minute, initiating or increasing I.V. fluids with 5% dextrose in lactated Ringer's solution (to enhance fluid volume and circulation), and sending blood for type and crossmatch (if this was not done on admission).
• Expect to assist in monitoring fetal heart tones with an internal fetal scalp electrode on the presenting part.
• Do not attempt to reinsert the cord if it protrudes from the vagina. Instead, lift it with gloved hands and gently wrap it in loose, sterile towels saturated with sterile saline solution.
• Keep the client informed throughout this emergency. Calmly convey the seriousness of the situation and emphasize the importance of cooperation. Reassure the client and her family that the medical and nursing staff will do everything possible to ensure a safe and successful delivery.
• Accompany the client to the operating room, continuing to keep pressure off the cord and monitoring for signs of maternal and fetal distress.

NURSING DIAGNOSIS

The nurse reviews all health history, physical assessment, and laboratory test findings and then formulates nursing diagnoses appropriate for the client. (For a partial list of applicable diagnoses, see Nursing Diagnoses: *Intrapartal complications,* page 285.)

PLANNING AND IMPLEMENTATION

In a client with vasa previa, the examiner may feel the cord vessels through the cervical os. Because rupture of these vessels could cause the fetus to exsanguinate before emergency cesarean delivery could be performed, the client should be kept on bed rest, and the cervical os should not be probed or manipulated. Expect a cesarean delivery.

Abnormal cord length can lead to other complications, such as cord prolapse or abruptio placentae; know the proper nursing care for these complications.

In a client with potential cord prolapse, a vaginal examination is performed if any signs of fetal distress exist or when the membranes rupture, especially in a client with twins, a malpositioned fetus, or an immature fetus. A nursing diagnosis for a client with a prolapsed cord might be *high risk for fetal compromise related to alteration in the fetal-placental unit.*

EVALUATION

The following examples illustrate appropriate evaluation statements:
• The client and her fetus completed labor and delivery safely with little or no additional complications.
• The client and her support person and family received regular updates about her condition and the status of the fetus, as the situation allowed.
• The client and her support person received support and encouragement from the nursing staff during complications.

DOCUMENTATION

Documentation should include the following:
• maternal vital signs
• maternal contraction rate and intensity
• maternal fluid intake and output
• medications given, time of administration, and effectiveness
• vaginal examinations and results
• vaginal discharge, type, and amount

• laboratory studies and their values
• fetal heart tones, variability, and any abnormal patterns
• interventions used to correct umbilical cord prolapse.

PLACENTAL DISORDERS

Placental abnormalities may become apparent during pregnancy, or they may remain undetected until labor or just after delivery (the puerperium). During any stage, they present a major risk to the client and fetus. The most common placental complications include placenta previa, abruptio placentae, and failure of placental separation.

Placenta previa

When the placenta forms near or over the cervical os instead of taking a position higher in the body of the uterus, the client risks mild to potentially life-threatening hemorrhage, depending on the location of the placenta. Four classifications describe this abnormality:
• Complete (or total) placenta previa, where the placenta covers the cervical os completely
• Partial placenta previa, where the placenta covers the os partially
• Marginal placenta previa, where an edge of the placenta meets the rim of the cervical os but does not occlude it
• Low-lying placenta, where the placenta implants in the lower uterine segment and a placental edge lies close to the cervical os.

Placenta previa occurs in 0.4% to 0.6% of pregnancies (Cunningham, MacDonald, and Gant, 1989). Incidence increases with multiparity, previous cesarean delivery, advanced maternal age, twin fetuses, and abnormal fetal lie (Ouimette, 1986).

The main symptom of placenta previa is painless vaginal bleeding after the twentieth week of pregnancy. In some clients, bleeding may not occur until labor begins. When bleeding begins before the onset of labor, it tends to be episodic, beginning without warning, stopping spontaneously, and beginning again later. The client may experience slow, steady bleeding that could affect blood count. Typically, the uterus is soft and nontender.

Diagnosis of placenta previa is based on the client's history, ultrasound examination, and physical assessment. Any pregnant client who reports an episode of painless, vaginal bleeding of sudden onset requires hospitalization and ultrasonography to display the location of the placenta. Laboratory studies should include a complete blood count, coagulation studies, and a type and crossmatch if bleeding is severe. To avoid potentially severe hemorrhage, the client should not have a manual pelvic examination until results of the ultrasound examination are available, especially if the fetus is premature. Severe hemorrhage warrants immediate emergency delivery. (See "Cesarean delivery" later in this chapter.)

Abruptio placentae

In approximately 1 in 75 to 90 pregnancies, some or all of the placenta separates from the uterine wall after the twentieth week of gestation and before delivery (Abdella, Sibae, Hays, and Anderson, 1984). Called abruptio placentae, this condition may threaten the life of the client and fetus. (For more information, see *Comparing placenta previa and abruptio placentae.*)

Although the primary cause of abruptio placentae is unknown, the following conditions may contribute to it: maternal hypertension, a short umbilical cord that places traction on the placenta, trauma, a uterine anomaly or tumor, sudden decompression of the uterus, pressure on the vena cava from the enlarged uterus, and dietary deficiency (Cunningham, MacDonald, and Gant, 1989).

Whether an abruption involves a small area of the placenta or total separation, vaginal bleeding after the twentieth week of pregnancy and constant abdominal pain are its classic signs. Additional signs may also include uterine tenderness or back pain, fetal distress, frequent contractions, hypertonic uterus, preterm labor, and fetal demise. Reliance on bleeding alone for diagnosis may be misleading because the presence and severity of vaginal bleeding may vary with the extent and location of placental separation. For example, vaginal bleeding will occur when a placental edge separates and blood flows between the placenta and uterine wall, escaping through the cervix. Vaginal bleeding will not occur when the center of the placenta separates but the edges remain attached. In this case, hemorrhage severe enough to cause fetal death could be concealed between the placenta and the uterine wall.

Diagnosis of abruptio placentae should be based on the client's history, physical assessment, and ultrasound examination. Most often, a client will report an episode of vaginal bleeding, typically accompanied by continuous abdominal pain. In some cases, she may report uterine contractions. Fetal monitoring may show distress; ultrasound examination may reveal a retroplacental hematoma. Even if ultrasound reveals no bleeding, a tentative diagnosis of abruptio placentae should be made if the client does not have placenta previa (which also would be revealed by ultrasound) and preparations must be made for immediate delivery.

COMPARING PLACENTA PREVIA AND ABRUPTIO PLACENTAE

By distinguishing between similar placental abnormalities, the nurse can anticipate care measures that the health care team must take.

PLACENTA PREVIA	ABRUPTIO PLACENTAE
Description	
Development of the placenta in the lower uterine segment. Classified according to the degree that it obstructs the cervical os.	Premature separation of some or all of the normally implanted placenta from the uterine wall. Classified according to the type of hemorrhage and degree of separation.
Signs and symptoms	
Abdomen appears normal; painless bleeding; uterus soft, except during contractions; fetus palpable; fetal heart tones almost always present; fetal movement not affected.	Abdomen distended, tense, and painful (boardlike); possible concealed hemorrhage; fetus nonpalpable; possible signs of fetal distress; if fetus has died, fetal heart tones absent, no fetal movement.
Management	
Bed rest; vaginal or cesarean delivery; vaginal examinations are contraindicated; Trendelenburg position to prevent shock.	Immediate cesarean or vaginal delivery to preserve the life of a live fetus or prevent further bleeding with a dead fetus.
Complications	
Hemorrhage; shock; infection; maternal or fetal death.	Hemorrhagic shock; hypofibrinogenemia; disseminated intravascular coagulation; hemorrhage into the myometrium; renal failure (acute tubular necrosis); maternal or fetal death.

Failure of placental separation

The placenta normally separates from the uterine wall within 10 minutes after fetal delivery. Occasionally, however, placental separation may be delayed – a condition known as retained placenta. Separation may not occur at all – a condition known as abnormal adherence that takes one of three forms: placenta accreta, placenta increta, or placenta percreta.

Retained placenta. When spontaneous placental separation does not occur within 30 minutes after fetal delivery, the nurse-midwife or physician may attempt to remove the retained placenta manually.

Abnormal adherence. In some clients, absence of the decidua basalis allows the placenta to adhere too firmly to the uterine wall. Known as placenta accreta, this condition may occur over the entire placenta or only in a portion of it (Cunningham, MacDonald, and Gant, 1989). In placenta increta, the placental villi invade the myometrium. In placenta percreta, the villi penetrate to the peritoneal covering of the uterus, sometimes causing uterine rupture.

Although the etiology of these conditions is unknown, predisposing factors may include placenta previa, previous cesarean delivery, previous curettage, and multiparity. Incidence of these abnormalities is unknown as well, but placenta accreta is the most commonly reported of the three conditions.

ASSESSMENT

Assessment of a client with placenta previa includes careful monitoring of bleeding, fetal status, vital signs, and laboratory test results. Assess vaginal bleeding by monitoring the client's perineal and bed pads. Continuous bleeding calls for I.V. fluid replacement; blood transfusions may be needed if hemorrhage occurs. Fetal monitoring may be continuous. Vital signs, level of consciousness, skin color and temperature, and pain as well as events preceding the bleeding also are necessary assessment data. Monitor the results of all laboratory tests, which will be performed more frequently if bleeding becomes more severe.

Assessment of a client with abruptio placentae is similar to that for placenta previa. However, because fetal distress is much more likely to occur, fetal assessment must be continuous for a suspected abruption. Also, abruptio placentae can lead to DIC; therefore, monitor the client for signs of this condition. (For more information, see "Systemic disorders" later in this chapter.)

Retained placenta is assessed by measuring the time between fetal and placental delivery; an interval of 30 minutes or more indicates retained placenta. The nurse-midwife or physician assesses for placenta accreta, increta, or percreta.

History data of the client with any of these conditions may show previous intrauterine fetal death, placenta previa, abruptio placentae, or preeclampsia or eclampsia.

NURSING DIAGNOSIS

The nurse reviews all health history, physical assessment, and laboratory test findings and then formulates nursing diagnoses appropriate for the client. (For a partial list of applicable diagnoses, see Nursing Diagnoses: *Intrapartal complications,* page 285.)

PLANNING AND IMPLEMENTATION

Placental problems can cause unexpected complications or profuse bleeding that may alarm the client. If placenta previa is diagnosed and the fetus is immature, the client may be hospitalized and on prolonged bed rest. If further bleeding episodes occur, the client may receive an intravenous line with a large-bore intra-catheter for fluid replacement and possible blood product transfusion. She may be transferred to a high-risk perinatal center for further care. The client with placenta previa may have a nursing diagnosis of *anxiety related to uncertain perinatal outcome.* Continuously provide the client and family with updated information to allay anxiety. Assess the coping mechanisms of the client and her family and determine the strength of their support systems; assist family members in verbalizing fears and concerns. Share information to clarify misconceptions and to make them feel involved.

Be aware of the anxiety that is experienced by the client with placenta previa and her family. The client and family may have a nursing diagnosis of *anxiety related to uncertain maternal outcome.* These feelings will occur not only during an episode of bleeding but until delivery because of the possibility of additional episodes of bleeding. Guidance and teaching will assist the family in dealing with these fears and will provide an understanding of the complication and the necessary interventions.

Complete and partial previas always warrant cesarean delivery; with marginal previa or a low-lying placenta, a vaginal delivery may be possible. Monitor the client closely during labor because marginal previa may develop into a partial obstruction as the cervix dilates; prepare the client and her family for either method of delivery.

The client may develop a nursing diagnosis of *high risk for alteration in maternal hemodynamic status caused by hemorrhage.* Expect immediate cesarean delivery regardless of the fetus's gestational age. However, if hemorrhage is not severe, bed rest may allow the pregnancy to continue until the fetus is viable or mature. Delivery then may be cesarean or vaginal, depending on the type of previa involved. If hemorrhage occurs, expect to monitor vital signs and fetal status and to administer fluids and blood, as prescribed.

Treatment and interventions for the client with abruptio placentae will depend on the degree of the abruption. Nursing interventions are similar to those for a client with placenta previa; however, fetal status must be monitored continually because rapid onset of fetal distress is more likely with abruptio placentae. In addition, monitor coagulation studies closely because of the risk of DIC.

If the client with abruptio placentae requires emergency procedures, keep the family informed as they occur, and be sensitive to the family's needs during the crisis.

Prepare the client and her family if a cesarean delivery is necessary. They may see' it as a disappointment or failure, but that feeling may be balanced by the delivery of a healthy neonate.

Treatment and interventions for the client with abruptio placentae depend on the degrees of abruption, hemorrhage, and resulting fetal distress. If abruption, hemorrhage, and fetal distress are severe, an appropriate nursing diagnosis would be *high risk for fetal compromise related to premature delivery and inadequate placental perfusion.* Emergency delivery is performed regardless of the fetus's gestational age. Support the client and inform her about the measures that will be taken.

When blood loss is not severe and no evidence of fetal distress is found, interventions may be less urgent. If the client is in labor with a full-term fetus, a vaginal delivery may be possible.

If a client's placenta fails to separate spontaneously within 30 minutes after fetal delivery, the physician may attempt to remove it manually (after administering adequate anesthesia or analgesia) by inserting one hand into the uterus and gently peeling the placenta away from the uterine wall. The client may require a dilatation and curretage (D&C) procedure afterward to ensure that all fragments have been removed. She also may receive an oxytocic drug to promote uterine contractions and reduce bleeding.

The treatment of a client with placenta accreta depends on the amount of placenta adhering to the uterine wall and subsequent hemorrhage. A small accreta may be managed by D&C; an oxytocic drug may be used to control bleeding. Total accreta, increta, or percreta require hysterectomy. Nursing care also depends on the amount of adhering placenta, the severity of blood loss, and whether hysterectomy was performed.

Cesarean delivery

Surgical incision of the abdominal and uterine walls allows cesarean delivery. The reasons for cesarean delivery encompass five general categories (Cunningham, MacDonald, and Gant, 1989).

• Dystocia (difficult or abnormal delivery) accounts for about 29% of all cesarean deliveries. The most common cause of dystocia is CPD, which results from a large fetus, malpresentation, a contracted pelvis, or—in rare cases—a tumor that blocks the birth canal.

• Previous cesarean delivery is the cause in 35% of all cesarean deliveries.

• Breech presentation prompts 10% of cesarean deliveries. This indication is becoming more common, particularly in nulliparous clients. Although vaginal delivery is still the method of choice, many practitioners consider cesarean delivery safer for breech fetuses.

• Fetal distress is the indication in 8% of all cases.

• Other indications account for the remaining 18% of cesarean deliveries. These include herpes simplex type 2 or condylomata acuminata lesions in the birth canal. Both are potentially dangerous if transmitted to the fetus during delivery. Condylomatous lesions also may obstruct the birth canal.

All methods of obstetric anesthesia pose some risks for the client and fetus that must be weighed against benefits when choosing an anesthetic agent. Choice of an agent should reflect the circumstances and the client's desires. If the client wishes to witness the delivery, the choice typically is spinal or epidural anesthesia. In an emergency requiring immediate cesarean delivery, a rapid-induction general anesthesia may be the type of choice.

Once the client is anesthetized, the physician selects one of several methods to section the skin of the lower abdomen and the uterine wall. (For more information, see *Types of incisions for cesarean delivery,* page 316.) If time is adequate and the client and fetus are normal, the physician makes a transverse incision at or just below the pubic hairline.

Much less common today is the classical incision, in which the physician cuts vertically through the body of the uterus. This type of incision increases the possibility of rupture during subsequent pregnancies.

Prepare for cesarean delivery. A client who discovers that she must undergo cesarean delivery may have a nursing diagnosis of *fear related to real or potential threat to fetus or self.* To prepare the client and her family for surgery, begin by explaining all steps in the procedure and ensuring that the client has given her written consent.

Next, take the client to the labor and delivery area or surgical unit, according to facility policy, for physical preparation. This typically includes:

• *Abdominal preparation or shaving.* Although the actual area of incision may vary, facility policy may instruct the nurse to shave the entire abdomen, beginning below the nipple line and including the pubic area.

• *Catheterization.* Establish an indwelling urinary catheter with a gravity flow drainage system to prevent bladder distention during surgery.

• *Laboratory tests.* Obtain the tests ordered by the physician, possibly including complete blood count, electrolytes, and type and cross match for blood replacement.

• *I.V. infusion.* Begin an infusion with the prescribed solution using a 16G to 18G needle.

• *Antacid administration.* As prescribed, administer an antacid 15 minutes before anesthesia administration to reduce the complications associated with possible aspiration of gastric contents.

• *Positioning.* Assist the client into an appropriate position on the delivery or surgical table. Manipulate the table position to prevent the gravid uterus from compressing the inferior vena cava and to help maintain adequate placental perfusion.

• *Preparation.* Clean the operation site using the recommended antiseptic solution, prepare the support person if one is to attend the delivery, notify the nursery staff and pediatrician, gown and glove the physicians and scrub nurses, check suction and other delivery room equipment for proper functioning, and perform an initial sponge count.

• *Assistance.* During the procedure itself, assist the surgical team as needed and maintain records as required. Document the starting time of the procedure, the time of delivery, and the completion time. Immediately after delivery, assist in caring for the neonate as needed. (See Chapter 14, The Second Stage of Labor, for more information.)

TYPES OF INCISIONS FOR CESAREAN DELIVERY

Skin incisions for cesarean delivery are either vertical or transverse. Uterine incisions are either vertical through the body of the uterus, vertical through the lower uterine segment, or transverse through the lower uterine segment.

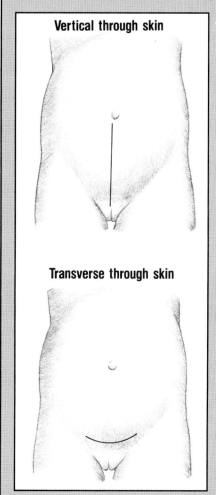

Vertical through skin

Transverse through skin

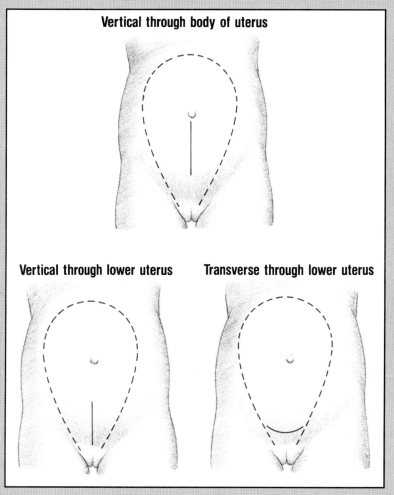

Vertical through body of uterus

Vertical through lower uterus

Transverse through lower uterus

EVALUATION

The following examples illustrate appropriate evaluation statements:
- The client expressed decreased anxiety when discussing the usual outcomes of cesarean delivery.
- The support person provided psychological support for the client during cesarean delivery.
- The client and support person expressed acceptance and understanding of the need for the procedure.
- The client and her fetus completed labor and delivery safely with little or no additional complications.
- The client and her support person and family received regular updates about her condition and the status of the fetus, as the situation allowed.
- The client and her support person received support and encouragement from the nursing staff during complications.

DOCUMENTATION

Documentation should include the following:
- maternal vital signs
- maternal contraction rate and intensity
- maternal fluid intake and output
- medications given, time of administration, and effectiveness
- laboratory studies and their values
- fetal heart tones, variability, and any abnormal patterns
- specific steps taken to prepare the client for cesarean delivery.

PELVIC DISORDERS

Critical to normal fetal descent is the relationship between the size of the pelvis and the size and presentation of the fetus. Complications develop when the pelvis is too small (contracted) to allow normal fetal descent. Additional complications involving obstructed fetal descent include lacerations of the vaginal canal and surrounding soft tissues. For this reason, the physician or nurse-midwife may elect an episiotomy.

Structural contractures

The pelvis may be contracted at the inlet, midpelvis, or outlet, or it may be generally small. This may not be a problem with a small fetus. With a fetus of normal or above-normal size, however, contracture may prevent passage.

The client has a contracted pelvic inlet when the anteroposterior diameter measures less than 10 cm or when the diagonal conjugate measures less than 11.5 cm. The client has a contracted midpelvis when the interspinous diameter measures less than 10 cm and a contracted outlet when the interischial tuberous diameter measures 8 cm or less. A contracted outlet rarely occurs without a contracted midpelvis.

With a normal fetopelvic relationship, uterine contractions gradually rotate the fetus's head to an anterior position that provides the most favorable adaptation between the head and the pelvis. A contracted pelvis may prevent this internal rotation, possibly placing the fetus's head in the transverse position. As with other causes of arrested fetal descent, this abnormal rotation will impair cervical dilation and may lead to a decrease in the frequency and intensity of uterine contractions. This would lead to a cesarean delivery after a diagnosis of arrest of cervical dilation is made.

Lacerations

During delivery, the soft tissues of the birth canal commonly sustain trauma and lacerations of the cervix, vagina, or perineum.

If the client is bleeding heavily after expelling the placenta and her fundus is firm, suspect a cervical laceration. Small cervical lacerations occur commonly during delivery and may not need repair. Severe lacerations, possibly affecting the upper vagina, will require surgical attention. Expect the cervix to be examined after a difficult vaginal delivery.

Lacerations of the lower portion of the birth canal may be classified by severity:

- First-degree lacerations involve the fourchette, perineal skin, and vaginal mucous membranes.
- Second-degree lacerations extend to the fascia and muscles of the perineal body.
- Third-degree lacerations extend to the anal sphincter.
- Fourth-degree lacerations extend to the anal canal.

ASSESSMENT

For a client with structural contractures, assess labor progress, particularly cervical dilation and the frequency and intensity of uterine contractions. Because prolonged labor can endanger the fetus, monitor fetal status closely.

During the postpartal period, assess for abnormal bleeding in the client with perineal lacerations.

NURSING DIAGNOSIS

The nurse reviews all health history, physical assessment, and laboratory test findings and then formulates nursing diagnoses appropriate for the client. (For a partial list of applicable diagnoses, see Nursing Diagnoses: *Intrapartal complications,* page 285.)

PLANNING AND IMPLEMENTATION

When caring for a client in labor who has a pelvic condition that may prolong labor, be supportive and alert for impending complications. The client with a contracted pelvis will need constant monitoring of maternal and fetal status because her labor may be arrested. Such a client may have a nursing diagnosis of *fatigue related to prolonged labor.* Keep the client informed of labor progress.

The client with a contracted pelvis may have a nursing diagnosis of *anxiety related to uncertain perinatal outcome.* The client and her support person will need constant updating of the status of her labor. Providing support and reassurance will help them to cope with the possibility of a cesarean delivery. They also will need support and reassurance that they have not failed if a vaginal delivery is impossible.

The client with a contracted pelvis may have a nursing diagnosis of *ineffective individual coping related to exhaustion and anxiety.* When a client has a contracted pelvis, the fetus's presenting part may not engage in the inlet, making cesarean delivery necessary. Even if the presenting part can engage, the fetus may not descend adequately and the cervix may not dilate normally. Rupture of the membranes without adequate engagement creates an open space between the fetus and pelvis, increasing the risk of uterine cord prolapse.

FORCEPS DELIVERY

The physician positions and then locks the blades over the parietal bones in the fetus's skull and pulls the fetus downward and outward through the birth canal during uterine contractions. Once the fetus's head clears the perineum, the rest of the body emerges easily.

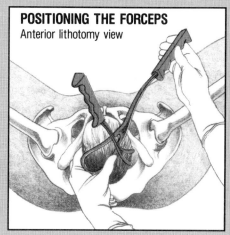

POSITIONING THE FORCEPS
Anterior lithotomy view

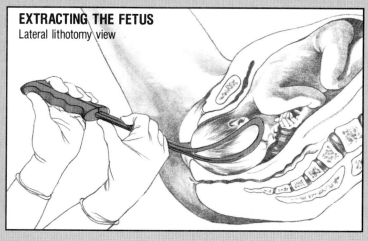

EXTRACTING THE FETUS
Lateral lithotomy view

Because labor is prolonged, the client risks exhaustion and intrauterine infection; she also may have a nursing diagnosis of *high risk for fetal injury secondary to fetal hypoxia and traumatic delivery*. If the fetus passes through the contracted area, cranial molding can be excessive. Vaginal delivery may require forceps or vacuum extraction.

Lacerations of the birth canal may be prevented or minimized by episiotomy. Episiotomy may be accomplished by two methods. The most common in the United States is a median episiotomy. Using round-tipped scissors, the physician or nurse-midwife cuts straight downward from the vaginal orifice. In the alternative method— mediolateral episiotomy—the cut is oblique, angling away from the anus.

Before episiotomy takes place, the fetus's head (or buttocks in a breech presentation) should be low enough to keep the perineum stretched. Ideally, it should be bulging and thinned. Waiting until this stage to perform the procedure lessens bleeding because thinner tissue contains fewer blood vessels. However, the physician or nurse-midwife should make the incision before the muscles supporting the rectum and bladder are severely stretched.

Even with an episiotomy, delivery may extend the incision to the anal sphincter (a third-degree laceration) or to the anal canal (a fourth-degree laceration). These extensions can cause pain, excessive blood loss, suture separation, fistula formation, or even permanent sphincter dysfunction (Borgetta, Piening, and Cohen, 1989). Blood loss usually is greater and repair more difficult and pain-

ful with the mediolateral episiotomy because the incision is through thicker tissue.

Research suggests that clients who massage the perineum during the 6 weeks before delivery may decrease the risk of laceration and the need for episiotomy.

A client with lacerations receives the same treatment as one who has had an episiotomy. If the lacerations are third- or fourth-degree, the client should receive nothing by rectum, including postpartal suppositories and enemas.

Forceps delivery

In this procedure, the physician uses two curved, articulated, blunt metal blades to extract the fetus from the birth canal or to rotate the fetus. (For more information, see *Forceps delivery*.)

Fetal station determines the type of forceps used. Low or outlet forceps may be appropriate when the head has reached the perineum (+2 station) and is visibly separating the labia. Forceps can help the client push the fetus out, shortening the second stage of labor. Use of low forceps is relatively safe; complications usually are limited to bruising of the fetus's head and minor perineal, vaginal, or cervical trauma.

If the head is engaged but not visible at the perineum and the vertex of the skull is at the ischial tuberosities, the physician may use mid forceps. However, use of mid forceps is rare because it endangers the client and fetus. Use of high forceps—when the head is unengaged and the vertex of the skull is located above the ischial spines—is extremely rare because of considerable risk to the client and fetus (Oxorn, 1986). Mid or high forceps can fracture the fetus's skull (Korones, 1986). Furthermore, use of forceps does not always guarantee delivery. Today, most physicians perform a cesarean delivery rather than using mid or high forceps (Laub, 1985).

Vacuum extraction

This procedure is popular in Europe but less common in the United States (Galvan and Broekhuizen, 1987). To accomplish vacuum extraction, the physician uses a suction-cup device known as a ventouse. Ventouses are available in several diameters, including 30, 40, 50, and 60 mm. The physician uses the largest cup size possible to minimize trauma to the fetus's scalp, especially to a suture line or fontanel.

The ventouse is attached by tubing to a suction pump. After positioning the ventouse on the fetus's scalp, air is pumped out of the space between the cup and the scalp, creating a vacuum. By pulling a chain or cord attached to the ventouse, the physician draws the fetus through the birth canal.

Those who favor vacuum extraction believe that it decreases delivery time. They also point out that the procedure does not require additional space inside the vaginal canal, as forceps do.

Vaginal birth after cesarean delivery

In vaginal birth after cesarean delivery (VBAC), a client who has had a cesarean delivery attempts to deliver vaginally. This approach offers several advantages over repeated cesarean deliveries:
• family experience of a normal childbirth
• reduced risk of infection and death
• less discomfort than cesarean delivery
• less recovery time than cesarean delivery
• less cost than cesarean delivery (Laufer, et al., 1987).

Physicians disagree about the extent of the disadvantages in attempting vaginal delivery after an earlier cesarean delivery. One complicating issue is that the reasons for the first cesarean delivery may still be valid. Another is the risk of uterine rupture. Early studies showed that vaginal delivery after an earlier cesarean delivery performed with a low vertical uterine incision commonly led to rupture, massive maternal shock, and extrusion of the fetus into the abdomen. Over the past two decades, however, physicians have used the low transverse incision almost exclusively. Only 0.25% to 0.5% of these scars rupture and, of those that do, about 90% involve only separation of the myometrial covering of the uterus. These ruptures cause no symptoms and little or no bleeding. No

deaths have been reported from such a rupture in more than 20 years (Laufer, et al., 1987).

The American College of Obstetricians and Gynecologists (1988) established specific criteria and guidelines for the client attempting VBAC. Although some physicians and facilities continue to avoid the procedure, it has become more common.

Criteria for VBAC include:
• previous uterine incision made in the low transverse position
• client desire to try vaginal delivery
• early notification of client's wishes to the physician
• available blood for transfusion
• an obstetric team prepared to perform cesarean delivery if necessary
• physician available during the entire labor
• no client medical problems that contraindicate VBAC.

EVALUATION

The following examples illustrate appropriate evaluation statements:
• Edema of the neonate's scalp resolved within 48 hours after vacuum extraction.
• The client and support person expressed acceptance and understanding of the need for the procedure.
• The client and her fetus completed labor and delivery safely with little or no additional complications.
• The client and her support person and family received regular updates about her condition and the status of the fetus, as the situation allowed.
• The client and her support person received support and encouragement from the nursing staff during complications.

DOCUMENTATION

Documentation should include the following:
• maternal vital signs
• maternal contraction rate and intensity
• maternal fluid intake and output
• medications given, time of administration, and effectiveness
• laboratory studies and their values
• fetal heart tones, variability, and any abnormal patterns
• I.V. administration of fluids or medications
• description and location of marks left on the neonate's head from forceps delivery
• perineal care delivered after episiotomy
• the client's expressed wish to attempt VBAC.

SYSTEMIC DISORDERS

Complications involving hemorrhage, shock, and disseminated intravascular coagulation (DIC) can occur at any time during labor and delivery.

Hemorrhage and shock

Many factors predispose the client to hemorrhage and subsequent shock, including placenta previa, abruptio placentae, uterine rupture, and lacerations during delivery. (See Chapter 25, Postpartal Complications, for a more detailed description.)

Disseminated intravascular coagulation

A pathological form of diffuse rather than localized clotting, DIC leads to massive internal and external hemorrhage as clotting factors (such as fibrinogen) are consumed. Intrauterine fetal death, abruptio placentae, septic shock, or amniotic fluid embolism can initiate normal clotting mechanisms. If these clotting factors are depleted, DIC may occur.

Diagnosis of DIC usually is made by laboratory studies that show a decreased fibrinogen and platelet count, increased prothrombin and partial thromboplastin times, and increased fibrinogen degradation products.

ASSESSMENT

To assess a client who may have DIC, observe for signs of excessive or abnormal vaginal bleeding, hematuria, bleeding from the gums or nose, prolonged bleeding from injection or other trauma sites, petechiae, and ecchymoses. Determine if the client has a history of intrauterine fetal death, abruptio placentae, or preeclampsia or eclampsia. Carefully monitor laboratory test results, particularly coagulation studies.

To assess for hemorrhage and shock, check maternal vital signs frequently for increased heart rate, decreased blood pressure, or widening pulse pressure. Assess vaginal discharge and any increase in vaginal bleeding that would indicate hemorrhage.

NURSING DIAGNOSIS

The nurse reviews all health history, physical assessment, and laboratory test findings and then formulates nursing diagnoses appropriate for the client. (For a partial list of applicable diagnoses, see Nursing Diagnoses: *Intrapartal complications,* page 285.)

PLANNING AND IMPLEMENTATION

The client with potential for hemorrhage and shock and possibly DIC is at risk, as is her fetus. She may have a nursing diagnosis of *high risk for alteration in maternal hemodynamic status caused by hemorrhage.* The client with any bleeding condition that could possibly progress to hemorrhage, shock, and DIC should be monitored for coagulation studies.

Treatment of a client with DIC must include treatment of the causative factor as well as aggressive support of blood volume and pressure. The client may require replacement of blood components, such as platelets or fresh frozen plasma (Weiner, 1987). Diagnosis of DIC typically is made by laboratory studies that indicate decreased fibrinogen and platelet count; increased bleeding, prothrombin, and partial thromboplastin times; and increased levels of fibrinogen and fibrin degradation products. Vigilant monitoring of laboratory studies is essential. Prepare the client for the possibility of blood transfusions and component replacement.

A client who understands the seriousness of her condition may have a nursing diagnosis of *anxiety related to uncertain perinatal outcome.* Provide emotional support during emergency procedures.

EVALUATION

The following examples illustrate appropriate evaluation statements:
- The client and her fetus completed labor and delivery safely with little or no additional complications.
- The client and her support person and family received regular updates about her condition and the status of the fetus, as the situation allowed.
- The client's coagulation studies remained within normal limits despite bleeding problems, and DIC was avoided.
- The client and her support person received support and encouragement from the nursing staff during complications.

DOCUMENTATION

Documentation should include the following:
- maternal vital signs
- maternal contraction rate and intensity
- maternal fluid intake and output
- medications given, time of administration, and effectiveness
- vaginal examinations and results
- vaginal discharge, type, and amount

- laboratory studies, including coagulation studies, and their values
- fetal heart tones, variability, and any abnormal patterns.

FETAL COMPLICATIONS

Many fetal factors can affect the progress of labor, including malpresentation, malposition, macrosomia, shoulder dystocia, and intrauterine fetal death. (For more information, see Emergency Alert: *Signs of fetal distress.*)

Malpresentation

When the fetal presenting part is not the head, the condition is known as a malpresentation. Examples of malpresentations include breech, shoulder, and face.

The most common malpresentation is breech, which occurs in 3% to 4% of births and more frequently in twins (Cunningham, MacDonald, and Gant, 1989; Oxorn, 1986). Currently in the United States, approximately 80% of breech fetuses that reach term are delivered by cesarean (Flanagan, Mulchahey, Korenbrot, Green, and Laros, 1987). However, opinions vary widely on whether cesarean delivery is necessary for such a large percentage of breech fetuses. Many studies have been performed but with no consensus on the proper management of this obstetric problem (Perkins, 1987). Some physicians attempt external version to convert the breech to a vertex presentation.

Breech presentation is associated with increased incidence of preterm labor, congenital anomalies, and birth trauma. The major risk to vaginal delivery of a breech fetus is lack of adequate cervical dilation because the buttocks are smaller than the head.

When the head is hyperextended into a face presentation, the chin becomes the presenting part. Although vaginal delivery is possible, the neonate's face will develop marked edema. Internal fetal monitoring is contraindicated because of potential damage to the face, such as skin tearing, infection, scarring, and eye injuries. When the head is midway between extension and flexion, the brow becomes the presenting part. This is a rare presentation and, because it presents the largest cephalic diameter, usually requires cesarean delivery. A transverse lie occurs when the long axis of the mother is perpendicular to that of the fetus and includes shoulder and arm presentations. Either one requires cesarean delivery (Perkins, 1987).

Malposition

Malposition occurs when the fetus's presenting part enters the birth canal in an abnormal position that makes deliv-

---

EMERGENCY ALERT

SIGNS OF FETAL DISTRESS

Signs of fetal distress indicate that the health—and possibly the life—of the fetus is in jeopardy. For example, meconium-stained or yellow amniotic fluid signals fetal hypoxia, which can lead to anoxia, central nervous system damage, or death. The nurse can use the following chart to identify signs of fetal distress and appropriate interventions.

Signs
- Abnormal fetal heart rate pattern, including a heart rate below 120 or above 160 beats/minute, decreased or increased variability, or periodic changes, such as late decelerations or deep, wide, variable decelerations
- Increased or decreased fetal activity
- Meconium-stained or yellow amniotic fluid after membrane rupture

Nursing considerations
- Help the client into the lateral or knee-chest position to relieve fetal pressure on the vena cava, aorta, or umbilical cord and improve maternal and fetal circulation.
- Supply oxygen to improve oxygenation of the client and the fetus. Administer by face mask at 8 to 10 liters/minute.
- Notify the physician and the surgical team.
- Expect to assist with initiating or increasing I.V. fluids, such as lactated Ringer's solution, to manage hypotension or hypovolemia.
- Expect to discontinue oxytocin immediately (if it is being administered) to improve uteroplacental perfusion.
- Be calm and purposeful when caring for the client. This will help prevent undue fear and anxiety, which could adversely affect uteroplacental perfusion.
- Explain what is happening, and reassure the client to help her gain control and cooperate fully. Keep her family informed and encourage their support.

---

ery difficult. An example is the persistent occiput posterior position where the occiput of the fetus's head is in one of the posterior quadrants of the maternal pelvis. (See Chapter 13, The First Stage of Labor, for more information.) If the occiput fails to rotate spontaneously to the anterior position, the physician may use forceps to complete the rotation and facilitate delivery. However, forceps deliveries may put the client and fetus at unacceptable risk.

Macrosomia

The classic definition of macrosomia is a fetus that weighs more than 4,500 g. This occurs in approximately 1% of births (Oxorn, 1986).

A large fetus does not necessarily preclude vaginal delivery; in fact, many are delivered vaginally or with low forceps. The fetopelvic relationship must be assessed for each client. Predisposing factors for macrosomia include maternal diabetes, multiparity, maternal age over 34, previous macrosomia, maternal height over 67" (170 cm), and maternal weight over 154 lb (70 kg) (Oxorn, 1986).

Shoulder dystocia

In shoulder dystocia, the fetus's head emerges but the anterior shoulder catches on the pubic arch—a rare and usually unexpected condition. Typically in shoulder dystocia, the head emerges and is immediately pulled back tightly against the vulva (Lee, 1987). Predisposing factors include macrosomia, a prolonged second stage of labor, multiparity, prolonged pregnancy, and previous delivery of a neonate weighing more than 4,000 g (Lee, 1987). Because this condition has the potential to cause fetal trauma or death, interventions must be immediate.

Intrauterine fetal death

If fetal activity fails to begin or if it ceases after 20 weeks' gestation, the client should be monitored for fetal heart tones. Absence of fetal heart tones warrants a real-time ultrasound examination to detect heart wall motion. Absence of such motion offers reliable evidence of fetal death.

In more than half the cases of fetal death, the cause cannot be determined. Where the cause is known, however, it may be associated with severe maternal disease, diabetes mellitus, hypertension, abruptio placentae, erythroblastosis fetalis, and umbilical cord accidents.

The death of a fetus is a tragic loss for the couple, possibly compounded by the need to go through labor. Labor usually occurs spontaneously within 2 weeks of the fetus's death. However, an increased risk of a coagulation defect and the severe psychological stress of carrying a dead fetus may prompt the physician to induce labor within a few days of the death. Throughout this time, coagulation studies must be carefully monitored.

ASSESSMENT

Once malposition, malpresentation, and macrosomia have been diagnosed, continue with careful monitoring of the labor for any further complications while a plan of medical management is established. Although shoulder dystocia does not occur until delivery, the nurse may assist the nurse-midwife or physician with maneuvers to deliver the shoulders.

If a client of 20 weeks' gestation or more reports that fetal activity has ceased, monitor fetal heart tones. If none are heard, a real-time ultrasonography is performed to

check for heart wall motion. Lack of such motion is reliable evidence of intrauterine fetal death.

NURSING DIAGNOSIS

The nurse reviews all health history, physical assessment, and laboratory test findings and then formulates nursing diagnoses appropriate for the client. (For a partial list of applicable diagnoses, see Nursing Diagnoses: *Intrapartal complications,* page 285.)

PLANNING AND IMPLEMENTATION

The client with a labor complication of fetal malpresentation may have a cesarean delivery, although some breech presentations can be delivered vaginally. An appropriate nursing diagnosis for such a client may be *anxiety related to uncertain perinatal outcome.* For a client with a fetal malposition, nursing interventions may assist with these problems. In some cases, version may be performed to avoid surgical intervention.

Two types of version may be performed: external, which is used to rotate the fetus from a breech or shoulder presentation to a cephalic presentation; and internal, which is used to deliver an unengaged second twin by grasping the feet.

When external version is performed, the client receives a drug to relax the uterus (such as ritodrine hydrochloride or terbutaline sulfate) and the physician repositions the fetus by manipulating the client's abdomen. The physician uses slow steady pressure against the client's abdomen to push the fetus's head toward the pelvic inlet while pushing the buttocks upward. Excessive force may harm the client or fetus. The procedure should be accompanied by continuous external fetal monitoring. Expect the physician to use sonography before and during external version to verify the position of the fetus and placenta. Also expect that the client will receive no anesthetic agent because it may mask possible trauma.

Rotating the fetus to a cephalic presentation increases the likelihood of successful vaginal delivery and reduces the probability of cesarean delivery. Performed properly and gently, external version carries little risk for the client or fetus.

External version is more easily accomplished in multiparous clients because their abdominal walls are more relaxed than those of nulliparous clients (Cunningham, MacDonald, and Gant, 1989).

Internal version may be performed to deliver a second twin when the occiput or breech is not over the pelvic inlet and external pressure fails to position a presenting part, or when uterine bleeding occurs. The physician inserts one sterile, gloved hand through the completely dilated cervix and draws one or both of the fetus's feet toward the birth canal. The physician's other hand applies gentle pressure to the client's abdomen to shift the fetus's head upward. Breech delivery occurs immediately thereafter. Expect the client to receive an anesthetic agent. The physician will attempt internal version as a last resort because it places the client and fetus at serious risk for trauma. Failure of either internal or external version may require an emergency cesarean delivery. (For more information on external and internal version as well as other obstetric procedures, see *Summary of selected obstetric procedures,* pages 324 to 326.)

A client who knows that her fetus is in a breech position before labor begins may be able to perform version on her own. In one study, women assumed a knee-chest position for 15 minutes, three times a day, for 7 days. In 41% of the women studied, the fetus shifted from a breech to cephalic presentation (Chenia and Crowther, 1987).

For a client with shoulder dystocia, the nurse-midwife or physician may attempt one of several maneuvers to deliver the shoulders, which may require assistance from the nurse. Downward traction may be applied to the head while an assistant applies moderate suprapubic pressure (Cunningham, MacDonald, and Gant, 1989). If this fails to move the shoulder, the client in a lithotomy position may remove her legs from the stirrups and flex them sharply (with assistance) against her abdomen (McRobert's maneuver) to straighten the sacrum relative to the lumbar spine and possibly free the shoulder (Lee, 1987).

A client experiencing any fetal complication requires sensitive, supportive nursing care. The client experiencing a labor complicated with fetal malposition, malpresentation, and macrosomia may have a nursing diagnosis of *pain related to abnormally prolonged labor* or *high risk for fetal injury secondary to fetal hypoxia and traumatic delivery.*

Providing nursing care for the client who has experienced a stillbirth is difficult. Be prepared for widely varying responses from the client and family members. If the client does not display grief, explore her personal feelings of anger and sadness.

A client may have begun labor when she is told her fetus is dead, or she may have known for some time before labor begins. An applicable nursing diagnosis may be *situational low self-esteem related to the inability to have a normal pregnancy.* Be extremely sensitive to the needs of the parents and take cues from them to meet their emotional needs. For example, some parents may need to talk about their loss; others may not. Providing any support or opportunities for grieving that the parents may need is essential. A nursing diagnosis of *dysfunctional grieving related to the death of the fetus* may apply.

Provide the same nursing care to a client in labor with a known stillbirth as to a client undergoing labor induction. In addition, continuously monitor the client's coagulation studies. Because of the death of the fetus, she may be at risk for DIC.

The death of a fetus is a tragic loss for the parents that can be compounded because the client must still go through labor. A nursing diagnosis of *powerlessness related to having to carry a dead fetus* may apply. Labor usually occurs spontaneously within 2 weeks of the fetus's death. However, the client faces some risks during this period, especially one of developing a coagulation defect. This risk, combined with the psychological stress of carrying a dead fetus, may necessitate inducing labor within a few days of the intrauterine fetal death. Throughout this time, carefully monitor the results of coagulation studies.

Give the parents an opportunity to see and hold their dead child if they wish. Wrap the child in a blanket and prepare the parents for its appearance. Give them as much time as they wish to spend with their child. Offer to provide a lock of hair, footprints, and bracelets; even if the parents decline, gather these things in case they change their minds. A polaroid picture of the child also may be appropriate. Many parents appreciate these simple gestures, which may provide them with the only mementos of their child that they will have.

The parents may want to have their child baptized. All nurses, regardless of their religion, can perform this rite.

EVALUATION

The following examples illustrate appropriate evaluation statements:

- The client and her fetus completed labor and delivery safely with little or no additional complications.
- The client and her support person and family received regular updates about her condition and the status of the fetus, as the situation allowed.
- The client and her support person received support and encouragement from the nursing staff during complications.

DOCUMENTATION

Documentation should include the following:

- maternal vital signs
- maternal contraction rate and intensity
- maternal fluid intake and output

(Text continues on page 326.)

SUMMARY OF SELECTED OBSTETRIC PROCEDURES

The following chart outlines some indications, contraindications, and risks and complications for the procedures discussed in this chapter.

PROCEDURE	INDICATIONS	CONTRAINDICATIONS	RISKS AND COMPLICATIONS
Version (external)	• Fetus in noncephalic (shoulder or breech) presentation	• Ruptured amniotic membrane • Cephalopelvic disproportion (CPD) • Oligohydramnios • History of premature labor • Abnormal fetus • Placenta previa • More than one fetus • Maternal obesity	• Fetus's possible return to non-cephalic presentation • Client discomfort • Decreased fetal heart rate (FHR) • Premature labor, hemorrhage, premature rupture of membranes • Abruptio placentae • Compression of fetus's spinal cord
Version (internal)	• Emergency need for rapid delivery in breech position only used with second twin	• Lack of anesthesia • No health care team member skilled in internal podalic version (cesarean delivery preferred) • Retracted cervix or contracted, thickened uterus	• Uterine trauma • Lacerations of perineum, vagina, or cervix • Postpartal hemorrhage • Fetal injury
Induction of labor (oxytocin)	• Maternal diabetes • Pregnancy-induced hypertension • Premature rupture of the membranes • Postterm pregnancy • Fetal hemolytic disease • Dead fetus • History of precipitous delivery • Ineffective uterine contractions (only after efforts to reduce tension and promote comfort have failed) • Uterine hypotonia or hypo-activity	• Preterm fetus (unless benefits outweigh risks) • Unripe cervix • Grand multiparity (five or more previous births) • No medical or obstetric need • CPD • Overly distended uterus, as from hydramnios or multiparity • Incoordinate or abnormal contractions • Hypersensitivity to drug • Severe fetal distress • Decreased FHR during contractions • Fetal malposition or malpresentation • Congenital fetal anomalies • Conditions that are contraindications for vaginal delivery, such as placenta previa, invasive cervical carcinoma, herpes simplex type 2 in the birth canal, and cord prolapse	• Excessive (tetanic) uterine contractions • Water intoxication with excessive amounts of fluid • Hypersensitivity to drug, resulting in hypertonia • Failure to initiate labor • With laminaria tents, mild pelvic cramping • Small risk of infection with prolonged laminaria insertion
Induction of labor (amniotomy)	• Postterm pregnancy • Insufficient uterine contractions • Medical or obstetric complications	• Preterm fetus, uncertain estimated delivery date • Unripe cervix • CPD • Presenting part unengaged • Placenta previa • Herpes simplex type 2 in birth canal • Fetal malposition or malpresentation • Multiple gestation (more than one fetus) • Hydramnios • Grand multiparity	• Umbilical cord prolapse • Amnionitis • Compression and molding of fetus's head • Failure to initiate labor • Infection

SUMMARY OF SELECTED OBSTETRIC PROCEDURES *(continued)*

PROCEDURE	INDICATIONS	CONTRAINDICATIONS	RISKS AND COMPLICATIONS
Forceps delivery	• Maternal cardiac or pulmonary disorder • Infection • Maternal exhaustion • Motor innervation from epidural or spinal anesthesia • Premature placental separation • Fetal distress • Prolapsed umbilical cord • Failure of descent or rotation	• Incomplete cervical dilation • Unengaged presenting part • Fetal malposition or malpresentation • Intact membranes • CPD • Full bowel or bladder	*Low forceps* • Bruises to fetus's head • Trauma to perineum, vagina, or cervix *Mid forceps* • *Fetal:* fractured skull, epilepsy, cerebral palsy, mental retardation, cephalohematoma, brain damage, intracranial bleeding, respiratory depression and asphyxia, facial paralysis or other neurologic problems, brachial palsy, bruising, cord compression, death • *Maternal:* fractured coccyx; ruptured uterus; lacerations of perineum, vagina, or cervix; hemorrhage; uterine atony; rectal trauma; genital tract infection; bladder injury, atony, or infection
Vacuum extraction	• Similar to forceps delivery	• Preterm fetus • Fetal malposition or malpresentation • Face presentation • CPD • Hydrocephalus or other congenital anomaly • Dead fetus • Incomplete cervical dilation (possible contraindication) • Unengaged head (possible contraindication)	• Lacerations and abrasions of scalp • Cephalohematoma • Intracranial hematoma • Distortion of fetus's head • Caput succedaneum
Vaginal birth after cesarean delivery	• Client desire • Absence of contraindications	• Vertical uterine scar • Multiple gestation • CPD or other medical problem incompatible with vaginal delivery • Estimated fetal weight above 4,000 g	• Uterine rupture with vertical scar • Reasons for previous cesarean may still exist • Infection if membranes have been ruptured 12 hours or more without delivery and without prophylactic antibiotics
Episiotomy	• Insufficient perineal stretching • Rapid, progressive labor • Narrow suprapublic arch and outlet • Preterm fetus weighing under 200 g • Fetus weighing over 4,000 g • Malpresentation	• Presenting part not descended far enough to stretch the perineum	• Pain • Dyspareunia • Infection • Increased blood loss • Altered vaginal shape or size • Extension to anal sphincter or anal canal *(continued)*

SUMMARY OF SELECTED OBSTETRIC PROCEDURES *(continued)*

PROCEDURE	INDICATIONS	CONTRAINDICATIONS	RISKS AND COMPLICATIONS
Cesarean delivery	• Breech presentation • Fetal distress • Dystocia, possibly caused by CPD, malpresentation, or (rarely) a tumor blocking the birth canal • Previous cesarean delivery • Herpes simplex type 2 in birth canal • Condylomata acuminata in birth canal • Placenta previa, abruptio placentae • Prolapsed umbilical cord • Unsuccessful induction of labor	• Dead fetus • Fetus too premature to survive	• Preterm birth • Anesthesia risk • Aspiration pneumonia • Injury to urinary tract organs or bowel • Bowel obstruction • Dehiscence of surgical wound, leading to evisceration • Infection • Hemorrhage • Thromboemboli

• medications given, time of administration, and effectiveness
• procedures performed, including external and internal version
• vaginal examinations and results
• vaginal discharge, type, and amount
• laboratory studies and their values
• fetal heart tones, variability, and any abnormal patterns.

CHAPTER SUMMARY

Chapter 16 discussed various intrapartal complications and their effects on nursing care of the intrapartal client. Here are the chapter highlights.

Conditions associated with the intrapartal client and complications include: age-related concerns; chronic disorders, such as cardiac disease, diabetes mellitus, infection, and substance abuse; pregnancy-related conditions, such as pregnancy-induced hypertension (PIH) and Rh isoimmunization; reproductive system disorders related to uterine, membrane, amniotic, umbilical cord, placental, and pelvic factors; systemic disorders of the pregnant client; and fetal complications.

The intrapartal client at risk for or with a complication faces the stress of childbirth compounded with concerns related to the condition. Because of this, she and her family are likely to be more anxious about her safety and that of her fetus or neonate.

Many intrapartal clients at risk may have undergone intense prenatal care and vigilant maternal and fetal surveillance. However, skilled, knowledgeable nursing care is essential in calming a client's and family's fears and anxieties as they realize that labor is not progressing normally.

Typically, nursing care of a intrapartal client at risk for or with a complication requires sophisticated nursing skills. It also requires a sound knowledge of the client's condition, including its etiology, pathophysiology, anticipated medical management, and effects on the client, fetus, and neonate.

When caring for a intrapartal client at risk for or with a complication, the nurse obtains a health history, assists with a physical assessment, and collects laboratory test results as for any client who seeks admission for labor and delivery. In addition, the nurse must make specific assessments and be prepared to notify the physician of significant findings. For example, when obtaining a mature client's health history, the nurse may ask if she received infertility treatments, which can cause multiple gestation and attending risks, such as premature labor, malpresentation, and dystocia. During the physical assessment of a client with cardiac disease, the nurse should be alert for dependent edema and other signs of cardiac decompensation. When testing a diabetic client, the nurse should check blood glucose levels carefully, as prescribed. When assessing the client with dysfunctional labor, the nurse must continuously monitor labor progress and fetal status.

Some nursing interventions for the intrapartal client at risk for or with a complication resemble those for any other intrapartal client. For example, the nurse must monitor the client and fetus, assess labor progress, promote comfort, prepare for delivery, provide emotional support, promote bonding, perform client teaching, and care for the client's family. In addition, the nurse must be prepared to respond quickly to intrapartal emergencies – such as diabetic ketoacidosis (DKA), eclampsia, umbilical cord prolapse, placenta previa, or abruptio placenta – and may need to approach the usual tasks differently and modify normal intrapartal care.

During labor and delivery, the nurse may need to assist with special obstetric procedures, including version, infusion of synthetic oxytocin, amniotomy, forceps delivery, vacuum extraction, episiotomy, cesarean delivery, and vaginal birth after cesarean delivery. The nurse plays a major role in providing guidance and information and in supporting the client and her partner.

Alterations to usual nursing tasks may result from participation as a member of a perinatal team. The nurse works closely with the physician when restricting analgesia for an isoimmunized client, preventing or arresting seizures in a client with PIH, isolating an infected client from her neonate, providing support to a substance abuser who may be afraid that a social service agency will take away her neonate, and assisting and comforting the family when fetal death occurs.

The nurse may need to coordinate the perinatal team and must anticipate the care that will be required for the intrapartal client and her neonate.

Documentation is critical to nursing care of the intrapartal client at risk for or with a complication. In addition to recording basic information required by the health care facility, the nurse should document specific interventions related to the client and her neonate.

STUDY QUESTIONS

1. Mrs. Gloria Mann, age 41, comes to the labor and delivery area prepared to give birth to her first child. What should the nurse assess for?

2. Maria Jenkins, a 32-year-old client with a history of gestational diabetes and pregnant with her third child, arrives at the labor and delivery area at 9:00 AM. She reports that her membranes ruptured spontaneously at 4:00 AM. Mrs. Jenkins has been monitoring her blood glucose four times a day and injecting herself with 20 units of NPH insulin at bedtime. What should the nurse anticipate doing for this client?

3. A client admitted to the labor and delivery area reports that she has used cocaine regularly during her pregnancy. How can the nurse promote bonding between the client and her neonate?

4. Mrs. Elaine Crump, age 35, is admitted to the labor and delivery area with suspected PIH. Her blood pressure is 140/96 mm Hg. What other assessments by the nurse would help to confirm PIH?

5. Immediately after a physician performs an amniotomy, what actions should the nurse take?

6. Mrs. Joan Olds is pregnant with her second child. Her previous delivery was by cesarean delivery. Now she expresses a desire to attempt vaginal delivery. What information does the nurse need to know about VBAC?

7. Beverly Dugas, age 24, is brought to the emergency department with vaginal bleeding that started suddenly. She is 33 weeks' pregnant and she reports no abdominal pain. What information should the nurse obtain during her assessment and how should the nurse intervene?

8. What are the immediate nursing interventions for a client with an umbilical cord prolapse?

BIBLIOGRAPHY

Abdella, T.N., Sibae, B.M., Hays, J.M., and Anderson, G.D. (1984). Perinatal outcome in abruptio placentae. *Obstetrics and Gynecology, 63*(4), 365-369.

American College of Obstetricians and Gynecologists (November 1987). Induction and augmentation of labor. *Technical Bulletin,* No. 110.

Borgetta, L., Piening, S., and Cohen, W. (1989). Association of episiotomy and delivery position with deep perineal laceration during spontaneous delivery in nulliparous women. *American Journal of Obstetrical Gynecology, 160*(2), 294-297.

Bowes, C., and Bowes, W. (1987). Insults to the fetus. In L. Sonstegard, K. Kowalski, and B. Jennings (Eds.), *Women's health: Volume three, Crisis and illness in childbearing* (pp. 91-102). Philadelphia: Saunders.

Brown, S. (1988). Preventing low birthweight. In H. Wallace, G. Ryan, and A. Oglesby (Eds.), *Maternal and child health practices* (3rd ed.; pp. 307-324). Oakland, CA: Third Party Pub.

Chenia, F., and Crowther, M. (1987). Does advice to assume the knee-chest position reduce the incidence of breech presentation at delivery? A randomized clinical trial. *Birth, 14*(2), 75-80.

Clark, S.L. (1987). Amniotic fluid embolism. In S.L. Clark, J.P. Phelen, and D.B. Cotton (Eds.), *Critical care obstetrics.* Oradell, NJ: Medical Economics.

Cohen, H., Green, J., and Cromblehome, W. (1988). Society of Perinatal Obstetrician Abstract Presentation, Las Vegas, Nevada.

Cohen, W. (1989). Preterm labor. In W. Cohen, D. Acket, and E Freidman (Eds.), *Management of labor* (2nd ed.; pp. 333-367). Rockville, MD: Aspen.

Cunningham, F.G., MacDonald, P.C., and Gant, N. (1989). *Williams obstetrics* (18th ed.). East Norwalk, CT: Appleton & Lange.

Flanagan, T., Mulchahey, K., Korenbrot, C., Green J., and Laros, R. (1987). Management of term breech presentation. *American Journal of Obstetrics and Gynecology, 156*(6), 1492-1502.

Friedman, E. (1987). Midforceps delivery: No? *Clinical Obstetrics and Gynecology, 30*(1), 93-105.

Friedman, E. (1989). Normal and dysfunctional labor. In W.R. Cohen, D. Acker, and E. Friedman (Eds.), *Management of labor* (pp. 1-18). Rockville, MD: Aspen.

Gabbe, S., and Main, D. (1988). Reproductive problems associated with lifestyle, work, and hazards in the workplace. In D. Hollingsworth and R. Resnik (Eds.), *Medical counseling before pregnancy* (pp. 97-122). New York: Churchill-Livingstone.

Hacker, N., and Moore, J. (1986). *Essentials of obstetrics and gynecology.* Philadelphia: Saunders.

Hill, L.M., Breckle, R., Thomas, M.L., and Fries, J.K. (1987). Polyhydramnios: Ultrasonically detected prevalence and neonatal outcome. *Obstetrics and Gynecology, 69*(1), 2125.

Hurd, W.W., Midovnik, M., Hertzberg, V., and Levin, J.P. (1983). Selective management of abruptio placentae: A prospective study. *Obstetrics and Gynecology, 61*(4), 467473.

Jackson, V. (1990). The uterus. In R. Lichtman and S. Papera (Eds.), *Gynecology: Well-woman care* (pp. 261-272). East Norwalk, CT: Appleton & Lange.

Kemp, V., and Page, C. (1986). The psychosocial impact of a high-risk pregnancy on the family. *JOGNN, 15*(3), 232-236.

Knupple, R., and Drukker, J. (Eds.) (1986). *High-risk pregnancy: A team approach.* Philadelphia: Saunders.

Korones, S.B. (1986). *High-risk newborn infants* (4th ed.). St. Louis: Mosby.

Lee, C.Y. (1987). Shoulder dystocia. *Clinical Obstetrics and Gynecology, 30*(1), 77-82.

McRae, M., and Mervyn, F. (1989). Contemporary issues in childbirth. In W. Cohen, D. Acker, and E. Friedman, *Management of labor* (2nd ed.; pp. 535-548). Rockville, MD: Aspen.

Ouimette, J. (1986). *Perinatal nursing: Care of the high-risk infant.* Boston: Jones and Bartlett.

Oxorn, H. (1986). *Human labor and birth.* (5th ed.). East Norwalk, CT: Appleton & Lange.

Perkins, R.P. (1987). Fetal dystocia. *Clinical Obstetrics and Gynecology, 30*(1), 56-58.

Petrie, R.H., and Williams, A.M. (1986). Induction of labor. In R. Knupple and J. Drukker (Eds.), *High-risk pregnancy: A team approach.* Philadelphia: Saunders.

Rochat, R., Koonin, L., Atrash, H., and Jewett, J. (1988) Maternal mortality in the United States: Report from the maternal mortality collaborative. *Obstetrics and Gynecology, 72*(1), 90-97.

Usher, R.H., Boyd, M.E., McLean, F.H., and Kramer, M.S. (1988). Assessment of fetal risk in postdate pregnancies. *American Journal of Obstetrics and Gynecology, 158*(2), 259-264.

Weiner, C.P. (1987). Disseminate intravascular coagulopathy. In S.L. Clark, J.P. Phalen, and D.B. Cotton (Eds.), *Critical care obstetrics.* Oradell, NJ: Medical Economics.

Age-related concerns

Acker, D. (1987). Elderly gravida. In E. Friedman, D. Acker, and B. Sachs (Eds.), *Obstetrical decision making* (2nd ed.; pp. 20-21). Philadelphia: B.C. Decker.

Berkowitz, G., Skovron, M., Lapinski, R., and Berkowitz, R. (1990). Delayed childbearing and the outcome of pregnancy. *New England Journal of Medicine, 322*(10), 659-664.

Brucker, M., and Muellner, M. (1985). Nurse-midwifery care of adolescents. *Journal of Nurse-Midwifery, 30*(5), 277-279.

Calandra, C., Abell, D., and Beischer, N. (1981). Maternal obesity in pregnancy. *Obstetrics and Gynecology, 57*(1), 8-12.

Corbett, M., and Meyer, J. (1987). *The adolescent and pregnancy.* Boston: Blackwell Scientific Pubs.

Friede, A., Baldwin, W., Rhodes, P., Buehler, J., and Strauss, L. (1988). Older maternal age and infant mortality in the United States. *Obstetrics and Gynecology, 72*(2), 152-157.

Halfar, M. (1985). Frequency of labor dysfunction in nulliparas over the age of thirty. *Journal of Nurse-Midwifery, 30*(6), 333-339.

Hollingsworth, D., Kotchen, J., and Felice, M. (1985). Impact of gynecologic age on outcome of adolescent pregnancy. In J. Queenan (Ed.), *Management of high-risk pregnancy.* Oradell, NJ: Medical Economics Books.

Institute of Medicine (1985). *Preventing low birthweight.* Washington, DC: National Academy Press.

Jennings, B. (1987). Mature childbearing. In L. Sonstegard, K. Kowalski, and B. Jennings (Eds.), *Women's health: Volume three, Crisis and illness in childbearing* (pp. 59-64). Philadelphia: Saunders.

Kirz, D., Dorchester, W., and Freeman, R. (1985). Advanced maternal age: The mature gravida. *American Journal of Obstetrics and Gynecology, 152*(1), 7-12.

Mansfield, P. (1986). Reevaluating the medical risks of late childbearing. *Women's Health, 11*(2), 37-60.

Mercer, R. (1987). Adolescent pregnancy. In L. Sonstegard, K. Kowalski, and B. Jennings (Eds.), *Women's health: Volume three, Crisis and illness in childbearing* (pp. 47-58). Philadelphia: Saunders.

Moore, M. (1989). Recurrent teen pregnancy: Making it less desirable. *MCN, 14*(2), 104-108.

Naeye, R. (1983). Maternal age, obstetric complications and the outcome of pregnancy. *Obstetrics and Gynecology, 61*(2), 210-215.

Oats, J., Abell, D., Andersen, H., and Beischer, N. (1983). Obesity in pregnancy. *Comprehensive Therapy, 9*(4), 51-55.

Queenan, J., Freeman, R., Niebyl, J., Resnik, R., and Simpson, J. (1987). Symposium: Managing pregnancy in patients over 35. *Contemporary OB/GYN, 29*(5), 180-198.

Resnik, R. (1988). Pregnancy in women aged 35 years or older. In D. Hollingsworth and R. Resnik (Eds.), *Medical counseling before pregnancy* (pp. 14-18). New York: Churchill Livingstone.

Slap, G., and Schwartz, J. (1989) Risk factors for low birth weight to adolescent mothers. *Journal of Adolescent Health Care, 10*(4), 267-274.

Winick, M. (1989). *Nutrition, pregnancy, and early intervention.* Baltimore: Williams & Wilkins.

Winslow, W. (1987a). Gravida over thirty-five years of age. In E. Knor (Ed.), *Decision making in obstetrical nursing* (p. 28). Philadelphia: B.C. Decker.

Winslow, W. (1987b). First pregnancy after 35: What is the experience? *MCN, 12*(2), 92-96.

Cardiac disease

Anderson, J. (1970). The effect of diuretics in late pregnancy on the newborn infant. *ACTA Paediatra Scandinavia, 59*(6), 659-663.

Greenspoon, J. (1988.) Heart disease in pregnancy. In D. Mishell and P. Brenner (Eds.), *Management of common problems in OB/GYN* (pp. 33-40). Oradell, NJ: Medical Economics.

Hall, J., Pauli, R., and Wilson, K. (1980). Maternal and fetal sequelae of anticoagulation during pregnancy. *American Journal of Medicine,* 68(1), 122-140.

Rubin, P., Butters, L., Clark, E., Summer, D., Phil, D., Belfield, A., Pledger, D., Low, R., and Reid, J. (1984). Obstetrical aspects of the use in pregnancy-associated hypertension of the beta-adrenoceptor against atenolol. *American Journal of Obstetrics and Gynecology,* 150(4), 389.

Samuels, P., and Landon, M. (1986). Medical complications. In S. Gabbe, J. Niebyl, and J. Simpson (Eds.), *Obstetrics: Normal and problem pregnancies* (pp. 856-978). New York: Churchill Livingstone.

Sullivan, J., and Ramanathan, K. (1985). Management of medical problems in pregnancy: Severe cardiac disease. *New England Journal of Medicine,* 313(5), 304-309.

Ueland, K. (1989). Cardiac disease. In R. Creasy and R. Resnik (Eds.), *Maternal-fetal medicine: Principles and practice* (2nd ed.; pp. 746-762). Philadelphia: Saunders.

Diabetes mellitus

Cousins, L. (1987). Pregnancy complications among diabetic women: Review 1965-1985. *Obstetrical and Gynecological Survey,* 42(3), 140-149.

Freinkel, N. (1980). Gestational diabetes 1979. *Diabetes Care,* 3, 399.

Hollingsworth, D., and Moore, T. (1989). Diabetes and pregnancy. In R. Creasy and R. Resnik (Eds.), *Maternal-fetal medicine: Principles and practice* (2nd ed.; pp. 925-988). Philadelphia: Saunders.

Jovanovic, L., and Peterson, C. (1982). Optimal insulin delivery for the pregnant diabetic patient. *Diabetes Care,* 5(Suppl. 1), 24-37.

Marble, A., Krall, L., Bradley, R., Christlieb, A., and Soeldner, J. (1985). *Joslin's diabetes mellitus* (12th ed.). Philadelphia: Lea & Febiger.

Mills, J., et al. (1988). Lack of relation of malformation rates in infants of diabetic mothers to glycemic control during organogenesis. *New England Journal of Medicine,* 318(11), 671-676.

Ryan, E., O'Sullivan, M., Skyler, J., and Mintz, D. (1982). Glucose control during labor and delivery. In J. Skyler (Ed.), *Insulin update 1982* (pp. 290-294). Princeton, NJ: Excerpta Medica.

Infection

Balgobin, B. (1987). Fever in labor. In E. Friedman, D. Acker, and B. Sachs (Eds.), *Obstetrical decision making* (2nd ed.; pp. 232-233). Philadelphia: B.C. Decker.

Benoit, J. (1988). Sexually transmitted diseases in pregnancy. *Nursing Clinics of North America,* 23(4), 937-945.

Cates, W., and Holmes, K. (1987). Sexually transmitted diseases. In J. Last (Ed.), *Public health and preventive medicine* (12th ed.). East Norwalk, CT: Appleton & Lange.

Centers for Disease Control (1987). Recommendations for prevention of HIV transmission in health care settings. *MMWR,* 36(31), 25-185.

Committee on Infectious Diseases (1985). Prevention of hepatitis B virus infections. *Pediatrics,* 75(2), 362-364.

Eschenbach, D. (1988). Infections and sexually transmitted diseases. In D. Hollingsworth and R. Resnik (Eds.), *Medical counseling before pregnancy* (pp. 249-269). New York: Churchill Livingstone.

Faro, S., and Pastorek, J. (1986). Perinatal infections. In R. Knupple and J. Drukker (Eds.), *High-risk pregnancy: A team approach* (pp. 74-111). Philadelphia: Saunders.

Gilstrap, L., and Cox, S. (1989). Acute chorioamnionitis. *Obstetrics and Gynecology Clinics of North America.* 16(2), 373-379.

Haggerty, L. (1985). TORCH: A literature review and implications for practice. *JOGNN,* 14(2), 124-129.

Hauer, L., and Dattel, B. (1988). Management of the pregnant women infected with the human imunodeficiency virus. *Journal of Perinatology,* 8(3), 258-262.

Krieger, J. (1984). Biology of sexually transmitted diseases. *Urology Clinics of North America,* 11(1), 15-25.

Quinn, P., Butany, J., and Taylor, J. (1987). Chorioamnionitis: Its association with pregnancy outcome and microbial infection. *American Journal of Obstetrics and Gynecology,* 156(2), 379-387.

Spence, M. (1989). Epidemiology of sexually transmitted diseases. *Obstetrics and Gynecology Clinics of North America,* 16(3), 453-470.

Wiley K., and Grohar, J. (1988). Human immunodeficiency virus and precautions for obstetric, gynecologic and neonatal nurses. *JOGNN,* 17(3), 165-168.

Wilson, D. (1988). An overview of sexually transmissible diseases in the perinatal period. *Journal of Nurse-Midwifery,* 33(3), 115-128.

Substance abuse

Burkett, G., Banstra, E., Cohn, J., Steele, B., and Palow, D. (1990). Cocaine-related maternal death. *American Journal of Obstetrics and Gynecology,* 163(1), 40-41.

Florida Child Abuse Statute 415.503, March 1987.

Frank, D., et al. (1988). Cocaine use during pregnancy: Prevalence and correlates. *Pediatrics,* 82(6), 888-895.

Landry, M., and Smith, D.E. (1987). Crack: Anatomy of an addiction, part 2. *California Nursing Review,* 9(3), 28.

Lynch, M., and McKeon, V. (1990). Cocaine use during pregnancy: Research findings and clinical implications. *JOGNN,* 19(4), 285-292.

MacGregor, S., Keith, L., Chasnoff, I., Rosner, M., Chisum, G., Shaw, P., and Minogue, J. (1987). Cocaine use during pregnancy: Adverse perinatal outcome. *American Journal of Obstetrics and Gynecology,* 157(3), 686-690.

Miller, G. (1989). Addicted infants and their mothers. *National Center for Clinical Infant Programs,* 9(5), 20.

Pregnancy-induced hypertension

Hayashi, R. (1986). Emergency care in pregnancy. In J. Queenan (Ed.), *Medical management of high-risk pregnancy* (pp. 447-469). Oradell, NJ: Medical Economics Books.

Knupple, R., and Drukker, J. (1986). Hypertension in pregnancy. In R. Knupple and J. Drukker (Eds.), *High-risk pregnancy: A team approach* (pp. 362-398). Philadelphia: Saunders.

Roberts, J. (1989). Pregnancy related hypertension. In R. Creasy and R. Resnik (Eds.), *Maternal-fetal medicine: Principles and practice* (2nd ed.; pp. 777-823). Philadelphia: Saunders.

Sibai, B., Lipshitz, J., and Anderson, G. (1981). Reassessment of intravenous MgSO₄ therapy in preeclampsia-eclampsia. *Obstetrics and Gynecology*, 57(2), 199-202.

Rh isoimmunization

Arias, F., and Johnson, D. (1984). Erythroblastosis fetalis. In F. Arias (Ed.), *High-risk pregnancy and delivery* (pp. 75-90). St. Louis: Mosby.

Lloyd, T. (1987). Rh factor incompatibility: A primer for prevention. *Journal of Nurse-Midwifery*, 32(5), 297-307.

Queenan, J. (1985). Rh and other blood group immunizations. In J. Queenan (Ed.), *Management of high-risk pregnancy* (pp. 505-520). Oradell, NJ: Medical Economic Books.

Sachs, B. (1987). Nonimmune hydrops fetalis. In E. Friedman, D. Acker, and B. Sachs (Eds.), *Obstetrical decision making* (2nd ed.; pp. 140-141). Philadelphia: B.C. Decker.

Induction of labor

Boyan, P., and MacDonald, D. (1988). Commentary—Oxytocin: The need to distinguish between induction and augmentation and between multiparous and primiparous. *Birth*, 15(4), 203.

Curtis, P., and Sofransky, N. (1988). Rethinking oxytocin protocols in the augmentation of labor. *Birth*, 15(4), 199-202.

Food and Drug Administration. New restrictions on oxytocin use. *FDA Bulletin*, 8(5).

Henderson, C. (1987). Artificial rupture of the membranes. *Nursing Times*, 83(38), 63-64.

Johnson, G. (1981). Oxytocics for the induction of labor. March of Dimes, Series 3, Module 2.

Marshall, C. (1985). The art of induction/augmentation of labor. *JOGNN*, 14(1), 22.

Rayburn, W. (March, 1989). Prostaglandin E₂ gel for cervical ripening and induction of labor: A critical analysis. *American Journal of Obstetrics and Gynecology*, 160(3), 529-534.

Forceps

Laub, D.W. (1985). Forceps delivery. *Clinical Obstetrical Gynecology*, June 29, 286.

Vacuum extraction

Galvan, B., and Broekhuizen, F. (1987). Obstetric vacuum extraction. *JOGNN*, 15(4), 242-248.

Episiotomy

Avery, M., and Von Arsdale, L. (1987). Perineal massage effect on the incidence of episiotomy and laceration in a nulliparous population. *Journal of Nurse-Midwifery*, 32(3), 181-184.

Cesarean delivery

Dansforth, D.N. (1985). Cesarean section. *JAMA*, 253(6), 811-818.

Leach, L., and Sproule, V. (1984). Meeting the challenge of cesarean births. *JOGNN*, 13(3), 191-199.

Schroder-Zwelling, E. (1988). The unexpected childbirth experience. In F. Nichols and S. Humenick (Eds.), *Childbirth and education: Practice, research, and theory*. Philadelphia: Saunders.

Shearer, E., Shiono, P., and Rhoads, G. (1988). Recent trends in family-centered maternity care for cesarean-birth families. *Birth*, 15(1), 3-7.

Vaginal birth after cesarean delivery

American College of Obstetricians and Gynecologists (October 1988). Committee on Maternal and Fetal Medicine. *Guidelines for vaginal delivery after cesarean birth.*

Flamm, B.L. (1985). Vaginal birth after cesarean section: Controversies old and new. *Clinical and Obstetrical Gynecology*, December 28, 735.

Hemminki, E. (1987). Pregnancy and birth after cesarean section: A survey based on the Swedish birth register. *Birth*, 14(1), 12-17.

Laufer, A., Hodenius, V., Friedman, L., Duncan, N., Guy, C.M., MacPherson, S., and Barrows, N. (1987). Vaginal birth after cesarean section. *Journal of Nurse-Midwifery*, 32(1), 41-47.

Miller, C. and Sonnemann-Sutter, C. (1985). Vaginal birth after cesarean. *JOGNN*, 14(5), 383-389.

UNIT IV
THE NEONATE

NEONATAL ADAPTATION

OBJECTIVES

After reading and studying this chapter, the student should be able to:

1. Compare and contrast fetal and neonatal circulation.
2. Identify the unique anatomic structures of fetal circulation.
3. Discuss the status of the integumentary, neurologic, and reproductive systems at birth.
4. Identify the neonate's four defenses against heat loss.
5. Describe the biological adaptations necessary in the hematopoietic, renal, gastrointestinal (GI), hepatic, and endocrine systems to ensure successful transition to extrauterine life.
6. Discuss the capacity of the neonate's immune system to prevent infection.
7. Identify the sensory capacities of the normal neonate.
8. Describe the periods of neonatal reactivity and the physiologic characteristics associated with each.

INTRODUCTION

Immediately after delivery, the neonate must assume the life-support functions performed by the placenta in utero. Birth begins a critical 24-hour phase, called the *transitional period,* that encompasses the neonate's adaptation from intrauterine to extrauterine life.

To survive outside the womb, the neonate must successfully navigate the transitional period. Statistics reflect the difficulty of this task: Mortality is higher during this period than at any other time; two-thirds of all neonatal deaths occur in the first 4 weeks after birth (Avery, 1987; March of Dimes, 1985).

The transitional period imposes changes in all body systems and exposes the neonate to a wide range of ex-ternal stimuli. Conditions that prevent successful adaptation to extrauterine life pose a serious threat. By becoming familiar with the normal events of transition, the nurse may recognize signs of poor adaptation and intervene promptly when they occur.

This chapter begins with a review of the biological characteristics of adaptation during the transitional period, including major changes in every body system. The first section also discusses the importance of neonatal thermoregulation. Next, the chapter describes the behavioral characteristics of adaptation, reviewing the neonate's response to environmental stimulation as well as neonatal sensory capacities. The chapter concludes with a discussion of the periods of neonatal reactivity (a series of behavioral and physiologic characteristics) and neonatal sleep and awake states.

BIOLOGICAL CHARACTERISTICS OF ADAPTATION

Crucial physiologic adjustments take place in all body systems after birth. The cardiovascular and pulmonary systems undergo immediate drastic changes as soon as the umbilical cord is clamped and respiration begins. Although cardiovascular and pulmonary changes occur simultaneously, they are discussed separately to facilitate understanding.

CARDIOVASCULAR SYSTEM

To ensure the neonate's survival, fetal circulation must convert to neonatal circulation during the transitional period. Fetal circulation involves four unique anatomic features that shunt most blood away from the liver and lungs.

The *placenta* serves as an exchange organ through which the fetus absorbs oxygen, nutrients, and other substances and excretes wastes (such as carbon dioxide). The *ductus venosus* links the inferior vena cava with the umbilical vein, permitting most placental blood to bypass the liver. The *foramen ovale* and *ductus arteriosus* direct most blood away from the pulmonary circuit. Although a small portion of pulmonary arterial blood enters the pulmonary circuit to perfuse the lungs, the ductus arteriosus shunts most to the aorta to supply oxygen and nutrients to the trunk and lower extremities.

Conversion from fetal to neonatal circulation

Beginning at birth, fetal shunts undergo changes that establish neonatal circulation. (For an illustration of blood flow in the neonate, see *Tracing neonatal circulation,* page 334.) As the umbilical cord is clamped and the neonate draws the first breath, systemic vascular resistance increases and blood flow through the ductus arteriosus declines. Most of the right ventricular output flows through the lungs, boosting pulmonary venous return to the left atrium. In response to increased blood volume in the lungs and heart, left atrial pressure rises. Combined with increased systemic resistance, this pressure rise results in functional closure of the foramen ovale. (*Functional closure* refers to cessation of blood flow, resulting from pressure changes, that renders a structure nonfunctional.) Within several months, the foramen ovale undergoes *anatomic closure* (structural obliteration from constriction or tissue growth).

Onset of respiratory effort and the effects of increased partial pressure of arterial oxygen (PaO_2) constrict the ductus arteriosus, which functionally closes 15 to 24 hours after birth. By age 3 to 4 weeks, this shunt undergoes anatomic closure.

Clamping of the umbilical cord halts blood flow through the ductus venosus, functionally closing this structure. The ductus venosus closes anatomically by the first or second week. After birth, the umbilical vein and arteries no longer transport blood and are obliterated.

Because anatomic closure lags behind functional closure, fetal shunts may open intermittently before closing completely. Intermittent shunt opening most commonly stems from conditions causing increased vena caval and right atrial pressure (such as crying); clinically insignificant functional murmurs may result. Also, because shunts allow unoxygenated blood to pass from the right to left side of the heart, bypassing the pulmonary circuit, they may cause transient cyanosis. Both cyanosis and murmurs in the neonate should be carefully monitored and evaluated so that any underlying abnormalities can be detected. (See Chapter 18, Neonatal Assessment, for more information about assessing the neonate's cardiovascular system.)

Blood volume

The blood volume of the full-term neonate ranges from 80 to 90 ml/kg of body weight, depending on the amount of blood transferred from the placenta after delivery. Delayed umbilical cord clamping increases blood volume by up to 100 ml (1 dl), possibly increasing heart rate, respiratory rate, and systolic blood pressure. Changes caused by increased blood volume may persist for about 48 hours, possibly leading to crackles and cyanosis.

RESPIRATORY SYSTEM

Throughout gestation, biochemical and anatomic respiratory features develop progressively, preparing the fetus for the abrupt respiratory changes brought on by birth. Between weeks 25 and 30 of gestation, Type II pneumocytes (alveolar cells) begin limited secretion of surfactant. A phospholipid, surfactant decreases the surface tension of pulmonary fluids and prevents alveolar collapse at the end of expiration. Reduction of surface tension facilitates gas exchange, decreases inflation pressures needed to open the airways, improves lung compliance, and decreases labor of breathing.

Onset of neonatal respiration

The fetal lungs contain fluid secreted by the lungs, amniotic cavity, and trachea. The fluid volume, which correlates with the neonate's functional residual capacity (FRC), typically reaches 30 to 25 ml/kg of body weight (West, 1985). For the neonate to assume the tasks of ventilation and oxygenation, air must rapidly replace lung fluid. In the healthy neonate, replacement occurs with the first few breaths.

As the neonate's chest squeezes through the birth canal, compression forces out roughly one-third of the lung fluid through the nose and mouth. The pulmonary circulation and lymphatic system absorb the remaining two-thirds after respiration begins.

After the neonate's chest clears the birth canal, elastic recoil pulls 7 to 42 ml of air into the lungs to replace the fluid that was forced out. Consequently, the neonate may cough before the first inspiration. Glossopharyngeal or frog breathing, which involves involuntary muscle contraction, pulls another 5 to 10 ml of air into the lungs. Each breath increases the neonate's FRC.

The time needed to clear the lungs varies from 6 to 24 hours after vaginal delivery of a healthy, full-term neonate

TRACING NEONATAL CIRCULATION

With birth comes functional closure of the fetal shunts (ductus venosus, foramen ovale, and ductus arteriosus) that direct blood flow away from the lungs and liver and separate the systemic and pulmonary circulations. As the shunts close, blood flows from the pulmonary arteries to the lungs and through the portal system to the liver. In the large illustration, the darker areas represent regions of high arterial oxygen saturation; the lighter areas, regions of low saturation. The boxed illustrations show the shunts as they previously existed.

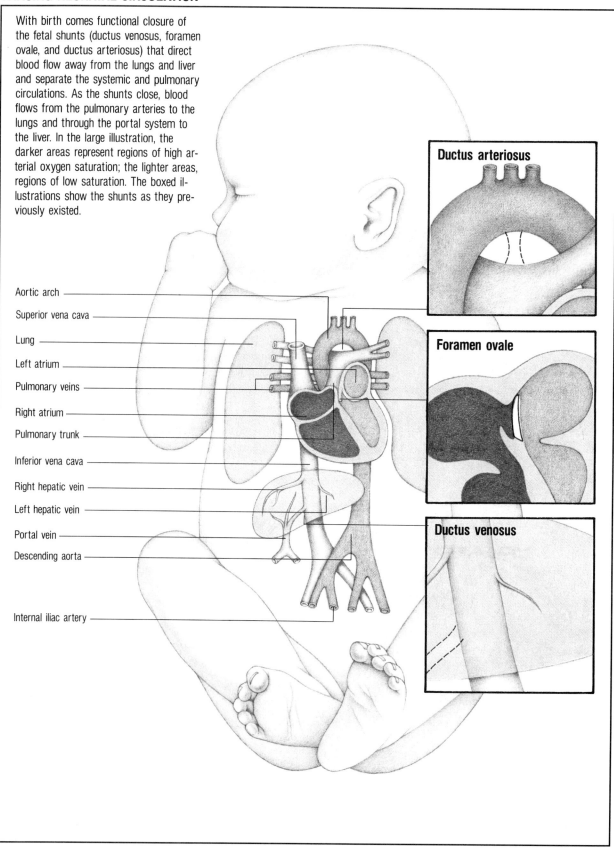

Aortic arch

Superior vena cava

Lung

Left atrium

Pulmonary veins

Right atrium

Pulmonary trunk

Inferior vena cava

Right hepatic vein

Left hepatic vein

Portal vein

Descending aorta

Internal iliac artery

Ductus arteriosus

Foramen ovale

Ductus venosus

(West, 1985). Inadequate lung fluid removal may cause transient tachypnea, a common problem in neonates.

Normally, the neonate breathes within 20 seconds of delivery, stimulated by the medullary respiratory center. (For an overview of the factors leading to respiration, see *Stimuli for respiration*.)

Asphyxia—the combination of hypoxemia, hypercapnia, and acidosis—provides the strongest stimulus for the first breath. Before the first breath, the neonate has an arterial oxygen saturation (SaO_2) of only 10% to 20%, reflecting hypoxemia; a partial pressure of arterial carbon dioxide ($PaCO_2$) of approximately 58 mm Hg, reflecting hypercapnia; and an arterial pH of approximately 7.28, reflecting acidosis.

Because the final stage of delivery interrupts gas exchange, even the healthy neonate has some degree of asphyxia at birth. Asphyxia stimulates chemoreceptors in the carotid bodies and aorta. As this stimulation increases, efferent impulses travel to the diaphragm, contracting it. The negative intrathoracic pressure that results draws air into the lungs, increasing intrathoracic volume.

Other stimuli that help trigger breathing include cord occlusion, thermal changes (from rapid heat loss caused by increased energy expenditure), tactile stimulation, and other environmental changes (such as bright lights and noise).

The onset of respiration and lung expansion indirectly decreases pulmonary vascular resistance because of the direct effect of oxygen and carbon dioxide on vessels. As oxygen saturation increases and the $PaCO_2$ value declines, the decrease in pulmonary vascular resistance leads to increased pulmonary blood flow. This further improves oxygen saturation.

Neonatal respiratory function

The respiratory rate varies over the first day, stabilizing by about 24 hours after birth. Maintained by the effects of biochemical and environmental stimulation, the neonate's respiratory function requires:

STIMULI FOR RESPIRATION

In response to various stimuli, the neonate draws the first breath within about 20 seconds of delivery. Asphyxia is the most important stimulus for neonatal respiration. However, as the flowchart below shows, other biochemical stimuli also come into play, as do various mechanical, thermal, and sensory factors.

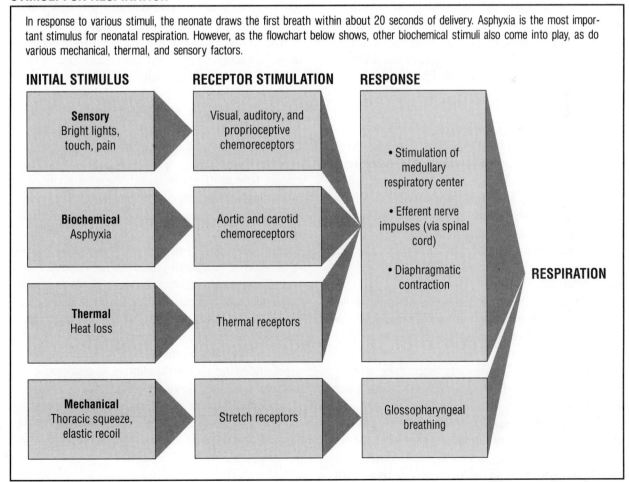

- a patent airway
- a functioning respiratory center
- intact nerves from the brain to chest muscles
- adequate calories to supply energy for labor of breathing.

HEMATOPOIETIC SYSTEM

Like other body systems, the hematopoietic system is not fully developed at birth. The hematologic features that ensured adequate tissue oxygenation in utero must be replaced by more mature elements after birth.

Red blood cells

Erythropoiesis – production of erythrocytes, or red blood cells (RBCs) – is stimulated by the renal hormone erythropoietin. In the fetus, low oxygen saturation causes erythropoietin release to rise; to ensure adequate tissue oxygenation, RBC production increases. At birth, the increased oxygen saturation that follows the onset of respiration inhibits erythropoietin release, reducing RBC production.

Fetal RBCs have a life span of about 90 days, compared to 120 days for normal RBCs. As fetal RBCs deteriorate, the neonate's RBC count decreases, sometimes resulting in physiologic anemia before stabilization. By age 2 to 3 months, however, the RBC count rises to within acceptable neonatal limits. (For normal neonatal laboratory values, see Chapter 18, Neonatal Assessment.)

Hemoglobin

Blood's oxygen-carrying component, hemoglobin is produced by developing RBCs. After birth, the hemoglobin value decreases simultaneously with the RBC count. Fetal RBCs produce hemoglobin F (fetal hemoglobin), which has a higher affinity for oxygen than hemoglobin A (produced by adult RBCs). This compensatory mechanism helps ensure adequate oxygenation in utero. As RBCs are replaced, hemoglobin A replaces hemoglobin F.

White blood cells

White blood cells (WBCs), or leukocytes, serve as the neonate's major defense against infection. WBCs exist in five types: neutrophils, eosinophils, basophils, lymphocytes, and monocytes. Neutrophils account for 40% to 80% of total WBCs at birth; lymphocytes account for roughly 30%. However, by age 1 month, lymphocytes outnumber neutrophils.

Neutrophils and monocytes are phagocytes – cells that engulf and ingest foreign substances. They form part of the mononuclear phagocytic system, which defends the body against infection and disposes of cell breakdown products. Despite the presence of these phagocytic properties, however, the neonate's immature inflammatory tissue response may not localize an infection.

Thrombocytes

Thrombocytes (platelets) are crucial to blood coagulation. The neonate usually has an adequate platelet count and function (Brown, 1988).

HEPATIC SYSTEM

The neonate's hepatic system – responsible for bilirubin clearance, blood coagulation, carbohydrate metabolism, and iron storage – is immature. Nonetheless, under normal circumstances, it functions adequately.

Bilirubin clearance

A yellow bile pigment, bilirubin is a by-product of heme after RBC breakdown. As RBCs age, they become fragile and eventually are cleared from the circulation by the mononuclear phagocytic system. The iron and protein portions are removed and recycled for further use. After leaving the mononuclear phagocytic system, bilirubin binds to plasma albumin. In this water-insoluble state, it is called indirect (unconjugated) bilirubin.

Indirect bilirubin must be conjugated – converted to direct bilirubin – for excretion. Conjugation occurs in the liver as bilirubin combines with glucuronic acid with the assistance of the enzyme glucuronyl transferase; a water-soluble bilirubin form results. Urobilinogen and stercobilinogen, the bilirubin compounds resulting from breakdown, can be excreted in the urine and stool.

Jaundice (icterus). If unconjugated bilirubin accumulates faster than the liver can clear it, the neonate may develop the yellow pallor known as jaundice. Slow or ineffective bilirubin clearance results in some degree of jaundice in approximately half of full-term neonates and 90% of preterm neonates. Fortunately, most full-term neonates avoid toxic bilirubin accumulation because they have adequate serum albumin binding sites and sufficient liver production of glucuronyl transferase. Factors that may increase the risk of unconjugated hyperbilirubinemia (an elevated serum unconjugated bilirubin level) include asphyxia, cold stress (ineffective heat maintenance), hypoglycemia, and maternal salicylate ingestion (Avery, 1987).

Ineffective excretion of conjugated bilirubin may cause conjugated hyperbilirubinemia (an elevated serum conjugated bilirubin level). Always abnormal in the neonate, this condition warrants evaluation.

Four types of jaundice occur in the neonate—physiologic jaundice, pathologic jaundice, breast milk jaundice (BMJ), and breast-feeding–associated jaundice (BFAJ).

Physiologic jaundice arises 48 to 72 hours after birth. The serum bilirubin level peaks at 4 to 12 mg/dl by the third to fifth day after birth. On average, the bilirubin level increases by less than 5 mg/dl/day. Physiologic jaundice normally disappears by the end of the seventh day (Wilkerson, 1988). Five conditions that may cause physiologic jaundice are decreased hepatic circulation, increased bilirubin load, reduced hepatic bilirubin uptake from the plasma, decreased bilirubin conjugation, and decreased bilirubin excretion.

In contrast, pathologic jaundice occurs within the first 24 hours after birth; the serum bilirubin level rises above 13 mg/dl. Pathologic jaundice may stem from such conditions as blood group or blood type incompatibilities; hepatic, biliary, or metabolic abnormalities; or infection.

BMJ was first identified in the 1960s. Although various causes have been suggested, current theory focuses on increased breast milk levels of the enzyme beta-glucuronidase. Researchers believe this enzyme causes increased intestinal bilirubin absorption in the neonate, thus blocking bilirubin excretion. BMJ appears as physiologic jaundice subsides (after the seventh day). The serum bilirubin level peaks at 15 to 25 mg/dl between days 10 and 15. BMJ may persist for several weeks or, rarely, several months. A serum bilirubin level that decreases 24 to 48 hours after discontinuation of breast-feeding confirms the diagnosis.

Controversy exists over whether BMJ warrants treatment. Some physicians and breast-feeding advocates consider treatment unnecessary. Conservative treatment involves temporarily stopping breast-feeding until the bilirubin level declines; this usually takes 24 to 48 hours. The mother should maintain lactation by expressing milk by hand or pump.

BFAJ correlates with the neonate's breast-feeding patterns. The underlying cause of BFAJ is poor caloric intake that leads to decreased hepatic transport and removal of bilirubin from the body. Typically, the neonate who develops BFAJ has not been able to stimulate an early and adequate supply of breast milk. BFAJ usually appears 48 to 72 hours after birth. The serum bilirubin level peaks at 15 to 19 mg/dl by 72 hours. The average serum bilirubin level increases by less than 5 mg/dl/day. Treatment of BMAJ involves measures that ensure an adequate breast milk supply. Wilkerson (1988) recommends breast-feeding the neonate every 2 hours to stimulate the mother's milk production and the neonate's intestinal motility.

The mother who quickly identifies signs of hunger in her infant should initiate feeding instead of waiting for the infant to cry vigorously. If the bilirubin level approaches 18 to 20 mg/dl, phototherapy may be necessary. (See Chapter 21, Care of High-Risk Neonates and Their Families, for more information on phototherapy.)

Bilirubin encephalopathy (kernicterus). Unconjugated serum bilirubin levels of approximately 20 mg/dl or higher may lead to bilirubin encephalopathy, a life-threatening condition characterized by bilirubin deposition in the basal ganglia of the brain. To assess the risk for bilirubin encephalopathy, the neonate's condition and gestational and chronological ages must be considered in conjunction with the bilirubin level. The condition may be treated with phototherapy or exchange transfusions.

Blood coagulation

For the first few days after birth, the GI tract lacks the bacterial action to synthesize adequate vitamin K. Vitamin K catalyzes synthesis of prothrombin by the liver, thereby activating four coagulation factors (II, VII, IX, and X). Consequently, the neonate is at special risk for hemorrhage (hemorrhagic disease of the neonate). All neonates now receive a prophylactic injection of vitamin K soon after delivery to help prevent hemorrhage (Putnam, 1984).

Carbohydrate metabolism

The major energy source during the first 4 to 6 hours after birth, glucose is stored in the liver as glycogen. The increased metabolic demands of labor, delivery, and the first few hours after birth cause rapid glycogen depletion (approximately 90% of liver glycogen is used within the first 3 hours). Skeletal muscle glycogen stores also decline rapidly (Streeter, 1986). If the neonate does not receive exogenous glucose, glycogenolysis (breakdown of glycogen into a usable glucose form) occurs. Until the neonate takes in sufficient glucose, glycogenolysis causes release of sufficient glucose into the bloodstream to maintain a serum glucose level of approximately 60 mg/dl. However, such stresses as hypothermia, hypoxia, and delayed feeding may rapidly exhaust glycogen stores, leading to hypoglycemia (Korones, 1986).

Iron storage

By term, the liver contains enough iron to produce RBCs until about age 5 months (provided the mother ingested adequate iron during pregnancy). Removed from destroyed RBCs, iron is stored in the liver, then recycled into new RBCs. The neonate must ingest sufficient dietary iron to maintain adequate RBC production.

RENAL SYSTEM

A relatively immature renal system makes the neonate susceptible to dehydration, acidosis, and electrolyte imbalance if vomiting and diarrhea occur (Gomella, 1988). The neonate's short, narrow renal tubules inhibit urine concentration and acidification and increase the fraction of excreted amino acids, phosphates, and bicarbonate. Also, the neonate's kidneys are relatively inefficient at secreting hydrogen ions in the tubule to promote acid-base balance.

Glomerular filtration rate

In utero, glomerular perfusion pressure is relatively low and arteriolar resistance high. These conditions contribute to a low fetal glomerular filtration rate (GFR), defined as the volume of glomerular filtrate formed over a specific period. A low GFR limits the capacity of the kidneys to excrete excess solutes and regulate body water composition.

In the last trimester of pregnancy, the fetal kidneys undergo tremendous growth and maturation. At 34 weeks of gestation, the GFR – and consequently renal function – improve markedly (Avery, 1987). Thus, neonatal GFR varies with gestational age; the full-term neonate has a higher GFR than the preterm neonate. The GFR reaches 30% of adult values within the first 2 days of extrauterine life, but it does not attain full adult values until about age 2.

Fluid balance

During the neonate's transition after birth, changes occur in extracellular, intracellular, and total body water volume. At birth, water makes up approximately 70% of the body composition, compared to approximately 58% by adulthood. Extracellular fluid accounts for about 40% of the neonate's total body water. As cell mass increases, this percentage drops; by adulthood, extracellular fluid accounts for 20% of total body water.

The neonate usually voids within 24 hours of birth. The first urine may be dark red and cloudy from urate and mucus (the slight reddish stain has no clinical significance). The neonate's urine usually is odorless; specific gravity ranges from 1.005 to 1.015.

As the neonate's fluid intake increases, urine output increases and urine becomes clear or light straw in color. The breast-fed neonate may require 10 to 12 diaper changes daily. The bottle-fed neonate typically requires about 6 diaper changes daily.

Loss of fluid through urine, feces, insensible (imperceptible) losses, intake restrictions related to small gastric capacity, and increased metabolic rate contributes to a reduction of 5% to 15% of the birth weight over the first 5 days of extrauterine life. However, in the period before the mother's milk supply is established, increased extracellular fluid volume protects the breast-fed neonate from dehydration. The neonate should regain the birth weight within 10 days (Avery, 1987). Typically, the infant doubles the birth weight by age 5 to 6 months and triples it by the first birthday.

GI SYSTEM

At birth, the neonate must assume the digestive functions previously performed by the placenta – including metabolism of sufficient amounts of water, proteins, carbohydrates, fats, vitamins, and minerals for adequate growth and development.

Gastric capacity

Despite a relatively immature GI system, the healthy neonate can ingest, absorb, and digest nutrients. Gastric capacity is between 40 and 60 ml on the first day after birth; it increases with subsequent feedings. Because of this limited capacity, nutrient needs must be met through frequent small-volume feedings. Gastric emptying time – typically 2 to 4 hours – varies with the volume of the feeding and the neonate's age. Peristalsis is rapid.

Many neonates regurgitate a small amount of ingested matter (1 to 2 ml) after feedings because of an immature cardiac sphincter (a muscular ring constricting the esophagus). Persistent, forceful, or large-volume regurgitation is abnormal and warrants investigation.

GI enzymes

Compared to the adult's intestine, the neonate's is longer relative to body size and has more secretory glands and a larger absorptive surface. The neonate's ability to digest nutrients depends on enzyme action and gastric acidity. The stomach lining consists of chief cells (which secrete pepsinogen and promote protein digestion) and parietal cells (which secrete hydrochloric acid to maintain gastric acidity). Salivary glands secrete only minimal amounts of saliva until age 2 to 3 months, when drooling becomes apparent. Milk digestion begins in the stomach and continues in the small intestine. Secretions from the pancreas, liver, and duodenum aid digestion.

Enzyme deficiencies limit the neonate's absorption of complex carbohydrates and fats. Deficiency of amylase, an enzyme produced in the salivary glands and pancreas, persists until age 3 to 6 months, restricting the conversion of starch to maltose. Deficiency of lipase, which the pancreas secretes in minimal amounts, impedes fat digestion (Avery, 1987). Lipase production increases in the first few weeks after birth.

Vitamin K synthesis

Synthesis of vitamin K through bacterial action is another important GI function. Although initially sterile, the GI tract establishes normal colonic bacteria within the first week after birth, allowing adequate vitamin K synthesis.

Initiation of feedings

In most cases, feedings should begin as soon as the neonate is physiologically stable and exhibits adequate coordination of the sucking and swallowing reflexes. An extended delay before feedings may deplete the neonate's limited glycogen reserves – already taxed by the increased energy demands of the transitional period. This may result in hypoglycemia (reflected by a serum glucose level below 35 mg/dl), which poses a threat to the glucose-dependent brain.

Feedings should be offered by breast or bottle. In some health care facilities, the neonate receives sterile water as the first feeding to verify the sucking and swallowing reflexes without risking aspiration of formula into the airway.

Neonatal stools

Initially, the neonate's intestines contain meconium, a thick, dark-green, odorless fecal substance consisting of amniotic fluid, bile, epithelial cells, and hair (from in utero shedding of lanugo – the fine, soft hair covering the fetus's shoulders and back). Typically, the neonate passes the first meconium stool within 24 hours of birth.

After enteric feedings begin, fecal color, odor, and consistency change. Transitional stools usually appear on the second or third day after feedings begin. These greenish brown stools have a higher water content than meconium.

The type of feeding determines the characteristics of subsequent stools. The formula-fed neonate passes pasty, pale-yellow stools with a strong odor. Stools from the breast-fed neonate are golden-yellow, sweet smelling, and more liquid.

The gastric distention that results from food ingestion causes relaxation and contraction of colonic muscles, commonly leading to a bowel movement during or after a feeding. Typically, the breast-fed neonate has more fre-

quent bowel movements than the formula-fed neonate because breast milk digests more rapidly than formula.

IMMUNE SYSTEM

The immune system is deficient at birth. With delivery comes exposure to substances (for example, bacteria) not normally present in utero. Such exposure activates components of the immune response. The first year is the period of greatest vulnerability to such serious infections as *Haemophilus influenzae*. Bacterial infections (including those caused by group B streptococci and staphylococci) occur in about 2% of neonates; viral infections – such as varicella and cytomegalovirus (CMV) – in about 8% (Berkowitz, 1984).

Immune response

The various elements of the immune system recognize, remember, respond to, and eliminate foreign substances called antigens. Primarily proteins, antigens may invade the body's protective barriers (such as the skin and mucous membranes) or arise from malignant cell transformation.

When local barriers and inflammation fail to fight off antigenic invasion, the immune system initiates a humoral or cell-mediated response. The response is carried out by the mononuclear phagocytic system, which includes cells in the thymus, lymphoid tissue, liver, spleen, and bone marrow. Cells involved in the immune response include lymphocytes (specifically, T cells and B cells), granulocytes, monocytes, RBCs, and platelets.

Humoral immunity. This response is mediated by humoral antibodies. Also called immunoglobulins, these proteins are synthesized in response to a specific antigen. B cells, coated with immunoglobulins, recognize invaders and produce antibodies, which are molecules that react specifically with a matching site on a corresponding antigen. This antigen-antibody reaction activates the complement system, a series of chemical reactions that removes the antigen from the body. Humoral immunity is most important against bacterial and viral reinfections.

Immunoglobulins have one or more molecules, each of which consists of four polypeptide chains. Properties of these chains determine the immunoglobulin's classification.

Immunoglobulin G (IgG). The most abundant immunoglobulin, IgG (gamma globulin) is synthesized in response to bacteria, viruses, and fungal organisms. Maternal IgG, transferred to the fetus via the placenta, confers passive acquired immunity (a short-lived immunity in which no antibodies are produced). Fetal IgG appears by the twelfth week of gestation, with levels increasing significantly during the last trimester.

IgG is active against gram-positive cocci (pneumococci and streptococci), meningococci, *H. influenzae,* some viruses, and diphtheria and tetanus toxins (if the mother has been exposed to these agents). The neonate also has protection against most childhood diseases – including diphtheria, measles, and smallpox – provided the mother has antibodies to these diseases. Because IgG does not act against gram-negative rods (such as *Escherichia coli* and *Enterobacter*), the neonate is more susceptible to infection by these agents.

Passive immunity may interfere with infant immunization by preventing a challenge to the infant's immune system, which ordinarily would cause the immune system to make antibodies to the disease for which the immunization was given. Thus, when the IgG level drops, the infant may contract the disease. For example, an infant may contract pertussis despite receiving the first DPT (diphtheria, pertussis, tetanus) injection.

By about age 3 months, maternally acquired IgG is depleted. By then, however, the body usually produces enough IgG to replace the lost antibodies.

Immunoglobulin M (IgM). The first immunoglobulin produced by antigenic challenge, IgM is the major antibody in blood type incompatibilities and gram-negative bacterial infections. Maternal IgM does not cross the placenta. By the twentieth week of gestation, however, the fetus produces IgM in response to antigenic exposure. IgM provides active immunity (a long-lasting or permanent immunity resulting from antigenic stimulation through inoculation or natural immunity). High IgM levels in the neonate may signal perinatal infection.

Immunoglobulin A (IgA). The major antibody in the mucosal linings of the intestines and bronchi, IgA appears in all body secretions. It does not cross the placenta and normally is absent in the neonate. Combining with a mucosal protein, IgA is secreted onto mucosal surfaces as a secretory antibody (secretory IgA). Present in breast milk, this substance confers some passive immunity on the breast-fed infant. Secretory IgA also limits bacterial growth in the GI tract.

Cell-mediated immunity. This immune response is most apparent in localized inflammations triggered by fungi, viruses, tissue transplants, and tumors. Various types of T cells carry out cell-mediated immunity. Recognizing a foreign antigen, T cells mobilize tissue macrophages in the presence of migration inhibitory factor. This substance triggers chemical reactions that convert local macrophages into phagocytes and prevent macrophages from leaving the invasion site until they have destroyed the antigen. The breast-fed infant may acquire passive immunity to such diseases as polio, mumps, influenza, and chicken pox through the cell-mediated response.

Congenital infections

Usually, congenital infections – those acquired in utero – result from exposure to such viruses as CMV, rubella, hepatitis B, herpes simplex, herpes zoster, varicella, and Epstein-Barr. However, they also may stem from such nonviral agents as toxoplasmosis, syphilis, tuberculosis, trypanosomiasis, and malaria. Collectively, these viral and nonviral agents are called TORCH – an acronym for toxoplasmosis, others, rubella, CMV, and herpes.

Fetal infection by a TORCH agent follows a systemic maternal infection with placental involvement and fetal spread. TORCH infections can cause a wide range of sequelae, from spontaneous abortion and fetal death to overt or asymptomatic infection at birth. In the early prenatal period, infection by certain TORCH agents (such as rubella and toxoplasmosis) causes disruption of embryogenesis, resulting in severe congenital anomalies (Avery, 1987).

Congenital bacterial infections may arise from bacterial organisms that travel to the fetus through the placenta. Organisms causing such infections include *Listeria monocytogenes, E. coli, Klebsiella,* and *Streptococcus pneumoniae.* The fetus also may become infected by organisms that reach the amniotic cavity via the mother's cervix. Other routes of infection include the fetal skin and mucous membranes, intervillous placental spaces, umbilical cord to the fetal circulation, and respiratory airways (via aspiration). Infectious agents that may take these routes include group B streptococci, *E. coli, L. monocytogenes,* and herpes simplex. An infected neonate may be acutely ill at birth with septicemia, pneumonia, or both (Berkowitz, 1984).

NEUROLOGIC SYSTEM

Although not fully developed, the neonate's neurologic system can perform the complex functions required to regulate neonatal adaptation – stimulate initial respirations, maintain acid-base balance, and regulate body temperature. The neonate's neurologic function is controlled primarily by the brain stem and spinal cord. The autonomic nervous system and brain stem coordinate respiratory and cardiac functions. All cranial nerves are present at birth; however, the nerves are not yet fully sheathed with myelin, a substance essential for smooth nerve impulse transmission.

The neonate has a functioning cerebral cortex, although the degree to which it is used remains unknown. At birth, the brain measures about one-fourth the size of the adult brain. The brain grows and matures in a cephalocaudal (head-to-toe) direction.

The brain needs a constant supply of glucose for energy and a relatively high oxygen level to maintain adequate cellular metabolism (Volpe and Hill, 1987). For this reason, the neonate's oxygenation status and serum glucose levels must be assessed and monitored carefully to detect impaired gas exchange or signs of hypoglycemia.

Nerve tract development

Sensory, cerebellar, and extrapyramidal nerve pathways are the first to develop. This accounts for the neonate's strong sense of hearing, taste, and smell. The cerebellum governs gross voluntary movement and helps maintain equilibrium. The extrapyramidal tract controls reflexive gross motor movement and postural adjustment by regulating reciprocal flexion and extension of muscle groups, thus maintaining smooth, coordinated movement.

Neonatal reflexes

The neonate's reflexes—categorized as feeding, protective, postural, and social—include such primitive reflexes as sucking and rooting (which causes the neonate to turn toward and search for the nipple). Crucial to survival, these reflexes serve as the basis for neonatal neurologic examination. Persistence of the neonatal reflexes beyond the age at which they normally disappear may indicate a neurologic abnormality.

ENDOCRINE AND METABOLIC SYSTEMS

At birth, the endocrine system is anatomically mature but functionally immature. Complex interactions between the neurologic and endocrine systems help coordinate adaptation to extrauterine life. Such interactions take place along three major feedback pathways:
- the parasympathetic–adrenal medulla pathway
- the hypothalamic–anterior pituitary pathway
- the hypothalamic–posterior pituitary pathway (Volpe and Hill, 1987).

Hormonal role in transition

Many extrauterine adaptations are regulated by hormones secreted by the endocrine glands, including growth hormone, thyroid-stimulating hormone, adrenocorticotropic hormone, cortisol, and catecholamines. However, the posterior pituitary gland secretes only a limited amount of antidiuretic hormone (ADH), a substance that limits urine production. Insufficient ADH contributes to the neonate's increased risk of dehydration.

Metabolic changes at birth

Interruption of placental circulation at birth halts the supply of oxygen, nutrients, electrolytes, and other vital substances to the neonate. Withdrawal of maternally supplied glucose and calcium necessitates significant and immediate metabolic changes to ensure successful neonatal adaptation. During the first few hours after birth, serum glucose and calcium levels change rapidly.

Glucose. At birth, the neonate's serum glucose level usually measures 60% to 70% of the maternal serum glucose level. Over the next 2 hours, this level falls, stabilizing between 35 and 40 mg/dl. By 6 hours after birth, however, it usually rises to about 60 mg/dl, unless the neonate experiences cold stress, delayed feeding, metabolic abnormalities, or sepsis.

Calcium. The serum calcium level decreases at birth but usually stabilizes between 24 and 48 hours after birth. A level below 7 mg/dl reflects hypocalcemia. Most commonly, hypocalcemia arises within the first 2 days or at 6 to 10 days after birth. Hypocalcemia may result from hypoxemia, interrupted maternal calcium transfer (early-onset hypocalcemia), or infant formula with an improper calcium-to-phosphorus ratio (later-onset hypocalcemia). In most cases, the full-term neonate given sufficient amounts of the proper formula or breast milk achieves the normal calcium-to-phosphorus ratio of 2:1 (Philip, 1987).

Thermoregulation

Body temperature maintenance—essential for successful extrauterine adaptation—is regulated by complex interactions between environmental temperature and body heat loss and production. The understanding and appropriate management of thermoregulation were among the earliest advances in neonatology.

The neonate has limited thermoregulatory capacity, achieved by body heating and cooling mechanisms. When the neonate no longer can maintain body temperature, cooling or overheating results; exhaustion of thermoregulatory mechanisms brings death. (For a depiction of the progressive effects of hypothermia, see *Dangers of untreated hypothermia,* page 342.)

As the neonate makes the transition to extrauterine life, the core temperature decreases by an amount that

DANGERS OF UNTREATED HYPOTHERMIA

Hypothermia prevention ranks among the most important goals of neonatal nursing care. As shown, untreated hypothermia can have grave consequences—culminating in death.

HYPOTHERMIA

Norepinephrine release

Peripheral vasoconstriction

DEATH

Pulmonary vasoconstriction

Increased acidosis

Increased pulmonary vascular resistance

Anaerobic metabolism

Increased right-to-left shunt

Hypoxia

---

varies with the environmental temperature and the neonate's condition. Initially, the full-term neonate's core temperature falls by approximately 0.54° F (0.3° C) per minute. Thus, under normal delivery conditions, it may drop 5.4° F (3° C) before the neonate leaves the delivery room.

Maintaining normal body temperature in the neonate can contribute significantly to successful adaptation. Neonatal morbidity and mortality can be favorably influenced by the nurse who takes steps to prevent cold stress.

Neutral thermal environment (NTE). Encompassing a narrow range of environmental temperatures, NTE requires the least amount of energy to maintain a stable core temperature. For an unclothed, full-term neonate on the first day after birth, NTE ranges from 89.6° to 93.2° F (32° to 34° C). Within this temperature range, oxygen consumption and carbon dioxide production are lowest and core temperature is normal. To maintain body temperature within the NTE, the neonate makes vasomotor adjustments—vasoconstriction to conserve heat and vasodilation to release heat. Environmental temperatures below or above the NTE increase oxygen consumption and boost the metabolic rate—the amount of energy expended over a given unit of time (Gomella, 1988).

The following characteristics place the neonate at a physiologic disadvantage for thermoregulation, increasing the risk of hypothermia:
• a large body surface relative to mass
• limited subcutaneous fat deposition to provide insulation
• vasomotor instability
• limited metabolic capacity.

Mechanisms of heat loss. Heat loss, which begins at delivery, can occur through the following four mechanisms:

Evaporation. Evaporative heat loss occurs when fluids (insensible water, visible perspiration, and pulmonary fluids) turn to vapor in dry air. The drier the environment, the greater the evaporative heat loss. The pronounced evaporative heat loss occurring with delivery can be minimized by immediately drying the neonate and discarding the wet towels.

Conduction. This form of heat loss takes place when the skin directly contacts a cooler object—for example, a cold bed or scale. Therefore, any metal surface on which the neonate will be placed should be padded.

Radiation. A cooler solid surface not in direct contact with the neonate can cause heat loss through radiation. Common sources of radiant heat loss include incubator walls and windows. Occurring even with warm air temperatures, radiant heat loss may be minimized through the use of a thermoplastic heat shield (such as Plexiglas).

Convection. Heat loss from the body surface to cooler surrounding air occurs through convection. It increases in drafty environments. Thus, a delivery room cooled for the comfort of personnel may cause significant convective heat loss in the neonate.

Defenses against hypothermia. In a cold environment or in other stressful circumstances, the neonate defends against heat loss through vasomotor control, thermal insulation, muscle activity, and nonshivering thermogenesis.

Vasomotor control. Peripheral nervous stimulation activates vasomotor control and metabolic processes to regulate thermal control. The neonate conserves heat through peripheral vasoconstriction and dissipates heat through peripheral vasodilation.

Thermal insulation. Provided by subcutaneous (white) fat, thermal insulation guards against rapid heat loss. The amount of subcutaneous fat determines the degree of thermal insulation. (Subcutaneous fat commonly accounts for 11% to 17% of the full-term neonate's weight.)

Muscle activity. Muscle activity increases heat production. Initially, the neonate reacts to a cold environment with increased movements (often perceived as irritability). For instance, the neonate may assume a tightly flexed posture that reduces heat loss by limiting body surface area.

Whether the neonate can produce heat by shivering remains unknown. Experts now believe the neonate may have some shivering ability. Nonetheless, even if shivering does occur in response to severe cold stress, it does not serve as a major heat source (Avery, 1987).

Nonshivering thermogenesis. Defined as the production of heat through lipolysis of brown fat, nonshivering thermogenesis is the neonate's most efficient heat production mechanism because it increases the metabolic rate minimally. A type of adipose tissue, brown fat accounts for up to 1.5% of a full-term neonate's total weight. Named for its brown color—a result of its rich vascular supply, dense cellular content, and numerous nerve endings—brown fat is deposited around the neck, head, heart, great vessels, kidneys, and adrenal glands; between the scapula; behind the sternum; and in the axillae.

The brain, liver, and skeletal muscles take part in nonshivering thermogenesis. In response to heat loss, sympathetic nerves stimulate the release of norepinephrine, the major mediator of nonshivering thermogenesis. Norepinephrine stimulates oxidation of brown fat, causing increased heat production. Heat produced by brown fat oxidation is distributed throughout the body by the blood, which absorbs heat as it flows through fatty tissue.

INTEGUMENTARY SYSTEM

The healthy neonate is moist and warm to the touch. Lanugo—fine, downy hair—may appear over the shoulders and back.

As with adults, the neonate's skin serves as the first line of defense against infection. The outermost skin layer, the stratum corneum, is fused with the vernix caseosa. A greasy white substance produced by sebaceous glands, the vernix caseosa coats the fetal skin and protects it from the amniotic fluid. (Because of its protective properties, the vernix caseosa should not be scrubbed off.) With maturation, the stratum corneum becomes an effective protective barrier (Guyton, 1985).

The full-term neonate's skin may appear erythematous (beefy red) for several hours after birth but soon takes on a normal color. In many neonates, vasomotor instability, capillary stasis, and high hemoglobin levels lead to acrocyanosis, characterized by bluish discoloration of the hands and feet. Skin color and circulation usually improve with warming of the hands and feet. (Acrocyanosis, a common condition, should not be confused with central cyanosis, which reflects impaired gas exchange. In central cyanosis, the neonate's skin and mucous membranes turn blue.)

MUSCULOSKELETAL SYSTEM

Ossification (bone development) is incomplete at birth but proceeds rapidly afterward. The neonate's skeleton consists mainly of bone.

Six thin, unjoined bones form the neonate's skull; these bones accommodate subsequent brain and head development. Separating the skull bones are sutures—fibrous joints in which the apposed bones are joined by a thin layer of fibrous connective tissue. Fontanels, soft-tissue areas covered with tough membranes, separate the sutures. Typically, vaginal delivery causes overriding sutures, a spontaneously resolving condition in which the sutures appear to be pushed together.

The muscles are anatomically complete at term birth. With age, muscle mass, strength, and size increase. Increasing muscle strength is crucial to the development of postural control and mobility (Lawrence, 1984).

REPRODUCTIVE SYSTEM

The reproductive system is anatomically and functionally immature at birth. However, the female's ovaries contain all potential ova, which decrease in number from birth to maturity by roughly 90%. In approximately 90% of males, the testes have descended into the scrotum by birth, although no sperm appear until puberty.

High maternal estrogen levels may cause transient adverse effects in the neonate. For example, breast hypertrophy with or without witch's milk (a thin, watery secretion similar to colostrum) may appear in both the male and female neonate. The female may have pseudomenstruation, a mucoid or blood-tinged vaginal discharge caused by the sudden drop in hormone levels after birth (Gomella, 1988). Clinically insignificant, breast hypertrophy and pseudomenstruation resolve spontaneously as the influence of maternal hormones subsides.

Normally, the male neonate has adhesions of the prepuce (penile foreskin) that prevent separation of the prepuce and glans. During fetal development, prepuce tissue is continuous with the epidermal glans covering.

BEHAVIORAL CHARACTERISTICS OF ADAPTATION

Research on neonatal development in the past 10 to 20 years has shown that the neonate has remarkable sensory, cognitive, and social abilities.

Neonate-environment interactions

The full-term neonate not only perceives the environment but attempts to control it through behavior. Able to see, hear, and differentiate among tastes and smells, the neonate responds to touch and movement, defends against stimulation, and gives signals that, when interpreted by a responsive caregiver, can satisfy the neonate's needs. For example, a neonate uncomfortable in a wet diaper cries; the mother responds by changing the diaper.

Neonatal sensory capacities

Using the sensory capacities—vision, hearing, touch, taste, and smell—the neonate perceives, interacts with, modifies, and learns from the environment. Combined with the neonate's attractive physical features, these sensory capacities play a major role in parent-infant bonding (sometimes called attachment).

Vision. Although the neonate can see, visual acuity is limited to a distance of approximately 9″ to 12″. The neonate has a preference for geometric shapes, such as squares, rectangles, or circles roughly 3″ in diameter. Black and white images hold the neonate's gaze longer than color images (Ludington-Hoe, 1983).

The neonate can conjugate the eyes (move them in unison) at or just after birth. However, immature neuro-

muscular control limits visual accommodation (the ability to adjust for distance) for the first 4 weeks after birth. Incomplete muscle control of ocular movements sometimes causes transient strabismus (deviation of the eyes, or "crossed" eyes). Also, the epicanthal fold covering the inner canthus of the eye may narrow the visible width of the sclera beside the iris, giving a neonate the appearance of having crossed eyes (pseudostrabismus).

The neonate apparently finds the human face intriguing and typically fixes the eyes and gazes intently at a face in proximity, as during feeding or cuddling. Such behavior strongly reinforces parent-infant bonding.

Visual acuity improves quickly; by age 6 months, adult level visual acuity is achieved. In the neonate exposed to various pleasing objects in a range of colors, shapes, and contrasts, visual acuity may improve even more rapidly. Placing crib gyms, mobiles, and pictures within view may help stimulate visual development. Because the neonate prefers more color, greater contrast, and more interesting patterns than the light pastels of the traditional nursery, a change in nursery decor and infant clothing may be warranted.

Sensitive to light, the neonate grimaces or frowns and turns the head away from a bright light directed toward the eyes and opens the eyes more readily in a dimly lit room. Thus, by dimming the lights, parents may improve eye contact with the neonate, facilitating bonding.

The neonate responds to movement in the environment, fixing on and following bright or shiny objects soon after birth. For instance, the neonate fixes on and follows a parent's eyes; while gazing at a parent's face, the neonate may appear to imitate that parent's facial expressions, thereby rewarding the parent's response. The ability to fix on and gaze at objects improves rapidly.

Hearing. The neonate can hear at birth. In fact, hearing begins even earlier: The fetus can hear extrauterine sounds (for instance, voices or music) as well as noises originating in maternal body systems, including variable low-pitched sounds in the maternal cardiovascular and GI systems (Kramer and Pierpont, 1976).

Hearing is well established after aeration of the eustachian tube and drainage of blood, vernix caseosa, amniotic fluid, and mucus from the outer ear. Shortly after birth, the neonate turns toward sounds and startles in response to loud noises, such as a ringing telephone, dropped chart, or slammed door. Able to differentiate sounds on the basis of frequency, intensity, and pattern, the neonate responds more readily to sounds below 4,000 Hz. (Human speech usually is between 500 and 900 Hz.)

The neonate responds variously to different vocal pitches. Most women have higher-pitched voices than men and instinctively raise their pitch when talking to an infant. A high-pitched voice attracts the attention of the neonate, who turns toward the sound with increased alertness. In contrast, the lower-pitched male voice seems to have a soothing effect. Mothers commonly make use of this effect by talking in a much lower pitch when trying to calm or console the neonate (Redshaw, Rivers, and Rosenblatt, 1985).

Touch. The neonate has well-developed tactile perception, which serves as a stimulus for the first breath. The most sensitive body areas include the face (especially around the mouth), hands, and soles.

Until recently, experts believed that incomplete nerve myelination prevented the neonate from experiencing pain, except perhaps to a limited degree. Current knowledge, however, refutes this assumption. Anand and Hickey (1987) concluded that the pain pathways and cortical and subcortical centers crucial to pain perception are well developed and that the neurochemical systems associated with pain transmission are intact and functional as term approaches. Physiologic changes associated with pain in the neonate include increased blood pressure and pulse during and after a painful procedure. During such a procedure, the neonate's PaCO$_2$ level fluctuates widely and palmar sweating increases. In neonates undergoing painful procedures, researchers also have documented marked hormonal changes—including increased plasma renin levels soon after venipuncture and elevated plasma cortisol levels during and after circumcision without anesthesia. Also, painful stimuli have elicited simple motor responses (flexion and adduction of extremities); distinct facial expressions (pain, sadness, surprise); and characteristic crying. Some preliminary studies suggest that neonates have pain memory as well as pain perception.

Pleasant cutaneous stimulation, on the other hand, induces muscle relaxation—another key factor in parent-infant bonding. As the mother becomes acquainted with the neonate by lightly touching the face, extremities, and trunk, the neonate's muscle tone and movement decrease and crying stops or declines, reinforcing the mother's attachment (Redshaw, Rivers, and Rosenblatt, 1985).

Handling of the neonate provides sensory stimulation from motion as well as from touch. Such stimulation elicits alertness and orienting responses. These responses, in turn, influence neonatal development and parent-neonate interaction. However, the neonate may tire if handled too much.

Taste. The neonate differentiates among tastes by the first or second day after birth. In response to a tasteless solution (such as sterile water), the neonate's facial expression remains unchanged. A sweet solution, on the other hand, elicits satisfied sucking; a sour solution induces a grimace and cessation of sucking; and a bitter solution provokes an angry facial expression, cessation of sucking, and in many cases, turning away of the head. Breast-feeding mothers also find that neonates prefer bottled breast milk to commercial formula during periods when they cannot nurse (Als, 1982).

Smell. Although little research has been conducted on neonatal olfaction, the neonate is known to react to strong or noxious odors by averting the head from the odor. Sensitivity to olfactory stimuli increases over the first 4 days after birth.

CHARACTERISTIC PATTERNS OF SLEEP AND ACTIVITY

During the transitional period, the neonate experiences a series of changes encompassing state of consciousness, behavioral response to stimuli, and physiologic parameters. Various neonatal sleep and awake states also have been identified.

Periods of neonatal reactivity

The neonate's initial hours are characterized by a predictable, identifiable series of behavioral and physiologic characteristics (Arnold, Putman, Barnard, Desmond, and Rudolph, 1965). Desmond and Associates (1966) described this series collectively as the periods of neonatal reactivity.

All neonates experience the same sequence of periods. However, when each period begins and how long it lasts varies from one neonate to another. Maternal medication, anesthesia, labor duration, and any stress affecting the neonate may influence the duration of a given period.

First period of reactivity. Beginning just after birth, this period lasts roughly 60 minutes. In this phase of intense activity and awareness of external stimuli, the neonate is alert and attentive to the environment and may exhibit vigorous activity, crying, and rapid respiratory and heart rates. The neonate has a strong desire to suckle during this period, so breast-feeding may be initiated. Gradually, the neonate becomes less alert and active and falls asleep.

Neonatal adaptations during this initial period are regulated mainly by the sympathetic nervous system. Irregular respirations, tachypnea, and nasal flaring unrelated to respiratory distress may occur. Other visible features of this period include spontaneous startles, the Moro reflex (in which the neonate extends and moves the limbs away from the body when the head is dropped backward suddenly), grimacing, sucking motions, sudden cries that stop abruptly, fine tremors of the jaw or extremities, blinking, and jerking eye movements.

The first period of reactivity provides a good opportunity for early parent-infant interaction. Studying the attachment of mothers and neonates, Klaus and Kennell (1976) concluded that this is the optimal time for promoting mother-infant bonding. They referred to this phase as a sensitive period, necessary to some degree for successful mother-infant bonding. Although the importance of this period to bonding has since been questioned, the work of Klaus and Kennell led to changes in routine obstetric and neonatal nursery care to prevent unnecessary separation of parents and neonate.

The nurse can enhance bonding by allowing the mother and neonate to remain together during this period (provided the neonate is healthy). After drying the neonate and performing initial care, the nurse should allow the parents to see and hold their child. Instillation of prophylactic eye medication should be delayed until after this period so that the neonate's heightened visual awareness can enhance parent-infant bonding.

Temperature must be monitored and maintained carefully during this period to prevent cold stress. For example, the nurse should carefully dry the neonate or use warmed blankets or overhead warming lights to supply heat and prevent heat loss. Although temperature maintenance should never be forfeited to allow parent-infant contact, the nurse should keep in mind that skin-to-skin contact between parent and neonate usually maintains the neonate's temperature adequately.

Sleep stage. The neonate typically falls asleeep about 2 to 3 hours after birth and remains asleep for a few minutes to 2 to 4 hours. Some authorities classify sleep as a distinct, self-contained period of reactivity. Others consider it a transitional phase bridging the first and second periods.

While asleep, the neonate's respiratory rate increases while the heart rate ranges from 120 to 140 beats/minute. Skin color improves, although some acrocyanosis persists. Because the neonate has little response to external stimuli during the sleep period, attempts at breast-feeding will elicit no response. However, the mother may wish to hold and cuddle her child.

Second period of reactivity. Beginning when the neonate awakens, this period is characterized by an exaggerated response to internal and external stimuli. The heart rate is labile, and episodes of bradycardia and tachycardia occur. The neonate's skin usually appears pink-tinged or ruddy (although skin color naturally varies with racial background). Thick oral secretions frequently cause gagging and emesis. The respiratory rate, ranging from about 30 to 60 breaths/minute, is irregular and may include brief apneic pauses and periodic tachypnea. The neonate usually expels meconium from the GI tract during this period.

The second period may last from 4 to 6 hours. As it ends, the neonate becomes more stable and the respiratory and cardiac rates normalize. A dynamic equilibrium emerges, with the neonate alternating between alert activity and sleep and establishing a pattern of sleeping, crying, activity, and feeding. Although the environment influences the neonate's diurnal and circadian rhythms, temperament also strongly affects behavior.

Nursing measures appropriate for this period include monitoring vital signs, maintaining temperature, and ensuring a patent airway. The nurse also should encourage the parents to get acquainted with their infant at this time. The neonate may exhibit vigorous sucking motions and may appear hungry. (For a discussion of assessment during the two periods of reactivity, see Chapter 18, Neonatal Assessment.)

Sleep and awake states of the neonate

Brazelton (1979) classified the neonate's state of consciousness into six states—two sleep states and four awake states. The sleep and awake states encompass the behavioral states used in the Brazelton Neonatal Behavioral Assessment Scale (BNBAS). Developed by Brazelton to measure a neonate's capabilities, the BNBAS assesses neonatal behavioral responses and elicited responses as well as behavioral states. (For details on the BNBAS, see Chapter 18, Neonatal Assessment.)

The neonate's ability to regulate the state of consciousness reflects central nervous system integrity. The state of consciousness may be affected by medication, hunger, diurnal cycles, stress (such as from noise, pain, and bright lights), and any other physical discomfort. Normally, the neonate in a sleep state responds to stimuli with increased activity, whereas a neonate in the crying state responds with decreased activity.

According to Brazelton, when confronted with external interferences (such as a heel prick or another painful stimulus), the neonate attempts to control the state of consciousness in one of four ways:

- by trying to withdraw physically
- by trying to push away the stimulus with the hands or feet
- by trying to withdraw emotionally (for example, turning away from the stimulus or falling asleep)
- by crying or fussing in an effort to interrupt the stimulus.

State of consciousness serves as a key focus of nursing assessment and as the basis for care of both neonate and parents. The nurse must be sufficiently familiar with neonatal sleep and awake states to recognize the neonate's state and any changes in it. By using this information, the nurse may more skillfully assess the neonate, plan neonatal care, and help promote parent-neonate interaction. (See Chapter 18, Neonatal Assessment, for details on assessing specific sleep and awake states.)

Deep sleep. In this sleep state, the neonate's eyes are closed and no rapid eye movements (REMs) appear. Except for occasional startle reflexes, no spontaneous activity occurs. Respirations are even and regular. The neonate in deep sleep usually cannot be aroused by external stimuli and will not breast-feed. Attempts by the mother to feed the neonate will cause frustration.

Light sleep. During this period, the neonate's eyes are closed and REMs occur. Variable breathing patterns, random movements, and sucking motions typify light sleep. External stimuli may arouse the neonate in this state.

Drowsy state. In this transitional state, the neonate attempts to become fully alert. The eyes may be open or closed and the eyelids may flutter frequently. Muscle movements are smooth, with intermittent spontaneous activity and startles. Tactile or auditory stimuli may evoke a response, but the response may be sluggish until the neonate approaches the next state.

Alert state. In this state, the eyes are open, bright, and shining and the neonate focuses on the source of stimulation. Aware of and responsive to the environment, the neonate makes purposeful movements and shows good eye-hand coordination. The neonate attempts to attain and maintain this state.

The alert state is considered the optimal state of arousal, ideal for parent-neonate contact or breast-feeding initiation. Although only minimally active, the neonate remains alert and responsive to visual and auditory stimulation for prolonged periods. Additional stimulation may cause a change of state (although the response to external stimulation is delayed).

Active state. The neonate's movements increase in this state, and external stimuli cause eye and body movements. The level of this activity increases as the next state approaches.

Crying state. In this state, the neonate responds to both internal and external stimuli. Usually beginning with slight whimpering and minimal activity, the neonate in the crying state typically progresses to increased motor activity, with thrusting movements of the extremities and spontaneous startles. The chance for successful feeding or interaction may improve if the parents or nurse can calm the neonate through such motions as rocking.

CHAPTER SUMMARY

Chapter 17 discussed neonatal adaptation, the transitional period that follows delivery. By becoming familiar with the neonate's normal adaptations during this period, the nurse can more easily identify signs of abnormal adaptation. Here are the chapter highlights.

During the first 24 hours after birth, called the transitional period, the neonate experiences many biological and behavioral adaptations to extrauterine life.

At birth, the four unique anatomic features of fetal circulation (the placenta, ductus venosus, foramen ovale, and ductus arteriosus) undergo changes that establish neonatal circulation. The placenta is removed at birth. The ductus venosus functionally closes as clamping of the umbilical cord eliminates its blood flow. Hemodynamic events triggered by the neonate's initial respirations lead to functional closure of the foramen ovale. The effects of the neonate's initial respirations also cause functional closure of the ductus arteriosus.

The full term neonate's blood volume typically is 80 to 90 ml/kg of body weight.

Asphyxia is the strongest stimulus for the first breath. Other breathing stimuli include hypoxia, acidosis, cord occlusion, thermal changes, and tactile stimulation.

Fetal erythrocytes contain fetal hemoglobin (hemoglobin F), which has a higher affinity for oxygen than adult hemoglobin (hemoglobin A). Leukocytes serve as the neonate's main internal defense against infection.

For several days after birth, Vitamin K levels are low because of insufficient bacterial action in the GI tract to synthesize vitamin K. Consequently, the neonate lacks several vitamin K–dependent coagulation factors.

Before feedings begin, glucose serves as the neonate's major energy source.

Because of a relatively immature renal system, the neonate is at risk for acidosis, dehydration, and electrolyte imbalance.

Like the adult, the neonate has two specific immune responses—humoral and cell-mediated. The three major classes of immunoglobulins are IgG, IgM, and IgA.

Neonatal defenses against heat loss include vasomotor control, thermal insulation, muscle activity, and nonshivering thermogenesis.

Acrocyanosis, a condition characterized by bluish discoloration of the hands and feet, results from vasomotor instability, capillary stasis, and a high hemoglobin level.

The typical neonate's visual acuity is limited to a distance of 9″ to 12″. The neonate has a preference for black and white geometric shapes.

Neonatal hearing is well established once the eustachian tube is aerated and the outer ear cleared of vernix, blood, mucus, and amniotic fluid.

The neonate reacts to pain with physiologic, hormonal, and motor responses.

The stages of neonatal reactivity represent a predictable series of behaviors and physiologic characteristics.

The neonate's state of consciousness consists of six states—two sleep states and four awake states. Knowledge of the characteristics of each state improves nursing assessment and care of the neonate and family.

STUDY QUESTIONS

1. What conditions occur to trigger the functional closure of the foramen ovale?

2. What is the action and function of pulmonary surfactant?

3. What stimuli are responsible for initiating respiration?

4. How does RBC production change after birth?

5. What is breast-feeding-associated jaundice (BFAJ), and how is it treated?

6. Which characteristics place the neonate at an increased risk of hypothermia?

7. What are the three periods of neonatal reactivity and what are the characteristics of each period?

8. How does the neonate attempt to control the state of consciousness when confronted by external interference?

BIBLIOGRAPHY

Avery, G.B. (1987). *Neonatology: Pathophysiology and management of the newborn* (3rd ed.). Philadelphia: Lippincott.

Brown, B.A. (1988). *Hematology: Principles and procedures.* Philadelphia: Lea & Febiger.

Cloherty, J.P., and Stark, A.R. (1985). *Manual of neonatal care (The Boston manual)* (2nd ed.). Boston: Little, Brown.

Gomella, T.L. (1988). *Neonatology: Procedures, "on-call" problems, diseases, drugs.* Norwalk, CT: Appleton & Lange.

Guyton, A. (1985). *Textbook of medical physiology* (7th ed.). Philadelphia: Saunders.

Klaus, M.H., and Kennell, J.H. (1976). *Maternal infant bonding.* St. Louis: Mosby.

Korones, S.B. (1986). *High-risk newborn infants: The basis for intensive nursing care* (3rd ed.). St. Louis: Mosby.

Kramer, L., and Piermont, M. (1976). Rocking waterbeds and auditory stimuli to enhance growth of preterm infants. *Journal of Pediatrics*, 88(2), 297-299.

March of Dimes (1985). *Report on child health.* White Plains, NY.

Philip, A.G. (1987). *Neonatology: A practical guide.* Philadelphia: Saunders.

Redshaw, M.E., Rivers, R.P.A., and Rosenblatt, D.B. (1985). *Born too early: Special care for your preterm baby.* New York: Oxford University Press.

Streeter, N.S. (1986). *High-risk neonatal care.* Rockville, MD: Aspen.

West, J.B. (1985). *Respiratory physiology—the essentials* (3rd ed.). Baltimore: Williams & Wilkins.

Neonatal assessment

Berkowitz, I.D. (1984). Infections in the newborn. In M. Ziai, T. Clarke, and T. Merritt (Eds.), *Assessment of the newborn: A guide for the practitioner* (pp. 59-80). Boston: Little, Brown.

Brazelton, T.B. (1973). Neonatal behavior assessment scale. *Clinics in Developmental Medicine*, No. 50. Philadelphia: Lippincott.

Brazelton, T.B. (1979). Behavioral competence of the newborn infant. *Seminars in Perinatology*, 3(1), 35-44.

Eisenberg, R. (1965). Auditory behaviors in the human neonate: Methodological problems. *Journal of Research*, 5, 159-177.

Ingelfinger, J.R. (1985). Renal conditions in the newborn period. In J.P. Cloherty and A.R. Stark (Eds.), *Manual of neonatal care* (2nd ed.; pp. 377-394). Boston: Little, Brown.

Lawrence, R. (1984). Physical examination. In M. Ziai, T. Clarke, and T. Merritt (Eds.), *Assessment of the newborn: A guide for the practitioner* (pp. 86-111). Boston: Little, Brown.

Ludington-Hoe, S.M. (1983). What can newborns really see? *AJN*, (9), 1286-1289.

Putnam, T.C. (1984). Gastrointestinal bleeding. In M. Ziai, T. Clarke, and T. Merritt (Eds.), *Assessment of the newborn: A guide for the practitioner* (pp. 207-209). Boston: Little, Brown.

Volpe, J.J., and Hill, A. (1987). Neurologic disorders. In G.B. Avery (Ed.), *Neonatology, pathophysiology, and management of the newborn* (pp. 1073-1132). Philadelphia: Lippincott.

Nursing management during transition

Als, H. (1982). Toward a synactive theory of development. Promise for the assessment and support of infant individuality. *Infant Mental Health Journal,* 3(4), 229-243.

Anand, K., and Hickey, P.R. (1987). Pain and its effects in the human neonate and fetus. *New England Journal of Medicine,* 317(21), 1321-1329.

Arnold, H.W., Putman, N.J., Barnard, B.L., Desmond, M.M., and Rudolph, A.J. (1965). Transition to extrauterine life. *AJN,* 65(10), 77-80.

Desmond, M.M., and Associates (1966). The transitional care nursery. *Pediatric Clinics of North America,* 13(3), 651-668.

Maisels, I. (1987). Neonatal jaundice. In G.B. Avery (Ed.), *Neonatology: Pathophysiology and management of the newborn* (3rd ed.; pp. 86-111). Philadelphia: Lippincott.

Wilkerson, N. (1988). A comprehensive look at hyperbilirubinemia. *MCN,* 13(5), 360-364.

CHAPTER 18

NEONATAL ASSESSMENT

OBJECTIVES

After reading and studying this chapter, the student should be able to:

1. Describe general guidelines to follow when assessing the neonate.

2. Discuss the characteristics of each period of neonatal reactivity and understand how these characteristics may affect assessment findings.

3. Identify the proper sequence to use for the comprehensive assessment.

4. Discuss the essential elements of neonatal gestational-age, physical, and behavioral assessments.

5. Describe the techniques used to conduct neonatal gestational-age, physical, and behavioral assessments.

6. Discuss the benefits of allowing parents to observe the neonatal assessment.

7. Describe how the neonate interacts with the environment.

INTRODUCTION

The neonate undergoes many physiologic changes during the neonatal period—the first 28 days after birth. To make a successful transition to the extrauterine environment, the neonate must adapt to these changes as smoothly as possible. The nurse plays a critical role in the neonate's transition by conducting a thorough, systematic assessment that provides baseline information about the neonate's physiologic status and the adequacy of neonatal adaptation.

Besides knowing how to conduct such an assessment, the nurse also must understand the significance of assessment findings. For example, by identifying gestational age, the nurse can determine whether the neonate has a gestational-age variation necessitating special care. Early detection of a potential or actual problem reduces the risk of complications; in some cases, it may mean the difference between life and death.

This chapter begins with an overview of neonatal assessment, including the timing of the various types of assessments—gestational-age assessment, physical assessment, and behavioral assessment. Next, it describes the essential components of these assessments and discusses the techniques used for each. The chapter includes a detailed chart that presents normal and abnormal physical assessment findings.

GENERAL ASSESSMENT GUIDELINES

The nurse must adapt the assessment to the neonate's tolerance, delaying any maneuvers that could compromise the neonate and combining overlapping portions of the various assessments to help conserve the neonate's energy. For instance, gestational-age assessment includes certain characteristics also evaluated during the physical and behavioral assessments; the nurse should examine these characteristics only once. Also, the nurse should allow a neonate who falls asleep during the assessment to sleep undisturbed to recuperate from the stress of birth, then resume the assessment when the neonate awakens.

Assessment sequence

Neonatal assessment proceeds from an immediate determination of the Apgar score to a complete physical assessment.

The immediate assessment—determination of the Apgar score—takes place in the delivery area. Once stabilized in the delivery area, the neonate is transferred to the nursery for observation. Some facilities have rooming-in privileges for the mother and neonate after a brief observation. Regardless of the setting, however, the ensuing assessment steps remain the same.

Within the next few hours, the nurse should conduct a complete physical assessment to determine how well the neonate is adapting to the extrauterine environment and to check for obvious problems and major anomalies. This assessment includes evaluation of general appearance, vital sign measurement, and anthropometric measurements.

The nurse then estimates the neonate's gestational age and, if necessary, conducts a formal gestational-age assessment, using a special assessment tool, to determine gestational age precisely. Based on education and experience, the nurse may assist with a behavioral assessment.

Health history

The nurse should obtain a complete history of the antepartal and intrapartal periods from the maternal and delivery room records, then review it for any problems that the client might have experienced during pregnancy.

Determination of preterm or postterm status usually is established by the time of delivery. However, the nurse may want to review the maternal history for factors that increase the risk of a gestational-age variation so that the health care team can anticipate potential perinatal problems more accurately. For instance, the risk of preterm delivery increases with:

- various intrapartal factors, such as multiple gestation (more than one fetus), fetal infection, preeclampsia, premature rupture of the membranes, abruptio placentae, hydramnios (excessive amniotic fluid), placenta previa, and poor prenatal care
- chronic maternal disease, such as cardiovascular disease, renal disease, or diabetes mellitus
- maternal history of abdominal surgery, trauma, uterine anomalies, cervical incompetency, infection, or previous preterm delivery
- maternal age under 19.

With a postterm neonate, the intrapartal history may include weight loss, decreased abdominal circumference, and reduced uterine size – signs of an altered fetal growth pattern (fetal dysmaturity).

The prenatal and intrapartal history also may suggest a birth-weight variation. Such variations include small for gestational age (SGA), defined as a birth weight that falls below the tenth percentile for gestational age on the Colorado intrauterine growth chart, and large for gestational age (LGA), defined as a birth weight that exceeds the ninetieth percentile for gestational age on the growth chart.

Like a gestational-age variation, a birth-weight variation increases the risk of perinatal problems. Women identified as high risk by history or clinical assessment deliver about two-thirds of SGA neonates (Cassady and Strange, 1987). Risk factors for delivery of an SGA neonate include low socioeconomic status, an age under 19 or over 34, multiparity, short stature, low prepregnancy weight, and previous delivery of an SGA neonate.

Typically, the diagnosis of LGA is established during the antepartal period, when fundal height appears disproportionate to gestational weeks. Also, because diabetes mellitus is a leading cause of accelerated intrauterine growth, an elevated maternal serum glucose level may result in an LGA fetus.

Periods of neonatal reactivity

During the first hours after birth, the neonate experiences gradual, predictable changes in physiologic characteristics and behavioral responses, reflecting the periods of neonatal reactivity. The two reactivity periods are separated by a sleep stage (considered a discrete period of reactivity by some authorities).

With each period of reactivity, vital signs, state of alertness, and responsiveness to external stimuli change. The nurse must be able to recognize the characteristics of each period and use them when interpreting assessment findings. (For key features associated with each reactivity period, see *Assessment findings during periods of reactivity,* page 352.) Although a specific assessment for the periods of reactivity is not necessary, the nurse should stay alert for deviations from normal findings because such deviations may signify a disorder. (For more information on the periods of reactivity, see Chapter 17, Neonatal Adaptation.)

INITIAL PHYSICAL ASSESSMENT

During the initial physical assessment of the neonate, the nurse evaluates the neonate's general appearance, assesses vital signs, and takes anthropometric measurements. To prevent the neonate from becoming tired or stressed, the nurse should conduct this assessment as swiftly and systematically as possible.

General appearance

By assessing general appearance, the nurse quickly gauges the neonate's maturity level (a reflection of gestational age) and may detect obvious problems. Features to assess in the general survey include posture, head size, skin color and tone, activity, maturity, body symmetry,

ASSESSMENT FINDINGS DURING PERIODS OF REACTIVITY

The nurse should consider the period of reactivity when assessing the neonate—especially when using the Brazelton neonatal behavioral assessment scale to evaluate behavior. This chart shows the normal assessment findings associated with each reactivity period.

PARAMETER	FIRST PERIOD	SECOND PERIOD
Skin color	Fluctuates from pale pink to cyanotic (blue)	Fluctuates from pale pink to cyanotic, with periods of mottling
Alertness level	Awake and alert, progressing to sleep	Hyperactive, with exaggerated responses
Cry	Rigorous, diminishing as sleep begins	Periodic
Respiratory rate	Up to 80 breaths/minute when crying	40 to 60 breaths/minute, with periods of more rapid respirations
Respiratory effort	Irregular and labored, with nasal flaring, expiratory grunts, and retractions	Usually unlabored
Heart rate	Up to 180 beats/minute when crying	120 to 160 beats/minute, with periods of more rapid beating
Heart rhythm	Fluctuating, progressing to regular	Fluctuating as the neonate falls asleep, progressing to regular
Bowel sounds	Absent	Present
Stool	May not be passed	Meconium stool passed
Voiding	Rare	Usually begins
Mucus production	Minimal, diminishing gradually	Present, may be excessive
Sucking reflex	Strong, diminishing as sleep begins	Strong

cry, and state of alertness. (For details on evaluating general appearance, see "Complete physical assessment" later in this chapter.)

Vital signs and blood pressure

After assessing general appearance, the nurse measures vital signs (temperature, respiratory rate, and pulse rate) and blood pressure—not a routine vital sign but usually included. (For details on how to take neonatal vital signs, see Psychomotor Skills: *Taking vital signs.*)

First measure the neonate's core (internal) temperature. The axillary temperature is preferred; taking the neonate's rectal temperature may cause rectal mucosal irritation and bowel perforation. Axillary temperature accurately reflects core temperature, but many health care professionals have questioned the reliability of axillary temperature in the first 24 hours after birth because of poor peripheral perfusion during this time. However, research has found that rectal and axillary temperatures differed by only 0.2 degree F (Bliss-Holtz, 1989).

Axillary temperature should measure 96.8° F to 98.6° F (36° to 37° C), although the more acceptable range is 97.5 to 99° F (36.4° to 37.2° C). Axillary temperature above 99° F (37.2° C) reflects hyperthermia or fever; below 96° F (35.5° C), poor peripheral perfusion or prematurity.

External heat or cooling sources may affect the neonate's temperature. Many neonates are poikilotherms, taking on the temperature of the environment. For example, a neonate who is exposed to direct sunlight may experience a rapid increase in core and skin temperatures, becoming restless and irritable. Consequently, room temperature must be kept constant to prevent overheating or excessive cooling of the neonate.

The respiratory rate varies with the state of alertness and period of reactivity; thus, it may fluctuate widely in the first hours after birth. After the first period of reactivity, the respiratory rate typically measures 40 to 60 breaths per minute. If it exceeds 60 breaths per minute, or if the neonate has apneic episodes lasting longer than 15 seconds accompanied by duskiness or cyanosis, the nurse should suspect prematurity, respiratory distress, sepsis, or transient tachypnea.

In the first few hours after birth, the pulse rate fluctuates from 120 to 160 beats per minute, but may increase to 180 beats per minute when crying.

The neonate's cardiopulmonary rates and rhythms may be irregular and high during the periods of reactivity, especially during the first few minutes after birth. Even nasal flaring and grunting may be noted immediately following birth. The neonate may or may not be

TAKING VITAL SIGNS

The nurse should measure the neonate's vital signs every 15 minutes for the first hour after birth. If they remain stable during this time, measure them at least every hour for the next 6 hours, then at least once every 8 hours until discharge.

Measuring temperature

Place the thermometer in the axilla and hold it along the outer aspect of the neonate's chest, between the axillary line and the arm. Keep the thermometer in place for at least 3 minutes (axillary temperature takes this long to register).

If the measured axillary temperature is outside the normal range—97.5° to 99° F (36.4° to 37.2° C)—check it again 15 to 30 minutes later. If the temperature still is abnormal, report this finding. A subnormal temperature may indicate infection; an elevated temperature, dehydration. (To ensure consistency of subsequent measurements, document the route used to take the temperature.)

Measuring respiratory rate

Count respirations for at least 1 minute. Depending on the neonate's period of reactivity, the respiratory rate should range from 40 to 80 breaths/minute. An abnormally rapid rate (tachypnea) may signal a perinatal problem. A lapse of 15 seconds or more after a complete respiratory cycle (one expiration and inspiration) indicates apnea.

Assess the neonate's breathing pattern for regularity. An irregular pattern may indicate respiratory dysfunction. Also check for signs of labored breathing, such as uneven chest expansion, nasal flaring, visible chest retractions, expiratory grunts, and inspiratory stridor (a high-pitched sound audible without a stethoscope). In some cases, labored breathing indicates blockage of nasal passages (the neonate is an obligate nose breather).

To evaluate breath sounds, auscultate the anterior and posterior lung fields, placing the stethoscope over each lung lobe for at least 5 seconds (for a total time of 1 minute). Normally, breath sounds are clear and equal bilaterally. However, immediately after birth, a few crackles (rales) may be audible because of retained fetal lung fluid. Document any abnormal breath sounds.

Observe the movement of the chest as it rises and falls; it should be symmetrical. Also determine the ratio between the anterior and posterior diameters of the chest. A ratio exceeding 1 suggests lung hyperinflation or respiratory distress.

Assessing pulse

Place the stethoscope over the apical impulse on the fourth to fifth intercostal space at the left midclavicular line over the cardiac apex. Listen for 1 minute to count the pulse and detect any abnormalities in the quality or rhythm of the heartbeat.

If heart rhythm is irregular, assess whether the irregularity is regular (follows an identifiable pattern) or irregular (lacks an identifiable pattern). This helps identify the type of abnormality present; for example, atrial fibrillation is an irregular rhythm with an irregular pattern.

Also auscultate for variations from the normal sounds ("lub-dub") of systole and diastole. Determine if the first and second heart sounds are separate and distinct or split into two sounds. Also assess for extra heart sounds and for sounds that seem to stretch into the next sound. Such abnormal sounds may signify a heart murmur, such as from a patent ductus arteriosus (in which blood rushes through the abnormal opening).

Taking blood pressure

When using a Doppler probe (an electronic blood pressure monitor), place the cuff directly over the brachial or popliteal artery to ensure an accurate reading; the machine automatically inflates the cuff. For the most accurate reading, keep the cuffed arm or leg extended during cuff inflation. Also observe the color of the extremity; duskiness signifies reduced blood flow.

When measuring blood pressure by the cuff-and-stethoscope method, make sure to choose the correct cuff size. Cuff width should be half the circumference of the neonate's arm. A cuff that is too large or too small may cause a misleading reading.

Place the cuff one to two fingerbreadths above the antecubital or popliteal area. With the stethoscope held directly over the chosen artery, hold the cuffed extremity firmly to keep it extended, then inflate the cuff.

To determine if blood pressure is within the neonate's normal range, compare the readings to baseline values; report any significant deviation.

crying. The nurse must report these irregularities if they continue, even though they represent only the normal transition to postnatal life for some neonates. For other neonates, however, they may be the earliest signs of respiratory difficulties or cardiac problems.

Neonatal blood pressure rises during periods of heightened activity; usually, it is relatively high for the first two weeks. The most accurate way to measure blood pressure is with a Doppler probe, an electronic instrument that eliminates the need for a stethoscope.

Average systolic blood pressure varies with gestational age. In the term neonate, systolic blood pressure ranges from 63 to 70 mm Hg. In the preterm neonate of 28 to 32 weeks' gestation, it averages about 52 mm Hg; in the preterm neonate of 33 to 36 weeks' gestation, 56 mm Hg. Diastolic pressure in the term neonate ranges from 40 to 50 mm Hg. (For the preterm neonate, the diastolic reading is not a useful parameter because pulse sounds are audible all the way to the zero point on the gauge.)

The nurse should measure blood pressure in both arms and legs to detect any discrepancy between the two sides or between upper and lower body. A discrepancy of 10 mm Hg or more between the arms and legs may signal a cardiac defect, such as coarctation of the aorta.

Anthropometric measurements

To take anthropometric measurements (weight, head-to-heel length, head and chest circumference, and crown-to-rump length), the nurse weighs and measures the neonate (as described in Psychomotor Skills: *Obtaining anthropometric measurements*). Birth weight averages 2,500 to 4,000 g (5 lb, 8 oz to 8 lb, 13 oz).

In the term neonate, head-to-heel length ranges from 45 to 55 cm (18″ to 22″); head circumference averages 33 to 35.5 cm (13″ to 14″), with a range of 32 to 36.8 cm (12½″ to 14½″). Chest circumference usually measures about 2 cm less than head circumference, averaging 30 to 33 cm (12″ to 13″). Crown-to-rump length approximates head circumference.

GESTATIONAL-AGE ASSESSMENT

Gestational-age assessment determines the neonate's physical and neuromuscular maturity, helping health care providers anticipate perinatal problems associated with preterm or postterm status. Correlation of gestational age with birth weight may suggest perinatal problems related to SGA or LGA status.

The average full-term gestation lasts about 38 weeks from fertilization, or 40 weeks from the first day of the last menstrual period. Traditionally, gestational age has been calculated from the latter. However, irregular menstrual cycles and fetal growth variations can lead to erroneous calculation.

Previously, health care professionals used birth weight alone to classify neonates. However, in the past few decades, as experts recognized the importance of gestational age, new classifications have been developed and mortality and morbidity rates identified for each classification. (For more information, see *Classifying the neonate by gestational age and birth weight,* page 356.)

Gestational age should be assessed for any neonate, but especially one who weighs less than 2,500 g (5½ lb) or who has a suspected alteration in the intrauterine growth pattern. Gestational-age assessment tools rely on external physical features and neurologic maturity—not birth weight—as indices of growth and maturation. Developing in an orderly manner during gestation, external physical features usually are not affected by labor and delivery and

OBTAINING ANTHROPOMETRIC MEASUREMENTS

Anthropometric measurements include weight, head-to-heel length, head and chest circumference, and crown-to-rump length. If abnormal, these measurements may indicate a significant problem or anomaly. The nurse should follow the illustrated procedures for taking anthropometric measurements.

1 **Measuring weight.** Take this measurement before—not after—a feeding, preferably with the neonate undressed. If the neonate must be weighed with clothing or equipment (such as an I.V. armboard), make sure to note this information.

Before the weighing, place one or two pieces of disposable scale paper over the scale to prevent cold stress. When taking the measurement, keep one hand directly above the neonate. However, avoid touching the neonate, which could affect the accuracy of the measurement.

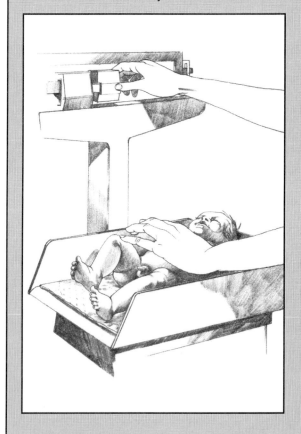

2 **Measuring head-to-heel length.** Position the neonate supine with legs extended and measure from head to heel. To make this measurement easier, use a length board.

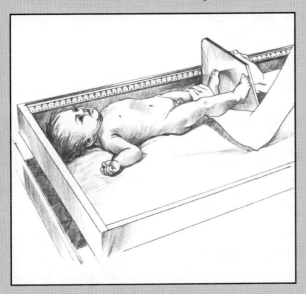

3 **Measuring head circumference.** Place a tape measure securely around the fullest part of the caput, from the middle of the forehead to the midline of the back of the skull. Record the result. Keep in mind that if delivery caused molding or swelling of the head, the measured head circumference may be misleading.

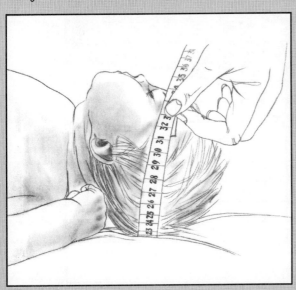

4 **Measuring chest circumference.** Place a tape measure around the neonate's chest at the nipples. Take the measurement after the neonate inspires, before expiration begins.

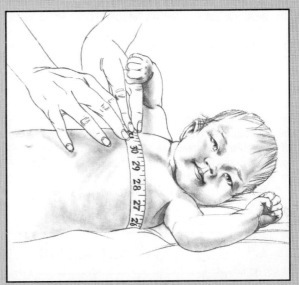

5 **Measuring crown-to-rump length.** With the neonate lying on one side, measure from the crown of the head to the buttocks. This measurement should approximate head circumference.

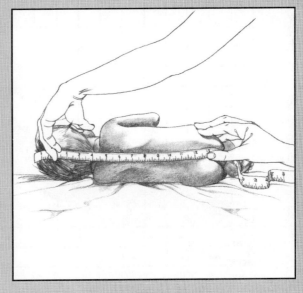

CLASSIFYING THE NEONATE BY GESTATIONAL AGE AND BIRTH WEIGHT

Organ system maturity depends largely on gestational age. Thus, the greater a neonate's gestational age, the more fully developed the organ systems. At the First World Health Assembly in 1948, the World Health Organization (WHO) defined an "immature" neonate as one weighing 5½ lb (2,500 g) or less; or, if the weight was not specified, one whose gestation lasted less than 37 weeks. In 1950, the WHO Expert Group on Prematurity defined the premature (preterm) neonate as one weighing 2,500 g or less.

However, health care professionals recognized that some neonates weighing less than 2,500 g were term or postterm but small for gestational age. Consequently, in 1961, the WHO Expert Committee on Maternal and Child Health redefined the premature neonate as one born before 37 weeks from the first day of the mother's last menstrual period. The committee defined low birth weight (LBW) as 2,500 g or less and subdivided neonates in this category into term and preterm LBW neonates.

In the 1980s, an additional classification—very low birth weight (VLBW)—was added to describe the neonate weighing 500 g to 1,499 g. Most VLBW neonates have a gestational age of 23 to 30 weeks. VLBW neonates have had a tremendous impact on medical research and have sparked important advances in neonatal care—even though they account for only a tiny percentage of neonates. (According to Usher [1987], only 0.87% of live births occur before 31 weeks; VLBW neonates make up just 0.85% of these births.)

Currently, neonates are classified according to the Colorado intrauterine growth chart. Developed by Battaglia and Lubchenco (1967), this chart correlates gestational age with birth weight. After weighing the neonate and determining gestational age, the examiner plots these two parameters on the graph. The neonate whose weight falls between the tenth and ninetieth percentiles for gestational age on this chart is classified as appropriate for gestational age. One whose birth weight falls outside this range is considered to be small or large for gestational age, with an increased risk for certain perinatal problems. Thanks largely to improved knowledge and technology, however, such a neonate has an improved chance for survival.

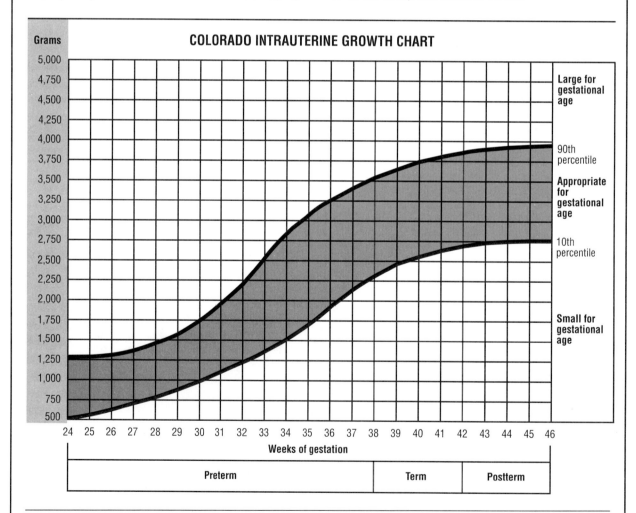

Battaglia, F.C., and Lubchenco, L.O. (1967). A practical classification of newborn infants by weight and gestational age. *Journal of Pediatrics, 71,* 159-163. Graph used with permission from Mosby-Year Book, Inc.

thus can be assessed immediately. Evaluation of neurologic maturity, however, may have to be postponed for 24 hours or so—especially if the neonate suffered fetal central nervous system depression, which may skew assessment findings.

The most common gestational-age assessment tools are the Dubowitz tool (1970) and the Ballard tool (revised in 1988). The Dubowitz tool includes 11 external and 10 neurologic signs. The examiner evaluates and scores each external sign, then totals the scores. After following the same procedure for neurologic signs, the examiner adds the two totals and plots the sum on a graph to identify the neonate's gestational age. (With early client discharge now routine, the Dubowitz tool has become somewhat impractical because the neurologic part of the examination must be delayed.)

The Ballard tool, an abbreviated version of the Dubowitz tool, consists of 7 physical maturity and 6 neuromuscular maturity criteria. This tool is refined periodically in response to research. The 1988 revision incorporates criteria for gestational-age assessment of neonates at 24 to 44 weeks' gestation. (For more information, see *Ballard gestational-age assessment tool,* pages 358 and 359.)

Assessment of physical features

Certain physical features vary with gestational age and thus reflect neonatal maturity. (These features are called external signs on the Dubowitz tool and physical maturity criteria on the Ballard tool.)

Skin texture, color, and opacity. The preterm neonate has thin, translucent, ruddy skin with easily seen veins and venules (especially over the abdomen). As term approaches, the skin thickens and becomes pinker; also, the number of large vessels visible over the abdomen decreases. The postterm neonate typically has thick, parchmentlike skin with peeling and cracking; few if any blood vessels appear over the abdomen.

Lanugo. Soft, downy hair, lanugo appears at approximately 20 weeks' gestation. From 21 to 33 weeks, it covers the entire body. It begins to vanish from the face at 34 weeks and by 38 weeks may appear only on the shoulders. Lanugo rarely appears after 42 weeks' gestation.

Plantar (sole) creases. Plantar creases should be assessed immediately after birth because the drying effect of environmental exposure causes additional creases to form. The preterm neonate of 34 to 35 weeks' gestation has one or two anterior creases; at 36 to 38 weeks' gestation, creases cover the anterior two-thirds of the sole. In the term neonate, creases appear over both the sole and heel. In the postterm neonate, deeper creases line the entire sole.

Breast size. The examiner assesses breast tissue through observation and palpation. To measure breast tissue, palpate the nipple gently between the second and third fingers. Do not use the thumb and index finger because surrounding skin may be measured inadvertently this way.

Breast tissue and areola size increase with gestation. The areola appears slightly elevated at 34 weeks' gestation. By week 36, a breast bud of 1 to 2 mm is visible; the bud may grow to 12 mm by week 42. Increased breast tissue may indicate subcutaneous fat accumulation from accelerated intrauterine growth (such as occurs in the LGA neonate). In contrast, the SGA or postterm neonate may have decreased breast tissue from inadequate fetal growth or lost fetal weight.

Ear form and firmness. In the preterm neonate of less than 28 weeks' gestation, decreased cartilage distribution prevents the ear from recoiling after it is folded forward against the side of the head and released. The ear appears flat and shapeless until 28 weeks' gestation when incurving of the pinna (the external part of the ear) begins. At 36 weeks' gestation, the upper two-thirds of the pinna are incurved and the pinna recoils instantly. In the term neonate, the pinna has well-defined incurving. The ear of the postterm neonate is firm and set apart slightly from the head.

Genitalia. In the male neonate, the genitalia should be assessed for testicular descent, scrotal size, and number of rugae (skin folds). In the preterm neonate of less than 28 weeks' gestation, the testes remain within the abdominal cavity and the scrotum appears high and close to the body. At 28 to 36 weeks' gestation, the testes can be palpated in the inguinal canal and a few rugae appear. At 36 to 40 weeks' gestation, the testes are palpable in the upper scrotum and rugae appear on the anterior portion. After 40 weeks' gestation, the testes can be palpated in the scrotum and rugae cover the scrotal sac. The postterm neonate has deep rugae and a pendulous scrotum.

The female preterm neonate of 30 to 36 weeks' gestation has a prominent clitoris extending from the labia minora and majora; the labia majora are small and widely separated. (This appearance occasionally complicates sex determination and may upset parents.) At 36 to 40 weeks' gestation, the labia majora are larger, almost covering the clitoris. Labia majora that cover the labia minora and clitoris suggest more than 40 weeks' gestation.

BALLARD GESTATIONAL-AGE ASSESSMENT TOOL

To use this tool, the examiner evaluates and scores the neuromuscular and physical maturity criteria, totals the scores, then plots the sum in the maturity rating box to determine gestational age. Unlike portions of the Dubowitz neurologic examination, the Ballard neuromuscular examination can be done even if the neonate is not alert.

	−1	0	1	2	3	4	5
Neuromuscular maturity							
Posture	–						–
Square window (wrist)	>90°	90°	60°	45°	30°	0°	–
Arm recoil	–	180°	140° to 180°	110° to 140°	90° to 110°	<90°	–
Popliteal angle	180°	160°	140°	120°	100°	90°	<90°
Scarf sign							–
Heel to ear							–

Adapted from Ballard, J.L., Khoury, J.C., Wedig, K., et al. (1991). New Ballard Score, expanded to include extremely premature infants. *Journal of Pediatrics*, 119(3), 417-423. Used with permission from Mosby-Year Book, Inc.

Assessment of neurologic maturity

Assessment of neurologic features (called neurologic signs on the Dubowitz tool and neuromuscular maturity criteria on the Ballard tool) determines the degree of neuromuscular tone – an index of neurologic maturity. Unlike other neurologic characteristics, which develop in a cephalocaudal (head-to-tail) direction, neuromuscular tone begins in the lower extremities and progresses upward.

The Dubowitz neurologic examination initially includes evaluation of posture and of arm and leg recoil. The remaining neurologic criteria are assessed 24 hours after birth to eliminate the effects of maternal analgesia, increased handling from additional assessments, and the normal physiologic fluctuations (such as vital sign changes) of the first few hours.

Correlating gestational age with birth weight and with length and head circumference

After determining the neonate's gestational age with an assessment tool, the examiner plots the age on the Colorado intrauterine growth chart to correlate it with birth weight. This reveals whether the neonate is SGA, LGA, or appropriate for gestational age – information that helps caregivers anticipate perinatal problems.

The examiner also plots gestational age against length and head circumference on an appropriate growth chart to determine whether these measurements fall within the normal range – the tenth to ninetieth percentile for the corresponding gestational age.

	−1	0	1	2	3	4	5
Physical maturity							
Skin	Sticky, friable, transparent	Gelatinous, red, translucent	Smooth, pink; visible vessels	Superficial peeling or rash; few visible vessels	Cracking; pale areas; rare visible vessels	Parchment-like; deep cracking; no visible vessels	Leathery, cracked, wrinkled
Lanugo	None	Sparse	Abundant	Thinning	Bald areas	Mostly bald	—
Plantar surface	Heel-toe 40 to 50 mm: −1; <40 mm: −2	>50 mm; no crease	Faint red marks	Anterior transverse crease only	Creases over anterior two-thirds	Creases over entire sole	—
Breast	Imperceptible	Barely perceptible	Flat areola, no bud	Stippled areola; 1- to 2-mm bud	Raised areola; 3- to 4-mm bud	Full areola; 5- to 10-mm bud	—
Eye and ear	Lids fused, loosely: −1; tightly: −2	Lids open; pinna flat, stays folded	Slightly curved pinna; soft, slow recoil	Well-curved pinna; soft but ready recoil	Formed and firm; instant recoil	Thick cartilage; ear stiff	—
Genitalia, male	Scrotum flat, smooth	Scrotum empty; faint rugae	Testes in upper canal; rare rugae	Testes descending; few rugae	Testes down; good rugae	Testes pendulous; deep rugae	—
Genitalia, female	Clitoris prominent; labia flat	Prominent clitoris; small labia minora	Prominent clitoris; enlarging minora	Majora and minora equally prominent	Majora large; minora small	Majora cover clitoris and minora	—
Maturity rating							

Score	−10	−5	0	5	10	15	20	25	30	35	40	45	50
Weeks	20	22	24	26	28	30	32	34	36	38	40	42	44

COMPLETE PHYSICAL ASSESSMENT

When conducting the complete physical assessment, the nurse may use a systematic, head-to-toe approach tailored to the neonate's size and age, or may assess heart and lung sounds first because these assessments require a quiet neonate. Ensure thermoregulation by placing the neonate under a radiant heat warmer and examining only one area at a time. For assessments requiring advanced skills, seek appropriate assistance.

Check vital signs before the examination begins; if they are unstable or if the neonate has a temperature below 96° F (35.5° C), do not proceed with the examination. Instead, swaddle the neonate, rewrapping securely. Because the period of reactivity affects assessment findings, record the neonate's behavioral state and age (in hours or days after birth) at the time of the examination.

Physical examination

Examine the neonate's skin for temperature, color, turgor, and variations. The skin should feel warm to the touch with a temperature ranging from 96° to 98° F (35.5° to 36.5° C), or 0.9° F (0.5° C) below core temperature. Palpate the neonate's skin for edema and document and report any generalized edema, which may indicate a cardiac or renal problem. Skin variations are common in neonates; most are minor and do not require treatment. Common variations include the following:

- *milia*—minute, white, epidermal cysts caused by sebaceous gland obstruction; commonly seen on the face
- *miliaria (prickly heat)*—rash consisting of minute vesicles and papules resulting from sweat duct blockage; occurs mainly on the forehead and in skin folds
- *erythema toxicum neonatorum*—pink, papular rash covering the thorax, back, abdomen, and groin; commonly occurs within 24 to 48 hours after birth
- *nevus flammeus (port wine stain)*—flat, capillary hemangioma; color of this permanent birthmark ranges from pale red to deep red-purple
- *telangiectatic nevi (stork bite)*—flat, deep pink, localized areas of capillary dilation; typically appear on the upper eyelids, across the nasal bridge and occipital bone, or along the neck.

Assess the neonate's head and neck for size, shape, and symmetry. Palpate the suture lines and the anterior and posterior fontanels. Examine the hair for distribution, texture, and color. To help assess cardiovascular status, palpate the carotid pulses, which should be equal and strong bilaterally.

Examine the neonate's face for symmetry of features. Observe the appearance of the mouth, chin, cheeks, and oral cavity. Inspect the oral mucous membranes, which should be moist, and inspect for the intactness of the hard and soft palates.

Evaluate the neonate's eyes for symmetry, spacing, and movement. Note the color of the sclerae and conjunctivae and the pupillary response to light.

Inspect the ears for symmetry, shape, and size. Also check the neonate's gross hearing ability; a loud noise should elicit the startle reflex or crying.

Assess the nose for location, size, and patency of nares (nostrils). Remember that the neonate is an obligate nose breather who depends on patent nares.

Assess the size and symmetry of the thoracic cavity and chest excursion. In the SGA or preterm neonate, expect decreased chest circumference.

Inspect the abdomen for shape and symmetry. Check the umbilical cord remnant, which should appear bluish-white, contain two arteries and one vein, and be free of drainage. Auscultate for bowel sounds, which normally begin a few hours after birth. Then palpate and percuss the abdomen for abnormalities.

Assess the neonate's back for spinal alignment, enlargement, or masses. Examine the sacrum for dimpling or a tuft of hair and observe for bulges. Palpate the vertebral column for enlargement and signs of pain.

Inspect the anus and genitalia for abnormalities. Keep in mind that genital appearance depends on gestational age. The urinary meatus should be midline, the perineum smooth, and the anus midline and patent. In the male neonate, palpate the scrotal sac to determine if the testes are descended.

Inspect the extremities for length, symmetry, and size—relative to each other and to the body as a whole. Test the neonate's range of motion. Inspect the hands and feet for number of digits, palmar and plantar creases, and such abnormalities as syndactyly (webbing). (For details on normal and abnormal assessment findings and their significance, see *Head-to-toe physical assessment findings*.)

When assessing neurologic status, keep in mind that some neurologic characteristics also are evaluated during the gestational age assessment, which precedes the complete physical assessment. To conserve the neonate's energy, do not reevaluate these characteristics during the complete physical assessment.

First, observe the neonate's posture, which typically reflects fetal positioning, gestational age, or delivery method. The healthy term neonate has a flexed posture and shows muscle resistance when the examiner extends the extremities. However, with breech delivery or in utero positioning, the legs may remain extended for a few days after birth. With some neonates born in a breech position, the legs are flexed back as far as the ears.

Also check for tremors of the extremities. Tremors may stem from hypoglycemia, cold stress, or neurologic immaturity. They may be hard to distinguish from a seizure, which sometimes manifests as a fixed gaze, yawning, or motions resembling sucking, swallowing, or chewing. To distinguish tremors from a seizure, attempt to halt the movement by grasping the involved extremity; tremors will stop, whereas a seizure will continue.

Next, assess reflexes—both localized and mass (full body) reflexes. Localized reflexes include the sucking, rooting, gag, blink, pupillary, grasp, and Babinski reflexes. Mass reflexes include the startle, Moro, fencing, Galant, and stepping reflexes. (For methods used to test reflexes, see Psychomotor Skills: *Assessing neonatal reflexes*, page 376.)

Finally, assess the neonate's cry. The cry should be loud and strong, even in a preterm neonate (unless respiratory problems are present). A high-pitched cry or cat-like cry suggests increased intracranial pressure; a grunting or low-pitched cry, respiratory distress syndrome; a weak, soft cry, brain damage. Duration of the cry varies with temperament.

HEAD-TO-TOE PHYSICAL ASSESSMENT FINDINGS

Comprehensive physical assessment of the neonate proceeds from head to toe. For each body area, the chart shows normal findings and common variations, and abnormal findings and their possible causes.

PARAMETER	NORMAL FINDINGS AND COMMON VARIATIONS	ABNORMAL FINDINGS	POSSIBLE CAUSES
General appearance and behavior			
Body shape and posture	Well-rounded torso with sufficient subcutaneous tissue and no obvious anomalies	Thin extremities, muscle wasting, loose skin, little or no subcutaneous tissue, obvious anomalies	Malnourishment, fetal stress, congenital defect (such as cleft lip or palate, omphalocele, gastroschisis, meningomyelocele)
	Flexed extremities, bowed legs	Fetal position (fists clenched, arms adducted and flexed, hips abducted, knees flexed)	Prematurity
		Frog position (flexed hips and thighs, extended arms)	Prematurity
		Opisthotonos (acute arching of back, with head bent back on neck, heels bent back on legs, and rigid arm and hand flexion)	Brain damage, birth asphyxia, neurologic abnormality
Muscle tone	Pronounced	Reduced or flaccid	Birth asphyxia, prematurity
	Spontaneous symmetrical movement (possibly slightly tremulous), bilaterally equal flexion and extension	No movement or asymmetrical, irregular, tremulous movement	Birth asphyxia, neurologic dysfunction, prematurity, drug-induced birth injury
Alertness level	Usually easy to console when upset	Decreased alertness, hard to arouse and console	Prematurity, stress, sepsis, neurologic disorder
Cry	Strong	Weak, high-pitched, or absent	Brain damage, neonatal drug addiction, increased intracranial pressure (ICP)
		Raspy	Upper airway problem
		Expiratory grunt during crying	Respiratory distress
Neuromuscular maturity			
Scarf sign	Elbow reaches midline when extended across chest	Elbow extends beyond midline	Prematurity
		Elbow does not reach midline	Postmaturity
Arm recoil	Brisk	Sluggish	Prematurity
Ankle dorsiflexion	0-degree angle	Angle greater than 0 degrees	Prematurity
Popliteal angle	90 degrees or less	Greater than 90 degrees	Prematurity
Heel-to-ear maneuver	Heel reaches only to shoulders	Heel approaches or reaches ear	Prematurity

(continued)

HEAD-TO-TOE PHYSICAL ASSESSMENT FINDINGS (continued)

PARAMETER	NORMAL FINDINGS AND COMMON VARIATIONS	ABNORMAL FINDINGS	POSSIBLE CAUSES
Skin			
Texture	Moist and warm	Gelatinous with visible veins	Prematurity
		Dry, peeling, cracking	Postmaturity
		Edematous, shiny, taut	Kidney dysfunction, cardiac or renal failure
Color	Varies with ethnic background; may deepen with crying and activity • Asian: pink or rosy red to yellow tinge • Black or Native American: pale pink to light brown with yellow or red tinge • Caucasian: pale pink to ruddy • Hispanic: pink with yellow tinge Cyanotic discoloration of hands and feet during first 24 hours after birth caused by transition to relatively cool extrauterine environment Reddish tinge just after birth caused by adjustment of central oxygen levels to extrauterine environment	Cyanotic discoloration of hands and feet lasting longer than first 24 hours	Poor peripheral circulation, possibly with cardiac compromise
		Dusky or cyanotic discoloration over entire body	Poor circulation, respiratory compromise
		Plethora (florid complexion), accompanied by elevated hematocrit or hemogloblin level	Polycythemia or blood hyperviscosity
		Pallor	Cardiopulmonary compromise or failure
		Mottling	Prematurity or cardiopulmonary disorder (if associated with cold stress, color changes, bradycardia, or apnea)
	Yellow discoloration (jaundice) arising in first 48 to 72 hours after birth and normally disappearing by the seventh day (physiologic jaundice)	Jaundice on first day after birth (pathologic jaundice)	Isoimmune hemolytic disease (such as Rh or ABO incompatibility), polycythemia, enzyme deficiency, excessive bruising or bleeding, Hirschsprung's disease, pyloric stenosis (or other intestinal obstruction that increases blood supply or shunts blood to liver), maternal diabetes, small-for-gestational-age (SGA) status
Vernix caseosa	Present over entire body	Absent	Severe prematurity
		Minimal or absent	Postmaturity
Lanugo (soft, downy hair)	Sparse or present only on shoulders	Abundant over entire body	Prematurity
		Absent	Postmaturity
Turgor	Adequate (indicated by brisk return of skin to original position after examiner pinches it between fingers)	Poor (indicated by tenting or sluggish return to original position)	Dehydration

HEAD-TO-TOE PHYSICAL ASSESSMENT FINDINGS *(continued)*

PARAMETER	NORMAL FINDINGS AND COMMON VARIATIONS	ABNORMAL FINDINGS	POSSIBLE CAUSES
Skin *(continued)*			
Skin variations	Ecchymosis of presenting part Harlequin (clown) sign (pink or reddish skin on one side of body, with color division at midline; caused by vasomotor instability) Mongolian spots (blue-black macules over buttocks, possibly extending to sacral region; most common in dark-skinned neonates)	Café-au-lait spots (small, light tan macules)	Possible early sign of neurofibromatosis, especially if appearing in group of seven or more
		Meconium staining	Fetal distress
		Petechiae	Hematopoietic disorder
		Cutaneous papilloma (small brownish or flesh-colored outgrowth of skin; also called skin tag)	Possible congenital anomaly
Respiratory system			
Respiratory effort and rhythm	Easy, unlabored effort; abdominal breathing; possible irregular rhythm and apneic episodes lasting less than 15 seconds	Dyspnea; substernal, supracostal, intercostal, or supraclavicular retractions; nasal flaring; stridor; grunting	Respiratory distress
Chest excursion	Symmetrical	Asymmetrical	Diaphragmatic hernia, pneumothorax, phrenic nerve damage
Anteroposterior (AP) diameter	1:1 ratio (almost round)	Ratio >1:1 (barrel chest)	Poorly developed rib cage and chest musculature, possible prematurity
Breath sounds	Clear; equal bilaterally, anteriorly, and posteriorly; crackles during first few hours after birth (unless accompanied by color changes or cyanosis)	Unequal	Pneumothorax or diaphragmatic hernia
		Crackles after first day, rhonchi, expiratory grunts, wheezing	Pulmonary congestion or edema, respiratory distress, pneumonia
Chest percussion	No increase in tympany over lung fields	Increased tympany over lung fields	Lung hyperinflation
Cardiovascular system			
Heart rate and rhythm	120 to 160 beats/minute (higher during active or crying periods); regular	Less than 100 beats/minute (bradycardia) or more than 160 beats/minute (tachycardia)	Prematurity, respiratory compromise, increased cardiac workload, sepsis, congenital heart defect
		Persistent arrhythmias	Congenital heart anomaly
Heart sounds	No audible murmur (however, slight murmur heard over base or left sternal border until foramen ovale closes)	Heart sounds on right side of chest	Possible dextrocardia
		Persistent murmur (usually heard at left sternal border or above apical impulse)	Persistent fetal circulation, congenital heart anomaly

(continued)

HEAD-TO-TOE PHYSICAL ASSESSMENT FINDINGS *(continued)*

PARAMETER	NORMAL FINDINGS AND COMMON VARIATIONS	ABNORMAL FINDINGS	POSSIBLE CAUSES
Cardiovascular system *(continued)*			
Apical impulse	Located at fourth or fifth intercostal space at midclavicular line; point of maximum impulse located at fourth intercostal space just right of midclavicular line (may shift to the right in first few hours after birth)	Displaced	Cardiac defect or cardiomegaly
Thrill	Absent (except for first few hours after birth)	Present beyond first few hours after birth	Increased cardiac activity
Head and neck			
Head size	Slightly large in proportion to body (average head circumference of term neonate is 32 to 35 cm)	Abnormally small	Microcephaly, caused by congenital syndrome or decreased brain development (such as from intrauterine growth retardation)
		Extremely small	Anencephaly (absent cerebral tissue or absent or minimal skull)
		Abnormally large	Macrocephaly, possibly caused by hydrocephalus (abnormal accumulation of cerebrospinal fluid within cranial vault) resulting from congenital anomaly (such as meningomyelocele, tumor, trauma, or infection)
Fontanels	Anterior fontanel open until age 12 to 18 months; diamond shaped; measures 2 x 3 x 5 cm; located at juncture of coronal, frontal, and sagittal sutures	Premature closure of anterior fontanel	Poor brain development
		Bulging fontanel (usually anterior fontanel)	Increased ICP
	Posterior fontanel open until age 2 to 3 months (may be closed at birth); triangular shaped; measures 1 x 1 x 1 cm; located at juncture of sagittal and lambdoidal sutures	Sunken fontanel	Dehydration
Head and scalp variations	Molding (cranial distortion lasting 5 to 7 days, caused by pressure on cranium during vaginal delivery)	Herniation of brain tissue through skull defect	Encephalocele (congenital or traumatic defect)
		Bradycephalus, premature closure of coronal suture line, increased AP diameter and lateral growth	Anomalies, such as congenital or traumatic defects
		Premature closure of skull sutures (craniosynostosis)	Genetic disorder

HEAD-TO-TOE PHYSICAL ASSESSMENT FINDINGS *(continued)*

PARAMETER	NORMAL FINDINGS AND COMMON VARIATIONS	ABNORMAL FINDINGS	POSSIBLE CAUSES
Head and neck *(continued)*			
Head and scalp variations *(continued)*		Overriding sutures, caused by excessive pressure on cranium during vaginal delivery	Prematurity
		Localized pitting edema of scalp, possibly extending over sutures	Caput succedaneum, caused by pressure on fetal occiput (as during extended labor)
		Forceps marks; edematous or reddened area	Forceps delivery
		Localized scalp swelling	Cephalhematoma (collection of blood between skull and periosteum that does not cross suture lines; commonly caused by forceps trauma; may last up to 8 weeks)
	No masses or soft areas over skull	Masses or soft areas (such as craniotabes) over parietal bones (may be insignificant if no other abnormality exists)	Possible anomaly of internal organs
	No bruits in temporal area over anterior or posterior fontanel	Bruits in vascular areas of head	Cerebral arteriovenous malformation
Head lag	No greater than 10 degrees	Greater than 10 degrees	Hypotonia or prematurity
Hair distribution and texture	Distributed over top of head; single identifiable strands of hair	Fine or fuzzy hair	Prematurity
Eyes and eyelids	Symmetrical; aligned with ears, face, nose midline	Wide-eyed, apprehensive look	Postmaturity, SGA status, intrauterine growth retardation
	Eyes spaced approximately 2.5 cm apart	Abnormally wide distance (greater than 2.5 cm) between eyes (hypertelorism)	Fetal hydantoin syndrome (from maternal hydantoin use during pregnancy)
		Abnormally small distance (less than 2.5 cm) between eyes (hypotelorism)	Trisomy 13
	Clear sclera	Yellow sclera	Jaundice (however, slight yellow tinge may reflect only ethnic influence)
		Blue sclera	Osteogenesis imperfecta (fatal genetic syndrome characterized by fragile bones and shortened limbs)
		Scleral hemorrhage	Birth trauma

(continued)

HEAD-TO-TOE PHYSICAL ASSESSMENT FINDINGS *(continued)*

PARAMETER	NORMAL FINDINGS AND COMMON VARIATIONS	ABNORMAL FINDINGS	POSSIBLE CAUSES
Head and neck *(continued)*			
Eyes and eyelids *(continued)*	Clear conjunctiva	Pink conjunctiva	Conjunctivitis (possibly resulting from silver nitrate or erythromycin instillation)
		Conjunctival hemorrhages	Birth trauma
	Even, bilateral iris color	Gold flecks in iris (Brushfield's spots)	Down's syndrome (trisomy 21), if accompanied by other anomalies
		Coloboma (cleft usually affecting iris, ciliary body, or choroid; extends inferiorly)	Possible congenital malformation of internal organs
	Bilaterally equal pupil reaction to light	Absent or bilaterally unequal pupil reaction to light	Brain damage or increased ICP
	Clear cornea	Hazy, milky cornea	Prematurity; congenital cataract (possibly from congenital rubella)
	Transparent, intact retina	Pigmented retinal areas; tortuous or poorly demarcated retinal vessels	Retinal damage or hemorrhage
	Patent, palpable lacrimal duct	Blocked or absent lacrimal duct	Congenital obstruction
	Positive blink reflex (eyes blink in response to bright light)	Absent blink reflex	Facial nerve paralysis or optic nerve damage
	Positive red reflex (luminous bilateral red appearance of retina)	Absent red reflex	Congenital cataract
	Positive doll's eye reflex (eyes remain stationary when head is moved to left or right)	Absent doll's eye reflex	Trochlear, oculomotor, or abducens nerve damage
	No eye slant or slant reflecting ethnic background	Pronounced upward eye slant	Down's syndrome
		Downward eye slant	Treacher Collins's syndrome (congenital syndrome characterized by small mandible, beaked nose, and lower lid and external ear malformations)
		"Sunset" eyes (upper lid retraction causing sclera to show above iris)	Hydrocephalus
		Edematous eyelids	Birth trauma or irritation from silver nitrate or erythromycin instillation

HEAD-TO-TOE PHYSICAL ASSESSMENT FINDINGS *(continued)*

PARAMETER	NORMAL FINDINGS AND COMMON VARIATIONS	ABNORMAL FINDINGS	POSSIBLE CAUSES
Head and neck *(continued)*			
Eyes and eyelids *(continued)*		Ptosis (drooping) of eyelids	Oculomotor nerve damage
		Epicanthal folds	Down's syndrome; cri du chat (cat's cry) syndrome
Nose	Located at midline	Located off midline	Congenital malformation or syndrome (such as Apert's syndrome, characterized by premature closure of sutures)
	Appropriate size for face	Beaked	Treacher Collins's syndrome
		Enlarged or bulbous	Trisomy 13
	Patent nares	Nonpatent nares	Nasal obstruction; choanal atresia
		Missing nares	Congenital syndrome or malformation (such as cleft lip)
	Grimace or cry in response to strong odors passed under nose	No response to strong odors passed under nose	Olfactory nerve damage
		Flattened nasal bridge	Congenital syndrome, such as arthrogryposis (characterized by persistent contractures)
	Positive sneeze reflex (indicated by sneezing when both nares are occluded for 1 to 2 seconds)	No response	Possible nonpatent nares
Ears	Symmetrical in size, shape, and placement; top of ear parallel to an imaginary line drawn through the outer and inner canthi of the eye	Low-set, slanted	Congenital syndrome (such as Down's syndrome)
		Pinpoint holes or sinus tracts along preauricular surface	Possible congenital renal anomaly
	Well-curved pinna; rigid cartilage; instant recoil after folding	Flattened or folded pinna; slow recoil	Prematurity
	Positive startle reflex (indicated by startling or crying in response to loud noise)	Absent or minimal startle reflex	Deafness or auditory nerve impairment
	Umbo (cone) of light visible on otoscopic examination; pearl gray, movable tympanic membrane with no bulges (membrane may be covered with vernix caseosa)	Umbo dull or absent; dull, immobile, or red tympanic membrane	Infection
		Blue tympanic membrane	Hemorrhage
		Bulging tympanic membrane	Otitis media (middle ear infection)

(continued)

HEAD-TO-TOE PHYSICAL ASSESSMENT FINDINGS *(continued)*

PARAMETER	NORMAL FINDINGS AND COMMON VARIATIONS	ABNORMAL FINDINGS	POSSIBLE CAUSES
Head and neck *(continued)*			
Mouth	Symmetrical; appropriate size for face; located at midline	Droops or slants unilaterally when neonate cries or moves mouth	Palsy or damage to seventh cranial or facial nerve, possibly resulting from birth trauma (such as from forceps delivery)
		Birdlike, with shortened vermilion border (exposed red portion of lips) and shortened philtrum (groove from upper lip to nose)	Fetal alcohol syndrome
		Extremely wide (macrostomia)	Metabolic disorder (such as hypothyroidism)
		Unusually small (microstomia)	Down's syndrome
	Lips pink, moist, and formed completely	One or more clefts in upper lip, possibly extending to nasal floor	Cleft lip (congenital anomaly in which maxillary and median nasal processes fail to fuse)
Mucous membranes	Moist and pink	Dry, dusky, or cyanotic	Dehydration, poor oxygenation
	Moderate salivation	Excessive salivation	Tracheoesophageal fistula, esophageal atresia
Palate	Intact with no arching or fissures	Markedly arched	Turner's syndrome
	Epstein's pearls (small, hard, white patches that resolve gradually)	Midline fissure	Cleft palate (congenital anomaly in which two sides of palate fail to fuse; may occur in conjunction with cleft lip)
Tongue	Appropriate size for face	Abnormally large (macroglossia)	Hypothyroidism
		Abnormally small (microglossia)	Congenital syndrome (such as Möbius's syndrome)
	Located at midline	Located off midline	Cranial nerve damage
	Juts forward when touched	Fails to jut forward when touched	Short frenulum
Uvula	Located at midline; rises with crying	Fails to rise with crying	Neurologic dysfunction
Chin	Slightly receding; appropriate size for face	Extremely receding; underdeveloped (micrognathia)	Congenital syndrome (such as Pierre Robin's syndrome)
Oral reflexes	Sucking, swallowing, rooting, and gag reflexes present; sucking and swallowing reflexes well coordinated	Absent gag reflex	Neurologic dysfunction
		Absent sucking or rooting reflex	Prematurity or neurologic dysfunction

HEAD-TO-TOE PHYSICAL ASSESSMENT FINDINGS *(continued)*

PARAMETER	NORMAL FINDINGS AND COMMON VARIATIONS	ABNORMAL FINDINGS	POSSIBLE CAUSES
Head and neck *(continued)*			
Neck	Symmetrical	Asymmetrical	Unusual fetal position
	Short, no webbing (excessive skin)	Short and webbed	Down's syndrome
	Full range of motion (head can turn to each side equally)	Partial range of motion or tilting of head to one side (torticollis)	Birth injury; muscle spasm resulting in contraction of sternocleidomastoid muscles
	Weak, asymmetrical tonic neck reflex	Strong, asymmetrical tonic neck reflex	Prematurity
		Symmetrical tonic neck reflex	Neurologic dysfunction
	Thyroid located at midline; appropriate in size	Enlarged thyroid	Goiter
		Palpable lymph nodes	Congenital infection
		Palpable neck masses	Cystic hygroma
	Regular, bilaterally equal, strong carotid pulses	Weak or irregular carotid pulses	Cardiac defect or circulatory problem
		Enlarged sternocleidomastoid muscle	Torticollis; birth or fetal injury resulting in sternocleidomastoid hematoma
Thorax			
Clavicles	Even; symmetrical; nontender; without masses or lumps	Uneven; asymmetrical; masses or lumps present	Clavicular fracture; shoulder dystocia (as from birth injury); brachial plexus damage or palsy
Chest circumference	30 to 33 cm (12″ to 13″)	Less than 30 cm	Prematurity or SGA status
		Barrel chest (circumference greater than 33 cm)	Respiratory compromise; large-for-gestational-age (LGA) status
Chest excursion	Bilaterally equal	Bilaterally unequal	Phrenic nerve damage
Ribs	Symmetrical, flexible, without masses or crepitus	Asymmetrical	Birth injury or congenital syndrome
		Masses or crepitus present	Fracture or subcutaneous air pocket caused by air leakage resulting from pulmonary dysfunction
Breasts	1 cm of palpable breast tissue	Less than 1 cm (possibly only 5 mm) of palpable breast tissue	Prematurity
	Raised areolas	Flat areolas	Prematurity

(continued)

HEAD-TO-TOE PHYSICAL ASSESSMENT FINDINGS *(continued)*

PARAMETER	NORMAL FINDINGS AND COMMON VARIATIONS	ABNORMAL FINDINGS	POSSIBLE CAUSES
Thorax *(continued)*			
Breasts *(continued)*	Horizontally aligned, well-spaced nipples; no extra nipples	Misaligned or supernumerary (more than two) nipples	Possible internal organ anomaly
	Breast hypertrophy, possibly with white nipple discharge (witch's milk) from maternal hormonal influence; appears within the first 2 to 3 days after birth, and usually diminishes during the first or second week	Purulent nipple discharge	Mastitis
Xiphoid process	Intact	Absent or depressed	Fracture (may result from resuscitation)
Abdomen			
Shape	Symmetrical; rounded	Asymmetrical	Abdominal mass
		Scaphoid	Diaphragmatic hernia
		Distended	Intestinal obstruction, renal disorder, ascites, edema resulting from congenital renal or cardiac defect, prematurity, fetal hydrops
		Distended left upper quadrant	Pyloric stenosis, duodenal or jejunal obstruction
Abdominal muscles	Strong	Weak	Prune-belly syndrome, possible renal problems (such as hypoplastic kidneys)
		Visible abdominal wall defect over bladder	Bladder exstrophy
	No visible peristaltic waves	Visible peristaltic waves moving in left-to-right direction	Intestinal obstruction (rarely manifests immediately after birth)
Umbilical cord remnant	Bluish white, three vessels (two arteries and one vein) present	Two vessels (one artery and one vein) present	Possible internal congenital anomalies (especially renal anomalies)
		Thick	LGA status
		Small	SGA status or malnourishment
		Red, with discharge	Infection
		Meconium-stained	Fetal distress
		Mass (hernia) present, with protrusion of abdominal viscera	Omphalocele

HEAD-TO-TOE PHYSICAL ASSESSMENT FINDINGS *(continued)*

PARAMETER	NORMAL FINDINGS AND COMMON VARIATIONS	ABNORMAL FINDINGS	POSSIBLE CAUSES
Abdomen *(continued)*			
Umbilical cord remnant *(continued)*		Hernia	Gastroschisis (congenital fissure of the abdominal wall, not located at umbilical cord insertion site, accompanied by intestinal protrusion)
Abdominal palpation	Abdomen soft, without tenderness or masses	Abdomen tense, rigid, and tender	Intestinal deformity or obstruction
		Masses present	Renal or urinary tract deformity
	Minor separation of rectus abdominis muscles	Wide separation of rectus abdominis muscles (diastasis recti abdominis)	Prematurity
Abdominal auscultation	Two to four bowel sounds per minute	Absent bowel sounds	Intestinal obstruction
		More than five bowel sounds per minute (except immediately after feeding)	Intestinal obstruction or hypermotility
	No audible bruit	Bruit over abdominal aorta	Arteriovenous malformation
		Bruit over kidneys	Renal artery stenosis
Abdominal percussion	Tympany over all areas except liver, spleen, and bladder (where dullness is heard)	Increased tympany	Increased fluid or air
		Increased areas of dullness (if liver or spleen is enlarged, dullness extends below costal margins; if bladder is enlarged, dullness extends toward umbilicus)	Mass or enlarged organ at increased area of dullness
	Tympany over gastric bubble, just below left costal margin toward midline	No tympany over gastric bubble	Esophageal atresia or gastric defect
Kidneys	Located in lumbar area; right kidney lower than left; 4 to 5 cm long	Enlarged	Polycystic kidney disease
		Both kidneys absent	Potter's syndrome
Liver	Firm	Hard	Liver damage or cardiopulmonary disorder
	Sharp edge of liver palpable just above right costal margin during inspiration	Sharp edge of liver palpable more than 1 cm below right costal margin during inspiration	Enlarged liver (from respiratory distress or congestive heart failure)
Spleen	Palpable 1 cm below left costal margin	Absent or not palpable	Congenital heart defect
		Enlarged	Erythroblastosis fetalis (ABO incompatibility)

(continued)

HEAD-TO-TOE PHYSICAL ASSESSMENT FINDINGS *(continued)*

PARAMETER	NORMAL FINDINGS AND COMMON VARIATIONS	ABNORMAL FINDINGS	POSSIBLE CAUSES
Abdomen *(continued)*			
Bladder	No visible distention (except just before voiding)	Distended (may be visible above pubic bone)	Urinary tract obstruction or full bladder
Groin	Smooth, no palpable masses	Masses present	Inguinal hernia
Back			
Spinal column	Straight	Curved	Vertebral misalignment (if caused by fetal position, condition usually resolves gradually)
	No visible deviations or defects	Visible defect, such as mass, dimple, or bulge (possibly with tuft of hair)	Spina bifida
		Hernial sac (may be open or covered with portion of spinal cord, meninges, and cerebrospinal fluid)	Meningomyelocele
		Sinus tracts or pinpoint holes	Pilonidal cysts
	No vertebral enlargement or tenderness	Vertebral bulge, mass, cyst, enlargement, or tenderness	Vertebral fracture, spina bifida, occult meningomyelocele, pilonidal cyst
Buttocks	Symmetrical midline crease	Asymmetrical midline crease	Congenital hip dysplasia
Anus and genitalia			
Anus	Patent, located at midline	Nonpatent or dimpled	Imperforate anus
		Shifted anteriorly or posteriorly	Anal defect
	Anal wink present (indicated by anal sphincter constriction in response to light stroking of anal area)	Anal wink absent	Neurologic deficit
Perineum	Smooth	Dimpled or with extra opening	Urinary or genital malformation; urinary fistula
Female genitalia	Distinguishable as female	Ambiguous genitalia; some structures resembling male genitalia (such as a greatly enlarged clitoris)	Trisomy 18; adrenocortical insufficiency
	Enlarged clitoris (from maternal hormonal influence)		
	Labia majora extend beyond labia minora	Labia majora smaller than labia minora	Prematurity
	Well-formed labia minora	Labia minora larger than labia majora	Prematurity

HEAD-TO-TOE PHYSICAL ASSESSMENT FINDINGS *(continued)*

PARAMETER	NORMAL FINDINGS AND COMMON VARIATIONS	ABNORMAL FINDINGS	POSSIBLE CAUSES
Anus and genitalia *(continued)*			
Female genitalia *(continued)*	Urethral meatus located anterior to vaginal orifice	Displaced urethral meatus	Urinary malformation
	Patent vagina, possibly with discharge or slight bleeding (pseudomenstruation)	Vagina opening completely covered by thickened hymen, possibly with slight bleeding (pseudomenstruation)	Vaginal malformation
Male genitalia	Penis straight; appropriate size for body (2.8 to 4.3 cm long)	Penis curved	Chordee (fibrous constriction of penis)
		Penis enlarged	Renal disorder
	Urinary meatus located at midline, at tip of glans	Urinary meatus displaced to ventral surface	Hypospadias
		Urinary meatus displaced to dorsal surface	Epispadias
	Urine stream flowing straight from penis	Crooked urine stream or urine leakage from patent urachus (abnormal fetal opening between bladder and umbilicus)	Urinary fistula; phimosis
	Full testes; numerous rugae	Smooth or few rugae	Prematurity
	Darkly pigmented testes	Bluish testes or scrotum	Testicular torsion
		Enlarged or edematous scrotum	Hydrocele or breech delivery
		Dimpled testes	Testicular torsion
	Testes descended on at least one side	Testes not palpable or found high in inguinal canal	Prematurity
Voiding onset	Within first 24 hours	Later than 24 hours	Renal or urinary obstruction or malformation
Arms			
General appearance	Of appropriate length relative to body; bilaterally equal; straight	Shortened or asymmetrical	Maternal diabetes or drug use, congenital syndrome
	Humerus, radius, and ulna symmetrical; no masses present	Humerus, radius, or ulna asymmetrical or absent	Possible syndrome, such as thrombocytopenia-absent radius syndrome
		Mass present on humerus, radius, or ulna	Fracture (as from birth injury)

(continued)

HEAD-TO-TOE PHYSICAL ASSESSMENT FINDINGS *(continued)*

PARAMETER	NORMAL FINDINGS AND COMMON VARIATIONS	ABNORMAL FINDINGS	POSSIBLE CAUSES
Arms *(continued)*			
Range of motion	Full	Limited	Birth injury or trauma
		Limited flexion	Prematurity
		Limited shoulder motion or flexion	Dystocia, brachial plexus damage or palsy
		Limited clavicular motion	Clavicular injury, osteogenesis imperfecta (genetic disorder resulting in fragile bones)
		Limited elbow, wrist, or hand motion	Possible birth injury
Hands and wrists	Hand straight	Hand turned outward	Possible congenital absence of radius
	No simian crease in palm	Simian crease in palm	Down's syndrome
	10 equally spaced fingers; no webbing	More than 10 fingers (polydactyly)	Possible congenital syndrome (such as trisomy 13)
		Webbed fingers, digital tags (syndactyly), unequal finger spacing	Congenital syndrome (such as Apert's syndrome)
	Nails extending beyond nail beds to tips of fingers	Spoon-shaped nails that do not reach beyond nail beds	Congenital syndrome (such as fetal alcohol syndrome)
		Absent nails	Possible congenital absence of radius
		Meconium-stained nails	Fetal distress
	Nail beds regain pink color equally bilaterally and briskly (within 3 seconds) during capillary refill test	Nail beds remain dusky or regain pink color unequally bilaterally or slowly (longer than 3 seconds)	Poor peripheral perfusion or oxygenation
	Carpal and metacarpal bones of bilaterally equal length; no masses	Carpal and metacarpal bones absent or bilaterally unequal; masses present	Fracture or absence of bone, possibly associated with congenital syndrome
	Strong palmar grasp	Weak palmar grasp	Prematurity
Pulses	Brachial and radial pulses strong and bilaterally equal; equal to femoral pulses	Brachial or radial pulse weak, absent, or bilaterally unequal	Poor peripheral perfusion, possible cardiac defect

HEAD-TO-TOE PHYSICAL ASSESSMENT FINDINGS *(continued)*

PARAMETER	NORMAL FINDINGS AND COMMON VARIATIONS	ABNORMAL FINDINGS	POSSIBLE CAUSES
Legs			
General appearance	Of apportionate length relative to body; bilaterally equal; straight	Disproportionate length relative to body, short or bilaterally unequal, crooked, internally rotated or bowed	Congenital hip dysplasia
	Fibula, tibia, trochanter, and femur bilaterally symmetrical	Fibula, tibia, trochanter, or femur absent or bilaterally asymmetrical	Fracture or absence of bone (may be associated with congenital syndrome)
		Limited hip motion; audible click heard with Ortolani's or Barlow's maneuver	Congenital hip dysplasia
Femoral pulses	Strong and bilaterally regular	Weak or bilaterally absent	Coarctation of the aorta
		Bounding	Patent ductus arteriosus
Feet	Straight	Turned out (valgus deformity)	Absent fibula, fetal positioning (apparent clubfoot), true clubfoot
		Turned in (varus deformity)	Absent tibia, fetal positioning (apparent clubfoot), true clubfoot
		Pedal edema	Pressure caused by fetal positioning, poor peripheral perfusion, or congenital syndrome (such as Turner's syndrome)
	Plantar creases covering sole	Few plantar creases; may cover only anterior third of sole	Prematurity
	Tarsal and metatarsal bones present and bilaterally equal	Tarsal and metatarsal bones absent or bilaterally unequal	Fracture or absence of bone (may be associated with congenital syndrome)
	10 equally spaced toes; no webbing	More than 10 toes; unequal toe spacing, webbing present	Possible congenital syndrome (such as trisomy 13)
Reflexes	Symmetrical plantar and patellar reflexes (knee jerk)	Absent, weak, or asymmetrical plantar reflex	Neurologic deficit, prematurity
		Absent, weak, or asymmetrical patellar reflex	Neurologic deficit, prematurity

ASSESSING NEONATAL REFLEXES

To evaluate neurologic status during the complete physical assessment, the nurse should test neonatal reflexes. The chart below describes testing methods and normal responses. A weak, absent, or asymmetrical response is considered abnormal. Some reflexes (such as the pupillary, blink, and gag reflexes) persist throughout life; others (including the doll's eye, sucking, grasp, Babinski, Moro, fencing, and Galant reflexes) normally disappear a few weeks or months after birth.

REFLEX	TESTING METHOD	NORMAL RESPONSE
Babinski	Stroke one side of the neonate's foot upward from the heel and across the ball of the foot.	Neonate hyperextends the toes, dorsiflexes the great toe, and fans the toes outward.
Blink (corneal)	Momentarily shine a bright light directly into the neonate's eyes.	Neonate blinks.
Crawl	Place the neonate prone on a flat surface.	Neonate attempts to crawl forward using the arms and legs.
Crossed extension	Position the neonate supine; extend one leg and stimulate the sole with a light pin prick or finger flick.	Neonate swiftly flexes and extends the opposite leg as though trying to push the stimulus away from the other foot.
Doll's eye	With the neonate supine, slowly turn the neonate's head to the left or right.	Neonate's eyes remain stationary.
Fencing (tonic neck)	With a swift motion, turn the neonate's head to either side.	Neonate extends the extremities on the side to which the head is turned and flexes the extremities on the opposite side.
Galant	Using a fingernail, gently stroke one side of the neonate's spinal column from the head to the buttocks.	Neonate's trunk curves toward the stimulated side.
Grasp	Palmar: Place a finger in the neonate's palm.	Neonate grasps the finger.
	Plantar: Place a finger against the base of the neonate's toe.	Neonate's toes curl downward and grasp the finger.
Moro	Suddenly but gently drop the neonate's head backward (relative to the trunk).	Neonate extends and abducts all extremities bilaterally and symmetrically; forms a "C" shape with the thumb and forefinger; and adducts, then flexes, the extremities.
Pupillary (light)	Darken the room and shine a penlight directly into the neonate's eye for several seconds.	Pupils constrict equally bilaterally.
Rooting	Touch a finger to the neonate's cheek or the corner of mouth. (The mother's nipple also should trigger this reflex.)	Neonate turns the head toward the stimulus, opens the mouth, and searches for the stimulus.
Startle	Make a loud noise near the neonate.	Neonate cries and abducts and flexes all extremities.
Stepping (automatic walking)	Hold the neonate in an upright position and touch one foot lightly to a flat surface (such as the bed).	Neonate makes walking motions with both feet.
Sucking	Place a finger in the neonate's mouth. (The mother's nipple also should trigger this reflex.)	Neonate sucks on the finger (or nipple) forcefully and rhythmically; sucking is coordinated with swallowing.

BEHAVIORAL ASSESSMENT

The behavioral assessment allows the nurse to evaluate the neonate's behavioral capacities and interaction with the environment.

Various tools are available for behavioral assessment. For best results, the assessment should be conducted in a quiet, softly lit setting. Findings must be interpreted in light of the period of reactivity and the neonate's gestational age.

If possible, the parents should observe the assessment so they can learn about their child's behavioral and interactional capacities. The nurse also can use this opportunity to assess the parents' behavior and determine the quality of parent-neonate interaction. For example, parental sensitivity and positive follow-up to cues (perceived signals) from the neonate indicate a reciprocal relationship that promotes bonding.

The Brazelton neonatal behavioral assessment scale (BNBAS), developed by pediatrician T. Berry Brazelton in 1973, is the most commonly used behavioral evaluation tool. To score the BNBAS reliably, the examiner must take an intensive 2-day course. The nurse without such preparation may want to use the BNBAS as a guideline for assessing neonatal behavior in a more general way, without scoring the neonate.

Areas evaluated by the BNBAS include the neonate's behavioral state (level of wakefulness) and behavioral responses, including elicited responses.

Behavioral state

The BNBAS assessment begins by observing the neonate's behavioral state (degree of alertness). The neonate experiences six behavioral states.

- Deep sleep is a quiet period during which the neonate makes few or no spontaneous movements; any movements that occur are brief and jerky. No rapid eye movements (REMs) are detected. Respirations are even and regular. The neonate can be aroused from this state only for a few moments.
- In light sleep, the neonate can be aroused and brought to wakefulness easily; REMs can be detected. The arms or legs may move occasionally, and movements are smoother than during deep sleep. The breathing pattern varies as the neonate drifts from light sleep to drowsiness.
- The drowsy state is characterized by an attempt to become fully alert. Movements become more frequent and regular and the eyes open periodically. Although the ne-

onate responds to auditory and tactile stimuli, the response may be sluggish until the next state approaches.
- In the alert state, the neonate seems to be transfixed by external stimuli and has limited motor activity.
- The active state is characterized by regular eye and body movements in response to external stimuli.
- In the crying state, the neonate responds to both internal and external stimuli, cries vigorously and without interruption, and makes thrusting movements.

The neonate should move successively through these states, although the time spent in each may vary widely from one neonate to the next. The sleep-awake pattern also varies, depending on gestational age and other factors. The typical neonate sleeps 10 to 20 hours daily, with deep sleep accounting for only about 4 hours of total sleep. A neonate affected by maternal drug use may have an extremely labile sleep-awake pattern (Blackburn, 1987).

Behavioral responses

Neonatal behavioral responses fall into six categories: habituation, orientation, motor maturity, variations, self-quieting ability, and social behaviors.

Habituation. A protective mechanism, habituation refers to the process of becoming accustomed (habituating) to environmental stimuli, such as noise and light. For example, if one neonate in the nursery starts to cry, a neonate in light sleep will startle initially. If a second neonate then cries, the neonate who was in light sleep may move about. As the other neonates continue crying, the neonate in light sleep gradually becomes less stimulated, reflecting habituation. Normally, habituation occurs after three consecutive presentations of a stimulus (in this example, the continued crying of both neonates is the third presentation).

A neonate's ability to become habituated to a stimulus varies with the behavioral state. Habituation should be tested only during deep sleep, light sleep, or the drowsy state. If habituation does not occur after three presentations of a stimulus, the neonate may be hyperresponsive to external stimuli. A slowed or diminished response from the outset of the first presentation (except during deep sleep) suggests lethargy or hyporesponsiveness. These variations commonly reflect neurologic immaturity or impaired neurologic function.

Orientation. This term refers to the neonate's responsiveness to visual and auditory stimuli. For best results, orientation should be tested while the neonate is in the alert or active state.

Normally, the neonate orients to (follows) a visual or auditory stimulus by moving both the head and eyes. No response or lack of head movement is abnormal. Also observe for nystagmus (rapid, darting eye movements) and for gaze aversion after direct eye contact—both normal responses.

A neonate is more responsive to a human face—either real or represented in a picture—than an inanimate object. (This especially is apparent when the neonate is held in the en face—face-to-face—position). If the parents are observing the behavioral assessment, show them how closely their child attends to visual stimuli by holding a brightly colored object, such as a ball, in front of the neonate. As the ball moves from side to side, the neonate's eyes will follow it and the head will turn from side to side.

In response to an auditory stimulus, such as a human voice or noise from a rattle, the neonate typically stops an activity to attend to the sound. If the sound comes from outside the visual field, the neonate will turn toward it. (If the neonate fails to respond, repeat the sound at a different pitch—many neonates alert better to higher pitches.) A sudden or loud stimulus usually causes crying.

Motor maturity. Best assessed with the neonate in the alert state, motor maturity refers to posture, muscle tone, muscle coordination and movements, and reflexes. Evaluate smoothness and equality of arm and leg movements. In the term neonate, asymmetrical or absent movement of an extremity calls for further investigation, as do muscle flaccidity or hypotonia, extreme tremors, and excessive jerking movements.

Keep in mind that the first 24 hours after birth represent a period of progressive changes; thus, motor responses may vary greatly. Neurologic stability typically is established by the third day. However, with early discharge, few neurologic assessments can be delayed until this time. If any abnormalities are detected, the examination must be repeated later.

Variations. This term refers to the frequency of changes in activity level, state, and skin color. Document these changes throughout the behavioral assessment.

Self-quieting ability. To test this, observe how soon and how effectively the neonate self-quiets when crying. Attempts to self-quiet include such behaviors as moving the hands toward the mouth, sucking on the fist, changing position, and attending to auditory or visual stimuli.

If the neonate does not attempt to self-quiet, the nurse or a parent should attempt to console the neonate by singing, talking, rocking, walking, cuddling, or facing the ne-

onate directly. The degree to which this attempt succeeds reflects the neonate's consolability. If the attempt fails to elicit self-quieting, the neonate may be hyperactive or hypersensitive to the environment.

Consolability is documented in terms of whether and to what degree the neonate self-quiets after introduction of a visual or an auditory stimulus.

Social behaviors. Neonatal social behaviors include reflexive smiling, cuddling, and other distinct behavioral cues. Such cues—signals that indicate the neonate's needs—include crying to be fed and stopping sucking when hunger has been sated. These behaviors should be tested with the neonate in the alert or active state.

Social behaviors are especially important to the parents, who commonly gauge their ability to provide care by their child's response to their actions. During this part of the behavioral assessment, the nurse can demonstrate to the parents that the neonate is an active partner in the relationship, giving as well as responding to cues from the parents.

Als's synactive theory of development
Extending Brazelton's work, Heidelise Als developed a theoretical model for assessing neonatal behavior based on developmental potential. Als's theory holds that the neonate both shapes and is shaped by the environment, of which the parents form a part. According to Als, whose work spans the past decade, the neonate's physiologic status depends on the environmental stimuli received and processed. Further, neonatal behavior consists of functional subsystems (autonomic-visceral, motoric [motor], and state-attentional), each with distinctive behavioral stress responses.

CHAPTER SUMMARY

Chapter 18 described the essential elements of neonatal assessment, including gestational-age, physical, and behavioral assessments. Here are the chapter highlights.

The nurse must adapt the assessment to the neonate's tolerance, delaying any examination that could compromise the neonate. Also, to conserve the neonate's energy, the nurse should integrate overlapping portions of the various assessments whenever possible.

In the first few hours after birth, the neonate experiences two distinct periods of reactivity, separated by a sleep stage. Because vital signs, alertness level, and responsiveness to external stimuli change as the neonate enters a new period, the nurse should interpret assessment findings in light of the specific period of reactivity.

The nurse should perform a brief physical assessment within a few hours after delivery. This assessment includes evaluation of general appearance, vital sign measurements, and anthropometric measurements.

Within the next few days, or before the neonate is discharged, a comprehensive assessment must be conducted. This assessment includes gestational-age assessment, a complete physical assessment, and behavioral assessment.

Gestational-age assessment determines the neonate's age in weeks from the time of conception. Gestational-age assessment tools, such as the Ballard and Dubowitz tools, include evaluation of physical and neurologic characteristics.

The complete physical assessment should proceed systematically from head to toe. To guard against cold stress during this assessment, the nurse should maintain thermoregulation by placing the neonate in a radiant warmer and uncovering only one part of the body at a time. The physical assessment also includes evaluation of neurologic characteristics, such as posture, muscle tone, reflexes, and cry.

Behavioral assessment reveals the neonate's behavioral capacities and the quality of the neonate's interaction with the environment. The specially prepared nurse may use the Brazelton neonatal behavioral assessment scale to assess neonatal behavior.

STUDY QUESTIONS

1. How do the periods of reactivity affect assessment findings?

2. How can the nurse help to ensure thermoregulation when assessing the neonate?

3. Under which circumstances should a neonate's gestational age be precisely determined?

4. What are the two major categories of criteria evaluated with the Dubowitz and Ballard gestational-age assessment tools?

5. Which response would the nurse consider normal when testing a neonate's Babinski reflex?

6. What are the six response categories assessed during a neonatal behavioral assessment?

BIBLIOGRAPHY

American Academy of Pediatrics and American College of Obstetricians and Gynecologists (1988). *Guidelines for Perinatal Care* (2nd ed.). Washington DC: Staff.

Beal, J.A. (1986). The Brazelton neonatal behavioral assessment scale: A tool to enhance parental attachment. *Journal of Pediatric Nursing,* 1(3), 170-177.

Jones, M.A. (1989). Identifying signs that nurses interpret as indicating pain in newborns. *Pediatric Nursing,* 15(1), 76-79.

Kimberlin, L.V., Kucera, V.S., Lawrence, P.B., Newkirk, A., and Stenske, J.E. (1989). The role of the neonatal intensive care nurse in the delivery room. *Clinics in Perinatology,* 16(4), 1021-1028.

Pigeon, H.M., McGrath, P.J., Lawrence, J., and MacMurray, S.B. (1989). Nurses' perceptions of pain in the neonatal intensive care unit. *Journal of Pain and Symptom Management,* 4(4), 179-183.

Shapiro, C. (1989). Pain in the neonate: Assessment and intervention. *Neonatal Network,* 8(1), 7-21.

Stevens, K.A. (1988). Nursing diagnoses in wellness childbearing settings. *JOGNN,* 17(5), 329-336.

Wilson, J.R.A. (1989). How neonatal nurses report infants' pain. *AJN,* 89(11), 1529-1530.

Behavioral assessment

Als, H. (1982). Toward a synactive theory of development: Promise for the assessment and support of infant individuality. *Infant Mental Health Journal,* 3(4), 229-243.

Brazelton, T. (1984). *Neonatal behavioral assessment scale* (2nd ed.). Philadelphia: Lippincott.

Davis, D.H., and Thoman, E.B. (1987). Behavioral states of premature infants: Implications for neural and behavioral development. *Developmental Psychobiology,* 20(1), 25-38.

Frankenburg, W.K. (1981). The newly abbreviated and revised Denver developmental screening test. *Journal of Pediatrics,* 99(6), 995-999.

Gestational-age assessment

Ballard, J.L. (1988). *Maturational assessment of gestational age.* Cincinnati: University of Cincinnati.

Ballard, J.L., Khoury, J.C., Wedig, K., et al. (1991). New Ballard Score, expanded to include extremely premature infants. *Journal of Pediatrics,* 119(3), 417-423.

Ballard, J.L., Novak, K.K., and Driver, M. (1979). A simplified score for assessment of fetal maturation of newly born infants. *Journal of Pediatrics,* 95(5, Pt.1), 769-774.

Battaglia, F.C., and Lubchenco, L.O. (1967). A practical classification of newborn infants by weight and gestational age. *Journal of Pediatrics,* 71, 159-163.

Cassady, G., and Strange, M. (1987). The small-for-gestational-age (SGA) infant. In G.B. Avery (Ed.), *Neonatology: Pathophysiology and management of the newborn* (3rd ed., pp. 299-378). Philadelphia: Lippincott.

Dubowitz, L., and Dubowitz, V. (1977). *Gestational age of the newborn.* Reading, MA: Addison-Wesley.

Dubowitz, L., Dubowitz, V., and Goldberg, C. (1970). Clinical assessment of gestational age in the newborn infant. *Journal of Pediatrics,* 77(1), 1-10.

Usher, R. (1987). Extreme prematurity. In G.B. Avery (Ed.), *Neonatology: Pathophysiology and management of the newborn* (3rd ed.). Philadelphia: Lippincott.

Physical assessment

Blackburn, S. (1987). Sleep and awake states of the newborn. In K. Barnard (Ed.), *NCAST learning resource manual* (pp. 25-28). Seattle: University of Washington.

Bliss-Holtz, J. (1989). Comparison of rectal, axillary, and inguinal temperatures in full-term newborn infants. *Nursing Research,* 38(2), 85-87.

Smith, D.W. (1988). Minor anomalies. In K.L. Jones (Ed.), *Smith's recognizable patterns of human malformation: Genetic, embryologic and clinical aspects* (4th ed., pp. 662-681). Philadelphia: Saunders.

CHAPTER 19

CARE OF THE NORMAL NEONATE

OBJECTIVES

After reading and studying this chapter, the student should be able to:

1. Identify the essential components of nursing care of the normal neonate.

2. Identify factors affecting neonatal thermoregulation.

3. Apply the nursing process to nursing care of the normal neonate.

4. Describe the information to include in a teaching plan for new parents to promote confidence in their caregiving abilities.

5. Discuss nursing strategies that promote a positive parent-infant interaction.

INTRODUCTION

The neonate undergoes various physiologic changes during the neonatal period—the first 28 days after birth. To make a successful transition from dependent fetus, the neonate must adapt to these changes effectively, especially during the first 24 hours (known as the transitional period).

The nurse plays a crucial role during the neonatal period by promoting a stable physiologic status. For instance, the nurse maintains oxygenation, hydration, nutrition, elimination, hygiene, and thermoregulation; prevents and detects complications; and ensures environmental safety.

Neonatal nursing care also calls for a family-centered approach that helps ease the neonate's transition to the home and promotes a positive parent-infant interaction.

The nurse must assess parent-teaching needs regarding neonatal care and identify risk factors for poor parent-infant bonding. Parent teaching can be enhanced if the nurse serves as a caregiver role model and provides positive reinforcement during the parents' supervised attempts at caring for their child.

While providing care, the nurse must remain aware of cultural differences that may affect the parents' neonatal care decisions—for example, cultural attitudes toward circumcision. Considering these differences when planning, promoting, and implementing holistic neonatal and family care is essential.

This chapter describes how the nurse manages these responsibilities using the nursing process. It begins by describing the data that the nurse collects during ongoing neonatal assessment. Then the chapter discusses how to plan and implement nursing care, highlighting measures that ensure neonatal thermoregulation, safety, and hygiene as well as routine care measures (for instance, umbilical cord care). After describing how the nurse evaluates this care, the chapter concludes with a brief discussion of documentation.

ASSESSMENT

During the first few days after the neonate's birth, the nurse should conduct a comprehensive assessment (as described in Chapter 18, Neonatal Assessment). Throughout the neonate's hospitalization, however, the nurse should conduct ongoing assessment to ensure optimal neonatal adaptation and to detect changes in the neonate's status.

NORMAL NEONATE

For the normal neonate, the nurse may find the following examples of nursing diagnoses appropriate.

- Altered family processes related to the neonatal feeding schedule
- Altered nutrition: less than body requirements, related to decreased oral intake and increased caloric expenditure
- Altered parenting related to the addition of a new family member
- Altered peripheral tissue perfusion related to transition to the extrauterine environment
- Altered urinary elimination related to inability to maintain fluid balance
- Altered urinary elimination related to renal immaturity
- Anxiety related to lack of confidence in parenting ability
- Constipation related to gastrointestinal (GI) immaturity
- Diarrhea related to GI immaturity
- Fluid volume excess related to renal immaturity
- High risk for altered body temperature related to radiant, conductive, convective, or evaporative heat loss
- High risk for infection related to immunologic immaturity
- High risk for infection related to the circumcision site
- High risk for infection related to transition to the extrauterine environment
- High risk for infection related to umbilical cord healing
- High risk for injury related to environmental influences during transition to the extrauterine environment
- High risk for injury related to slippage while bathing
- High risk for trauma related to inability to process vitamin K
- Hypothermia related to cold stress
- Ineffective airway clearance related to the presence of mucus
- Ineffective breathing pattern related to respiratory dysfunction
- Ineffective breathing pattern related to transition to the extrauterine environment
- Potential altered parenting related to lack of knowledge about neonatal care
- Potential altered parenting related to transition to the role of parent
- Potential fluid volume deficit related to insensible fluid loss
- Potential fluid volume deficit related to poor oral intake

The nurse evaluates the neonate continually for obvious or subtle changes from baseline clinical findings (including heart and respiratory rate and rhythm, skin color, cry, response to stimuli, alertness level, and irritability level) or laboratory values. The nurse also assesses for indications of neonatal distress. These include:
- abdominal distention
- apprehensive facial expression

- bile-stained emesis
- cyanosis (other than acrocyanosis or periorbital cyanosis)
- excessive mucus production or meconium in the nasal passages
- frequent apneic episodes
- hypotonia during active and alert periods
- jaundice
- labored respirations accompanied by skin or mucous membrane color changes
- lethargy during periods of expected activity
- meconium-stained skin
- persistent, pronounced increase or decrease in heart and respiratory rates from baseline vital signs
- temperature instability.

Such distress could lead to serious complications. (For information on the comprehensive neonatal assessment and a thorough discussion of other characteristics to assess, see Chapter 18, Neonatal Assessment.)

NURSING DIAGNOSIS

After gathering assessment data, the nurse reviews it carefully to identify pertinent nursing diagnoses for the neonate. (For a partial list of applicable diagnoses, see Nursing Diagnoses: *Normal neonate.*)

PLANNING AND IMPLEMENTATION

After assessing the neonate and formulating nursing diagnoses, the nurse develops and implements a plan of care. For the normal neonate, the plan centers on promoting optimal neonatal adaptation and parent-neonate interaction and includes such routine therapeutic interventions as umbilical cord care and vitamin K administration. Nursing goals include:
- ensuring oxygenation
- maintaining thermoregulation
- maintaining optimal hydration and nutrition
- promoting adequate urinary and bowel elimination
- providing hygienic care
- preventing and detecting complications
- ensuring environmental safety
- providing care for the family
- performing routine therapeutic interventions.

The American Academy of Pediatrics (1988) recommends that the neonate be kept in a transitional care or observation area in the nursery during the transition period to allow close observation. Then the neonate may be moved to the mother's room to avoid separating mother and neonate. This area should have oxygen and suction outlets, resuscitation equipment, and multiple electrical outlets with safety grounds.

Ensuring oxygenation

At birth, the neonate must begin breathing through the nose and drawing air into the lungs. Closure of the fetal shunts (ductus arteriosus, ductus venosus, and foramen ovale) after birth changes the circulatory direction and facilitates peripheral circulation and alveolar gas exchange. (See Chapter 17, Neonatal Adaptation, for more information on fetal shunt closure and neonatal respiration.) To ensure successful respiratory adaptation, maintaining adequate oxygenation is crucial.

A few hours after birth, the gastrointestinal (GI) tract begins secreting gastric juices; this leads to increased saliva and mucus production. Mucus production peaks in the first 2 to 3 days after birth. For the neonate with a nursing diagnosis of *ineffective airway clearance related to the presence of mucus,* suctioning with a bulb syringe or sterile catheter may be necessary to prevent aspiration of mucus. A bulb syringe may be kept at the bedside; clean it with warm, soapy water after each use to reduce the risk of bacterial growth. (For details on how to suction with a bulb syringe, see Psychomotor Skills: *Suctioning with a bulb syringe,* pages 384 and 385.)

A suction catheter should be used only if absolutely necessary because suctioning carries a risk of apnea, reflex bradycardia, cardiopulmonary arrest, and laryngospasm. For this procedure, the neonate is placed in a side-lying or prone position. Lubricate the end of the catheter with sterile water, then insert the catheter into the oral cavity without applying pressure. When the catheter reaches the pharynx, apply pressure for 5 seconds, then withdraw. After suctioning the pharynx, suction each naris (nostril). Before each new suctioning attempt, the catheter tip must be lubricated and the catheter rinsed with sterile water.

While suctioning, observe for skin and mucous membrane color changes. If the neonate is attached to a cardiopulmonary monitor, check for changes in the heart and respiratory rates. If the neonate becomes cyanotic (indicated by a bluish color), withdraw the catheter and stop suctioning. The amount and appearance of any secretions and the neonate's tolerance for the procedure should be documented.

An irregular respiratory pattern, including periodic breathing and slight chest retractions, is common in the first few hours after birth while the neonate adapts to the new environment. However, stay alert for changes in the respiratory pattern that persist for several hours or become increasingly severe; these may indicate respiratory distress. If skin or mucous membrane color changes from pink to dusky or cyanotic, check for grunting, nasal flaring, crackles, rhonchi, and other abnormal signs. The neonate with these signs may have a nursing diagnosis of *ineffective breathing pattern related to transition to the extrauterine environment.* Immediately report any significant deviations from normal cardiopulmonary parameters, and assess vital signs continually to help prevent complications.

Maintaining thermoregulation

The term neonate has protective mechanisms to promote heat conservation—layers of adipose tissue and areas of brown fat, most prominent over the scapula and flank. Brown fat supplies fatty acids for heat production (thermogenesis), a process that begins when the neonate starts to lose heat. To maintain a stable core temperature, the body breaks down fats, burns calories, consumes oxygen, and increases the metabolic rate.

The preterm neonate, in contrast, has insufficient adipose tissue and brown fat insulation and may suffer cold stress from heat loss. The posture of the preterm neonate also contributes to heat loss. Unlike the term neonate—who assumes a fetal position to reduce the exposed surface area and thus minimize convective heat loss—the preterm neonate lies flaccid with arms and legs extended, exposing a greater surface area.

Cold stress may occur in any neonate who is exposed to a cold environment without adequate protection or whose caloric expenditure exceeds caloric consumption. When oxygen and nutritional reserves are depleted, the neonate loses protein and muscle tissue as well as weight. Anabolic metabolism ensues, leading to metabolic acidosis.

To stabilize the neonate's body temperature and thus minimize oxygen, caloric, and fat expenditure, maintain a neutral thermal environment. This narrow temperature range maintains a stable core temperature with minimal caloric and oxygen consumption, allowing calories and oxygen to be used for growth and adaptation rather than thermoregulation. (For further information on the mechanisms of heat loss and gain, see Chapter 17, Neonatal Adaptation. For specific nursing measures that help prevent heat loss, see *Preventing heat loss,* page 386.)

Throughout the neonate's nursery stay, enforce measures to conserve body heat—especially for the neonate with a nursing diagnosis of *high risk for altered body temperature related to radiant, conductive, convective, or evaporative heat loss.* For example, always keep the neonate dry; a warm, wet neonate loses heat to the surrounding

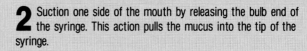

PSYCHOMOTOR SKILLS

SUCTIONING WITH A BULB SYRINGE

If the neonate has excess mucus in the respiratory tract, the nurse may need to aspirate the mouth and nasal passages using a bulb syringe. To perform this procedure, which demands skill and sensitivity to touch, follow these steps.

1 Depress the bulb to remove air. Then insert the tip of the syringe into the neonate's mouth until it reaches the pharyngeal area.

2 Suction one side of the mouth by releasing the bulb end of the syringe. This action pulls the mucus into the tip of the syringe.

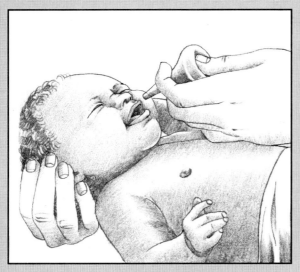

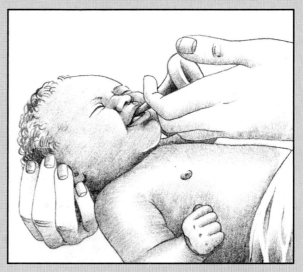

environment through evaporation and convection. Keep the neonate's head covered at all times. The head accounts for 25% of the neonate's total body surface; substantial heat can be lost to surrounding cool surfaces and air through radiation, conduction, and convection unless the head is covered with a blanket, hat, or stockinette. (For more information on neonatal head coverings, see Chapter 17, Neonatal Adaptation.)

Even if the neonate is placed under a radiant warmer and dried to reduce heat loss, wide temperature fluctuations are common in the first few hours after birth. If the neonate has been in an open warmer for 2 to 3 hours and the axillary temperature measures over 97.6° F (36.5° C), wrap the neonate in a blanket and place in an open, clear basinette. Monitor skin temperature, which should measure 97.5° to 99° F (36.4° to 37.2° C), or 0.2 to 0.9 degrees F below the core temperature.

Using an incubator or radiant warmer. If the core temperature drops below an acceptable level, keep the neonate in a thermally controlled environment. Depending on health care facility policy, this may necessitate use of an incubator or a radiant warmer. (An incubator is a fully enclosed, single-walled or double-walled bed containing a heating source and a humidification chamber. A radiant warmer is an open bed with an overhead radiant heat source.) Because the neonate requires close observation during the transitional period, keep the incubator or radiant warmer in clear view at all times.

With an incubator, temperature can be controlled externally or servo-controlled by taping a flat probe to the neonate's skin and setting the thermostat to maintain a skin temperature of 97.5° (36.4° C). Do not tape the probe to areas of brown fat, such as the scapula and flank; these areas generate more heat, causing a falsely elevated skin temperature reading. With a radiant warmer, control the temperature by positioning the skin probe, then setting the thermostat of the bed to maintain a stable skin temperature.

Observing and intervening for cold stress. Signs of cold stress include an accelerated respiratory rate, labored respirations, and an increased metabolic rate accompanied by hypoglycemia (indicating greater use of glucose stores). In the neonate with a nursing diagnosis of *hypothermia related to cold stress,* check for signs of hypoglycemia, such as a serum glucose level below 30 mg/dl before the third

3 Suction the other side of the mouth the same way. Be sure to avoid touching the midline of the throat because this could activate the gag reflex.

4 Finally, suction the nasal passages, one nostril at a time, using the same approach.

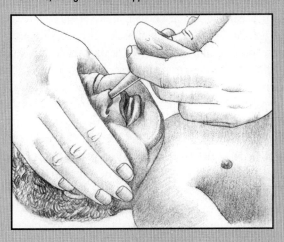

day after birth or below 40 mg/dl on or after the third day.

Other signs of hypoglycemia include tremors, seizures, irritability and lethargy (from breakdown of fats and proteins to maintain body heat), and apnea or bradycardia (from changes in arterial oxygen saturation and a shift to anaerobic metabolism). Neurologic immaturity may prevent homeostasis in the hypoglycemic neonate, leading to unstable vital signs.

If the neonate suffers cold stress, rewarm gradually to avoid hyperthermia and its complications; closely observe the neonate and check vital signs every 15 to 30 minutes. Hyperthermia may cause skin reddening, irritability, and an initial increase — then gradual drop — in the heart and respiratory rates, leading to apnea and bradycardia. To prevent complications, report any status changes immediately.

Maintaining optimal hydration and nutrition

Hydration and nutrition are vital to immune system development and maintenance. The American Academy of Pediatrics (1988) recommends that the initial feeding never be delayed more than 6 hours after birth. If the mother plans to breast-feed, the neonate can be put to the breast in the delivery room.

Assessing the adequacy of fluid intake. To maintain adequate output and hydration and help avert a nursing diagnosis of *potential fluid volume deficit related to poor oral intake,* assess fluid intake frequently and compare it to urine output. The term neonate requires a fluid intake of 140 to 160 ml/kg/day to maintain hydration (Streeter, 1986). This requirement increases with illness, preterm birth, and excessive evaporative or radiant fluid loss. Urine output should measure 1 to 2 ml/kg/hour. In the first 24 hours after birth, the neonate may void only once or twice, although output from these first voidings exceeds output from later voidings.

The bottle-fed neonate who requires a diaper change every 2 to 4 hours is receiving adequate fluids. (Diapers should be moderately saturated.) The breast-fed neonate usually voids less frequently but at least six to eight times a day. With any neonate, scanty or infrequent voiding (less than five times a day) suggests impaired fluid intake or a urinary problem. Document this finding and notify the physician.

Assessing for insensible fluid loss. The neonate experiences insensible fluid loss, such as radiant and evaporative fluid loss resulting from the transition to the relatively cool extrauterine environment. For the neonate with a nursing diagnosis of *potential fluid volume deficit related to insensible fluid loss,* assess for and guard against such loss, including that caused by environmental sources. For example, phototherapy (used to treat jaundice) increases GI motility, causing diarrhea and fluid loss in the stool. Also, phototherapy increases radiant fluid loss by warming the neonate. (For specific interventions to maintain thermoregulation, see the previous section on "Maintaining thermoregulation.")

Giving the first feeding. For the first feeding, the bottle-fed neonate usually is given sterile water because it is less irritating than formula or glucose water if it is aspirated. (Some facilities suggest an initial sterile water feeding for the breast-fed neonate as well to determine if the neonate is prone to aspiration or other complications.) If the neonate takes the sterile-water feeding without problems, glucose water or formula then may be given. In some facilities, the neonate is given a few milliliters of sterile water followed by 15 to 30 ml of glucose water to prevent hypoglycemia.

During the first feeding, assess the neonate's sucking ability and observe how well the neonate coordinates the

PREVENTING HEAT LOSS

Preventing heat loss is an important part of neonatal nursing care. Heat loss can occur through four mechanisms—conduction, convection, evaporation, and radiation. The chart below describes some nursing measures that help prevent heat loss by each mechanism.

Conductive heat loss
• Preheat the radiant warmer bed and linen.
• Warm the stethoscope before use.
• Wrap the neonate in a warm blanket or allow the mother to hold the neonate to provide the warming effect of skin contact.
• Pad the scale with paper or a preweighed, warmed sheet to weigh the neonate.
• Check the temperature of any surface before placing the neonate on it.

Convective heat loss
• Place the neonate's bed out of direct line with an open window, a fan, or an air-conditioning vent.
• Cover the neonate with a blanket when moving the neonate to another area.
• Raise the sides of the radiant warmer bed to prevent exposing the neonate to air currents.
• Avoid using fans in the delivery room or nursery.

Evaporative heat loss
• Dry the neonate immediately after delivery.
• When the neonate is not in a warming bed, keep the neonate dry and swaddled in warmed blankets.
• Remove wet blankets.
• Delay the bath until the neonate's temperature is stable.
• When bathing the neonate, expose only one body part at a time; wash each part thoroughly, then dry it immediately.
• When assessing the neonate, uncover only the specific area to be assessed.
• Place a cap on the neonate's head in the delivery room.

Radiant heat loss
• Use a radiant heat warmer for initial post-delivery stabilization.
• Place the neonate in a double-walled incubator.
• Keep the neonate away from areas with cold surfaces (such as a cold formula bottle or a window in winter).

sucking, swallowing, and gag reflexes. Immediately after the feeding, check for salivation, mucus production, aspiration, and regurgitation. The neonate produces more saliva and mucus in the first few hours after birth than at later times. Consequently, regurgitation—especially of a combination of mucus and feeding matter—is common. To promote digestion, place the neonate in a right side-lying position, which allows food to move more easily

through the stomach and into the GI tract for absorption. This intervention helps prevent a nursing diagnosis of *altered nutrition: less than body requirements, related to decreased oral intake and increased caloric expenditure.*

Continue to check for signs of excessive salivation or mucus production, which may indicate a blind esophageal pouch (esophageal atresia) or a fistula between the esophagus and trachea (tracheoesophageal fistula). A neonate who aspirates or regurgitates copious amounts of mucus or the entire feeding also may have esophageal atresia or a tracheoesophageal fistula.

Regurgitation after a feeding also may indicate an immature cardiac sphincter that allows reflux of feeding matter through the weak muscle. This condition may cause esophageal irritation from acidic gastric juices, possibly leading to aspiration. Projectile vomiting or bile-colored emesis indicates GI blockage. If the vomiting is accompanied by abdominal distention, suspect an intestinal obstruction—a condition that requires immediate intervention.

A neonate with excessive mucus production may require nasopharyngeal suctioning. Be sure to use caution when performing this procedure because it may trigger the gag reflex, causing aspiration.

To prevent aspiration and facilitate digestion, place the neonate in semi-Fowler's position after feeding. The neonate who becomes cyanotic or extremely fatigued during a feeding may have a cardiac or respiratory problem. A respiratory rate above 60 to 80 breaths/minute increases the risk of aspiration.

If aspiration or regurgitation occurs, stop the feeding immediately and allow the neonate to rest before attempting further feeding. Document the incident thoroughly, and report it for further assessment.

Supporting the parents' choice of feeding method. Optimal enteral nutrition may be achieved by breast-feeding, bottle-feeding, or both. Support the parents' choice of feeding method. Their choice may be based on such factors as economic and financial considerations, the mother's occupational status, and sociocultural influences as well as neonatal health implications. (For more information on feeding methods, see Chapter 20, Infant Nutrition.)

Promoting adequate urinary and bowel elimination
Urinary and bowel elimination must be adequate to maintain hydration and nutrition. Elimination patterns are established in the first few days after birth. Although the kidneys begin functioning in utero (fetal urine is the major component of amniotic fluid), the neonate's kidneys do not concentrate urine as effectively as an adult's. The ne-

onate also has an immature glomerular filtration system (restricting elimination of water and solutes) and limited tubular reabsorption (impairing the ability of bicarbonate ions and buffers to maintain the glomerular filtration system at a homeostatic pH).

Monitoring for voiding onset. Despite the limitations described above, voiding should begin by 48 hours after birth. (Some neonates even void on the delivery table.) Over 90% of term neonates void within 24 hours of birth; all but 1%, within 48 hours (Kim and Mandell, 1988). Failure to void within 48 hours may indicate a renal disorder, inadequate fluid intake, increased water loss, or fluid retention (edema). The neonate with any of these problems may have a nursing diagnosis of *altered urinary elimination related to renal immaturity.*

Assessing urine characteristics. Initially, urine should be cloudy and amber (from urinary protein, blood, and mucus); specific gravity should measure 1.005 to 1.015. In the female neonate, blood in the urine represents pseudomenstruation; in the circumcised male neonate, blood originates from the surgical site.

After the first 24 hours or so, urine should appear clear and amber. A specific gravity below 1.005 may indicate excessive fluid loss unless the neonate has been edematous and is eliminating excess fluids. A specific gravity above 1.025 may indicate fluid retention unless the neonate has been dehydrated (in which case it represents an attempt to restore fluid balance).

A deviation from the usual urinary pattern—too few or too many saturated diapers, a high specific gravity, or dilute urine—may warrant a nursing diagnosis of *altered urinary elimination related to inability to maintain fluid balance.* If the neonate is losing excessive fluids, check skin turgor and assess the fontanels and eye area. With dehydration, skin turgor is decreased and the anterior fontanel and eye orbits appear sunken. Edema, indicated by shiny, taut skin, may suggest fluid retention caused by a cardiac or renal disorder. All of these signs warrant further evaluation to help prevent complications.

Assessing bowel elimination patterns. The first stool (usually passed in the delivery room or within 48 hours after birth) consists of meconium, a thick, dark green, sticky, odorless material made up of amniotic fluid and shed GI mucosal cells. Failure to pass meconium within 48 hours may indicate anal or bowel malformation or Hirschsprung's disease (aganglionic megacolon), a congenital disorder characterized by incomplete bowel innervation.

Once feeding patterns have been established, stools change in color and consistency, the GI tract starts to secrete digestive enzymes, and intestinal bacteria (especially *Escherichia coli*) start to colonize. Transitional stools—thinner, lighter green, and seedier than meconium—then appear. After 2 or 3 days, stools change again, taking on distinctive characteristics that vary with the feeding method. (For details on characteristics of the neonate's stools, see Chapter 17, Neonatal Adaptation.)

Feeding method affects stool consistency and output. The stool of a breast-fed neonate is looser and paler yellow than that of a formula-fed neonate. Also, the breast-fed neonate typically passes 2 to 10 stools daily; the formula-fed neonate usually passes one stool daily or every other day.

Assess for deviations in stool pattern or consistency. A neonate with such a deviation may have a nursing diagnosis of *diarrhea related to GI immaturity* or *constipation related to GI immaturity.* If the neonate has diarrhea, a condition that increases fluid loss, assess for signs of dehydration (described above). If the neonate fails to pass stool or passes a hard, ribbon-like stool, suspect an intestinal obstruction. Also assess for abdominal distention, and palpate the abdomen for fecal masses. Observe the neonate during and just after feeding; an abdominal obstruction may cause vomiting and irritability at these times. Report any problem with stools, feedings, and related changes in the neonate's status so that prompt diagnosis and treatment can begin.

Providing hygienic care

Maintaining hygiene is an important aspect of neonatal care. The epidermal layer of the skin protects against traumatic injury, helps minimize heat loss, and serves as a barrier against bacterial infection by maintaining the pH of the skin at 4.9. (For more information and illustrated procedures for providing hygienic care, see Psychomotor Skills: *Cleaning the scalp and face,* page 388.)

Bathing the neonate. Because scented, medicated, and harsh soaps can alter the pH of the skin, use only mild soap (or the soap specified by the health care facility) when bathing the neonate. To prevent cross-contamination and bacterial growth, a soap dispenser should be assigned for each neonate. Avoid scrubbing the skin because this may cause abrasions through which microorganisms can enter.

To guard against heat loss during bathing, bathe the neonate only after temperature and vital signs have stabilized—especially if the core temperature is below normal. In the first hour or so after birth, use a soft sterile cotton pad soaked with warm water to remove dried

CLEANING THE SCALP AND FACE

The nurse who bathes a neonate should expose only one area at a time, washing and drying thoroughly before exposing the next area. Follow these steps to ensure safety when cleaning the scalp and face.

1 Hold the neonate in the football position, which supports the back and head and frees one hand for bathing.

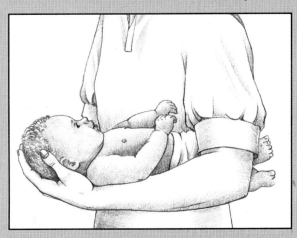

2 If shampooing is necessary, extend the neonate's head slightly while keeping the neonate supine, and tilt the head backward over a small basin. This position allows water to run from the front to the back of the head, preventing soapy water from getting into the eyes. Gently lather the scalp in a circular motion by hand or with a small cloth or soft brush containing mild, nonmedicated shampoo.

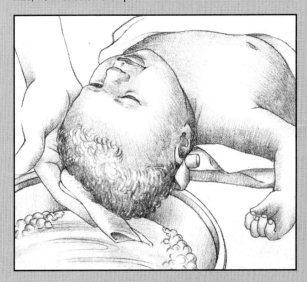

3 To rinse, fill a small cup with tepid water and pour the water over the scalp. Dry the hair quickly and thoroughly with a soft towel to minimize heat loss.

4 To wash the eyes, wrap a small washcloth around one hand so that no ends dangle. (This reduces the risk of dragging a wet cloth across the neonate, which could cause chilling from the dripping water or cross-contamination from contact with a soiled surface.) Moisten the washcloth with water, then gently stroke from the inner aspect of the lacrimal duct to the outer portion of the eyelid.

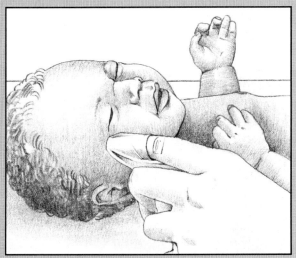

5 Wash the ears by wrapping a cloth around one finger and gently cleaning the external part of the ear (including the posterior portion). Never use a cotton-tipped applicator to clean the ears because this may damage the delicate internal ear structures and lead to infection.

6 To clean the nose, insert the twisted end of a washcloth into the naris (nostril). Remove any crusted matter or nasal secretions at the surface of the nostril. To help detect excessive nasal drainage (which may indicate infection), document any nasal drainage and secretions.

7 Wash each side of the face with mild soap.

blood, meconium, and debris arising from delivery; then dry the skin thoroughly. Removing these contaminants reduces the risk of infection by the hepatitis B, herpes simplex, and human immunodeficiency viruses (American Academy of Pediatrics, 1988). Also, gently wash off the vernix caseosa, the grayish white substance that covers the skin of the term neonate.

Proceed from head to toe, washing the cleanest areas first to reduce the risk of infection from any contaminated areas and help avoid a nursing diagnosis of *high risk for infection related to transition to the extrauterine environment.* Do not immerse the neonate in a tub; this could cause chilling or infection of the umbilical cord or an unhealed circumcision. During bathing, inspect the neonate's body for such variations as skin tags, unusual hair distribution, palmar creases, and other minor abnormalities. These variations may indicate more serious abnormalities. (For more information, see Chapter 18, Neonatal Assessment.)

Assess the neonate's response to each portion of the bath. For example, a change in appearance or skin color may indicate stress, fatigue, or chilling. (If any of these changes occurs, stop the bath immediately and dry the neonate.) Observe for drainage (exudate), discoloration, swelling, and redness around the eyes, which may signal infection or chemical irritation.

Washing the neonate's hair and scalp may decrease the risk of seborrheic dermatitis (cradle cap)—a potential cause of skin breakdown and infection. However, cradle cap also may occur in a neonate whose hair is washed frequently. The exact cause of this condition remains unknown.

Wash the neonate's face only after feedings, if milk or formula remains on the skin. If necessary, wash the chin and mouth more often.

After drying the neonate's head and face, wash the rest of the body one part at a time, covering each part immediately after drying it to avoid evaporative heat loss. In the female neonate, clean the perineal region from front to back, proceeding from the cleanest area to the most soiled. In the male neonate, gently clean the penis to remove smegma. Use plain warm water or soapy water followed by a plain warm water rinse. Gently pat the penis dry to avoid causing abrasions. Some health care facilities recommend applying a thin layer of petrolatum gauze or a bactericidal ointment over the circumcision site.

In the uncircumcised male, gently retract the foreskin until encountering resistance, then expose the glans penis. If the foreskin cannot be retracted, do not force it; simply wash the penis as is. Make sure to return a retracted foreskin to its natural position—the neonate's skin is so tight

that the foreskin rarely retracts on its own; the glans may become inflamed and swollen if the foreskin is left retracted. Next, lift the scrotal sac—a potential infection source because of accumulated stool—and wash the underlying surface.

Wash the anal region from front to back to avoid cross-contamination from stool and dry the area thoroughly. Also clean the buttocks and genitalia at each diaper change to prevent infection and skin irritation.

Excessive bathing—more frequently than every other day—may dry the skin, increasing the infection risk. Although relatively aggressive washing may be needed to remove the vernix caseosa and dried blood found in natural creases (such as the neck, axillae, and groin), always use care to keep the skin intact.

Ensuring safety during bathing. All neonates have a nursing diagnosis of *high risk for injury related to slippage while bathing.* Make sure to maintain a secure grip while bathing the neonate. Using the forearm, support the neonate's back and head; wash with the other hand. Then dry each body part thoroughly. Immediately place the neonate in a bath blanket, making sure the neonate is thoroughly dry. Then redress and swaddle in a dry blanket.

Preventing and detecting complications

To prevent and detect neonatal complications, assess continually, staying alert for subtle changes in the neonate's condition. Document and report any changes immediately. Also monitor laboratory values and report any deviations. (For more information, see *Normal laboratory values* and *Psychomotor Skills: Performing a heel stick,* page 390; for a more detailed discussion of complications occurring in neonates, see Chapter 21, Care of High-Risk Neonates and Their Families.)

Respiratory dysfunction. The most common neonatal complication, respiratory dysfunction may be mild (such as transient tachypnea) or severe (such as respiratory distress syndrome). In a neonate with a nursing diagnosis of *ineffective breathing pattern related to respiratory dysfunction,* stay alert for respiratory distress by assessing for changes in the respiratory rate and effort and checking for accompanying skin color changes, such as duskiness or cyanosis. If cyanosis is present, supplemental oxygen may be necessary. Be sure to allow the neonate to rest between nursing procedures to minimize oxygen consumption.

Hypocalcemia. The neonate who experienced birth asphyxia, is premature, or was born of an insulin-dependent diabetic mother is at risk for hypocalcemia (a serum calcium level below 7 mg/dl). Hypocalcemia also may occur if enteral feedings must be delayed (such as in the neurologically impaired neonate). Signs of hypocalcemia include twitching of extremities, cyanosis, apneic episodes, seizures, and listlessness. To detect hypocalcemia early and help prevent complications, monitor the serum calcium level. Expect to give enteral or parenteral calcium supplements to a hypocalcemic neonate.

Physiologic jaundice. Physiologic jaundice (yellow skin discoloration accompanied by an increased serum bilirubin level) is a common neonatal complication resulting from hepatic immaturity. It develops in the full-term neonate

NORMAL LABORATORY VALUES

The physician may order various laboratory tests to check for such neonatal complications as infection, hematologic problems, and metabolic disorders (such as hypoglycemia). The chart below shows normal laboratory values for commonly ordered tests. However, because values differ among laboratories, the nurse must check the values for the laboratory used.

TEST	NORMAL VALUES
Hematocrit	51% to 56%
Hemoglobin	16.5 g/dl (cord blood)
Platelets	192,000 to 290,000/mm³
Serum electrolytes	
Bicarbonate	18 to 23 mEq/liter
Calcium	7 to 12 mg/dl
Carbon dioxide	15 to 25 mEq/liter
Chloride	90 to 114 mEq/liter
Potassium	4 to 6 mEq/liter
Sodium	135 to 148 mEq/liter
Serum glucose	40 to 80 mg/dl
Total protein	4 to 7 g/dl
White blood cell total	18,000/mm³
White blood cell differential	
Band neutrophils	1,600/mm³ (9%)
Segmented neutrophils	9,400/mm³ (52%)
Eosinophils	400/mm³ (2.2%)
Basophils	100/mm³ (0.6%)
Lymphocytes	5,500/mm³ (31%)
Monocytes	1,050/mm³ (5.8%)

PERFORMING A HEEL STICK

In some facilities, the nurse who cares for normal neonates is required to perform a heel stick to obtain blood for measurement of glucose level and hematocrit. The blood also is used to test for phenylketonuria, galactosemia, and hypothyroidism.

1 Before beginning, wash the hands and put on gloves. Next, clean the neonate's heel with alcohol and dry with a sterile 2″ x 2″ gauze pad.

2 Choose a capillary site for venipuncture (as shown in the shaded area) to avoid the plantar artery.

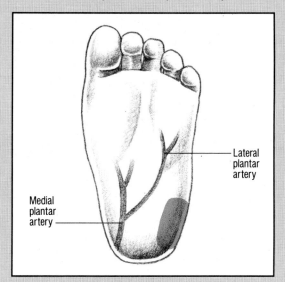

Lateral plantar artery

Medial plantar artery

3 Using the appropriate blade, quickly puncture the heel deeply enough to trigger a free flow of blood. Discard the first drop by wiping it away with another sterile gauze pad.

4 Collect blood into the appropriate capillary tubes. Clean the heel of any blood and cover with a bandage.

48 to 72 hours after birth. Suspect physiologic jaundice if the neonate's skin appears abnormally yellow. To verify the disorder, apply pressure to the tip of the neonate's nose. With jaundice, a yellow tinge appears instead of the normal blanching as circulation is impeded. (This test is accurate in dark-skinned as well as light-skinned neonates.)

If the neonate has jaundice, pathologic jaundice must be ruled out. Unlike physiologic jaundice, pathologic jaundice develops within 24 hours.

Infection. Infection, another common complication, stems from immunologic immaturity. Thorough hand washing significantly reduces the risk of neonatal infection and may help avoid a nursing diagnosis of *high risk for infection related to immunologic immaturity.* Before and after performing any nursing procedure, wash the hands. Also emphasize to parents the importance of frequent hand washing and proper hand-washing technique.

Because the neonate does not have localized immune reactions, infection causes only subtle, nonspecific signs. Such signs may include a high, low, or unstable body temperature; a weak or high-pitched cry; pallor; cyanosis; feeding problems or fatigue after feedings; diminished peripheral perfusion causing reduced skin temperature; sudden onset of apneic or bradycardic episodes; and jaundice.

If the neonate has signs that suggest infection, immediately document and report them. Obtain vital signs every 1 to 2 hours, observe closely for behavioral changes, and expect the physician to order a complete diagnostic workup for sepsis. Depending on health care facility policy and updated recommendations from the Centers for Disease Control, isolation procedures may be necessary.

Neonatal ophthalmia, an eye infection caused by *Neisseria gonorrhoea* or *Chlamydia trachomatis,* can be prevented if 1% silver nitrate solution, 1% tetracycline ointment, or 0.5% erythromycin ointment is applied to the eyes shortly after delivery. (Tetracycline and erythromycin are less irritating than silver nitrate.) Previously, the medication was administered in the delivery room. However, in many facilities, the procedure now is delayed until the neonate arrives in the nursery. This allows clear vision during the first period of reactivity, facilitating parent-infant bonding. (For details on administering eye medication, see Psychomotor Skills: *Administering eye medications.*)

Ensuring environmental safety

Environmental safety is an important concern of neonatal nursing, particularly for the neonate with a nursing diagnosis of *high risk for injury related to environmental influences during transition to the extrauterine environment.*

To ensure environmental safety, verify that room lighting is strong enough to allow accurate observation of skin color and respiratory effort, a clock is kept within easy view, and noise is held to the lowest level possible. Also, room temperature should be kept consistent and humidity maintained at 35% to 60% (American Academy of Pediatrics, 1988). Besides promoting thermoregulation, this intervention helps prevent drying of the mucous membranes, which can permit infectious agents to enter the respiratory tract. If necessary, drafts should be sealed off

ADMINISTERING EYE MEDICATIONS

Eye prophylaxis is an essential part of neonatal nursing care. Most states require the administration of 1% silver nitrate ophthalmic solution, 1% tetracycline ointment, or 0.5% erythromycin ointment to prevent ophthalmia neonatorum, a severe eye infection.

To administer the medication, wash the hands thoroughly. Position the neonate securely so that the head remains still. While holding the eyelid open, instill the medication into the conjunctival sac. Repeat with the other eye.

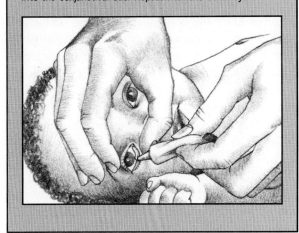

and the window shades drawn to minimize neonatal heat loss.

Consider safety when providing all care measures, such as feeding, bathing, and weighing. Never look away or leave the neonate unattended while bathing or weighing. Before leaving the neonate's bedside, make sure the crib side rails are up and in the locked position.

When the neonate is ready for discharge, confirm that an infant car seat (not a carrier seat, which cannot be locked into place) is available for the trip home. Most states require such seats for children under age 4.

Providing care for the family

Nursing care must involve the entire family—not just the neonate. By facilitating bonding and offering parent teaching, the nurse can help prepare the family for the neonate's discharge.

Promoting parent-infant bonding. Bonding—the reciprocal relationship between parents and infant—may begin even before delivery. For instance, many parents imagine how their child will look and act or may think of the child as male or female. This helps the parents adjust after the neonate's arrival.

How easily a couple makes the transition to parenthood depends on many variables, including their ages, length of time they have been together, previous experience with children, available social support, teaching needs, coping patterns, perception of the neonate, and knowledge of neonatal behavior. Various relationships—between the parents, among the parents and any existing children, and among siblings—also play a role in the assumption of the parenting role.

The parents' perceptions of their parenting abilities also affect bonding. Many new parents have doubts about their ability to care for a dependent person, leading to a nursing diagnosis of *potential altered parenting related to transition to the role of parent.* Call attention to the neonate's positive responses to the parents' initial caregiving attempts. Such responses include recognizing each parent's voice; smiling when a parent smiles; quieting in response to a parent's consoling efforts; and taking feedings well from parents.

Bonding between parents and neonate increases after delivery and continues to grow in the coming days through skin contact. The parents usually examine their child for physical features that link their child with the rest of the family. Putting the neonate to the breast and breast-feeding successfully reinforce the mother's confidence in her ability to nourish her child.

If the parents were unable to see or touch their child in the delivery room, reassure them that bonding will occur and that the neonate will be ready to interact with them when the sleep phase (which follows the first period of reactivity) ends and the second period of reactivity begins.

Ask the parents to describe the child they imagined during the pregnancy—for example, a son or daughter, or a light-haired or dark-haired child. If their child does not conform to this image, they may need to mourn the loss of the imagined child before they can bond with the real one.

Providing parent teaching. Ongoing parent teaching is an essential part of discharge planning. Such teaching includes bathing, providing cord and diaper rash care, changing diapers, observing stool and voiding patterns, ensuring environmental safety, and integrating the neonate into the family. (For details, see Parent Teaching: *Caring for your infant.* For information on discharge planning, see Chapter 22, Discharge Planning and Care at Home.)

The nurse also should serve as a caregiver role model for the parents and reinforce their caregiving behaviors. Steele (1987) found that active parental involvement in neonatal care before discharge led to a strong parent-infant bond. Encourage the parents to ask questions about their child or the required care. Also urge them to interact with their child to enhance bonding. For parents with a nursing diagnosis of *anxiety related to lack of confidence in parenting ability,* explain how to detect early signs of potential problems, such as cold stress, infection, and dehydration, to help prevent life-threatening complications. The parents may be eager for their child to establish regular sleep-awake and eating patterns. However, inform them that a neonate typically sleeps 10 to 20 hours a day at first. Also emphasize that sleep patterns vary and that a deviation from the typical pattern does not necessarily indicate an abnormality.

Point out that the mother will have an increased need for support after discharge and would benefit by having relatives or friends available to help her. This is especially important for the single mother who may have to serve as the sole caregiver.

Performing routine therapeutic interventions

Routine nursing care of the normal neonate includes umbilical cord care, vitamin K administration, circumcision care, and collection of urine specimens.

Providing umbilical cord care. Immediately after birth, the umbilical cord is moist, making it an excellent breeding ground for bacteria. To avoid a nursing diagnosis of *high risk for infection related to umbilical cord healing,* aim to promote drying of the cord and prevent infection. Depending on health care facility policy, one of several methods may be used to clean the cord. The American Academy of Pediatrics does not recommend a particular method.

The first method entails cleaning the cord by wiping the surface gently with an alcohol swab or a cotton ball saturated with isopropyl alcohol. Pay particular attention to the base of the cord because this area is most likely to become infected. To ensure the base is coated with alcohol, lift the cord away from the abdomen when wiping.

The second method entails use of an antibiotic ointment (such as bacitracin) instead of alcohol to clean the cord. The antibiotic may prevent bacterial growth. However, not all physicians believe such treatment is necessary.

With either method, note any drainage, such as blood, urine, or pus, appearing at the cord. Document and report such drainage so that cultures can be taken and antibiotic therapy initiated, if necessary. Urine leakage may indicate a patent urachus (a fetal structure between the bladder and umbilicus), which requires surgical intervention.

Typically, the umbilical cord dries and falls off within 2 weeks after birth. Until this happens, fold down the disposable diaper below the cord, turning the plastic layer

PARENT TEACHING

CARING FOR YOUR INFANT

Basic infant care techniques include bathing, diaper changing, umbilical cord care, and environmental safety measures. These help ensure your infant's well-being, and they give you an opportunity to learn about your infant and to bond through close contact. The guidelines and techniques described below will help you provide the best possible care.

Bathing your infant

- Use only nonmedicated, unscented soap. A harsh soap may alter the skin's pH and impair the skin's ability to provide a barrier against infection. Also, be sure to use a mild shampoo, such as a baby shampoo or an unscented product, to reduce the risk of chemical irritation of your infant's eyes from the soap.
- Before bathing your infant, test bath water temperature; it should be warm to the touch.
- Use a firm grasp to hold your infant. Never let go, because the infant might slide down in the tub or fall out.
- Do not immerse your infant in a tub until the umbilical cord

and circumcision site (if present) have healed because these are potential infection sites. Wash the umbilical cord and circumcision site with water and pat dry gently. Avoid excessive rubbing.
- The use of powder after a bath is unnecessary and possibly unsafe. Powder particles that disperse into the air may enter the infant's lungs. If these particles are inhaled, they could cause irritation and infection.
- Baby oil is not recommended. The extra lubrication is unnecessary and may block pores. Also, it makes the infant harder to hold.

Providing umbilical cord care

- The umbilical cord dries gradually during the first week, then falls off. To clean the cord, gently rub its surface with alcohol swabs or cotton balls saturated with rubbing alcohol. As an alternate method, use an antibiotic ointment, if prescribed. Lift the cord away from the abdomen, then coat the stump or base with alcohol. (This is the area most likely to become infected.)

- Call the physician if you see pus or drainage at the base of the cord or if the cord remains moist. Pus or drainage may indicate infection. The physician may recommend a 1% silver nitrate solution to dry a moist cord.
- To keep the cord as dry and bacteria-free as possible, fold the diaper down below the cord and avoid giving your infant tub baths. Typically, the umbilical cord dries and falls off within the first 2 weeks after birth.

Changing diapers

- Clean and dry the perineal area, observing for diaper rash (for a girl, always clean the perineal area from front to back; for a boy, always be sure to clean and dry under and around the scrotum). Then place a diaper on the infant. For a snug fit, wrap the diaper from back to front, then check for gaps at the waist and abdominal areas and around the thighs. (If the diaper is not secure, stool or urine will leak, soiling the infant and bed and possibly causing chilling.) However, make sure the diaper is loose enough to allow the legs to move freely.
- For a boy wearing cloth diapers, fold the diaper so that a double thickness covers the penis. If the infant has been circumcised, allow enough room in front so that the cloth does not irritate the circumcision site.

- When diapering a girl, keep in mind that urine will fall to the front of the diaper when the infant lies on her stomach and to the back when she is on her back.
- If your infant develops a diaper rash after wearing disposable diapers, consider switching to cloth diapers, which allow air to reach the skin surface and promote healing. However, do not place a disposable diaper over a cloth diaper because this will seal in moisture and may promote bacterial growth.
- If your infant is wearing cloth diapers, use a mild detergent when laundering and rinse these items thoroughly to ensure soap removal.

Caring for your infant's circumcision site

- The circumcision site may appear yellow in light-skinned infants and lighter than the surrounding skin in dark-skinned infants. This signifies healing and is not a cause for concern. Observe the circumcision site regularly for pus or bloody discharge, which may indicate delayed healing or infection. If these signs appear, call the physician.
- The rim of the device used for circumcision may remain in

place after discharge. Do not be alarmed if you find the rim in your infant's bed; typically, it falls off 3 or 4 days after circumcision. If the rim does not come loose 1 week after the circumcision, call the physician. A retained rim may lead to infection.
- For the first 1 to 2 hours after circumcision, keep the neonate in a side-lying position with the diaper off.

(continued)

This teaching aid may be reproduced by office copier for distribution to clients. ©1993, Springhouse Corporation.

CARING FOR YOUR INFANT *(continued)*

Monitoring stool patterns

- Report any changes in your infant's stool pattern or appearance—especially if they are accompanied by fever or behavioral changes, such as irritability or fussiness.
- If your infant cries excessively with a bowel movement or produces small, hard fecal pellets, constipation may be the cause. This problem usually can be corrected by giving additional water between feedings or by introducing fruit juice (if the physician approves).
- In some cases, constipation results from iron supplements or from iron-containing infant formula. If this happens, the physician may recommend that you switch to another formula.

- Diarrhea may result from a particular infant formula, introduction of new foods, or—in the breast-fed infant—changes in the mother's diet. If your infant normally passes stool only once a day but begins to pass loose, watery stools more than 5 times in a 24-hour period, notify the physician. Diarrhea may lead to excess fluid loss.
- In a breast-fed infant, loose, watery stools or a water ring appearing in the diaper around more solid fecal matter may indicate infection. If this sign appears, call the physician. Loose, seedy, dark-green stools with a foul odor suggest an intestinal infection.

Monitoring voiding patterns

- The infant's urine should appear amber and clear. Although usually odorless, it occasionally may take on an ammonia-like odor, which is normal.

- Six diaper changes a day indicate adequate urine output. (The diapers should be at least moderately saturated.)

Ensuring environmental safety

- Maintain adequate lighting, temperature, and humidity in the infant's room. Keep room temperature at 80° F for the first week, then 75° F. Keep the humidity level at 35% to 70% to maintain moist mucous (nasal) membranes (which serve as an important infection barrier).
- If your infant has nasal secretions that must be removed, remove them with a bulb syringe. Depress the bulb to remove air, then insert the syringe in the infant's nostrils and release the bulb to withdraw the secretions. This technique adequately removes most nasal secretions without injuring the inside of the nostrils.

- Never prop a formula bottle against the infant because this may lead to inhalation of formula or otitis media (middle ear infection). Bottle propping also eliminates an opportunity for the closeness and touch between you and your infant that is necessary for bonding.
- Never look away or leave the neonate unattended during bathing or weighing. Before leaving the neonate, make sure crib side rails are up and locked in place.

Providing visual and auditory stimulation

- Keep in mind that your infant can see bright objects and will follow a brightly colored ball or a human face. To provide visual stimulation, hang a mobile over the infant's bed. A mobile that turns is better than a stationary mobile because it offers greater variation.

- To provide auditory stimulation or quiet the infant, place a radio (on low volume) or a music box in the infant's room.
- Because infants can become used to noise, you do not have to reduce the noise level in your home when the infant sleeps. Some infants even sleep better with quiet music in the room.

away from the skin. To keep the areas as dry and bacteria free as possible, avoid giving the neonate tub baths.

Administering vitamin K. The neonate has a vitamin K deficiency, which results partly from lack of intestinal bacterial flora necessary to synthesize vitamin K. Because only small amounts of bacterial flora cross the placenta, this deficiency continues until enteral feedings are established and milk or formula is digested. Without sufficient vitamin K, the liver cannot synthesize coagulation factors II, VII, IX, and X (Streeter, 1986), which predisposes the

neonate to hemorrhage and may lead to a nursing diagnosis of *high risk for trauma related to inability to process vitamin K.* The American Academy of Pediatrics (1988) recommends a prophylactic I.M. injection of 0.5 to 1 mg of vitamin K_1 (phytonadione) during the first hour after birth. (For an illustrated procedure of I.M. injection in the neonate, see Psychomotor Skills: *Giving an I.M. injection.*)

Caring for a circumcision site. Circumcision, the surgical removal of the prepuce (foreskin) that covers the glans penis, has become controversial. The traditional rationale for the

GIVING AN I.M. INJECTION

When caring for the normal neonate, the nurse may have to administer prophylactic vitamin K or other medications by I.M. injection. In most cases, a 25-gauge (25G), ⅝″ needle should be used to allow medication to reach the muscle without causing excessive pain or trauma.

Before administering any medication, confirm the route, dose, time, and medication, and cross-check the neonate's identification with the medication order and identification bracelet. Also check the neonate's history for reactions to previous medications; although rare, medication or allergic reactions do occur in neonates. Check the medication record for the previously used injection site. To minimize bruising and increase medication absorption, rotate the injection site from one leg to the other.

To administer the injection, follow these steps.

1 Put on clean gloves to guard against contamination from potentially infected blood. Then examine and palpate the neonate's leg above the knee and below the groin fold to determine how much muscle tissue is present. To find a safe injection site away from the bone and nerves, palpate along the femur. Place two fingers below the groin fold and two fingers above the knee. The thigh surface between these areas contains much muscle tissue and no major blood vessels or nerves, making it a good choice for injection.

The injection may be given along the top of the thigh or in the vastus lateralis, along the side of the thigh above the femur (the shaded area in the illustration). Do not give the injection in the buttocks; because the muscle mass here is not well developed, the needle or medication can enter a major vessel or nerve more easily.

2 To keep the neonate still and reduce tissue trauma, gently restrain the leg. If possible, ask an assistant to help with this; as one person holds the leg, the other can give the injection.

If a pinchable amount of muscle or a large, solid muscle mass is palpated (as in a term neonate), stretch the skin and hold it taut. This reduces the risk of medication entering the subcutaneous tissue. If the muscle is small and soft to a gentle pinch with little palpable mass, gently pinch about 1 cm of skin during needle insertion to allow the injection to reach the muscle mass.

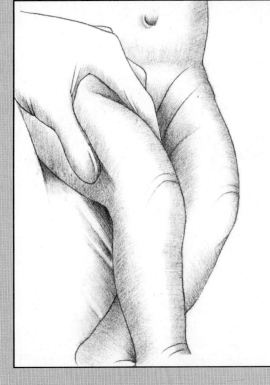

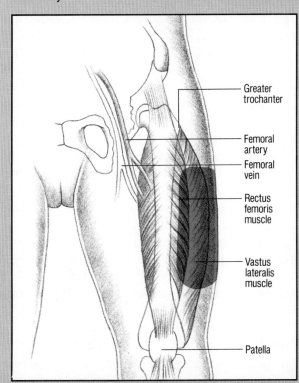

Greater trochanter

Femoral artery

Femoral vein

Rectus femoris muscle

Vastus lateralis muscle

Patella

(continued)

GIVING AN I.M. INJECTION *(continued)*

3 Without releasing the leg, aim the needle at a 90-degree angle toward the thigh. Then, using a quick, darting wrist motion, insert the needle almost down to the hub.

Next, release the skin that has been pinched or stretched. Gently aspirate the plunger to check for a flash of blood. Blood indicates that the needle has pricked a blood vessel; if the medication enters the vessel, an adverse reaction may result. If blood appears, withdraw the needle immediately. Then discard the needle and start the procedure over, using new medication and a new syringe and needle.

If no blood appears, inject the medication steadily by applying gentle pressure on the plunger. When the barrel is empty, withdraw the needle quickly by pulling it straight out (this makes the injection less painful). Do not recap the needle—this may lead to an accidental needle stick. Instead, keep it out of the neonate's reach until it can be discarded.

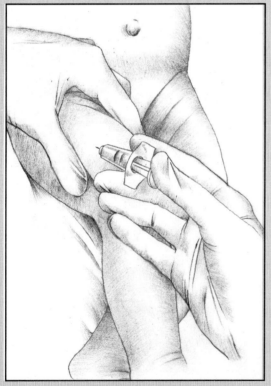

4 Massage the site with alcohol and soothe the neonate. Besides having a quieting effect, massage increases circulation and enhances medication absorption. In most cases, the site does not need to be covered by an adhesive bandage because any bleeding that occurs is minimal and stops rapidly. Also, removing the bandage might tear the skin, causing more pain than a small injection site.

procedure was that it promotes hygiene and helps prevent penile and cervical cancers, urinary tract infections, and sexually transmitted diseases. However, some medical authorities believe that no known medical reason exists for performing circumcision during the neonatal period. The American Academy of Pediatrics does not state that there is a medical indication for circumcision.

The main advantage of circumcision is hygienic. The circumcised penis is easier to keep clean and free of smegma, a sebaceous secretion that accumulates under the foreskin. Because the neonate's tight skin makes foreskin retraction difficult, bacterial growth is less common with a circumcised penis. Wiswell, Enzenauer, Holton, Cornish, and Hankins (1987) found an increase in urinary tract infections in male neonates as the circumcision rate declined.

The major disadvantage of circumcision is the pain and discomfort it causes. After circumcision, the neonate cries and has a disturbed sleep-awake pattern. To reduce pain, the neonate may receive a topical anesthetic (Stang, Gunnar, Snellman, Condon, and Kestenbaum, 1988).

Various factors may influence the parents' decision whether to circumcise their child, including religious beliefs, the perception that circumcision is a sign of manhood, and the fear that an uncircumcised male will be stigmatized.

For the first 1 to 2 hours after a circumcision, keep the neonate in a side-lying position and leave the diaper off to reduce irritation and observe the incision for bleeding. If bleeding occurs, grasp the penis gently but firmly with a sterile gauze pad, apply pressure until the bleeding stops, and notify the physician.

Apply petrolatum gauze over the penis to prevent bleeding and encrustation and to serve as a protective layer against abrasion from the diaper. To reduce the risk of contamination from fecal matter or urine—and thereby avoid a nursing diagnosis of *high risk for infection related to the circumcision site*—change the petrolatum gauze at each diaper change. The gauze is necessary for only 2 to 3 days after the procedure. The neonate should not be under a radiant warmer once the petrolatum gauze is in place because burning may occur.

Collecting urine specimens. When caring for the normal neonate, urine specimens sometimes must be collected for urine cultures, for routine urinalysis, or to determine urine specific gravity, pH (by dipstick testing), protein, ketones, glucose, bilirubin, or blood.

To obtain urine for a specific gravity measurement or dipstick test, withdraw the specimen from a collection bag (via the covered port at the bottom of the bag) or from a

PSYCHOMOTOR SKILLS

OBTAINING A URINE SPECIMEN FROM A URINE COLLECTION BAG

The nurse may collect a urine specimen from a neonate for routine urinalysis, cultures, specific gravity measurement, or other studies. Follow these steps when using a urine collection bag to obtain the specimen.

1 Remove the diaper and place the neonate in the supine position. With a male neonate, clean the urinary meatus, if soiled, with water and a towelette. Then clean the meatus with povidone-iodine swabs, using one swab for each stroke.

With a female neonate, clean the labia from front to back to avoid contamination from the anal area. Next, clean the urinary meatus with water and a towelette, then with povidone-iodine swabs, again using a front-to-back motion.

2 In an uncircumcised male, retract the foreskin until resistance is met, then clean the glans with povidone-iodine swabs. Release the foreskin, returning it to its natural position. In the circumcised male, clean the glans penis in the same manner.

3 To place the urine collection bag over the urinary meatus, remove the tabs from either side of the bag and uncover the adhesive sides. With a female neonate, apply the bag one side at a time to the labia majora and extend the tab to the femoral (groin) fold.

With a male neonate, place the bag over the urinary meatus in the same manner, enclosing the penis and scrotum in the bag if possible.

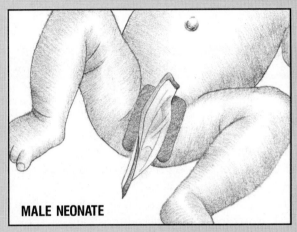

MALE NEONATE

With any neonate, make sure the bag does not cover the anus, because this may contaminate the specimen. After the bag has been positioned, press the tabs in place to ensure a secure fit. If the adhesive does not hold, apply a small amount of benzoin tincture to the skin under the tab to help keep the bag in place. However, use benzoin tincture only if absolutely necessary; the strong adhesion it provides may deter removal of the bag and can cause irritation.

4 Place a clean diaper over the bag and secure it. The diaper holds the bag in place and collects any stool or overflow from the bag.

5 When 1 to 2 ml of urine has been obtained, gently remove the bag and observe for skin irritation. Aspirate the specimen with a syringe, then place the specimen in a sterile plastic tube or culture bottle and send it to the laboratory immediately.

6 Document that a specimen was obtained and sent to the laboratory.

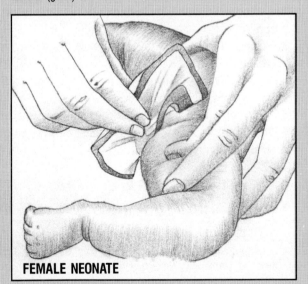

FEMALE NEONATE

disposable diaper. Both urine collection methods yield accurate results. (For an illustrated procedure of urine specimen collection from a collection bag, see Psychomotor Skills: *Obtaining a urine specimen from a urine collection bag.*)

EVALUATION

During this step of the nursing process, the nurse evaluates the effectiveness of the care plan by ongoing evaluation of subjective and objective criteria. Evaluation findings should be stated in terms of actions performed

or outcomes achieved for each goal. The following examples illustrate appropriate evaluation statements.
• The neonate did not appear cyanotic or dusky.
• The neonate maintained a stable axillary temperature of 97.7° F (36.5° C).
• The neonate voided clear amber urine six times in 24 hours.
• The neonate passed a meconium stool 24 hours after birth.
• The parents exhibited appropriate bonding behavior with their infant.

DOCUMENTATION

All steps of the nursing process should be documented as thoroughly and objectively as possible. Thorough documentation not only allows the nurse to evaluate the effectiveness of the care plan, but it also makes the data available to other members of the health care team, helping to ensure consistency of care.

Documentation for the normal neonate should include:
• vital signs, including temperature, heart rate and rhythm, and respiratory rate and rhythm
• strength and symmetry of peripheral pulses
• capillary refill time
• general appearance
• size and shape of fontanels
• umbilical cord description
• circumcision site description (as appropriate)
• stool and urine passage, including times, amounts, and characteristics
• any abnormal physical or behavioral findings
• parent teaching provided.

CHAPTER SUMMARY

Chapter 19 described nursing care of the normal neonate. Here are the chapter highlights.

The nurse conducts ongoing assessment of the neonate to ensure optimal neonatal adaptation and to detect changes in the neonate's status.

Nursing goals for the normal neonate include ensuring oxygenation, thermoregulation, hydration, and nutrition; promoting adequate urinary and bowel elimination patterns; providing hygienic care; preventing and detecting complications; ensuring environmental safety; providing care for the family; and performing routine therapeutic interventions.

To promote bonding, the nurse helps the parents identify their child's unique personality and recognize the neonate's responses to the parents. For example, the nurse may point out when the neonate smiles in response to a parent's smile or quiets in response to a parent's attempt at consoling.

The nurse can ensure sound discharge planning and the neonate's smooth transition to home by assessing the parents' readiness to provide proper cord care, bathing, diaper changes, and environmental safety. Other parent-teaching points include observing for diaper rash and monitoring stool and urine patterns. To help the parents develop confidence in their caregiving abilities, the nurse should have them practice these skills in a supervised setting before the neonate's discharge.

The nurse must consider cultural and social factors that might influence the parents' attitude toward circumcision and other aspects of neonatal care.

STUDY QUESTIONS

1. What is a neutral thermal environment?
2. The nurse is planning to suction a neonate with a suction catheter. What should the nurse assess for during this procedure?
3. What measures should the nurse take to prevent heat loss during a neonate's bath?
4. What information should the nurse collect when assessing a neonate's hydration status?
5. How soon after birth should a neonate begin voiding?
6. Which nursing interventions promote a positive parent-neonate interaction?

BIBLIOGRAPHY

American Academy of Pediatrics (1988). *Guidelines for perinatal care* (2nd ed.). Washington, DC: American Academy of Pediatrics and American College of Obstetricians and Gynecologists.

Carlo, W.A., and Chatburn, R.L. (1988). *Neonatal respiratory care* (2nd ed.). Chicago: Year Book.

Kim, M., and Mandell, J. (1988). Renal function in the fetus and neonate. In L.R. King (Ed.), *Urologic surgery in neonates and young infants* (pp. 59-76). Philadelphia: Saunders.

Harris, C.C. (1986). Cultural values and the decision to circumcise. *Image: Journal of Nursing Scholarship*, 18(3), 98-104.

Stang, H., Gunnar, M.R., Snellman, L., Condon, L.M., and Kestenbaum, R. (1988). Local anesthesia for neonatal circumcision. *JAMA*, 259(10), 1507-1511.

Steele, K.H. (1987). Caring for parents of critically ill neonates during hospitalization: Strategies for health care professionals. *MCN,* 16(1), 13-27.

Streeter, N.S. (1986). *High-risk neonatal care.* Rockville, MD: Aspen.

Wiswell, T.E., Enzenauer, R.W., Holton, M.E., Cornish, J.D., and Hankins, C.T. (1987). Declining frequency of circumcision: Implications for changes in the absolute incidence and male to female sex ratio of urinary tract infections in early infancy. *Pediatrics,* 79(3), 338-342.

CHAPTER 20

INFANT NUTRITION

OBJECTIVES

After reading and studying this chapter, the student should be able to:

1. Determine the learning needs of the childbearing family regarding infant nutrition.

2. Teach the client how breast milk and infant formula differ in composition and nutritional value.

3. Discuss the impact of nursing interventions on successful feeding outcome.

4. Teach the client positioning techniques that help prevent infant feeding problems.

5. Describe the nurse's role in identifying and reducing barriers to successful breast-feeding.

INTRODUCTION

The rapid physical and developmental growth of the first year necessitates optimal nutrition. Besides playing a crucial part in infant health, nutrition also provides an opportunity for positive feeding experiences and important interactions between infant and caregiver. Parents may view positive feeding experiences and a satisfied infant as a measure of their parenting ability; for the infant, repeated pleasurable feeding experiences help develop trust in the caregiver.

Teaching about infant nutrition is a major role of the nurse who works with young families. By understanding the nutritional needs of the first year, the nurse can provide the client with accurate and practical rationales for feeding recommendations.

This chapter considers the nurse's role in promoting optimal infant nutrition. It begins by describing the infant's nutritional needs. Then it focuses on breast-feeding, highlighting such topics as the physiology of lactation and breast milk composition. Next, the chapter discusses infant formula, including preparation and sucking dynamics. The last section demonstrates how to follow the nursing process steps—assessment, nursing diagnosis, planning, implementation, and evaluation—to individualize nursing care.

INFANT NUTRITIONAL NEEDS

The neonate's immature organ systems and the unparalleled growth of the first year impose special requirements for nutrients and fluids. These factors also limit the types and amounts of foods a neonate can ingest and digest. Recommendations for the introduction of solid foods are based on these limitations.

Nutrient and fluid requirements

As with all diets, the neonate's must contain sufficient amounts of carbohydrates, proteins, fats, vitamins, minerals, and fluids.

Energy. Three basic nutrients—carbohydrates, proteins, and fats—supply the body's caloric needs. Carbohydrates should serve as the body's main source of calories. Proteins promote cellular growth and maintenance, aid metabolism, and contribute to many protective substances. Fats provide a concentrated energy storage form, transport essential nutrients (such as fatty acids needed for neurologic growth and development), and insulate vital organs. Carbohydrates, which contain 4 calories per gram, should provide 35% to 55% of the neonate's total calories; fats, which contain 9 calories per gram, 30% to 55%; and proteins, which contain 4 calories per gram, the remaining calories.

Vitamins and minerals. Vitamins regulate metabolic processes and promote growth and maintenance of body tissues. Fat-soluble vitamins (A, D, E, and K) in excess of needs can be stored in the body to some extent and normally are not excreted; therefore, reserves may accumulate. Water-soluble vitamins (C, B_1, B_2, B_6, B_{12}, niacin, folic acid, pantothenic acid, and biotin) are stored only in small amounts. Consequently, if these vitamins are not ingested regularly, deficiencies may develop relatively quickly.

All major minerals and most trace minerals are essential for a wide range of body functions, including regulation of enzyme metabolism, acid-base balance, and nerve and muscle integrity. Calcium and iron are particularly important for growth, calcium for the rapid bone mineralization of the first year and iron for hemoglobin synthesis.

Fluids. The neonate's difficulty concentrating urine plus a high extracellular water content result in a much greater need for fluids (150 ml/kg/day) compared to the adult (20 to 30 ml/kg/day). By age 1, the daily fluid requirement is roughly 700 ml.

Special considerations

The neonate has limited gastric capacity. Also, fat absorption does not reach adult levels until ages 6 to 9 months. For the first 3 months, limited synthesis of the starch-splitting salivary enzyme ptyalin and absence of pancreatic amylase restrict digestion of complex starches found in solid foods. Because of the neonate's low glomerular filtration rate (GFR) and difficulty concentrating urine, high renal solute loads may cause fluid imbalance. (Renal solute load is a collective term for solutes that must be excreted by the kidneys.) The major solutes are sodium, potassium, and urea (an end product of protein metabolism). Some commercial infant formulas have a higher renal solute load than breast milk. Coupled with the neonate's low GFR, the solutes can cause too much fluid to be excreted, increasing the neonate's fluid needs even more.

Although the basic components of the neurologic system are present at birth, myelinization (development of the myelin sheath that protects nerve fibers) is incomplete. Only breast milk, infant formula, and whole milk contain enough linoleic acid to facilitate myelinization; for this reason, milk that contains less than 2% milk fat is not recommended before age 1.

Sleeping through the night, a significant developmental milestone, usually occurs earlier in the formula-fed infant than in the breast-fed infant. Parents may feel compelled to introduce solid foods early, believing this will lengthen the infant's sleep and help this milestone occur sooner (Wright, 1987). However, before age 3 months, the infant is ill-equipped to ingest solids. The extrusion reflex, in which the tongue pushes out food placed on it, does not diminish until approximately age 4 months. Also, an infant under age 3 months lacks the tongue motion needed to pass solids from the front to the back of the mouth. These limitations indicate unreadiness for solid foods.

Nutritional assessment

Weight, length, and head circumference are the major nutritional assessment indices in the infant. In North America, growth charts with standardized measurements for these indices are used to compare an infant to others of the same age. Repeat measurements at various ages show whether the infant is growing at the expected rate. However, current charts are based on formula-fed infants and may be unreliable for exclusively breast-fed infants, who grow rapidly during the first 3 months and more slowly from ages 3 to 6 months (Wood, Isaacs, Jensen, and Hilton, 1988).

The neonate typically loses an average of 10% of the birth weight in the first few days. This may alarm parents, who commonly view weight as a reflection of their infant's health status. However, the formula-fed neonate usually returns to birth weight by day 10 and the breast-fed neonate by 3 weeks (Lauwers and Woessner, 1989). Birth weight typically doubles by ages 5 to 6 months and triples by age 1 year. Body length increases by about 50% by age 1; head circumference expands along with the rapidly growing brain.

INFANT FEEDING METHODS

Choice of an infant feeding method involves more than a simple comparison of the biophysical properties of breast milk and formula. Cultural, psychosocial, and other factors also come into play. Although various health groups have endorsed breast-feeding, many women still choose to use infant formula or to breast-feed only briefly. Consequently, the nurse must be familiar with the basic techniques of both breast-feeding and formula-feeding. Also, the nurse must recognize any personal biases toward a particular feeding method and make sure they do not influence the interaction with the family.

Because many clients make infant feeding decisions during pregnancy, the nurse should be prepared to offer guidance at that time to ensure an informed decision.

Working with the client after delivery, the nurse helps her gain skills and confidence in the method she has chosen.

BREAST-FEEDING

Breast-feeding is an evolving, interdependent, and reciprocal relationship between mother and infant. Although the reflexes involved are natural, many of the techniques of breast-feeding must be learned by both mother and infant. The nurse who strives to work successfully with the breast-feeding client must have a comprehensive understanding of the physiology of lactation and a genuine commitment to facilitating practices that promote breast-feeding.

Breast-feeding has preventive health potential in both developing and industrialized countries. It has been endorsed officially by the World Health Organization (WHO), the International Pediatrics Association, the American Academy of Pediatrics, and the Canadian Pediatric Society. Nearly all researchers agree that breast-feeding has health benefits, although they do not concur on the extent of such benefits (Cunningham, 1988; Jason, Nieburg, and Marks, 1984; Kovar, Serdula, Marks, and Fraser, 1984; Kramer, 1988; Leventhal, Shapiro, Aten, Berg, and Egerter, 1986). Several studies show that breast milk has distinct advantages over formulas; in contrast, no studies have reached the opposite conclusion (Baer, 1981). In North America, an increasing percentage of women are breast-feeding their neonates. Approximately 60% of American women breast-fed in 1985, compared to 25% in 1971 (Fomon, 1987). The trend is similar in Canada, where 79% of women breast-fed in 1984, compared to roughly 25% in the 1970s (Myres, 1988). Internationally, a marketing code for breast milk substitutes established by WHO in 1979 helped promote breast-feeding in developing countries.

The U.S. Surgeon General has established as a goal for 1990 that 75% of American women breast-feed at the time of discharge after delivery and that 35% continue to breast-feed by the infant's sixth month (U.S. Department of Health and Human Services, 1984). Canada developed a national program to promote breast-feeding in 1978 (Myres, Watson, and Harrison, 1981).

Physiology of lactation

Lactation operates on a supply-meets-demand basis: The more milk the infant removes, the more milk the breast produces. Hormones control milk production and ejection to make milk available to the infant.

Milk production. Milk is produced in the breast alveoli—tiny sacs made up of epithelial cells. The female breast has a rich blood supply from which the alveoli extract nutrients to produce milk. The alveoli are situated in lobules—clusters leading to ductules that merge into lactiferous ducts. These larger ducts widen further into ampullae, or lactiferous sinuses, located behind the nipple and areola.

Lactogenesis—initiation of milk production—begins during the third trimester of pregnancy under the influence of human placental lactogen, a hormone secreted by the placenta. The lactating breast functions in synchrony with maternal hormones; along with effective infant attachment on the breast, these hormones mediate milk flow through the alveoli and ductules.

After delivery of the placenta and the resultant decrease in circulating estrogen and progesterone, the anterior pituitary gland releases prolactin, one of many hormones that stimulate mammary gland growth and development. In response, alveolar secretory cells begin extracting nutrients from the blood and converting them to milk. Initial prolactin production also hinges on tactile stimulation of the nipple-areola junction by infant sucking or milk expression (Neville, 1983).

Prolactin is secreted intermittently throughout the day, with secretion rising markedly during sleep (Neville, 1983) and night feedings (Glasier, McNeilly, and Howie, 1984). Thus, frequent feeding over the entire 24-hour period enhances prolactin secretion and significantly increases milk production (Klaus, 1987). Prolactin secretion also creates a calm, relaxed feeling in the mother, which may enhance mother-infant bonding.

Milk ejection. The hormone oxytocin makes breast milk available to the infant through the let-down reflex. In this reflex, nipple stimulation or an emotional response to the infant causes the hypothalamus to trigger release of oxytocin by the posterior pituitary gland. Myoepithelial cells surrounding the alveoli then contract and eject milk into the ductules and sinuses, making milk available through nipple openings. A conditioned reflex, let-down occurs after 2 to 3 minutes of sucking during the first days of breast-feeding; several let-downs occur over the course of a feeding.

Some women have no symptoms of let-down. Others experience it as a tingling sensation, a momentary pain in the nipple, or a warm rush from the chest wall toward the nipple. In the early postpartal period, other let-down symptoms may include uterine cramps (afterpains), caused by the action of oxytocin on the involuting uterus, and a slight increase in lochia (the vaginal discharge emitted after delivery). Also, the breasts may leak. However, let-down may occur even in the absence of milk leakage. In some women, the sphincters controlling milk expulsion from the lactiferous sinuses to the nipple function so effectively that only active sucking on the breast leads to milk release.

Restricting sucking time, a practice based on the erroneous notion that prolonged sucking causes nipple soreness, can disrupt optimal function of the let-down reflex by preventing the infant from completely emptying the milk ducts. This, in turn, leads to milk buildup and signals the body to stop producing milk. The breasts become engorged and harden; the nipples may become flat, hindering proper infant attachment. The body responds to engorgement by halting milk production. In the early days of breast-feeding, restricted sucking time may establish a negative feedback system that can lead to insufficient milk production. Also, it may force the infant to feed more often to satisfy hunger.

Breast milk composition and digestion

The composition of breast milk undergoes various changes. Initial feedings provide colostrum, a thin, serous fluid. Unlike mature breast milk, which has a bluish cast, colostrum is yellow (Casey and Hambridge, 1983). However, its color may vary considerably from one woman to the next.

Colostrum contains high concentrations of protein, fat-soluble vitamins, minerals, and immunoglobulins, which function as antibodies. (For more on the immunologic properties of breast milk, see Chapter 17, Neonatal Adaptation.) Colostrum's laxative effect promotes early passage of meconium. Also, the low colostrum volumes produced do not tax the neonate's limited gastric capacity or cause fluid overload.

The breasts may contain colostrum for up to 96 hours after delivery. The maturation rate from colostrum to breast milk varies (Humenick, 1987). With increased breast-feeding frequency and duration in the first 48 hours, colostrum matures to milk more rapidly (Humenick, 1987). This discovery helped disprove the theory that breast-feeding frequency should be limited until mature milk comes in. (However, in some cultures, infants never receive colostrum, as described in Cultural Considerations: *Cultural aspects of infant feeding.*)

Breast milk composition also changes over the course of a feeding. The foremilk—thin, watery milk secreted when a feeding begins—is low in calories but contains abundant water-soluble vitamins. It accounts for about 60% of the total volume of a feeding. Next, whole milk is released. The hindmilk, available 10 to 15 minutes after the initial let-down, has the highest concentration of cal-

CULTURAL CONSIDERATIONS

CULTURAL ASPECTS OF INFANT FEEDING

When caring for a client whose background is different from yours, keep the following cultural considerations in mind.

Infant feeding practices vary with geography and culture. In Finland, where no infant formula is manufactured, breast-feeding is the norm (Carr, 1989). Some developing countries (for example, Colombia, Brazil, Thailand, and New Guinea) have reversed the recent decline in breast-feeding through vigorous breast-feeding promotion.

Filipinos, Mexican Americans, Vietnamese, and some Nigerians do not give colostrum to neonates; mothers in these groups begin breast-feeding only after milk ejection begins. Some Korean women delay breast-feeding until 3 days after delivery; others begin breast-feeding immediately and breast-feed whenever the infant cries (Choi, 1986).

In Kenya, mothers feed premature neonates only by breast and begin breast-feeding them much earlier than in North America. Kenyans never use gavage tubes and feed neonates from small cups until they are ready to suck (Armstrong, 1987).

ories for satisfying hunger between feedings. The rate of milk transfer to the infant varies among mother-infant couples (Woolridge, 1989). Consequently, limiting feeding times or insisting that the woman use both breasts at each feeding may prevent the infant from obtaining the maximum benefit of variable breast milk content.

The whey proteins that predominate in breast milk lead to formation of soft, easily digested curds. The infant typically digests breast milk within 2 to 3 hours after a feeding and thus may become hungry more often than the formula-fed infant, who typically feeds every 4 hours. In the first few weeks after birth, the breast-fed neonate may feed eight to twelve times every 24 hours.

Infant sucking

The dynamics of sucking on a breast and sucking on an artificial nipple differ dramatically. No frictional movement occurs during breast-feeding (Woolridge, 1986); therefore, it should be painless, provided the infant is properly attached (Royal College of Midwives, 1988). Misinformation about the dynamics of sucking has led to such practices as limiting feeding times. Incorrect infant sucking technique, not prolonged feeding, causes nipple soreness. Some infants must be taught to suck correctly.

Using images generated by real-time ultrasound studies, investigators have observed the dynamics of breast sucking. Smith, Erenberg, and Nowak (1988) found that the human nipple is a highly elastic structure that elongates to nearly twice its resting length during active feeding. Little change occurs in the nipple's lateral dimension, confirming the theory that the cheeks serve as a passive seal. The researchers also observed that nipple compression between the infant's tongue and palate reduces the tongue's height by half and causes milk ejection. This sucking pattern was confirmed by Weber, Woolridge, and Baum (1986), who found that the breast-fed infant uses a rolling or peristaltic tongue action in contrast to the squeezing or pistonlike tongue action of the bottle-fed infant. The researchers also noted that the tongue's resting position between bursts of sucking differs in breast-fed and bottle-fed infants.

Intake requirements

A breast-fed infant typically needs to be fed every 2 to 3 hours. During the first 3 to 4 weeks, before the feeding pattern is established fully, parents may wonder if the neonate is receiving adequate nourishment. Signs of adequate intake include 10 to 12 wet diapers in 24 hours, steady weight gain, and contentedness after feeding.

Duration

Despite an increase in breast-feeding rates of women at the time of discharge after delivery, 65% of American women who breast-feed stop before 4 months (Fomon, 1987); 23% of Canadian women stop before 3 months (Tanaka, Yeung, and Anderson, 1987). By anticipating the reasons why a client may choose to stop breast-feeding, the nurse can identify strategies that may help reduce barriers to continued breast-feeding.

Lactation insufficiency (lack of milk) is the most common reason for stopping breast-feeding in the early weeks (Newman, 1986). The incidence of primary lactation insufficiency is unknown. However, lactation insufficiency most commonly stems from mismanagement of lactation (Neifert and Seacat, 1987); this in turn may result from such institutional practices as routine supplementation with bottled glucose and water, omission of night breast-feeding until mature milk comes in, and arbitrary feeding schedules. These practices may strain the adaptability of the mother-infant couple and interrupt the interactions necessary for successful breast-feeding (Winikoff, Laukaran, Myers, and Stone, 1986). Also, indiscriminate use of bottles to supplement breast-feeding in the neonate's first days may cause nipple confusion, making the neonate refuse the breast the next time it is offered. When such problems occur, ready availability of an alternative infant food source may cause the mother to switch to formula rather than try to correct the problems.

Like the client's decision to breast-feed initially, her decision to stop involves many factors, including her age, family or social attitudes toward breast-feeding, and her socioeconomic status or educational level. For example, an adolescent mother may stop breast-feeding when she realizes how much time and energy it requires; a new mother who is the first woman in her family to breast-feed may feel pressured to stop if problems arise. Maternal ambivalence toward breast-feeding also may play a role (Jones, West, and Newcombe, 1986). However, with proper antepartal teaching, a client may learn to adjust her expectations about breast-feeding and thus avoid becoming so discouraged that she stops when problems occur. For instance, she can learn to anticipate ambivalence and doubt about her ability to breast-feed and to expect such physical discomforts as leaking breasts and frequent feedings.

Hewat and Ellis (1986) compared women who breast-fed for prolonged periods with those who discontinued breast-feeding early. They concluded that those who continued:
• fed their neonates more frequently in the early days of breast-feedings
• showed less anxiety about initial neonatal weight loss and interpreted neonatal behavior in a positive light
• demonstrated a greater ability to relax
• showed more flexibility in their daily routines
• more readily incorporated siblings into the feeding experience
• received more support from their partner.

The nurse can help prevent a poor breast-feeding outcome by teaching the client about the physiology of lactation, providing anticipatory guidance about the normal course of breast-feeding, and making sure the client knows how to obtain information and support after discharge. Although the availability of follow-up support varies, some community health nurses make routine home visits after a neonate's birth. Also, the assistance of a lactation nurse has significantly prolonged breast-feeding during the first 4 weeks and among women of lower socioeconomic status (Jones and West, 1985). Professional and lay breast-feeding support may be available from a lactation consultant or a local LaLeche League group.

FORMULA-FEEDING

Because of the current emphasis on breast-feeding, the client who chooses formula-feeding may feel uncertain about her choice and react defensively if she feels it is being questioned. By recognizing the many factors that go into infant feeding decisions, the nurse can convey respect and offer support to the client who has made an in-

NUTRITIONAL OPTIONS FOR THE FORMULA-FED INFANT

Commercial formulas are recommended for non-breast-feeding infants. The table below compares three major types of commercial formulas.

OPTION	RECOMMENDATIONS FOR USE	FORM AND ENERGY CONTENT
Milk-based commercial formula (Enfalac, Similac, SMA, Milumil)	• Infants with no family history of food allergy who receive little or no breast milk	Liquid concentrate, powdered concentrate, ready-to-serve Energy content: 68 kcal/dl
Soy-based commercial formula (Isomil, Nursoy, ProSobee)	• Infants with galactosemia or primary lactase deficiency • Infants recovering from secondary lactose intolerance • Infants with a family history of food allergy but no clinical manifestations • Infants in strict vegetarian families that wish to avoid animal protein formulas	Liquid concentrate, powdered concentrate, ready-to-serve Energy content: 68 kcal/dl
Casein hydrolysate–based commercial formula (Nutramigen, Pregestimil, Alimentum)	• Infants with clinical manifestations of food allergy	Liquid or powdered concentrate Energy content: 68 kcal/dl

Adapted with the permission of the Minister of the Supply and Services Canada, 1992, from Health and Welfare Canada publication *Feeding babies: A counselling guide on practical solutions to common infant feeding questions,* 1986.

formed decision to formula-feed. Also, by working with the client in the antepartal period, the nurse can help ensure that she receives relevant information in a way that would allow her to revise her choice (Gabriel, Gabriel, and Lawrence, 1986).

Although choice of specific formula and preparation method are important aspects of formula-feeding, the feeding process goes beyond simply giving the infant a bottle. As with breast-feeding, formula-feeding involves a developing relationship between mother and infant. The nurse who remains aware of this added dimension can provide the family with appropriate anticipatory guidance during the early learning period of infant feeding.

Commercial formulas and equipment

Commercial infant formulas fall into three categories: milk-based, soy-based, and casein hydrolysate–based. (For a comparison of these formula types, see *Nutritional options for the formula-fed infant.*) The American Academy of Pediatrics recommends commercially prepared formulas over other formulas for infants up to age 1 year. Commercial formulas provide all necessary vitamins, so infants receiving them do not require vitamin supplements. However, use of noncommercial formulas necessitates vitamin supplementation.

Product convenience, personal preference, and economic status influence the client's choice of formula equipment. Commercially available equipment includes glass bottles, boilable plastic bottles, disposable plastic bags (which the preparer places in a hollow plastic holder), and artificial nipples. Because sucking action on the NUK nipple (which is flat and broad) most closely resembles sucking action on the human nipple, some authorities recommend this nipple for breast-fed infants who receive an occasional supplemental bottle.

Infant sucking

Sucking on a regular latex nipple is largely a squeezing action. The bottle-fed infant tends to swallow with every suck at the beginning of a feeding. If milk flow is restricted (for instance, from vacuum buildup that makes the nipple collapse), the suck-swallow ratio may rise to 2:1 or even higher, until sucking stops completely.

Intake requirements

The amount and frequency of formula-feedings vary with infant size, maturity, and activity level. Daily formula intake averages 180 ml/kg. Like parents of the breast-fed infant, parents of the formula-fed infant may believe all crying signals hunger. The nurse can help them interpret infant behavior more accurately by reviewing guidelines on feeding frequency.

Digestion

The casein proteins predominating in formula result in tougher, less digestible curds than the whey in breast milk. Consequently, infant formula takes more time and energy to digest than breast milk. (However, homogenization and heat treatment of commercially prepared formulas have improved curd digestibility somewhat.)

ASSESSMENT

The nurse should begin client assessment by collecting general data and then make specific assessments related to the feeding method.

The breast-feeding client

Ideally, assessment should begin in the early antepartal period as the nurse determines how much the client knows about infant nutrition and breast-feeding techniques. Also, the nurse should evaluate nipple grasp ability and protractility by determining whether the nipples are slightly everted, flat, or inverted. The slightly everted nipple, the most common type, becomes more graspable when stimulated. A flat nipple is hard to distinguish from the areola and changes shape only slightly when stimulated. Inverted nipples fall into three categories. A pseudoinverted nipple appears inverted but becomes erect with stimulation. A semi-inverted nipple initially appears graspable but retracts with stimulation. A truly inverted nipple is inverted both at rest and when stimulated.

For the client in the postpartal period, after breastfeeding has begun, the nurse should assess:
• consistency of the breasts (softness, mobility, engorgement, and warmth)
• condition of the nipples (tenderness, abrasions, and discoloration)
• sensations experienced during breast-feeding (such as tingling).

For the breast-feeding neonate, the nurse should assess the sucking reflex before the first feeding because improper sucking will prevent adequate feeding. Clues that the neonate is sucking properly include puffing out of the cheeks and absence of biting. Also assess for signs of lactose intolerance, including abdominal cramps and distention and severe diarrhea. The major carbohydrate in milk, lactose normally is broken down by the enzyme lactase. Lactose intolerance occurs from the absence of lactase in the border of the intestinal villi. Most common among non-Caucasian neonates, lactose intolerance may warrant the use of a soy-based formula, which provides corn syrup solids and sucrose as the primary carbohydrates. The nurse also should assess for proper client and infant positioning. The client may assume a sitting or reclining position, bringing the infant to her. A pillow can be placed under the arms to prevent shoulder elevation, which could cause muscle tension. The client should hold the infant facing her and level with the breast so that the infant's neck need not twist or flex.

The nurse should assess the client and infant during a feeding to determine if the infant is correctly attached on the breast, as indicated by a wide open mouth with lips curved backward.

Assessment of the client and infant after discharge can promote breast-feeding success. Many life-style adjustments must be made when a neonate joins the family. These adjustments may cause role strain and conflict. Postdischarge nursing assessment may reveal breastfeeding problems caused by such role strain and conflict.

The client using infant formula

For the client in the antepartal period, the nurse should assess for:
• knowledge of proper feeding techniques
• understanding of types of formula
• previous experience with infant formula.

Also, the nurse should find out what equipment and facilities the client will use to prepare formula and determine if the client will need financial aid to meet the infant's nutritional needs. (For information on sources of financial aid for mothers of young children, see *Nutritional aid for mothers and infants.*)

For the client in the postpartal period, the nurse should assess bottle and infant positioning during feeding and the client's ability to adjust feeding technique in response to infant cues. The nurse also should inspect the client's breasts for signs of engorgement, such as tenderness, swelling, warmth, hardness, shininess, and redness.

Infant factors to assess for include:
• excessive drooling, coughing, gagging, or respiratory distress during feeding (which may indicate tracheal or esophageal fistula, as discussed in Chapter 21, Care of High-Risk Neonates and Their Families)
• amount of formula the infant takes
• regurgitation after feeding
• mucus in regurgitated matter
• how readily the infant burps
• signs of lactose intolerance (discussed under "The breast-feeding client")

NUTRITIONAL AID FOR MOTHERS AND INFANTS

In the United States, a government program called the Women, Infants, and Children Nutrition Program (WIC) provides supplemental foods, access to health care, and nutrition education during critical stages of growth and development. Those eligible include pregnant and postpartal women, infants up to age 1 year, and children up to age 5 whom a health care professional has classified as being at nutritional risk. Although federally funded, WIC is administered by states; consequently, eligibility requirements may vary. Further information can be obtained from the Department of Agriculture or from state health departments.

In Canada, access to health care is universal. However, no universal social assistance program exists specifically for mothers and infants. Instead, each Canadian province has its own program. In special cases, government subsidies are available for infant feeding equipment and formulas. Otherwise, a woman receiving social assistance is expected to meet her and her child's nutritional needs with the monthly allowance she receives. Provincial community health nurses employed by the government can provide specific information about health care for Canadian mothers with infants.

• presence of circumoral cyanosis (bluish skin around the mouth) during feeding. This may reflect insufficient oxygen to meet the infant's increased metabolic needs.

NURSING DIAGNOSIS

After gathering all assessment data, the nurse must review it carefully to identify pertinent nursing diagnoses for the client or neonate. (For a partial list of applicable diagnoses, see Nursing Diagnoses: *Infant nutrition,* page 408.)

PLANNING AND IMPLEMENTATION

After assessing the client and formulating nursing diagnoses, the nurse develops and implements a plan of care. For example, if the client has a nursing diagnosis of *knowledge deficit related to breast-feeding,* the nurse should plan what and how to teach her about breast-feeding.

Although the plan will depend on the client's abilities, it may include written materials, discussion of proper feeding methods and infant positioning, and client demonstration of breast-feeding.

CARE FOR THE BREAST-FEEDING CLIENT

The nurse's role in working with the breast-feeding client includes teaching of proper feeding techniques and intervention to correct any related problems. The nurse also helps the client deal with physiologic or psychosocial problems related to breast-feeding.

Client teaching

Ideally, teaching about breast-feeding should begin in the antepartal period and continue postpartum until breast-feeding is well established.

Antepartum. In the antepartal period, teaching should focus on practical knowledge that will help the client establish and maintain lactation after delivery. Some general topics that could be incorporated into antepartal teaching include:
• physiologic, emotional, and social factors that influence lactation
• the role of the neonate and the client's partner in breast-feeding outcome
• common breast-feeding problems and possible solutions
• the possibility of continuing to breast-feed after the client returns to work
• the role of support groups or professional services and how to gain access to them.

Antepartal teaching also can help prepare the client to deal with incorrect advice about breast-feeding. Such advice, which may come from friends, relatives, or even health care professionals, typically is based on emotion rather than scientific principles that promote a positive breast-feeding outcome. When initiating breast-feeding, the client is especially vulnerable to such outside interference. To make her less vulnerable, the nurse can establish credibility as a knowledgeable professional during the pregnancy. Then, the nurse may use role-playing techniques, asking the client to predict who might offer advice and having her play the role of each of those persons. Practicing this technique in the antepartal period prepares the client to react rationally to incorrect advice once she begins breast-feeding.

Postpartum. The nurse should encourage the client to take advantage of the neonate's early responsiveness by breast-feeding as soon as possible. For the healthy full-term neonate, no contraindications exist to feeding immediately after delivery. In the first 30 minutes or so after birth, the neonate is highly responsive and eager to suck. Many neonates breast-feed shortly after delivery; all at least make licking or nuzzling motions, helping to stimulate the

INFANT NUTRITION

The following are potential nursing diagnoses for problems and etiologies that a nurse may encounter when caring for a client as she begins to nourish her neonate. Specific nursing interventions for many of these diagnoses are provided in the "Planning and implementation" section of this chapter.

- Altered family processes related to breast-feeding
- Altered family processes related to infant feeding
- Altered nutrition: high risk for more than body requirements, related to breast-feeding
- Altered parenting related to infant prematurity and the mother's wish to breast-feed
- Altered role performance related to the new task of breast-feeding
- Altered sexuality patterns related to requirements of the breast-feeding infant
- Anxiety related to change in infant feeding pattern secondary to a growth spurt
- Anxiety related to the ability to breast-feed multiple infants
- Anxiety related to the ability to properly feed the infant
- Body image disturbance related to physiologic changes secondary to breast-feeding
- High risk for infection related to improper expression and storage of breast milk
- High risk for injury related to improper nipple care
- Ineffective breast-feeding related to improper positioning of the infant at the breast
- Ineffective infant feeding pattern related to inadequate milk supply
- Interrupted breast-feeding related to maternal illness
- Knowledge deficit related to breast-feeding
- Knowledge deficit related to formula-feeding
- Pain related to breast engorgement
- Potential fluid volume deficit related to breast-feeding
- Sleep pattern disturbance related to the infant's nutritional needs

mother's prolactin production. Also, during this time the client's breasts may be soft and easily manipulated, facilitating proper attachment. Immediate breast-feeding also offers the chance for intimate contact that can enhance mother-infant bonding and have a positive psychological effect on the parents.

Valid reasons for delaying breast-feeding immediately after delivery include such obvious contraindications as life-threatening illness of the mother or neonate. In less obvious cases, the nurse must exercise good judgment. For example, immediate breast-feeding may be inappropriate if the neonate has anomalies that warrant evaluation, if the mother is heavily sedated or fatigued, or if the neonate has a 5-minute Apgar score of 6 or less.

General breast-feeding guidelines

Although lactation is a natural process, breast-feeding skills must be learned and practiced. The nurse can promote breast-feeding success through timely intervention to correct any problems. (See Client Teaching: *Breast-feeding your infant.*)

Helping the client initiate breast-feeding. In many cases, the nurse must help the client initiate feeding. However, the client who believes breast-feeding should be entirely natural may feel like a failure for needing help. Especially for a client with a nursing diagnosis of *knowledge deficit related to breast-feeding,* the nurse should point out that some infants must learn to breast-feed. Others may need to be wakened for every feeding.

Providing comfort measures and promoting hygiene. Before a feeding begins, the nurse should meet the client's comfort needs – for example, by having her void or by administering an analgesic, if prescribed. Also, the nurse should encourage her always to wash her hands just before breast-feeding.

Ensuring proper positioning. The nurse should emphasize the importance of correct positioning. The client may breast-feed in three different positions: cradle position, side-lying position, or football hold. Whichever position the client uses, her back and arms should be firmly supported; pillows may be placed under the arm on the breast-feeding side to keep the infant close to the breast. Help the client into the chosen position and instruct her to hold the infant so that the infant looks down on her breast, then tilt the breast so that the nipple points toward the roof of the infant's mouth. This position typically places the infant's lower lip and jaw well below the nipple.

In the client's eagerness to ensure that breast-feeding goes well, she may lean in toward the infant, believing this facilitates attachment. However, to avoid discomfort, the client should bring the infant toward her instead.

For a client with a nursing diagnosis of *ineffective breast-feeding related to improper positioning of the infant at the breast,* the nurse should check for common positioning mistakes, such as placing the infant so low that the neck must hyperextend to grasp the nipple or so high that the neck must flex to grasp it.

Ensuring correct infant attachment. To ensure that the infant is correctly attached on the breast and getting enough nipple

BREAST-FEEDING YOUR INFANT

Before you begin breast-feeding, review the guidelines below to gain confidence and help both you and your infant get the most from the experience.

STARTING TO BREAST-FEED

The first time you breast-feed your infant can be exciting, especially if the infant sucks and feeds properly at once. If your infant does not, however, breast-feeding still can succeed.

During the first days, you and your infant are getting to know each other. Here are some tips that may help.

- No hard and fast rules exist for the first feeding. Do not follow rigid guidelines for feeding times or frequency because these can impede milk production.
- Do not offer the infant a bottle when establishing breast-feeding. Sucking on a nipple differs from sucking on a bottle; nipple confusion may make the infant refuse the breast the next time you offer it.
- Keep the infant in the room with you and breast-feed every 2 to 3 hours or on demand—whichever comes first.
- Feed the infant through the night to help increase milk production.
- Let the infant decide when to stop breast-feeding rather than breaking suction yourself and pulling the infant off your breast. Also, let the infant finish feeding on one breast before offering the other. Keep in mind that reducing breast-feeding time will not prevent sore nipples and may cause milk drainage problems.
- Give yourself and your infant time to develop a mutually satisfying breast-feeding pattern.
- Keep in mind that a breast-fed infant usually needs to be fed more often than a formula-fed infant, so avoid comparing your infant's feeding pattern to that of a formula-fed infant.

BREAST-FEEDING POSITIONS

You may use the cradle position, side-lying position, or football hold to breast-feed your infant. By alternating positions, you rotate the infant's position on the nipple to avoid constant friction on the same area.

Cradle position
To use this position—the most common one—sit in a comfortable chair and rest the infant's head in the bend of your arm. You may want to place pillows under your elbow to minimize tension and fatigue. Tuck the infant's lower arm alongside your body so it stays out of the way. The infant's mouth should remain even with your nipple and the stomach should face and touch your stomach.

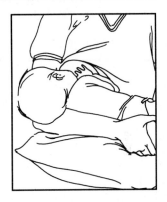

Side-lying position
You may find this position useful for night feedings or if you are recovering from a cesarean delivery. Lie on your side with your stomach facing the infant's stomach and the infant's head near your breast. Lift your breast; as the infant's mouth opens, pull the infant toward your nipple.

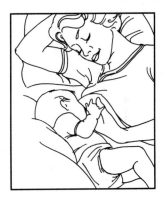

Football hold
This may be the most comfortable position if you have large breasts, if the infant is very small or premature, or if you have had a cesarean delivery and find other positions uncomfortable. Sit in a chair with a pillow under your arm on the nursing side. Place your hand under the infant's head and bring it close to your breast; place the fingers of your other hand above and below the nipple. As the infant's mouth opens wide, pull the head close to your breast.

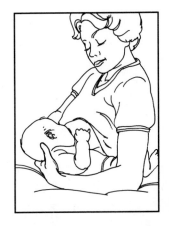

(continued)

BREAST-FEEDING YOUR INFANT *(continued)*

REMOVING THE INFANT FROM THE BREAST

When removing the infant from the breast to feed from the other breast or to end the feeding, you can use a special technique to minimize pulling or tension on the nipple. Place your little finger in the corner of the infant's mouth, as shown here, and release suction before pulling the infant away.

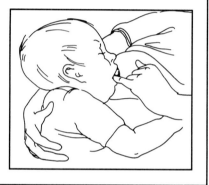

BURPING YOUR INFANT

You may burp your infant in any of the three positions described below. Be sure to place a cloth diaper or pad under the infant's mouth to protect your clothing from any expelled matter.

Upright position
Position the infant upright, with the head resting on your shoulder. Supporting the infant with one hand, pat or rub the infant's back with your other hand.

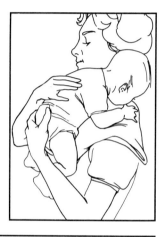

Across your lap
Place the infant face down across your lap. While holding the infant's head with one hand, rub or pat the infant's back with the other.

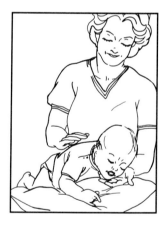

Upright on your lap
With the infant upright on your lap, hold the head from the front with one hand while patting or rubbing the back with the other hand. To help bring up air, gently rock the infant back and forth.

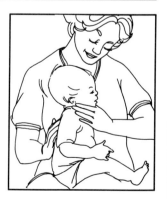

tissue to suck properly, instruct the client to cup the breast with her thumb well away from the nipple and fingers. After tickling the infant's lip with the nipple to stimulate rooting, the client should wait for the infant to open the mouth wide (with the tongue pointing downward), then center the nipple in the mouth and pull the infant toward her breast. Sometimes a slight delay before bringing the infant to the breast makes the infant open the mouth wider.

Assess the infant's jaw action to confirm proper attachment. The jaws should move rhythmically (possibly accompanied by slight ear movement). Gumming jaw motions and a clicking sound signal improper attachment. The let-down reflex also confirms proper attachment. If the client lacks the experience to recognize let-down internally from the drawing sensation in the ducts, teach her to place her finger lightly across the top of her breast; with proper attachment, she will feel the drawing sensation externally with her finger.

Establishing a breast-feeding pattern. Advise the client that the infant may need to feed for at least 15 minutes on each breast at each feeding. The client should let the infant complete a feeding on one breast before offering the other (Woolridge, 1989). As milk volume adjusts to the infant's needs, the client may change this pattern several times, offering only one breast at a feeding, then offering both breasts again.

The nurse also should tell the client to expect to breast-feed every 2 to 3 hours during the day and every 4 to 5 hours at night (or sooner, if the infant awakens). On average, the neonate should feed at least once every 3 to 4 hours. Unless feeding time is extremely long (which may indicate inadequate attachment and let-down), the client should let the infant determine the length of a feeding by continuing to breast-feed until the infant begins to release the nipple.

Encouraging night feedings. Because more prolactin is released during night feedings than day feedings, the client should breast-feed at night to take advantage of the nocturnal boost in milk production. This boost proves especially important in the early postpartal period when milk production begins. Early postpartal night feedings also give the mother added experience in handling her breasts and attaching the infant while the breasts are still relatively soft and easily manipulated. Also, increased breast-feeding frequency helps widen and stretch the lactiferous ducts, promoting breast drainage and emptying.

Helping the client cope with growth spurts. Occurring at ages 10 to 14 days, 6 weeks, 3 to 4 months, and 6 months, growth spurts seem much more noticeable in the breast-fed than the formula-fed infant. During a growth spurt, a previously satisfied infant will want to feed much more frequently. The infant's behavior, chewing on fists, crying, and settling down only for short periods, may make the client fear that her milk supply is inadequate and that the infant is malnourished. If a growth spurt coincides with the client's return to work, this may raise particular concern about milk supply.

To minimize these fears in the client with a nursing diagnosis of *anxiety related to change in infant feeding pattern secondary to a growth spurt,* point out that the breasts may take up to 48 hours to produce enough milk to meet the increased demands of a growth spurt. The required time may vary somewhat, however, depending on how efficiently the infant feeds and how the client's body responds. (For more information on helping the client deal with fears about her milk supply, see Client Teaching: *Coping with fears about your milk supply,* page 412.)

Providing nipple and breast care. Usually, the breasts require no care other than daily cleaning with clear water. However, the nipples may become sore, especially during the first days of breast-feeding, necessitating special care.

Nipple soreness. Although proper infant attachment and sucking help prevent nipple soreness, some soreness is common in the first few days or weeks of breast-feeding until the nipples become more elastic. For the client with a nursing diagnosis of *high risk for injury related to improper nipple care,* teach about proper infant attachment.

These measures can help relieve sore nipples:
- Apply ice compresses just before feeding (this numbs the nipples and makes them firmer and more graspable).
- Lubricate the nipples with a few drops of expressed milk before the feeding. This helps prevent tenderness as effectively as lanolin-based creams (Adcock, Burleigh, and Scott-Heads, 1988). Also, such creams have come under question because of possible contamination with pesticides resulting from sheep dipping (Food and Drug Administration, 1988).
- Let the nipples air dry thoroughly after feeding to promote healing and comfort.
- Avoid applying soaps directly to the nipples when washing the breasts.

The value of antepartal nipple preparation in reducing nipple tenderness is controversial. Some breast-feeding experts do not recommend it (Lauwers and Woessner,

COPING WITH FEARS ABOUT YOUR MILK SUPPLY

While breast-feeding, you may worry that you are not producing enough milk. At times, you may even fear that your milk supply has stopped. Anxiety about adequacy of milk supply is most common during the first few days of breast-feeding and during your infant's growth spurts, which occur at ages 10 to 14 days, 6 weeks, 3 to 4 months, and 6 months. To prepare for growth spurts, mark them on your calendar so that you can build up your milk supply in advance. Also keep in mind the following points about breast milk.

- Milk supply grows in response to demand: The more milk your infant removes, the more you will produce.
- Expect to breast-feed every 2 to 3 hours while building up your milk supply.
- Use the number of wet diapers to gauge your infant's milk intake. An infant who wets 10 to 12 diapers daily is getting adequate intake.
- Do not skip feedings because that tells your body it does not need to make milk.
- Breast-feed long enough for your infant to receive the rich, more filling hindmilk—about 15 minutes on each breast in the early days.
- Rest as often as possible to increase your milk production. Especially try to rest when your infant is sleeping.
- Accept all offers of help in caring for the infant and doing household chores.
- Offer both breasts at a feeding even if your infant has lately been feeding only at one breast.
- Review your fluid and nutrient intake to ensure that your own needs are met. Remember to drink fluids each time your infant breast-feeds.
- Remember that the need to increase your milk supply during a growth spurt is only temporary.
- Motivate yourself by keeping in mind how much your infant benefits from breast-feeding.

1989). Others have found the practice helpful (Storr, 1988).

Breast engorgement. Breast engorgement may involve excessive fullness of the breast veins or alveoli. Vascular engorgement occurs in all lactating women as blood flow to the breasts increases to prepare for breast-feeding. However, vascular engorgement commonly is confused with alveolar (milk) engorgement, which refers to alveolar overdistention with milk. Initially, vascular and alveolar engorgement may coincide.

If breast milk is insufficiently removed (as through restricted sucking time, incorrect infant attachment, or improper sucking technique), milk volume will exceed alveolar storage capacity, causing extreme discomfort. For a client with a nursing diagnosis of *pain related to breast engorgement,* encourage frequent feeding throughout the day and night in the initial days to alleviate engorgement. One study demonstrated that prophylactic breast massage after each feeding in the first 4 days after delivery also helped prevent breast engorgement (Storr, 1988).

Determine the cause of breast engorgement by assessing the client's breast-feeding technique and frequency. Suggest any necessary changes. Because milk engorgement can create serious drainage problems unless treated, teach the client what causes milk engorgement and remind her not to limit feeding time at the first breast offered in the mistaken belief that this will relieve engorgement. If the infant does not feed at the second breast, advise the client to express milk from the second breast, then offer this breast at the next feeding.

To help soften the breasts and facilitate attachment, the client with engorged breasts should express some milk gently before a feeding. Also, the client may massage her breasts after a warm shower or bath (applying mineral oil or a similar lubricant to the hands may make breast massage easier and reduce any discomfort it causes). Cold compresses applied to the breasts between feedings also may reduce discomfort, although no evidence shows that this relieves engorgement (Royal College of Midwives, 1988).

Milk expression. Milk expression by hand or pump may be indicated for a client who needs relief from breast engorgement or who is separated from the infant by infant illness or prematurity or by employment outside the home. Also, milk expression by pump helps improve graspability of flat or retracted nipples. Hopkinson, Schanler, and Garza (1988) found that women who express their milk can improve milk volume in the early postpartal period by minimizing the interval between delivery and the start of milk expression. They also linked optimal milk production with five or more milk expressions and total pumping time exceeding 100 minutes daily.

Warn the client who has a nursing diagnosis of *high risk for infection related to improper expression and storage of breast milk* that expressed milk probably is not sterile. Urge her to minimize bacterial contamination through frequent hand washing, aseptic handling of equipment, and aseptic transfer of her milk to storage containers (McCoy, Kadowski, Wilks, Engstrom, and Meier, 1988).

Breast pumps are available as hand-operated, battery-operated, and electric models. (For more information about expressing milk by hand and pump, see Client Teaching: *Expressing your milk,* pages 414 and 415.)

Advising the client about supplemental bottles. Some health care facilities continue the outmoded, unscientific practice of giving supplemental bottled fluids to breast-feeding neonates. Besides causing nipple confusion, supplemental bottles given in the early weeks of breast-feeding may interfere with the fragile dynamics of milk supply and demand. The nurse should advise the client to avoid giving supplemental bottles until her milk supply is well established (which typically takes 4 to 6 weeks).

Although some mothers have successfully combined breast-feeding and formula-feeding (Morse and Harrison, 1988), a client who feels she must use formula supplements should be advised to give bottles at a separate time from breast-feeding. This will disrupt the milk supply less than giving a bottle just after breast-feeding. (Parents with a family history of food allergies may wish to avoid any use of formula until the infant's gastrointestinal mucosa has matured and is less susceptible to allergic reactions.)

Ensuring adequate maternal fluid and food intake. Advise the breast-feeding client to maintain a fluid intake sufficient to keep her urine clear and amber. For a client with a nursing diagnosis of *potential fluid volume deficit related to breast-feeding,* provide fluids at each feeding. Also advise the client to restrict intake of caffeine-containing fluids because caffeine accumulates in the body and transfers to the infant in breast milk, possibly making the infant fussy in the evening.

Although many obstetricians still advise lactating women to consume 500 extra calories daily, the Royal College of Midwives (1988) now recommends that hunger—rather than a rigid caloric requirement—should guide food intake during breast-feeding.

When counseling the client with a nursing diagnosis of *altered nutrition: high risk for more than body requirements, related to breast-feeding,* help her establish a well-balanced diet and assure her that she can consume any food in moderation. However, if the infant develops symptoms of food allergy, she may have to restrict some foods. The client with a family history of food allergy may need to modify her diet (ideally, modification should begin during pregnancy).

Advising the client about drug use. Almost any drug the client consumes potentially transfers to the infant through breast milk. However, the client need not necessarily stop breast-feeding during drug therapy. Instead, she should seek her physician's advice. Usually, the breast-feeding woman can safely use therapeutic doses of such drugs as analgesics, antibiotics, stool softeners, and bulk-forming laxatives. On the other hand, potent diuretics, antineoplastic drugs, stimulant laxatives, and radioactive drugs nearly always warrant temporary discontinuation of breast-feeding. Use of oral contraceptives during breast-feeding is controversial.

Promoting family support. The breast-feeding client needs practical and emotional support from those close to her. The client's partner can play an especially key role. Hewat and Ellis (1986) found that mothers of neonates view three types of support from the father as important: physical support (such as helping with housework or other children), verbal reinforcement (such as ensuring the mother that breast-feeding is progressing well), and psychological support or sensitivity to the mother's feelings.

Childbirth education groups can serve as a source of support for new parents dealing with role adjustment. For a family with a nursing diagnosis of *altered family processes related to breast-feeding,* urge the partner to provide physical support by helping the client rest when she is establishing her milk supply. Also, encourage the partner to prevent visitors from overwhelming the client in the early breast-feeding days. Further, incorporate the partner in client teaching about such topics as infant positioning and attachment and determining if the infant is getting adequate nourishment.

Grandparents also may be expected to provide support. However, many of today's grandparents formula-fed their infants and thus know little about breast-feeding. Promote grandparent involvement in breast-feeding by developing teaching materials designed specifically for them.

Encouraging cuddling and eye contact. Breast-feeding brings the infant into close contact with the mother, allowing interaction that facilitates attachment. The nurse can encourage such interaction, for example, by suggesting that the client stroke the infant during feeding (especially if the client breast-feeds while lying down, which frees both hands). If the client breast-feeds while sitting, she can make eye contact with the infant.

Breast-feeding in special situations

Few circumstances completely rule out breast-feeding. The nurse with limited exposure to special breast-feeding

(Text continues on page 416.)

EXPRESSING YOUR MILK

You may express milk when your breasts are engorged, when weaning your infant, or when you want to provide breast milk during periods of separation from your infant. Refer to the guidelines below for milk expression by hand or pump.

EXPRESSING MILK BY HAND

You may want to practice expressing milk by hand at a time when you feel relaxed. The illustrated steps below show the proper expression sequence. Keep in mind that you must squeeze milk from the back of the milk reservoirs forward.

To push milk out of nipple openings, start the squeezing motion well behind the areola and move forward. For the final squeeze, keep your fingers behind the areola's outer edge—not on the areola or nipple.

1 Form a "U" with your fingers, as shown here, by placing your thumb above the areola and the other fingers below it.

2 While pushing your fingers away from the nipple, squeeze your thumb and fingers together.

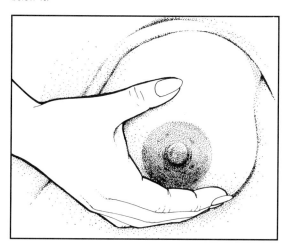

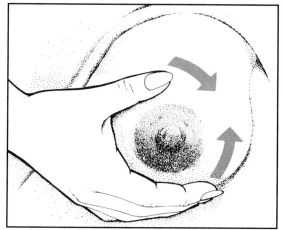

3 Now change direction by squeezing toward the nipple.

4 Rotate the thumb and fingers a quarter turn around the breast, then return to step 1 and continue until you have rotated 360 degrees around the breast.

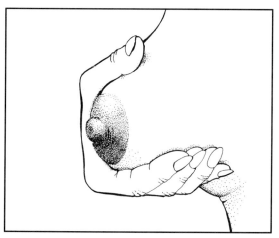

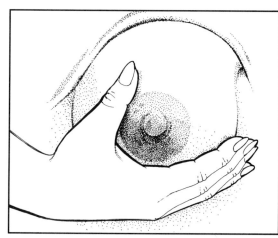

EXPRESSING YOUR MILK *(continued)*

PUMPING AND STORING BREAST MILK

Breast pumps generate a suck-release action via an adapter (flange) placed over the areola. The adapter presses on milk reservoirs, pushing out milk. Breast pumps come in several varieties. Here are some guidelines to follow.

You can begin pumping breast milk as soon after delivery as you feel well enough. (If your infant was born prematurely, you may begin pumping within 24 hours after delivery.)

Wash your hands and gather all equipment (make sure the equipment is clean). You may want to apply warm, wet washcloths to your breasts or take a warm shower to help release the milk. Stimulate the nipple and areola by rolling the nipple between your thumb and forefinger for a minute or two.

Pump each breast for at least 10 minutes every 3 to 4 hours during the day; at night, pump only if you are awake. Try to pump for a total of at least 100 minutes every 24 hours.

To obtain the most milk, switch breasts several times while pumping. For example, pump each breast for 5 to 8 minutes, then for 3 to 5 minutes, and finally for 2 to 3 minutes.

Transfer milk from the collection bottle to a sterile container (preferably plastic) and refrigerate it immediately. Breast milk can be kept refrigerated for 24 to 48 hours before use.

For longer storage periods (up to 6 months), breast milk must be frozen. Let frozen breast milk thaw in the refrigerator or at room temperature, or set the container in warm water. However, be careful not to overheat it. Once thawed, it must be used within 24 hours. Also, it must not be refrozen.

If you must transport your milk to the hospital, store it in the refrigerator to prevent bacterial growth. (Some health care facilities may request that you freeze your milk. Others freeze it after it arrives.)

TYPES OF BREAST PUMPS

Battery-operated pump
This pump has a battery-operated motor and can be used with one hand. Easy to clean, it is a good choice if you work outside the home or need a breast pump only for short-term use.

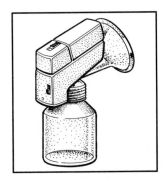

Electric pump
Usually used in hospitals, this pump is efficient and gentle and requires only one hand for operation. It is available as a small, 2-lb model or as a larger model about the size of a small sewing machine (the latter can be rented from a pharmacy or medical supply company).

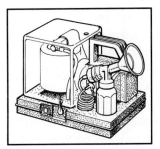

Cylinder pump
This pump has two plastic cylinders, one inside the other, that create gentle suction as you move the cylinder back and forth. Because you must use two hands to operate it, you may find it tiring. Easily cleaned and portable, this pump proves relatively efficient for short-term or intermittent use.

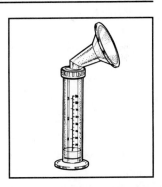

Rubber bulb or bicycle horn pump
To operate this pump, squeeze the rubber bulb, then release it slowly. This pump usually is not recommended because it is inefficient and tends to cause nipple and areola trauma. Also, sterility cannot be maintained because milk commonly becomes trapped inside the bulb.

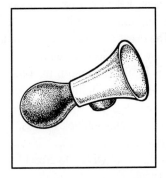

situations should develop contacts with such groups as the International Lactation Consultant Association (ILCA) or the LaLeche League for information or client referral.

The premature infant. Many premature infants can be breast-fed. Providing breast milk may be the only role the mother of a premature infant is permitted or able to perform; doing so may help her feel she is mothering her infant (Driscoll and Sheehan, 1985). For a client with a nursing diagnosis of *altered parenting related to infant prematurity and the mother's wish to breast-feed,* provide accurate information and ongoing support.

In North America, feeding schedules for premature infants typically are based on infant weight, gestational age, and ability to bottle-feed without signs of distress. However, none of these parameters is a research-based index of readiness to breast-feed (McCoy, Kadowski, Wilks, Engstrom, and Meier, 1988). Some data suggest that the premature infant can coordinate sucking and swallowing earlier for breast-feeding than for bottle-feeding (Meier and Pugh, 1985) and that breast-feeding creates less physiologic stress than bottle-feeding (Meier, 1988). However, most premature infants breast-feed for shorter durations than full-term neonates (Neifert and Seacat, 1988).

Besides coping with the stress of premature delivery, the client who wishes to breast-feed her premature infant but who cannot do so directly must establish and maintain a milk supply by expressing milk.

Multiple infants. Many mothers have successfully breast-fed twins and even triplets and quadruplets (Keith, McInnes, and Keith, 1982). For a client with a nursing diagnosis of *anxiety related to the ability to breast-feed multiple infants,* help instill confidence by relating these findings. However, also promote realistic expectations about the additional time needed to initiate and maintain a milk supply for multiple infants. If the client chooses to breast-feed the infants simultaneously, she may need help in positioning them. Refer her to a Parents of Twins group for support and information if the community has one.

The client with premature multiple infants may have to delay breast-feeding until the infants can tolerate it (Storr, 1989). However, if the infants were born close to term and are permitted to breast-feed, the client should keep them together while breast-feeding to accustom her to breast-feeding multiple infants (Lauwers and Woessner, 1989).

If the client wishes to breast-feed exclusively, this pattern should be initiated in the health care facility. If she plans to supplement breast-feeding with formula, however, advise her that this practice will decrease breast milk production and may create nipple confusion in the infants.

Working outside the home. The client who plans to continue breast-feeding after returning to work will need guidance and support. Although breast-feeding in this circumstance calls for extra commitment and effort, both mother and infant may reap rewards. For instance, knowing that her breast milk is meeting the infant's nutritional and immunologic needs may help ease any misgivings she has about returning to work.

The client may breast-feed at home and pump milk at work, schedule work around feeding times, or wean the infant from work-time feedings. Weaning should be done gradually to avoid adverse effects in both infant and mother. The client who wants to wean may decrease milk production by pumping only minimally, for comfort; as the demand for milk drops, so does milk production. Instruct the client to give the infant a bottle for the feeding that will be eliminated and warn her that her body will probably need several days to adjust to the elimination of each feeding.

Help the working mother devise a breast-feeding schedule that meets her individual needs, especially if she has a nursing diagnosis of *altered role performance related to the new task of breast-feeding.*

The client's work wardrobe should include clothes that can be easily unbuttoned or pulled aside to express milk to feed to the infant later. Breasts may leak in the first few weeks after she returns to work as they readjust to the new schedule. To help prevent or minimize breast leakage, the client can press against the breasts when she feels the tingling that signals let-down. Instruct her to place breast pads in her bra so that milk will not stain clothing and to change the pads frequently to avoid skin irritation from milk. She may prefer to wear patterned fabrics, which disguise milk stains better than solid colors. Taking a sweater and a spare blouse to work will avoid embarrassment caused by milk stains.

Warn the client that anxiety and fatigue caused by her return to work may reduce her milk production for a week or so. Maintaining an adequate fluid intake at work may minimize this problem.

CARE FOR THE CLIENT USING INFANT FORMULA

For the client who plans to formula-feed her infant, teaching on such topics as formula preparation can begin in the antepartal period. As with breast-feeding, initial formula-feeding experiences can prove crucial for both mother and infant. A positive first feeding experience can enhance maternal confidence and set the right tone for subsequent feedings. The nurse who observes early feedings has a unique opportunity to assess client-infant interaction and, if necessary, provide timely intervention.

Client teaching

The nurse should consider both short-term and long-term goals to anticipate guidance needed by the client who chooses formula-feeding. In the antepartal period, develop varied client teaching methods (perhaps using such items as films and books) to present current recommendations about formula-feeding. Discuss with the client specific feeding situations that might arise and plan a strategy for handling them. For example, ask the client what she would do if a friend or relative told her the infant was not eating enough or if the infant did not sleep through the night as early as a friend's did. Usually, antepartal discussion of growth spurts, of alternatives to early introduction of solid foods, and of support systems is more effective than discussion during the postpartal period, when the client may be fatigued from sleep deprivation and anxiety accompanying new parenthood.

Ensuring proper formula preparation

To teach the client about formula preparation, find out what preparation facilities and equipment will be available as well as which formula the client will use. Where water and refrigeration are readily available, rigorous sterilization practices largely have been replaced with an emphasis on cleanliness of the equipment and preparer. However, a client who lacks easy access to refrigeration and running water may have to modify preparation procedures.

Preparation methods. Four basic methods may be used to prepare infant formula.

Aseptic method. In this method, the preparer sterilizes formula equipment (including the mixing pitcher, measuring spoons, tongs, bottles, nipples, and nipple caps) by boiling it for 10 minutes. After reconstituting the formula according to manufacturer's instructions, the preparer pours the specified amount into each bottle, applies nipples and caps, and stores the bottles in the refrigerator until needed.

Terminal method. The preparer thoroughly washes the equipment and prepares the formula under clean (not sterile) conditions. After pouring reconstituted formula into bottles (with nipples and caps applied loosely), the preparer places the bottles in a pot with a tightly covered lid and boils them for 25 minutes. Once the bottles have cooled slightly, the preparer screws the caps down tightly and refrigerates them. Formula prepared by this method may take up to 2 hours to cool sufficiently to give to the infant.

One-bottle method. Using clean equipment, the preparer reconstitutes enough formula for one feeding, then pours it in a bottle. Prepared formula should be used within 30 minutes; the can containing the remaining unreconstituted formula must be refrigerated.

Clean method. With this method, an entire day's formula is prepared at one time and placed in clean bottles. The preparer reconstitutes the formula, applies clean nipples and caps, and refrigerates the bottles immediately.

General principles. Some common principles are basic to all formula preparation methods. The preparer must use good hand-washing technique—a point to reinforce frequently. Also, before opening the can, the preparer should wash the can opener and the top of the formula can with soap and water.

Prepared formula should be used within 24 hours (or 30 minutes with the one-bottle method). Opened formula cans should be covered with plastic or foil and refrigerated. Equipment used in formula preparation may be cleaned in an automatic dishwasher (providing the temperature reaches 140° F) or in warm, soapy water. However, latex nipples cleaned in a dishwasher may need to be replaced frequently because repeated exposure to heat weakens them. Instruct the client to place latex nipples in a covered basket in the dishwasher to prevent their displacement to the heating element, where they could melt. Also instruct the client to inspect nipples regularly to ensure that no milk particles block the opening, forming a bacterial breeding ground.

Giving the first feeding

No research-based guidelines support delaying formula-feeding. Nonetheless, in many health care facilities, the first feeding is given when the neonate is about 4 hours old. In other facilities, it is given when physiologic and behavioral cues suggest the neonate is ready to feed. Such cues include active bowel sounds, lack of abdominal distention, and sucking and rooting responses to stimulation of the lips. Neonates fed according to these cues are less likely to gag during the first feeding because their sucking and rooting responses are active. In some health care facilities, a nurse—rather than the mother—gives the first bottle (usually sterile water). However, this practice is based on tradition rather than research.

Helping the client with early feedings

Contrary to popular belief, the client using infant formula may require help with early feedings, especially if she has a nursing diagnosis of *knowledge deficit related to formula-feeding.*

Provide comfort measures (such as encouraging voiding and administering an analgesic, if prescribed) and have the client wash her hands before preparing the formula and feeding the infant. Then, help the client to a comfortable position with good back support and instruct her to hold the infant close to her in a semi-reclining position, with the bottle tilted so that the nipple always is filled with formula. This position minimizes air swallowing and permits air to rise to the top of the infant's stomach.

Some neonates will take an artificial nipple into the mouth readily; others must be coaxed. Instruct the client to stroke the infant's lips gently with the nipple; usually, this causes the mouth to open wide enough for nipple insertion. The first-time mother may be reluctant to place more than the tip of the nipple in the infant's mouth; urge her to insert the nipple further to trigger the sucking reflex.

Instruct the client to check nipple openings by holding the bottle upside down and noting whether formula drips freely from the nipple. (Formula that runs in a continuous stream is flowing too quickly.) The client can assume that nipple openings are the correct size if feedings take roughly 15 to 20 minutes, long enough to meet the infant's nutritional needs without causing fatigue. Warn the client to discard any formula left in the bottle at the end of a feeding because of the risk of bacterial contamination.

Most health care facilities use glass bottles with standard latex nipples; when the infant sucks, air bubbles may appear in these bottles, indicating that the infant is obtaining milk. However, point out that at home, the client may use a feeding system with a collapsible bag in which she cannot see air bubbles move. Instead, she should watch for the bag to collapse gradually, as a sign that the infant is obtaining formula.

Ensuring good burping technique.

The infant should be burped after every ounce of formula and again at the end of the feeding. Burping can be done in three positions: upright, across the lap, or upright on the lap. Because a neonate's cardiac sphincter does not function fully, the infant may expel milk along with air; a towel or cloth diaper placed in front of the infant will protect the client's clothing.

Helping the client establish a feeding pattern. Like the breast-fed infant, the formula-fed infant should be fed on a flexible demand schedule, not a rigid regimen. The formula-fed infant may awaken for feedings as often as every 2 hours or as infrequently as every 5 hours; many feed satisfactorily on a 3- or 4-hour schedule. If the client worries that the infant is not getting enough nourishment, explain that the initial feeding pattern does not necessarily indicate the pattern that will emerge later.

Promoting physical contact. Although formula-feeding allows less intimate contact than breast-feeding, it still provides an opportunity to cuddle the infant. Encourage the client to make eye contact and to vocalize with the infant during feeding.

Encouraging family support. A commonly cited benefit of formula-feeding is that it allows other family members to help with feedings. This help can be particularly valuable if the mother is fatigued. However, encourage family members to do such chores as preparing formula and cleaning formula equipment rather than insisting on giving the infant the bottle—an activity the mother may find relaxing. Siblings may or may not want to assist with feedings; parents should let them decide for themselves, especially in the early feeding days.

For the client with a nursing diagnosis of *altered family processes related to infant feeding,* discuss how to spend adequate time with the infant while obtaining help for more tiring chores.

EVALUATION

Evaluation findings should be stated in terms of actions performed or outcomes achieved for each goal. The following examples illustrate appropriate evaluation statements for the breast-feeding client:

• The client demonstrated appropriate techniques for attaching the infant to the breast.
• The client showed no signs of breast problems, such as sore nipples or excessive engorgement.
• The client expressed an understanding of breast-feeding dynamics.
• The client expressed confidence in her ability to seek help for breast-feeding problems.

The following examples illustrate appropriate evaluation statements for the client who uses infant formula:

• The client expressed an understanding of formula preparation and feeding techniques.

• The client maintained close contact with the neonate during feeding.
• The client expressed confidence in her ability to seek support for feeding problems.

Objective infant criteria include hydration status and weight-gain pattern.

DOCUMENTATION

When assisting a client with breast-feeding, include the following points in the documentation:
• maternal vital signs
• maternal fluid intake and output
• maternal position and comfort level during feeding
• maternal understanding of breast-feeding technique
• maternal understanding of proper infant positioning and ability to achieve proper positioning
• maternal attitude toward breast-feeding
• maternal understanding of dietary needs and breast care
• condition of the nipples and breasts
• infant sucking ability.

When assisting a client with formula-feeding, include the following points in the documentation:
• maternal vital signs
• maternal comfort level when feeding the infant
• maternal understanding of formula preparation
• maternal understanding of normal infant feeding patterns, including amount of formula taken and feeding frequency
• infant sucking ability.

CHAPTER SUMMARY

Chapter 20 described the needs of the childbearing family regarding infant nutrition. Here are the chapter highlights.

Feeding is an important part of infant care, not only because it provides nutrition but because the reciprocal interactions that take place are important to the infant's psychosocial development and the parent-infant relationship.

Breast milk and infant formula differ in nutritional value and immunologic properties.

Unparalleled physical growth takes place during the infant's first year; throughout this period, nutritional requirements change dramatically.

Feeding methods include breast-feeding and formula-feeding. The nurse should provide the client with appro-

priate information so that she can make a choice appropriate to her beliefs and life-style.

Infant feeding can be an emotionally charged issue; many traditional infant feeding practices may not reflect updated knowledge.

To make breast-feeding mutually satisfying, mother and infant must adjust and integrate their differing and sometimes opposing needs.

Nipple abrasion in the breast-feeding client usually can be avoided through correct infant attachment and positioning.

In the United States and Canada, breast-feeding only recently has become common once again. Thus, the client who breast-feeds may need support and guidance, especially in recognizing the breast-fed infant's frequent feeding requirements.

The client who chooses formula-feeding may need assistance with early feedings as well as continued support and guidance on infant behavior and feeding recommendations.

STUDY QUESTIONS

1. The nurse is performing a nutritional assessment on Jane Gray, who is 4 hours old. What information should the nurse include?

2. Compare the protein, fat, cholesterol, carbohydrate, and iron contents of breast milk and formula and their health implications.

3. During an antepartal visit, Mrs. Clay, a 25-year-old primiparous client, asks the nurse whether she should breast-feed or formula-feed her infant. What client-teaching information should the nurse discuss with Mrs. Clay?

4. Describe the two processes involved in lactation.

5. What assessments should the nurse make for the postpartal breast-feeding client and her neonate?

6. Describe the nursing interventions that the nurse can institute for the client with breast engorgement.

7. Mrs. Jones, who is breast-feeding her infant, plans to return to work outside the home in approximately 8 weeks and continue breast-feeding her infant. What information should the nurse discuss with Mrs. Jones?

8. Which topics should the nurse discuss with a new mother preparing to formula-feed her infant?

BIBLIOGRAPHY

Health and Welfare Canada (1986). *Feeding babies: A counselling guide on practical solutions to common infant feeding questions.* Minister of Supply and Services, Canada.

Lewis, C. (1986). *Nutrition and nutritional therapy in nursing.* Norwalk, CT: Appleton & Lang.

Marieb, E. (1989). *Human anatomy and physiology.* Redwood City, CA: Benjamin-Cummings.

Meier, P. (1988). Bottle and breast feeding: Effects on transcutaneous oxygen pressure and temperature in small preterm infants. *Nursing Research, 37*(1), 36-41.

Morse, J., and Harrison, M. (1988). Patterns of mixed feeding. *Midwifery, 4*(1), 19-23.

Myres, A. (1988). Tradition and technology in infant feeding, achieving the best of both worlds. *Canadian Journal of Public Health, 79*(2), 78-80.

Seeley, R., Stephens, T., and Tate, P. (1989). *Anatomy and physiology.* Redwood City, CA: Benjamin-Cummings.

Shapiro, A., Jacobson, L., Armon, M., Manco-Johnson, M., Hulac, P., Lane, P., and Hathaway, W. (1986). Vitamin K deficiency in the newborn infant: Prevalence and perinatal risk factors. *Journal of Pediatrics, 109*(4), 675-680.

Storr, G.B. (1988). Prevention of nipple tenderness and breast engorgement in the postpartal period. *JOGNN, 17*(3), 203-209.

Tanaka, P., Yeung, D., and Anderson, G. H. (1987). Infant feeding practices: 1984-85 versus 1977-78. *Canadian Medical Association Journal, 136*(9), 940-944.

Winikoff, B., Laukaran, V., Myers, S., and Stone, R. (1986). Dynamics of feeding: Mothers, professionals, and the institutional context in a large urban hospital. *Pediatrics, 77*(3), 357-365.

World Health Organization (1981). International code of marketing of breast-milk substitutes. *WHO Chronicle, 35,* 112-117.

Wright, P. (1987). Hunger, satiety and feeding behavior in early infancy. In R. Boakes, D. Popplewell, and M. Burton (Eds.), *Eating habits, food, physiology and learned behavior* (pp. 75-106). New York: Wiley.

Breast-feeding

Adcock, A., Burleigh, A., and Scott-Heads, D. (1988). Hind milk as an effective topical application in nipple care in the postpartum period. *Breastfeeding Review, 13,* Abstract 68.

American Academy of Pediatrics (1978). Breast-feeding. *Pediatrics, 62,* 591-601.

Baer, E. (1981). Promoting breastfeeding: A national responsibility. *Studies in Family Planning, 12,* 198-206.

Canadian Pediatric Society (1978). Breast-feeding: What is left besides the poetry? *Canadian Journal of Public Health, 69,* 13-20.

Casey, C., and Hambridge, K. (1983). Nutritional aspects of human lactation. In M. Neville and M. Neifert (Eds.), *Lactation physiology, nutrition and breast-feeding* (pp. 199-248). New York: Plenum.

Cunningham, A. (1988). Studies of breastfeeding and infections. How good is the evidence? *Journal of Human Lactation, 4,* 54-56.

Driscoll, J., and Sheehan, C. (1985). Breast-feeding and premature babies: Guidelines for nurses. *Neonatal Network, 5*(1), 18-24.

Food and Drug Administration (1988, September 13). *Lanolin contaminated with pesticides.* Talk paper. (T-88-66).

Glasier, A., McNeilly, A., and Howie, P. (1984). The prolactin response to suckling. *Clinical Endocrinology, 21*(2), 109-116.

Goldman, A., Garza, C., Nichols, B., and Goldblum, R. (1982). Immunologic factors in human milk during the first year of lactation. *Journal of Pediatrics, 100*(4), 563-567.

Hanson, L., Adlerberth, L., Carlsson, B., Castrignano, S., Hahn-Zoric, M., Dahlgren, U., Jalil, F., Nilsson, K., and Robertson, D. (1988). Breastfeeding protects against infections and allergy. *Breastfeeding Review, 13,* 19-22.

Hartman, P., and Kent, J. (1988). The subtlety of breast milk. *Breastfeeding Review, 13,* 14-18.

Hayward, A. (1983). The immunology of breast milk. In M. Aleville and M. Neifert (Eds.), *Lactation physiology, nutrition and breast-feeding* (pp. 249-270). New York: Plenum.

Hewat, R., and Ellis, D. (1986). Similarities and differences between women who breastfeed for short and long duration. *Midwifery, 2*(1), 37-43.

Hewat, R., and Ellis, D. (1987). A comparison of the effectiveness of two methods of nipple care. *Birth, 14*(1), 41-45.

Hopkinson, J., Schanler, R., and Garza, C. (1988). Milk production by mothers of premature infants. *Pediatrics, 81*(6), 815-820.

Humenick, S. (1987). The clinical significance of breast milk maturation rates. *Birth, 14,* 174-181.

Jones, D., and West, R. (1985). Lactation nurse increases duration of breast-feeding. *Archives of Disease in Childhood, 60*(8), 772-774.

Jones, D., West, R., and Newcombe, R. (1986). Maternal characteristics associated with duration of breast-feeding. *Midwifery, 2*(3), 141-146.

Keith, D., McInnes, S., and Keith, L. (1982). *Breastfeeding twins, triplets and quadruplets: 195 practical hints for success.* Chicago: Center for the Study of Multiple Birth.

Klaus, M. (1987). The frequency of suckling: A neglected but essential ingredient of breast-feeding. *Obstetrics and Gynecology Clinics of North America, 14*(3), 623-633.

Lauwers, J., and Woessner, C. (1989). *Counselling the nursing mother* (2nd ed.). Wayne, NJ: Avery.

Lawrence, R. (1989). *Breastfeeding: A guide for the medical profession* (3rd ed.). St. Louis: Mosby.

Leventhal, J., Shapiro, E., Aten, C., Berg, A., and Egerter, S. (1986). Does breast-feeding protect against infections in infants less than 3 months of age? *Pediatrics, 78,* 896-903.

McCoy, R., Kadowski, C., Wilks, S., Engstrom, J., and Meier, P. (1988). Nursing management of breastfeeding for preterm infants. *Journal of Perinatal Neonatal Nursing, 2*(1), 42-55.

Meier, P., and Pugh, E. (1985). Breastfeeding behavior of small preterm infants. *MCN, 10*(6), 396-401.

Minchin, M. (1985). *Breastfeeding matters.* Sydney, Australia: George Allen & Unwin.

Myres, A., Watson, J., and Harrison, C. (1981). The national breast-feeding promotion program: Professional phase—a note on its development, distribution and impact. *Canadian Journal of Public Health, 72*(5), 307-311.

Neifert, M., and Seacat, J. (1987). Lactation insufficiency: A rational approach. *Birth,* 14(4), 182-190.

Neifert, M., and Seacat, J. (1988). Practical aspects of breast-feeding the premature infant. *Perinatology-Neonatology,* 12(1), 24-31.

Neville, M. (1983). Regulation of mammary development and lactation. In M. Neville and M. Neifert (Eds.), *Lactation physiology, nutrition and breast-feeding* (pp. 103-140). New York: Plenum.

Newman, J. (1986). Breast-feeding: The problem of 'not enough milk'. *Canadian Family Physician,* 32, 571-574.

Ogra, P., and Greene, H. (1982). Human milk and breast feeding: An update on the state of the art. *Pediatric Research,* 16(41), 266-271.

Royal College of Midwives (1988). *Successful breastfeeding—a practical guide for midwives.* Oxford: Holywell Press.

Rumball, S. (1988). Structure and function of the human milk protein lactoferrin. *Breastfeeding Review,* 13, 31-32.

Smith, W., Erenberg, A., and Nowak, A. (1988). Imaging evaluation of the human nipple during breast-feeding. *American Journal of Diseases in Children,* 142(1), 76-78.

Storr, G.B. (1989). Breastfeeding premature triplets: one woman's experience. *Journal of Human Lactation,* 5(2), 74-77.

U.S. Department of Health and Human Services (1984). *Report on the surgeon general's workshop on breastfeeding and human lactation* (DDHS Publication No. HRS-D-MC 84-2). Washington, DC: U.S. Government Printing Office.

Weber, F., Woolridge, M., and Baum, J. (1986). An ultrasonographic study of the organization of sucking and swallowing by newborn infants. *Developmental Medicine & Child Neurology,* 28(1), 19-24.

Wood, C., Isaacs, P., Jensen, M., and Hilton, H.G. (1988). Exclusively breast-fed infants: Growth and caloric intake. *Pediatric Nursing,* 14(2), 117-124.

Woolridge, M. (1986). The anatomy of infant sucking. *Midwifery,* 2(4), 164-171.

Woolridge, M. (1989, July 8). *The physiology of suckling and milk transfer.* Paper presented at ILCA Conference, Toronto.

Formula-feeding

Fomon, S. (1987). Reflections on infant feeding in the 1970s and 1980s. *American Journal of Clinical Nutrition,* 46, 171-82.

Jason, J., Nieburg, P., and Marks, J. (1984). Mortality and infectious disease associated with infant-feeding practices in developing countries. *Pediatrics,* 74(4, Pt. 2), 702-727.

Kovar, M., Serdula, M., Marks, J., and Fraser, D. (1984). Review of epidemiologic evidence for an association between infant feeding and infant health. *Pediatrics,* 74(4, Pt. 2), 615-638.

Kramer, M. (1988). Infant feeding, infection and public health.

Ross Laboratories (1985). *Formula intake guidelines.* Columbus, OH.

Cultural references

Armstrong, H. (1987). Breastfeeding and low birth weight babies: Advances in Kenya. *Journal of Human Lactation,* 3, 34-37.

Carr, C. (1989). A four-week observation of maternity care in Finland. *JOGNN,* 18(2), 100-104.

Choi, E.C. (1986). Unique aspects of Korean-American mothers. *JOGNN,* 15(5), 394-400.

Gabriel, A., Gabriel, K. R., and Lawrence, R. (1986). Cultural values and biomedical knowledge: Choices in infant feeding. *Social Science and Medicine,* 23(5), 501-509.

CHAPTER 21

CARE OF HIGH-RISK NEONATES AND THEIR FAMILIES

OBJECTIVES

After reading and studying this chapter, the student should be able to:

1. Explain the concept of regionalized neonatal care.
2. Identify the goals of neonatal intensive care.
3. Discuss the ethical and legal issues associated with neonatal intensive care.
4. Discuss the nursing goals applicable to all high-risk neonates.
5. Identify the measures used to resuscitate a neonate at delivery.
6. Discuss the concerns of the family of a high-risk neonate.
7. Describe nursing interventions that help the family cope with a high-risk neonate.
8. Identify strategies used to encourage parent interaction with a high-risk neonate.
9. Describe interventions that provide support to the family of a neonate who dies.
10. Identify maternal, antepartal, intrapartal, and fetal factors that increase the risk of perinatal problems.
11. Identify perinatal problems commonly seen in preterm neonates.
12. Discuss the physiologic basis for such perinatal problems as hypothermia, fluid imbalance, and hyperbilirubinemia.
13. Apply the nursing process when caring for a high-risk neonate.

INTRODUCTION

The high-risk neonate is one who has an increased chance of dying during or shortly after delivery or who has a congenital or perinatal problem necessitating prompt intervention. As medicine continues to develop more treatments for perinatal problems, many high-risk neonates who formerly would have died after mere hours or days now survive; many have few or no residual effects of the crisis that marked their first hours after birth.

With the birth of a high-risk neonate (one who is preterm or very ill), family members experience a sense of loss. Even the family of a preterm neonate who becomes healthy enough to leave the neonatal intensive care unit (NICU) within a few weeks must work through some grief at the loss of the expected "perfect" child before they can bond strongly to the imperfect one. The family of a neonate with a chronic illness or congenital anomaly must find ways to cope with long-term grief and develop strategies to provide the special care the condition will require (and perhaps to balance these care needs with those of other children). If the neonate is stillborn or dies within a few hours or days after birth, family members must complete their bonding with the neonate, then detach themselves gradually so they can focus again on the family's life and needs.

To provide care in the first weeks after the birth of a high-risk neonate, the nurse must:
• understand the function of grief
• recognize the stages of grief in individual family members

- assess how family members are responding to and coping with the crisis of the high-risk neonate
- identify and implement strategies to help family members cope
- help family members identify support systems that can provide further help
- teach family members about the condition and care of the high-risk neonate
- maintain empathetic contact with family members as they work to integrate care of the high-risk neonate into family life.

This chapter begins by describing the levels and regionalization of neonatal care and discussing some ethical and legal concerns surrounding such care. Next, the chapter discusses the nursing care of the high-risk neonate, highlighting the goals common to all high-risk neonates. The chapter then explains how the nurse can care for the family of the high-risk neonate, including how to deal with their own needs as well as those of the neonate, describing typical responses of family members to the birth of a high-risk neonate, and explaining how family members progress through the stages of grief and how grief expressions may vary. The chapter then discusses the nursing care of the family, focusing on helping the family cope with the birth of the high-risk neonate, forming a bond with the neonate, beginning to deal with long-term concerns, and dealing with perinatal and fetal death. Next, the chapter describes the etiology and pathophysiology of common perinatal problems. Finally, the chapter shows how to plan and implement nursing care for these common perinatal problems. Throughout the chapter, the nursing process is used as a framework for discussing nursing care.

NEONATAL INTENSIVE CARE

Many high-risk neonates require care in a neonatal intensive care unit. Besides a highly skilled, round-the-clock medical and nursing staff, the NICU offers full life-support, resuscitation, and monitoring equipment and extensive ancillary support staff and services.

Regionalization of care

To ensure the highest quality of care for high-risk neonates, the American Academy of Pediatrics (1988) has established a system of "leveled" regionalized care in which a neonate is referred to the facility with the most appropriate staff and equipment to manage the neonate's specific problems. Ideally, regionalized care allows the most efficient use of resources by eliminating the need for all facilities to acquire the expensive equipment and staff for an NICU.

Every hospital in the United States is assigned to a region and classified according to the level of neonatal care provided. Level 1 care (as in the normal neonatal nursery) is most appropriate for uncomplicated deliveries; level 2 care, for neonates with mild to moderate problems; level 3 (NICU) care, for more serious problems.

Some neonatal care regions cross state lines; others include only a portion of a single state. Based on their needs and interdependence, facilities within each region are clustered to form referral networks. Within each region, one facility (or, in some cases, two) is designated as a regional referral center (a level 3 facility). Depending on the specific problems involved, a high-risk neonate who is delivered at a level 1 facility will be transported to a level 2 or level 3 facility.

Obstetric facilities also are classified according to the level of care provided; in some cases, this means that a mother may be cared for in a different facility than her neonate. For example, when no perinatal problems are anticipated, a woman may deliver in a level 1 obstetric facility with a level 1 nursery; if her neonate develops unexpected problems, he or she will require transport to a level 3 neonatal facility. (When a high-risk delivery is anticipated, however, the mother may be transported before delivery to a facility with level 3 neonatal care so that she and her neonate can be together.)

Sometimes a neonate is returned to the referring facility after treatment in a regional center; this is referred to as reverse transport. Candidates for reverse transport include neonates in whom the problem has resolved completely or neonates who have recovered sufficiently to be managed by the referring facility. Benefits of reverse transport include a decrease in the level 3 neonatal population and, in many cases, closer proximity to the family.

Goals of neonatal intensive care

The goals of neonatal intensive care include averting or minimizing complications, subjecting the neonate to as little stress as possible, and furthering parent-infant bonding. To achieve these goals, the NICU staff:

- anticipates, prevents, and detects potential or actual perinatal problems
- intervenes early for identified problems
- carries out care procedures in a way that minimizes disturbance to the neonate
- uses a family-centered approach.

Ethical and legal issues

As treatment advances increase the survival odds for high-risk neonates, debate over various ethical and legal issues grows. Economic factors are intertwined with these issues; as the financial burden of providing medical care for high-risk neonates increases, economic considerations may influence the treatment measures used for a particular neonate.

Resuscitation and life-support decisions. A major ethical and legal dilemma centers on which neonates should be resuscitated—specifically, the gestational age limit below which delivery room resuscitation or other aggressive measures should not be attempted. For example, before 23 weeks' gestation, the respiratory system is too immature to sustain extrauterine survival; thus, some care providers may forgo aggressive measures for a neonate born before this time. Most clinicians use 24 weeks' gestation as the cutoff point because the distance between the fetus's alveoli and arterial capillaries makes gas exchange—and thus extrauterine survival—difficult before this time. However, in some cases, fetal stress (for instance, from intrauterine growth retardation and certain other conditions) stimulates respiratory development, making extrauterine survival possible and increasing the chance that resuscitation will succeed.

Other specific topics of debate are the number of rounds of resuscitative drugs to administer and the circumstances that warrant ventilatory support and experimental therapies. Some facilities have protocols to address these issues; others rely on physicians to make judgments in individual cases.

A closely related issue concerns the "Do not resuscitate" order, which specifies the circumstances under which life support can be withheld legally. In some states, technological support may be discontinued when well-documented evidence strongly suggests that the neonate's condition will not improve. Other states require evidence that supports the poor prognosis, including a flat electroencephalogram for 24 hours in the absence of drugs that depress the central nervous system (CNS).

Quality-of-life considerations. Quality of life becomes a consideration for some high-risk neonates. Many congenital anomalies, for instance, can be corrected by surgery; however, the child may be left with serious disabilities that necessitate costly, lifelong care. For example, neonates with meningomyelocele, a congenital neurologic anomaly, may suffer paralysis despite surgery. In some cases, the physician or parents may believe that the poor quality of life that awaits the child justifies withholding treatment; the expense of lifelong care is a complicating issue.

Decision-making power. Further clouding such dilemmas is the question of who should make care decisions for a neonate. For instance, the choice to allow a severely disabled neonate to die formerly was left mainly to the parents. Now, however, the child's rights sometimes are weighed against the parents'. If caregivers believe that the parents are acting in their own best interests rather than the child's, they may ask the courts to remove the parents as legal guardians. As technology advances, decision making becomes increasingly complex.

NURSING CARE OF THE HIGH-RISK NEONATE

In many—perhaps most—cases, delivery of a high-risk neonate can be predicted from the maternal health history or from antepartal or intrapartal data. For instance, fetal distress (signaled by an abnormal fetal heart rate, meconium-stained amniotic fluid, or a fetal scalp blood pH below 7.25) warns strongly of a high-risk delivery. Thus, anticipation and preparation can help prevent or minimize perinatal problems. When a client is due to deliver, check the calculated date of delivery and review the history for factors that help predict neonatal outcome. (For more information, see *Risk factors for perinatal problems.*)

Although the neonate's condition will dictate the specifics of nursing care, the same nursing goals apply to all high-risk neonates: to ensure oxygenation, ventilation, thermoregulation, nutrition, and fluid and electrolyte balance; prevent and control infection; and provide developmental care.

ASSESSMENT

If a high-risk neonate is expected, a brief assessment immediately after delivery verifies the endangered status, as when the neonate fails to breathe spontaneously or has central cyanosis or an inadequate heart rate. Poor 1-minute and 5-minute Apgar scores also may confirm or suggest high-risk status. In some cases, however, a perinatal problem is not discovered until a complete examination is conducted several hours or days later. (For a detailed discussion of neonatal assessment, see Chapter 18, Neonatal Assessment.)

RISK FACTORS FOR PERINATAL PROBLEMS

The health care team can anticipate a neonate's high-risk status from the maternal, antepartal, or intrapartal history or from certain neonatal conditions present at birth.

Maternal risk factors
- Age over 34 or under 19
- Alcohol or drug use during pregnancy
- Chronic illness (including diabetes mellitus, anemia, hypertension, kidney disease, or heart disease)
- Cigarette smoking
- Death of a previous fetus
- Death or illness of a previous neonate
- Exposure to toxic chemicals, radiation, or other hazardous substances or conditions
- Exposure to infection during pregnancy
- Family history of a genetic disease
- Hereditary disease
- Isoimmunization
- Low socioeconomic status
- More than seven previous pregnancies
- Poor prenatal care
- Previous multiple fetuses
- Short interval between pregnancies (less than 12 months)

Antepartal risk factors
- Abruptio placentae
- Accelerated fetal growth
- Fetal surgery
- First-trimester bleeding
- Hydramnios
- Intrauterine growth retardation
- Multiple fetuses
- Placenta previa
- Pregnancy-induced hypertension
- Premature rupture of the membranes

Intrapartal risk factors
- Abnormal fetal presentation
- Cesarean delivery
- Fetal distress
- Maternal anesthetics or analgesics
- Prolonged labor
- Umbilical cord prolapse
- Use of forceps during delivery

Neonatal risk factors
- Abnormal placental weight or appearance
- Cardiorespiratory depression
- Congenital anomaly
- Low Apgar score
- Lack of spontaneous respirations
- Meconium-stained amniotic fluid
- Prematurity or postmaturity
- Small or large size for gestational age
- Unusual number of umbilical vessels

NURSING DIAGNOSIS

After gathering all assessment data, the nurse must review it carefully to identify pertinent nursing diagnoses for the neonate. (For a partial list of applicable diagnoses, see Nursing Diagnoses: *High-risk neonates and their families,* page 426.)

PLANNING AND IMPLEMENTATION

Once a fetus or neonate is identified as high risk (such as when fetal distress has been detected late in pregnancy), initial intervention should focus on preventing complications and death. Some high-risk neonates require emergency interventions; others, such as those with relatively minor congenital anomalies, are fairly stable at birth but require prompt treatment to prevent complications.

Performing emergency intervention

In most cases, the need for resuscitation at delivery can be anticipated from maternal, antepartal, or intrapartal factors. Immediately after delivery, the neonate must be evaluated to determine the need for resuscitation. Depending on the neonate's condition and response to each resuscitative measure, neonatal resuscitation typically involves some combination of the following:
- free-flow oxygen
- positive-pressure ventilation (PPV)
- closed-chest cardiac massage
- gastric decompression
- emergency drugs
- endotracheal intubation.

Preparation for resuscitation. Before every delivery, verify that emergency equipment and supplies are present, in working order, and ready to use; ideally, all items should be double-checked. This helps avert problems during resuscitation, when replacement of a missing supply or malfunctioning part could cause a dangerous treatment delay. (For a list of equipment and supplies, see *Resuscitation equipment, techniques, and drugs,* pages 427 to 430.)

Resuscitation personnel. Every delivery should be attended by at least one person skilled in all resuscitation techniques and another person who is an experienced resuscitation assistant. When asphyxia is likely, a third person also should be present in the delivery room to manage the mother so that the resuscitators can attend solely to the neonate.

Before performing resuscitation on a neonate, an inexperienced nurse should observe a skilled nurse per-

HIGH-RISK NEONATES AND THEIR FAMILIES

The following are potential nursing diagnoses for problems and etiologies that a nurse may encounter when caring for high-risk neonates and their families. Specific nursing interventions for many of these diagnoses are provided in the "Planning and implementation" sections of this chapter.

- Altered family processes related to the birth of a high-risk neonate and the adjustments necessitated by the neonate's condition and hospitalization
- Altered growth and development related to functional immaturity, prolonged environmental stress, and lack of stimulation appropriate for gestational age and physical status
- Altered nutrition: less than body requirements, related to increased caloric requirements, respiratory distress, gastrointestinal immaturity, a weak sucking reflex, or metabolic dysfunction
- Anticipatory grieving related to the prospect of the neonate's death
- Anxiety related to the neonate's condition and unknown outcome
- Caregiver role strain related to neonate status and transfer to NICU
- Defensive coping related to the seriousness of the neonate's condition and long-term implications
- Fluid volume deficit related to renal immaturity or increased fluid loss
- High risk for aspiration related to meconium in the respiratory tract
- High risk for infection related to immunologic immaturity, altered ventilation, ineffective airway clearance, or frequent invasive procedures
- High risk for injury related to lack of cushioning from inadequate subcutaneous fat
- Hypothermia related to an immature temperature-regulating center, decreased body mass-to-surface ratio, reduced subcutaneous fat, inability to shiver or sweat, and inadequate metabolic reserves

- Impaired gas exchange related to surfactant deficiency and altered alveolar function
- Ineffective airway clearance related to inability to expel excess secretions
- Ineffective breathing pattern related to respiratory and neurologic immaturity
- Ineffective denial related to the immediate and long-term implications of the neonate's condition
- Ineffective family coping: compromised, related to family disorganization secondary to the neonate's condition
- Ineffective individual coping related to family disorganization secondary to the neonate's condition
- Ineffective individual coping related to the stress of a preterm birth
- Interrupted breast-feeding related to surgery for congenital anomaly
- Knowledge deficit related to the hospital course and care of a high-risk neonate
- Parental role conflict related to limited opportunities to care for the neonate
- Potential altered parenting related to poor parent-infant bonding
- Potential altered parenting related to the neonate's condition, difficulty coping with a less-than-perfect neonate, and enforced separation
- Potential impaired skin integrity related to frequent invasive procedures
- Powerlessness related to the health care environment and limited interaction with the neonate

forming the procedures, then practice on a mannequin to the point of proficiency. The first few times the nurse resuscitates a neonate, close supervision is mandatory.

Resuscitation procedure. Initial neonatal evaluation and subsequent resuscitative measures are based on respirations, heart rate, and skin color—not on the 1-minute Apgar score (American Heart Association and American Academy of Pediatrics, 1987). Waiting until the end of the first minute to start resuscitation makes the procedure more difficult and increases the chance for brain damage and death. With a severely asphyxiated neonate, a delay is especially dangerous. (However, Apgar scores should be used to help determine whether resuscitative measures are effective.)

Like any resuscitation, the goal of neonatal resuscitation is to ensure the ABCs—airway, breathing, and circulation. Resuscitation follows an orderly sequence; after each intervention, the team quickly evaluates the neonate's condition and response to the intervention, then decides which further measures, if any, are necessary.

Respirations. If the neonate lacks spontaneous respirations, PPV with a bag and mask must begin immediately. If the neonate is breathing (as indicated by chest movements), the resuscitation team moves on, evaluating heart rate.

Heart rate. If the heart rate is below 60 beats/minute or between 60 and 80 beats/minute and not increasing,

(Text continues on page 430.)

RESUSCITATION EQUIPMENT, TECHNIQUES, AND DRUGS

RESUSCITATION EQUIPMENT AND SUPPLIES

To help ensure the most effective resuscitation, the nurse should be familiar with the delivery room equipment and supplies listed below.

Bag-and-mask equipment
- Face masks (sizes 0 and 1)
- Infant resuscitation bag (anesthesia bag or self-inflating bag) capable of delivering 90% to 100% oxygen
- Oxygen delivery unit with adjustable fraction of inspired oxygen, humidification source, flowmeter, tubing, and pressure gauge or pressure-release (pop-off) valve (40 to 60 cm H_2O)
- Oropharyngeal airway (sizes 000, 00, and 0)

Emergency drugs and solutions
- Dextrose 10% in water
- Epinephrine 1:10,000
- Naloxone 0.02 mg/ml
- Normal saline solution
- Sodium bicarbonate 4.2% (5 mEq/10 ml)
- Volume expander, such as albumin

Intubation equipment
- Endotracheal tubes with adapters (sizes 2.5, 3, 3.5, and 4 mm)
- Extra bulbs and batteries
- Laryngoscope with straight blades (sizes 0 and 1)
- Magill forceps
- Wire stylet for tubes
- Scissors

Suction equipment (80 to 100 mm Hg)
- Bulb syringe
- DeLee mucus trap
- Mechanical suction machine
- Suction catheters (#5, #6, #8, and #10 Fr.)

Other items
- Adhesive tape
- Blood pressure cuff and gauge
- Cardiorespiratory monitor
- Clock or timer
- Electrocardiograph electrodes
- I.V. solution and tubing
- Water-soluble lubricating jelly (such as K-Y jelly)
- Nasogastric tube
- Radiant warmer resuscitation bed (preheated)
- Gloves
- Sterile water
- Stethoscope
- Syringes (tuberculin 3, 5, and 10 ml)
- Umbilical artery catheter tray (including #3.5 and #5 Fr.)

RESUSCITATING A NEONATE

The neonate with birth asphyxia or another form of cardiopulmonary compromise needs immediate resuscitation after delivery. The guidelines below, which describe the essential steps in neonatal resuscitation, reflect the recommendations of the American Heart Association and American Academy of Pediatrics (1987).

Suctioning the airway

1 Dry the neonate and place on a firm surface under a preheated radiant warmer. Extend the neck slightly to the "sniff" position. To maintain this position, place a rolled towel or blanket under the shoulders to raise them ¾" to 1" off the surface.

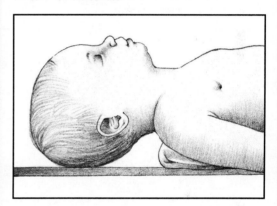

2 Using a soft catheter, mechanical suction, or a bulb syringe, suction the mouth, then the nose, to remove blood, meconium, or other matter. If the neonate has copious oral secretions, turn the head to the side to facilitate suctioning. To avoid stimulating the vagal reflex, which could cause bradycardia or apnea, avoid suctioning too vigorously or for more than 10 seconds.

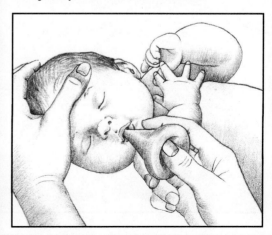

(continued)

RESUSCITATION EQUIPMENT, TECHNIQUES, AND DRUGS *(continued)*

RESUSCITATING A NEONATE *(continued)*

Administering positive-pressure ventilation

1 If drying, suctioning, or other tactile stimulation (such as tapping the soles or rubbing the back) does not induce respirations immediately, begin positive-pressure ventilation with a bag and mask at once. Attach the resuscitation bag to an oxygen source and select a mask of the correct size (size 0 for the preterm neonate, size 1 for the term neonate). Connect the mask to the resuscitation bag.

2 Standing at the neonate's side or head, apply the mask so that it covers the neonate's nose and mouth, with the edge of the neonate's chin resting within the rim of the mask. To obtain an airtight seal, use light downward pressure on the rim to apply the mask.

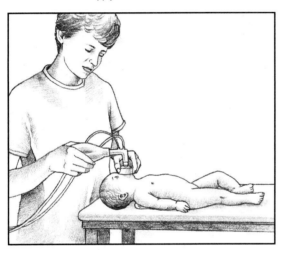

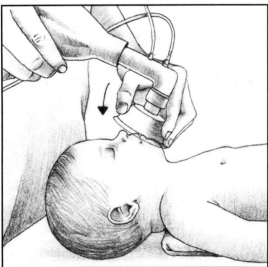

3 Check the seal and the ventilation technique by ventilating two or three times and watching for chest movement. (Make sure to squeeze the bag with the fingertips only, not the entire palm.) The neonate's chest should rise slightly, as in a shallow breath. A deep breath indicates that the lungs are being overinflated from excessive pressure on the bag.

If the neonate's chest does not rise, suspect an inadequate seal, a blocked airway, or insufficient pressure delivered by the bag. Correct these problems by reapplying the mask; repositioning the neonate's head; checking for secretions and suctioning, if necessary; or increasing the pressure to 20 to 40 cm H_2O or until the pop-off valve activates.

4 If the chest rises slightly, give an initial ventilation of 15 to 30 seconds with 100% oxygen at a rate of 40 ventilations/minute. Initial breaths may require a pressure of up to 40 cm H_2O; for subsequent ventilations, use only the minimum pressure necessary to move the chest.

5 Subsequent actions depend on the heart rate. Check the heart rate with a cardiac monitor (if a monitor is not available, listen to the apical beat with a stethoscope or feel the umbilical pulse at the base of the cord). To estimate the 1-minute heart rate, count the heartbeat for 6 seconds and multiply by 10.
- If the heart rate is above 100 beats/minute and the neonate is breathing spontaneously, discontinue bag-and-mask ventilation and provide gentle stimulation (for instance, by rubbing the skin). Monitor the neonate to assess for stabilization.
- If the heart rate is above 100 beats/minute but the neonate is not breathing spontaneously, continue to ventilate at a rate of 40 breaths/minute.
- If the heart rate is 60 to 100 beats/minute and increasing, continue to ventilate. If the heart rate is between 60 and 100 but *not* increasing, continue to ventilate and verify that the chest is moving properly and that 100% oxygen is being delivered.
- If the heart rate is less than 60 beats/minute or between 60 and 80 beats/minute and *not* increasing, another member of the team must start closed-chest cardiac massage (chest compressions) at once while the first resuscitator continues to ventilate.

Performing chest compressions

1 To ensure the best outcome, resuscitation team members should position themselves so that each can work effectively without hindering the other.

For the **two-finger method,** place the tips of the middle finger and the ring or index finger over the midsternum in the midline while supporting the neonate's back with the other hand.

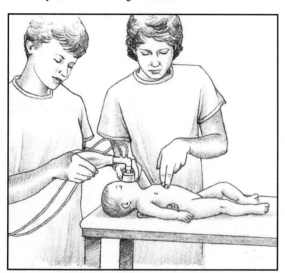

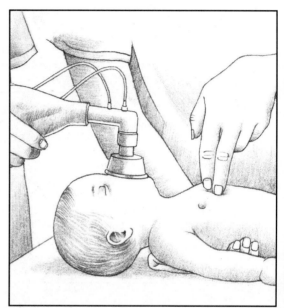

2 The resuscitator who administers chest compressions may use either the thumb method or the two-finger method.

For the **thumb method,** place both thumbs side-by-side over the midsternum, with the hands encircling the chest and the fingers supporting the neonate's back (illustration at left). If the neonate is very small, one thumb can be placed over the other (illustration at right).

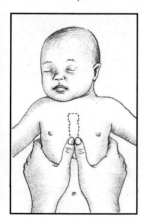
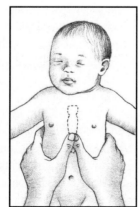

3 With either method, depress the sternum ½″ to ¾″, then release the pressure to allow the heart to refill; keep the thumbs or fingertips in contact with the sternum at all times, even during the release. Deliver 120 compressions/minute (one compression equals the downward stroke plus the release). When delivering compressions, take care not to squeeze the chest with the whole hand or apply pressure to the xiphoid process.

4 To determine if chest compressions are effective, one resuscitator should check the pulse after 30 seconds of compressions, then periodically (by counting for 6 seconds). Once the neonate's heart rate reaches 80 beats/minute, chest compressions should be discontinued. However, ventilations should continue until the heart rate exceeds 100 beats/minute and the neonate is breathing spontaneously.

If the heart rate is below 80 beats/minute, chest compressions and ventilation must continue; in some cases, emergency drugs are administered at this point. If the neonate still shows no response, resuscitation continues until the physician decides to stop it.

RESUSCITATION EQUIPMENT, TECHNIQUES, AND DRUGS *(continued)*

RESUSCITATION DRUGS

For the neonate with no detectable heartbeat at delivery, the physician typically orders emergency drugs immediately (along with bag-and-mask ventilation and chest compressions). Drugs also are indicated for a neonate whose heart rate remains below 80 beats/minute despite adequate bag-and-mask ventilation and chest compressions. The chart below summarizes indications and nursing considerations for drugs recommended for neonatal resuscitation by the American Heart Association and American Academy of Pediatrics (1987).

DRUG	INDICATIONS	NURSING CONSIDERATIONS
dopamine	Poor peripheral perfusion, thready pulses, and continuing signs of shock after administration of epinephrine, a volume expander, and sodium bicarbonate	• Administer as a continuous I.V. infusion in a prepared solution. • Use an infusion pump to control the infusion rate.
epinephrine	Heart rate of 0 or heart rate below 80 beats/minute after 30 seconds of ventilation with 100% oxygen and chest compressions	• Prepare 1 ml of 1:10,000 dilution in a syringe for I.V. or endotracheal administration. • Administer rapidly.
sodium bicarbonate	Metabolic acidosis	• Prepare two prefilled syringes (10 ml) or draw 20 ml into a syringe for I.V. administration. • Give over at least 2 minutes.
naloxone hydrochloride	Severe respiratory depression in a neonate whose mother received a narcotic no more than 4 hours earlier	• Draw 2 ml of 0.02 mg/ml dilution into a syringe for I.V., I.M., subcutaneous, or endotracheal administration. • Inject rapidly.

closed-chest cardiac massage (chest compression) typically begins as PPV continues. (PPV should be initiated whenever the heart rate is below 100, even if the neonate has spontaneous respirations.) If the heart rate is above 100 beats/minute, the team evaluates skin color.

Skin color. If the neonate has central cyanosis, reflecting lack of oxygen in the blood, the team administers free-flow oxygen by holding the end of an oxygen tube close to the neonate's nose or by holding an oxygen mask over the neonate's mouth and nose.

Special considerations. Although most neonates respond to PPV and chest compressions, some require other measures.

Gastric decompression. Bag-and-mask ventilation forces air to enter the stomach, which can prevent full lung expansion, cause aspiration of gastric contents, and lead to abdominal distention (which impedes breathing). Consequently, when bag-and-mask ventilation is required for more than 2 minutes, an orogastric tube must be inserted to suction gastric contents; the tube is left in place throughout resuscitation to vent air.

Emergency drugs. Drugs may be administered if the neonate fails to respond to bag-and-mask ventilation and chest compressions. Such drugs typically are administered via the umbilical vein or, in some cases, through a peripheral vein (such as a scalp or extremity vein) or an endotracheal tube.

Endotracheal intubation. This intervention, which should be performed only by an experienced intubator, is indicated when diaphragmatic hernia is suspected, when the neonate requires prolonged ventilation, or when prolonged bag-and-mask ventilation proves ineffective.

Endotracheal intubation also is necessary when meconium aspiration syndrome (MAS) is suspected. If the amniotic fluid contains thick meconium—a sign of asphyxia experienced in utero—the neonate has a nursing diagnosis of *high risk for aspiration related to meconium in respiratory tract.* As soon as the neonate's head is delivered, the mouth, oropharynx, and hypopharynx must be suctioned with a flexible suction catheter. Immediately after delivery, an experienced intubator visualizes the larynx with a laryngoscope, then intubates the trachea and suctions any meconium from the lower airway — preferably by applying suction to an endotracheal tube. After the tube has been inserted, continuous suction is applied as the tube is withdrawn. This procedure is repeated until no more meconium is suctioned.

Post-resuscitation care. After resuscitation, observe the neonate closely for signs of respiratory distress, including cyanosis, apnea, tachypnea, and inspiratory retractions. Blood pressure and cardiac perfusion are other key indicators; if either is inadequate, expect to administer volume expanders to reverse shock.

If an endotracheal tube is in place, observe for tube dislodgement, signs of tube obstruction, and associated complications, such as pneumothorax. To monitor tube placement, check tube length (from the point where it leaves the mouth to the connection point) and assess for equal bilateral breath sounds and symmetrical chest expansion.

If the neonate was severely asphyxiated at delivery, the physician may want to maintain the serum glucose level at 100 to 150 mg/dl; expect to administer dextrose 10% in water and monitor the serum glucose level. Also monitor the hematocrit and assess renal status by measuring fluid intake and checking for abrupt weight changes, which may signal renal complications of asphyxia. Ensure thermoregulation by keeping the neonate under a radiant warmer and monitoring skin temperature.

If the neonate requires transport to a level 3 nursery, make preparations according to institutional protocol and notify the nursery of the impending admission as soon as possible so that staff and necessary equipment can be mobilized.

Supporting oxygenation and ventilation

Most neonates who have been successfully resuscitated — as well as many other high-risk neonates — need supplemental oxygen to prevent or correct hypoxia. Supplemental oxygen can be administered by hood, nasal cannula, or continuous positive-airway pressure (CPAP); it always should be warmed and humidified. To avoid a nursing diagnosis of *impaired gas exchange related to surfactant deficiency and altered alveolar function* or *ineffective breathing pattern related to respiratory and neurologic immaturity,* be alert to neonates who require additional ventilatory support in the form of mechanical ventilation.

The goal of supplemental oxygen therapy is to maintain a partial pressure of arterial oxygen (PaO_2) of 60 to 80 mm Hg. A higher level may lead to retinopathy of prematurity (ROP); a lower level, to profound hypoxia and CNS problems (including cerebral hemorrhage and brain damage). Record the fraction of inspired oxygen (FiO_2) as a percentage (however, for the older neonate who is receiving oxygen by nasal cannula, FiO_2 may be recorded in liters/minute). FiO_2 ranges from 21% (the oxygen concentration in room air) to 100%.

Because oxygen is a drug, the nurse must be familiar with its potential adverse effects and ways to avoid them. For instance, to prevent or minimize the risk of ROP, always administer oxygen at the lowest concentration that will correct hypoxia, using an oxygen analyzer to determine the actual concentration of delivered oxygen.

To ensure therapeutic efficacy and avoid oxygen toxicity, monitor the neonate's oxygenation status continuously with a noninvasive technique, such as transcutaneous oxygen pressure ($tcPO_2$) monitoring or pulse oximetry. With a $tcPO_2$ monitor, the probe measures oxygen diffusion and carbon dioxide perfusion across the skin; with pulse oximetry, the probe measures beat-to-beat arterial oxygen saturation. Be sure to place the probe in a well-perfused area. $TcPO_2$ readings should range from 50 to 80 mm Hg; oximetry readings can range from 88% to 94% (Harbold, 1989).

However, $tcPO_2$ or oximetry values alone are not adequate; they must be correlated with simultaneously obtained arterial blood gas (ABG) samples drawn every 3 to 4 hours. To obtain ABG samples, use a heparinized syringe; place the samples on ice to prevent oxygen and carbon dioxide diffusion.

Oxygen hood and nasal cannula. An oxygen hood, which fits over the neonate's head, can deliver up to 100% oxygen and allows easy access to the rest of the neonate's body for care procedures. A nasal cannula delivers oxygen concentrations above room air (21%); typically, it is used for a neonate with bronchopulmonary dysplasia (BPD) or a congenital cardiac defect (the minimal equipment involved allows frequent cuddling and other stimulation).

CPAP. CPAP usually is implemented if the neonate requires an FiO_2 of 60% or greater to maintain a PaO_2 level of 60 mm Hg. CPAP delivers air at a constant pressure throughout the respiratory cycle, keeping the lungs expanded at all times to reduce shunting and improve oxygenation. CPAP may be delivered via a nasopharyngeal tube or an endotracheal tube inserted through the mouth or nose. Some neonatologists believe a nasal tube is more secure than an oral tube. However, prolonged nasal intubation may cause anterior naris (nostril) damage and deviation or nasal septal erosion. An excessively long oral tube, on the other hand, may become kinked. With either tube, take steps to avoid accidental extubation.

During CPAP therapy, monitor the neonate's vital signs, blood pressure, and respiratory effort; stay especially alert for tachycardia, tachypnea, and arrhythmias.

Mechanical ventilation. Mechanical ventilation usually is used instead of CPAP if any of the following criteria are present:
- PaO_2 level below 50 mm Hg with administration of 100% oxygen (Goldsmith and Karotkin, 1988)
- $PaCO_2$ level above 60 mm Hg
- arterial pH below 7.2.

During mechanical ventilation, assess the neonate's vital signs, breath sounds, chest movement, respiratory effort, and oxygenation status every hour. When assessing breath sounds, keep in mind that in a mechanically ventilated neonate, breath sounds normally are loud and high-pitched. However, extremely high-pitched sounds may signal excessive secretions. A pitch decrease, in contrast, may reflect atelectasis or pulmonary air leakage.

As necessary, suction the endotracheal tube to maintain a patent airway, making sure to apply suction only while removing the catheter. If possible, use a suctioning method that does not necessitate interruption of mechanical ventilation. Report any change in the amount or consistency of secretions.

Be sure to assess endotracheal tube positioning and patency regularly; a tube resting along the tracheal wall may impair ventilation. Also check ventilator function periodically, making sure all alarms are working. Assess the system for leaks.

Maintaining thermoregulation

An essential part of care for all neonates, thermoregulation is particularly crucial to the high-risk neonate, whose oxygen and energy reserves may be depleted rapidly by illness. The preterm neonate especially is at risk for cold stress because of limited subcutaneous fat, an extremely high surface-to-mass ratio, inability to shiver, and minimal brown fat (a type of fat that provides body heat).

Heat loss may result from radiation, conduction, evaporation, or convection (as discussed in Chapter 17, Neonatal Adaptation). A neonate who suffers heat loss and progressive cold stress may experience peripheral vasoconstriction, hypoglycemia, reduced cerebral perfusion, metabolic acidosis, exacerbation of respiratory distress syndrome (RDS), decreased surfactant production, impaired kidney function, gastrointestinal (GI) disturbances, hypoglycemia, and, ultimately, death.

A first step in preventing hypothermia is to minimize cooling at delivery; such cooling may delay adequate thermoregulation for hours. During the initial examination and resuscitation, the neonate should be placed under a radiant heat warmer. Wrap the neonate with a plastic bag or thermal foil blanket as soon as possible after resuscitation, and then transfer the neonate to an incubator or radiant warmer bed.

Because heat loss from the neonate's head is considerable, keep the neonate's head covered at all times. Also, warm the hands before touching the neonate to prevent conductive heat loss through handling.

Neutral thermal environment. Throughout care, aim for a neutral thermal environment (NTE), a narrow range of environmental temperature (89.6° to 93.2° F [32° to 34° C]) that maintains a stable core temperature with minimal caloric and oxygen expenditure. Although NTE may prove hard to achieve, certain measures may help prevent a nursing diagnosis of *hypothermia related to an immature temperature-regulating center, decreased body mass-to-surface ratio, reduced subcutaneous fat, inability to shiver or sweat, and inadequate metabolic reserves.* For instance, use of a warmed, humidified incubator with an air temperature of 96.8° F (36° C) helps maintain proper skin temperature (Perlstein, 1988).

Thermoregulation during transport. Special measures must be taken if the neonate requires transport to another facility. Causes of heat loss during transport include poor heat retention in the transport bed, radiant heat loss within the transport vehicle, and drafts as the transport bed passes through unheated corridors or as the door or hood to the transport bed is opened to place the neonate inside. To help minimize the risk of cold stress from these causes, provide an NTE before transport (for instance, by protecting the neonate from heat loss during examinations or care procedures). Also, double-wrap the neonate before transport or place a warming mattress in the transport bed to enhance its heating capacity.

Providing adequate nutrition

The accelerated metabolic rate and energy expenditure of the high-risk neonate may lead to a nursing diagnosis of *altered nutrition: less than body requirements, related to increased caloric requirements, respiratory distress, GI immaturity, a weak sucking reflex, or metabolic dysfunction.* Respiratory distress, for instance, increases caloric requirements 50% to 75%; the metabolic response to surgery, by 30% (Kaempf, Bonnabel, and Hoy, 1989).

The preterm neonate may need 104 to 130 calories/kg/day, compared to the normal healthy neonate, who requires 100 to 120 calories/kg/day. However, caloric requirements change over time and should be adjusted depending on the neonate's tolerance.

For the high-risk neonate who can take nourishment by mouth, breast milk is the preferred nutritional form. If the neonate cannot receive breast milk, the physician may order a special high-calorie infant formula to provide 24 or 27 calories/oz (in contrast to the 20 calories/oz in standard formulas). In some cases, the neonate may begin feedings with half-strength formula and gradually increase to three-quarters-strength, then full-strength.

Enteral nutrition (gavage feedings). To avoid aspiration resulting from a weak sucking reflex, uncoordinated sucking and swallowing, or respiratory distress, many high-risk neonates must be fed enterally, typically through a tube passed through the nose or mouth into the stomach. (However, some neonates must be fed through a surgically placed gastrostomy tube.)

Although a nasogastric tube typically is used to provide enteral feedings, some neonatologists prefer a nasojejunal or orojejunal tube. A nasojejunal tube is passed from the nose through the stomach to the jejunum; an orojejunal tube is passed from the mouth to the jejunum. Because of a possible link between jejunal tubes and NEC, some authorities do not recommend them for neonates weighing less than 2,000 g (Moyer-Mileur, 1986). Nonetheless, jejunal tubes may be used in neonates with gastric reflux and a high risk for aspiration pneumonia. With either tube, placement usually is confirmed by X-ray and aspirate pH values.

If intermittent bolus feedings are prescribed, a tube is passed with each feeding; continuous feedings are administered through an indwelling tube. Typically, the delivery rate for enteral feedings is increased at 12-hour intervals; the increase must be gradual to avoid complications associated with poor feeding tolerance, such as dehydration, diarrhea, vomiting, and abdominal distention. Monitor the neonate closely for these signs.

Check tube placement every 4 hours; remove the tube immediately if the neonate begins to choke or cough or becomes cyanotic—signs that the tube has entered the trachea. To prevent aspiration, keep the mattress elevated 30 degrees for 30 minutes after intermittent bolus feedings and at all times for continuous feedings.

To check gastric residual matter, aspirate gastric contents every 4 hours by attaching a syringe containing 0.5 to 1 ml of air to the tubing. Inject the air while listening through a stethoscope over the epigastric area for a rush of air. Note the color, amount, and consistency of gastric contents; more than 15 ml of matter aspirated before a feeding may signal poor tolerance of feedings.

Parenteral nutrition. This method, in which nutrients are administered by the I.V. route, may be required by the preterm or postsurgical neonate who cannot tolerate oral or enteral feedings. Parenteral nutrition requirements depend on birth weight and diagnosis. For many high-risk neonates, a solution of dextrose 5% or 10% in water (80 to 100 ml/kg/day) is initiated in the delivery room or soon after transfer to the NICU. Electrolytes typically are added to the solution 24 hours after delivery; the most commonly administered electrolytes are sodium and potassium chloride.

Monitor urine and serum glucose levels carefully during parenteral nutrition to prevent glycosuria and hyperglycemia; if these conditions develop, expect to reduce the dextrose concentration. For the preterm neonate, hyperglycemia is confirmed by a glucose oxidase dipstick or heelstick glucose value above 150 mg/100 ml.

If the neonate will not be fed orally for more than 3 days, expect the physician to order total parenteral nutrition (TPN), which provides adequate carbohydrates, amino acids, lipids, glucose, vitamins, and electrolytes for growth and development. When caring for the neonate who is receiving TPN, monitor the serum glucose level with a glucose oxidase dipstick and the urine glucose level with a copper reduction tablet or glucose oxidase dipstick. Obtain hematocrit and serum electrolyte and urea levels to assess how well the neonate is tolerating TPN. (Required laboratory values vary from one facility to another; however, expect to obtain calcium, phosphate, magnesium, alkaline phosphate, protein, and transaminase levels at least weekly.)

Any substance with a dextrose concentration above 12.5% must be administered via a central line (such as an umbilical vessel catheter); peripheral administration of fluids with a higher dextrose concentration can cause tissue swelling, necrosis, and cellular death at the infusion site. When administering parenteral nutrition via a central line, maintain meticulous aseptic technique and clean the infusion site according to facility protocol to minimize the risk of contamination. Also make sure the line remains intact to prevent the introduction of organisms that may cause systemic infection. Keep the dressing over the insertion site occlusive; if it appears loose, change it immediately.

In some facilities, blood cultures and cultures from the infusion site are obtained routinely; in others, cultures are required only if infection is suspected. With the extremely preterm neonate, who has limited vascular volume, avoid obtaining blood cultures unless an infection is suspected.

Maintaining fluid and electrolyte balance

Renal immaturity, small fluid reserves, a high metabolic rate, and pronounced insensible fluid losses make even the normal, healthy neonate susceptible to fluid and electrolyte imbalance. Perinatal problems—especially those causing diarrhea, vomiting, or high fever—and surgery can further upset fluid balance in the high-risk neonate, leading to a nursing diagnosis of *fluid volume deficit related to renal immaturity or increased fluid loss.*

Both clinical and environmental conditions influence fluid requirements. For example, congenital heart failure (CHF), certain renal disorders, and use of a thermal blanket or mist tent reduce the fluid requirement. On the other hand, the neonate who is receiving phototherapy has a greater need for fluid, as does one with respiratory distress or blood loss. Likewise, use of a radiant warmer increases fluid needs by enhancing insensible fluid losses. After surgery, a neonate is particularly vulnerable to fluid volume deficit—not only is hypovolemia a natural response to surgery, but the neonate loses blood during surgery and loses insensible fluids in the cool, dry operating room. To counter environmental conditions that promote insensible fluid loss, provide an NTE whenever possible.

I.V. fluid requirements for the high-risk neonate range from 60 to 150 ml/kg/day. To maintain fluid balance, give sufficient fluids to maintain a urine output of about 1 ml/kg/hour and a specific gravity of 1.005 to 1.012. However, if gastric compression is used, give additional fluids, as prescribed, to counter gastric fluid losses.

Measure fluid intake and urine output hourly for each shift, and at 24-hour intervals by using a urine collection bag or by weighing diapers. Weigh the neonate daily, using the same scale if possible, and compare fluid intake to output for each shift and at 24-hour intervals. Also monitor laboratory data (hematocrit, blood pH, and serum electrolyte, blood urea nitrogen, creatinine, and uric acid levels) to evaluate acid-base status. Assess urine specific gravity with each voiding or at least every 4 hours.

Stay alert for signs of fluid deficit and fluid excess; the latter is most likely with a cardiac or renal problem. (For signs of fluid deficit and excess, see *Assessing fluid status.*)

Assess the neonate's electrolyte status by monitoring serum electrolyte levels. As a general rule, serum sodium should approximate 133 to 146 mmol/liter; serum cal-

---

ASSESSING FLUID STATUS

Various factors place the high-risk neonate in danger of fluid imbalance—particularly fluid volume deficit. To assess for fluid volume deficit or excess, check for the signs listed below.

Signs of fluid volume deficit (dehydration)
- Dry mucous membranes
- Elevated hematocrit, hemoglobin level, and blood urea nitrogen value
- Increasing heart and respiratory rates
- Low-grade fever
- Poor skin turgor
- Slightly decreased blood pressure
- Sunken eyeballs or fontanels
- Urine output less than 1 ml/kg/hour
- Urine specific gravity above 1.013
- Weight loss

Signs of fluid volume excess (overhydration)
- Chronic cough
- Crackles
- Dyspnea
- Edema
- Increasing central venous pressure
- Rhonchi
- Tachypnea
- Urine output exceeding 5 ml/kg/hour

---

cium, 9.0 to 11.6 mg/dl; serum potassium, 4.6 to 6.7 mmol/liter; and serum chloride, 100 to 117 mmol/liter.

Preventing and controlling infection

Nearly all high-risk neonates have a nursing diagnosis of *high risk for infection related to immunologic immaturity, altered ventilation, ineffective airway clearance, or frequent invasive procedures.* Consequently, take the following precautions to help minimize the risk of infection.

Practice meticulous hand washing. Scrub for 3 minutes before entering the nursery and wash hands frequently throughout caregiving activities. After providing care for each neonate, perform a 1-minute scrub.

Pay meticulous attention to asepsis during all care procedures. Maintain sterile technique during invasive procedures, such as suctioning and drawing blood from arterial lines. As permitted by facility protocol, use triple-dye alcohol or an antimicrobial agent when caring for the umbilical cord and any puncture sites.

Make sure all equipment used for neonatal care is sterile or has been cleaned thoroughly. A stethoscope should be assigned to each neonate to prevent cross-contamination, and health care providers should refrain from using their own equipment when providing neonatal care.

Avoid wearing rings and other jewelry. Many facilities also prohibit nursery staff from using hand lotions, which serve as a breeding ground for pathogenic organisms.

Wear gloves and follow other universal precautions when changing diapers and performing other activities involving contact with body secretions.

If an I.V. line is in place, document the appearance of the I.V. site every 30 minutes to 1 hour, depending on the solution being given. If redness or swelling appears, indicating infiltration, the infusion site may have to be changed. However, never stop a glucose or calcium infusion abruptly without immediately restarting it because this may cause serum glucose or calcium levels to fluctuate widely.

When bathing the neonate, use mild soap and wash only creases and soiled areas. Avoid harsh chemicals, such as alcohol and povidone-iodine, and carefully rinse the neonate's skin after using any irritating substance.

Maintain an intact skin barrier—especially if the neonate has a nursing diagnosis of *potential impaired skin integrity related to frequent invasive procedures*—by using as little tape as possible to secure I.V. catheters, urine collection containers, feeding tubes, and other equipment (tape removal may peel off the epidermis). Also, first apply an adhesive removal pad when removing ECG leads.

To help prevent pressure-point breakdown, change the neonate's position, provide range-of-motion exercises, and place the neonate on sheepskin or a waterbed. Assess the skin for redness (especially over bony prominences), which indicates poor circulation to the reddened area. To guard against skin tears and scrapes when turning or moving the neonate, apply a protective transparent covering over elbows, knees, and other vulnerable joints.

Evaluate all visitors for signs of infection. Any staff member with active herpes simplex lesions (those that have not reached the crusting stage) should refrain from working in the nursery. Even after lesions have crusted, the person should wear gloves and wash hands before and after contact.

To detect infection early, assess the neonate regularly for such systemic signs as hypothermia or hyperthermia, lethargy, jaundice, petechiae, respiratory distress, purulent drainage from the eyes or umbilical site, and subtle behavioral changes. Also check for signs of localized infection from the umbilical and I.V. sites.

If the neonate has potential signs of infection, place in an incubator and, if possible, an isolation room to protect other neonates. Expect the physician to prescribe prophylactic antibiotics (typically ampicillin and gentamicin)

and a septic workup, which routinely includes cultures of blood, cerebrospinal fluid (CSF), and urine; a chest X-ray; serum electrolyte analysis; and a complete blood count (CBC) with differential.

Once culture and sensitivity test results determine the infectious organism, the physician may change the antibiotic prescribed; in most cases, a combination of antibiotics is used. If the physician prescribes gentamicin, expect to obtain peak and trough serum blood levels after the third dose to detect or prevent adverse drug reactions; obtain a trough level 30 minutes before administering the next dose and a peak level 30 to 45 minutes afterward, as ordered. Antibiotic therapy typically continues for 10 days, with reevaluation at the end of the course.

During antibiotic therapy, assess the neonate for signs of drug-induced nerve damage, including palsy, decreased arm or leg mobility, and tremors; also check for behavioral changes, which could signal decreased tolerance of antibiotic therapy. Monitor fluid intake and output every 4 to 8 hours, and notify the physician if output falls below normal.

For a group B streptococcal infection, monitor blood pressure, including mean arterial pressure. Decreasing blood pressure may warrant administration of plasma protein fraction to expand blood volume and correct the shock response resulting from this infection. Unless immediate aggressive interventions begin, this infection carries a mortality rate as high as 90% (Nelson, Merenstein, and Pierce, 1986).

Providing developmental care and environmental support

Research from the past 20 years shows that the neonate is aware of surroundings and responds to sensory stimulation. Within the past decade, health care providers increasingly have aimed to establish a developmentally appropriate environment for the high-risk neonate by reducing detrimental stimulation, providing appropriate stimulation during caregiving activities, and teaching parents how to provide appropriate stimulation.

To reduce environmental noise, for example, eliminate loud music and loud talking near the neonate and make sure doors, trash-can bottoms, and incubator portholes are padded. Also, dim the lights and minimize handling of the neonate. When trying to arouse the neonate, use a soft voice and call the neonate by name.

For the neonate with a nursing diagnosis of *altered growth and development related to functional immaturity, prolonged environmental stress, and lack of stimulation appropriate for gestational age and physical status*, nursing interventions include:

- initiating direct-care procedures only when the neonate is alert
- providing rest periods between activities
- encouraging parents to interact with the neonate in ways that promote optimal development
- providing tactile, auditory, visual, and vestibular stimulation (handling) according to the neonate's tolerance. Activities that provide such stimulation include gentle stroking, caressing (especially during feeding), talking, singing, calling the neonate by name, playing a tape of the parents' voices, promoting eye contact with visitors, displaying pictures and designs near the neonate, holding the neonate in a ventral (face-down) position during burping, and stroking the back until the neonate burps. Also, continually assess the neonate's response to stimulation.

Ensuring preoperative and postoperative care

For the neonate who requires surgery, preoperative nursing care includes monitoring vital signs, maintaining a patent airway, assessing respiratory status, ensuring fluid balance, and maintaining adequate nutrition (as with enteral or parenteral feedings). Depending on the neonate's specific problems, other measures may be warranted—for example, providing gastric decompression via a nasogastric tube; preventing trauma, heat loss, and infection at a defect site (such as with encephalocele or gastroschisis); and administering broad-spectrum antibiotics.

After surgery, check vital signs for the first 24 hours—every 15 minutes for the first hour, every 30 minutes for the next 2 hours, every hour for the next 4 hours, then every 2 hours. Maintain patency of the airway and any airway tubes by suctioning frequently and checking for signs of respiratory distress. Support oxygenation and ventilation by giving supplemental oxygen or maintaining mechanical ventilation, as appropriate, and by turning the neonate from side to side every few hours.

Ensure fluid and electrolyte balance by monitoring fluid intake and output and checking serum electrolyte levels. If the neonate must be fed through a gastrostomy tube, give feedings by slow gravity drip. If possible, have the neonate suck on a pacifier to stimulate the sucking and swallowing reflexes.

Maintain skin integrity at the surgical site by cleaning frequently (as specified by facility protocol) and observing for signs of infection, such as skin breakdown, erythema, edema, or bloody or purulent drainage. To prevent disruption of the suture line, use restraints if necessary.

If a nasogastric tube is present for postoperative gastric decompression (to prevent stress on the surgical site), tape the tube to the neonate's face. Irrigate the tube frequently to ensure patency and drainage, and connect it to low-intermittent suction.

If a chest tube is present, check for patency of the system by observing for a consistent flow of bubbles in the underwater seal container. Auscultate breath sounds frequently; diminishing breath sounds may signal a developing pneumothorax.

If a colostomy was performed (as with certain GI defects), check the amount, color, and consistency of stools. When changing dressings, avoid applying undue friction when cleaning around the stoma. Check for skin breakdown and bleeding near the stoma.

For the neonate recovering from surgery for a neurologic anomaly, check neurologic status frequently by assessing pupil size and response, level of consciousness, behavior and activity levels, motor function, and firmness of fontanels. Also evaluate for signs of increased intracranial pressure (such as lethargy, a high-pitched cry, and sunset eyes) and measure head circumference daily. Monitor fluid intake and output and observe extremities for mottling and poor capillary refill.

After surgery for a cardiac anomaly, frequently assess vital signs, breath sounds, and results of ABG analysis and blood tests (especialy hematocrit and hemoglobin values). Maintain electronic cardiorespiratory monitoring and assess urine output hourly.

Carrying out special procedures

Many high-risk neonates require phototherapy or exchange transfusion to treat hyperbilirubinemia; a few require extracorporeal membrane oxygenation (ECMO). General nursing measures during phototherapy and exchange transfusions focus on maintaining body temperature, proper timing of care to avoid unnecessary stress, and assessing oral intake, urine output, and stools. With any of the procedures described in this section, observe the neonate closely for respiratory compromise. The neonate with hyperbilirubinemia is at risk for asphyxia and respiratory distress; the neonate who requires ECMO commonly has preexisting respiratory distress.

Phototherapy. In this procedure, used to treat hyperbilirubinemia, the neonate is placed unclothed approximately 18″ under a bank of lights for several hours or days until the serum bilirubin level drops to within acceptable limits. Phototherapy lights decompose bilirubin in the skin through oxidation, facilitating biliary excretion of unconjugated bilirubin.

To prevent retinal damage, an opaque mask must be placed over the neonate's eyes. Make sure that the mask is tight enough to stay in place but not so tight that it impedes circulation or puts pressure on the eyeballs (direct pressure may cause reflex bradycardia). Also keep the genitals covered with a mask or small diaper to catch urine and stool while leaving the skin surface open to the light. Observe for signs of pressure caused by eye and genital coverings. Turn the neonate every 2 hours to relieve pressure on the knees, hips, and other joints and to allow exposure of all skin surfaces.

Turn off the phototherapy lights for 2 to 5 minutes at least every 8 hours to assess the eyes for irritation or redness and help the neonate establish a normal sleep-awake pattern (phototherapy may lengthen sleep). Monitor the number and consistency of stools; bilirubin breakdown increases gastric motility, resulting in loose stools that can cause skin excoriation and breakdown. Be sure to clean the neonate's buttocks after each stool to help maintain skin integrity.

Check the serum bilirubin level every 4 to 8 hours as ordered to determine if phototherapy is effective, and frequently assess skin and sclera color to check the degree of jaundice. Also estimate fluid losses and check for dehydration, which occurs as GI hypermotility pulls fluids into the intestines; if dehydration occurs, notify the physician. To minimize insensible fluid losses, place the neonate in an incubator if possible, and provide I.V. fluids, as prescribed.

Complete exchange transfusion. Hyperbilirubinemia that does not respond to phototherapy may necessitate a complete exchange transfusion. In this procedure, the neonate's blood is removed via an umbilical catheter and replaced with fresh whole donor blood to remove the unconjugated bilirubin in the serum. The procedure carries a risk of transfusion reaction and subsequent death.

To minimize the risk of cardiovascular complications, isovolumetric exchange transfusion may be used. In this method, both the umbilical vein and umbilical artery are catheterized. A three-way stopcock is placed at the end of each catheter and a syringe is connected to the arterial catheter at the junction of the stopcock; the arterial catheter serves as the site for blood withdrawal. After the neonate's blood is withdrawn, warmed whole blood is administered via the venous catheter.

In the most common isovolumetric technique, 5 to 10 ml of the neonate's blood are removed and the same amount of warmed donor blood administered via the venous catheter over at least 2 minutes. Withdrawing or administering blood at a faster rate may lead to life-threatening arrhythmias. Half-way through the exchange transfusion, calcium gluconate is administered to prevent hypocalcemia and consequent cardiac irritability.

The procedure takes 1 to 2 hours, depending on the volume of blood exchanged and the neonate's condition. (The volume of blood to be exchanged typically is calculated by multiplying kilograms of body weight by 180 ml.) An exchange transfusion may be repeated if the serum bilirubin level continues to rise.

For several hours before an exchange transfusion, withhold oral intake to decrease the risk of aspirating saliva or feeding matter (the neonate must be strapped into a supine position during the procedure, increasing the risk of aspiration). Also obtain a blood sample for laboratory analysis of the total and conjugated serum bilirubin levels, as ordered.

Donor blood should be checked by two staff members to verify that it is the correct blood. During the transfusion, vital signs are assessed every 5 to 15 minutes; a running total of the amount of blood administered and withdrawn is kept. The best way to accomplish this is for an assistant to call out the amounts—for example, by stating "5 ml of blood out" and "5 ml of blood in." The exact time of blood administration and withdrawal should be documented. The heart and respiratory rates displayed on the monitor should be noted and the cardiac monitor observed for arrhythmias, which may signal poor tolerance of the transfusion.

When the procedure is completed and the catheter is withdrawn, assess the infusion site for bleeding; expect to transfer the neonate to the phototherapy unit. For the next several hours, monitor the neonate closely for signs of complications, such as metabolic acidosis, hypothermia, circulatory overload, electrolyte disturbances, air embolism, arrhythmias, infection, and hypoglycemia.

Check serum bilirubin levels every 4 to 8 hours as ordered to determine if the exchange transfusion was effective. (Always draw blood with the phototherapy lights off to prevent misleading laboratory results.) Approximately 4 hours after the transfusion, check serum electrolyte and glucose levels; if these levels are below normal, a corrective I.V. solution may be ordered.

ECMO. In major neonatal centers, ECMO may be used to maintain gas exchange and perfusion during preoperative management of diaphragmatic hernia or for selected neonates with refractory respiratory failure or meconium aspiration syndrome (MAS). In this technique, the neonate's blood is oxygenated outside the body through an arterial shunt to maintain ventilation and oxygenation; this permits cardiopulmonary recovery at low FiO$_2$ levels and ventilator settings.

In the neonate, ECMO usually involves venoarterial bypass, in which a cannula is inserted into the right atrium via the right internal jugular vein and the aortic arch is cannulated via the right common carotid artery. Blood circulates through tubing via a pumping device, then through a membrane oxygenator. After blood is oxygenated, it flows through a heating device and into the carotid cannula. The neonate continues on mechanical ventilation during ECMO, with ventilator settings reduced to the minimum level required.

A specially trained nurse perfusionist typically manages the neonate during ECMO, drawing blood samples for ABG analysis hourly from the neonate and at specified intervals from the ECMO circuit. This nurse also monitors laboratory values (including CBC, platelet count, hemoglobin, hematocrit, and serum electrolytes) and adjusts the heparin drip, as needed, to maintain optimal clotting times.

The nurse assigned to the neonate should change the neonate's position and check vital signs frequently. Weigh dressings under the neonate's neck and assess for blood leakage at the cannulation site. Be sure to monitor fluid intake and output and $tcPO_2$ or pulse oximetry readings frequently. Also, check neurologic status hourly; suction the endotracheal tube and collect tracheal aspirate, as prescribed.

Supporting the family and promoting parent-infant bonding

The birth of a critically ill neonate creates a crisis for family members. Provide emotional support to the family throughout the neonate's stay but especially during each parent's first visit to the NICU—a potentially overwhelming experience. Explain the use of monitors and other supportive equipment to lessen the intimidating effect these machines can have. To help the parents adjust to their child's appearance, emphasize the neonate's normal features.

The parents may be especially anxious if their child is being cared for in a regional center located far from their home. For the family with a nursing diagnosis of *potential altered parenting related to the neonate's condition, difficulty coping with a less-than-perfect neonate, and enforced separation,* make sure to keep communications open and pay special attention to the family's needs. Encourage the parents to visit frequently; if this is not possible, ask them to keep in touch with the NICU staff by telephone. Give them the names and telephone numbers of the physician, primary nurse, social worker, and other contact persons.

To promote parent-infant bonding, encourage the parents to contribute to their child's environment by attaching a small family item, such as a family photograph, to the neonate's bed. Allow the parents to touch and hold

their child whenever possible and provide them with simple caregiving tasks, such as diaper changes. Point out how their child responds to their presence, voice, and touch, and show them how to offer appropriate sensory stimulation so that they can take an active role in their child's development—a measure that enhances their self-esteem.

If the neonate's problem has an underlying genetic cause, refer the parents for genetic testing, as appropriate. Throughout nursing care, consider the neonate's discharge planning needs to ease the transition to the home.

EVALUATION

During this step of the nursing process, the nurse evaluates the effectiveness of the care plan by ongoing evaluation of subjective and objective criteria. Evaluation findings should be stated in terms of actions performed or outcomes achieved for each goal. The following examples illustrate appropriate evaluation statements for the high-risk neonate:

• The neonate's vital signs improved.
• The neonate maintained an adequate core temperature.
• The neonate's cardiopulmonary status improved or remained within acceptable limits.
• The neonate maintained fluid and electrolyte balance, as evidenced by adequate urine output, no signs of dehydration or fluid overload, and acceptable serum electrolyte levels.
• The neonate tolerated feedings.
• The I.V. infusion site remained free of signs of infiltration.
• Skin integrity remained intact.
• The neonate's parents showed positive coping mechanisms in response to their child's problem.
• The neonate's parents know how to obtain appropriate counseling and support.

For the neonate who underwent surgery, these additional evaluation statements may be appropriate:

• The neonate's vital signs remained normal.
• No signs of postoperative complications appeared.
• The suture line remained intact.
• The incision site remained clean and free of redness or swelling.

DOCUMENTATION

All steps of the nursing process should be documented as thoroughly and objectively as possible. Thorough documentation not only allows the nurse to evaluate the effectiveness of the care plan, but it also makes this information available to other members of the health care team, helping to ensure consistency of care.

Documentation for the high-risk neonate should include:
• vital signs and alertness level
• changes in status
• serum bilirubin, calcium, and glucose levels
• fluid intake and output
• stool characteristics
• tolerance for feedings
• location and appearance of any I.V. infusion site
• presence of any gastric distention
• presence of an indwelling nasogastric tube
• amount and appearance of secretions obtained by suctioning
• tolerance for medical and nursing procedures
• parents' level of acceptance of their child's problem.

For the neonate receiving phototherapy, documentation also should include:
• number of stools
• skin turgor
• skin and sclera color
• amount and color of urine.

For the neonate who underwent exchange transfusion, documentation also should include:
• tolerance for the procedure
• neurologic status.

For the neonate who underwent surgery, documentation also should include:
• preoperative and postoperative vital signs
• the time when feedings were instituted
• tolerance for feedings
• respiratory effort
• appearance and amount of drainage from the incision site
• appearance of the suture line
• presence of bladder distention
• need for Credé's maneuver.

NURSING CARE OF THE FAMILY

To the family, the birth of a high-risk neonate may seem like a tragedy. Over the course of the pregnancy, they built expectations of a child whose features would reflect their own, whose abilities they could nurture, and whose interests they would share. With the neonate's birth, the family experiences the loss of the "perfect" child of their dreams. They must deal with that loss and the grief it causes and find ways of adjusting their expectations and plans to match the reality of the child born to them.

Because of the enormity of a perinatal loss, parents and other family members must adapt slowly to the situation – or experience overwhelming anxiety and pain. The degree of parental feelings of grief do not correlate with the severity of the neonate's condition (Benefield, Leib, and Reuter, 1976).

Before the family can accept their loss, they must progress through several stages of grief. Various researchers and theorists have developed concepts of grieving. Among the most influential is that of Kübler-Ross (1969), who proposed that a person encountering death or another type of loss progresses through five stages: denial, anger, bargaining, depression, and acceptance. Sahu (1981) and other authorities apply these stages specifically to perinatal loss. Based on studies by Bowlby (1961) and Parkes (1970) as well as on original research, thanatologist Glen Davidson (1984) describes four phases, or dimensions, of grief that survivors of loss may move among: shock and numbness, yearning and searching, disorientation, and reorganization.

Regardless of the grief model used, the nurse should regard the stages of grief as descriptive rather than clearly defined. Rather than progressing through the stages in an orderly manner, the parents and other family members may experience aspects of several stages at once or may regress to a stage previously experienced.

ASSESSMENT

During the assessment, the nurse should keep in mind the various stages of grief; this helps identify the family's need for practical and emotional support. Because parents usually are the family members most closely involved with the neonate, this chapter focuses mainly on them. However, the nurse should not overlook the neonate's siblings, grandparents, and other close family members.

Assessing the parents
Already upset by the arrival of a high-risk neonate, parents may feel further stress within the NICU, with its sophisticated equipment, flashing monitors, buzzing alarms, and hurrying staff members. For this reason, the nurse should try to conduct the assessment in a quiet, unhurried, and straightforward manner.

Assessment of the parents should include the following:
• age, experience as parents, and history of previous childbirths
• understanding of and feelings about the neonate's condition
• concerns about the neonate's care
• family and home care arrangements

• response to the NICU
• grieving behavior and coping mechanisms.

Age, experience, and history. Find out the parents' age and their experience as parents. Young or first-time parents may have little experience dealing with illness. Especially if they are young enough to require parenting themselves, they may feel particularly inadequate about coping with a high-risk neonate.

Ask about any family history of problem pregnancies or deliveries. Parents who have experienced a previous perinatal illness or death may fear or believe that the past problem and this one are related. Even if their anxiety is inappropriate, it may impair their ability to cope with their neonate. On the other hand, parents whose earlier pregnancies and deliveries were problem-free may have trouble accepting that this delivery has produced a high-risk neonate.

To determine whether genetic counseling might be advisable eventually, look for indications of a genetic cause for the neonate's condition. Ask about the presence, in this or previous generations, of such conditions as inherited disorders, metabolic disorders, or chromosomal disorders. Even if parents are not aware of any history of these problems, such a condition in the neonate suggests a genetic link.

Understanding and feelings. Ask the parents what they understand about their child's condition and how it makes them feel. Although grief and anxiety are natural reactions to the delivery of a neonate who is preterm or born with a severe illness or an obvious physical anomaly, parents may feel perinatal loss for other reasons as well. Because of the value society places on physical beauty, any physical irregularity may cause great anxiety. Knowing the cause of the parents' grief is essential in planning interventions to help them deal with it; even if their grief seems out of proportion, it is real and must be addressed. Here and throughout the assessment, stay alert for signs of stress developing between the parents.

Concerns about care of the neonate and its effects. To determine where counseling and teaching can decrease anxiety, explore the parents' feelings about their ability to care for their child. They may express doubt about being able to care for their child at home and may worry about financial consequences of giving up work days to spend time with their child and about long-term medical expenses.

Also look and listen for signs of emotional discomfort. A parent who feels anxious and powerless may have trouble absorbing and putting into practice information about caregiving. A parent who hesitates to participate in simple neonatal care may be establishing emotional distance from the neonate.

Family and home care arrangements. Ask the parents about arrangements they have made for care of other children at home and other family concerns. Even parents who have made adequate care arrangements may worry that they are short-changing their other children. Assess whether they need help allocating their time or arranging care for the children.

Also ask them how their other children are responding to the birth of a high-risk neonate. Under these circumstances, an older child's relationship with the parents may change (Trahd, 1986). However, parents may not be aware of this in the first days and weeks, when the neonate holds so much of their attention. Most parents probably realize that siblings are likely to feel neglected or jealous because of the disruptions in routine and the time parents spend at the NICU. However, parents may not be aware of other feelings the high-risk neonate may evoke, including fear and guilt that they somehow are responsible for the neonate's illness. Asking what responses parents have noticed may help them relate better with their other children and also will help focus teaching plans for preparing the neonate's siblings to visit the NICU.

Response to the NICU. Find out what previous experience the parents have had with health care facilities. The less experience they have, or the less recent their experience, the more unsettling they may find the NICU and the more help they may need in understanding that many of the procedures and equipment that seem extraordinary actually are routine.

The apparent ease with which the NICU staff functions may increase parents' doubts about their own ability to provide care, especially if no one explains what is happening and why. To plan ways to make parents more comfortable in the NICU, ask how much they understand about the equipment being used to help their child and invite questions about the care being given.

Also assess the effect of the NICU location on the developing parent-infant bond and on the relationship between the parents. For most parents, the ideal situation is an NICU located within the mother's obstetric unit. Here, both parents can visit the neonate in the first few days after delivery with little or no trouble. However, if the neonate must be transferred to a distant tertiary care center, only the father may be able to visit for the first several days. Ask whether the mother was able to spend time with the neonate before the transfer and what effect the transfer has had on each parent. Particularly if the mother did not see the neonate before the transfer, she may feel isolated and resentful of the father's greater contact (Consolvo, 1984); the father, meanwhile, may feel uncomfortable in the primary parent role in which circumstances have placed him.

If the NICU is relatively far from the home, neither parent may be able to visit frequently. Assess for signs that the parents' lack of physical contact is delaying parent-infant bonding. Without such bonding, their interest and motivation may not be strong enough to meet their child's long-term needs.

Grieving behavior and coping mechanisms. Throughout the neonate's hospitalization, parents typically exhibit signs of grief. Determine each parent's grief stage. Keep in mind that grief expression may depend somewhat on cultural background, but avoid drawing conclusions based on culture alone. (For more information on grief expression, see Cultural Considerations: *Variations in grief expression.*)

Also determine which coping mechanism each parent is using – denial, anger, guilt, intellectualizing, or withdrawal. (Remember, though, that coping mechanisms may vary from day to day or even moment to moment.) Accurately identifying the coping mechanisms that parents use is crucial to planning nursing interventions that respond to their needs.

To assess for denial, look for signs that parents are denying the reality of the neonate's condition. Normally, parents move beyond denial on their own, so assess for signs that this transition is occurring; if it is not, they may require help.

If parents exhibit anger or hostility (such as toward the health care team), assess for any misunderstanding of the neonate's condition. Keep in mind that angry parents usually are reacting to the situation and rarely feel real hostility toward health care personnel.

Clues that a parent is using guilt to cope include such obvious statements as, "It's all my fault" as well as more subtle indications, such as utterances beginning with "If only I . . ." In guilt statements, listen for misunderstandings of the causes of the neonate's condition.

Parents who focus on the cause of their child's condition more than on the neonate as a person are using intellectualizing as a coping mechanism. These parents may ask many questions about their child's treatment and seem hesitant to focus on the child.

Assess for withdrawal by observing how the parents relate to their child. Withdrawn parents may not touch or hold their child or may look away while doing so.

CULTURAL CONSIDERATIONS

VARIATIONS IN GRIEF EXPRESSION

To evaluate grieving behavior accurately in a family that has experienced or anticipates a neonate's death, the nurse must be aware of any cultural customs that may affect grief expression. However, the nurse should assess carefully before drawing conclusions. Although some cultures are associated with characteristic grieving behaviors, practices change over time. Also, a person born into one culture but socialized in another may be influenced by elements of both.

Black Americans, Mexican Americans, and Arabs tend to display grief openly. Chinese and Japanese cultures frown on public display of emotion; consequently, members of a traditional Chinese or Japanese family may not respond to the nurse's encouragement to communicate their feelings, although they may grieve quietly at home. Members of certain Native American tribes also may not express grief openly. Also, some may refuse to visit a dying neonate out of fear of modern medicine or "evil spirits" (York and Stichler, 1985).

Some Hispanic cultures regard public expression of grief as acceptable for the mother but not the father, in whom such expression is considered a sign of weakness. (Of course, such attitudes may show up in any family, regardless of culture.) In a few cultures, handling of the body is part of the formalized expression of grief.

In certain Asian cultures, where one does not give up hope for survival until death has occurred, anticipatory grief (sadness in anticipation of a neonate's expected death) is considered inappropriate (Manio and Hall, 1987). Also, not all cultures perceive a neonate's death as a tragic event (York and Stichler, 1985). For example, in Korean tradition, more concern is focused on the parents than on the dead neonate; as adults, the parents are considered more important members of the family and society than the neonate, whose life had just begun (Choi, 1986).

Although both individual and culturally shaped expressions of grief deserve respect and support, family members occasionally need guidance to avoid manifestations or attitudes that might harm themselves or others. For example, in some Asian cultures, the mother may be blamed for causing the neonate's condition by something she did or ate (Manio and Hall, 1987); in such a case, the nurse and physician must do their best to help the mother and family understand the true cause and to dissolve any feelings of guilt or blame.

The following religious beliefs can affect the amount of grief family members feel and the practices they follow after a neonate's death:
• belief in an afterlife
• acceptance of death as God's will
• belief that the soul returns to the ancestors or reincarnates in another body
• belief that spirits control illness and death
• belief in the value of religious rituals for the dead.

Assessing support systems

Coping with the birth of a high-risk neonate is not something that one parent – or even both – can handle alone. Parents need help from various sources.

Family and friends. For most parents, the first line of support comes from within the family. In a two-parent family, the partners typically form each other's base of support. If one parent is unavailable – for example, as in the case of a single mother – another family member or a close friend may assume the support role. Assess parents to determine which family members or close friends make up their support base and how nursing care can assist the supporters.

Ask about the relationship between the neonate's parents and grandparents. In many cases, grandparents can provide both emotional and practical support.

Other support sources. Beyond the circle of family and friends, additional support may be available to parents through religious practices, cultural customs, and support groups consisting of other parents.

The birth of a high-risk neonate may pull the parents back to their religious roots. They may find comfort in speaking with a member of the clergy, reading scripture, or participating in religious services. Assess parents for their interest in seeing a chaplain or their own priest, minister, or rabbi. Ask whether they would like any religious practices to be observed for their neonate; members of some Christian churches, for example, may wish to have their child baptized. Even parents who might not think of asking for such support may use it if they know it is available.

If cultural identity is important to the family, they may derive additional support from observing traditional care customs with their child. In assessing cultural customs, however, bear in mind that although cultural norms exist, variations do occur. Also, the beliefs one generation holds to strongly may be less important to a second or third generation. Although an overall awareness of such beliefs is helpful, assess the parents for their own beliefs as individuals.

Begin the cultural assessment by asking about the main elements of values and beliefs the parents hold and the customs these values dictate regarding childbirth in general and the birth of a high-risk neonate in particular. Then focus on specific care concerns parents may want addressed.

Assess parents for their awareness of parent-to-parent support groups – including national organizations, local groups, and groups associated with the health care facility.

NURSING DIAGNOSIS

After gathering assessment data, the nurse must review it carefully to identify pertinent nursing diagnoses for the family. (For a partial list of applicable diagnoses, see Nursing Diagnoses: *High-risk neonates and their families,* page 426.)

PLANNING AND IMPLEMENTATION

The goal of nursing care is to help the family develop the understanding, skills, and confidence to give competent care after the neonate's discharge. Thus, the nurse should plan interventions to help them deal with the crisis of a high-risk neonate and to meet the neonate's needs. Such interventions should focus on the neonate's physical and developmental needs and the family's practical and emotional needs.

Whenever possible, involve family members in planning. This not only helps ensure that they can carry out the planned interventions, but it also makes them active participants in their child's care. Such involvement particularly helps the family with a nursing diagnosis of *powerlessness related to the health care environment and limited interaction with the neonate.*

Interventions for the family of a high-risk neonate fall into four main categories:
• providing information
• strengthening support systems
• teaching caregiving skills
• enhancing parent-infant bonding.

Depending on the neonate's status, the nurse also may need to help the family plan for their child's discharge or help them cope with their child's death.

Provide information

Two nursing diagnoses that apply to almost every family of a high-risk neonate are *knowledge deficit related to the hospital course and care of a high-risk neonate* and *anxiety related to the neonate's condition and unknown outcome.* Nursing care is essential in helping the family with either diagnosis. In many cases, the family relies mainly on the nurse – not just for information but for help in understanding that information. Although the physician initially may identify the neonate's medical condition to the parents and may speak with them regularly, the nurse typically provides daily reports and thus may be the person to whom parents turn with questions.

The more thorough the parents' understanding, the better equipped they will be to cope with the crisis and achieve the eventual goal of adequate caregiving at home.

To give them the most complete picture possible, cover the following topics:
• the neonate's medical condition, its cause (if known), and its long-term implications
• potential length of stay and probable course of treatment in the NICU
• ways parents can enhance their contact with their child
• ways parents can participate in their child's care.

Present, reinforce, and reinterpret. Such factors as familiarity with health care facilities, previous experience with health problems, and emotional state affect parents' ability to comprehend information the health care team gives them. Thus, adapt teaching strategies to parents' needs and assess the parents' comprehension frequently.

Especially during denial, the first stage of grief, parents may not absorb all the information they receive about their child's condition. Although parents with a nursing diagnosis of *ineffective denial related to the immediate and long-term implications of the neonate's condition* can be frustrating to work with, the problem arises from grief. Acknowledge the parents' feelings, but persist, presenting the information in small chunks and reinforcing it patiently. Eventually, parents will move beyond denial and begin to take in the facts.

Even after progressing past denial, parents may need help to grasp their child's condition fully. Try to be present whenever the physician talks with them, and review any new information with them afterward to clarify uncertainties and correct misunderstandings. Invite their questions, and encourage them to talk over what they have learned.

Once parents become hungry for information, they may seek it constantly—for example, in conversation with other parents with children in the NICU. Listen for such conversations, and intervene if necessary to clarify differences so that parents do not expect their child to have the same course of illness as another with a different diagnosis or maturity level.

In seeking information, parents' main concerns may differ from those of the health care team. For example, they may focus on their child's long-term problems before short-term problems have been overcome.

To give parents a clearer idea of neonatal care procedures, use any available illustrations or photographs. Also provide information booklets, written in lay terms, that address the neonate's condition. (Several national support groups, such as the March of Dimes, publish such booklets.) As they read this material at home, they may develop a better understanding of what they have been told.

Parents may need help in understanding what is happening to them emotionally. Explain that anxiety, fear, anger, and guilt are common among parents of high-risk neonates. To provide further reassurance and help them deal with their feelings, discuss the stages of grief.

Familiarize parents with the NICU. To most parents, the NICU is an alien and frightening environment. To make them feel more comfortable, describe the neonate's care routine, identifying each piece of equipment used and explaining its purpose. Be aware that anything attached to the neonate—even a temperature probe taped to the abdomen—may look threatening. If a new piece of equipment is introduced after the parents' first visit, explain its purpose and operation. Also encourage parents to enliven their child's surroundings with photographs or toys. If they have other children, suggest that they have the children draw pictures to tape near the neonate's incubator or crib. Be especially alert to the cultural customs of the family. (For further suggestions on personalizing the NICU, see Cultural Considerations: *Incorporating cultural customs into the neonate's care routine,* page 444.)

As far as possible, explain the probable course the neonate's treatment will take and the time that may be involved. Prepare parents for the chance that their child may need oxygen therapy or assisted ventilation at some point.

An insistent question among parents of high-risk neonates is whether their child will survive. A problem that the health care team regards as minor may seem to parents like a sign of impending death. While not playing down the likelihood of death if the neonate's condition is life-threatening, do not minimize the chance for survival, either. Advise parents that although the usual hospital course of a high-risk neonate is unstable at best, the health care team may be surprised by the amount of fight in even the smallest and sickest neonate.

For the parents with a nursing diagnosis of *potential altered parenting related to poor parent-infant bonding,* foster attachment and reduce anxiety by letting them know by frequent communication that they are welcome partners in their child's care. Even if the parents visit frequently, encourage them to phone daily. Initiate calls to them from time to time simply to give progress reports or to check with them about points brought up in their last visit. Include news of milestones achieved by their child, such as a weight gain, as well as a condition update.

If parents live so far away that daily phone calls are too costly, write them a note every few days to give them a sense of their child's course between one visit and the next. If possible, occasionally include a photograph of their child.

INCORPORATING CULTURAL CUSTOMS INTO THE NEONATE'S CARE ROUTINE

When caring for a client from a different culture, the nurse should keep the following considerations in mind.

Although nearly all parents feel intimidated during their first visit to the neonatal intensive care unit (NICU), those who have deep religious beliefs or belong to an ethnic group with strong cultural identity and traditional health practices may feel particularly uncomfortable. To help reduce their anxiety, the nurse should find out if their customs include any health-related practices (for example, folk remedies). Practices that pose no health threat, or that can be modified so they do not, can be incorporated fairly easily into the neonate's care routine.

For instance, to prevent the escape of spirits or the entrance of "bad air" into the body, mothers in some Hispanic cultures wrap their child in an abdominal binder or cover the umbilical stump with a coin (Zepeda, 1982). Neither custom can be permitted as is—the binder could restrict breathing or cause vomiting, and a coin covering an incompletely healed stump could cause infection. However, the nurse may suggest covering the stump with a dry, sterile dressing; if necessary, a cauterizing agent, such as silver nitrate, can be applied to heal the stump rapidly before the neonate's discharge.

Various folk remedies involve protection from evil spirits by such means as medallions, crosses, special clothes, prayer cards, and candles. If having such items near their child would comfort the parents, the nurse may tape them to the wall, hang them on the outside of the crib, or place them on a nearby table. As long as the candles remain unlit, even they can be placed near the neonate.

Parents with deep religious beliefs may welcome the opportunity to place devotional objects near their child. The nurse may tape religious medals or scapulars to an armboard, diaper, or crib frame or place pictures or books on a nearby table.

Strengthen support systems

The family of a high-risk neonate needs a tremendous amount of support. The nurse should plan interventions that help parents make good use of the support sources they know of and identify other potential sources.

Ensure that parents make the best possible use of familiar support systems by encouraging them to communicate with each other and by providing opportunities for them to discuss their feelings.

Even if the parents normally serve as each other's greatest source of emotional support, their ability to meet each other's needs may fall short in a crisis. Also, they may move through grief at vastly different rates. However, one parent may assume that the other is at the same stage; when that assumption proves wrong, anger and resentment on both sides may result. To counter this potential, urge them to keep communication open.

When parents visit their child, invite them to express their feelings. Such a comment as, "You must feel overwhelmed by all this" may release a flood of feelings. If one parent speaks but not the other, ask the silent parent what his or her reactions are.

Given an opening for honest discussion, parents may find common ground in their concerns and a sense of relief at not being alone. Even if they are not at the same stage of grief, one may be able to affirm the other's feelings as something he or she went through. If parents cannot reach common ground in their perceptions, urge them to find another family member—a grandparent, for example—who is understanding and supportive. Likewise, encourage a single parent to look to another family member or close friend for support.

Especially in the first few days after the neonate's birth, the parents' needs may differ. The mother, physically weakened and perhaps feeling isolated from other family members and from her child while in the maternity unit, may not have her usual control of her feelings. She may depend heavily on the father's visits for emotional support; between these visits, she may feel particularly alone. Even after her discharge, such feelings may persist because of her separation from her hospitalized child.

The father, too, needs support. The comfort he provides to the mother may drain his reserves. Should he believe he must be strong in crisis, he may be reluctant to reach out to other family members. His sense of isolation may increase further if friends and coworkers lack sympathy for any life-style changes he makes in response to family needs (Battles, 1988).

Each parent may feel so overwhelmed by the situation as to be unaware of the emotional drain made on the other. Help them open up to each other and discuss their feelings, which can strengthen understanding between them.

Also encourage parents to find time alone together—perhaps something as simple as a regular stop at a coffee shop on the way home from a visit to the NICU. Such an occasion, away from the pressures of home and hospital, may help them replenish their mental and emotional reserves.

Among the most important interventions by the nurse caring for the family of a high-risk neonate are those that promote interaction among all family members. The family can be the strongest source of support for individual family members in a crisis. Conversely, physical or emotional isolation of any one member from the rest may put tremendous stress on all members and on the family as a whole.

Unless their needs receive attention, siblings of a high-risk neonate may face lifelong problems in dealing with the changes such a birth creates. Communication problems may develop (Scheiber, 1989), and siblings may experience conflicting feelings about the neonate.

Besides helping parents balance the needs of the neonate and siblings for attention, make sure they are aware of the feelings siblings may be experiencing. For example, siblings may become fearful as they sense their parents' fear. If they are not old enough to understand the neonate's health problem or if no one explains it to them, they may fear "catching" the same ailment. In many cases, siblings fear that the neonate will take their mother away from them.

Siblings also may feel guilt over the neonate's condition. Not wanting to share the parents' attention with another child, for example, a sibling earlier may have wished that the birth would not occur and now may fear that the neonate's condition is a punishment for that wish. Preschool-age children, who believe that their thoughts have the power of actions (Gardner and Merenstein, 1989), are particularly likely to feel guilty.

Jealousy and anger may occur as siblings see how much of the parents' time and energy the neonate has captured. To regain some attention for themselves, they may display signs and symptoms similar to those of the ill neonate. If the siblings are staying with friends or relatives while the mother is hospitalized, they may be angry with the neonate for disrupting their home life.

Using terms the siblings can understand, explain to them the neonate's condition. Also, urge the parents to let siblings visit and care for the neonate and reassure them that their lives will not change drastically. (For more information about nursing interventions for siblings, see *Caring for the siblings of a high-risk neonate,* page 446.)

Let parents know that they are not expected to spend every possible moment with the neonate. Discuss with them their own needs and those of children at home, and help them set priorities for meeting these needs along with the neonate's.

For a family with a nursing diagnosis of *ineffective family coping: compromised, related to family disorganization secondary to the neonate's condition,* help parents explore ways of scheduling regular family time together at home and of making sure that birthdays and other special occasions are not neglected. Suggest, for example, that parents ask grandparents or other relatives to help with housekeeping chores so that when parents are home they can devote attention and energy to family interaction, not just to home care.

Help parents plan ways to include grandparents, siblings, and other family members in visits to the NICU. If the neonate is stable and the facility's physical layout and policies permit, suggest bringing the whole family together in a private area near the NICU. If no such area is available but sibling visits are permitted, family members can take turns visiting the neonate; the time they spend together in the waiting area may provide the chance for them to interact with and support one another. Grandparents and older, responsible siblings also may take part in the neonate's care.

Inform parents of support groups available within the facility, locally, and nationally. Many facilities with NICUs have parent or family support groups, organized by parents or the nursing or social services staff. Parent-to-parent support groups in particular can provide emotional support and practical advice. Parents who take part in these groups can discuss their concerns, learn how parents of neonates with similar problems have coped, and find out about available community resources. If an in-house support group is available, let parents know its meeting time and place.

National support groups include those tied to a specific problem, such as spina bifida, and those with a more general scope, such as the March of Dimes. Provide parents with names, addresses, and phone numbers for local chapters (or, if no local group exists, national headquarters). Many national groups provide practical help. For instance, the United Way and the March of Dimes may provide funding for medical care, equipment, and transportation for follow-up care. Encourage parents to talk with the facility's social worker about applying for such assistance.

Teach caregiving skills

To promote parenting skills and parent-infant bonding, the nurse should involve parents in their child's care. With few exceptions, parents can provide some care for even the sickest neonate (Kelting, 1986). Although some parents welcome the chance to do this, others express doubts. These doubts may reflect insecurity about their own abilities or reluctance to establish a relationship with the neonate. If parents are uncomfortable with the idea of becoming caregivers, recognize their fears and work toward overcoming them. To do this, begin with the simplest procedures and increase the parents' participation only as they indicate readiness.

To help the parents feel comfortable around their child, arrange for the neonate and parents to be together

CARING FOR THE SIBLINGS OF A HIGH-RISK NEONATE

Siblings of a high-risk neonate need special attention to make them feel like important family members. To help siblings cope with a visit to the neonatal intensive care unit (NICU) or the death of the neonate, the nurse may refer to the guidelines below.

When siblings visit the NICU

Many facilities permit siblings to visit the NICU in an effort to help them understand and feel more sympathetic about the neonate's special needs. Contrary to popular belief, sibling visits do not increase the incidence of infection in neonates (Wranesh, 1982); nor do siblings develop emotional problems from visiting (Consolvo, 1987).

Before the visit, siblings should be prepared through a joint teaching effort by the nurse and the parents. For preschoolers (ages 2 through 4), the nurse should concentrate on explaining basic information about the neonate's condition and the NICU in simple, direct terms. For children ages 5 and older, the scope can be widened to include possible ways their roles in the family may change (parents should offer specific ideas about this) and how they may be able to participate in the neonate's care. Parents may want to show older children how to perform simple caregiving tasks during their visit.

For siblings of any age, the nurse may suggest that they contribute an item to the neonate's environment—perhaps a drawing or toy—that can be placed near the neonate's crib. This helps siblings develop an attachment to the neonate and reinforces their own identity within the family.

Any time siblings visit, the nurse should make sure they have an opportunity afterward to express their thoughts and ask follow-up questions. The more matter-of-fact their understanding becomes, the better they will be able to cope and the less of a stranger the neonate will seem to them when the neonate is discharged.

Helping siblings cope with a neonate's death

Although children mourn when a neonate sibling dies, they do so differently from an adult. Even though they may feel sad, for instance, they may continue to play (Trouy and Ward-Larson, 1987). For various reasons—unresolved fears of abandonment, guilt over the neonate's death, and inability to understand their parents' expressions of grief—children typically have a harder time than adults in expressing grief. Consequently, they may need help in understanding what has happened and in dealing with it.

Although the nurse or social worker can provide advice and perhaps written materials to help siblings deal with death, the nurse should urge parents to take charge of explaining the neonate's death to siblings. Doing so can help parents regain confidence in their parenting ability (Gardner and Merenstein, 1989) and can reassure siblings that their parents still care and watch out for them.

In helping siblings understand a neonate's death, the nurse should keep in mind their limitations and needs. Preschoolers do not view death as permanent; no matter how often they are told that their little brother or sister is not coming back, the point may not sink in completely. Also, they may believe that a bad thought they had about the neonate caused the death. In contrast, school-age children may understand the permanence of death but probably will have many questions about death itself.

All children, but especially younger ones, may be shaken to see a parent crying. If this occurs, reassure them that grown-ups can feel sad and that letting the sadness out by crying or talking about it is beneficial.

Children may ask the same questions repeatedly, either because they need confirmation of what they were told or because some new angle for looking at the neonate's death and its consequences has occurred to them. All children have a basic need for clear, honest information about the neonate's death and for straightforward answers to their questions. Thus, the nurse and parents should avoid evasive explanations that the neonate has been "taken away" or "gone to sleep"; these explanations can create misunderstandings and nightmares that the same thing may happen to them.

---

as much as possible. Take the mother to the NICU as soon as she has recovered sufficiently from delivery; if the neonate's health status permits, let the mother hold as well as see her child for a few minutes. Encourage her to touch her child if she seems hesitant.

Whenever parents come to the NICU, help them feel physically close to their child—for instance, by arranging chairs to let them comfortably see and touch their child. When their child is in a quiet but alert state, in which interaction is least stressful, encourage the parents to use gentle touch to get acquainted. Try to provide privacy and minimize interruptions at this time.

As the neonate's condition permits, encourage the parents to perform basic care. For instance, if the neonate is stable, invite the parents to participate in feeding. Show

them how to hold their child during and after feeding, and explain how to perform simple mouth care. If the mother is considering breast-feeding, explain that giving breast milk may be beneficial physically and psychologically to her child and to her (Steele, 1987). Even if the neonate cannot suckle, the mother can provide breast milk she has pumped.

If the neonate must be gavage-fed, show the parents how to assist by holding the feeding tube or cylinder or by pouring the milk into the container. Invite them to supply a pacifier for their child to use between feedings.

Bathing the neonate can be a special time for parents. For the first bath with parents present, explain any special precautions they must take and encourage parents to watch their child respond to gentle touch; on future occasions, parents may give the bath with minimal supervision.

Diapering provides another opportunity for parents to strengthen their caregiving skills and perhaps also a chance to make some care decisions. Even if the neonate's fecal output must be monitored carefully, parents can change the diaper, weighing it themselves or saving it for a staff member to weigh. Offer parents their choice of several diaper ointments and creams, and encourage them to apply whatever they choose with a gentle touch.

As parents become more familiar with neonatal care needs, encourage them to rely less on staff supervision during caregiving—for example, suggest that they perform routine bottle- or breast-feeding on their own. The more successfully they function on their own as caregivers, the more confident they will feel when caring for their child at home.

An ideal way to enhance and evaluate parents' caregiving ability is to observe them as they care for their child. Such supervision also may decrease anxiety in parents before discharge and may prove particularly helpful if the neonate has complex care needs. Many facilities provide this experience by means of a care-by-parent unit. In this arrangement, one or both parents live with the neonate for 18 to 36 hours in a private room within or near the NICU.

To help parents participate in developmental care, which can reduce some physical and mental limitations resulting from high-risk birth, suggest that they bring in items that stimulate vision and hearing, such as brightly colored toys or mobiles, tape recordings of family members' voices, or toys that make soothingly rhythmic sounds. Devices that mimic the sound of the maternal heartbeat are especially effective in calming a fussy neonate.

Ask parents how they would like their child's daily care routine to be adjusted to give them maximum participation. For example, they may ask that bath time be set for when they can be present and routine medical procedures scheduled to avoid interfering with visiting time. Accommodate the parents' desires as much as possible; if something will not fit in, explain the problem to them.

Involve parents in decision making on as many levels as possible, both simple and complex. Even when the physician must make the final decision, help them to understand the options and the reason for the physician's choice so that they become partners in the decision.

Enhance parent-infant bonding

Parents whose neonate is critically ill or separated from them for long periods may show poor bonding with the neonate for several years (Plunkett, Meisels, Stiefel, Pasick, and Roloff, 1986). However, to withstand the rigors of caregiving for a high-risk neonate, they must develop a strong bond. The nurse can promote bonding by continuing to encourage frequent visiting, caregiving, phone calls, and other interaction. Also, give the parents the fullest possible picture of their child's characteristic behavior, including patterns of fussiness and wakefulness, so that they know what to expect once their child is discharged. Such advance knowledge minimizes strains on parent-infant bonding.

Plan for the neonate's discharge

As technological advances have increased survival rates, many high-risk neonates who only a few years ago would have lived hours or days now survive and eventually go home with their parents. However, some require complex, demanding, and expensive care for years—perhaps the rest of their lives. Nursing care for the family of a high-risk neonate should aim to ensure that the family will know how to provide this level of care. (For details on discharge planning, see Chapter 22, Discharge Planning and Care at Home.)

Preparation of the family for the neonate's discharge requires an evaluation of their concerns and any weaknesses in their caregiving ability. The nurse must look not only for the skills they demonstrate but for any persisting fears—understandable as they face the prospect of taking over care of a neonate whose life so far has been supported by advanced equipment. For example, they may fear that they will not recognize signs of a sudden downturn until too late.

To determine whether the family needs further nursing intervention before the neonate's discharge, evaluate the parents for their emotional and practical readiness to assume primary care. Discharge to a poorly prepared family could result in such problems as failure to thrive or abuse of the neonate by a family member.

Although careful teaching can prepare most parents to be effective caregivers, some parents need more than this. Carefully evaluate the parents' ability and motivation to care for their child, and inform the physician if they display any of the following behaviors as the neonate's discharge date nears:

• delay in arranging for medical-support equipment in the home
• infrequent calls or visits to the NICU
• apparent lack of interest in giving simple care to their child in the NICU.

Make sure parents understand which kinds of continuing care their child will require after discharge. For parents whose child is likely to remain technologically dependent for life, the availability of health services is a major concern—not just whether they exist but whether they are affordable and available nearby. Help parents identify facilities in their area that offer continuing support, and encourage them to enlist the social worker's help in applying for funds from institutional, governmental, and support-group sources.

Help the family deal with death

If the neonate has a poor prognosis or if death appears imminent, the nurse can help the family deal with the prospect of death as well as the event itself. Fetal loss and stillbirth also warrant special nursing interventions.

Perinatal death. The kinds of interventions family members need before and after a neonate's death depend somewhat on the relationship they have formed with the neonate and on the stage of grief they are in. To facilitate a healthy resolution of grief, carry out measures that help family members complete their bond with the neonate. Some family members experience a brief denial phase after the death of a high-risk neonate; others skip denial and show signs of anger, guilt, or despair.

Even if the parents have spent little time with their child, their emotional bond probably has been developing since pregnancy. To resolve their grief, they must complete their bonding with the neonate as their child and a member of their family, building memories to sustain them in the future.

To promote bonding, encourage the parents to name their child (if they have not done so already). As they look at the child, point out physical features that resemble those of family members; this may help them put their thoughts about their child into words (Krone and Harris, 1988). Find out whether they want the child to be baptized or to receive some other blessing, and make appropriate arrangements. If possible, let them hold their child; otherwise, encourage gentle touching and stroking.

Also plan interventions to help family members deal with their grief. For family members in denial, do not attempt to force them past denial, but provide and reinforce clear, accurate information about the child's condition.

For family members feeling anger, provide the opportunity to vent feelings. However, if one family member blames another for the child's condition, point out that in most cases, preterm birth, neonatal illness, and birth defects result from a combination of factors. Even if the action of one or both parents seems to have been the immediate cause, laying blame serves no purpose.

Use similar reasoning to help family members put aside guilt, a form of self-targeting anger. Although the mother is more likely to express feelings of guilt—remembering a week of unauthorized dieting or a single glass of wine—the father may feel guilt for not being committed enough to the mother's care while she was pregnant.

Anticipatory grieving can occur during the fourth stage of grief—depression and withdrawal. If the neonate is in critical condition and not expected to live, the parents may begin grieving by withdrawing from the neonate (Lindemann, 1944). Even if the parents say nothing, reduced attention to their child may signal that they have begun to withdraw.

Anticipatory grieving and emotional withdrawal may occur briefly or continue throughout the neonate's hospitalization. Although these behaviors can ease pain when an anticipated perinatal death occurs, they also can create problems in bonding if the neonate survives. For the family with a nursing diagnosis of *anticipatory grieving related to the prospect of the neonate's death,* make sure the parents' understanding of their child's condition is not bleaker than the situation warrants, and inform them that even critically ill neonates may recover.

Keep parents informed of changes in their child's condition. Assure them that the staff will do its best to let them know when death appears near so that they can be with their child.

Before the family arrives, dress the neonate in regular baby clothing (some units keep a supply of baby clothes to use if the parents have not provided any). If family members will be permitted to hold their child, have a receiving blanket ready for wrapping the neonate; later, parents may wish to have the blanket as a keepsake.

When the family arrives, provide as much privacy as possible. Move the neonate to a private area (or at least to the quietest corner of the NICU). Post a sign near the entrance to this area, alerting staff to the family's need for quiet. When no additional medical intervention is planned, let the family spend the last few moments alone with the neonate.

Family members need support to cope with the immediate reality of their child's death and to deal with their grief. After the neonate has died, the nurse should give family members all the time they need to say goodbye to and hold the child.

If the family was absent at the time of death, check with the physician about notification procedure. Some physicians prefer to inform the family personally rather than by telephone. Offer to be present to give support when the family is notified. (For information about organiza-

RESOURCES FOR DEALING WITH PERINATAL LOSS

The grief and loss experienced by the family of a neonate who dies last far longer than the brief time most neonatal nurses are in contact with the family. Consequently, the nurse should be aware of support groups that can help family members deal with their loss in the months and years to come.

Pregnancy and Infant Loss Center (PILC)
1421 E. Wayzata Boulevard, Suite 40
Wayzata, MN 55391
612-473-9372

Resolve Through Sharing
La Crosse Lutheran Hospital
1910 South Avenue
La Crosse, WI 54601
608-791-4747

**Source of Help in Airing and Resolving
Experiences (SHARE)**
St. Elizabeth's Hospital
211 South 3rd Street
Belleville, IL 62222
618-234-2415

tions that help bereaved parents cope with perinatal loss, see *Resources for dealing with perinatal loss.*)

If the family arrives after the neonate has died, prepare the body for them to see. Wash, dress, and wrap the neonate in a way that displays positive features and covers disfigurements. With the physician's permission, remove all tubes and lines (except where removal might affect the outcome of an autopsy); disconnect, tie off, and secure those lines under the clothing while the family visits. Remove drainage stains and tape marks; cover surgical wounds or puncture sites with small dressings.

Place the wrapped body in a cool area until just before the family arrives. Then, before presenting the body to them, wrap it in warmed linens, which will transfer some of the warmth to the neonate's skin.

To provide the family with tangible memories of the neonate, assemble a memory packet, including such items as photographs, a lock of hair, the identification bracelet, a footprint, caps, and blankets. If the family does not wish to take these items home, let them know that the packet will be kept in case they want it later; when they are past the initial shock, these mementos may help them through grief.

For some parents, making funeral arrangements for their child is calming; focusing on the task at hand helps them accept their loss and deal with their grief. Recog-

nize, however, that parents who have never before experienced the death of a close relative may need help to identify what needs to be done; particularly distraught parents may be unable to face the task at all. Discuss with them—or have the chaplain or social worker discuss—possible funeral and burial choices (including having the hospital take care of the body, if that option is available).

If the parents' reactions to the death are so intense that they cannot make arrangements, call on a family support source, such as a grandparent, to help out. (However, do not seek help if parents can do their own planning; a well-meaning relative or friend who takes over may deprive parents of tasks that would help them resolve grief.)

Even if the parents can make their own arrangements, talk with other family members about ways to help them out at home. Relatives may think they should remove all signs of preparation for the child's birth—crib, toys, clothing—and keep the mother so busy once she comes home that she has no chance to think about her loss. Explain that such tasks as packing up these items may help parents come to terms with their loss. Suggest that offering an afternoon's child care or other practical help might be more appropriate.

Between experiencing and accepting their child's death, parents go through a lengthy internal struggle. The aim of nursing interventions during this period is twofold: help maintain basic family functioning and help family members work through grief to a healthy resolution.

Be familar with signs of dysfunctional grief. After their child's death, parents may experience disorganization and physical ailments. For instance, various studies show that the risk of disease increases during bereavement. Parkes (1970) described psychosomatic pain, especially chest pain, among bereaved adults. Mourners also have a higher risk of serious illness than nonmourners (Rees and Lutkins, 1967). Lynch (1979) found a twofold risk of myocardial infarction in mourners compared to nonmourners and, depending on the region in which they lived, a threefold risk of GI cancer.

Some bereaved parents may be unable to eat, sleep, or make decisions; they may seem caught up in anger at the health care team or in depression about their inability to produce a healthy child. In some cases, they may fail to cope with everyday experiences or to meet their own and their children's basic needs.

To assess for these problems, monitor the parents' physical appearance, if possible. Also talk with them frequently about how they are managing home affairs, and be ready to call in a friend or relative who can help keep the family functioning until the parents can resume their

PATHOLOGIC MOURNING

Ultimately, grief results in healing. When the process is completed, family members can resume normal functioning, remembering the dead neonate with sorrow but able to move on. In a few cases, however, mourning (the outward expression of grief) becomes pathologic—most commonly when a parent tries to suppress grief (Gardner and Merenstein, 1989) instead of letting the process work through. The family member may never reach resolution without intervention by a professional skilled in grief counseling.

The nurse who cares for the family of a neonate who has died should stay alert for indications that a family member is fighting recognition of grief. If any of the following signs or symptoms appear, alert other members of the health care team and refer the family member to an expert:
• agitated depression
• changes in relationships with family or friends
• hostility toward specific individuals
• illness that may be psychosomatic (for example, chronic fatigue and headache)
• inability to function productively
• loss of social-interaction patterns
• overactivity with no sense of loss
• schizophrenia-like formality of manner
• symptoms resembling those of the neonate.

normal roles. Suggest that they undergo a physical examination approximately 4 months after the loss to ensure early detection of any physical problems associated with bereavement. (For more information about dysfunctional grief, see *Pathologic mourning*.)

Because family members may pass through the stages of grief at different rates, misunderstandings may arise. Most commonly, the mother's grief takes longer to resolve. Her attachment may be greater because of the special bond she developed with the fetus during pregnancy. Thus she may find grief resolution more difficult. The father, meanwhile, may seem to have distanced himself from the dead child. His grief may not be evident, even though his sense of loss may be great.

To help reduce misunderstandings, teach the parents about the grief stages and encourage them to communicate with each other about their feelings—not only about the loss of their child, but about the pressures they feel in its aftermath. The father, for example, may explain that although the loss is painful for him, he feels he must be stoic, fearing that the same people who sympathize with the mother's expression of grief would disapprove of his. If the parents have trouble understanding each other, suggest that they talk together with the social worker, chaplain, or another counselor.

Also talk with other family members. As they reach their own points of grief resolution, they may become impatient with the mother (or both parents) for being "preoccupied" with the child's death. When the mother attempts to discuss her feelings, for example, other family members may urge her to stop dwelling in the past. They even may encourage her to start a "replacement" child before she is ready to consider another pregnancy.

To avert such well-meaning intrusion, discuss with other family members the individuality of grieving. Assure them that 6 weeks of acute mourning are by no means unusual, that full resolution of grief may take 2 years, and that accepting the mother's feelings will help her resolve her grief.

Fetal death. Because parents can begin bonding with a child as soon as they are aware of a pregnancy, the death of a fetus can be as traumatic as the death of a neonate. Nursing interventions similar to those provided after a neonate's death can help parents who suffer a fetal loss; however, depending on when in the pregnancy the fetal loss occurs, opportunity to provide such interventions may be limited. Thus the timing and circumstances of the fetal loss guide nursing interventions.

With a first-trimester loss (usually a spontaneous abortion), the mother may have been unaware of the pregnancy—and she may not be hospitalized for treatment. If she simply is treated in the physician's office, little opportunity exists for nursing intervention; yet she may need such intervention.

On the other hand, if the mother was aware of the pregnancy, she and her partner may have begun their emotional investment; if so, they will need to grieve. Unfortunately, family and friends may minimize a first-trimester fetal loss, believing that the pregnancy cannot have meant that much yet and thus fail to give parents support. Nursing interventions in this situation include affirming the parents' right and need to grieve, explaining the stages of grief to them, and encouraging them to communicate with and support each other.

Fetal death during the second trimester typically results in spontaneous abortion. In most cases, the parents were aware of the pregnancy and had invested themselves emotionally in the forthcoming birth. Nursing interventions include helping the parents express their grief, explaining the stages of grief, and encouraging them to communicate with each other and other family members.

As pregnancy progresses and parents invest more time and energy in the fetus, bonding with the expected child increases. Thus third-trimester fetal loss may be quite traumatic. The mother may have to go through labor to expel the fetus, adding to the trauma. Parents in this situation need much support from each other, other family members, and friends. Nursing interventions may include suggesting that they pack up whatever clothes, toys, and other items they had begun accumulating to help them complete their bonding with the expected child. Although this may be a difficult task, it can help parents face their loss and express their feelings (Limbo and Wheeler, 1986).

Stillbirth. Stillbirth—the death shortly before or during delivery of a fetus that had been expected to live—is a wrenching experience as happy anticipation suddenly vanishes. If fetal death occurs before labor begins, the parents also must deal with feelings of helplessness as they wait for delivery to occur. Because grieving will be easier if they complete their bonding with the child, encourage the parents to look at, touch, and hold the stillborn neonate. Also, provide solitude as they say goodbye to their child.

EVALUATION

During this step of the nursing process, the nurse evaluates the effectiveness of the care plan by ongoing evaluation of subjective and objective criteria. Evaluation findings should be stated in terms of actions performed or outcomes achieved for each goal. Keep in mind that while the neonate is hospitalized, the nurse may have difficulty evaluating the effect of care for the family because full results of some interventions may not be apparent until after the neonate is discharged.

The following examples illustrate appropriate evaluation statements for the family of a high-risk neonate:
• The parents demonstrated specific caregiving skills required by their neonate during and after hospitalization.
• The parents identified and used available support sources during and after the neonate's hospitalization.
• The parents' verbal and nonverbal behaviors reflected at least a moderate level of comfort in meeting the neonate's physical and emotional needs.
• The parents demonstrated an understanding of and used appropriate coping mechanisms.
• The parents expressed grief in a constructive manner.
• The parents demonstrated an accurate perception of the neonate's condition and have realistic expectations.

DOCUMENTATION

Documentation for the parents of a high-risk neonate should include:
• signs of individual expressions of grief

• length and frequency of visits to the neonate
• nature of the interaction with the neonate
• ability to express feelings about the neonate
• ability to identify and provide for the neonate's care needs
• ability to accept help and advice from the health care team
• verbal expression of coping ability
• expression of comfort with caring for the neonate at home
• willingness to make necessary arrangements for home care
• ability to identify appropriate follow-up medical care for the neonate
• contact with the deceased neonate if perinatal death has occurred.

Documentation for the neonate with regard to family interaction should include:
• physiologic response to parents' care, including response to feeding and simple caregiving activities
• eye contact and other signs of interaction with parents
• response to interaction by the parents (for example, "Takes feeding easily from mother; no vomiting after eating; quiet after feeding").

PERINATAL PROBLEMS

The most common problems seen in NICUs are prematurity and its sequelae, congenital heart defects, and congenital anomalies requiring emergency surgery (such as omphalocele and tracheoesophageal fistula).

GESTATIONAL-AGE AND BIRTH-WEIGHT ABNORMALITIES

Abnormalities in gestational age (prematurity and postmaturity) and birth weight (small or large size for gestational age) predispose the neonate to various problems. (For information on the causes and consequences of these abnormalities, see *Gestational-age variations*, pages 452 and 453, and *Birth-weight variations*, pages 454 and 455.)

Assessment

In many cases, maternal, antepartal, and intrapartal factors give advance warning of these problems—particularly preterm or postterm status.

GESTATIONAL-AGE VARIATIONS

Birth before or after full-term gestation markedly increases the risk of perinatal problems. In the past 25 years, advances in research and technology have improved the survival rate dramatically for neonates with gestational-age variations—even extremely preterm neonates.

PRETERM NEONATE

The preterm neonate—the classic high-risk neonate—is one born before completion of week 37 of gestation. The risks of preterm birth and the associated economic burden are tremendous. Neonatal mortality and morbidity are highest among preterm neonates; each day of prematurity can represent thousands of dollars in medical care and significantly reduces the chance for a positive outcome.

Delivery of a preterm neonate is more likely with any of the following maternal conditions:
- age extreme (under 19 or over 34)
- low socioeconomic status
- poor nutritional status
- poor prenatal care
- exposure to known teratogens (including drugs, alcohol, cigarette smoke, and hazardous chemicals)
- chronic disease (such as cardiovascular disease, renal disease, or diabetes mellitus)
- antepartal trauma, infection, or pregnancy-induced hypertension
- uterine anomalies or cervical incompetency

- a history of previous preterm delivery.

Other predisposing factors include more than one fetus, hydramnios (excessive amniotic fluid), fetal infection, premature rupture of the membranes, abruptio placentae, and placenta previa.

Perinatal problems

General immaturity can lead to dysfunction in any organ or body system. Thus, the preterm neonate risks a wide range of problems, including respiratory distress syndrome, apnea, bronchopulmonary dysplasia, patent ductus arteriosus, ineffective thermoregulation, hypoglycemia, intraventricular hemorrhage, gastrointestinal dysfunction, retinopathy, hyperbilirubinemia, and infection. The preterm neonate also may suffer ineffective development from the effects of intensive medical treatment (such as sensory overload and environmental stress); an immature central nervous system compounds this risk. Also, mother-infant bonding may be jeopardized. (The pathophysiology, assessment, and treatment of the problems listed above are discussed in detail throughout this chapter.)

POSTTERM NEONATE

The postterm neonate is one whose gestation exceeds 294 days or 42 weeks. Typically, the neonate's weight falls above the ninetieth percentile on the Colorado intrauterine growth chart (discussed in Chapter 18, Neonatal Assessment).

Perinatal problems

Problems associated with postmaturity include fetal dysmaturity syndrome, asphyxia, meconium aspiration, polycythemia, hypothermia, and birth trauma (Fanaroff and Martin, 1987).

Fetal dysmaturity syndrome. Some 20% to 40% of postterm neonates experience placental insufficiency leading to fetal dysmaturity syndrome and a diagnosis of small for gestational age (SGA). After 280 days of gestation, the risk of placental insufficiency, fetal growth retardation, and chronic hypoxia increases. Fetal weight plateaus around the term date until week 42 (typically from placental lesion formation and decreased placental weight), then drops rapidly. Placental dysfunction after week 42 impairs fetal oxygenation and nutrition and exhausts placental reserves, retarding fetal growth (Resnick, 1989).

Fetal dysmaturity occurs in three forms: chronic, acute, and subacute placental insufficiency. Each form has distinctive manifestations. With *chronic placental insufficiency,* no meconium staining occurs but the neonate appears malnourished, with skin defects and an apprehensive look reflecting hypoxia. *Acute placental insufficiency* leads to a malnourished and apprehensive appearance and green meconium staining of the skin, umbilical cord, and placental membranes. With *subacute placental insuffi-*

ciency, the skin and nails are stained bright yellow (from breakdown of green-bile meconium stain), and the umbilical cord, placenta, and placental membranes may be stained greenish brown (Vorherr, 1975).

Asphyxia and meconium aspiration. The postterm neonate has a high risk of birth asphyxia and meconium aspiration. Usher, Boyd, McLean, and Kramer (1988) found that meconium release (defecation) occurs twice as frequently and meconium aspiration syndrome eight times as frequently in postterm neonates than in other neonates. Some researchers suggest that the postterm fetus reacts more dramatically than the term fetus to episodes of asphyxia, experiencing fetal heart abnormalities, gasping, and meconium release.

Oligohydramnios (presence of less than 300 ml of amniotic fluid at term) increases the risk of asphyxia and aspiration by making meconium less diluted and thus unusually thick (Eden, Seifert, Winegar, and Spellacy, 1987). Normally, amniotic fluid volume peaks at 1,000 to 1,200 ml at about 38 weeks' gestation, then decreases rapidly. By week 42, it drops to approximately 300 ml; further decreases occur at 43 and 44 weeks. In the neonate with no congenital anomalies, oligohydramnios confirms postmaturity and has been linked to fetal decelerations (as shown on fetal monitoring strips), bradycardia, or both (Phelan, Plah, Yeh, Broussard, and Paul, 1985).

Other perinatal problems. Intrauterine hypoxia in the postterm fetus may trigger increased red blood cell production, causing polycythemia; this in turn may lead to sluggish perfusion and

GESTATIONAL-AGE VARIATIONS *(continued)*

POSTTERM NEONATE *(continued)*

complications associated with hyperviscosity. Subcutaneous fat deficiency caused by skin wasting predisposes the postterm neonate to hypothermia, despite a mature thermoregulatory system. Thus, a postterm neonate exposed to cold stress may develop respiratory compromise and hypoglycemia (Fanaroff and Martin, 1987).

Delivery complications
The risk of delivery complications increases after 280 days (40 weeks) of gestation. Excessive size may cause a dysfunctional labor and shoulder dystocia, possibly necessitating cesarean delivery. Because of maternal uterine inefficiency and cephalopelvic disproportion, postterm neonates have a higher-than-average rate of surgical deliveries (Boyd, Usher, McLean, and Kramer, 1988).

Maternal, antepartal, and intrapartal history. The preterm neonate is the classic high-risk neonate, making prematurity the leading predictor of high-risk status. Prematurity and postmaturity usually can be anticipated from maternal, antepartal, and intrapartal data; the calculated delivery date; and ultrasound evaluation. For example, maternal weight loss, decreased abdominal circumference, and reduced uterine size during pregnancy may indicate an altered fetal growth pattern reflecting postterm gestation; ultrasound can be used to estimate gestational weeks.

The diagnosis of large for gestational age (LGA) typically comes during the antepartal period, when fundal height appears disproportionate to gestational weeks (and ultrasound determines exact fetal size). Also, because maternal diabetes mellitus is a leading cause of accelerated intrauterine growth, this condition is a risk factor for LGA status.

About two-thirds of neonates diagnosed as small for gestational age (SGA) are born to women with SGA-associated risk factors (Cassady and Strange, 1987). Consequently, check the maternal history for such factors as low socioeconomic status, age extreme, increased parity, short stature, low prepregnancy weight, and previous delivery of an SGA neonate.

Neonatal findings. After delivery, assess the neonate for physical signs of gestational-age and birth-weight variations as well as perinatal problems associated with these variations. For example, the preterm neonate may appear inactive, with extended positioning at rest, splayed legs, and arms held away from the body. The respiratory pattern typically is irregular, possibly with apneic episodes. Other signs of prematurity include translucent, ruddy skin; visible blood vessels; absent skin folds (from decreased subcutaneous fat); thick vernix caseosa, especially around the neck and thighs; prominent lanugo across the back and face; long, thin fingers with soft, pliable nails; sparse or absent breast tissue; and immature external genitalia.

Physical examination of the postterm neonate typically reveals macrosomic (excessively large) features. Some postterm neonates also have green, brown, or yellow meconium staining of the skin, nails, umbilical cord, or placental membranes. A postterm LGA neonate may show signs of birth trauma and hypoglycemia. With a postterm SGA neonate, expect dry, cracked, wrinkled skin with decreased subcutaneous fat; no visible vernix caseosa or lanugo; skin maceration; long, thin arms and legs; long nails; and full hair growth.

Although birth weight must be correlated with gestational age to verify SGA or LGA status, assess for associated physical signs and perinatal problems if either problem is suspected. The typical SGA neonate has loose, dry skin with diminished skinfold thickness; reduced breast tissue (from soft-tissue wasting); skin wasting in the buttocks and thighs; widened skull sutures with large fontanels; and shortened crown-to-heel, femoral, and foot lengths (from bone growth failure). In a neonate with these findings, also check for congenital anomalies, which are 10 to 20 times more common in SGA neonates than normal neonates.

With the LGA neonate, assess for signs of birth injury, congenital anomalies, hypoglycemia, and polycythemia. If the LGA neonate is preterm, check for signs of respiratory distress and hyperbilirubinemia. With a postterm LGA neonate, expect respiratory distress from meconium aspiration syndrome (MAS) or asphyxiation. With the LGA neonate of a diabetic mother, check for signs of hypoglycemia and hypocalcemia.

Nursing diagnosis

For a partial list of applicable diagnoses, see Nursing Diagnoses: *High-risk neonates and their families,* page 426.

BIRTH-WEIGHT VARIATIONS

Like the neonate with a gestational-age variation, one whose weight is inappropriate for the estimated gestational age is at high risk for perinatal problems.

SMALL-FOR-GESTATIONAL-AGE (SGA) NEONATE

The SGA neonate is one whose birth weight falls below the tenth percentile for gestational age. SGA status results from intrauterine growth retardation (IUGR), an abnormal process in which fetal development and maturation are delayed or impeded. After prematurity, IUGR is the leading cause of death during the perinatal period (Cassady and Strange, 1987).

Causes of IUGR
IUGR may result from maternal conditions, genetic factors (for example, trisomies), fetal and placental abnormalities, infection, fetal malnutrition caused by placental insufficiency, or exposure to such teratogens as drugs and alcohol.

Maternal conditions. The most common causes of IUGR are maternal conditions that reduce uteroplacental perfusion, such as toxemia, chronic hypertensive vascular disease, and renovascular and cardiac disorders. Maternal hypertension, smoking, renal disease, and diabetes mellitus that progresses to renovascular compromise also can result in IUGR. Ounsted, Moar, and Scott (1985) estimate that the SGA incidence could be reduced by 60% by eliminating such risk factors as smoking and hypertensive disorders.

During early pregnancy, smoking is the most important risk factor for IUGR. Typically, the neonate of a woman who smokes weighs 150 to 200 g less than other neonates. Fetal hypoxia, carbon monoxide poisoning of hemoglobin, and the vascular effects of nicotine have been suggested as smoking-related factors that contribute to IUGR.

The role of maternal nutrition in fetal growth remains unclear. Some researchers minimize its importance while others emphasize it. Those who minimize it point out that despite the high incidence of infertility and spontaneous abortion during famines and wars, only severe maternal starvation during the last trimester has reduced birth weight.

Fetal and placental abnormalities. IUGR can result from infarction, hemangiomas, aberrant cord insertion, single umbilical artery, and umbilical vascular thrombosis. Premature placental separation and other conditions that diminish placental surface area and thus decrease fetal-placental exchange capability also may cause IUGR.

Placental insufficiency. Placental insufficiency is the inadequate or improper functioning of the placenta, leading to a compromised intrauterine environment. Causes of placental insufficiency include systemic diseases (such as diabetes mellitus and infection) and placental abnormalities that impair fetal circulation and compromise fetal nutrition and oxygenation (such as abnormal placental implantation, abnormal cord attachment, and placental membrane abnormalities). Although placental insufficiency is most common in the postterm period, it may occur at any time during gestation. The severity of IUGR arising from placental insufficiency depends on the duration of fetal distress.

Exposure to drugs and alcohol. Maternal use of heroin, cocaine, and methadone significantly reduces the neonate's weight, length, and head circumference at birth (Chasnoff, Bussey, Savich, and Stack, 1986). The neonate of a heroin-addicted mother, for instance, typically is SGA, preterm, and weighs less than 2,500 g. Maternal alcohol consumption may cause fetal alcohol syndrome (FAS). Some neonates show severe manifestations whereas others appear normal. Besides mental retardation—the most serious and common effect—FAS may reduce the neonate's weight and length at birth (Wright, 1986).

Perinatal problems
Although the SGA neonate may avoid the problems stemming from organ system immaturity seen in the preterm neonate, other perinatal problems may arise.

Asphyxia and meconium aspiration. The SGA neonate who suffered placental insufficiency risks asphyxiation during labor and delivery, as the flow of oxygen and nutrients slows and uterine contractions reduce placental perfusion. Also, the neonate may aspirate meconium that has entered the amniotic sac. Respiratory distress, cyanosis, pulmonary air trapping, pneumothorax, and pulmonary hypertension may result, along with severe asphyxia and cerebral hypoxia (Fanaroff and Martin, 1987).

Organ size variations. Relative to body weight, the SGA neonate has a larger brain and heart than the preterm neonate but smaller adrenal glands and a smaller liver, spleen, thymus, and placenta.

Hematologic and metabolic problems. The SGA neonate may experience hematologic changes from chronic fetal hypoxia, a condition that triggers compensation through increases in red blood cell (RBC) volume (polycythemia) and erythropoietin levels. Polycythemia, in turn, may cause hyperviscosity and sluggish microcirculation perfusion.

Disturbed carbohydrate metabolism and inefficient hepatic gluconeogenesis and glycogenolysis may lead to hypoglycemia. With increased energy requirements but inadequate glycogen and fat reserves, the SGA neonate is predisposed to hypoglycemia (Lubchenco and Koops, 1987). A stressful labor may further deplete already deficient energy reserves.

Long-term problems
An SGA neonate later may suffer developmental, immunologic, and neurologic problems.

Slowed growth and immunologic deficiencies. Growth rate depends on when IUGR occurred and how long it lasted. Commonly, the child who was SGA at birth remains slimmer and shorter than other children of the same gestational age or birth weight. The rate of catch-up growth depends on causative factors and postnatal events. Head growth may equal or exceed weight and height increases.

BIRTH-WEIGHT VARIATIONS *(continued)*

SMALL-FOR-GESTATIONAL-AGE (SGA) NEONATE *(continued)*

Impaired fetal skeletal growth may contribute to delayed tooth eruption and enamel hypoplasia. Severely growth-retarded neonates also have an increased incidence of infection, possibly from immunologic deficiency.

Neurologic impairment. IUGR-induced brain damage and its potential effect on neurologic development remains a major medical concern. Most investigators believe IUGR has more serious neurologic consequences in the preterm than the term SGA neonate. Follow-up evaluations in children who experienced IUGR in utero have revealed defects in speech and language comprehension; outcome studies have described hyperactivity, short attention span, poor fine-motor coordination, hyperreflexia, and learning problems. Stunted growth and delayed intellectual or neurologic development were found in children who experienced both short and long periods of IUGR. Other factors that worsen the neurologic prognosis include male sex and low socioeconomic status, regardless of the severity of compromise (Teberg, Walther, and Pena, 1988).

LARGE-FOR-GESTATIONAL-AGE (LGA) NEONATE

The LGA neonate is one whose birth weight exceeds the ninetieth percentile for gestational age. A neonate delivered at term is considered to be LGA if the birth weight exceeds 4,000 g (8 lb, 13 oz). The leading cause of LGA status is maternal diabetes mellitus.

Traditionally, the large neonate was considered a healthy one. However, clinicians now know that the accelerated intrauterine growth of the LGA fetus poses a threat to both mother and neonate during delivery and increases the risk of complications and death in the early neonatal period.

Intrapartal problems
When the membranes rupture, large fetal size and possible high station may result in umbilical cord prolapse. Uterine overdistention from an LGA fetus increases the risk of premature labor. Usually, the physician will initiate labor and delivery before term (once fetal lung maturity has been confirmed) because of the high incidence of unexplained death among term LGA fetuses. If the mother has an adequate pelvis, the physician typically administers oxytocin to induce labor; otherwise, cesarean delivery may be necessary. Shoulder dystocia stemming from cephalopelvic disproportion also may necessitate cesarean delivery, with all the inherent risks.

During vaginal delivery, the neonate's large size may cause birth injury, such as clavicular fracture resulting from shoulder dystocia, skull fracture from increased head size, or other traumatic head injuries (such as cephalhematomas, facial nerve damage, and intracranial bleeding). A difficult delivery also may lead to phrenic nerve damage or brachial plexus palsy.

Perinatal problems
If the mother is diabetic, the neonate may suffer hypocalcemia (possibly from depressed parathyroid function), hypoglycemia (from maternal hyperglycemia that stimulates fetal hyperinsulinism), and polycythemia (from RBC overproduction). Other problems associated with excessive size include congenital anomalies (such as transposition of the great vessels), erythroblastosis fetalis (hemolytic anemia), and Beckwith's syndrome (a hereditary disorder associated with neonatal hypoglycemia and hyperinsulinemia).

If the mother had postconceptional bleeding causing an error in the calculated delivery date, the LGA neonate may be delivered postterm and thus experience respiratory distress from meconium aspiration or intrauterine asphyxiation. The LGA neonate delivered before term to prevent fetal death or intrapartal complications of excessive size may suffer respiratory distress syndrome, hyperbilirubinemia, and other problems linked to prematurity.

Planning and implementation
Nursing care of the neonate with gestational-age or birth-weight variations is similar to that for any high-risk neonate. (For more information, see "Nursing care of the high-risk neonate" and "Nursing care of the family" earlier in this chapter.)

Evaluation
During this step of the nursing process, the nurse evaluates the effectiveness of the care plan by ongoing evaluation of subjective and objective criteria. Evaluation findings should be stated in terms of actions performed or outcomes achieved for each goal. For examples of appropriate evaluation statements, see the general ones listed in "Nursing care of the high-risk neonate" earlier in this chapter.

Documentation
All steps of the nursing process should be documented as thoroughly and objectively as possible. Thorough documentation not only allows the nurse to evaluate the effectiveness of the care, but it also makes this information available to other members of the health care team, helping ensure consistency of care.

For information about appropriate documentation, see the general points listed in "Nursing care of the high-risk neonate" earlier in this chapter.

RESPIRATORY PROBLEMS

In utero, the placenta supplies oxygen to body tissues; the respiratory arterioles remain partially closed so that blood is diverted through the ductus arteriosus and away from the lungs. At birth, the neonate's lungs must take over the task of providing oxygen for body tissues. For this to happen, lung fluid must be replaced by air and the arterioles must dilate to allow more blood into the lungs. The healthy neonate accomplishes this within seconds.

However, some neonates have trouble initiating respirations or develop respiratory distress after breathing is established. For instance, problems may arise if fluid remains in the lungs or if the blood perfusion of the lungs does not increase; neonates with apnea at birth or a weak respiratory effort (from such conditions as prematurity, asphyxia, or maternal anesthesia) are predisposed to respiratory distress.

Asphyxia and apnea. Asphyxia may occur late in gestation or during delivery. Chemically, this condition is defined as insufficient oxygen in the blood (hypoxemia), excessive carbon dioxide in the blood, and a decreased blood pH. As carbon dioxide accumulates, respiratory acidosis occurs; poor tissue oxygenation leads to buildup of lactic acid, resulting in metabolic acidosis. If hypoxia is prolonged, the foramen ovale and ductus arteriosus — fetal shunts that normally close shortly after delivery — may reopen. This causes a return to fetal circulatory pathways to maintain circulation to the heart and brain.

Asphyxia causes rapid breathing at first. If asphyxia continues, apnea (absence of respirations) ensues, respiratory movements cease, and the heart rate starts to drop. Deep, gasping respirations then begin, the heart rate continues to fall, and blood pressure drops. Respirations weaken progressively until they stop altogether. Because hypoxemia and acidosis cause arteriolar constriction, lung perfusion is poor; consequently, the body cannot be oxygenated.

Without immediate resuscitation, the neonate will die. Complications of prolonged asphyxia include cerebral hypoxia, seizures, intraventricular hemorrhage (IVH), renal failure, necrotizing enterocolitis (NEC), and metabolic imbalances.

Several days after delivery, apneic episodes (cessation of breathing for more than 15 seconds) are common among preterm neonates, many of whom have irregular respiratory patterns from neuronal immaturity. Such episodes may result from acidosis, anemia, hypoglycemia, hyperglycemia, hypothermia, hyperthermia, patent ductus arteriosus (PDA), abdominal distention, regurgitation, sepsis, or IVH. Central apnea (caused by insufficient neural impulses from the respiratory center) and obstructive apnea (resulting from upper airway obstruction) also occur in some preterm and low-birth-weight neonates.

Meconium aspiration syndrome. A lung inflammation, meconium aspiration syndrome (MAS) results from aspiration of meconium-stained amniotic fluid in utero or as the neonate takes the first few breaths after delivery. Meconium staining of amniotic fluid results from fetal asphyxia: In response to asphyxia, intestinal peristalsis increases, the anal sphincter relaxes, and meconium enters the amniotic fluid.

As meconium obstructs the bronchi and bronchioles, it creates a ball-valve effect: Air can enter but not exit the bronchi and bronchioles because meconium acts as a ball, plugging the alveolar sac. Alveoli then become overdistended; pneumothorax, bacterial pneumonia, or pulmonary hypertension may develop secondarily.

Respiratory distress syndrome. Respiratory distress syndrome (RDS, also called hyaline membrane disease) is characterized by respiratory distress and impaired gas exchange. RDS affects mainly preterm neonates, who have highly pliable and easily overinflated thoracic muscles, weak intercostal muscles, and insufficient surfactant. A lipoprotein synthesized by type II alveolar cells, surfactant is necessary to keep alveoli expanded. Although surfactant production begins at around 22 to 24 weeks of gestation, it is inadequate at this time to prevent alveolar collapse. Surfactant production probably becomes sufficient only after about 35 weeks.

Insufficient surfactant causes alveolar collapse, leading to decreased lung volume and compliance. The resulting atelectasis causes hypoxia and acidosis, which in turn lead to anaerobic metabolism. As lactic acid accumulates in body tissues, myocardial contractility diminishes, impairing cardiac output and arterial blood pressure. Organ perfusion then diminishes; eventually respiratory failure occurs.

Transient tachypnea. This disorder, characterized by transient episodes of tachypnea (accelerated breathing), stems from incomplete removal of fetal lung fluid. Usually accompanied by cyanosis, it affects mainly full-term or nearly full-term neonates born by cesarean delivery (this delivery method eliminates fetal lung compression by the birth canal, which normally helps expel lung fluid).

Bronchopulmonary dysplasia (BPD). In this lung disease, the bronchiolar epithelial lining and alveolar walls become necrotic; in some cases, right-sided heart failure develops as a complication. BPD occurs mainly in preterm neonates as a complication of oxygen therapy or assisted mechanical ventilation—common treatments for RDS. The neonate with BPD typically becomes ventilator-dependent. Low birth weight and overhydration (in a neonate with PDA) may contribute to BPD.

Assessment

Signs of a respiratory problem may be obvious, immediate, and life-threatening, such as with birth asphyxia or apnea, or may arise hours, days, or even weeks later.

The cardinal sign of asphyxia is deep gasping or failure to breathe spontaneously at delivery. Associated signs include a slow heart rate, abnormally low blood pressure, poor muscle tone, and poor reflexes. To help anticipate birth asphyxia, check for such risk factors as maternal diabetes, infection, pregnancy-induced hypertension, or anesthesia; more than one fetus; prolonged labor; prolapsed umbilical cord; abruptio placentae; placenta previa; prolonged rupture of the membranes; meconium-stained amniotic fluid; oligohydramnios; hydramnios; umbilical cord compression; placental insufficiency; abnormal fetal heart rate patterns; isoimmunization; delivery complications; excessive fetal size; abnormal presentation; or neonatal prematurity, postmaturity, or congenital anomalies.

Apneic episodes commonly manifest as rapid respirations punctuated by brief pauses. Hypoxemia, cyanosis, and bradycardia may ensue. With central apnea, expect absence of respiratory efforts and muscle flaccidity. With obstructive apnea, expect respiratory motions accompanied by hypoxemia and bradycardia (from inability to draw air into the lungs).

In MAS, signs of respiratory distress may be mild, moderate, or severe. The neonate typically appears barrel chested because of an increased anteroposterior chest diameter (from bronchial obstruction by meconium or tension pneumothorax). Skin and nails may be meconium stained.

Signs of RDS may appear at delivery or within a few hours. They include tachypnea (a respiratory rate over 60 breaths/minute), labored respirations, grunting, nasal flaring, cyanosis, and chest retractions. The neonate may become restless and agitated (probably from the increasing $PaCO_2$ level) and show fatigue even after simple care procedures. Complex procedures, such as endotracheal suctioning, may thoroughly exhaust the neonate's limited energy reserves, leading to bradycardia and hypoxia.

The likelihood of RDS may be determined antenatally from analysis of amniotic fluid lipids; a lecithin-sphingomyelin ratio below 2 and a phosphatidylglycerol level below 3% suggest fetal lung immaturity and a high risk for RDS.

RDS affects mainly preterm neonates. Other risk factors include maternal diabetes mellitus, infection, or hemorrhage; maternal steroid or analgesic use; more than one fetus; abruptio placentae; umbilical cord prolapse; meconium-stained amniotic fluid; fetal distress; and breech presentation.

Tachypnea—alone or accompanied by hypoxemia, cyanosis, grunting, and chest retractions—is the hallmark of transient tachypnea. Cesarean delivery and term or near-term gestation are common history findings.

Because BPD typically occurs as a complication of treatment for RDS, signs usually arise after supplemental oxygen administration or mechanical ventilation. The severity of these signs reflects the degree of disease progression and pulmonary dysfunction. Expect nasal flaring, retractions, tachypnea, and grunting. However, the first clue to BPD may be difficulty weaning the neonate from a ventilator. As the disease progresses, carbon dioxide retention and pulmonary secretions increase and crackles can be auscultated. Bronchospasm may result from bronchial smooth muscle hypertrophy. Typically, the neonate's condition worsens and oxygen dependency occurs. (Conversely, decreased oxygen dependency may be the earliest sign of recovery.)

Nursing diagnosis

For a partial list of applicable diagnoses, see Nursing Diagnoses: *High-risk neonates and their families,* page 426.

Planning and implementation

Serious respiratory depression at birth calls for immediate resuscitation (as discussed in "Nursing care of the high-risk neonate" earlier in this chapter). After resuscitation, monitor the neonate's cardiopulmonary status and skin temperature. Expect to obtain blood samples for ABG analysis at least every 4 hours (or as needed); obtain samples for serum electrolyte analysis on admission and 24 hours after delivery, as ordered. Monitor arterial blood pressure at least every 2 hours; stay alert for subtle changes, which may signal an impending change in respiratory status.

For RDS, standard interventions include administration of supplemental oxygen and positive-pressure ventilation. If the severity of RDS has not been determined, the neonate typically is given supplemental oxygen or positive-pressure ventilation (CPAP or positive end-expiratory pressure). Assess the neonate every 30 minutes during this therapy.

To help prevent RDS, exogenous surfactants may be administered to preterm neonates via an endotracheal tube to stimulate surfactant production (Jobe, 1988). However, this experimental treatment is available only in selected regional centers. Antenatally, several approaches are available. For instance, ritodrine may be administered to prevent premature labor and delivery before the fetal lungs have matured; subsequent lecithin-sphingomyelin ratios are determined to assess fetal lung maturity. If the pregnancy is threatened at 28 to 32 weeks, betamethasone or another glucocorticoid may be given 24 hours before delivery to stimulate fetal surfactant production. (For more information on medical management of respiratory and other perinatal problems, see *Medical management of perinatal problems.*)

Evaluation

For examples of appropriate evaluation statements, see the general ones listed in "Nursing care of the high-risk neonate" earlier in this chapter. For the neonate with respiratory problems, these additional evaluation statements may be appropriate:
• Signs of increased breathing effort diminished.
• The neonate's ABG and tcPO$_2$ or pulse oximetry values approached normal limits.
• The neonate had no episodes of apnea.

Documentation

For information about appropriate documentation, see the general points listed in "Nursing care of the high-risk neonate" earlier in this chapter. For the neonate with respiratory problems, documentation also should include:
• breathing effort
• any apneic episodes
• administration route and FiO$_2$ of supplemental oxygen (if given)
• ABG and tcPO$_2$ or pulse oximetry values
• ventilator pressure, rate, and positive end-expiratory pressure settings (if the neonate is on a mechanical ventilator).

RETINOPATHY OF PREMATURITY

Retinopathy of prematurity (ROP; formerly called retrolental fibroplasia) may lead to blindness. It begins with retinal vasoconstriction, which eventually causes vessels in some portions of the retina to become ischemic. To compensate for ischemia, new capillaries develop to provide oxygen and nutrients to the damaged tissue. However, lacking sufficient structural integrity, the new vessels rupture and hemorrhage. This leads to formation of scar tis-

sue, which grows rigid and shortens, causing traction that results in retinal detachment and eventual blindness. In some cases, however, early retinal changes revert spontaneously, sparing the neonate's vision.

Immature retinal vessels are particularly vulnerable to ROP; the disorder is most common in the preterm neonate of less than 35 weeks' gestation who receives supplemental oxygen. Most experts attribute ROP to high concentrations of administered oxygen leading to an elevated PaO$_2$; even brief PaO$_2$ elevations have been linked with ROP. However, researchers suspect that coexisting factors must be present. These may include prematurity, blood transfusions, IVH, PDA, apnea, infection, vitamin E deficiency, lactic acidosis, administration of prostaglandin synthetase inhibitors, and prenatal and genetic factors. A study conducted by Subramanian, et al. (1985) shows a link between ROP and continuous exposure to bright lights in the nursery.

Assessment

Ophthalmoscopic examination of the neonate with ROP reveals a proliferation of dilated, tortuous retinal vessels; edema; and retinal detachment.

Nursing diagnosis

For a partial list of applicable diagnoses, see Nursing Diagnoses: *High-risk neonates and their families,* page 426.

Planning and implementation

All preterm neonates who have received supplemental oxygen should have their eyes examined by the physician before discharge. Abnormal findings are graded I through IV, with I signifying minimal change and IV indicating severe retinal damage and blindness.

The precise PaO$_2$ level and the duration of the elevation that may cause ROP have not been determined. To minimize the risk, neonatologists now recommend that the PaO$_2$ level of a neonate receiving oxygen be kept at 60 to 80 mm Hg. (For more information on monitoring the neonate receiving supplemental oxygen, see "Nursing care of the high-risk neonate" earlier in this chapter.)

Evaluation

For examples of appropriate evaluation statements, see the general ones listed in "Nursing care of the high-risk neonate" earlier in this chapter. For the neonate with ROP, this additional evaluation statement may be appropriate:
• The neonate's PaO$_2$ level was maintained at 60 to 80 mm Hg.

MEDICAL MANAGEMENT OF PERINATAL PROBLEMS

Management of a perinatal problem may involve any or all of the measures specified in the chart below. (For details on nursing care for a neonate with some of these problems, see the "Planning and implementation" sections of this chapter.)

Birth asphyxia
- Immediate resuscitation followed by supplemental oxygen, continuous positive-airway pressure (CPAP), or mechanical ventilation

Meconium aspiration syndrome
- Immediate resuscitation, with endotracheal intubation and suctioning of the lower airway

Episodic apnea
- Treatment of the underlying disorder (such as intracranial hemorrhage or hypoglycemia)
- Aminophylline or theophylline to stimulate respirations
- CPAP

Respiratory distress syndrome
- Supplemental oxygen, CPAP, or mechanical ventilation, with close monitoring of oxygenation status
- Preventive therapies, such as maternal betamethasone administration to stimulate fetal surfactant production or administration of exogenous surfactant to the neonate

Transient tachypnea
- Oxygen administration (or, rarely, CPAP or mechanical ventilation) with close monitoring of oxygenation status

Bronchopulmonary dysplasia
- Close monitoring of oxygenation status during supplemental oxygen therapy
- Gradual weaning from mechanical ventilation
- Nutritional support (typically enteral or parenteral feedings)
- Fluid restriction and diuretics to prevent pulmonary edema

Retinopathy of prematurity
- Close monitoring of oxygenation status during supplemental oxygen therapy
- Frequent ophthalmologic evaluations
- Reduced intensity of nursery lighting
- Cryosurgery

Intraventricular hemorrhage
- Supportive treatment, typically including vitamin K, platelets, and anticonvulsant medication
- Reduced environmental stimulation and handling
- Close monitoring of neurologic status

Necrotizing enterocolitis
- Colostomy
- Parenteral nutrition
- Antibiotics

Neonate of a diabetic mother
- Treatment of associated birth trauma
- Correction of associated metabolic and electrolyte imbalances

Hypoglycemia
- Early oral feedings or I.V. glucose (typically as dextrose 10% in water)
- Close monitoring of serum glucose level

Hypocalcemia
- Supplemental calcium (typically as I.V. or oral calcium gluconate)

Hyperbilirubinemia and jaundice
- Early, frequent feedings
- Phototherapy
- Exchange transfusion

Polycythemia
- Partial exchange transfusion

Ineffective thermoregulation
- Maintenance of neutral thermal environment
- Gradual rewarming (1 F degree [0.6 C degree/hour])

Rh incompatibility
- Complete exchange transfusion with Rh-negative red blood cells, sometimes followed by phototherapy
- Close monitoring of hematocrit and serum bilirubin level

ABO blood group incompatibility
- Correction of hyperbilirubinemia (as with phototherapy)
- Close monitoring of hematocrit and serum bilirubin level

Fetal alcohol syndrome
- Developmental care
- Reduced environmental stimulation
- Enteral feedings if the neonate has poorly coordinated sucking and swallowing

Drug exposure, addiction, or withdrawal
- Developmental care
- Reduced environmental stimulation
- Enteral feedings, if the neonate has incoordinated sucking and swallowing
- Swaddling and frequent feedings to decrease irritability and tremors
- Phenobarbitol to control seizures (for a neonate going through drug withdrawal)

(continued)

MEDICAL MANAGEMENT OF PERINATAL PROBLEMS (continued)

Infection
- Antibiotics
- Infection control measures (including universal precautions)

Meningomyelocele
- Surgery
- Proper positioning

Encephalocele
- Surgery
- Proper positioning

Congenital hydrocephalus
- Surgical placement of a ventriculoperitoneal or ventriculoatrial shunt
- Proper positioning

Microcephaly
- Supportive treatment
- Anticonvulsant medications

Teratoma
- Surgical tumor excision
- Proper positioning

Cardiac anomalies
- Palliative or corrective surgery
- Diuretics or digoxin to control congestive heart failure
- Supportive therapy (such as I.V. fluids and iron supplements to correct anemia)

Diaphragmatic hernia
- Respiratory support
- Gastric decompression
- Extracorporeal membrane oxygenation
- Surgical restoration of abdominal contents to their proper anatomic position
- Postsurgical endotracheal intubation and chest tube placement
- Antibiotics

Tracheoesophageal malformations
- Surgical separation of the trachea and esophagus (with gastrostomy tube placement to prevent aspiration and provide access for feedings)
- Continuous low-pressure suction of blind pouch
- Oxygen therapy

Omphalocele or gastroschisis
- Oxygen therapy
- Immediate positive-pressure ventilation followed by I.V. fluid administration
- Coverage of defect with sterile dressings (to keep tissues moist and reduce heat loss)
- Gastric decompression
- Surgical reduction of defect or creation of pouch around herniated abdominal contents to reduce tissue swelling (with placement of gastrostomy tube to provide access for feedings)

Meconium ileus
- Enemas and fluid administration
- Ileostomy

Imperforate anus
- Gastric decompression
- Colostomy

Cleft palate and cleft lip
- Later surgical repair
- Use of special nipple for feeding
- Close monitoring for ear infection

Unilateral renal agenesis
- Surgical removal of affected kidney (may not be necessary if other kidney is functional)

Polycystic kidney disease
- Surgical removal of the affected kidney
- Gastric decompression
- Dialysis
- Antibiotics for urinary tract infection

Posterior urethral valves
- Surgical correction of the obstruction
- Placement of nephrostomy tube or stent for drainage
- Open fetal surgery for temporary relief of obstruction (if diagnosed antepartally)

Genital ambiguity
- Hydrocortisone (if caused by congenital adrenal hyperplasia)
- Later surgical reconstruction of external genitalia

Clubfoot
- Corrective shoes, casts, or braces
- Later corrective surgery, if necessary

Documentation

For information about appropriate documentation, see the general points listed in "Nursing care of the high-risk neonate" earlier in this chapter. For the neonate with ROP, documentation also should include:
- oxygen flow rate and concentration
- laboratory studies, including PaO_2 levels.

INTRAVENTRICULAR HEMORRHAGE

Fragile periventricular capillaries predispose the preterm neonate to IVH, or bleeding into the ventricles of the brain. IVH is associated with increased venous pressure and increased blood osmolarity. RDS also may lead to IVH because it typically causes hypoxia and hypercapnia. (Hypoxia can lead to vessel damage because it interrupts the brain's autonomic regulatory functions, hypercapnia because it causes cerebral vasodilation.)

Assessment

Typically, IVH causes bulging fontanels, increasing head size, hypotonia, forceful vomiting, downward eye deviation, seizures, lethargy, and extreme irritability. Also assess for generalized signs of hemorrhage, including temperature instability, bradycardia, increasing respiratory distress, apnea, and hypotension.

Nursing diagnosis

For a partial list of applicable diagnoses, see Nursing Diagnoses: *High-risk neonates and their families*, page 426.

Planning and implementation

For the neonate with IVH, supportive care is essential. Nursing care includes close monitoring of the neonate's neurologic status, including level of consciousness, fontanels, and head circumference measurements. In addition, the nurse must continually monitor the neonate for signs of bleeding and institute measures to prevent its occurrence.

Evaluation

For examples of appropriate evaluation statements, see the general ones listed in "Nursing care of the high-risk neonate" earlier in this chapter.

Documentation

For information about appropriate documentation, see the general points listed in "Nursing care of the high-risk neonate" earlier in this chapter. For the neonate with IVH, documentation also should include:
• status of fontanels
• head circumference measurements
• neurologic status, including level of consciousness
• seizures, including type, frequency, and duration
• supportive treatment measures.

NECROTIZING ENTEROCOLITIS

An acute inflammatory GI mucosal disease, NEC may develop after hypoxic injury to the bowel at birth or during the early neonatal period. (Most commonly, it arises within the first 2 weeks after birth.) Hypoxia causes shunting of blood away from the GI tract to vital organs; the resulting intestinal ischemia predisposes the bowel to bacterial invasion, leading to necrotic lesions and possible perforation.

NEC has been linked to prematurity, which may predispose the neonate to anoxia and subsequent bowel ischemia. Intrauterine infection, maternal diabetes, multiple gestation (more than one fetus), and other conditions that cause fetal stress also may contribute to NEC.

Assessment

Signs of NEC may be generalized — for instance, apnea, hypothermia, lethargy, and irritability — or restricted to the GI tract. GI signs include abdominal distention and tenderness; absent bowel sounds; visible distended, rope-like bowel loops; vomiting; increased gastric residual matter; bloody stools; and feeding problems. Also, stools may contain positive reducing substances — various forms of glucose in abnormal amounts — which indicate impaired intestinal carbohydrate absorption caused by NEC-induced tissue damage.

Determine the neonate's glucose level from a copper reduction tablet test and perform a guaiac test to check for occult blood in the stool. X-ray evidence of pneumatosis (air within the intestinal walls), adynamic ileus (intestinal obstruction caused by reduced intestinal motility), thickened bowel walls, and free air in the peritoneum or portal system confirm the diagnosis.

Nursing diagnosis

For a partial list of applicable diagnoses, see Nursing Diagnoses: *High-risk neonates and their families*, page 426.

Planning and implementation

For NEC, parenteral nutrition is necessary to allow the bowel to rest. A temporary colostomy may be performed. A portion of localized necrotic bowel may be excised; widespread bowel necrosis may necessitate massive bowel resection, with resulting short-gut syndrome, a condition characterized by impaired nutrient digestion. Expect to administer antibiotics to control secondary infection.

Evaluation

For examples of appropriate evaluation statements, see the general ones listed in "Nursing care of the high-risk neonate" earlier in this chapter.

Documentation

For information about appropriate documentation, see the general points listed in "Nursing care of the high-risk neonate" earlier in this chapter.

NEONATE OF A DIABETIC MOTHER

Long-standing maternal diabetes mellitus or gestational diabetes mellitus (diabetes that arises during pregnancy) may cause various fetal and neonatal complications. Maternal serum insulin and glucose levels typically increase during pregnancy from increased tissue resistance to insulin in response to secretion of human placental lactogen and rising estrogen and progesterone levels. If the glucose level remains elevated, as in poorly controlled diabetes, the fetus responds by producing more insulin to combat hyperglycemia. Continued glucose elevation results in fetal hyperinsulinism, leading to changes in fetal glucose metabolism, growth, and development. Exposure to high glucose levels early in gestational development may have a teratogenic effect, causing various congenital anomalies, including heart defects, sacral agenesis, renal vein thrombosis, and small left colon (Fanaroff and Martin, 1987).

The neonate of a woman with diabetes (sometimes called an infant of a diabetic mother, or IDM) also has an increased risk of asphyxia, prematurity, infection, respiratory distress, severe hypoglycemia, hypocalcemia, hyperbilirubinemia, polycythemia, and neonatal death; unexplained fetal death also is higher than normal in IDMs. Typically, the IDM is large for gestational age (with a birth weight exceeding the ninetieth percentile for gestational age) and thus may suffer birth trauma, such as shoulder dystocia, cephalhematoma, subdural hemorrhage, ocular hemorrhage, or brachial plexus injury (Fanaroff and Martin, 1987).

Previously, large fetal size and the high incidence of fetal death late in gestation led many obstetricians to advise early delivery for pregnant diabetic clients. However, that approach has changed slightly, partly because the fetus affected by maternal diabetes has delayed alveolar maturation and thus cannot synthesize adequate surfactant to establish respirations after delivery. If early delivery is mandatory, however, it typically is scheduled for the thirty-seventh week of gestation.

Assessment

Typically, this neonate is macrosomic, with a birth weight in the upper percentile range for gestational age. The face is round with chubby cheeks and the skin is ruddy to bright red. Signs of hypoglycemia and hypocalcemia may be present (see "Metabolic disorders" later in this chapter for details); however, over half of neonates of diabetic mothers have asymptomatic hypoglycemia. Assess for signs of birth trauma, such as bruising, ecchymosis, and shoulder dystocia (sometimes manifested as a flaccid or unusually positioned arm).

For the neonate whose mother had questionably or poorly controlled diabetes during pregnancy, assess for signs of hypoglycemia and check blood glucose levels using a glucose oxidase dipstick at delivery and 30 minutes afterward.

Nursing diagnosis

For a partial list of applicable diagnoses, see Nursing Diagnoses: *High-risk neonates and their families,* page 426.

Planning and implementation

Assess for signs of birth trauma (for example, by evaluating mobility, especially in the upper extremities), correct any fluid or electrolyte imbalances, and assess for complications stemming from widely fluctuating serum glucose, calcium, and bilirubin levels. Also monitor the neonate's vital signs as well as tcPO$_2$ or pulse oximetry values and ABG values, as ordered. (For specific interventions associated with hypoglycemia, hypocalcemia, and hyperbilirubinemia, see "Metabolic disorders" later in this chapter.)

Evaluation

For examples of appropriate evaluation statements, see the general ones listed in "Nursing care of the high-risk neonate" earlier in this chapter.

Documentation

For information about appropriate documentation, see the general points listed in "Nursing care of the high-risk neonate" earlier in this chapter.

METABOLIC DISORDERS

The most common metabolic disorders in high-risk neonates are hypoglycemia, hypocalcemia, and hyperbilirubinemia and jaundice.

Hypoglycemia. This condition is defined as two serum glucose levels below 35 mg/dl in the first 3 hours, less than 40 mg/dl from 4 to 24 hours, or less than 45 mg/dl from 24 hours to 7 days of age in a term neonate. In a preterm neonate, hypoglycemia is diagnosed when two serum glucose values are below 25 mg/dl during the first 72 hours. Hypoglycemia typically results from prematurity, low birth weight, severe fetal or neonatal stress, or maternal diabetes. Because fetal glycogen is deposited during the last few gestational months, the preterm neonate has deficient glycogen stores; if a stressful event, such as respiratory distress, develops at birth, these stores quickly become depleted. The low-birth-weight neonate has a high metabolic rate and inadequate enzyme supplies to activate glucogenesis — conditions that contribute to hypoglycemia.

Poorly controlled maternal diabetes, on the other hand, triggers increased insulin production by the fetal pancreas. After birth, the neonate continues to produce high levels of insulin; this facilitates the entry of glucose into muscle and fat cells, rapidly depleting serum glucose. Glucose expenditure during the transition to the extrauterine environment and sudden cessation of maternal glucose when the umbilical cord is clamped further tax the neonate's glucose stores.

Hypocalcemia. Defined as a serum calcium level below 7 mg/100 ml, hypocalcemia typically arises within the first 2 days or at 6 to 10 days after birth. It affects about half of neonates born to women with type I (insulin-dependent) diabetes mellitus. Other risk factors include small-for-gestational-age (SGA) status, prematurity, and birth asphyxia.

During pregnancy, the maternal parathyroid glands attempt to increase the maternal serum calcium level to compensate for loss of the calcium transferred to the fetus. The fetal parathyroid glands respond to this increase by a reduction in function; this in turn may cause hypoparathyroidism and subsequent hypocalcemia. After delivery, the neonatal serum calcium level drops further.

Hyperbilirubinemia and jaundice. Hyperbilirubinemia — an elevated serum level of unconjugated bilirubin — is common among both low-risk and high-risk neonates. It results from overproduction or underexcretion of bilirubin, as from liver immaturity or increased hemolysis. The disorder sometimes leads to jaundice, a yellow discoloration of the skin and sclerae. Types of jaundice include physiologic jaundice, which commonly arises 48 to 72 hours after birth and peaks by the third to fifth day; and pathologic jaundice, which arises secondary to another disorder, appears within the first 24 hours, and is char-

acterized by a serum bilirubin level above 20 mg/dl. Pathologic jaundice, seen mainly in high-risk neonates, results from blood type or blood group incompatibility; infection; or biliary, hepatic, or metabolic abnormalities. (For more information on bilirubin production and excretion and physiologic jaundice, see Chapter 17, Neonatal Adaptation, and Chapter 19, Care of the Normal Neonate.)

The risk of hyperbilirubinemia is greatest in preterm neonates, those who are ill, those with isoimmune hemolytic anemia, and those who experienced a traumatic delivery leading to bruising and polycythemia. Such conditions as hypoxia and hypoglycemia (characterized by bilirubin displacement from binding sites) predispose the preterm neonate to hyperbilirubinemia (Fanaroff and Martin, 1987).

A serum bilirubin level of 18 to 20 mg/dl (or even lower in the preterm or low-birth-weight neonate) may lead to bilirubin encephalopathy (kernicterus), a condition in which unconjugated bilirubin crosses the blood-brain barrier and accumulates in the brain. This may result in damage to the brain and other organs, such as the kidneys, intestines, and pancreas (Fanaroff and Martin, 1987).

Assessment

Signs of metabolic disorders range from extremely mild to severe.

Hypoglycemia. Signs of hypoglycemia include apnea or bradycardia, seizures, irregular respirations, cyanosis, irritability, listlessness, lethargy, tremors, feeding problems, vomiting, hypotonia, and a high-pitched cry. Also, neurologic immaturity may prevent homeostasis in the hypoglycemic neonate, leading to unstable vital signs. However, some hypoglycemic neonates are asymptomatic.

Besides maternal diabetes, risk factors for hypoglycemia include prematurity, SGA status, severe isoimmune hemolytic anemia, and birth asphyxia.

A glucose oxidase dipstick value below 25 mg/100 ml indicates hypoglycemia and warrants a venous blood sample to confirm the diagnosis. Hypoglycemia is confirmed by a blood glucose level below 40 mg/dl before the first day after birth or below 45 mg/dl on or after the third day.

Hypocalcemia. The hypocalcemic neonate may have seizures, irritability, hypotonia, poor feeding, a high-pitched cry, and signs associated with hypoglycemia. Suspect hypocalcemia in the neonate of a diabetic mother. Other at-risk neonates include those who are preterm or SGA and those who experienced birth asphyxia.

To assess for hypocalcemia, attempt to elicit Chvostek's sign by tapping the skin over the sixth cranial nerve (in front of the ear); unilateral contraction of the muscles surrounding the eye, nose, and mouth indicates tetany, a sign of hypocalcemia. A serum calcium level below 7 mg/100 ml confirms the diagnosis.

Hyperbilirubinemia and jaundice. The neonate with hyperbilirubinemia has yellow skin and sclerae. For the most accurate assessment, apply pressure over the tip of the neonate's nose; a yellow tinge appearing as circulation returns indicates jaundice.

With pathologic jaundice (the more dangerous jaundice form), the serum bilirubin level rises above 13 mg/dl within the first 24 hours after delivery. Transcutaneous bilirubinometry (reflective photometry) sometimes is used as a screening tool for hyperbilirubinemia. This method detects bilirubin levels through the skin and is considered superior to observation of the skin or sclera color alone. However, its accuracy may be reduced in neonates with dark skin.

With severe hyperbilirubinemia (bilirubin encephalopathy), signs vary with the disease phase. Phase 1 signs include hypotonia, vomiting, lethargy, a high-pitched cry, a poor sucking reflex, a decreased or absent Moro reflex, and diminished flexion. During phase 2, spasticity develops; this may take the form of opisthotonus, a prolonged, severe muscle spasm in which the back arches acutely, the head bends back on the neck, the heels bend back on the leg, and the arms and hands flex rigidly at the joints.

In phase 3, spasticity diminishes, the sclera shows above the iris (a condition called sunset eyes), and seizures may occur. During phase 4, gastric, pulmonary, and CNS hemorrhages may develop (these problems also may occur during phase 2). A neonate who survives phase 4 usually has residual effects, such as mental retardation, cerebral palsy, and such sensory alterations as deafness and poor visual acuity or blindness.

Nursing diagnosis

For a partial list of applicable diagnoses, see Nursing Diagnoses: *High-risk neonates and their families,* page 426.

Planning and implementation

For hypoglycemia, if the neonate has no other problems, early feedings may be initiated to counteract the glucose imbalance. In other cases, expect to give glucose I.V., as 3 ml/kg of dextrose 10% in water. (The use of dextrose 25% to 50% in solution is contraindicated because it can cause vascular damage leading to ischemic necrosis.)

For hypocalcemia, expect to administer I.V. or oral supplemental calcium. The typical I.V. dosage is 24 mg/kg/day; the typical oral dosage, 75 mg/kg/day (Kliegman and Wald, 1986). When administering calcium by slow infusion, check the pulse frequently to detect bradycardia. Assess the infusion site every 30 minutes for signs of infiltration, which may cause tissue necrosis and sloughing. Monitor the serum calcium level every few hours, or according to facility policy. Once the serum calcium level stabilizes, draw daily blood samples.

For hyperbilirubinemia, the treatment depends on the serum bilirubin level. If the level is elevated only moderately or begins to fall by the fourth or fifth day after birth, the physician may order only early, frequent feedings, which increase intestinal motility and thus speed bilirubin excretion. However, persistent or severe hyperbilirubinemia commonly warrants phototherapy or complete exchange transfusion to prevent bilirubin encephalopathy.

The serum bilirubin level at which these treatments are ordered depends on the physician, facility policy, and the neonate's gestational age and condition. Some physicians initiate treatment when the bilirubin level measures 15 to 20 mg/100 ml; others wait until it reaches 20 mg/100 ml. (However, the preterm neonate may receive prophylactic phototherapy.) The nurse caring for a neonate undergoing phototherapy or exchange transfusion should perform the measures described earlier under "Nursing care of the high-risk neonate."

Evaluation

For examples of appropriate evaluation statements, see the general ones listed in "Nursing care of the high-risk neonate" earlier in this chapter. For the neonate with hyperbilirubinemia, these additional evaluation statements may be appropriate:
- The serum bilirubin level decreased to normal or near-normal limits.
- Jaundice diminished, as evidenced by improved skin and sclera color.
- The neonate was free of complications, such as transfusion reaction or infection, after exchange transfusion.

Documentation

For information about appropriate documentation, see the general points listed in "Nursing care of the high-risk neonate" earlier in this chapter.

INEFFECTIVE THERMOREGULATION

All neonates are in danger of ineffective thermoregulation—particularly hypothermia (an abnormally low body temperature). However, the risk is greatest in the preterm neonate, who has an immature temperature-regulating center, reduced body mass-to-surface ratio, decreased subcutaneous fat, inability to shiver or sweat, and inadequate metabolic reserves.

Hypothermia or hyperthermia (an abnormally high body temperature) can cause dramatic changes in vital signs (including tachycardia or bradycardia, tachypnea, and apnea) and increase energy consumption—especially dangerous in a high-risk neonate. Hypothermia increases oxygen consumption, predisposing the neonate to hypoxia. When hypothermia begins, skin temperature decreases first; without intervention, the core temperature falls and irreversible hypothermia may ensue, leading to death.

The body attempts to compensate for hypothermia by increasing the basal metabolic rate (BMR). If the BMR increases above the normal baseline level, however, energy supplies may become depleted, leading to acidosis. This, in turn, causes changes in subcutaneous tissue; decreased peripheral perfusion may lead to tissue damage and necrosis in the cheeks and buttocks, cessation of GI motility, and internal hemorrhage. Hypoglycemia may occur as glucose is metabolized in an effort to meet cellular energy demands. Less commonly, hypothermia causes coagulation changes (Fanaroff and Martin, 1987).

Other changes that may result from hypothermia include pulmonary vasoconstriction, decreased surfactant production, exacerbation of RDS, and impaired weight gain (Fanaroff and Martin, 1987).

Assessment
Hypothermia (a body temperature below 99.5° F [37.5° C]) causes an accelerated respiratory rate, labored respirations, an increased metabolic rate, and signs of hypoglycemia (indicating greater use of glucose stores).

Hyperthermia (a core temperature above 99.5° F) may cause skin reddening, dehydration, irritability, and an initial rise, then gradual drop, in the heart and respiratory rates.

Nursing diagnosis
For a partial list of applicable diagnoses, see Nursing Diagnoses: *High-risk neonates and their families,* page 426.

Planning and implementation
A first step in preventing hypothermia is to minimize cooling at delivery; such cooling may delay adequate thermoregulation for hours. Wrap the neonate in a plastic bag or thermal foil blanket as soon as possible after resusci-

tation, and then transfer the neonate to an incubator or radiant warmer bed.

Because heat loss from the neonate's head is considerable, keep the neonate's head covered at all times. Also, warm the hands before touching the neonate to prevent conductive heat loss through handling. For more information about preventing hypothermia, see the section on thermoregulation under "Nursing care in the high-risk neonate" earlier in this chapter.

Evaluation
For examples of appropriate evaluation statements, see the general ones listed in "Nursing care of the high-risk neonate" earlier in this chapter.

Documentation
For information about appropriate documentation, see the general points listed in "Nursing care of the high-risk neonate" earlier in this chapter.

POLYCYTHEMIA

In this disorder, the number of red blood cells (RBCs) increases, as reflected by a hematocrit elevation. Polycythemia can result from maternal-fetal transfusion, delayed umbilical cord clamping, or placental insufficiency.

As RBCs increase, blood viscosity increases, leading to impaired blood pumping through vessels. Respiratory compromise, cardiac problems, and thrombosis may ensue; hyperbilirubinemia may develop as the excess RBCs are destroyed.

Assessment
The neonate with polycythemia may have such signs as tachypnea, cyanosis, seizures, jaundice, and pleural and scrotal effusions. However, most polycythemic neonates are asymptomatic (Cassady and Strange, 1987).

Nursing diagnosis
For a partial list of applicable diagnoses, see Nursing Diagnoses: *High-risk neonates and their families,* page 426.

Planning and implementation
For an asymptomatic neonate, the physician may order only close observation and monitoring of the serum bilirubin level and fluid status. For a symptomatic neonate, a partial exchange transfusion may be ordered.

Evaluation

For examples of appropriate evaluation statements, see the general ones listed in "Nursing care of the high-risk neonate" earlier in this chapter.

Documentation

For information about appropriate documentation, see the general points listed in "Nursing care of the high-risk neonate" earlier in this chapter.

ISOIMMUNE HEMOLYTIC ANEMIAS

In these disorders (also called erythroblastosis fetalis), RBCs are destroyed prematurely. Two hemolytic anemias occurring in neonates are Rhesus (Rh) incompatibility and ABO blood group incompatibility.

Rh incompatibility. This blood incompatibility, which may cause critical illness in the neonate, occurs when an Rh-negative woman (one who lacks the Rh factor in the blood) carries an Rh-positive fetus. If maternal and fetal blood mix (as from a placental tear, prenatal bleeding, or a previous delivery), the mother may develop antibodies against fetal Rh antigens – a response called Rh sensitization. The antibodies cross the placenta, causing hemolysis of fetal RBCs. The resulting anemia may stimulate release of immature RBCs into the circulation; hemoglobin from hemolyzed RBCs breaks down to bilirubin.

In the fetus, the liver may enlarge to the point where it compresses the umbilical vein, compromising circulation and oxygen delivery. If hypoxia arises, the cardiovascular reserve is depleted rapidly and fluid accumulates, causing ascites. Also, as the liver becomes congested, hepatic protein synthesis may diminish, causing a life-threatening condition called hydrops fetalis, characterized by massive fetal edema (Nicholaides, 1989).

RBC destruction continues after delivery, causing severe anemia and jaundice in the neonate. Fortunately, Rh-negative women now receive $Rh_o(D)$ immune globulin (RhoGAM) within 3 days of a delivery or an abortion. Thus, Rh incompatibility now is rare.

ABO blood group incompatibility. This condition results from an antigen-antibody reaction by maternal RBCs, causing hemolysis of fetal RBCs. ABO incompatibility is most common when the mother has type O blood and the fetus has type A, B, or AB blood. Usually, it causes signs and symptoms similar to but far less severe than those seen in Rh incompatibility.

Assessment

When isoimmunization has occurred in utero, antepartal ultrasound evaluation may reveal fetal hepatomegaly and hydramnios; fetal monitoring may detect an abnormal heart rate pattern caused by tissue hypoxia at the level of the medulla oblongata (which controls cardiac function via the autonomic nervous system).

The neonate with Rh incompatibility typically is anemic at birth, as indicated by pale mucous membranes, and has massive generalized edema; with severe disease, expect pathologic jaundice, congestive heart failure (CHF), an enlarged liver and spleen, and generalized ascites. The neonate with ABO incompatibility may have anemia at birth and develop hyperbilirubinemia after delivery.

Nursing diagnosis

For a partial list of applicable diagnoses, see Nursing Diagnoses: *High-risk neonates and their families,* page 426.

Planning and implementation

Care for the neonate with Rh or ABO incompatibility centers on correcting anemia, managing hyperbilirubinemia, and preventing complications. Typically, these disorders warrant exchange transfusion followed by phototherapy.

To prevent Rh isoimmunization, expect the physician to administer prophylactic anti-D immunoglobulin (RhoGAM) to a woman with Rh-negative blood during the twenty-eighth week of pregnancy (Fanaroff and Martin, 1987) and within 48 to 72 hours of delivery of an Rh-positive neonate.

Evaluation

For examples of appropriate evaluation statements, see the general ones listed in "Nursing care of the high-risk neonate" earlier in this chapter. For the neonate with isoimmune hemolytic anemia, these additional evaluation statements may be appropriate:

• The serum bilirubin level decreased to normal or near-normal limits.
• Jaundice diminished, as evidenced by improved skin and sclera color.
• The neonate was free of complications, such as transfusion reaction or infection, after exchange transfusion.

Documentation

For information about appropriate documentation, see the general points listed in "Nursing care of the high-risk neonate" earlier in this chapter.

EFFECTS OF MATERNAL SUBSTANCE ABUSE

Maternal use of alcohol, narcotics, and other chemical substances during pregnancy can have devastating effects on the fetus and neonate. Maternal substance use during pregnancy is a serious and growing problem. Most drugs cross the palcenta, with potentially devastating effects on the fetus.

Fetal alcohol syndrome. This syndrome involves alterations in intrauterine growth and development. A common finding in the NICU, fetal alcohol syndrome (FAS) may lead to growth deficiency, microcephaly, mental retardation, poor coordination, facial abnormalities, behavioral deviations (such as irritability), and cardiac and joint anomalies.

Alcohol crosses the placenta in the same concentration as is present in the maternal circulation. Damage to fetal cells may result from alcohol itself or from acetaldehyde, an alcohol oxidation product. Such damage is not limited to a particular gestational period. Also, researchers cannot pinpoint a safe level of alcohol consumption; even moderate drinking during the first trimester can cause physical characteristics of FAS. Consequently, pregnant women should be advised to avoid all alcohol (Jones, 1986). (Alcoholic beverages now carry labels warning that alcohol ingestion during pregnancy may affect the fetus.)

Drug exposure, addiction, and withdrawal. Depending on the stage of fetal development during exposure, maternal narcotic use may cause subtle or profound effects, including congenital anomalies, asphyxia, prematurity, respiratory and cardiac disorders, CNS abnormalities, and death. Intrauterine growth retardation leading to low birth weight also may occur, possibly from drug-induced slowing of blood flow to the placenta, which reduces nutrient delivery to the fetus. A fetus exposed to such drugs as heroin, methadone, or barbiturates also may become addicted and must go through withdrawal after birth.

A pregnant woman who uses drugs also puts her fetus in jeopardy by increasing her risk of poor nutrition, anemia, systemic or local infection, preeclampsia, and exposure to such diseases as human immunodeficiency virus (HIV), the virus that causes acquired immunodeficiency syndrome (AIDS). Intrapartal effects of maternal drug use include fetal distress and preterm delivery. After delivery, the neonate who is going through withdrawal may exhibit behavioral deviations that hinder parent-infant bonding, including irritability, continual crying, and poor feeding.

Ironically, the fetal stress caused by maternal heroin use has one positive consequence: It accelerates respiratory maturation. Consequently, the incidence of respiratory infections and RDS is relatively low among neonates of heroin users (Flandermeyer, 1987).

Maternal use of cocaine—a powerful CNS stimulant causing vasoconstriction, hypertension, and tachycardia—may result in various perinatal problems, depending on the gestational period and duration of exposure. These problems include profound congenital anomalies (such as urogenital anomalies in male neonates), abruptio placentae, altered brain-wave activity, cerebral infarcts (which may develop as late as 40 weeks' gestation), and prune-belly syndrome (characterized by a protruding, thin-walled abdomen; bladder and ureter dilation; small, dysplastic kidneys; undescended testes; and absence of a portion of the rectus abdominis muscle). Death also may occur (Kennard, 1990).

Assessment

The neonate with FAS may have cardiac anomalies, decreased joint mobility, behavioral deviations, kidney defects, labial hypoplasia, and distinctive facial features. The latter include short palpebral fissures (eye openings); ptosis (drooping eyelids); strabismus (eye muscle deviation); a thin, smooth upper lip with a long philtrum (vertical groove) above it; a short, upturned nose; and a receding jaw. Behavioral deviations include irritability, excessive crying, and poor feeding.

The neonate affected by maternal drug abuse may have muscle tremors, twitching, or rigidity, with inability to extend the muscles; seizures; temperature instability; GI disturbances, including vomiting and diarrhea; tachycardia; tachypnea; diaphoresis with mottling over the extremities; and excessive sneezing and yawning. If the mother used heroin or methadone during pregnancy, the neonate may be SGA or have a low birth weight with cardiorespiratory depression at delivery.

Typically, the behavior pattern of the drug-addicted neonate is disorganized, with marked fussiness and irritability (which may be exacerbated by eye contact), prolonged periods of high-pitched crying, and poor consolability. Normal neonatal reflexes, especially the Moro reflex, are highly exaggerated. The sucking reflex is strong and the neonate may suck on the hands and fists frequently. However, sucking may be poorly coordinated with swallowing, impairing feeding. Sleep periods may be abnormally short; unlike the normal neonate, who spends more time asleep than awake, the addicted neonate may have a sleep-awake ratio of 1 to 3.

Signs of drug withdrawal typically begin about 12 to 48 hours after birth. (For a list of these signs, see *As-*

ASSESSING FOR DRUG WITHDRAWAL

The neonate whose mother used such drugs as narcotics, barbiturates, or cocaine during pregnancy may be addicted at birth and go through withdrawal. Classic signs of neonatal drug withdrawal are listed below.

Vital sign deviations
- Profound diaphoresis
- Skin mottling
- Tachycardia or bradycardia (depending on the drug involved)
- Tachypnea
- Temperature instability (fever followed by hypothermia)

Neuromuscular signs
- Absent or strong sucking reflex (may be poorly coordinated with swallowing reflex)
- Exaggeration of other neonatal reflexes
- Difficulty extending muscles
- Jerky movements
- Muscle rigidity with flexion
- Muscle twitching
- Seizures
- Tremors

Behavioral signs
- Decreased sleep periods and lengthened awake periods
- Dislike for cuddling and close body contact
- Frequent or prolonged sneezing or yawning
- High-pitched or weak cry, inconsolability
- Irritability

Gastrointestinal signs
- Frequent vomiting
- Increased gastrointestinal motility, with diarrhea and rapid (possibly visible) peristalsis

sessing for drug withdrawal.) As withdrawal progresses, these signs worsen. Try to verify that the mother used drugs during pregnancy if neonatal drug addiction or withdrawal is suspected. However, keep in mind that some women may deny or misrepresent drug use.

If the neonate's mother used I.V. drugs, an HIV test should be done. Maternally conferred IgG may interfere with the accuracy of an HIV antibody test for the first few months after birth; therefore, an HIV antigen test is preferred. Assess for signs of HIV infection, including facial dysmorphism, hepatosplenomegaly, interstitial pneumonia, subtle neurologic abnormalities, behavioral changes, and recurrent infection.

Nursing diagnosis

For a partial list of applicable diagnoses, see Nursing Diagnoses: *High-risk neonates and their families,* page 426.

Planning and implementation

For FAS, no treatment exists because the structural damage occurs in utero. Supportive management focuses on developmental care and environmental support. If the neonate has poorly coordinated sucking and swallowing reflexes, expect to give enteral feedings to prevent aspiration; physical therapy also may be implemented to help alleviate this problem.

For the neonate who is addicted to maternal drugs or going through drug withdrawal, nursing goals include:
- ensuring adequate nutritional intake
- improving coordination of the sucking and swallowing reflexes
- reducing irritability by minimizing environmental stimulation
- avoiding abrupt movements near the neonate
- promoting a normal sleep-awake cycle to prolong sleep
- stabilizing body temperature.

To reduce tremors and extraneous movement, swaddle the neonate and touch the tremulous area firmly and calmly. To minimize muscle rigidity or hypertonicity, bathe the neonate in warm water, massage gently, and swaddle in a flexed position. Do not leave the neonate in a supine position that maintains muscle extension or stiffness.

For the neonate going through withdrawal, treatment varies with the health care facility and the substance involved. Seizures may be controlled with phenobarbital (5 to 8 mg/kg/day).

Evaluation

For examples of appropriate evaluation statements, see the general ones listed in "Nursing care of the high-risk neonate" earlier in this chapter.

Documentation

For information about appropriate documentation, see the general points listed in "Nursing care of the high-risk neonate" earlier in this chapter. For the neonate suffering the effects of maternal substance abuse, documentation also should include:
- vital sign deviations
- reflexes
- muscle twitching or rigidity
- seizures

- behavioral status, including crying, irritability, and sleep and awake periods
- gastrointestinal status, including vomiting, diarrhea, and increased peristalsis.

INFECTION

An infection can be acquired in utero, during labor and delivery, or after birth. The preterm neonate is especially vulnerable to postnatal infection because of reduced transmission of maternal immunoglobulins, including IgM and IgA. Unable to produce antibodies, the preterm neonate also cannot effectively phagocytose foreign proteins or mount a sufficient inflammatory response.

Agents that can infect the fetus or neonate, causing potentially morbid effects, are referred to as TORCH agents. This acronym stands for toxoplasmosis, others, rubella, cytomegalovirus, and herpes. Most TORCH infections are acquired in utero.

Cytomegalovirus (CMV) is the most common transplacentally acquired infection; it also can be acquired during delivery. CMV may result in CNS damage, although typically it causes no detectable signs at birth. Rubella, another transplacentally acquired infection, also causes serious sequelae. If acquired during the first trimester, it may result in CNS damage and cardiac defects; after the fourteenth week of gestation, the major sequela is deafness. Other transplacentally acquired infections include measles, chickenpox, smallpox, vaccinia, hepatitis B, HIV, toxoplasmosis, and syphilis.

Bacterial pneumonia, which can lead to intrauterine death, may be acquired by the fetus after prolonged rupture of the membranes (more than 24 hours), in which vaginal organisms may migrate upward. Bacterial organisms that can cause intrauterine bacteria pneumonia include nonhemolytic streptococci, *Escherichia coli* and other gram-negative organisms, *Listeria monocytogenes,* and *Candida.*

HIV can be acquired transplacentally at various times in gestation, intrapartally through contact with maternal blood and secretions, and postnatally through breast milk. The neonate with HIV typically has a distinctive facial dysmorphism (malformation) and suffers such problems as interstitial pneumonia, hepatosplenomegaly, recurrent infections, behavioral deviations, and neurologic abnormalities. In many cases, the neonate with HIV is small for gestational age and suffers failure to thrive. (For information on this problem, see *Child abuse and failure to thrive in the high-risk neonate,* page 470.)

Infections that can be acquired as the fetus passes through the birth canal include:

- *Chlamydia trachomatis,* which may lead to conjunctivitis or pneumonia (if secretions pass into the eyes or oropharynx)
- *Neisseria gonorrhoeae,* which may cause ophthalmia neonatorum, an acute purulent conjunctivitis
- herpes simplex virus, which may result in skin vesicles, lethargy, respiratory problems, convulsions, disseminated vascular coagulation, hepatitis, keratoconjunctivitis, and death.

A pregnant client with known herpes simplex virus should be observed closely through frequent cervical cultures to determine whether the virus is active. Active virus at the time of delivery usually warrants cesarean delivery—an approach that has reduced the number of neonatal herpes cases (Hager, 1983).

Assessment

The neonate with an infection may be SGA at birth, with a nonspecific rash, pallor, hypotonia, jaundice, lethargy, hyperthermia, or hypothermia. Other common signs accompanying infection include apnea or tachypnea, tachycardia or bradycardia, abdominal distention, hepatomegaly, splenomegaly, seizures, diarrhea, occult blood in the stool, and bleeding disorders. The behavior pattern may be abnormal and the reflexes diminished; poor feeding may cause failure to thrive.

With an intrapartally acquired infection, the neonate may not appear ill at birth but will show gradual deterioration in vital signs over the next 6 to 12 hours. However, with group B streptococcal infection—a commonly acquired intrapartal infection—the neonate may have dyspnea and cyanosis and appear quite ill. However, RDS and congenital cardiac anomalies can cause similar signs and must be ruled out. The following laboratory results suggest perinatal infection:

- an increased number of immature cells, as shown by the white blood cell (WBC) differential
- a WBC count above 20,000/mm³, reflecting leukocytosis (an abnormal increase in the number of WBCs)
- an absolute neutrophil count exceeding 60%
- a thrombocyte count below 100,000/mm³ with an abnormally high reticulocyte count.

A neonate who acquired HIV intrapartally may be preterm or SGA, with an abnormally small head and distinctive facial features. Disorders seen in neonates with HIV infection include oral candidiasis (thrush) and lymphoid interstitial pneumonitis. Later, such problems as lymphadenopathy, chronic diarrhea, viral and bacterial infections, *Pneumocystis carinii* pneumonia, and parotid gland enlargement may occur.

CHILD ABUSE AND FAILURE TO THRIVE IN THE HIGH-RISK NEONATE

Potential long-term effects of high-risk status at birth include child abuse and failure to thrive.

Child abuse

Although studies have failed to show a clear link between child abuse and preterm birth or chronic illness, both preterm status and congenital anomalies are associated with child abuse. However, the actual cause of abuse usually is secondary; for instance, frustration brought on by the combined pressures of the child's high-risk status and other family circumstances, such as poor financial resources (White, Benedict, Wulff, and Kelley, 1987). Therefore, identifying potential sources of stress and planning interventions to help parents deal with them is a crucial focus of nursing care.

If other factors with a high incidence in child-abuse cases also are present in a high-risk neonate's family, the potential for abuse—and thus the need for further assessment and intervention—may increase. These factors include:

- family or social isolation
- history of family abuse or neglect
- marital problems
- insufficient child-care arrangements
- siblings close in age
- decreased parent-neonate contact in the neonatal intensive care unit (Hunter, Kilstrom, Kraybill, and Loda, 1978).

If indications of a potential problem appear, the nurse should assess further and, as necessary, arrange for follow-up counseling with a nurse specialist in family therapy, a social worker, or other professional to help family members deal with pressures before they lead to child abuse. The nurse who suspects that abuse already has occurred should follow legal requirements and facility policy for reporting suspected child abuse.

Failure to thrive

In a full-term neonate or infant, failure to thrive is defined as a length and weight below the third percentile. For a preterm neonate or infant whose birth weight was significantly below normal, failure to thrive must be judged in terms of progress; the term should not be applied as long as the infant gains steadily over time, even if length and weight are below the third percentile.

Failure to thrive occurs because the neonate or infant cannot grow and develop normally—for organic reasons, inorganic reasons, or a combination of the two. In *organic* failure to thrive, physiologic problems (some of which may be associated with a high-risk birth) prevent the neonate or infant from digesting or ingesting sufficient nutrients to maintain normal growth. In *inorganic* failure to thrive, diagnosed when no organic cause can be found, the neonate or infant does not develop a bond with the caregiver; even with sufficient intake, the child has poor weight gain and may fail to achieve developmental milestones.

Failure to thrive occurs in high-risk neonates for both organic and inorganic reasons. Not only may a physical defect or repeated illness interfere with growth, but lengthy hospitalization may prevent the formation of a trusting relationship with a permanent caregiver. Likewise, parents who fear that their seriously ill child will die may hold back from forming a normal parent-infant bond.

In the high-risk neonate or infant, lack of steady growth progress, poor eye contact, decreased interaction with the environment, and heightened irritability or lethargy may indicate failure to thrive. If such signs appear, the nurse should report them to the physician while working with the parents to strengthen their bond with the child.

Because maternal HIV antibodies are transferred to the fetus, a neonate whose mother has the virus may test positive for HIV antibodies even when not infected. Consequently, an HIV culture or antigen test must be used to confirm infection.

Nursing diagnosis

For a partial list of applicable diagnoses, see Nursing Diagnoses: *High-risk neonates and their families,* page 426.

Planning and implementation

When caring for a neonate with an infection, practice meticulous hand washing and asepsis. For more information, see "Preventing and controlling infection" in this chapter.

Evaluation

For examples of appropriate evaluation statements, see the general ones listed in "Nursing care of the high-risk ne-onate" earlier in this chapter. For the neonate with infection, this additional evaluation statement may be appropriate:

- The neonate showed a positive response to antibiotic therapy, as evidenced by improved vital signs and reductions in behavioral deviations, high-pitched crying, and temperature instability.

Documentation

For information about appropriate documentation, see the general points listed in "Nursing care of the high-risk neonate" earlier in this chapter. For the neonate with a diagnosed infection, documentation also should include:

- behavioral and physical changes indicative of infection
- the time when antibiotic therapy began and ended
- response to and tolerance of antibiotic therapy
- any cultures or blood samples taken.

CONGENITAL ANOMALIES

Many congenital anomalies are life-threatening and warrant immediate intervention and referral to a level 3 nursery. Such disorders include tracheoesophageal malformations, diaphragmatic hernia, omphalocele, gastroschisis, meningomyelocele, encephalocele, and imperforate anus. Other anomalies do not require immediate treatment but may lead to chronic disability or deformity.

The exact cause of many congenital anomalies remains unknown. Some have been linked to genetic or chromosomal disorders, congenital rubella, exposure to radiation, maternal diabetes, and maternal drug use. Increased maternal age also has been associated with certain anomalies, including the trisomy disorders.

CNS anomalies. More congenital anomalies involve the CNS than any other body system. Some CNS anomalies result in only minimal dysfunction; others have devastating consequences.

Meningomyelocele. In this anomaly (also called spina bifida), part of the meninges and spinal cord substance protrude through the vertebral column; the defect may be covered by a thin membrane. (When only the meninges protrude, the anomaly is called a meningocele.) Meningomyelocele results from defective neural tube formation during embryonic development. Hydrocephalus (discussed below) commonly accompanies the anomaly.

Consequences of meningomyelocele may be severe—for instance, paralysis below the defect. The child's appearance may be noticeably abnormal even after surgical correction.

Encephalocele. In this anomaly, the meninges and portions of brain tissue protrude through the cranium, usually in the occipital area. Typically, it occurs at the midline, through a suture line. Like meningomyelocele, encephalocele results from failure of the neural tube to close during embryonic development, may be accompanied by hydrocephalus, and may lead to paralysis.

Congenital hydrocephalus. In this disorder, excessive CSF accumulates within the cranial vault, leading to suture expansion and ventricular dilation. This anomaly may result from obstruction of the foramen of Monro—a passage allowing communication between the lateral and third ventricles. Hydrocephalus sometimes is associated with meningomyelocele and other neural tube defects, intrauterine infection, meningitis, cerebral hemorrhage, head trauma, or Arnold-Chiari malformation (herniation of the brain stem and lower cerebellum through the foramen magnum into the cervical vertebral canal).

Anencephaly and microcephaly. In anencephaly, the cephalic end of the spinal cord fails to close, causing absence of the cerebral hemispheres. Anencephaly commonly causes stillbirth; if not, the neonate typically lives only a few days.

In microcephaly, the head is abnormally small and the brain underdeveloped, usually resulting in severe mental retardation and motor dysfunction. Microcephaly may result from an inborn error of metabolism (such as uncontrolled maternal phenylketonuria), intrauterine infection, or severe prolonged intrauterine hypoxia. (For a description of some inborn errors of metabolism, see *Inborn errors of metabolism,* pages 472 and 473.)

Teratoma. This neoplasm, which may be solid or fluid-filled, consists of various cell types, none of which normally occur together. The most common site is the sacrococcygeal area, although it may occur anywhere. Teratoma develops if the primitive streak (a dense area on the central posterior region of the embryonic disk) fails to disappear. This gives rise to a mass that may contain calcium and other tissue fragments (visible on X-ray).

Cardiac anomalies. Congenital cardiac anomalies—structural defects of the heart and great vessels—can occur during any stage of embryonic development. Cardiac structures are most susceptible to defects from the third to ninth weeks of gestation. In most cases, the cause remains unknown, although researchers believe that genetic and environmental factors play a role. Defects become noticeable after delivery when fetal circulation normally changes to neonatal circulation.

Congenital cardiac anomalies are classified as acyanotic or cyanotic. Acyanotic defects include atrial septal defect, ventricular septal defect, coarctation of the aorta, pulmonic stenosis, and PDA. These anomalies do not interfere with shunting of oxygenated blood from the left to the right side of the heart; the left side continues to eject oxygenated blood, preventing cyanosis. However, pulmonary blood flow to the right ventricle increases, placing the neonate at risk for pulmonary edema and CHF.

Cyanotic defects include tetralogy of Fallot, transposition of the great vessels, and tricuspid atresia. In such defects, abnormally high pressure in the right side of the heart permits left-to-right shunting of unoxygenated blood. As this blood mixes with oxygenated blood, arterial blood oxygen becomes desaturated. Peripheral perfusion then decreases and cyanosis develops. (For descriptions

INBORN ERRORS OF METABOLISM

An inborn error of metabolism is a genetic condition in which a defect of a specific enzyme disrupts metabolism and nutrient use. The involved enzyme may not be produced or its action may be blocked by lack of a precursor necessary for a crucial chemical reaction.

The nursing goal for a neonate with an inborn error of metabolism is early detection and prevention of complications. The chart below describes these disorders and presents nursing implications for each.

CONDITION	DESCRIPTION	NURSING IMPLICATIONS
Congenital hypothyroidism	Deficiency of thyroid hormone secretion during fetal development or early infancy. The condition (also known as cretinism) typically stems from defective embryonic development causing absence or underdevelopment of the thyroid gland or severe maternal iodine deficiency; in some cases, it is inherited as an autosomal recessive disorder involving an enzymatic defect in the synthesis of the thyroid hormone thyroxine. Untreated, congenital hypothyroidism can lead to respiratory compromise and persistent physiologic jaundice.	• Signs of congenital hypothyroidism in the neonate include inactivity, jaundice, excessive sleep, hoarse cry, constipation, and feeding problems. • Many states require measurement of thyroid hormone levels at birth to detect congenital hypothyroidism early and thus help minimize mental and physical retardation. The disorder is confirmed by an elevated serum level of thyroid-stimulating hormone (TSH) and a low serum thyroxine (T_4) level. (However, test results may be misleading in the preterm neonate—especially one with respiratory distress syndrome, who typically has abnormal TSH and T_4 levels.) • Treatment involves lifelong administration of L-thyroxine, with periodic dosage adjustments to meet the demands of rapid growth periods. During the neonatal period, thyroxine can be given mixed with several milliliters of formula or crushed and mixed with rice cereal or applesauce when the infant begins eating solid foods.
Galactosemia	Hereditary autosomal recessive disorder in which deficiency of the enzyme galactose-1-phosphate uridyltransferase leads to inability to convert galactose to glucose and subsequent galactose accumulation in the blood. The disorder can be fatal if not detected and treated within the first few days after birth.	• Because the affected neonate cannot tolerate lactose, feeding problems may be the first sign of the disorder. Such problems may include anorexia, diarrhea, vomiting, jaundice, hepatomegaly, growth failure, lack of a red light reflex during eye examination, cataracts, and mental retardation (from elevated fetal galactose levels). Also, birth weight may be somewhat low. With early detection and treatment, these problems may subside. • Diagnosis is confirmed by the galactosemia tolerance test and examination of red blood cells revealing deficient galactose-1-phosphate uridyltransferase activity. • In some cases, galactosemia may be detected in utero by amniocentesis. In such cases, the mother should be placed on a galactose-restricted diet to prevent fetal complications and mental retardation. • Treatment involves lifelong avoidance of galactose-containing foods (milk and milk products).
Maple syrup urine disease	Autosomal recessive disorder characterized by an enzyme deficiency in the second step of branched-chain amino acid (BCAA) catabolism. BCAAs accumulate in the blood and urine, causing severe ketoacidosis soon after birth. Without intervention, the neonate progresses rapidly to death (usually from pneumonia and respiratory failure).	• The neonate typically appears normal at birth but deteriorates within 1 week as respirations become rapid and shallow and the level of consciousness declines. Other signs of the disorder include lethargy, alternating muscle hypotonicity and hypertonicity, brief tonic (rigid) seizures, hypoglycemic manifestations (from altered glucose metabolism), and a maple syrup odor to the urine. • Diagnosis is confirmed by a 2,4-dinitrophenylhydrazine test and serum elevation of the essential amino acids leucine, isoleucine, and valine. • Management involves lifelong dietary restriction of BCAAs and close monitoring of serum leucine, isoleucine, and valine levels. An acute episode warrants peritoneal dialysis.

INBORN ERRORS OF METABOLISM *(continued)*

CONDITION	DESCRIPTION	NURSING IMPLICATIONS
Phenylketonuria (PKU)	Autosomal recessive disorder characterized by the abnormal presence of metabolites of phenylalanine (such as phenylketone) in the urine. It results from deficiency of phenylalanine hydroxylase, the enzyme responsible for converting the amino acid phenylalanine to tyrosine. Phenylalanine is transaminated to phenylpyruvic acid or decarboxylated to phenylthalanine, which then accumulates in the blood. Prolonged exposure to high serum levels of phenylalanine may cause severe brain damage and mental retardation.	• Most states require PKU screening at birth. The test usually is done within the first 24 to 48 hours after birth. If results are positive, re-testing and referral should take place immediately to ensure early treatment. • Obtain blood for the screening test by heel stick. To prevent a false-negative test result, make sure the neonate has received adequate dietary protein and had no contraindications for oral feedings for 24 to 48 hours before the test. • Immediately after diagnosis, the neonate should be given Lafenalac (if the overall condition permits). This formula has a phenylalanine concentration of about 0.5% (in contrast to the 5% found in most infant formulas). • Usually, Lafenalac must be substituted for milk throughout the child's growing periods. Dietary restriction of phenylalanine must continue lifelong. Serum phenylalanine blood levels must be monitored closely throughout childhood. • Provide teaching, nutritional counseling, and emotional support to the neonate's family. Emphasize that the neonate cannot be given substitutions for prescribed food products, especially for Lafenalac. Refer the family to any available support groups for help in coping with the disease. • A woman with PKU who contemplates pregnancy should be warned about the possible effects of an elevated maternal phenylalanine level on the developing fetus (including congenital anomalies and mental retardation).

and illustrations of specific acyanotic and cyanotic defects, see *Congenital cardiac anomalies,* pages 474 and 475.)

Respiratory tract anomalies. The most common respiratory tract anomaly is diaphragmatic hernia. In this defect, the various segments of the diaphragm fail to fuse during embryonic development, causing the abdominal contents to protrude from the abdominal cavity into the thoracic cavity at birth. Diaphragmatic hernia occurs in 1 of every 2,000 births. In the United States, it is twice as common in males as in females (Harjo, Kenner, and Brueggemeyer, 1988).

The defect may be unilateral or bilateral; most commonly, it occurs on the posterolateral aspect of the diaphragm on the left side. In a left-sided defect, the stomach and intestines typically protrude into the thoracic cavity; protrusion of the liver, spleen, and other abdominal organs is rare.

Most neonates with diaphragmatic hernia have impaired lung development—typically only a lung bud is present (a condition known as hypoplastic lung). This may lead to profound respiratory compromise and death if intervention does not begin immediately after delivery.

GI tract anomalies. These anomalies include tracheoesophageal malformations, abdominal wall defects (omphalocele and gastroschisis), meconium ileus, imperforate anus, and cleft palate and lip.

Tracheoesophageal malformations. Tracheoesophageal malformations, which occur in 1 of every 1,500 live births (Harjo, Kenner, and Brueggemeyer, 1988), result from altered embryonic development of the trachea and esophagus. These anomalies sometimes occur as part of the VACTERL syndrome—vertebral, anal, cardiac, tracheal, esophageal, renal, and limb anomalies. Types of tracheoesophageal anomalies include tracheoesophageal fistula (an abnormal connection between the trachea and esophagus), esophageal atresia (closure of the esophagus at some point), and absence of the esophagus. Usually, tracheoesophageal fistula occurs in tandem with esophageal atresia. In the most common tracheoesophageal malformation, esophageal atresia accompanies distal tracheoesophageal fistula; the upper esophageal section ends in a blind pouch (atresia) that does not connect with the stomach. (For an illustration of this and other types of tracheoesophageal malformations, see *Tracheoesophageal malformations,* page 476.)

CONGENITAL CARDIAC ANOMALIES

Abnormalities during fetal development may cause structural defects of the heart and great vessels. These defects probably stem from a combination of genetic or chromosomal disorders and environmental factors. Maternal alcoholism, malnutrition, rubella, or diabetes mellitus may contribute to cardiac anomalies. In the illustrations, blood flow is indicated by arrows—red arrows for oxygenated blood, black arrows for deoxygenated blood, and dotted arrows for mixed blood.

Atrial septal defect

In this defect, an abnormal opening in the atrial septum allows oxygenated blood from the left atrium to shunt to the right atrium where it mixes with deoxygenated blood; thus, blood in the right heart and the pulmonary arteries is mixed. The increased blood flow to the right heart and pulmonary arteries causes the right ventricle and atrium to enlarge. In many cases, this defect results from failure of the foramen ovale to close.

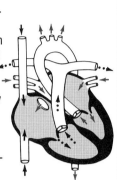

Coarctation of the aorta

This anomaly obstructs preductal or postductal blood flow. The more commonly encountered postductal coarctation illustrated here causes increased pressure in the left ventricle. To compensate, collateral circulation develops, enhancing blood flow from the proximal arteries and bypassing the obstructed area.

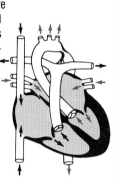

Pulmonic stenosis

This defect may be characterized by poststenotic dilation of the pulmonary trunk and concentric hypertrophy of the right ventricle, which cause a systolic pressure differential between the right ventricular cavity and pulmonary artery.

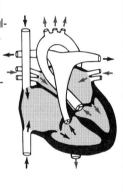

Tetralogy of Fallot

This anomaly consists of four defects—ventricular septal defect, overriding aorta, pulmonic stenosis, and right ventricular hypertrophy. Hemodynamic changes depend on the severity of these defects and typically involve a right-to-left shunt, in which deoxygenated blood from the right ventricle enters the overriding aorta directly. The blood in the aorta is mixed (deoxygenated blood from the right ventricle and oxygenated blood from the left ventricle).

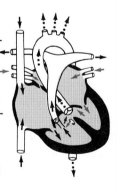

Transposition of the great vessels

In this anomaly, the pulmonary artery arises from the left ventricle and the aorta from the right ventricle, preventing the pulmonary and systemic circulations from mixing. Without associated defects that allow these circulatory systems to mix—such as a patent ductus arteriosus or septal defect—the neonate will die.

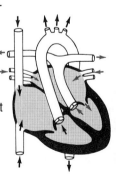

Ventricular septal defect

In this defect, an abnormal opening in the ventricular septum allows oxygenated blood to flow from the left to right ventricle, resulting in recirculation of mixed blood through the lungs and pulmonary artery. If the defect is large, pulmonary vascular resistance increases, causing elevated pulmonary and right ventricular pressures.

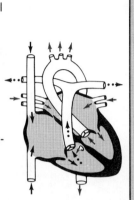

Patent ductus arteriosus

This anomaly occurs when the ductus arteriosus—a tubular connection that shunts blood away from the fetus's pulmonary circulation—fails to close after birth. Oxygenated blood then shunts from the aorta to the pulmonary artery, resulting in mixed blood distal to the ductus arteriosus.

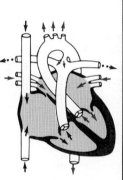

Tricuspid atresia

In this defect, which usually is accompanied by an atrial or ventricular septal defect (both shown), the tricuspid valve is absent or incomplete, preventing the flow of blood from the right atrium to the right ventricle. Right atrial blood then shunts through an atrial septal defect into the left atrium, resulting in mixed blood in the left atrium, left ventricle, and aorta.

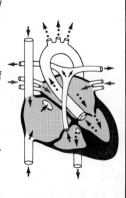

Abdominal wall defects. Omphalocele and gastroschisis occur in approximately 1 of every 7,000 births (Harjo, Kenner, and Brueggemeyer, 1988). In omphalocele, a portion of the intestine protrudes through a defect in the abdominal wall at the umbilicus, in the midline. A thin, transparent membrane composed of amnion and peritoneum typically covers the protruding part. (The membrane sometimes ruptures during delivery and thus may not be visible by the time the neonate is admitted to the NICU.) The defect may be quite large—or small enough to elude detection on brief inspection.

Omphalocele arises during embryonic development when the abdominal contents migrate into the umbilical cord. Normally, at 9 weeks' gestation, the abdominal contents recede from the umbilical cord, regressing into the abdominal cavity; if the contents fail to recede, omphalocele occurs.

Gasproschisis refers to incomplete abdominal wall closure not involving the site of the umbilical cord insertion. Usually, the small intestine and part of the large intestine protrude. No membranous sac covers the protrusion.

Meconium ileus. This intestinal obstruction results from obstruction of the terminal ileum by viscous meconium. Beyond the ileal obstruction, the colon atrophies and narrows in diameter. In at least 95% of cases, it is a sign of cystic fibrosis, a genetic disease resulting from a pancreatic enzyme deficiency.

Imperforate anus. In this malformation, the anus is closed abnormally. Occurring in 1 of every 20,000 live births, the disorder is more common in males than females (Harjo, Kenner, and Brueggemeyer, 1988). It results from persistence of the membrane that separates the lower rectum from the lower aspect of the large intestine. (Normally, this membrane disappears by the ninth week of gestation, leading to formation of a patent tube from the intestine to the rectum.) In many cases, imperforate anus is associated with other defects, such as rectourethral and rectovaginal fistula (both of which permit abnormal evacuation of fecal matter from the rectum).

Imperforate anus occurs as several variants. In anal agenesis, the most common variant, the rectal pouch ends blindly above the surface of the perineum; an anal fistula commonly is present. In anal stenosis, the anal aperture is abnormally small. In anal membrane atresia, the anal membrane covers the aperture, creating an obstruction.

Imperforate anus also may be classified as high or low. In the high form, a fistula links the upper rectal pouch to the bladder, urethra, or vagina. If a fistula is absent, bowel obstruction occurs and the neonate has a large, distended

TRACHEOESOPHAGEAL MALFORMATIONS

Tracheoesophageal malformations result from incomplete separation of the trachea and esophagus during the first trimester of pregnancy. Among the most serious surgical emergencies in neonates, they require immediate correction. In many cases, they are accompanied by other congenital anomalies. Common variations of tracheoesophageal malformations are illustrated here.

Esophageal atresia with distal tracheoesophageal fistula is the most common variation.

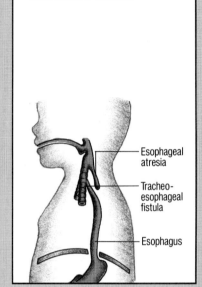

Esophageal atresia

Tracheo-esophageal fistula

Esophagus

In **esophageal atresia without tracheoesophageal fistula,** the upper esophageal portion ends in a blind pouch, the upper and lower esophageal portions do not connect, and the trachea and esophagus are not linked by a fistula.

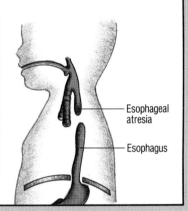

Esophageal atresia

Esophagus

Tracheoesophageal fistula without esophageal atresia (sometimes called an H-type tracheoesophageal fistula) is characterized by an intact esophagus and a connection between the trachea and esophagus.

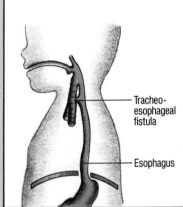

Tracheo-esophageal fistula

Esophagus

In some cases, **esophageal atresia** occurs with a **proximal fistula.**

Esophageal atresia

Tracheo-esophageal fistula

Esophagus

Esophageal atresia sometimes occurs with a **double** (proximal and distal) **fistula.**

Double tracheo-esophageal fistula

Esophagus

abdomen. In low imperforate anus, intestinal patency may be compromised by a membrane at the anal sphincter level.

Cleft palate and cleft lip. These congenital defects, which occur in 1 of every 1,000 live births (Harjo, Kenner, and Brueggemeyer, 1988), sometimes result from chromo-somal abnormalities. Cleft palate occurs when the sides of the palate fail to fuse during embryonic development, leading to a fissure in the palatal midline. The fissure may be complete, extending through both the hard and soft palates into the nasal cavities, or incomplete.

In cleft lip (harelip), one or more clefts appear in the upper lip resulting from failure of the maxillary and median nasal processes to close during embryonic development. The defect, which is more common in males than females, may be unilateral or bilateral and sometimes occurs in conjunction with other anomalies. It commonly accompanies cleft palate.

Genitourinary tract anomalies. Genitourinary tract anomalies include renal agenesis, polycystic kidney disease, posterior urethral valves, and external genital ambiguity.

Renal agenesis. One of the most common congenital anomalies in males, renal agenesis may be unilateral (absence of one kidney) or bilateral (absence of both kidneys). The bilateral form (also called Potter's association) is incompatible with life and typically causes stillbirth or death during the neonatal period; autopsies of neonates with bilateral renal agenesis show hypoplastic lung and multiple pneumothoraces. With unilateral agenesis, the single kidney enlarges to maintain normal renal function.

Polycystic kidney disease. In this disorder, which occurs as an autosomal recessive disease in the neonate and as an acquired disease in the adult, multiple cysts form within the kidney. As the cysts enlarge, adjacent tissue is destroyed. At birth, the neonate with polycystic kidney disease typically suffers renal failure, respiratory distress, CHF, and hypertension.

Posterior urethral valves. This anomaly, which occurs only in males, causes urinary tract obstruction, hydronephrosis, impaired urine flow, and (when untreated) profound renal damage. Typically, the obstructing valves are exaggerations of two mucosal folds that normally are continuous with the lower end of the urethera where the ejaculatory ducts open.

External genital ambiguity. This problem may reflect a developmental defect, genetic abnormality, or hormonal influences. In some cases, it complicates determination of the neonate's sex. In males, genital ambiguity typically stems from a developmental abnormality. In females, a common cause is congenital adrenal hyperplasia, a condition stemming from blockage of cortisol precursors (enzymes that convert cholesterol to cortisol). The resulting corticotropin deficiency leads to increased secretion of cortisol precursors and androgens and subsequent masculinization of the female external genitalia.

Musculoskeletal anomalies. The most common congenital musculoskeletal anomaly is clubfoot (talipes). This deformity involves unilateral or bilateral deviation of the meta-

tarsal bones; talus deformation and a shortened Achilles tendon give the foot a clublike appearance. Clubfoot sometimes is associated with other anomalies, such as meningomyelocele.

The second most common musculoskeletal disorder is congenital hip dysplasia. This disorder occurs more commonly in females.

Assessment

Antepartal factors suggesting congenital abnormalities include increased or decreased amniotic fluid volume. For example, hydramnios (excess amniotic fluid) may accompany tracheoesophageal anomalies; oligohydramnios (insufficient amniotic fluid) may signify a genitourinary tract anomaly. If a congenital anomaly is discovered in one body system, other systems should be investigated thoroughly because congenital anomalies commonly occur in tandem.

CNS anomalies. Most CNS anomalies are apparent even on rapid inspection.

Meningomyelocele. Most commonly, this anomaly appears in the lumbosacral region of the vertebral column. CSF may leak through the defect. Sometimes it is covered only by a thin, membranous sac; otherwise, nerve tissue is exposed. In less obvious cases, the defect manifests as a slight indentation or dimple over the lumbosacral region, detected on palpation; sometimes the indentation is covered by a mole with hair follicles. Such a dimple or mole should be reported for further evaluation. If meningomyelocele is detected, also check for associated anomalies, such as hip dislocation, knee and foot deformities, and hydrocephalus.

If the defect appears above the lumbosacral region, the lower extremities may lack sensation and movement and the bladder and bowel may lack innervation, causing impaired bladder and bowel function. To assess bowel innervation, test for an anal wink by lightly stroking the anus with a cotton-tipped applicator; absence of anal sphincter constriction indicates lack of bowel innervation.

Encephalocele. Suspect this defect when the meninges protrude through the cranium. The defect may be covered with skin or membrane and may be accompanied by hydrocephalus, paralysis, and seizures.

Hydrocephalus. The neonate with hydrocephalus has an enlarged head with an excessive diameter (the occipitofrontal circumference typically exceeds the ninetieth percentile by 2 cm). Wide or bulging fontanels, a shiny scalp with prominent veins, and possible separation of the suture lines are common. Also check for downward eye slanting caused by increased intracranial pressure, and for sunset eyes (appearance of the sclera above the iris), reflecting upper lid retraction.

Associated findings include an abnormal heart rate (usually bradycardia), apneic episodes, vomiting, irritability, excessive crying, and reduced alertness.

Anencephaly and microcephaly. Suspect anencephaly if the neonate lacks a forehead and has a minimal posterior cranium. Suspect microcephaly if head circumference is more than three standard deviations below the average for age, sex, race, and gestational age (Brann and Schwartz, 1987); the forehead is narrow and receding; the occiput (back of the head) is flattened; and the vertex (top of the head) is pointed.

Teratoma. This tumor may be visible on inspection of the sacral area; it may be completely or partly external.

Cardiac anomalies. A heart murmur, which can be assessed on auscultation, is common to most cardiac anomalies. Other general signs of cardiac anomalies include diminished capillary refill time, tachypnea, dyspnea, and tachycardia.

With acyanotic defects, cyanosis usually is absent. Atrial and ventricular septal defects may cause no signs at birth (although a systolic murmur is possible with the atrial defect). PDA causes a continuous or systolic heart murmur, increased heart pulsation (a heartbeat palpable over the precordium), tachycardia, tachypnea, hepatomegaly, bounding pulses, a palpable thrill over the suprasternal notch, bounding peripheral pulses, widened pulse pressure, and signs of respiratory distress or CHF, such as increasing respiratory effort, crackles or other moist breath sounds, feeding intolerance, fatigue, and decreasing urine output.

Coarctation of the aorta also may cause CHF as well as systolic hypertension in the arms, systolic hypotension in the legs, weak or absent femoral pulses, and a systolic ejection murmur at the left sternal border.

With cyanotic cardiac defects, expect cyanosis, especially during hypoxic spells. With tetralogy of Fallot, also expect dyspnea and a continuous murmur heard across the back. Transposition of the great vessels may cause tachypnea, poor feeding, dyspnea, and a soft murmur at the midsternal border. With tricuspid atresia, a systolic murmur at the second intercostal space along the left border may be auscultated. Expect signs of CHF with transposition and tricuspid atresia.

Respiratory tract anomalies. Cyanosis and respiratory compromise are the first signs of diaphragmatic hernia; the more severe the defect, the greater the respiratory compromise. The chest typically appears asymmetrical and the abdomen concave (from lack of abdominal contents). Substernal, intercostal, and suprascapular retractions usually occur over the unaffected side. The neonate usually is tachypneic, with a respiratory rate of at least 80 breaths/minute.

Record the neonate's temperature and assess pulse and respirations. Also, auscultate breath sounds over the entire chest wall; expect diminished or absent breath sounds on the affected side. A decrease or other change in breath sounds usually signifies gastric distention, which can lead to further respiratory compromise. Depending on the extent of the defect, heart sounds may be displaced.

GI tract anomalies. Except for meconium ileus, signs of these anomalies are obvious.

Tracheoesophageal malformations. In almost half of affected neonates, the maternal history includes hydramnios. After delivery, suspect a tracheoesopagheal malformation if the neonate has labored breathing, chest retractions, nasal flaring, cyanosis, or frothy secretions. Difficulty inserting a nasogastric tube and choking or aspiration during oral feedings are other suggestive signs.

Abdominal wall defects. Omphalocele and gastroschisis are apparent from the protruding intestine. Evaluate the abdominal wall defect for signs that the exposed viscera are becoming dry or infected. Also observe for fluid loss through the defect, which may be considerable, and for signs of gastric distention (such as a distended abdomen). If the neonate has omphalocele, examine carefully for associated anomalies.

Meconium ileus. This disorder manifests as abdominal distention, bilious vomiting, and distended bowel loops in the right lower quadrant (found on palpation).

Imperforate anus. This anomaly usually is obvious at delivery, although in some cases it is detected only during an attempt to take a rectal temperature. With a complete defect, the anus appears as a dimple in the perineal skin; an incomplete defect may manifest as a narrow opening where the anus should appear. If this anomaly is accompanied by bowel obstruction, the abdomen will be distended. The neonate typically does not pass meconium;

however, sometimes meconium passes through a fistula or misplaced anus.

The level of the defect commonly is diagnosed by abdominal X-rays. A lateral abdominal X-ray with the neonate inverted distinguishes high from low imperforate anus. If air appears below a line drawn from the pubis to the sacrococcygeal junction (with a marker placed over the rectum), the defect is low. Air appearing above the line indicates a high defect.

Cleft palate and cleft lip. Except when the cleft affects the soft palate only, these anomalies are obvious. The neonate may have difficulty sucking, with expulsion of milk or formula through the nose. With cleft lip, the neonate may have signs of localized infection in the oral cavity, causing a fever, crying, and irritability.

Genitourinary tract anomalies. An anomaly involving the kidneys commonly causes acute renal failure, as reflected by oliguria or anuria. In many cases, the neonate has associated signs, such as hypoplastic lungs or GI defects.

Renal agenesis. Maternal oligohydramnios during pregnancy is a predictor of renal agenesis; fetal ultrasound examination can confirm it before delivery. With bilateral renal agenesis, stillbirth occurs or the neonate dies within a few days after birth. Check for Potter facies: low-set ears; prominent skin folds beneath the eyes; a small, flattened nose; and a small chin and mandible with excessive skin folds. Oliguria or anuria within the first 48 hours after birth is diagnostic of this disorder. Skeletal anomalies that sometimes accompany renal agenesis include bowed legs and flat or broad hands and feet.

Polycystic kidneys. A protruding abdomen and greatly enlarged kidneys suggest this disorder; the liver also is enlarged. Fluid buildup may cause signs of acute renal failure, such as oliguria or anuria, edema, and blood pressure fluctuations.

Posterior urethral valves. A dribbling urine stream in a male neonate suggests this defect.

Genital ambiguity. In the affected female, androgen hypersecretion may cause such genital abnormalities as a small penis and the beginning of a scrotal sac. In the male, genital abnormalities may include abnormally small or undescended testes, hypospadias, and incomplete scrotal fusion.

The nurse who detects ambiguous genitalia should notify the physician immediately so that genetic evaluation can begin. Sex determination not only permits prompt treatment of the underlying adrenal disorder but may help reduce parental anxiety. Definitive sex determination may take up to 2 weeks. Meanwhile, review the prenatal history, especially noting any maternal exposure to hazardous environmental substances, and check the family history for associated problems.

Musculoskeletal anomalies. Clubfoot may be mild to severe and occurs in several variations. In equinovarus, the most common form, the heel turns inward from the midline of the leg, the foot is plantarflexed, the inner border of the foot is raised, and the anterior part of the foot is displaced so that it lies medial to the vertical axis of the leg. Other forms of clubfoot include calcaneovalgus, metatarsus adductus, and metatarsus varus.

If the neonate has an obvious foot deformity, first rule out "apparent clubfoot" (caused by fetal positioning) by taking the foot through the full range of motion. If the foot does not revert to a natural position with manipulation, suspect true clubfoot.

Nursing diagnosis
For a partial list of applicable diagnoses, see Nursing Diagnoses: *High-risk neonates and their families,* page 426.

Planning and implementation
For a potentially life-threatening congenital anomaly, immediate interventions must begin; the neonate may require corrective surgery within hours. Specific management varies with the anomaly and the neonate's condition.

CNS anomalies. These defects usually warrant surgery, commonly soon after childbirth.

Meningomyelocele. This disorder calls for surgery—perhaps within a few hours after birth. The surgeon removes the herniated tissue and covers the defect with surrounding skin.

Before surgery, if the defect is open, cover it immediately with warm saline-solution compresses and plastic wrap. To reduce pressure on the defect and minimize tissue damage, position the neonate to avoid pressure on the defect; be sure to support the defect when moving the neonate.

After surgery, place a rolled towel under the neonate's hips to maintain the legs in a relaxed position. Observe the suture line for signs of CSF leakage and infection, indicated by redness or swelling. Closely monitor neurologic status and assess movement; lack of movement suggests neurologic damage (from the anomaly or surgery). Also monitor for skin mottling, coolness of the legs and arms, decreased capillary refill, and reduced muscle tone.

Prevent contamination of and trauma to the wound and stay alert for signs of infection (particularly meningitis). To prevent fecal contamination of the suture line, tape a cup or a plastic diaper lining to the lower part of the surgical dressing to cover the anus. Because surgery for this disorder may cause hydrocephalus, check head circumference daily.

If the neonate's bladder function is disturbed, monitor fluid intake and output and observe for bladder distention. With lack of innervation (neurogenic bladder), an indwelling catheter may be necessary both before and after surgery. However, in some facilities, the Credé method is used to remove urine from the urethra. In this method, gently roll the fingers from the umbilicus toward the symphysis pubis; pushing on the bladder forces urine into the urethra for elimination. (However, be aware that this method may cause infection from reflux of urine from the lower urinary tract to the bladder.)

Encephalocele. This defect must be closed surgically, necessitating removal of external brain tissue. Surgery may cause such problems as paralysis, mental retardation, or even death.

Preoperatively, position the neonate to avoid pressure on the defect. To prevent infection at the defect, administer antibiotics, as prescribed; cover the defect if CSF leakage occurs. Postoperatively, monitor neurologic status and vital signs frequently; assess motor function in all extremities. If the neonate cannot breathe independently, support respirations by maintaining mechanical ventilation. Inspect the dressing for drainage or CSF leakage; to avoid serious neurologic complications, maintain its sterility. Avoid placing the neonate on the suture site.

Congenital hydrocephalus. This condition typically warrants surgical placement of a ventriculoperitoneal shunt (or, rarely, a ventriculoatrial shunt). The shunt drains CSF from the dilated ventricle into the peritoneal cavity or atrium for absorption and removal; it must be revised periodically as the child grows.

Preoperatively, keep the neonate comfortable. To prevent apnea caused by backward head movement, position the neonate on one side and keep the head of the bed flat or slightly elevated. Postoperatively, maintain suture line integrity and observe for signs of CSF leakage and infection.

To monitor for increasing intracranial pressure, measure and record head circumference once during each shift. As head circumference decreases, discomfort should subside and oral feedings may begin slowly. Also assess for suture line integrity, check the alertness level, and note how well the neonate tolerates enteral or oral feedings.

Teratoma. In most cases, the tumor is excised within the first 28 days after birth. The surgical procedure depends on the tissue involved and the amount of associated tissue. If the tumor is in the sacrococcygeal area, the coccyx may be removed along with the tumor to avoid tumor recurrence. (The nursing measures described below apply mainly to a neonate with a sacrococcygeal tumor.)

Before surgery, position the neonate to minimize pressure on the affected area. After surgery, assess neurologic function by observing movement and color of the legs. Also assess the appearance and amount of drainage from the incision site. Keep the neonate prone, and place sheepskin under the knees to prevent skin irritation and breakdown. To assess for urine retention, measure urine by weighing diapers; if urine output diminishes, notify the physician. Take measures to help prevent infection and minimize stress on the incision line; if necessary, use loose leg restraints to prevent suture line trauma.

Cardiac anomalies. Treatment may be medical or surgical, depending on the specific defect. For an acyanotic defect, corrective surgery may be delayed in favor of symptomatic treatment. For instance, indomethacin, a synthetic prostaglandin inhibitor, may be administered I.V. to close a PDA. However, if this defect is accompanied by severe CHF, the duct is ligated surgically.

For temporary or palliative surgical treatment of an atrial or ventricular septal defect, a band may be placed around the pulmonary artery to decrease blood flow into the pulmonary circulation and alleviate CHF. Other treatments are aimed at managing CHF and include diuretic therapy and digoxin to support cardiac output. When the child is older, a patch graft may be placed to correct the defect.

Surgical correction of coarctation of the aorta, attempted during the toddler or preschool years, involves resection of obstructed blood flow through placement of a graft over the stenotic area; the two segments then are anastomosed on either side of the stenosis.

With a cyanotic defect, palliative surgery typically is performed during the neonatal period. For example, balloon septostomy may be used to open atrial shunts or an artificial graft may be placed. Palliative medical treatments aim to prevent complications of hypoxemia—for instance, iron supplements may be given to correct anemia and fluids and nutritional therapy to prevent fluid overload or dehydration. (Oxygen administration will not improve the neonate's color because cyanosis does not result from pulmonary compromise.) A temporary shunt may be placed to increase pulmonary blood flow.

Nursing goals for the neonate with a congenital cardiac anomaly include maintaining adequate cardiopulmonary function and preventing complications. The neonate will require intensive, expert care and close monitoring. Assess for cyanosis, heart murmurs, arrythmias, absent or unequal pulses, and respiratory distress, and monitor daily weight and fluid intake and output.

Respiratory tract anomalies. Although recent changes in surgical technique have decreased mortality from diaphragmatic hernia, the neonate with this anomaly poses a challenge for the health care team. Gastric decompression is necessary to relieve gastric distention caused by pressure over the stomach and decreased intestinal motility. The sooner the defect is corrected, the better the prognosis. Surgery for diaphragmatic hernia involves a transthoracic or transabdominal incision to restore the abdominal contents to their proper anatomic position. The surgeon pulls the outer skin layers to cover the abdominal wall defect.

Unfortunately, surgical repair does not guarantee survival. If the neonate has respiratory complications or if the unaffected lung is compromised and the affected lung is hypoplastic, the prognosis is guarded at best.

Preoperatively, the main nursing goal is to stabilize and support respiration. Expect to administer prophylactic antibiotics and I.V. fluids; as prescribed, give dextrose 10% in water for the first 24 hours after birth. As appropriate, obtain samples for CBC, WBC differential, serum electrolyte levels, and ABG analysis.

Postoperatively, stay alert for signs of complications, such as a right-to-left shunt, pneumothorax, and pulmonary arterial hypertension. Maintain airway patency, respiratory support, and fluid and electrolyte balance. Auscultate breath sounds every 1 to 2 hours to detect a developing pneumothorax, indicated by diminished breath sounds. Check the incision site every 1 to 2 hours for signs of leakage or infection. As prescribed, institute feedings gradually once the neonate no longer requires ventilatory assistance.

The neonate probably will require endotracheal intubation; perform endotracheal suctioning and maintain ventilatory support, as needed. To help reinflate the lung on the affected side, a chest tube also is inserted. Maintain chest tube patency by monitoring tube drainage every hour and moving the contents away from the chest wall toward the collection system. Be sure to monitor the amount and color of drainage. If chest tube patency appears questionable or drainage suddenly increases or decreases markedly, notify the physician.

GI tract anomalies. Management of GI tract anomalies usually requires surgical intervention. Nursing care for the neonate with a GI tract anomaly focuses on thorough preoperative and postoperative care.

Tracheoesophageal malformations. Surgical intervention is necessary to separate the trachea and esophagus and to maintain the patency of each structure. The surgical procedure used depends on the specific malformation. A gastrostomy tube commonly is inserted during surgery to prevent gastric reflux and aspiration pneumonia. Some neonates also require cervical esophagostomy to drain saliva and mucus from an atretic area (this procedure is performed only when no tracheoesophageal fistula is present).

Nursing goals include maintaining a patent airway and ensuring fluid and electrolyte balance before and after surgery. Preoperatively, if a blind pouch has been diagnosed, observe secretions for color and amount. As requested, insert a nasogastric tube and connect it to the blind pouch to provide continuous low-pressure suction and prevent aspiration. Check tube patency hourly, and assess vital signs every 1 to 2 hours.

Oxygen therapy may be required if the neonate's breathing effort increases or if cyanosis develops. A warmed mist, delivered by an oxygen hood or through a closed incubator, may be used to thin secretions. Monitor vital signs, respiratory effort, skin color, appearance of the I.V. infusion site, and the amount of secretions suctioned.

Postoperative nursing interventions resemble those used for the neonate with diaphragmatic hernia, except that no chest tube is present. Turn the neonate every 2 hours to prevent atelectasis. If the neonate can tolerate it, perform nasopharyngeal suctioning with a marked catheter, as ordered, to a depth just short of the suture line to help prevent suture perforation during suctioning.

If the nasogastric tube remains in place for gastric decompression, maintain its patency by inserting 2 ml of air every 2 hours. If cervical esophagostomy was performed, maintain skin integrity by cleaning the skin, applying petroleum jelly to create a waterproof barrier, and applying a secretion-absorbing dressing every 4 hours. Diminished secretions suggest that the stoma is closing, necessitating surgical dilatation with a soft rubber catheter.

Keep the neonate in an upright position before and after surgery—for instance, by using a cholasia chair, which allows the neonate to remain upright after feeding to prevent reflux of secretions. Maintain patency of the gastrostomy tube by inserting 2 ml of air every 2 to 4 hours (gravity drainage typically is used). Also, note how well the neonate tolerated medical and nursing procedures, and assess the appearance of secretions, the neonate's breathing effort, and skin color.

Once enteral feedings begin, assess the neonate's tolerance for them. Any aspirate found before the next feeding may indicate impaired intestinal activity; make sure to document and report this finding.

Bottle feedings typically can begin once an intact suture line is verified. Expect to begin bottle feedings gradually with a clear electrolyte solution, such as Pedialyte. Give feedings slowly to prevent aspiration and gastric distention. Methylene blue, a dye, commonly is added to feedings to reveal suture line leakage. If a fistula is present, this dye appears in the chest tube; dye appearing only in the gastrostomy tube means that the suture line is intact.

If the esophagus has been pulled taut and stretched to make the ends meet, gastrostomy feedings may be needed and the surgeon may perform dilatation with increasing catheter sizes several weeks after surgery. When these feedings begin, evaluate how well the neonate tolerates them. A dusky skin color or choking during feedings may indicate fistula leakage; increased mucus may indicate stenosis around the surgical site.

Abdominal wall defects. The neonate with gastroschisis or omphalocele requires immediate intervention in the delivery room – ventilatory support followed by peripheral line placement for I.V. fluid administration. As soon as possible, cover the defect with sterile gauze dressings moistened with warm normal saline solution; place plastic wrap on top of the dressings to help keep tissues moist and reduce heat loss. Maintain gastric decompression with a nasogastric tube.

Corrective treatment of a small defect involves complete or primary surgical reduction. In the operating room, the bowel and protruding tissues are inspected for trauma that could cause loss of GI contents and bacterial wound contamination. If the protruding contents are too large to return to the abdominal cavity, a silastic pouch is placed around them. Later, keep this pouch (now referred to as a silo) suspended from the top of the incubator to help reduce tissue swelling and facilitate eventual return of the abdominal contents to the abdominal cavity. Position the neonate supine and moisten the silo with povidone-iodine every 8 hours (or as specified by facility protocol).

If the defect is large, the reduction must be performed in stages to prevent excessive pressure on the diaphragm and resulting complications, such as respiratory compro-

mise and tissue hypoxia. In some cases, reduction may be performed in the NICU; in others, the neonate must return to the operating room.

The nursing goal is to minimize the risk of infection and maintain the herniated tissue and organs in optimal condition. Be sure to maintain sterile technique throughout caregiving procedures. Before surgery, keep the dressings sterile and moist and evaluate for skin breakdown from supine positioning. If appropriate, place an air mattress or sheepskin under the neonate to minimize skin breakdown.

After the neonate's final surgical closure, expect to administer feedings through a gastrostomy tube. Begin feedings gradually and increase the volume based on the neonate's tolerance. Usually, a central line also must be inserted for administration of parenteral nutrition, which will continue for several days or weeks.

Monitor for changes in respiratory status and vital signs (especially during the immediate postoperative period), and assess tolerance of feedings once these begin. Also evaluate the appearance of the defect, checking closely for signs of infection. To assess for circulatory compromise caused by pressure from the defect, check capillary refill in the legs.

Imperforate anus. The neonate with this anomaly requires surgical restoration of the anal canal to achieve urinary and bowel continence. For a low defect, a peripheral anoplasty typically is performed during the neonatal period. For an intermediate defect, a colostomy is performed in most cases, with further surgery performed several months later. A high defect always necessitates a colostomy.

Nursing goals include preventing gastric distention and dehydration. Preoperatively, nursing measures depend on the severity of the defect. Expect to maintain gastric decompression and initiate I.V. therapy.

Postoperatively, position the neonate on the stomach or side. Maintain gastric decompression until 24 hours before feedings are to begin. If anoplasty was performed, assess the site for skin breakdown, redness, and drainage. Clean it regularly and after every stool; avoid taking rectal temperatures or examining the rectum. To minimize stool formation until the incision heals, delay feedings at least 24 hours after surgery.

If the neonate has a colostomy, assess the suture line and skin around the stoma for color, swelling, and drainage; check for separation of the suture line. As needed, change the dressing to prevent infection, and change the colostomy bag to prevent leakage.

Cleft palate and cleft lip. Surgical repair of these anomalies usually is delayed to prevent disruption of facial growth and tooth-bud formation. However, it must occur early enough so that the defect does not interfere with speech development. Repair of cleft lip (cheilorrhaphy, or Z-plasty) commonly takes place when the child is 3 months old; repair of cleft palate (by joining of the palatal segments) typically is performed when the child is 9 to 15 months old.

Ensure adequate nutrition before and after surgery because air leaks around the cleft and nasal regurgitation typically cause feeding problems. Many neonates with cleft lip can be breast-fed (except after surgery); the mother may provide breast milk she has pumped. With cleft palate, a feeding neonate requires a syringe or cleft palate feed or a special elongated nipple (such as a Martin's nipple). When using an elongated nipple, be sure to place it far into the mouth—but not far enough to induce gagging. Burp the neonate frequently while feeding because cleft lip or palate causes swallowing of much air during feeding. To prevent aspiration of feeding matter through the palatal opening and the nares, elevate the head of the bed or place the neonate in an infant seat or on the stomach after feedings.

The neonate's abnormally short eustachian tubes provide easy access for nasal and oral bacteria, increasing the risk of ear infection. To help reduce this risk, clean the nose and oral cavities after feedings, and assess frequently for fever, irritability, and other signs of ear infection. To remove excess formula, rinse the neonate's mouth with water after feedings.

Be sure to teach the parents how to provide the special care their child requires. Cleft palate and lip can cause long-term speech, dental, hearing, and other problems, so the nurse should refer parents to appropriate professionals for follow-up care.

Genitourinary tract anomalies. Management of genitourinary tract anomalies involves strict maintenance of fluid and electrolyte imbalance and thorough preoperative and postoperative care.

Polycystic kidney disease and posterior urethral valves. A polycystic kidney is removed surgically. Before surgery, monitor the neonate for infection (especially of the urinary tract). Afterward, maintain gastric decompression and monitor urine output, urine specific gravity, and dipstick for blood every 2 hours. Report any decrease in urine output.

With posterior urethral valves, the obstruction is corrected surgically and a nephrostomy tube or stent is placed to drain the ureter that has been anastomosed around the stenotic area. Sometimes, temporary relief of the obstruction is achieved antenatally with open fetal surgery. This procedure has the highest reported success rate of any fetal surgery attempted (Pringle, 1989).

Nursing goals include maintaining fluid and electrolyte balance and supporting respiration (hypoplastic lungs accompany some renal problems). If surgery is scheduled, preoperative nursing care centers on maintaining fluid and electrolyte balance. Assess intake and output every 4 to 8 hours, and check urine specific gravity every 4 hours. Support respiratory efforts, as needed, by maintaining oxygen therapy or assisted ventilation.

Assess the neonate before and after surgery for signs of acute renal failure, such as oliguria or anuria, edema, blood pressure fluctuations, and cardiopulmonary compromise secondary to fluid accumulation. Take postoperative measures to prevent infection. Also, assess for signs of respiratory compromise, decreased urine output, and drainage from the nephrostomy tube or stent. Evaluate renal status by comparing vital sign measurements with baseline values. Also compare fluid intake and output from the previous 24 hours to detect any difference.

Observe and evaluate output from any nephrostomy tube or stent. To help prevent infection, protect the dressing at the suture line and observe this site closely. Keep all dressings dry; as needed, replace dressings at the suture line and around tubes.

Genital ambiguity. If genital ambiguity stems from congenital adrenal hyperplasia, hydrocortisone is given to arrest the disorder; with severe adrenal hyperplasia, hydrocortisone must be administered immediately to prevent acute adrenocorticol failure—a fatal condition. Later, surgical reconstruction of the external genitalia may be attempted.

Expect to assist in genetic testing and determination of the neonate's underlying problem if this has not been established. Providing support to the family is a nursing priority. Refer them to a psychiatrist or other professional for help in coping with this problem. Also, advise them to select a unisex name for their child. Some professionals encourage parents to delay the announcement of their child's birth until the sex can be determined; others believe that a delay exacerbates parental anxiety.

Musculoskeletal anomalies. For clubfoot, corrective shoes, casts, or braces typically are used as soon as possible to correct the deformity. If these measures fail, surgery may be performed when the child is several years old. Inform the parents of the need for early and continual medical evaluation to avoid problems when the child begins to walk.

Treatment for congenital hip dysplasia involves pressing the femoral head against and into the acetabulum. This pressure allows formation of an adequate socket before ossification is complete. To abduct and externally rotate the leg and flex the hip, a triangular pillow is applied over the diaper. At a later date, the neonate typically is placed in a spica cast.

Evaluation

For examples of appropriate evaluation statements, see the general ones listed in "Nursing care of the high-risk neonate" earlier in this chapter.

Documentation

For information about appropriate documentation, see the general points listed in "Nursing care of the high-risk neonate" earlier in this chapter.

CHAPTER SUMMARY

Chapter 21 described nursing care for high-risk neonates and their families. Here are the chapter highlights.

Neonatal care is delivered in level 1, 2, and 3 nurseries; the level reflects the intensity of care provided. Many high-risk neonates require level 3 (NICU) care.

Regionalization of neonatal care promotes high-quality care and allows the most efficient use of resources.

The goals of neonatal intensive care include anticipation of perinatal problems, early intervention, and minimal disturbance of the neonate.

In many cases, the birth of a high-risk neonate can be anticipated from maternal history findings or from antepartal, intrapartal, or fetal factors. Prompt recognition of actual or potential perinatal problems in the delivery room helps avert long-term complications.

Immediately after delivery, the neonate is evaluated to determine the need for resuscitation. Neonatal resuscitation proceeds in an orderly sequence, with each succeeding step based on the neonate's condition and response to the previous measure.

When caring for a neonate receiving supplemental oxygen or mechanical ventilation, the nurse should monitor the neonate's oxygenation status continuously.

Maintaining thermoregulation and ensuring fluid balance are particularly important for the high-risk neonate, who is at increased risk for hypothermia and fluid volume deficit.

The nurse caring for a high-risk neonate must follow strict infection control guidelines.

Developmental care has taken on increasing importance in the NICU. To provide such care, the nurse should reduce detrimental stimulation and provide appropriate stimulation according to the neonate's tolerance.

Loss and grief occur in families that experience a real or perceived loss of the neonate. Death of the neonate or birth of a neonate who is preterm, severely ill, or afflicted with a physical or mental anomaly or disability may trigger these responses.

The stages of grief described by Kübler-Ross include denial, anger, bargaining, depression, and acceptance. Completion of grieving can take a year or more; family members may progress through the stages at different rates and may experience facets of two or more stages at once.

Initially, the nurse must assess the parents, grandparents, and siblings for ability to cope emotionally and practically with the birth of a high-risk neonate. Factors to assess include family history, understanding of the neonate's condition, familiarity with the health care environment, home and family needs, and support from such sources as other family members, religious practices, and cultural customs.

Later nursing assessment focuses on the developing relationship between the family and the neonate, the family's acquisition of neonatal care skills, and use of coping mechanisms.

Nursing intervention includes providing accurate, consistent information to family members; establishing communication with them; strengthening family support systems and interaction between family members and the neonate; teaching caregiving skills; enhancing parent-infant bonding; and planning for the neonate's discharge.

In the event of a neonate's death, nursing interventions include providing emotional support, arranging a quiet area for the family to say goodbye to the neonate, collecting mementos for the family, and encouraging the family to complete their bonding with the neonate.

A gestational-age or birth-weight abnormality predisposes the neonate to perinatal problems. The preterm neonate is particularly at risk because general immaturity can cause dysfunction in any organ or system.

Common problems seen among high-risk neonates include respiratory dysfunction, metabolic disorders, and congenital anomalies of the CNS, cardiovascular system, respiratory tract, GI tract, genitourinary tract, and musculoskeletal system.

The nurse should evaluate all care to determine the neonate's response to interventions and progress toward goals and must document assessment findings and nursing activities thoroughly.

STUDY QUESTIONS

1. Which antepartal history findings suggest a potential perinatal problem?

2. Brenda Jergens, born 3 hours ago, is exhibiting classic signs of respiratory distress. What are these signs?

3. Which nursing interventions are appropriate to prevent complications of oxygen therapy in neonates?

4. Linda Leach was born at 45 weeks' gestation weighing only 1,500 g. What types of problems may she face as a postterm SGA neonate?

5. Born at 34 weeks' gestation, Martin Glick is a preterm neonate and is thus predisposed to hypothermia. Which nursing interventions can help prevent hypothermia?

6. How should the nurse position the neonate's head during resuscitation?

7. Carol Becker is crying at the bedside of her child, whose encephalocele will necessitate repeated hospitalizations and lifelong care. Which interventions can the nurse use to help Mrs. Becker express her grief?

8. Timmy Clark is transferred to an NICU 100 miles away from his parents' home. Which interventions might the nurse suggest to encourage parent-infant bonding for the parents, who can only visit once a week?

9. Which signs and symptoms of pathologic mourning should the nurse be alert for when assessing the parents of a stillborn neonate?

BIBLIOGRAPHY

American Academy of Pediatrics (1988). *Guidelines for perinatal care* (2nd ed.). Chicago: Author.

American Heart Association and American Academy of Pediatrics (1987). *Textbook of neonatal resuscitation.* Dallas.

Brann, A., and Schwartz, J.F. (1987). Developmental anomalies and neuromuscular disorders. In A.A. Fanaroff and R.J. Martin (Eds.), *Behrman's neonatal-perinatal medicine: Diseases of the fetus or infant.* St. Louis: Mosby.

Chatburn, R.L., and Carlo, W.A. (1988). Assessment of neonatal gas exchange. In W.A. Carlo and M. Lough (Eds.), *Neonatal respiratory care* (2nd ed.). Chicago: Year Book.

Fanaroff, A.A., and Martin, R.J. (1987). *Behrman's neonatal-perinatal medicine: Diseases of the fetus or infant.* St. Louis: Mosby.

Goldsmith, J.P., and Karotkin, E.H. (1988). *Assisted ventilation of the neonate* (2nd ed.). Philadelphia: Saunders.

Hager, J.J. (1983). Characteristics and management of pregnancy in women with genital herpes simplex virus infection. *American Journal of Obstetrics and Gynecology, 145,* 784.

Harbold, L. (1989). A protocol for neonatal use of pulse oximetry. *Neonatal Network,* 8(1), 41, 42, 55-57.

Harjo, J., Kenner, C., and Brueggemeyer, A. (1988). Alterations in effective breathing patterns. In C. Kenner, J. Harjo, and A. Brueggemeyer (Eds.), *Neonatal surgery: A nursing perspective* (pp. 79-120). Orlando, FL: Grune & Stratton.

Harjo, J., Kenner, C., and Brueggermeyer, A. (1988). Alterations in the gastrointestinal system. In C. Kenner, J. Harjo, and A. Brueggemeyer (Eds.), *Neonatal surgery: A nursing perspective* (pp. 121-189). Orlando, FL: Grune & Stratton.

Jobe, A. (1988). *Surfactant replacement therapy.* Workshop presented at the National Perinatal Association Conference, Perinatal Health: Facing the 21st Century. San Diego, CA.

Kaempf, J.W., Bonnabel, C., and Hoy, W.W. (1989). Neonatal nutrition. In G.B. Merenstein and S.L. Gardner (Eds.), *Handbook of neonatal care* (p. 185). St. Louis: Mosby.

Kliegman, R.M., and Wald, M.K. (1986). Problems in metabolic adaptation: Glucose, calcium, and magnesium. In M.H. Klaus and A.A. Fanaroff (Eds.), *Care of the high risk neonate* (3rd ed.). Philadelphia: Saunders.

Moyer-Mileur, L.J. (1986). Nutrition. In N.S. Streeter (Ed.), *High-risk neonatal care* (p. 276). Rockville, MD: Aspen.

Nelson, S.N., Merenstein, G.B., and Pierce, J.R. (1986). Early onset group B streptococcal disease. *Journal of Perinatology, 6,* 234.

Nicolaides, K.H. (1989). Studies on fetal physiology and pathophysiology in Rhesus disease. *Seminars in Perinatology,* 13(4), 328-337.

Perlstein, P.H. (1988). The thermal environment. In A.A. Fanaroff and R.J. Martin (Eds.), *Behrman's neonatal-perinatal medicine: Diseases of the fetus or infant.* St. Louis: Mosby.

Plunkett, J.W., Meisels, S.J., Stiefel, G.S., Pasick, P.L., and Roloff, D.W. (1986). Patterns of attachment among preterm infants of varying biological risk. *Journal of the American Academy of Child Psychiatry,* 25(6), 794-800.

Pringle, K.C. (1989). Fetal diagnosis and fetal surgery. *Clinics in Perinatology,* 16(1), 13-22.

Subramanian, K.N.S., Glass, P., Avery, G.B., Kolinjavadi, N., Keys, M.P., Sostek, A.M., and Friendly, D.S. (1985). Effect of bright light in the hospital nursery on the incidence of retinopathy of prematurity. *New England Journal of Medicine,* 313(7), 401-404.

Wranesh, B.L. (1982). The effect of sibling visitation on bacterial colonization rate in neonates. *JOGNN,* 11(4), 211-213.

Families in crisis

Battles, R.S. (1988). Factors influencing men's transition into parenthood. *Neonatal Network,* 6(5), 63-66.

Consolvo, C.A. (1984). Nurturing the fathers of high-risk neonates. *Neonatal Network,* 2(6), 27-30.

Kelting, S. (1986). Supporting parents in the NICU. *Neonatal Network,* 4(6), 14-18.

Lemons, P.M. (1986). Beyond the birth of a defective child. *Neonatal Network,* 5(3), 13-20.

Scheiber, K.K. (1989). Developmentally delayed children: Effects on the normal sibling. *Pediatric Nursing,* 15(1), 42-44.

Steele, K.H. (1987). Caring for parents of critically ill neonates during hospitalization: Strategies for health-care professionals. *MCN,* 16(1), 13-27.

Tarbert, K.C. (1985). The impact of a high-risk infant upon the family. *Neonatal Network,* 3(4), 20-23.

Trahd, G.E. (1986). Siblings of chronically ill children: Helping them cope. *Pediatric Nursing,* 12(3), 191-193.

Grief

Benefield, D.G., Leib, S.A., and Reuter, J. (1976). Grief response of parents after referral of the critically ill newborn to a regional center. *New England Journal of Medicine,* 294(18), 975-978.

Bowlby, J. (1961). Process of mourning. *International Journal of Psychoanalysis,* 42, 317-340.

Cordell, A.S., and Apolito, R. (1981). Family support in infant death. *JOGNN,* 10(4), 281-285.

Davidson, G.W. (1984). *Understanding mourning: A guide for those who grieve.* Minneapolis: Augsburg Publishing House.

Gardner, S.L., and Merenstein, G.B. (1989). *Handbook of neonatal intensive care.* St. Louis: Mosby.

Krone, C., and Harris, C.C. (1988). The importance of infant gender and family resemblance within parents' perinatal bereavement process: Establishing personhood. *Journal of Perinatal and Neonatal Nursing,* 2(2), 1-11.

Kübler-Ross, E. (1969). *On death and dying.* New York: Macmillan.

Limbo, R.K., and Wheeler, S.R. (1986). *When a baby dies: A handbook for healing and helping.* Holmen, WI: Harsand Press.

Lindemann, E. (1944). Symptomatology and management of acute grief. *American Journal of Psychiatry,* 101, 141-148.

Lynch, J.J. (1979). *The broken heart: The medical consequences of loneliness.* New York: Basic Books.

Olshansky, S. (1962, April). Chronic sorrow: A response to having a mentally defective child. *Social Casework,* 43, 190-193.

Parkes, C.M. (1970). "Seeking" and "finding" a lost object: Evidence from recent studies of the reaction to bereavement. *Social Science and Medicine,* 4(2), 187-201.

Rees, W.D., and Lutkins, S.G. (1967). The mortality of bereavement. *British Medical Journal,* 4(570), 13-16.

Sahu, S. (1981). Coping with perinatal death. *Journal of Reproductive Medicine,* 26(3), 129-132.

Trouy, M.B., and Ward-Larson, C. (1987). Sibling grief. *Neonatal Network,* 5(4), 35-40.

Neonatal mortality

National Center for Health Statistics (1989, March 28). Monthly vital statistics report – Births, marriages, divorces, and deaths for 1988. *U.S. Dept. of Health and Human Services Publication No. (PHS) 89-1120.* Hyattsville, MD: U.S. Public Health Service.

National Center for Health Statistics (1989, June 29). Monthly vital statistics report – Advance report of final natality statistics, 1987. *U.S. Dept. of Health and Human Services,* 38, (3). Hyattsville, MD: U.S. Public Health Service.

Birth-weight and gestational-age abnormalities

Boyd, M.E., Usher, R.H., McLean, F.H., and Kramer, M.S. (1988). Obstetric consequences of postmaturity. *American Journal of Obstetrics and Gynecology,* 158(2), 334-338.

Cassady, G., and Strange, M. (1987). The small-for-gestational-age (SGA) infant. In G.B. Avery (Ed.), *Neonatology: Pathophysiology and management of the newborn* (pp. 299-378). Philadelphia: Lippincott.

Chasnoff, I.J., Bussey, M.E., Savich, R., and Stack, C.M. (1986). Perinatal cerebral infarction and maternal cocaine use. *Journal of Pediatrics,* 108(3), 456-459.

Eden, R.D., Seifert, L.S., Winegar, A., and Spellacy, W.N. (1987). Perinatal characteristics of uncomplicated postdate pregnancies. *Obstetrics and Gynecology,* 69, 296-299.

Lubchenco, L.O., and Koops, B.L. (1987). Assessment of weight and gestational age. In G.B. Avery (Ed.), *Neonatology: Pathophysiology and management of the newborn* (3rd ed.; pp. 235-257). Philadelphia: Lippincott.

Ounsted, M., Moar, V.A., and Scott, A. (1985). Risk factors associated with small-for-date and large-for-date infants. *British Journal of Obstetrics and Gynecology,* 92, 226-232.

Phelan, J.P., Plah, L.P., Yeh, S.Y., Broussard, P., and Paul, R.H. (1985). The role of ultrasound assessment of amniotic fluid volume in the management of the post-date pregnancy. *American Journal of Obstetrics and Gynecology,* 151, 304-308.

Resnick, R. (1989). Post-term pregnancy. In R.K. Creasy and R. Resnick (Eds.), *Maternal-fetal medicine: Principles and practice* (2nd ed.; pp. 505-509). Philadelphia: Saunders.

Teberg, A.J., Walther, F.J., and Pena, I.C. (1988). Mortality, morbidity, and outcome of the small-for-gestational age infant. *Seminars in Perinatology,* 12, 84-94.

Usher, R.H., Boyd, M.E., McLean, F.H., and Kramer, M.S. (1988). Assessment of fetal risk in postdate pregnancies. *American Journal of Obstetrics and Gynecology,* 158, 259-264.

Vorherr, H. (1975). Placental insufficiency in relation to postterm pregnancy and fetal postmaturity. *American Journal of Obstetrics and Gynecology,* 123(1), 67-103.

Maternal substance abuse

Flandermeyer, A.A. (1987). A comparison of the effects of heroin and cocaine abuse upon the neonate. *Neonatal Network,* 6(3), 42-48.

Jones, K.L. (1986). Fetal alcohol syndrome. *Pediatrics in Review,* 8(4), 122-126.

Kennard, M.J. (1990). Cocaine use during pregnancy: Fetal and neonatal effects. *Journal of Perinatal and Neonatal Nursing,* 3(9), 53-63.

Failure to thrive and child abuse

Hunter, R.S., Kilstrum, N., Kraybill, E.N., and Loda, F. (1978). Antecedents of child abuse and neglect in premature infants: A prospective study in a newborn intensive care unit. *Pediatrics,* 61(4), 629-635.

White, R., Benedict, M.I., Wulff, L., and Kelley, M. (1987). Physical disabilities as risk factors for child maltreatment: A selected review. *American Journal of Orthopsychiatry,* 57(1), 93-101.

Cultural references

Choi, E. (1986). Unique aspects of Korean-American mothers. *JOGNN,* 15(5), 394-400.

Leininger, M.M. (1985). Transcultural care diversity and universality: A theory of nursing. *Nursing and Health Care,* 6(4), 208-212.

Manio, E.B., and Hall, R.R. (1987). Asian family traditions and their influence in transcultural health care delivery. *Children's Health Care,* 15(3), 172-177.

Tripp-Reimer, T., Brink, P.J., and Saunders, J.M. (1984). Cultural assessment: Content and process. *Nursing Outlook,* 32(2), 78-82.

York, C.R., and Stichler, J.F. (1985). Cultural grief expressions following infant death. *Dimensions of Critical Care Nursing,* 4(2), 120-127.

Zepeda, M. (1982). Selected maternal-infant care practices of Spanish-speaking women. *JOGNN,* 11(6), 371-374.

CHAPTER 22

DISCHARGE PLANNING AND CARE AT HOME

OBJECTIVES

After reading and studying this chapter, the student should be able to:

1. Describe why the demand for home health care for neonates has increased in the past decade.

2. Define discharge planning, describe its goals, and identify the personnel and resources typically involved in planning for a neonate's discharge.

3. Identify the discharge planning needs of both the neonate and the family.

4. Discuss the financial implications of home health care for the family.

5. Describe methods the nurse may use to prepare parents for the neonate's discharge.

6. Describe the home health care needs of neonates with specific perinatal problems.

7. Discuss community resources that support home health care for neonates.

INTRODUCTION

For increasing numbers of neonates, health care has been extended to the home. In the past decade, dramatic changes in health care — economic pressures, advances in the treatment of high-risk neonates, and the desire by families for more active participation in health care — have led to a growing demand for home health care and other community-based services.

Philosophical changes within the neonatal health care community also have played a role. For example, early discharge is now standard for normal healthy neonates. For the nurse working within the setting of a health care facility, early discharge means less time to plan for the neonate's discharge — yet a greater need for thorough discharge planning. For the nurse who makes postdischarge visits to the home, early discharge may mean a longer period of follow-up with a greater need for family support and individualized attention.

Also, high-risk neonates who survive their initial problems and become medically stable commonly require further treatment at home. Many have multiple chronic problems that call for specialized, complex home care; some depend on monitors and other technological devices. In 1988, for example, an estimated 10,000 American families experienced the birth of a catastrophically ill child (National Association of Children's Hospitals and Related Industries, Inc., 1989). Thus, home health care for neonates has become increasingly complex as well as common. The long-term success of the sophisticated technology now available for home use may hinge on how effectively the nurse and other health care professionals can extend their specialized knowledge and skills to the home.

To meet the challenges of home health care, the nurse must have expert assessment skills — sophisticated and holistic in scope, yet specific. Discharge planning must be the focus of care from the time of the neonate's admission to the nursery. As the main liaison between the family and health care providers, the nurse must possess a wealth of knowledge about neonatal and pediatric home health care and act as family advocate in determining the appropriateness of this care.

This chapter discusses both preparation for and delivery of home health care for neonates. The chapter begins by describing discharge planning, which takes place within the health care facility. It delineates the nurse's role in discharge planning, discusses resources the nurse uses in discharge planning, and explains how to identify the discharge planning needs of the neonate and family. Then the chapter describes how the nurse provides health care in the home for both the normal and special-needs neonate. After describing the concept of case management and selection of home health care services and suppliers, the chapter uses the nursing process steps – assessment, nursing diagnosis, planning, implementation, and evaluation – to provide care for a neonate at home. The chapter concludes with a brief discussion of documentation.

DISCHARGE PLANNING

Discharge planning involves the formulation of a program by the health care team, client, family, and appropriate outside agencies to meet the client's physical and psychosocial needs after discharge. Discharge planning for a neonate prepares the neonate and family (or other primary caregivers) for care at home or in another health care facility.

The American Nurses' Association (1975) defines discharge planning as "that part of the continuity of care . . . designed to prepare the client for the next phase of care, whether it be self care, care by family members, or care by an organized health care provider."

All clients have the right to planned continuity of care after discharge. When effective, discharge planning improves both the continuity and cost-effectiveness of care. In response to fiscal restraints and pressure from third-party payers, most health care facilities now emphasize discharge planning.

NURSE'S ROLE

The nurse's role in discharge planning is delineated in the standards of neonatal nursing established in 1986 by NAACOG, the organization for obstetric, gynecologic, and neonatal nurses.
• The nurse develops the discharge plan, making referrals as necessary to help the family cope with the neonate's condition.
• The nurse helps integrate the neonate into the family.
• The nurse provides the family with health education to promote neonatal and infant care.
• The nurse initiates and participates in neonatal care conferences with the family and other members of the health care team.

DISCHARGE PLANNING SYSTEMS

Although nurses are responsible for the health care aspects of discharge planning, some health care facilities have centralized discharge planning conducted by social workers or by a combination of social workers and nurses. With this system, the discharge planning department receives a list of new admissions every morning and identifies those neonates who will need extensive discharge planning.

Other facilities have a decentralized system, in which the nurse who works most closely with the client is responsible for discharge planning; as necessary, this nurse consults with other professionals for help with special aspects of planning, such as obtaining financial assistance.

The high-risk screen, a popular tool used by admitting offices, categorizes clients according to the intensity of their discharge planning needs. Most commonly, it is used in centralized discharge planning systems to "red-flag" and prioritize clients. In primary or secondary perinatal care facilities, the high-risk screen is used at nursery admission to identify:
• preterm neonates
• neonates of adolescent mothers
• neonates of mothers who used drugs or other substances during pregnancy
• neonates with no insurance coverage.

The use of high-risk screens is less helpful in a tertiary (intensive care) facility, where almost every neonate fits the high-risk category.

DISCHARGE PLANNING RESOURCES

Discharge planning requires close collaboration among health care team members. In most cases, the nurse can refer the family to any professional for discharge planning assistance (although in some cases a physician's order is required for a referral to a specialist from another discipline). Typically, in-facility resource personnel involved in discharge planning include:
• clinical nurse specialist
• physician
• social worker
• financial counselor
• speech, hearing, occupational, and physical therapists
• utilization review nurse
• dietitian
• respiratory therapist
• child life therapist.

For example, the nurse would collaborate with a social worker when planning the discharge of a preterm neonate

DISCHARGE PLANNING QUESTIONNAIRE

To help assess discharge planning needs, the nurse may ask the parents (or other primary caregiver) to complete a questionnaire, such as the one shown here.

1. What is your name and your relationship to the infant?

_____

2. During which times of day will you be able to visit your infant here at the health care facility?

_____ Mornings   _____ Nights

_____ Afternoons   _____ Not sure

_____ Evenings

3. How will you get here to visit your infant?

_____ Own car   _____ Relative or friend

_____ Public transpor-   will bring

tation   _____ Other

4. Who will be caring for your infant after discharge?

_____ Mother   _____ Friend

_____ Father   _____ Day care

_____ Babysitter   _____ Other

_____ Relative

5. Who will be able to help you with your infant's care at home?

_____ Spouse   _____ Other

_____ Relative   _____ No one available

_____ Friend

6. What kinds of help do you think your family will need to care for your infant at home?

_____

7. Would you like to see a social worker who can help your family work out problems you might be having while your infant is in the health care facility?

_____ Yes   _____ No

8. Do you have any questions about your insurance coverage for your infant's home care?

_____ Yes   _____ No

9. Would you like to see a financial counselor to discuss your insurance coverage or to obtain information on applying for financial assistance?

_____ Yes   _____ No

10. Please indicate if you would like to see any of these professionals.

_____ Chaplain   _____ Dietitian

_____ Child life therapist   _____ Other

Adapted with permission from Children's Hospital Medical Center, Cincinnati.

of an unwed mother who rarely visits and is undecided about keeping her child. In this case, the nurse documents lack of visits by the mother and any conversations with other family members; the social worker determines whether the child should be discharged to another family member or to foster care if the mother chooses not to keep the child.

Complex discharge

For help with a complex discharge, particularly on weekends or holidays when other resource personnel may be unavailable, the nurse may refer to unit discharge planning manuals. Also, some facilities have parent libraries that offer information at the layperson's level on diseases, medical procedures, child development, and community resources; toy libraries may be available to lend toys adapted for children with special needs. For help in identifying appropriate home care resources within the community, a community nurse may prove invaluable.

Nurses and other professionals who are experts in discharge planning may belong to the American Association for Continuity of Care. This organization holds annual conferences and state-level meetings where members share information. The legislative arm lobbies for continuity-of-care issues at the national level.

Family involvement

To enhance their commitment to and confidence in the discharge plan, the neonate's parents should be allowed to participate actively in discharge planning and set realistic goals mutually with the health care team. The Joint Commission for Accreditation of Healthcare Organizations (JCAHO) stipulates that the medical record document the parents' involvement in discharge planning (1989). To help ensure parental involvement, the nurse may use a questionnaire, such as the one shown in *Discharge planning questionnaire*.

IDENTIFYING DISCHARGE PLANNING NEEDS

To help avoid a delay in discharge once the neonate is medically ready, the nurse or other discharge planner should begin family preparation and arrangements for needed services at the time of delivery or, at the latest, by the time the neonate is admitted to the nursery. The nurse assesses the discharge planning needs of both the neonate and parents, using information from the nursing admission assessment and from ongoing assessment. (For details on gathering relevant data from admission information, see *Assessing discharge planning needs.*)

Neonatal needs

Assess the scope and complexity of the neonate's physical care needs, which may vary from routine care and arrangements for follow-up medical visits for the normal neonate to complex, high-technology care for the special-needs neonate. Identify the neonate's primary caregiver and at least one secondary caregiver who will be responsible for care in the primary caregiver's absence. Also determine which community agencies may need to be involved in home health care, which equipment and supplies will be required at home, and whether the home is adequate and safe for health care. To determine the latter, consider arranging for a predischarge home visit by a community health nurse.

Parental needs

To determine the parents' discharge planning needs, assess their:
• ability and willingness to care for the neonate at home
• ability to bond with the neonate
• understanding of growth and development
• knowledge of neonatal and infant care techniques
• physical and psychosocial support systems
• need for additional caregivers
• stress level
• medical insurance and financial resources
• psychosocial adaptation to the changing family structure.

Assessing the feasibility of home care

Although caring for the neonate at home may sound ideal, this is not always best for the neonate or family. The parents and health care team must consider many factors when determining the most appropriate postdischarge care setting, especially if the neonate has special needs.

Neonate's health status. Usually, the neonate must be in stable condition to be cared for at home. If the neonate will need

ASSESSING DISCHARGE PLANNING NEEDS

To obtain sufficient information to formulate a discharge plan, the nurse may want to use information obtained from the neonate's parents by an admission assessment tool, such as the one shown here. Each question is accompanied by a rationale that explains how the answer might affect the neonate's discharge planning needs.

Is this your first child?
Rationale: For parents of a first child, teaching of routine neonatal care is essential. However, all parents can benefit from a review of routine neonatal care.

Where does your family live?
Rationale: A family living in a rural area may have trouble obtaining follow-up care at a tertiary perinatal center for a special-needs neonate. Also, certain high-technology home care services may not be available in isolated areas.

Who will be the caregiver at different times of the day?
Rationale: Secondary caregivers and babysitters may need to learn special care techniques.

How do you plan on paying for home health care?
Rationale: For the neonate with a chronic illness or an anticipated long-term need for home health care, public and private insurers may cover only some costs, if any. Thus, the family will need financial counseling about alternative financial sources.

Is your family experiencing much stress right now? How extensive is your family's support system?
Rationale: To provide a safe environment for home care, the family may need help to minimize stress or enhance their support systems before the neonate's discharge. For the family with significant stress or little support, a referral to a social service agency may be necessary.

How much do you know about your child's medical condition?
Rationale: General teaching usually can begin soon after the neonate's admission to the nursery. (However, predicting what the neonate's condition will be at discharge or exactly which equipment and services will be needed at home may be impossible.)

high-technology equipment or extensive professional services, a final decision on the suitability of home care should be delayed until the neonate is medically stable. Continuing instability or the need for frequent laboratory tests usually necessitates institutional care.

Parental willingness and ability. For home care to succeed, the parents must be willing and able to take on primary responsibility for the neonate's health care. Some parents—those who are ill themselves, for instance—are unable physically to care for a child. Others cannot afford to quit a job to stay home with the neonate, particularly if the employer pays for medical insurance. Home care also may be out of the question if the neonate needs complex or frequent care—a situation requiring two or more caregivers so that one can relieve the other.

The nurse should not assume that all parents want to care for a special-needs child at home. Some parents feel intimidated by medical equipment and overwhelmed by the demands of providing complex care. Some are unwilling to add the burden of health care to their other responsibilities or to make the necessary life-style changes to accommodate complex home care. A few parents, unable to cope with an uncertain future, are unsuited psychologically to caring for a special-needs child.

In some cases, parents express the desire to care for the neonate at home but repeatedly fail to attend learning sessions; this may indicate that they have unexpressed concerns about their ability to provide home care. Other parents are willing but lack the ability to learn caregiving skills.

Practical and psychosocial support. The parents of a special-needs child must have sufficient physical and psychosocial support to cope with home health care. Yet these parents may not get the support they need. The U.S. General Accounting Office (1989) identified lack of information about available services or a resource person to contact when parents need help with home care as among the most common reasons why families with special-needs children have trouble obtaining support services.

Ideally, friends and other family members should be available to help care for other children and perform household chores. Respite for the parents also is crucial; a secondary caregiver who is trained in the required skills should be available to relieve the parents periodically from caregiving.

Psychosocial support is particularly important; parents of chronically ill children perceive less social support than parents of well children (Ferrari, 1986). Knowing that someone understands what the parents are going through, cares about them, and is available to offer emotional support can help the parents withstand the emotional rigors of caring for a special-needs child.

Cost considerations. In the United States, cost is a major issue when planning for discharge. Most major insurers provide only minimal coverage, if any, for home care even though home care usually costs significantly less than institutional care of comparable duration. Also, few insurers will pay for home care if it costs more than institutional care—a situation that may occur with a special-needs child who requires one-to-one nursing care.

When home care is covered by insurance, the family may have to pay a yearly deductible of $100 to $500 before the insurer will begin to reimburse 80% of the charges. Also, some insurers cover only certain types of equipment; for instance, they may pay for durable medical equipment, such as enteral feeding pumps, but not for disposables, such as the feeding bags and tubes used with such pumps. Moreover, most third-party payers limit the amount they will reimburse yearly for home nursing services; the average $5,000 limit would cover just 1 week of around-the-clock nursing care at $30/hour (this amount includes indirect costs as well as the nurse's wage). Many special-needs children nearly exhaust their lifetime maximum insurance benefits before discharge; further medical costs may devastate the family financially. This is a major concern for U.S. citizens, legislators, and health care providers and has sparked the introduction of catastrophic health care legislation.

Hidden costs usually are not reported in comparisons of institutional and home health care expenses; however, such costs can be substantial. Hidden costs include lost income when a family member must take time off from work to care for the child, higher home electricity bills (such as when the neonate requires mechanical ventilation), modifications of the home or family vehicle to accommodate special equipment, and transportation to and from physician appointments.

Other factors. The family considering home care must have transportation for follow-up medical visits. Also, the home environment must be suitable for caregiving, with adequate space to store supplies and set up equipment. Preferably, it also should have indoor plumbing, refrigeration, electricity, and a telephone (or easy access to one). Availability of services also must be considered. For instance, private-duty nurses may not be available in rural areas.

Supporting the family's decision. The nurse and other members of the health team must be willing to support the family's informed decision regarding the neonate's placement. This is particularly important if the parents are considering an alternative care setting and have unresolved doubts about their moral, ethical, and legal obligations to their child; reinforcement of these doubts by the nurse could cause overwhelming parental guilt.

Likewise, the nurse should avoid imposing personal values on the parents. A parent's unkempt appearance or unhealthful life-style, for instance, may offend the nurse;

lack of toilets and running water in the home may not conform to the nurse's view of a safe, healthful home environment. However, make an effort to maintain objectivity when considering whether such deficiencies represent real threats to the child's health and safety. After all, many children thrive even in the harshest environments. Also, the nurse who tries to "make the picture perfect" stands a good chance of encountering repeated disappointments and may have trouble establishing a positive relationship with the family. In any event, making referrals to the appropriate social service agencies and other resources fulfills the nurse's responsibility.

On the other hand, if the parents seem incapable of responsible parenting and their behavior or attitude suggests that the neonate will be neglected or abused after discharge, the nurse should consider notifying a social worker, who may attempt to have the court place the neonate in protective custody.

Ongoing assessment of discharge planning needs

Obviously, the nurse cannot assess all discharge planning needs at the time of nursery admission but must continue to assess these needs throughout the neonate's stay in the health care facility. As new needs arise, they must be incorporated into the discharge plan.

Many health care facilities conduct ongoing assessment of discharge planning needs during weekly discharge planning rounds and regularly scheduled client care conferences in addition to daily nurse-physician rounds. Topics discussed in these forums typically include the parents' understanding of and attitude toward the neonate's condition, the parents' coping ability and capacity to provide adequate care at home, the home environment, the family's need for support services and community resources, and the neonate's readiness for discharge.

Discharge planning rounds. During discharge planning rounds, each client on the unit is discussed briefly by a multidisciplinary team consisting of a nurse, physician, social worker, occupational or physical therapist, dietitian, child life therapist, and perhaps a utilization review nurse and financial counselor. The team discusses assessment findings and ways to meet the neonate's and family's discharge planning needs.

Each team member is assigned specific tasks. The physician, for instance, typically will record which pediatrician or other primary care physician the parents have chosen for postdischarge care. The nurse will provide parent teaching (such as how to perform cardiopulmonary resuscitation [CPR], if appropriate) and make referrals to home health care companies. The social worker will de-

termine if friends or other family members will be available to help with household tasks. The financial counselor will determine if the family's medical insurance covers private-duty home nursing care and, if so, to what dollar limit.

This discussion is documented in the client progress notes. In subsequent days or weeks, members of the health care team report on their assignments and work to finalize the discharge plan.

Client care conference. This forum, usually used to discuss a single client in depth, aids in the development and implementation of the discharge plan for the neonate who requires special planning. For some special-needs neonates, several such conferences may be required. The nurse may call the conference to conduct prospective planning or to discuss a new development or health crisis. To minimize the miscommunication and differences of opinion that can arise when several professionals are involved in a client's care, all major health care team members should take part in the conference; to help ensure continuity of care, the neonate's private physician also should attend. Usually, the parents are invited to attend, at least for the summary.

The physician or primary nurse usually chairs the conference, describing the neonate's current situation and requesting clarification and consensus on the plan of care. The nurse should ensure that the parents are supported rather than intimidated at the conference and that any questions or concerns they bring up are addressed adequately. As with discharge planning rounds, the client care conference is summarized by the primary nurse and recorded in the neonate's medical record.

IMPLEMENTING THE DISCHARGE PLAN

To implement the discharge plan, the nurse prepares the parents by teaching them about the care the child will require, helps them select a home health agency and order medical equipment and supplies, arranges for follow-up medical visits, makes appropriate referrals to community health services and other resources, and verifies that a family support system is in place by the time the neonate is discharged.

For the neonate with special needs, the American Academy of Pediatrics (1984) recommends that the discharge plan include a primary care physician, a case coordinator, a defined backup system for medical emergency care, verification of family access to a telephone, and a means of monitoring and adjusting the care plan as necessary. If the neonate requires special equipment, some health care facilities require that the equipment be brought there and used to check its operation and familiarize the parents with it.

Preparing the parents for the neonate's discharge

The nurse must ensure that the parents learn caregiving skills before the neonate's discharge. Besides routine neonatal and infant caregiving techniques, teaching topics may include emergency interventions, signs and symptoms of medical problems, use of special equipment, the purpose and adverse effects of medications, and names of people to contact when the parents have questions.

Use of written, standardized teaching plans ensures that teaching content is congruent over time and among professionals; however, when using such plans, make sure to individualize them so that they are relevant to the family's unique situation. Also, provide adequate learning time, making allowances for such problems as tardiness or missed appointments because of work responsibilities, lack of transportation, or difficulty finding a babysitter.

During parent preparation, keep in mind the various factors that can affect a parent's readiness and ability to learn: anxiety, previous experiences with illness, physical and mental capacities, cultural and ethnic background, language, family relationships, and motivation. As necessary, adjust the teaching plan around these factors. Because many parents are under stress when learning new information or skills and may not absorb information completely, be sure to reinforce verbal teaching with printed materials written at a fourth-grade reading level; preferably, these materials should have pictures or diagrams. Topics covered in such handouts should include illnesses, medications, special procedures, and well-baby care. (Use of written teaching materials also makes documentation of teaching more efficient and consistent.)

Besides verbal and written instruction, another useful teaching strategy is demonstration. Asking for a return demonstration of skills demonstrated by the nurse gives parents the chance to practice these skills and allows the nurse to check for evidence of their caregiving competence and confidence.

Videotapes are increasingly used as a teaching tool because they allow demonstration of skills with maximum consistency of content. Many nurses find that one-on-one teaching time is reduced when parents have seen a videotape. Many videotaped teaching resources are available for parents.

Selecting home health care services

Over the past 10 years, the home health care industry has seen phenomenal growth. However, not every agency or company that describes itself as a home health care service specializes in neonatal or pediatric care. The discharge planning staff should steer the parents toward agencies and companies with neonatal and pediatric expertise.

To avoid problems with reimbursement that could delay the neonate's discharge, the nurse should aim for early identification of the home health care services the neonate will need. (For specific information on home health care services, see the "Home health care" section of this chapter.)

Planning for payment of home health care

If third-party payment is unavailable, refer the family to a financial counselor for information on alternative funding sources, such as private, religious, local, and national associations and foundations, as well as specialized support groups, such as the March of Dimes Foundation.

Arranging for follow-up care

Verify that the parents know the dates and times of scheduled follow-up medical visits; this information should be supplied to them in writing. Also make sure they will have transportation for these visits. If they do not have transportation, refer them to a social worker, who can inform them of transportation services. Also make sure the parents know whom to call with questions and concerns about the child's health care. To evaluate the effectiveness of the discharge plan and to provide emotional support, arrange to call the parents a few days after the neonate's discharge.

Preparing discharge instructions

Discharge instructions may take the form of written materials, such as booklets and printed instruction sheets for specific diseases, medication, or equipment; however, be sure to individualize such materials. Give discharge information to the parents early enough to allow them to read it, absorb it, and come up with questions that can be answered before the neonate's discharge, while the health care team is most accessible. Make sure to give parents emergency numbers to keep by the telephone at home. However, tell them that they are welcome to place non-emergency calls to ask any questions that may arise.

Send a copy of the discharge instructions and information about the neonate's status at discharge to the private physician's office and to the health care agency that will follow the child at home. If the parents received teaching handouts, also send a copy of these to the home health care agency to ensure continuity of care.

DOCUMENTING THE DISCHARGE PLAN

The JCAHO (1989) stipulates that the discharge plan be recorded in the client's medical record; this promotes continuity of care, provides a communication link for other team members, and serves as a reference for legal and other purposes. Make sure the medical record includes:
• assessment of the neonate's needs, problems, capabilities, and limitations
• evidence of parental participation in discharge planning
• evidence of parental learning of information provided
• availability of recommended services for the family
• the neonate's medical status at discharge
• the actual discharge plan, including prescribed medications, follow-up medical appointments, and any referrals to community agencies.

HOME HEALTH CARE

Home health care—the services, supplies, and equipment provided to a client at home—helps to maintain or promote a client's physical, mental, or emotional health. Home health care can reduce the cost of infant care while providing support to the family.

Studies show that home health care can be safe and cost-effective even for high-risk children. Brooten, et al. (1986) randomly assigned low-birth-weight neonates to two groups. One group was discharged according to routine nursery criteria. The second group was discharged an average of 11 days earlier and weighed 200 g (7 oz) less; a perinatal nurse specialist provided evaluation and parent teaching and support for this group before discharge, during home visits 1 week after discharge, and periodically afterward. The researchers found no difference between the groups in number of rehospitalizations or in physical and mental growth and development, but health care costs per neonate in the group discharged earlier were $18,560 lower than for the other group.

Home health care also may improve mother-infant interaction. Norr, Nacion, and Abramson (1989) studied interaction between low-income, inner-city mothers and their neonates in three groups:
• simultaneous early discharge of mother and neonate (24 to 47 hours after delivery)
• early discharge of the mother, with discharge of the neonate after 48 hours
• simultaneous conventional discharge of mother and neonate (48 to 72 hours after delivery).

The selection criteria ensured that only low-risk mothers and neonates were discharged early. A nurse and community aide visited the simultaneous early-discharge group 1 to 2 days after discharge to conduct physical examinations and phenylketonuria and bilirubin testing; provide standard teaching on health, safety, and infant growth and development; and discuss the mothers' concerns. The researchers found stronger mother-infant bonding, fewer maternal concerns, and greater maternal satisfaction with postpartal care in this group, with no increase in maternal or neonatal morbidity in the first 2 weeks after discharge. However, all of the subjects in this study required careful health monitoring, and the mothers needed considerable teaching during the first month at home.

As these studies suggest, including a perinatal nurse specialist in a home health care program helps ensure that the parents receive expert advice and that neonatal problems are prevented or detected early through comprehensive assessment. In regions where perinatal nurse specialists are not available, home nurse generalists must maintain conscientious communication with nurse specialists and physicians to provide continuity of care.

Home health care services may be provided by public agencies or private companies. Equipment, supplies, and other products used for home care typically are obtained from private companies. The tremendous expansion in home health care has led to increased competition among providers of services and products. However, many services are geared to geriatric clients; therefore, careful selection is crucial.

Services
Formerly, home health care was the nearly exclusive province of the public health nurse, who provided not only illness care but health promotion and comprehensive family care. However, the passage of Medicare and Medicaid legislation led to dramatic changes in payment and provision systems and in client eligibility for home care. As physicians' roles in home care enlarged, such care became less comprehensive and more narrowly focused on illness care. Currently, professionals who may provide home health care include nurses, physicians, social workers, dietitians, and speech, hearing, occupational, and physical therapists. Many clients also require home health aides and homemaker services.

Nurses involved in home health care include public or community health nurses, private-duty nurses, and nurses from home care departments of local hospitals or for-profit (proprietary) home health care companies. These nurses and other professionals can be hired through a public, proprietary, or hospital-based agency.

CRITERIA FOR HOME MECHANICAL VENTILATION

The decision to care for a mechanically ventilated infant at home is a difficult one. The parents must undergo extensive predischarge teaching, and the child's prolonged need for complex care creates an enormous emotional and financial drain on the family. Also, home assessment of the mechanically ventilated infant can be challenging. In the health care facility, blood gas analysis, transcutaneous monitoring, and pulse oximetry help the health care team assess the neonate's ventilatory requirements. At home, where these evaluative mechanisms usually are not available, management is based on skin color, absence or presence of signs of respiratory compromise, and, in some cases, apnea monitoring.

On the other hand, the ventilator-dependent infant who is cared for at home usually has a decreased infection risk, greater socialization, and better stimulation for growth and development (Donar, 1988).

Ahmann (1986) identifies the following criteria for mechanical ventilation at home.

- The infant must have a stable underlying disease and continued inability to be weaned from mechanical ventilation.
- The infant must be able to maintain an adequate nutritional intake, as measured by consistent growth and development.
- The parents must have a positive attitude, motivation, and willingness to make a 24-hour commitment to their child's care.
- The family must have access to a community source for equipment and supplies, emergency care, and home nursing personnel and must have the financial resources to support the cost of prolonged, complex care.
- The home must support the mechanical and electrical needs of the ventilator and have adequate space for caregiving activities and storage of equipment and supplies.

A certified home care nursing agency (which may be run privately or publicly) is one that is subject to certain standards of care and has been certified for Medicare reimbursement. Such an agency can provide nurses for intermittent visits and also may provide speech, hearing, occupational, and physical therapists; homemakers; and home health aides. Many certified agencies also can supply private-duty or hourly nurses for families who have private insurance or can pay directly for nursing care.

Equipment and supplies

Home health care equipment and supplies can be obtained from durable medical equipment companies, surgical pharmacies, and home infusion therapy services. Selection of a vendor should take into account the company's pediatric experience and the range of equipment and supplies provided. Optimally, the vendor should offer preventive maintenance, free loaner equipment during repairs, 24-hour availability for emergency service, and prompt response to service calls.

Durable medical equipment companies provide respiratory equipment, such as oxygen tanks, mechanical ventilators, and apnea monitors; most also can supply hospital beds (but usually not cribs), wheelchairs, phototherapy equipment, enteral feeding pumps, and other supplies for home use. These companies usually employ a nurse or respiratory therapist to manage the home use of their equipment. Home infusion therapy services can provide home chemotherapy, pain control therapy, antibiotic therapy, and enteral feedings. For neonates and infants, home infusion therapy is used mainly to deliver total parenteral nutrition.

CASE MANAGEMENT

Case management is a system whereby a single person manages a client's care, helping to prevent duplication of services, to decrease costs (by ensuring timely services and preventing complications), and to promote continuity of care. In the home care setting, the case manager may be responsible for advising the family on the services they need, arranging for nurses and equipment, arranging for payment of services, solving problems, and visiting the family regularly. For home care, the community health nurse is especially well-suited to serve as case manager.

Ironically, case management has become so popular that several case managers may be assigned to a family—perhaps one from the insurance company, another from the home health agency, and yet another from developmental services. However, not every family requires case management; many need information only and can act as their own case managers. Case management is most helpful for parents who lack the ability or means to coordinate their child's care and for those whose child has multiple needs necessitating the involvement of several agencies and support services (U.S. General Accounting Office, 1989).

HOME HEALTH CARE NEEDS

The trend toward early discharge has increased the need for home health care for both normal, healthy neonates and special-needs neonates. (For information on when mechanical ventilation may be appropriate, see *Criteria for home mechanical ventilation;* for indications for nutritional therapy and applicable nursing considerations, see *Home nutrition therapy.*)

HOME NUTRITION THERAPY

The infant who cannot ingest sufficient nutrients orally or whose gastrointestinal (GI) tract cannot be used for nutritional replenishment may require enteral or parenteral (I.V.) nutrition therapy at home to ensure adequate nutrition.

ENTERAL NUTRITION

The preferred method for nutritional support, enteral nutrition is the administration of nutrients through a feeding tube to the GI tract. Besides helping to maintain GI function, enteral therapy has fewer risks and costs less than parenteral nutrition. Enteral therapy may be required to supplement oral feedings or to supply the total caloric intake for the infant with a vomiting disorder (such as gastroesophageal reflux), an inadequate sucking reflex (for instance, from prolonged mechanical ventilation), or a respiratory or cardiac disorder that reduces the energy available for oral feeding.

Administration routes

High-risk infants usually receive enteral nutrition through a nasogastric (NG) tube or an orogastric tube—methods known as gavage feeding. In some cases, however, a gastrostomy tube is used. Gavage feeding commonly is used for intermittent or short-term home use but also may be appropriate for long-term home use. The tube may be made of polyurethane, polyvinyl chloride, or silicone (Silastic) material. Although Silastic tubes are more expensive than ones made of harder plastic, they are preferred for home use because they are easier to insert and cause less irritation to the GI mucosa. For home use, they can be reused after washing with soap and water.

Gastrostomy feedings necessitate surgical placement of a tube in the abdomen to deposit feedings directly into the stomach. Gastrostomy feedings are the preferred method for long-term home enteral nutrition.

Administration methods

The method used to administer gavage or gastrostomy feedings depends on the infant's GI tolerance. Bolus feedings can be given by gravity through a syringe attached to the tube; larger volumes are introduced into the stomach at a rate similar to that of normal sucking on a breast or bottle. Some high-risk infants given bolus feedings experience feeding intolerance, manifested as diarrhea or vomiting. Bolus feedings are contraindicated in neonates or infants with a history of gastroesophageal reflux (unless the cardiac sphincter has been repaired) because they may precipitate regurgitation or aspiration.

With continuous feedings, a pump and administration set are used to deliver small volumes of formula continuously. Although continuous feedings usually are tolerated better than bolus feedings, they restrict the infant's mobility because the pump and tubing must remain attached. However, scheduling most feedings at night minimizes the need to restrict daytime activities (if appropriate, oral feedings can be given during the day). Because the family must rent the pump and buy the tubing, continuous feedings are relatively expensive.

Enteral nutrition formulas

The high-risk infant may need a high-calorie enteral nutrition formula (27 to 30 calories/oz) to meet energy and growth demands. Some of these formulas are hyperosmolar, however, and may cause diarrhea and subsequent weight loss.

PARENTERAL NUTRITION

Parenteral nutrition refers to the I.V. administration of fluids containing glucose, amino acids, electrolytes, vitamins, and minerals in specific proportions necessary for growth. In most cases, parenteral nutrition is administered as total parenteral nutrition (TPN), a nutritionally complete form usually delivered through a central venous catheter inserted into a large neck or chest vessel. Many neonates and infants receive a combination of TPN and enteral nutrition.

Candidates for parenteral therapy include infants who cannot receive adequate food through the GI tract. For instance, those with congenital GI anomalies, such as omphalocele (protrusion of an intestinal portion through an abdominal wall defect at the umbilicus) or gastroschisis (protrusion of an intestinal portion through a defect elsewhere in the abdominal wall), may have suffered significant small intestine loss during surgery or may have developed multiple obstructions secondary to adhesions. Thus, they may be unable to tolerate any enteral formula.

NURSING CONSIDERATIONS

- For enteral feedings, teach the parents to position the infant prone, with the shoulders at least 30 degrees higher than the feet, and to maintain this position for at least 20 minutes after the feeding.
- If the infant has gastroesophageal reflux, inform the parents that the head must remain higher than the stomach to reduce the risk of aspiration. If appropriate, teach them how to use a special harness to maintain proper positioning, with the head of the crib elevated 30 to 45 degrees.

- To help prevent aspiration of enteral feedings, show the parents how to aspirate stomach contents to check for residual matter before feedings. Also teach them how to use a stethoscope to auscultate air insertion through the tube when checking tube placement before feedings.
- Make sure the parents know how to prepare and administer feedings. For example, teach them to warm the formula to room temperature. Explain how to attach the filled drip set to

(continued)

HOME NUTRITION THERAPY *(continued)*

NURSING CONSIDERATIONS *(continued)*

the tube and regulate the flow using the clamp or pump. Advise them to burp the infant periodically and at the end of the feeding and to position the infant on the right side afterward.
- Instruct the parents to call the physician if the feeding tube becomes blocked or dislodged; insertion of a new tube may be necessary.
- Teach the parents how to provide skin care around the tube insertion site or stoma. Advise them to tape the NG tube without applying upward pressure against the nostril. Instruct them to clean the infant's nose or stoma with soap and water (or the prescribed solution) and to keep the area dry.
- Instruct the parents how to prepare a high-calorie enteral formula, if ordered; proper preparation helps minimize diarrhea.

Make sure they know how to assess for diarrhea and other complications of tube feedings, such as vomiting, aspiration of feeding matter (from improper tube position), abdominal cramps (from rapid feeding administration), and skin breakdown around the stoma of the gastrostomy tube.
- Mouth care is especially important for infants who are fed enterally or parenterally. Instruct the parents to swab the infant's mouth with moistened sponge-tipped swabs or gauze to keep it clean and moist and to apply white petrolatum to the lips to help prevent drying and cracking.
- Instruct the parents to weigh the infant regularly to monitor nutritional status.

Routine and basic care

For the normal, healthy neonate, home health care typically involves assessment of the neonate and teaching, counseling, and support for the family. Areas of particular interest to the nurse include the neonate's nutritional status, healing of the umbilicus and circumcision site, feeding patterns, urinary and bowel elimination patterns, and sleep-awake patterns. As necessary, the nurse may draw blood samples for various laboratory tests (such as serum bilirubin analysis).

The nurse also assesses the parents' ability to provide routine care (such as bathing, feeding, diapering, stimulation, and cord and circumcision care) and perform basic health care procedures (such as taking rectal temperature, administering vitamins and medications, and suctioning with a bulb syringe).

Some otherwise healthy neonates require phototherapy at home for the treatment of jaundice or an elevated serum unconjugated bilirubin level. Phototherapy, which involves exposure of the neonate's skin to various lights, previously necessitated continued hospitalization. The significant cost of the treatment in this setting and the enforced separation from parents led practitioners to attempt home phototherapy (Hartsell, 1986; Heiser, 1987). Home phototherapy with supportive teaching for parents is a safe, satisfactory intervention that produces substantial savings for families, health care facilities, and insurance providers (Heiser, 1987).

Candidates for home phototherapy typically include term neonates who tolerate oral feedings well and lack underlying hemolytic disease. Also, the parents must be willing and able to manage this treatment at home and to arrange for serial laboratory bilirubin testing.

Specialized care

Besides routine and basic care, the high-risk or special-needs child requires sophisticated, complex care at home. Such care may involve apnea monitoring, suctioning, chest physiotherapy, oxygen therapy, tracheostomy care, mechanical ventilation, enteral or parenteral nutrition, medication administration, and developmental stimulation programs.

The typical infant who requires specialized home care is preterm or low birth weight and has one or some combination of the following disorders: respiratory distress, bronchopulmonary dysplasia, apnea of prematurity, patent ductus arteriosus, hearing or visual impairment, hydrocephalus, intraventricular hemorrhage, seizures, or necrotizing enterocolitis. Congenital anomalies and the effects of maternal substance abuse also may necessitate specialized home care. (For information on the pathophysiology and management of these and other perinatal disorders, see Chapter 21, Care of High-Risk Neonates and Their Families.)

Psychosocial support is a key aspect of home care for the family of the special-needs child. The transition from the intensive care unit to the home can be stressful for parents; although they are relieved that their child is well enough to be discharged, they also may have doubts and fears about their ability to provide care at home.

ASSESSMENT

Before the first home visit, the nurse should review the discharge plan to become acquainted with the neonate's hospital course, discharge medications, and care instructions and to determine the parents' caregiving skills, confidence level, and teaching and support needs.

First home visit

Make every effort to establish a rapport so that the parents will feel free to discuss their concerns openly. Avoid medical jargon and be attentive and nonjudgmental as the parents discuss their concerns. Keep in mind that the home, unlike the health care facility, is the family's territory; an intrusive, domineering approach here could make the family resent the nurse's presence.

Obtain baseline information about the infant's physical status, growth, and development, and make a preliminary assessment of the parents' caregiving knowledge and skills and the family's support system. Also assess the home environment and the family's emergency plans, and confirm that any required equipment is functioning properly and that all needed supplies are present. Obtain information for insurance and other financial matters, and have the parents sign any necessary forms. At this visit and all subsequent visits, ask the parents what their main concerns are and then address these concerns.

Also obtain a health history and perform a physical assessment; however, if this will take more time than the family can spare, the history may be obtained gradually over subsequent visits. For the high-risk child, gear the physical assessment toward the specific condition, as described below under "Assessment of the special-needs child."

If the neonate is taking medications, review the dosages and schedules with the parents. If the schedules are inconvenient, with nighttime doses and many separate dosage times, consider asking the physician to modify them.

Parental caregiving knowledge and skills. Assess the parents' ability to perform routine and basic neonatal health care. Also evaluate their ability to provide any specific interventions, such as phototherapy, that the child requires. If specialized care is needed, such as enteral or parenteral feeding, apnea monitoring, or oxygen therapy, assess the parents' understanding of the purpose of this care and the proper operation of equipment and medical supplies; make sure they know how to examine the child for problems related to the use of such equipment. (For detailed assessment information, see *Assessment guidelines for the infant who requires special equipment,* pages 500 and 501.) If premixed solutions are required, such as for nutritional therapy, verify that the family has a refrigerator for solution storage; if not, find out if the home infusion therapy service can supply refrigeration, and if so, whether they will charge for this.

Support system. Although the hospital discharge planning staff makes a preliminary assessment of the support system that may be available to the family after discharge, the home health care nurse has the advantage of assessing the support system in action, determining its extent and reliability. The major support needs of the family caring for a special-needs child at home are physical support for caregiving and household tasks, respite care, and psychosocial support.

Assess how much physical support the parents need and how much they are receiving. Many parents of special-needs children must rely on help from friends and relatives because few community support agencies are geared toward the special-needs child. Meals On Wheels, for example, provides hot meals for people physically unable to cook for themselves but not for parents struggling with an ill child. Also, many insurance companies reimburse homemaker services for adults who cannot physically maintain their homes but not for parents of ill children, on the grounds that the parents are physically able to perform household tasks.

Also assess whether the parents have a realistic attitude toward their need for physical support. Many parents are reluctant to ask for help, feeling that they should be able to care for their special-needs child round the clock while keeping house, attending to other children, and meeting their personal needs.

Determine whether a secondary caregiver is available. The parents of a child who requires high-technology or other complex care need occasional respite, or relief, from caregiving but may have trouble finding it. Some regional perinatal centers provide respite care. Also, respite care is available through various community programs; however, the caregivers provided by these programs rarely are trained to care for special-needs neonates or infants. On the other hand, friends and relatives may be intimidated by the idea of caring for a child who depends on medical equipment; although wishing they could help, they may worry that they will not know what to do if something happens and that the child will die while in their care.

Thus, many parents of special-needs children discover that only a nurse is comfortable with, or capable of, caring for their child. But hiring a nurse to provide a few hours of respite care costs at least five times as much as a regular babysitter. Consequently, parents may forego respite care and never take a break from care-giving. Eventually, this can take a toll on the parents' health as well as the couple's relationship and other family relationships.

Determine if the parents are aware of support groups and other resources that can provide psychosocial support, especially if their child has special needs. Members

(Text continues on page 502.)

ASSESSMENT GUIDELINES FOR THE INFANT WHO REQUIRES SPECIAL EQUIPMENT

The chart below shows key assessment guidelines if the infant requires special medical equipment. Before the first home visit, the nurse should obtain the health history to review the reason for the equipment and the neonate's hospital course. On each home visit, verify that all equipment is functioning properly; conduct a rapid review of functional patterns and body systems, then focus the assessment on the infant's specific problem.

INDICATIONS	HEALTH HISTORY AND PHYSICAL ASSESSMENT DATA	PARENTAL KNOWLEDGE AND SKILLS	EQUIPMENT-RELATED DATA
Apnea monitor			
Apnea of prematurity, respiratory compromise, tracheostomy use, acute drug withdrawal, family history of apnea or sudden infant death	• Vital signs • Respiratory status • Frequency and duration of predischarge apneic episodes, need for resuscitation after an episode, and any associated signs or precipitating factors • Postdischarge history of pallor, cyanosis, or hypotonia • Postdischarge history of apnea or bradycardia alarms, their frequency and duration, and type of stimulation required to arouse the infant	• Understanding of apnea and purpose of monitor • Knowledge of correct monitor settings • Operation of monitor • Safety precautions; proper response to monitor alarms • Ability to keep an accurate apnea log • Knowledge of infant cardiopulmonary resuscitation (CPR) procedure	• Presence of all needed supplies in the home, including lead wires, patches, and an instruction manual • Use of grounded outlet for monitor • Appropriateness and accuracy of monitor settings • Proper monitor placement (on a hard surface at the bedside with sufficient ventilation behind and above monitor) • Correct placement of electrodes (contacting sides of chest wall)
Oxygen therapy			
Respiratory or cardiac disorder	• Vital signs • Respiratory status • Skin color changes, such as peripheral cyanosis and signs of respiratory distress	• Understanding of purpose and use of oxygen therapy • Competence and confidence in using equipment • Knowledge of safety precautions	• Accuracy of concentration and liter flow • Use of recommended equipment • Correct number of hours of daily oxygen therapy • Proper equipment function • Adequate supply level of oxygen source • Use of a humidification source (if prescribed) and proper humidifier function and settings • Proper use of prescribed delivery method
Tracheostomy			
Upper airway obstruction, respiratory failure from mechanical or neurologic problems, chronic aspiration, longterm mechanical ventilation	• Vital signs • Respiratory status • Quality, color, viscosity, and odor of tracheal secretions • Condition of skin at tracheostomy site	• Purpose of tracheostomy • Indications for suctioning (such as wheezing breath sounds and signs of respiratory distress) • Competence and confidence in performing tracheostomy care (such as routine daily cleaning of the tracheostomy site, suctioning, and tube insertion and removal) • Knowledge of modified CPR procedure	• Proper use of humidification source (such as compressor with a nebulizer or cascade, room humidifier, or tracheostomy humidifying filter) • Correct size of tracheostomy tubes and suction catheter

ASSESSMENT GUIDELINES FOR THE INFANT WHO REQUIRES SPECIAL EQUIPMENT (continued)

INDICATIONS	HEALTH HISTORY AND PHYSICAL ASSESSMENT DATA	PARENTAL KNOWLEDGE AND SKILLS	EQUIPMENT-RELATED DATA
Mechanical ventilator			
Respiratory disorder	• Vital signs (compare observed respiratory rate against ventilator rate) • Skin color, respiratory pattern, and rise and fall of chest with each breath	• Understanding purpose, function, and operation of ventilator • Ability to assess for signs of respiratory distress, fatigue, and periorbital edema • Ability to prevent atelectasis through frequent positioning changes, hyperinflation, chest physiotherapy, and suctioning • Ability to check for proper ventilator function and settings • Knowledge of proper response to ventilator alarms • Ability to use other required equipment (such as oxygen therapy or apnea monitor)	• Proper ventilator settings • Correct bellows functioning • Alarm lights on • Connections secure • Tubing unkinked • Humidifier filled • Availability of backup power supply (such as batteries or a generator)
Enteral or parenteral nutrition therapy			
Inability to ingest adequate calories by mouth	• Nutritional status (such as growth parameters and daily tube or I.V. intake) • Skin condition around tube or I.V. insertion site	• Knowledge and ability to prepare and administer feedings correctly • Ability to assess for proper tube placement before each tube feeding (using a stethoscope to auscultate air insertion through tube) • Ability to identify such problems as tube dislodgement and nasal irritation • Knowledge of proper interventions for tube dislodgement • Ability to identify and troubleshoot equipment problems • Ability to provide mouth care and assess and intervene for complications of tube feedings (such as vomiting, diarrhea, aspiration of feeding matter, and abdominal cramps) or parenteral nutrition (such as air embolism, infection, metabolic problems, and fluid extravasation) • Understanding of special positioning requirements during feedings	• Correct function of feeding pump • Appropriateness of feeding technique; enteral or I.V. formula; placement, size, and type of tube; administration method; feeding frequency and duration; and infant positioning • Availability of refrigeration for storage of feeding solutions • Adequate home sanitation to allow sterile procedures required for nutritional therapy

of parent support groups have had first-hand experience in caring for special-needs children and can offer advice on which problems to anticipate, how to cope with problems, and where to find special supplies or services. For instance, Sick Kids Need Involved People (SKIP) is a support group for families of technology-dependent children, particularly those requiring tracheostomies and ventilatory support. Founded in 1980, it promotes specialized pediatric home care for medically fragile children.

Home environment. Assess whether the home has adequate facilities and space for caregiving. For the special-needs child, check for sufficient electrical outlets and adequate shelving or other storage arrangements for supplies (however, make sure supplies are not stored directly over the child's bed). Determine whether the family might benefit by installing ramps to allow easier movement of the child and equipment into and out of the house. Also observe for evidence that home health care may be disrupting family functioning; if so, assess whether the parents should consider converting a downstairs room into the child's bedroom to give them privacy from home health personnel.

Emergency plan. Determine if the family has a good emergency plan. A telephone is essential; if the home lacks one, find out if the parents have made other arrangements for obtaining help in an emergency. To help ensure prompt emergency intervention, verify that they have notified the police and fire departments in writing about their child's condition, medications, and treatments as well as the names of the child's health care providers and the health care facility to transport the child to in an emergency. Likewise, the parents should notify the telephone and electric companies requesting placement on a priority service list, advance notification of anticipated interruptions, and priority reinstatement of service after unexpected interruptions.

Also make sure parents and all other caregivers know how to administer infant CPR correctly and when to seek immediate medical attention for a problem. Check whether CPR instructions are posted near the child's bed and a list of emergency telephone numbers is located near all telephones.

Subsequent home visits

Once the nurse has established a rapport with the family and made baseline assessments, assessment during later visits should focus on detecting changes in the infant's physical status, observing the parents' caregiving skills for improvement, and assessing parent-infant interaction. For the high-risk or special-needs child, also assess specific aspects of the neonate's condition (as described below under "Assessment of the special-needs child") and observe how the infant's care is affecting other family members.

Take vital signs and assess for changes in the infant's condition. For the neonate receiving phototherapy, assess for signs of treatment efficacy, such as improved color of the skin and mucous membranes. Also check for dehydration, an adverse effect of phototherapy, which may manifest as lethargy, poor feeding, and excessive, watery stools.

As the parents become more familiar and comfortable with infant care, expect their caregiving skills to improve. A deficiency in skills warrants additional teaching sessions.

The home is a good environment in which to observe parent-infant interaction, which is crucial to child growth and development. In some cases, the nurse may use a specific assessment tool to assess the mother-infant relationship. Also note the degree of eye contact between parent and infant and observe how frequently the mother fondles, kisses, and vocalizes with the neonate. Keep in mind that problems in parent-infant bonding sometimes manifest in neonatal or infant behavioral problems, such as sleep disturbances, feeding disorders, failure to gain weight, and refusal to cuddle or feed.

Assessment of the special-needs child

For the special-needs child, augment routine assessment with an investigation tailored to the specific problem.

Respiratory disorder. Measure the pulse, respiratory rate, and temperature. A change from baseline values when unrelated to crying, position changes, feeding, or activity may signal cardiac or respiratory compromise. Auscultate the lungs, noting the general quality of breath sounds and checking for adventitious sounds.

Assess the skin color and respiratory pattern, and note any signs of respiratory distress, such as pallor, cyanosis, nasal flaring, chest retractions, edema, or diaphoresis. Ask the parents if they have noted irritability, appetite loss, or other signs of respiratory distress, such as color changes. Assess respiratory secretions for amount, consistency, color, and odor; suspect infection if secretions are foul-smelling, yellowish green, or more copious or viscous than normal. Also assess for medication efficacy and adverse effects; be sure to ask the parents whether they have noticed the latter.

Determine whether the parents understand respiratory anatomy and physiology as well as the pathophysiology, signs and symptoms, and course of the underlying respiratory disease and the purpose of each intervention.

Also find out if they know how to assess the infant's respiratory status.

The infant with respiratory compromise is predisposed to respiratory infections; simple colds can rapidly progress to fulminant viral pneumonia, bronchopneumonia, respiratory syncytial virus, reactive airway disease, or bronchospasm. Assess whether the parents can identify signs of respiratory infection, such as irritability, fever, cyanosis, increased respiratory distress, pallor, tachypnea, increased oxygen requirements, increased secretions, cough, and poor feeding.

A respiratory disorder can compromise the infant's nutritional status; therefore, be sure to assess nutritional intake and growth.

If the infant is receiving nebulized medications, assess the parents' administration skills. Also, if appropriate, observe them as they perform chest physiotherapy, assessing whether they position the infant correctly and use proper percussion techniques. Also observe the parents as they suction the neonate (performed after chest physiotherapy). Suctioning may be done with a bulb syringe or a catheter. In some cases, a suction machine is used at home; assess whether the parents know how to use this equipment properly.

Neurologic problem. In hydrocephalus, excessive cerebrospinal fluid (CSF) accumulates within the cranial vault, leading to suture expansion and ventricular dilation. The infant discharged with hydrocephalus may have a surgically placed ventricular shunt to drain excess CSF from the ventricles to a distal compartment, such as the peritoneum.

Before the first home visit, review the infant's health history for shunt location, serial head circumference measurements, neurologic status, and prognosis. On each visit, measure head circumference, noting any abnormally rapid increase. Assess the infant's mental status (orientation level, alertness, and behavior). Check range of motion of the neck, and assess eye movements for nystagmus, convergence, and ability to follow. Also evaluate the fontanels, which should be flat and soft, and palpate the sutures, which should not be split or overlapped.

Assess for shunt obstruction and infection, which may manifest in fontanel tenseness or bulging, increased head circumference, irritability, vomiting, appetite changes, sleepiness, and sunset eyes (upper lid retraction causing the sclera to show above the iris). Infection may cause fever, erythema, and tenderness along the shunt tract.

Determine if the parents understand the purpose of the shunt and know how to check the fontanel to assess for shunt obstruction and infection. Also make sure they know when to call the physician (such as for rapidly increasing head circumference, irritability, vomiting, or hypoglycemia, hypocalcemia, and decreased alertness).

Preterm and low-birth-weight infants are predisposed to seizures. A symptom rather than a disease in itself, a seizure may stem from such conditions as intraventricular hemorrhage, head trauma, or drug withdrawal. An infant with seizures usually is discharged on anticonvulsant therapy, which typically continues until the child is at least age 6 months.

Before the first home visit, review the health history for the type of seizure the infant has experienced, seizure signs observed, postseizure behavior, and medications. During each visit, assess vital signs, alertness level, and motor and ocular responses to stimulation. Ask the parents whether they have observed signs of a seizure. (Preferably, they should keep a seizure log.) A subtle seizure may manifest as eyelid fluttering, nystagmus, drooling, tongue thrusting, lip smacking, tonic limb positioning, bicycling movements of the legs, or apnea. Also assess whether the parents can differentiate a seizure from jitteriness (unlike seizures, jittery movements commonly subside when the limbs are restrained.)

Determine whether the parents know how to assess the infant's neurologic status and behavior, care for the infant during a seizure, observe activity during and after the seizure, and provide emergency interventions (including CPR) for apnea. Also assess whether they know when to seek medical attention (such as when a seizure is prolonged), and evaluate their understanding of anticonvulsant medication—its regimen, potential adverse effects, and the need to avoid abrupt discontinuation (which could cause seizures). Make sure they know how often blood samples will be required for blood drug level monitoring and understand that stressful events (such as immunizations, infections, fever, and emotional stress) may trigger a seizure. Determine their knowledge of safety precautions, such as secure positioning, and make sure they understand that the child's neurologic outcome may remain undetermined for some time.

Visual or hearing impairment. Conditions leading to visual impairment include retinopathy of prematurity (ROP) and (rarely) congenital cataracts. A retinal disorder seen mainly in preterm and low-birth-weight neonates treated with oxygen therapy for respiratory distress, ROP can be detected as early as 6 weeks after birth. A congenital cataract is an opacification of the lens associated with such disorders as trisomy 13 and 18, galactosemia, and rubella syndrome. Many visually impaired neonates have multiple physiologic problems, including respiratory and neurologic compromise.

A neonate who receives oxygen therapy typically undergoes ophthalmologic examination before discharge. However, ROP usually is not detectable until after the neonatal period. Therefore, before the first home visit, be sure to review the medical records to determine if the neonate received oxygen therapy and is at risk for ROP.

During the first visit, perform a vision screening, examining the lids, pupils, sclera, and conjunctivae. Note any lesions, discharge, and unequal or absent pupillary reaction to light. Also assess for nystagmus, strabismus, and red reflex. Evaluate the neonate's ability to focus on an object placed 8″ to 10″ directly ahead and to follow objects moving horizontally. If the results of this screening suggest a problem, refer the child to an ophthalmologist.

For the infant with a previously diagnosed visual impairment, assess the parents' understanding of the condition and their awareness of home stimulation programs. Such programs may involve placement of mobiles and colorful toys in the crib, shaking a colorful noisemaker, or slowly moving an object from side to side in front of the neonate.

A hearing impairment is associated with such factors as low birth weight, congenital or perinatal infection, severe birth asphyxia, hyperbilirubinemia, exposure to high levels of environmental noise, chronic maternal illness, and malnutrition. The impairment may be unilateral or bilateral, may vary from mild to profound, and may involve low-frequency sound, high-frequency sound, or both. Depending on the auditory structures involved, a hearing impairment also may be classified as conductive (involving structures of the outer and middle ear), sensorineural (involving malformation of or damage to inner ear structures), or mixed (a combination of conductive and sensorineural).

A hearing impairment may not be detected before discharge. If a hearing problem is suspected, conduct an informal auditory behavioral screening, which determines responses to noisemakers with known intensity and frequency. If the results of this examination suggest a problem, refer the child for a complete audiologic and medical evaluation.

If a hearing impairment already has been diagnosed, find out if the child is wearing a hearing aid and whether the parents are aware of the benefits of a home stimulation program, which can teach them how to provide an optimal auditory environment and use alternative communication methods.

Acquired immunodeficiency syndrome (AIDS). Every neonate born to a woman infected with human immunodeficiency virus (HIV) carries the mother's HIV antibodies. This complicates neonatal diagnosis because a neonate who tests positive for HIV at birth may not actually be infected. To make a definitive diagnosis, the physician must determine if the child is producing HIV antibodies, indicating true HIV infection; this may take up to 15 months (Cruz, 1988).

Keep in mind that signs and symptoms of HIV infection may not appear until age 6 months to 2 years. A distinctive facial dysmorphism can help with early detection, as can persistent oral candida infections and diaper rash from diarrhea. Other suggestive findings include failure to thrive, severe bacterial infections, chronic parotid swelling, and pulmonary lymphoid interstitial pneumonitis. Sometimes central nervous system abnormalities are the only signs of HIV infection. For instance, the infant may be microencephalic with delayed cognitive and motor functioning. In some cases, the brain is affected directly; at least 50% of affected infants have encephalopathy (Cruz, 1988).

If AIDS is suspected, perform a complete physical assessment of the infant. If AIDS already has been diagnosed, assess the parents' ability and willingness to care for their child at home, especially if a parent also has AIDS or abuses drugs. Determine how much the parents know about the disease and the care required for the infant (such as management of life-threatening opportunistic infections). Also find out if they know which precautions are necessary to prevent disease spread to other family members; a misinformed caregiver may be afraid of catching the disease through casual contact and thus avoid the infant, placing the infant at risk for inadequate care and sensory deprivation. (For home care guidelines, see Parent Teaching: *When your infant has AIDS.*)

Effects of maternal substance abuse. The neonate affected by maternal substance abuse during pregnancy may remain in the health care facility until drug withdrawal is achieved. However, if this problem somehow eludes detection before discharge, the home health nurse who suspects it should check for such suggestive signs as abnormal reflex responses, marked irritability, continual high-pitched crying, poor feeding, muscle tremors, twitching, or rigidity with inability to extend the muscles. (For details on assessing for neonatal drug addiction or withdrawal, see Chapter 21, Care of High-Risk Neonates and Their Families.)

WHEN YOUR INFANT HAS A.I.D.S.

To care for your infant with AIDS, you will need to follow certain safeguards. Because of a weakened immune system, the child is more vulnerable to infection by germs that most children can fight off. Also, although AIDS cannot be transmitted through casual contact, you and other family members should avoid coming into direct contact with the infant's blood and body fluids. The precautions below can help ensure the safety of your infant as well as the rest of the family.

- Instruct all family members to wash their hands before eating and after using the toilet.
- To prevent the infant from developing an intestinal infection, use premixed commercial formulas, or prepare formula with pasteurized milk and milk products. Do not put the infant to bed with a bottle of milk or juice because bacteria grow rapidly in these fluids.
- Do not feed the infant directly from a jar; bacteria from the mouth may spoil the food that remains in the jar. Refrigerate opened jars and use the food within 24 hours.
- Cook or peel fruits and vegetables and cook meats thoroughly before giving them to the infant.
- Use a dishwasher or wash dishes in hot, sudsy water and air dry them.
- If possible, use disposable diapers. When changing diapers, wear disposable gloves; place used diapers in a sealed plastic bag.
- Keep diaper-changing areas separate from food preparation and serving areas. After each diaper change, clean the changing surface with a 1:10 solution of household bleach and water. (Be sure to wear disposable gloves when doing this.)
- Reserve separate towels and washcloths for the infant.
- Launder items soiled with the infant's blood or body fluids separately from the family laundry, and use hot sudsy water. The rest of the infant's laundry can be washed with other household laundry.
- Flush the infant's body wastes down the toilet and keep the infant's trash in a closed plastic container. Place needles and other sharp objects in an impenetrable container and arrange for their disposal.
- If you have a pet in the house, keep the animal's waste products away from the infant; do not allow animals that may bite or scratch to come near your child.

Assessment of the family of the special-needs child

For the family of the special-needs child, discharge may herald a new crisis. Already grieving over the loss of the anticipated "perfect" child, they must now confront the challenge of providing complex care on their own. To en-sure family-centered nursing care during this stressful transition, assess family members for the following factors, found by Wegener and Aday (1989) to increase the risk of stress in family members of special-needs children:
- discontinuous medical care of the infant
- financial problems
- many extended family members living in the household
- lack of a designated nurse–case manager at the time of the infant's discharge.

Also evaluate the parents for signs of grief and determine the coping mechanism each parent is using. Expect the parents to show signs of exhaustion and possibly marital strain. Assess siblings for overt or covert signs of jealousy and resentment of the neonate. Also explore family dynamics, strengths, and weaknesses.

Parental grief and coping mechanisms. The parents of a neonate with a chronic or disabling condition must pass through the stages of grief to deal with the loss of the "perfect" child and accept the real one. These stages typically include denial, anger, bargaining, depression, and acceptance. Like anyone faced with a stressful situation, parents of high-risk children also use certain coping mechanisms—denial, anger, withdrawal, guilt, and intellectualizing—to deal with their feelings. If possible, determine which stage of grief each parent is in and which coping mechanism each parent is using.

If the infant has a chronic condition, assessment of the parents in subsequent months or years may uncover chronic sorrow, a phenomenon first described by Olshansky (1962). The intensity of chronic sorrow varies from person to person and over time; it may disappear temporarily, only to recur. To assess for chronic sorrow, observe for sadness, fear, anxiety, anger, guilt, ambivalence, helplessness, or hopelessness. Keep in mind, however, that some parents conceal their sorrow; a few even try to suppress it to cope with the grim reality they face, seeming unduly optimistic about their child's condition.

Effect on the couple's relationship. Many parents of special-needs children report a strengthening of the marital relationship over time (Thomas, 1987). Also, studies show that parents of a special-needs child do not necessarily experience reduced marital satisfaction or have a shorter marriage duration. Nonetheless, the child's condition undoubtedly causes tremendous stress within the relationship, especially at first. Some couples may choose to stay together even though they do not derive support or enjoyment from the relationship.

Assess for both overt signs of marital stress, such as arguments, and more subtle indications, such as terse con-

INFANT RECEIVING NURSING CARE AT HOME

When caring for an infant at home, the nurse may find these examples of nursing diagnoses appropriate. Specific nursing interventions for many of these diagnoses are provided in the "Planning and implementation" section of this chapter.

For the infant
- Altered growth and development related to impaired oral feeding and inadequate caloric intake
- Altered nutrition: less than body requirements, related to immature gastrointestinal function
- High risk for infection related to respiratory compromise
- Impaired physical mobility related to restrictions imposed by feeding tubes or I.V. lines
- Ineffective airway clearance related to pooling of secretions
- Ineffective infant feeding pattern related to respiratory compromise
- Potential impaired skin integrity related to the presence of feeding tubes or I.V. lines
- Sensory-perceptual alterations: auditory, related to perinatal infection
- Sensory-perceptual alterations: visual, related to retinopathy of prematurity

For the family
- Altered family processes related to the arrival of a new family member or household disruption caused by the infant's care
- Anxiety related to the infant's constant care needs or the demands of delivering complex, specialized care
- Dysfunctional grieving related to loss of the anticipated healthy neonate
- High risk for caregiver role strain related to demands of delivering specialized infant care
- Ineffective individual coping related to the stress of caregiving procedures or fear that the infant will die
- Knowledge deficit related to the infant's medical condition or infant caregiving skills

versation and reluctance to acknowledge the partner's presence. If stress is apparent or suspected, consider tactfully suggesting that the couple see a marriage counselor.

Effect on siblings. Siblings of chronically ill children may be ill-informed about the nature of the infant's illness. Also, they may be unsure of what others expect of them and feel that their own identity is threatened. Anger, guilt, and resentment are common (Seligman, 1987). To help prevent or detect these problems, assess siblings for signs of behavioral changes and maladaptation – jealousy and re-

sentment of the infant, aggressive behavior, fear, guilt, and anger.

NURSING DIAGNOSIS

After gathering assessment data, the nurse must review it carefully to identify pertinent nursing diagnoses for the infant. (For a partial list of applicable diagnoses, see Nursing Diagnoses: *Infant receiving nursing care at home.*)

PLANNING AND IMPLEMENTATION

For the nurse who provides intermittent home visits, nursing goals include managing or correcting any problems detected during assessment and ensuring that the parents (or other primary caregivers) are providing safe, appropriate care.

Nursing care in the home calls for flexibility and innovation. Be patient and understanding about interruptions in teaching sessions and unanticipated household events. If the family has a diagnosis of *altered family processes related to the arrival of a new family member or household disruption caused by the infant's care,* help them devise individualized solutions to such problems as cramped quarters, inadequate storage space for equipment and supplies, and too few electrical outlets.

A key nursing intervention is to ensure that the infant has a source of primary pediatric care, that all of the infant's care is coordinated, and that the family's resources are adequate to provide appropriate, ongoing care. If necessary, help the family obtain a pediatrician; also facilitate communication and coordination among care providers. If the home lacks indoor plumbing, running water, hot water, or electricity, make sure a social service agency has been contacted. Besides city and county social services departments, resources for financial assistance include:
- state children services programs
- federal Special Supplemental Food Program for Women, Infants, and Children; Aid to Dependent Children program; and Aid to Dependent Families and Children program
- Salvation Army
- religious organizations and charities.

Be prepared to help the family through sudden financial crises triggered by the infant's care requirements. For example, mechanical ventilation may increase monthly electric bills substantially; if necessary, refer the family to a social service agency to arrange for emergency financial assistance to pay these bills, or help them contact the electric company to make special payment arrangements.

USING A HOME APNEA MONITOR

Because your infant has had problems breathing, the doctor has determined that a home apnea monitor is necessary. The monitor will alert you to changes in your infant's heart rate or absence of breathing. By following the steps below, you can help ensure your infant's well-being when the monitor is in use.

General guidelines
- Prepare the home environment for monitoring—for instance, by providing a sturdy surface for the monitor and by displaying emergency telephone numbers (such as for the doctor and monitor dealer or vendor) in a prominent place.
- Make sure other family members know how to use the monitor.
- If your monitor has electrodes, make sure the respirator indicator goes on each time your infant breathes. If it does not, move the electrodes slightly until it does.
- If the apnea or bradycardia alarm goes off, check the color on the inside of the infant's mouth. If it is bluish and the infant is not breathing, try to stimulate breathing by calling loudly, then touching the infant. Use gentle touch at first, then stronger stimulation as necessary; do not shake the infant. If the infant does not respond, begin cardiopulmonary resuscitation (CPR).
- A loose-lead alarm may indicate a dirty electrode, a loose electrode patch, a loose belt, a disconnected or malfunctioning wire, or monitor malfunction. If this alarm sounds, see the equipment manual for instructions.
- Periodically review CPR and other life-saving techniques you have been taught. Make sure that everyone who cares for your infant knows these techniques.
- Notify the local police, ambulance company, telephone company, and electric company that your infant is on an apnea monitor. Also make sure the pediatrician and visiting nurse know about the monitor.
- For two useful booklets—*A Manual for Home Monitoring* and *At Home with a Monitor*—write to the Sudden Infant Death Syndrome Alliance, 10500 Little Patuxent Parkway, Suite 420, Columbia, MD 21044 or call 1-800-221-SIDS.

This teaching aid may be reproduced by office copier for distribution to clients. ©1993, Springhouse Corporation.

Ensuring parental caregiving knowledge and skills. For parents with a nursing diagnosis of *knowledge deficit related to the infant's medical condition or infant caregiving skills,* reinforce discharge teaching about the underlying disease and the care required. An effective way to do this is to observe the parents as they care for the infant, then demonstrate any aspect of their care that is incorrect and ask for a return demonstration. (For more information about parent teaching, see Parent Teaching: *Using a home apnea monitor,* and Parent Teaching: *When your infant is receiving oxygen by nasal cannula,* page 508.)

A parent may feel overwhelmed by the responsibility of providing care, even when the infant's care needs seem fairly simple to the nurse. The parent's reaction may lead to a nursing diagnosis of *ineffective individual coping related to the stress of caregiving procedures or fear that the infant will die.* Even when the parents' caregiving skills are deficient, convey a sense of trust and confidence in their eventual ability to care for the child adequately at home.

Keep in mind that the addition of a dependent new family member can be enormously stressful, possibly resulting in a nursing diagnosis of *anxiety related to the infant's constant care needs or the demands of delivering complex, specialized care.* Reassure the parents that negative as well as positive feelings are bound to arise during the immediate postdischarge period; if necessary, refer them for counseling or other support resources to ease the neonate's transition to the home. Also, to reduce the burden presented by the infant's care demands, encourage the parents to seek and accept any offers of help.

Promoting positive parent-infant interaction. If parent-infant interaction suggests poor bonding, reinforce teaching about neonatal behavioral states, communication cues, growth and developmental patterns, and sleep-awake patterns. If poor interaction seems to stem from parental disappointment or grief over the infant's medical condition or physical appearance, encourage the parents to express their feelings freely, without fear of being judged as bad people or bad parents.

In some cases, poor parent-infant interaction or parental failure to provide proper care may reflect child neglect or abuse. The nurse who suspects this should contact the local child protective services agency.

Helping siblings adjust. The addition of a new family member may cause siblings to feel neglected and unloved, especially if the infant's care is demanding and time-consuming. If family assessment reveals sibling behavioral changes or maladaptation, urge the parents to help siblings understand the infant's condition and express their fears and concerns, and to reassure siblings that they are not the cause of the infant's illness. Also encourage the parents to let siblings participate in the infant's care at a level appropriate for each sibling's developmental stage; this can help the sibling feel more involved in and important to the family. (However, if a sibling is assuming too much caregiving responsibility, point out to the parents that the sibling may need more time to

WHEN YOUR INFANT IS RECEIVING OXYGEN BY NASAL CANNULA

The doctor has prescribed oxygen therapy by nasal cannula for your infant. To improve the safety and effectiveness of this treatment, refer to the guidelines below.

SETTING UP THE SYSTEM

1 Make sure you have a nasal cannula, tubing, skin tape, oxygen tank, and humidifier (if prescribed). Also, keep a spare cannula available to use when the original one is being cleaned.

2 Fill the humidifier with sterile distilled water and attach it to the flowmeter.

3 Attach the flowmeter to the oxygen source and connect the cannula to the system.

4 To apply the cannula, slip it over the infant's head so that the nasal prongs curve inward toward the face. Tape the cannula to each cheek to secure it.

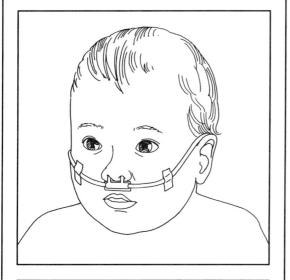

5 Adjust the flowmeter to the prescribed rate.

MAINTAINING HYGEINE

- Once a week, or whenever the cannula appears dirty, wash it with soap and water; let it dry for 24 hours. Make sure no water remains in the cannula after cleaning, because this could block the flow of oxygen.
- Every day, remove the humidifier from the oxygen source, empty the remaining water from the tank, and clean it with equal parts water and hydrogen peroxide.

ENSURING SAFETY

- Store the oxygen container upright and secure it to prevent it from falling (which may cause a leakage in the system).
- Keep the tank away from direct sunlight and do not store grease, oil, or other flammable materials nearby. Keep a fire extinguisher nearby.
- Keep the oxygen tank at least 5 feet from heat sources and electrical devices and ban smoking near the oxygen tank.
- Make sure the electrical equipment is properly grounded.
- Turn off both the volume regulator and flow regulator when oxygen is not in use to prevent oxygen leakage.
- Do not use alcohol-based or oil-based substances (such as petroleum jelly or baby oil) on your infant, because these substances are highly flammable.
- Dress the infant in flame-retardant clothing.
- Weaning from supplemental oxygen must be done gradually, as instructed by the doctor. Never discontinue oxygen therapy abruptly; this may cause serious harm to your infant.
- Notify the police and fire departments that oxygen tanks are in your home.

be a child.) Also urge the parents to spend some time alone with each sibling regularly to convey the feeling that the sibling has a special place in the family.

EVALUATION

During this step of the nursing process, the nurse evaluates the effectiveness of the care plan by ongoing evaluation of subjective and objective criteria. Evaluation findings should be stated in terms of actions performed or outcomes achieved for each goal. The following examples illustrate appropriate evaluation statements for the infant receiving care at home:

- The infant's physiologic status remained stable, with no changes in vital signs since the last visit.
- The infant maintained a satisfactory nutritional status based on a defined weight gain.

- The home environment is safe and adequate for the infant care required.
- The family has sufficient resources to care for the infant at home.
- All appropriate items required for the infant's care are present in the home.
- Medical equipment is functioning properly.
- The parents provide the required care in a competent and confident manner.
- The family shows a positive adjustment to the responsibility of providing complex care for their special-needs child.

DOCUMENTATION

All steps of the nursing process should be documented as thoroughly and objectively as possible. Thorough documentation not only allows the nurse to evaluate the effectiveness of the care plan, but it also makes this information available to other members of the health care team, helping to ensure consistency of care.

Documentation of a home nursing visit should include:
- the infant's physiologic status, including vital signs
- the infant's nutritional status based on a defined weight gain
- the parents' ability to provide the required care
- the parents' ability to cope with infant care responsibilities and the infant's condition
- the parents' understanding of the infant care required.

CHAPTER SUMMARY

Chapter 22 discussed preparation for and delivery of home health care for neonates and infants. Here are the chapter highlights.

Over the past decade, economic pressures, the move toward early discharge of neonates, the desire by families for more active participation in health care, and advances in the treatment of high-risk neonates have increased the need for home health care. Studies show that home care can be safe and cost-effective even for high-risk neonates.

The discharge plan is a joint effort by the health care team, client, family, and appropriate outside agencies to meet a client's physical and psychosocial needs after discharge.

Discharge planning should begin when the neonate is delivered or, at the latest, by nursery admission. The nurse continues to assess the discharge planning needs until discharge.

Within the health care facility, resource personnel used in discharge planning may include a clinical nurse specialist; physician; social worker; financial counselor; occupational, speech, hearing, and physical therapists; utilization review nurse; dietitian; respiratory therapist; and child life therapist.

To prepare the parents for discharge, the nurse teaches them caregiving skills, emergency interventions, signs and symptoms of medical problems, use of special equipment, and names of people to contact when they have questions. Teaching strategies may incorporate verbal and written instruction, demonstration, and videotapes.

Home health care needs range from routine well-baby care for the normal, healthy neonate to complex, high-technology care for the special-needs child. The latter may involve apnea monitoring, suctioning, chest physiotherapy, oxygen therapy, tracheostomy care, mechanical ventilation, enteral or parenteral nutrition, medication administration, and developmental stimulation programs.

Establishing a rapport with the family and avoiding a domineering approach are priorities for the home health nurse. Besides evaluating the infant's physical status, the nurse should assess the parents' caregiving knowledge and skills, parent-infant interaction, the home environment, the family's support system, the family's emergency plans, and the functioning of any required equipment.

The family of a special-needs child requires physical support (such as for caregiving and household tasks), respite care, and psychosocial support.

Goals for the home health nurse include managing or correcting any problems detected during assessment; ensuring that the parents (or other primary caregivers) are providing safe, appropriate care; supporting parent-infant interaction; and helping family members adjust to the child.

STUDY QUESTIONS

1. What role does the nurse play in discharge planning?
2. Which factors should the health care team and family consider when determining the feasibility of home care?
3. Which two methods might the health care team use to conduct ongoing assessment of discharge planning needs?
4. Sean Young, age 25 days, is scheduled for discharge. He will require a feeding tube and tracheostomy tube at home. Which items should the nurse include when documenting Sean's discharge plan?
5. Which interventions can the nurse take to help Sean's siblings adjust to his birth and arrival at home?

BIBLIOGRAPHY

Discharge planning and home health care

Ahmann, E. (1986). *Home care for the high risk infant: A holistic guide to using technology.* Rockville, MD: Aspen.

American Nurses' Association (1975). *Continuity of care and discharge planning programs* (p. 3). New York: Author.

Brooten, D., Kumar, S., Brown, L., Butts, P., Finkler, S., Bakewell-Sachs, S., Gibbons, A., and Delivoria-Papadopoulos, M. (1986). A randomized clinical trial of early hospital discharge and home follow-up of very-low-birth-weight infants. *New England Journal of Medicine,* 315(15), 934-939.

Joint Commission for Accreditation of Healthcare Organizations (1989). *The joint commission 1990 AMH accreditation manual for hospitals* (p. 131). Chicago: Author.

NAACOG (1986). *Standards for obstetric, gynecologic, and neonatal nursing* (3rd ed.; p. 32). Washington, DC: Author.

National Association of Children's Hospitals and Related Institutions, Inc. (1989). Fact sheet on catastrophically ill children. In *Pediatric nursing, forum on the future: Looking toward the 21st century.* Proceedings and report from an invitational conference, May 16-17, 1988 (p. 9). Pitman, NJ: Anthony J. Jannetti.

Norr, K., Nacion, K., and Abramson, R. (1989). Early discharge with home follow-up: Impacts on low-income mothers and infants. *JOGGN,* 18(2), 133-141.

Rawlins, P., and Horner, M. (1988). Does membership in a support group alter needs of parents of chronically ill children? *Pediatric Nursing,* 14(1), 70-72.

Wegener, D.J., and Aday, L.A. (1989). Home care for ventilator-assisted children: Predicting family stress. *Pediatric Nursing,* 15, 371-376.

Special-needs children

American Academy of Pediatrics Ad Hoc Task Forces on Home Care of Chronically Ill Infants and Children (1984). Guidelines for home care of infants, children, and adolescents with chronic disease. *Pediatrics,* 74, 434-436.

Cruz, L.D. (1988, November). Children with AIDS: Diagnosis, symptoms, care. *AORN Journal,* 48, 893-910.

Donar, M.E. (1988). Community care: Pediatric home mechanical ventilation. *Holistic Nursing Practice,* 2(2), 68-80.

Hartsell, M.B. (1986). Home phototherapy. *Journal of Pediatric Nursing,* 1(4), 282-283.

Heiser, C.A. (1987). Home phototherapy. *Pediatric Nursing,* 13(6), 425-427.

Olshansky, S. (1962, April). Chronic sorrow: A response to having a mentally defective child. *Social Casework,* 43, 190-193.

Seligman, M. (1987). Adaptation of children to a chronically ill or mentally handicapped sibling. *Canadian Medical Association Journal,* 136(12), 1249-1252.

Thomas, R.B. (1987). Family adaptation to a child with a chronic condition. In M.H. Rose and R.B. Thomas (Eds.), *Children with chronic conditions* (p. 39). Orlando: Grune & Stratton.

Family needs

Ferrari, M. (1986). Perceptions of social support by parents of chronically ill versus healthy children. *Children's Health Care,* 14, 26-31.

U.S. General Accounting Office (1989, June). *Health care—Home care experiences of families with chronically ill children* (GAO-HRD-89-73) (p. 3). Washington, DC: Author.

UNIT V
THE POSTPARTAL PERIOD

CHAPTER 23

PHYSIOLOGY OF THE POSTPARTAL PERIOD

OBJECTIVES

After reading and studying this chapter, the student should be able to:

1. Discuss the process of uterine involution.

2. Describe the normal progress of lochia.

3. Discuss the postpartal restoration of normal hypothalamic-pituitary-ovarian function.

4. Identify the hemodynamic events that restore blood volume to the nonpregnancy level.

5. Describe the postpartal return of normal physiologic function of all body systems.

6. Identify specific pregnancy- and delivery-related changes that may not resolve completely.

INTRODUCTION

Throughout pregnancy, gradual changes occur in all body systems. The most pronounced changes are those affecting the reproductive system and the hormonal processes that regulate its function. During the postpartal period (puerperium), these changes resolve; eventually, each body system returns to a nonpregnant state.

Although officially defined as a 6-week period, the postpartal period spans the time between delivery and the resumption of normal physiologic function. Thus it may vary greatly, especially among lactating clients. The client's physical capabilities and body image must adapt to postpartal changes and the restorative processes accompanying them. The nurse who understands such changes can assess the client more proficiently and make scientif-

ically grounded decisions, facilitating the client's return to optimal health.

This chapter describes the anatomic and physiologic alterations that restore the body to a nonpregnant state. It begins with the reproductive and endocrine systems, highlighting the dramatic postpartal uterine and hormonal changes. The chapter continues with a description of the postpartal status of each body system.

REPRODUCTIVE SYSTEM

The reproductive system recovers from pregnancy and childbirth in a unique and efficient manner. However, some structures retain permanent effects.

Uterus

After delivery of the fetus and placenta, the uterus undergoes profound and dramatic changes leading to its return to a nonpregnant state. These changes, which involve both the myometrium (uterine muscle) and endometrium (uterine lining), take place through physiologic mechanisms not common to other organs.

Involution. The myometrium resumes a normal size through involution. A gradual process, involution results from muscle contractions and autolysis—self-disintegration or self-digestion of cells or tissue.

Immediately after delivery of the placenta, strong myometrial contractions (afterpains) shrink the uterus to the size of a grapefruit—a reduction of roughly half from the immediate predelivery size. This rapid shrinkage forces the uterine walls into close proximity, causing the center cavity to flatten.

Myometrial contractions are irregular in both timing and strength. A multiparous client usually experiences stronger, more uncomfortable contractions than a primiparous client—probably because uterine muscles lose elasticity with each pregnancy. Also, a lactating client has stronger contractions than a nonlactating client because oxytocin, a hormone that helps regulate milk ejection, stimulates uterine muscles.

Uterine involution is rapid and steady. Just after delivery, the uterus weighs 1,000 to 1,200 g; 1 week later, it weighs 500 g. By 6 weeks postpartum, the uterus has returned to its normal nonpregnant weight of 50 to 70 g (Cunningham, MacDonald, and Gant, 1989).

Uterine size decreases along with uterine weight. One hour after delivery, the fundus of the uterus (the rounded portion above the level of the fallopian tube attachments) is palpable at or just above the umbilicus. Each day thereafter, the uterus becomes smaller so that the fundus is palpable about one fingerbreadth lower than on the previous day. (For more information, see *Postpartal changes in fundal height,* page 514.) By 2 weeks postpartum, the uterus has returned to the pelvic cavity and no longer can be palpated as an abdominal organ. Although never regaining its nulliparous size and shape, the uterus usually resumes a nonpregnant size and contour by 6 weeks postpartum.

Through autolysis—the second mechanism leading to involution—hypertrophic uterine cells return to a nonpregnant shape and size. The by-products of autolyzed cellular protein are absorbed and excreted by the renal system. Because autolysis reduces uterine cell size so efficiently, the number of uterine cells after delivery remains unchanged from pregnancy.

Endometrium. During the postpartal period, healing and regeneration restore normal endometrial structure and function. As the placenta and membranes separate from the uterine wall at delivery, the decidua basalis (the decidual portion directly beneath the implanted ovum attached to the myometrium) remains in the uterine cavity.

In the early stages of involution, myometrial contractions compress blood vessels throughout the decidua and at the placental site, leading to hemostasis (arrest of bleeding). Contractions in the arteriolar walls immediately after delivery enhance hemostasis. Veins and arterioles at the placental site also undergo hyalinization. Hyaline thickening narrows the vessel lumen, leading to microscopic vascular changes and a more stable hemostasis.

After the first 2 or 3 postparta[...] alis differentiates into two distinct layer[...] cidual blood vessels leads to necrosis of [...] layer, which is sloughed off as part of the lochia[...] (see "Lochia"). The deeper decidual layer (basal lay[...] mains attached to the uterine wall.

By 7 days postpartum, endometrial glands begin to regenerate within the basal layer; by 16 days postpartum, the endometrium is completely restored except at the placental site. Involution of the placental site and restoration of normal tissue here take longer than in the rest of the endometrium.

As the placental site heals, regenerating endometrial tissue slowly and progressively replaces the decidua basalis. Immediately after delivery, the decidua basalis at the placental site measures 8 to 9 mm thick; by 8 days postpartum, it has shrunk by half. At 6 weeks, it measures approximately 2 mm and typically is healed. Healing occurs gradually and without scarring. If healing were less efficient and the placental site became scarred, the area available for implantation of a fertilized ovum would be significantly reduced, limiting the number of future pregnancies.

Cervix. In a client who delivered vaginally, cervical muscle tone is poor and the cervix and lower uterine segment are thin and collapsed. Examination of the external os reveals lacerations and bruising—usually more pronounced in the primiparous than the multiparous client.

The external os contracts slowly; on the second and third days after delivery, it remains flaccid and open approximately 2 to 3 cm. By the end of the first week, the os has contracted to 1 cm and cervical tone has improved, making admission of one finger difficult. At this point, cervical edema and hemorrhage have subsided markedly and the cervical canal (the structure extending from the external os to the interior of the uterus) has begun to reform as the cervix thickens.

Although the cervix resumes its normal functional anatomy by 6 to 12 weeks postpartum, it never regains its nulliparous appearance. The external os remains widened and linear, compared to the tiny circular os of the nulliparous client. Occasionally, the os appears fishmouthed, particularly in cases of significant cervical trauma during delivery.

Lochia. The amount and duration of lochia—postpartal vaginal discharge—correlate with endometrial healing and regeneration. Generally, clients who have cesarean deliveries exhibit a lighter lochial flow of shorter duration than those who deliver vaginally—probably because some

EIGHT

...s that returns the uterus to a normal size—advances so rapidly that the level of the ...he previous day. Autolysis (self-destruction) of hypertrophic uterine muscle cells aids

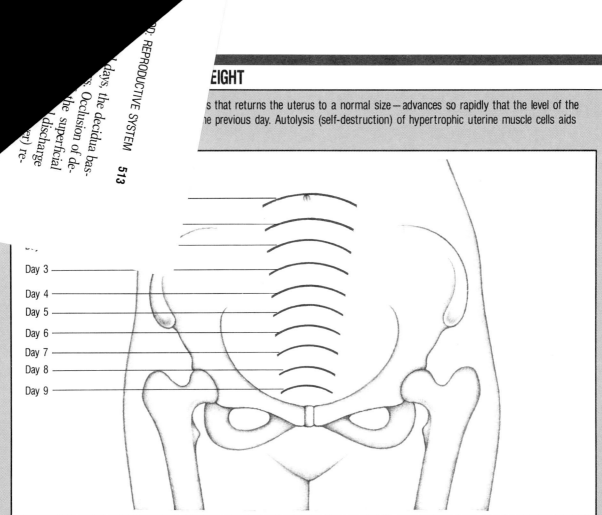

Day 3
Day 4
Day 5
Day 6
Day 7
Day 8
Day 9

UTERINE INVOLUTION

Day 1

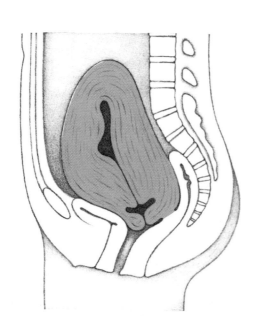

Day 6

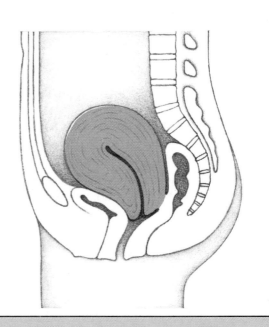

of the uterine debris found in lochia is removed manually during cesarean delivery.

In all clients, lochial flow occurs in three distinct stages. (For more information, see *Stages of lochia*.) Although rates of lochial discharge vary among clients, normal parameters for the amount and duration of lochia during each stage have been established. Lochia rubra, the first stage, typically lasts up to 4 postpartal days and contains a mixture of mucus, tissue debris, and blood.

As uterine bleeding subsides, lochia becomes paler and more serous, entering the second stage. Called lochia serosa, this pink or brownish discharge persists for 5 to 7 days postpartum.

Between 7 and 14 days postpartum, sloughing at the former placental site may cause a sudden temporary increase in lochial flow or even bleeding. This self-limiting condition should last no more than 1 to 2 hours.

The final stage of lochial discharge is lochia alba, a creamy white, brown, or colorless discharge consisting mainly of serum and white blood cells (WBCs). Lochia alba usually diminishes after the third postpartal week but may persist for 6 weeks or longer.

Lochia is considered abnormal if it contains large clots (as large as or larger than a fifty-cent piece) or tissue fragments (pieces of tissue, not the tissue debris normal to lochial flow). Also, lochia should not have a foul or offensive odor and should not relapse to a previous stage.

Fallopian tubes

Postpartal changes in the fallopian tubes take place mainly at the cellular level. During the first few weeks after delivery, many clients show acute inflammatory changes in the cells lining the fallopian tubes but lack symptoms of inflammation (such as fever and tenderness). Inflammation, which may stem from cellular debris that has collected within the lumen of the tubes, resolves without treatment and causes no damage.

The fallopian tubes also show the effects of changing hormone levels. With the sudden sharp drop in the estrogen level after delivery, epithelial cells lining the tubes take on a menopausal appearance, displaying atrophy and decreased numbers of ciliated cells. These changes are most pronounced at 2 weeks postpartum. With a gradual return to normal hormonal balance by 6 to 8 weeks postpartum, epithelial cells return to the condition seen in the early follicular phase of the menstrual cycle, with an increase in ciliated cells to help propel the ovum.

Vagina

After vaginal delivery, the vagina is smooth-walled and somewhat enlarged, with poor muscle tone and significant

STAGES OF LOCHIA

Lochia progresses through three stages, each with distinctive characteristics that reflect progressive endometrial healing.

STAGE	USUAL DURATION	DESCRIPTION
Lochia rubra	1 to 4 days postpartum	Bloody, possibly with some mucus, tissue debris, and small clots; may have a slightly fleshy odor
Lochia serosa	5 to 7 days postpartum	Pink-brown, serous, odorless
Lochia alba	1 to 3 weeks postpartum	Creamy white, brown, or almost colorless; may have a slightly stale odor

edema. Gradually, it shrinks and the edema subsides. By the third postpartal week, rugae reappear within the vaginal walls. These rugae may remain permanently flattened to varying degrees, never returning to the nulliparous state (characterized by numerous mucosal infoldings). Consequently, the vaginal canal rarely resumes its nulliparous size.

The vaginal epithelium also undergoes notable postpartal changes. Vascular and well-lubricated during pregnancy because of estrogen increase, the epithelium becomes fragile and atrophic by the third or fourth postpartal week. In the nonlactating client, atrophy resolves by 6 to 10 weeks postpartum as estrogen normalizes. However, because the estrogen level remains low during lactation, the breast-feeding client may continue to experience symptoms of vaginal atrophy, such as decreased vaginal lubrication and diminished sexual response.

External structures

The clitoris and labia may remain permanently enlarged to some extent—a residual effect of the cellular hypertrophy, enhanced vascularity, and increased fat deposits occurring with pregnancy. After vaginal delivery, the vaginal introitus remains edematous and sometimes ecchymotic. Lacerations may appear on the introitus and perineum, even if an episiotomy was not performed.

Without such complications as hematoma or infection, the perineum heals rapidly. Usually, the introitus and perineum resume a nonpregnant state by 6 weeks postpartum. However, in cases of extreme musculofascial

HOW NIPPLE STIMULATION AFFECTS MILK PRODUCTION

Nipple stimulation triggers a series of events leading to milk production, as shown in the diagram below.

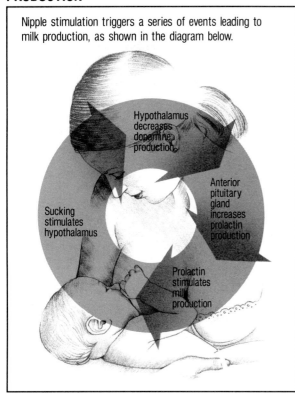

Hypothalamus decreases dopamine production

Anterior pituitary gland increases prolactin production

Sucking stimulates hypothalamus

Prolactin stimulates milk production

relaxation, extensive laceration, or inadequate perineal repair, the introitus may show residual gaping; typically, this change is permanent. Nonetheless, muscular contraction exercises, such as Kegel exercises, may help the introitus (as well as the vagina) approximate a nonpregnant state.

Pelvic muscular support structures

Uterine support structures, such as the broad and round ligaments, stretch significantly during pregnancy as the uterus expands. During vaginal delivery, the support structures of the uterus, vagina, urethra, and bladder undergo trauma. Although laxity of these structures improves gradually, some pelvic relaxation may persist beyond the postpartal period, causing any of the following conditions:

• uterine prolapse (sliding of the uterus into the vaginal canal)
• cystocele (herniation of the bladder into the vagina)
• rectocele (herniation of the rectum into the vagina)
• enterocele (herniation of the intestine into the posterior portion of the vagina).

Because the effects of stretching are cumulative, the likelihood of permanent relaxation of pelvic muscular support increases with each pregnancy and delivery.

Breasts

The breast changes initiated during pregnancy – nipple and areola enlargement, maturation of lobes and ducts, and increased vascularity – progress after delivery, particularly in the lactating client. The size of breast cells and the number of oxytocin receptors (cellular structures sensitive to the effects of oxytocin) also increase.

In the first 2 postpartal days, breast alveoli (tiny sacs made up of epithelial cells) enlarge and display substantial amounts of rough endoplasmic reticulum and Golgi bodies (membranous intracellular structures); the reticulum and Golgi bodies play key roles in milk production. The alveoli – the basic secretory units of the breast – are the site of milk production. Surrounded by a capillary network, alveoli cluster in groups of 10 to 100 to form lobules. Each lobule is drained by a lactiferous duct. The breast contains 15 to 20 lactiferous ducts, which merge at the nipple and areola to allow emptying of the breast.

Lactation – synthesis and secretion of breast milk – results from an interaction among several hormones. Alveolar growth and development is regulated by estrogen, progesterone, human placental lactogen (hPL), prolactin, cortisol, and insulin. Estrogen stimulates the release of prolactin and sensitizes the mammary gland to prolactin action. However, in combination with progesterone, estrogen inhibits prolactin. The profound drop in serum estrogen and progesterone levels after delivery of the placenta removes this inhibition, allowing prolactin to stimulate lactogenesis (initiation of milk secretion) within the alveoli.

Dopamine, a neurotransmitter originating in the hypothalamus, also inhibits prolactin (hence its alternate name, prolactin-inhibiting factor). However, nipple stimulation overcomes this inhibition. When the neonate sucks on the nipple, nerve endings in the areola transmit sensory messages to the hypothalamus that cause dopamine production to diminish; this removes prolactin inhibition. (For details on this hormonal interaction, see *How nipple stimulation affects milk production*.)

In some cases, such as when the client chooses to bottle-feed her neonate, lactation must be suppressed. With suppression, absence of sucking and emptying of the breasts usually leads to breast involution and cessation of lactation within 1 week. No longer stimulated, alveolar cells flatten and stop secreting milk; within 24 hours, cellular organelle structure begins to take on a more normal configuration, with a decrease in rough endoplasmic reticulum and Golgi bodies. Mammary blood flow decreases, leading to further involution. Over the next 3 months, connective and adipose tissue replaces glandular tissue, although the breast retains some increased glandular tissue. As involution nears completion, the breasts typically resume their nonpregnancy size. However, a mild alteration in breast shape may be permanent.

ENDOCRINE SYSTEM

Like the reproductive system, the endocrine system undergoes profound postpartal changes. Many of these changes interrelate with those of the reproductive system.

Placental hormones

With delivery of the placenta, levels of circulating placental hormones drop rapidly. The serum estrogen level plunges sharply in the first 3 hours after delivery, then more gradually until the seventh postpartal day, when it reaches its lowest level. In the nonlactating client, estrogen begins to rise to a normal level at approximately 2 weeks postpartum. In the lactating client, the rise is delayed, leading to such problems as vaginal mucosal atrophy (the estrogen level increases gradually when breast-feeding frequency decreases).

Serum progesterone falls below normal luteal-phase levels by the third postpartal day. After the first week, progesterone cannot be detected in the circulation until ovulation returns. Consequently, the first few postpartal menstrual cycles may be irregular and shorter than normal.

The two remaining placental hormones – hPL and human chorionic gonadotropin (hCG) – also rapidly diminish. Reyes, Winter, and Faiman (1985) found that circulating hCG – the hormone measured in most standard pregnancy tests – disappears within 8 to 24 hours after delivery in both lactating and nonlactating clients. The decline is so pronounced that by the end of the first postpartal week a urine pregnancy test is negative. Neither hCG nor hPL is produced until a subsequent pregnancy.

Pituitary hormones

Levels of thyrotropin and adrenocorticotrophic hormone, which increase during pregnancy to help maintain the corpus luteum, drop to nonpregnancy levels in the postpartal period. Antidiuretic hormone (ADH, or vasopressin), no longer needed in larger amounts to maintain fluid balance, also diminishes.

In the nonlactating client, serum prolactin typically drops to a nonpregnancy level by 3 weeks postpartum. In the lactating client, it remains elevated into the sixth week and sometimes beyond, depending on breast-feeding frequency. The client must breast-feed at least six times daily to maintain this elevation; otherwise, prolactin falls to a normal level within 6 months.

Levels of circulating follicle-stimulating hormone (FSH) and luteinizing hormone (LH) remain low for the first 2 weeks postpartum. FSH levels are identical in lactating and nonlactating clients. However, low estrogen levels in lactating clients reduce ovarian sensitivity to FSH, making ovulation less likely.

Hypothalamic-pituitary-ovarian function

Resumption of the menstrual cycle is coordinated by hormones secreted by the hypothalamus (gonadotropin-releasing hormone [GnRH]), pituitary gland (FSH and LH), and ovaries (estrogen and progesterone). Although a period of amenorrhea normally follows delivery, experts do not concur on its physiologic basis or the mechanism that reestablishes a normal cycle.

Among nonlactating clients, the average time before the return of ovulation is about 10 weeks; menstruation typically resumes by 7 to 9 weeks. Thus, for most nonlactating clients, the first postpartal menstrual period may be anovulatory.

Lactation delays the return of a normal menstrual cycle; the length of the delay depends on breast-feeding duration and frequency. Thus, a client who breast-feeds for 6 months will have longer-lasting amenorrhea than one who breast-feeds for 4 weeks. Likewise, six or more daily breast-feeding sessions decrease the chance for a normal menstrual cycle.

Return of ovulation in lactating clients also varies. For both lactating and nonlactating clients, an increased interval before the first postpartal menstrual period increases the likelihood of an ovulatory cycle. Thus, the longer a client breast-feeds, the greater the chance that the first postpartal cycle will be ovulatory. (However, poor nutritional status during lactation may delay resumption of normal hypothalamic-pituitary-ovarian function.)

Reversal of other changes

No longer stimulated by an increased estrogen level, the pituitary, thyroid, and parathyroid glands resume their normal size after delivery. Thyroxine, thyroxine-binding plasma proteins, and parathyroid hormone decrease to a nonpregnancy level. Corticosteroid levels, elevated during pregnancy by reduced renal excretion of cortisol, also fall. Nonpregnancy levels may resume as early as 1 week postpartum; by the sixth week, all clients have normal serum cortisol levels.

The rapid decline in estrogen, progesterone, cortisol, and hPL leaves insulin relatively unopposed (not blocked) in the early postpartal period compared to late pregnancy. Also, for the first few postpartal days, the serum glucose level, which decreases during pregnancy, remains low. Consequently, clients with diabetes mellitus have a greatly reduced need for exogenous insulin; some require none. As hormone levels begin to stabilize, the need for exogenous insulin returns and the insulin requirement approximates the nonpregnancy dosage.

RESPIRATORY SYSTEM

The postpartal period typically brings complete resolution of pregnancy-related respiratory changes and associated complaints, such as shortness of breath, chest and rib discomfort, and decreased tolerance for physical exertion.

Reversal of anatomic changes
Anatomic changes in the thoracic cavity and rib cage, caused by increasing uterine size, reverse gradually after delivery. Thus, full lung expansion returns and the rib cage regains a normal diameter. As the estrogen level declines, vascularization of the respiratory tract—increased by pregnancy—also resumes a nonpregnancy status.

Reversal of functional changes
As the serum progesterone level declines, oxygen demand decreases, and the uterus no longer impinges on the diaphragm, the following changes occur, restoring normal respiratory function.
- Tidal volume (the amount of air exchanged with each breath), minute volume (the amount of air expelled from the lungs per minute), and vital capacity (the amount of air expelled after maximum inspiration) decrease to nonpregnancy values.
- Functional residual capacity (the amount of air remaining in the lungs after normal, quiet inspiration) rises to nonpregnancy values.

Resumption of normal acid-base balance and oxygen saturation
Shifting hormone levels after delivery cause reversal of the mild hyperventilation of pregnancy. Thus, arterial oxygen partial pressure (PaO_2) decreases, arterial carbon dioxide partial pressure ($PaCO_2$) increases, and the bicarbonate level rises. As the respiratory rate falls to a nonpregnancy level, $PaCO_2$ elimination and red blood cell (RBC) oxygen-carrying capacity normalize, reducing serum pH.

Postpartal hormonal changes also restore a normal respiratory stimulus. Thus, the $PaCO_2$ threshold needed to stimulate respiration increases.

CARDIOVASCULAR SYSTEM

After delivery, the cardiovascular system exhibits few subjectively noticeable changes as it resumes a nonpregnancy status.

Reversal of anatomic and auscultatory changes
Cardiac enlargement and displacement reverse as the uterus resumes its normal size and position. Abnormal heart sounds—a result of the anatomic and hemodynamic changes caused by pregnancy—also resolve in the postpartal period.

Reversal of hemodynamic changes
Altered significantly by pregnancy, blood volume and cardiac output quickly resume a nonpregnancy status after delivery. Blood pressure and pulse undergo less dramatic changes.

Blood volume. Increased approximately 45% during pregnancy, blood volume drops sharply just after delivery. Within 4 weeks, it returns to a nonpregnancy level.

Blood loss during delivery immediately reduces blood volume. Normal vaginal delivery leads to an average blood loss up to 500 ml; cesarean delivery, 1,000 ml or more. The increase in blood volume during pregnancy allows the body to withstand this substantial loss. However, excessive blood loss at delivery may delay functional recovery.

After delivery, extravascular fluid shifts to the circulation, leading to a plasma volume increase that helps offset blood loss at delivery. This fluid then is excreted by the renal system—first in large amounts, later more gradually, as postpartal diuresis occurs.

Delivery of the placenta reduces the size of the maternal vascular bed by 10% to 15%. Thus, a smaller blood volume is needed for tissue perfusion.

The vasodilatory effects of hormonal tissue disappear after delivery, reducing the amount of blood required to maintain adequate tissue perfusion and blood pressure.

Cardiac output. Markedly increased during pregnancy, cardiac output remains high for 48 hours postpartum, then declines gradually to a nonpregnancy level. The decline is similar in lactating and nonlactating clients. Most of the decrease occurs as early as 2 weeks postpartum.

Blood pressure and pulse. Immediately after delivery, blood pressure readings should differ only slightly, if at all, from readings taken during the third trimester of pregnancy. A decrease may indicate uterine hemorrhage or excessive blood loss at delivery; an increase may signal a preeclamptic tendency, especially if accompanied by headache or visual changes. According to Robson, Hunter, Moore, and Dunlop (1987), blood pressure readings typically remain relatively stable in the first 12 weeks postpartum, then increase gradually until the twenty-fourth week when nonpregnancy readings return.

For 7 to 10 days after delivery, transient bradycardia (a heart rate of 50 to 70 beats/minute) may occur. This finding is normal and may result from the decrease in cardiac work load that follows delivery. On the other hand, tachycardia (a heart rate above 100 beats/minute) warrants investigation because it may reflect hypovolemia—especially in a client with a low RBC count or a decreasing hemoglobin level.

Reversal of varicose conditions
Varicose conditions of the legs, anus (hemorrhoids), or vulva may arise during pregnancy from diminished venous return of the legs, pressure exerted by the fetus, and straining during labor and delivery. In many clients, these conditions improve significantly or regress completely after delivery. However, signs and symptoms become more pronounced with each pregnancy. If problems persist after the postpartal period, surgery may be required.

HEMATOLOGIC SYSTEM

Levels of blood constituents may vary in the postpartal period. Coagulation, enhanced during pregnancy and delivery, normalizes gradually. However, coagulatory stimulation induced by labor and delivery increases the risk of thromboembolism.

Red blood cell parameters
Immediately after delivery, the hemoglobin level and hematocrit vary from one client to the next, as does the RBC count. Generally, for a client who delivered vaginally without complications, these values remain near predelivery levels despite normal blood loss at delivery. (This phenomenon results from hemoconcentration—packing of blood cells—which follows postpartal diuresis.) In a client who underwent cesarean delivery, increased blood loss may cause RBC parameters to fall slightly just after delivery.

In a healthy client with adequate nutrition, all RBC parameters typically will return to nonpregnancy levels by 6 weeks postpartum. A significant or progressive decrease in these parameters in the first few postpartal days is abnormal and may indicate excessive or continued blood loss.

White blood cell count
The WBC count increases in the first 10 to 12 days postpartum, possibly rising as high as 25,000/mm³ (the increase is mainly in granulocytes). Although this change reflects a normal stress response, it may complicate diagnosis of a postpartal infection, which also increases the WBC count.

Serum electrolyte levels
Serum potassium and calcium levels, which rise during pregnancy, fall rapidly to nonpregnancy values after delivery because of the fluid shift and subsequent diuresis.

Coagulation factor levels
Postpartal changes in coagulation factors are gradual. Throughout pregnancy, levels of coagulation factors I (fibrinogen), VII, IX, and X rise progressively; during late pregnancy, fibrinolysis (destruction of blood clots) diminishes. These circumstances place the pregnant client at a progressively increasing risk for thromboembolic disorders.

Delivery stimulates the coagulation system, increasing this risk even further in the early postpartal period. Studying the rate at which coagulation factors normalize after delivery, Dahlman, Hellgren, and Blomback (1985) found that these factors remain significantly elevated for the first 2 to 3 weeks postpartum, then fall gradually, approaching nonpregnancy levels after 6 weeks. The platelet count returns to a nonpregnancy level by 2 weeks postpartum. However, traumatic delivery, infection, or prolonged immobility may delay the return to normal levels.

URINARY SYSTEM

Pregnancy affects both the anatomic structure of the urinary tract and the function of the urinary system; delivery may contribute to certain anatomic changes. Unlike most other body systems, the urinary system may show the effects of pregnancy and delivery well into—and even beyond—the postpartal period.

Reversal of anatomic changes

At delivery, fetal passage through the pelvis and vagina causes varying degrees of trauma to the urethra and bladder. A normal amount of trauma leads to edema and microscopic bleeding. Delivery complications (such as precipitous delivery or forceps instrumentation) may cause increased trauma, leading to laceration of the urethra and meatus. With cesarean delivery, the potential for surgical trauma of the bladder is a possibility.

Delivery trauma accompanied by anesthesia (especially spinal or epidural anesthesia) may impair bladder tone. If this occurs, the bladder may lose sensitivity, resulting in a diminished voiding urge. This contributes to postpartal urine retention.

Postpartal diuresis may cause bladder overdistention, possibly resulting in muscle damage, atony, and urinary tract infection (from stasis and urine retention). Without such complications, however, the lower urinary tract resumes normal function within 1 or 2 weeks as edema and diuresis resolve, although bladder distention may persist for 3 months.

Typically, dilation of the renal pelvis, calyces, and ureters begins in the first trimester and progresses as pregnancy advances. Slowing urine passage through the ureters, dilation causes distention of the renal pelvis. Within the first 12 to 16 weeks postpartum, dilation resolves gradually, although some mild dilation may persist for years (Jaffe, 1985). Urinary frequency, urgency, and other symptoms caused by pressure on the bladder from increasing uterine size resolve after delivery.

Reversal of functional changes

Pregnancy increases the renal plasma flow and the glomerular filtration rate (GFR). In late pregnancy, the GFR begins a gradual decline that continues into the postpartal period. Usually, the GFR returns to a nonpregnancy level by 6 weeks postpartum. Renal plasma flow also normalizes.

Urinalysis

Mild proteinuria, caused by excretion of protein byproducts of uterine involution, is common after delivery but should disappear by 6 weeks postpartum. Glycosuria, another common postpartal finding, usually resolves by the end of the first week.

GASTROINTESTINAL SYSTEM

With the gastrointestinal (GI) tract no longer obstructed by the expanding uterus and hormone levels declining rapidly, the GI tract quickly resumes normal function after delivery.

Appetite

After vaginal delivery, most clients are extremely hungry from lack of food intake and the exertion of labor and delivery—especially if little or no anesthesia was used. Appetite tends to subside to a normal level in 1 to 2 days, although a breast-feeding client may maintain an increased appetite and food intake while breast-feeding.

After cesarean delivery, the client whose appetite return is less pronounced may be started on a clear liquid diet and gradually advanced to a regular diet as GI function returns.

Bowel motility and evacuation

During pregnancy, GI motility is inhibited by the high serum progesterone level (which relaxes intestinal smooth muscle, decreasing peristalsis) and by increasing uterine size (which compresses the intestines). With delivery resolving both factors, normal peristalsis and bowel function usually return rapidly. However, bowel motility may remain sluggish in cases of intestinal manipulation during cesarean delivery or use of anesthetic or analgesic agents.

Typically, bowel evacuation normalizes once bowel motility is restored. Nonetheless, the first bowel movement may be delayed until 2 to 3 days postpartum for reasons unrelated to intestinal function. For example, abdominal muscle tone may be so poor that the client cannot attain sufficient pressure to evacuate the bowel. Also, the client may avoid bowel evacuation, fearing it will cause pain or damage the episiotomy. Residual dehydration from labor and the subsequent decrease in the fluid content of the stool also may impair bowel evacuation. In many cases, a stool softener, laxative, suppository, or enema must be used to reestablish normal bowel function.

Reversal of other changes

Gallbladder emptying, slowed during pregnancy, increases after delivery, reducing the risk of gallstones. The bile flow, hepatic work load, and hepatic blood flow decrease to nonpregnancy levels, and liver function studies should no longer be abnormal.

MUSCULOSKELETAL SYSTEM

Although pregnancy-related changes in the musculoskeletal system reverse after delivery, joints and muscles may show some residual effects.

Reversal of postural and joint changes

As pregnancy advances, increasing body weight and the shift in the center of gravity subject the musculoskeletal system to significant stress. Also, estrogen, progesterone, and relaxin (a hormone released by the corpus luteum during pregnancy) relax the joints, decreasing their stability. Abdominal distention exaggerates the lordotic (forward) curvature of the lumbar spine and loosens pelvic joints.

Delivery removes the mechanical strain on the musculoskeletal system and halts secretion of relaxin. Over the first 6 to 8 postpartal weeks, posture returns to normal and structural changes reverse gradually. However, foot enlargement—caused by the effects of relaxin on foot joints as well as weight gain and dependent edema—may persist. Thus, increased foot and shoe size tend to be a permanent reminder of pregnancy.

Reversal of muscular changes

Enlargement of breast and abdominal wall muscles during pregnancy weakens these structures. Although the damage is not permanent, many clients have trouble regaining satisfactory muscle tone in these areas.

During the third trimester, the rectus abdominis muscles may separate, causing diastasis recti abdominis. This condition sometimes can be corrected by postpartal abdominal exercises. However, it may persist indefinitely unless adequate muscle tone is restored. Poor abdominal muscle tone may contribute to back strain and complaints of low backache.

Effects of regional anesthesia

Regional (spinal or epidural) anesthesia used during delivery may cause transient musculoskeletal effects, including decreased sensation and function in the lower extremities. However, these effects usually disappear within 8 to 12 hours.

INTEGUMENTARY SYSTEM

Pregnancy-related skin changes resolve completely or partially after delivery as hormone levels decrease and the skin no longer is stretched.

Reversal of hormone-related changes

During the postpartal period, pigmentation changes caused by pregnancy—including chloasma (also called melasma, or mask of pregnancy) and linea nigra (a dark midline streak on the abdomen)—reverse gradually. However, they may never disappear completely.

Pregnancy may stimulate pigmented nevi (colored moles), causing them to enlarge or change color or leading to formation of new nevi. These changes tend to regress after delivery. Nevi that do not resume their prepregnancy appearance warrant further evaluation. Nipple darkening, also caused by pregnancy, reverses partially in the postpartal period. Any increased acne associated with pregnancy also resolves as hormone levels stabilize.

Pregnancy-related hirsutism also regresses (however, coarse hairs that arose during pregnancy tend to remain). Some clients complain of excessive hair loss from the head after delivery. This is a compensation for the below-normal loss during pregnancy; the postpartal loss is merely catching up with the loss that would have taken place without pregnancy. The catch-up process ends roughly 6 to 12 months postpartum.

Some vascular skin conditions observed in pregnant clients mimic those accompanying liver disease, such as spider angiomas and palmar erythema. Stemming from enhanced subcutaneous blood flow (caused by the increased serum estrogen level), these conditions disappear soon after delivery as the estrogen level falls.

Changes in the mucous membranes during pregnancy—epistaxis (nosebleed), nasal edema with congestion, and bleeding of the gums—reverse as the estrogen level decreases. Some pregnant clients develop gingivitis, sometimes with small vascular nodules at the gum line. This condition, called epulis gravidarum, usually regresses within 1 to 2 months postpartum (Gabbe, Niebyl, and Simpson, 1986).

Striae (stretch marks) result from increased corticosteroid levels and mechanical stretching of the skin during pregnancy. These harmless marks commonly appear over the abdomen, back, thighs, and breasts. As body size normalizes, striae shrink and fade from dark red to silvery-white within a year after delivery. Although they become less apparent, they never disappear completely.

Diaphoresis

In the first 2 to 3 days postpartum, many clients experience episodes of profuse diaphoresis (sweating). Associated with the postpartal fluid shift, diaphoresis is a normal mechanism that helps the renal system excrete excess fluid and waste products. It should resolve within the first postpartal week.

OTHER SYSTEMS

Metabolic, neurologic, and immunologic changes brought on by pregnancy reverse rapidly after delivery.

Metabolic system

Throughout pregnancy, the basal metabolic rate (BMR) – the lowest rate of metabolism that preserves physiologic function – rises until delivery, when it measures approximately 20% above normal. (The increase primarily reflects fetoplacental demands and the greater cardiac work load.) After delivery, the BMR decreases rapidly, approaching nonpregnancy levels by 5 to 6 days postpartum.

Neurologic system

Neurologic effects of pregnancy, which may range from minor to extremely bothersome, rarely linger after delivery. Entrapment neuropathies – nerve compression disorders usually caused by fluid retention – are among the most common neurologic changes caused by pregnancy. As soft tissue becomes edematous, it exerts pressure on nerves within the tissue, causing such symptoms as numbness, tingling, and loss of function. For example, in carpal tunnel syndrome, the median nerve in the wrist is compressed. With the disappearance of edema after delivery, entrapment neuropathies usually resolve. In rare cases, surgery is required to release an entrapment.

Other neurologic complaints during pregnancy include tension headache and syncopal or near-syncopal episodes. These conditions are associated with stress, decreased rest, poor nutritional status, increased blood glucose levels, and hormonal changes accompanying pregnancy. As delivery eliminates these factors, tension headaches and syncopal episodes diminish. With proper postpartal nutrition and rest, they disappear completely.

Immunologic system

Inhibited during pregnancy to prevent the body from rejecting the fetus as foreign matter, the immune system resumes normal function during the postpartal period. However, a client lacking the Rh factor (an antigenic substance usually found in RBCs) who delivers an Rh-positive neonate may become sensitized to the Rh antigen in neonatal RBCs and may produce Rh antibodies directed against the sensitizing antigen; this could cause problems in subsequent pregnancies. To prevent this, an Rh-negative client must receive Rh_o (D) immune globulin (RhoGAM) at 28 weeks of pregnancy and again within 72 hours after delivery.

CHAPTER SUMMARY

Chapter 23 described the postpartal physiologic processes that restore the body to a nonpregnant state. Here are the chapter highlights.

Pregnancy affects all body systems to varying degrees. Each system returns to a nonpregnant state during the postpartal period. However, some pregnancy-related changes do not reverse completely.

The rapid drop in serum estrogen and progesterone levels after delivery triggers reversal of many pregnancy-related changes.

Within 6 weeks after delivery, the uterus returns to an approximately normal size and shape through involution. This process involves uterine muscle contractions and self-destruction of uterine cells.

The superficial lining of the uterus becomes necrotic and is sloughed off after delivery.

Lochia (postpartal vaginal discharge) progresses through three stages – lochia rubra, lochia serosa, and lochia alba.

In the nonlactating client, menstruation usually returns in 7 to 9 weeks, although the first period may be anovulatory. In the lactating client, the return of menstruation is delayed, depending on the duration and frequency of breast-feeding.

In a breast-feeding client, breast development continues after delivery. Prolactin stimulates milk production in the breast alveoli; oxytocin causes contraction of the alveoli, which leads to ejection of milk toward the nipple. In a nonlactating client or a client who discontinues breast-feeding, the breasts undergo involution, possibly becoming engorged for 1 to 2 days. With absence of sucking and emptying of the breast, milk production ceases within 1 week.

In the cardiovascular system, blood volume and cardiac output quickly resume a nonpregnancy status after delivery. Blood pressure and pulse undergo less dramatic changes.

Anatomic and functional changes in the respiratory system resolve with delivery as hormone levels decrease and the thoracic cavity and rib cage are no longer affected by the pregnant uterus.

The hematologic system, enhanced by pregnancy, is stimulated further in the early postpartal period, increasing the risk of thromboembolism.

Some changes in the urinary system, such as dilation of the renal pelvis, calyces, and ureters, may persist beyond the postpartal period.

Gastrointestinal function quickly returns to normal, although bowel evacuation may be delayed for several postpartal days.

Weakened breast and abdominal wall muscles require exercise to restore muscle tone in these areas.

Some integumentary changes caused by pregnancy, such as linea nigra and striae, may not reverse completely after delivery.

The metabolic, neurologic, and immunologic systems also undergo significant changes after delivery.

STUDY QUESTIONS

1. What condition of the uterus, breasts, and lochia should the nurse expect in a breast-feeding client 24 hours after delivery?

2. During a prenatal class, Mrs. Katz, a 29-year-old multiparous client, asks if she will experience the same changes during recovery from this delivery as she did with her first. After gathering information about her first postpartal experience, how should the nurse answer her?

3. Mrs. Davis, a postpartal client, experiences painful uterine contractions 36 hours after delivery. How should the nurse explain the reason for these contractions?

4. How is lactation affected by a neonate's sucking of the breast?

5. Ms. Burke, an 18-year-old nonlactating primiparous client, asks when her menstrual period will resume. How should the nurse respond?

BIBLIOGRAPHY

Cunningham, F., MacDonald, P., and Gant, N. (1989). *Williams obstetrics* (18th ed). East Norwalk, CT: Appleton & Lange.

Dahlman, T., Hellgren, M., and Blomback, M. (1985). Changes in blood coagulation and fibrinolysis in the normal puerperium. *Gynecologic Obstetric Investigation,* 20(1), 37-44.

Gabbe, S., Niebyl, J., and Simpson, J. (1986). *Obstetrics: Normal and problem pregnancies.* New York: Churchill Livingstone.

Jaffe, D. (1985). Postpartum evaluation of renal function. *Clinical Obstetrics and Gynecology,* 28(2), 298-309.

Karp, R., Greene, G., Smiciklas-Wright, H., and Scholl, T. (1988). Postpartum weight change: How much of the weight gained in pregnancy will be lost after delivery? *Obstetrics and Gynecology,* 71(5), 701-707.

Oppenheimer, L., Sherriff, E., Goodman, J., Shaw, D., and James, C. (1986). The duration of lochia. *British Journal of Obstetrics and Gynecology,* 93(7), 754-757.

Poindexter, A., Ritter, M., and Besch, P. (1983). The recovery of normal plasma progesterone levels in the postpartum female. *Fertility and Sterility,* 39(4), 494-498.

Reyes, F., Winter, J., and Faiman, C. (1985). Postpartum disappearance of chorionic gonadotropin from the maternal and neonatal circulations. *American Journal of Obstetrics and Gynecology,* 153(5), 486-489.

Robson, S., Hunter, S., Moore, M., and Dunlop, W. (1987). Hemodynamic changes during the puerperium: A Doppler and M-mode echocardiographic study. *British Journal of Obstetrics and Gynecology,* 94(11), 1028-1039.

CHAPTER 24

NORMAL POSTPARTAL ADAPTATION

OBJECTIVES

After reading and studying this chapter, the student should be able to:

1. Identify the physiologic and psychosocial components of postpartal nursing care.
2. Discuss the importance of parent-infant bonding.
3. Describe the optimal conditions for parent-neonate interaction.
4. Identify appropriate parental responses to neonatal communication cues.
5. Identify synchronous reciprocity in parent-neonate interaction.
6. Discuss the phases of maternal adaptation to parenthood.
7. Describe safety, comfort, rest, and exercise requirements for the postpartal client.
8. State the indications, actions, and dosages for specific medications used in the postpartal period.
9. Explain how to use the nursing process to provide appropriate and individualized care for the postpartal client and her family.
10. Design a teaching plan to meet the needs of the postpartal client and her family.
11. Describe the adjustment of the father, siblings, and grandparents to the birth of a new family member.

INTRODUCTION

The postpartal period is a time of both exhilaration and stress. Although the client is engrossed in her neonate and eager to share her good news with family and friends, she also faces new physical, emotional, and financial challenges. She may have concerns about the changes that motherhood will bring and may feel anxious about the new relationship she and her partner must develop as they adapt to their roles as parents.

The birth of a child creates major changes in the family. Family members—especially the parents—must adjust to changes in their roles, tasks, and responsibilities. The family as a whole also must adapt to meet the demands of the dependent neonate and the changing needs of individual members.

The nurse can help the postpartal family make a healthy transition to the changing family structure by offering knowledge, assistance, and support. Serving as a resource person, the nurse teaches the family about the components of healthy parent-neonate interaction, explains the neonate's characteristics and needs, helps the family meet those needs, and provides emotional support and guidance.

Caring for the postpartal client offers the nurse an opportunity to promote a full and healthy recovery from delivery while helping the client and her partner make an optimal adaptation to the birth of their child. As early discharge after delivery becomes increasingly common, skillful implementation of the nursing process takes on greater importance as a way for the nurse to meet the client's physiologic, psychosocial, and teaching needs.

This chapter discusses the nurse's role in caring for the postpartal client. It begins with a discussion of the transition to parenthood and parent-neonate interaction. Next, it discusses assessment of postpartal adaptation, including vital signs, body systems, and psychosocial status, identifying signs of poor postpartal recovery. Then it discusses how to plan and implement care, highlighting measures that help ensure the client's smooth transition to a nonpregnant status and parenthood as well as the family's adaptation to the birth of the neonate. It includes client teaching aimed at preventing postdischarge problems. After describing how to evaluate postpartal nursing care, the chapter concludes with a brief discussion of documentation.

TRANSITION TO PARENTHOOD

Parenting is a complex process encompassing various tasks, attitudes, and responsibilities through which a mature adult takes on the care of a dependent child. The parent-child dyad, or unit, is the most basic and complex relationship within the family, profoundly affecting the child's development.

The birth of a child impels a parent to put aside the role of perceived carefree person and move toward a more responsible, caregiving role. How successfully the parent does this determines how well parenting tasks and responsibilities are performed. Each person has a preconceived concept of parenting based on childhood experiences, values, cultural and ethnic background, philosophy, and desires.

Besides taking on the role of parent to the new child, a parent in a couple relationship must successfully negotiate parenting tasks and responsibilities with the partner to adapt to the changing family structure. Also, the couple's relationship must accommodate the parent-child relationship; if the couple have other children, they also must help them adjust to the arrival of a new family member. At the same time, the parents must redefine their relationship to each other to meet the family's changing needs; this can prove challenging because the birth of a child reduces the couple's time alone together.

ACQUAINTANCE, ATTACHMENT, AND BONDING

The development of a healthy parent-child relationship in the early postpartal days and weeks increases the chance for optimal child growth and development. Poor attachment and bonding can lead to such disorders as vulnerable child syndrome, child abuse, failure to thrive, and a disturbed parent-child relationship (Klaus and Kennell, 1982).

During the immediate postpartal period, parents and neonate typically become *acquainted* — they interact to gain information about each other. Acquaintance behaviors include eye contact, touching, verbalizing, and exploring (Klaus and Kennell, 1983). Acquaintance is a prerequisite of attachment and bonding.

Although the terms *attachment* and *bonding* now are used interchangeably to describe the process in which parent and child form an enduring relationship, earlier theorists offered varying definitions. For instance, Brazelton (1978) defined bonding as the initial mutual attraction between parent and child and attachment as the long-term process of maintaining the relationship. Klaus and Kennell (1976) described attachment as a unique relationship between two people that is specific and enduring.

Mercer (1983) defined attachment as a "process in which an affectional and emotional commitment or bonding...is formed and is facilitated by positive feedback to each partner through a mutually satisfying experience." According to Stevenson-Hinde and Parkers (1982), attachment begins during pregnancy and intensifies in the early postpartal period; once established, it is constant and consistent.

PARENT-NEONATE INTERACTION

Positive interaction between the parents and neonate promotes healthy bonding. Such interaction depends on the ability of both parties to send, receive, and interpret messages correctly.

Optimal conditions for interaction

The best time for interaction is when both the parent and neonate are rested, focused, and attentive; preferably, the neonate should be in a quiet, alert state. The first period of reactivity may be such a time.

Health also is important. Prematurity or illness may restrict the neonate's ability to interact. Likewise, if the mother is fatigued or suffering postpartal discomfort or complications, her desire, energy, and attention for interacting may be limited. Under these conditions, bonding may take longer to achieve.

Neonatal attentiveness and temperament

By altering the degree of attentiveness to stimuli, the neonate can affect the interaction with the parent. A neonate who is attentive and responsive rewards the parent's interactive efforts; this in turn encourages the parent to continue such interaction. Thus, the more attentive and responsive the neonate, the more frequently the parent will interact.

Temperament also plays a part. A neonate who smiles frequently, eats well, is easy to console, and remains alert for long periods is more pleasant to interact with than one who is irritable and hard to console.

Communication cues, reciprocity, and synchrony

The neonate presents predictable, behaviorally organized communication cues that reflect neonatal needs and normally elicit a response from the parent or other caregiver. Prematurity, illness, temperament, and other factors can affect a neonate's ability to send communication cues.

Parental sensitivity to neonatal cues is essential to the developing parent-child relationship. As part of this relationship, parents also exhibit communication cues that elicit a response from the neonate. Parents typically vary in their ability to interpret neonatal cues and respond appropriately.

Communication cues can be verbal or nonverbal. Verbal cues used by neonates include crying and cooing; nonverbal cues include reaching movements, facial expressions, staring, and gaze aversion. For example, a neonate who averts the gaze and turns away from a stimulus is indicating either boredom or overstimulation (Field, 1978). By refusing to focus on the person offering stimulation, the neonate signals that he or she does not want additional stimulation at that time.

The process by which the neonate gives cues and the parent interprets and responds to these cues is known as reciprocity. Through reciprocity, the interaction is maintained and the parent-neonate relationship develops. Reciprocity may take several weeks to develop. (For an example of reciprocity, see *Reciprocity in parent-neonate interaction.*)

Appropriate action and reaction to cues by parents and neonate is called synchrony (Censullo, Lester, and Hoffman, 1985.) A synchronous, reciprocal interaction is mutually rewarding. Ideally, mother and neonate establish synchrony within the first few weeks of delivery.

Verbal communication and entrainment

At first, parent-neonate communication takes on unique qualities. In most mother-neonate couples studied by Lang (1972), mothers spoke to their neonates in a high-pitched voice as they held them in the en face position. To soothe a neonate, parents frequently speak softly and slowly; to gain the neonate's attention, they use fast, high-pitched speech. Parents also use such games as "peek-a-boo" to communicate with their neonate verbally.

Healthy neonates move in rhythm with adult speech (Condon and Sander, 1974). This phenomenon, known as entrainment, is essential to parent-infant bonding, rewarding the parent and encouraging further communication. Entrainment continues as the child learns speech.

Nonverbal interaction

To interact nonverbally, parents may imitate the neonate's facial expressions. This helps the neonate develop communication skills by demonstrating that the parent responds to nonverbal interaction and that nonverbal behaviors have a meaning between people.

Rubin (1963) found that initial touching between mother and neonate progresses in a typical pattern. First, the mother touches the neonate with her fingertips only; then she progresses to whole-hand touching, and finally embraces the neonate with her arms. Primiparous and multiparous women demonstrate the same progression, although the latter progress to the embrace more rapidly.

Rodholm and Larsson (1979) found that fathers use the same touching pattern; in a later study, they found that medical students also used this pattern, even though they were not related to the neonates with whom they were interacting. These findings suggest that such touching is a human behavior pattern not restricted to parents.

PARENTAL ADAPTATION

As parents begin their relationship with the neonate, family relationships, interactions, and life-style must be adjusted. The adjustments each parent makes influence the welfare of the family as a whole.

Maternal adaptation

Many factors affect the mother's adaptation to the birth of a child. Energy level, attitude, degree of confidence in care-giving skills, and psychological status can help or hinder adaptation. For instance, a client who is exhausted from labor and delivery may lack the energy to interact with her neonate, and one who lacks experience with children may feel overwhelmed by the challenges of providing child care.

Rubin, one of the first nurses to study parental behavior, identified three phases of behavior that occur as a woman adapts to the parental role (1963): taking in, taking hold, and letting go. These phases establish a framework for understanding maternal adaptation; however, they must now be viewed from a wider perspective. Maternity and neonatal care policies and procedures have changed since Rubin conducted her research, as have family expectations about the childbirth experience. In particular, the length of time spent in each phase now is much shorter than Rubin observed it to be, especially if the mother has early contact with the neonate. Also, because of the current emphasis on early discharge, the nurse probably will not see clients progress to the third stage.

RECIPROCITY IN PARENT-NEONATE INTERACTION

The diagram shows how the neonate's communication cues trigger a response from the parent and the parent's cues trigger a response from the neonate. Known as reciprocity, this process helps maintain parent-neonate interaction and promotes a healthy parent-child relationship.

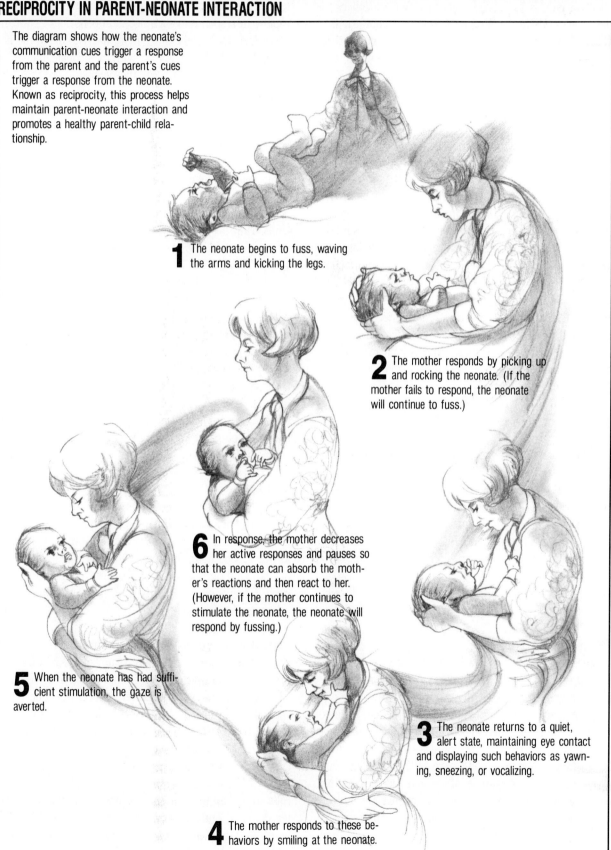

1 The neonate begins to fuss, waving the arms and kicking the legs.

2 The mother responds by picking up and rocking the neonate. (If the mother fails to respond, the neonate will continue to fuss.)

6 In response, the mother decreases her active responses and pauses so that the neonate can absorb the mother's reactions and then react to her. (However, if the mother continues to stimulate the neonate, the neonate will respond by fussing.)

5 When the neonate has had sufficient stimulation, the gaze is averted.

3 The neonate returns to a quiet, alert state, maintaining eye contact and displaying such behaviors as yawning, sneezing, or vocalizing.

4 The mother responds to these behaviors by smiling at the neonate.

Taking in (dependent phase). Immediately after delivery, the client usually is exhausted and dependent on others to meet her needs for nourishment, rest, and comfort. Because she focuses on her own needs, she may not initiate contact with the neonate. Also, she may be excited and eager to talk about the childbirth experience, reviewing the events and seeking details from others so that she can integrate them into reality. Rubin proposed that this phase lasts 1 to 2 days after delivery; today, the nurse should expect it to last just a few hours because of early discharge and other factors.

Taking hold (dependent-independent phase). In this phase, the client vacillates between seeking nurturing and acceptance for herself and seeking to resume an independent role. In an attempt to regain control of her body, she may express concerns about her breast-feeding ability and bowel and bladder control. As her energy and comfort levels increase, her focus shifts from herself to the neonate. She seeks positive feedback and reassurance about her caregiving skills and performance as a mother and responds to teaching with enthusiasm. However, she may become discouraged easily if she feels incompetent as a caregiver. According to Rubin, this phase lasts from 3 days to 8 weeks postpartum; however, its duration may be much shorter now.

Letting go (interdependent phase). During this final phase, the client gives up obsolete roles (such as that of a childless woman) and takes on the new role of mother. Also, she begins to accept the neonate as an individual separate from herself. As her mothering and care-giving abilities become more established, she gains confidence; her dependency on others lessens, and interdependency on family members or a support system takes over. This phase typically is marked by stress as the client and other family members reorganize tasks, responsibilities, and schedules.

Paternal adaptation

As the father's role and tasks within the family have evolved to include more active participation in child care and nurturing, researchers have begun to investigate paternal adaptation and father-neonate interaction. Results of recent studies of paternal adaptation refute earlier theories that minimized fathers' feelings for their neonates. For instance, Greenberg and Morris (1974) described engrossment between first-time fathers and neonates during early contact; observing their neonates en face, the fathers appeared to be preoccupied and absorbed. Engrossment may promote father-infant bonding.

As described earlier, fathers use the same progressive touching pattern typical of mothers. Also, they tend to talk rapidly in response to such neonatal behaviors as vocalization, whereas mothers are more likely to touch the neonate. When both parents are with the neonate, the father touches, vocalizes, and holds the neonate more than the mother does but smiles at the neonate less (Park, 1979).

The opportunity to attend care classes or otherwise receive instructions on bathing, feeding, and diapering helps acquaint fathers with their neonates. Bills (1980) and Giefer and Nelson (1981) found that participation in such classes increased fathers' comfort level in handling and caring for their neonates. Fathers who had attended classes also reported greater father-child affectional bonds (Bills, 1980).

ASSESSMENT

Postpartal assessment begins with a review of the client's antenatal, labor, and delivery records. The nurse on the postpartal unit should make sure this information has been included in the report from the nurse who transferred the client from the recovery unit. Then, throughout the client's stay, the nurse must measure vital signs, determine the client's comfort level, assess rest and sleep patterns, and evaluate the status of all body systems. In addition, the nurse assesses the client's and family's psychosocial status.

Vital signs

Obtain complete vital signs—temperature, pulse, and respiratory rate—and measure blood pressure every 15 minutes for the first hour after delivery, every 30 minutes for the second hour, then every hour for the next 4 hours or until vital signs are stable. Thereafter, obtain vital signs every 4 hours until 24 hours after delivery, then every 8 hours until discharge.

Temperature. Measure the client's temperature orally. A slight temperature elevation from mild dehydration, caused by labor and delivery, is common during the first 24 hours after delivery. However, suspect infection if the client has a morbid temperature, defined by the Joint Committee on Maternal Welfare as one that exceeds 100.4° F (38° C) for 2 successive days after delivery, excluding the first 24 hours (Gibbs and Weinstein, 1976).

Pulse. The pulse may remain normal for an hour or so after delivery. During the first postpartal rest or sleep, which usually occurs 2 to 4 hours after delivery, the pulse rate typically decreases, possibly slowing to 50 beats/minute (bradycardia). This condition may persist for several days without ill effects and probably results from supine positioning and such normal physiologic phenomena as the postpartal increase in stroke volume and reduction in vascular bed size.

On the other hand, an abnormally rapid pulse (tachycardia) may be an early sign of excessive blood loss—especially if the pulse is thready and the client has such signs as pallor, an increased respiratory rate, and diaphoresis. (However, transient tachycardia may occur during periods of excitement, incisional discomfort, or severe uterine contractions; usually, it is not a cause for concern.)

Respiratory rate. Although the respiratory rate rarely changes significantly after delivery, it may drop slightly (along with the pulse rate) during the first postpartal sleep or if the client received a narcotic during labor. Like the pulse rate, the respiratory rate increases slightly during periods of excitement or discomfort. If it increases significantly, however, suspect uterine hemorrhage.

Blood pressure. Postpartal blood pressure should not differ significantly from the client's average reading under normal circumstances. A gradual but persistent drop in blood pressure suggests excessive blood loss. A persistent elevation, especially when accompanied by edema, proteinuria, headache, blurred vision, and hyperactive reflexes, suggests pregnancy-induced hypertension (PIH), a potentially life-threatening disorder. Although most common during the antepartal period, PIH sometimes arises after delivery. To ensure prompt intervention, immediately report suspicious signs and symptoms to the physician.

Keep in mind that certain drugs used during labor and delivery or the postpartal period may affect blood pressure. For instance, oxytocin, ergonovine, and methylergonovine may increase blood pressure; bromocriptine, used to suppress lactation, may decrease it.

Comfort level

Comfort is essential to the client's postpartal recovery and adaptation to the role of new mother. However, even if she has uterine cramps, breast tenderness, or perineal discomfort, she may be too excited by the birth of her child to complain of discomfort. Stay alert for covert clues to discomfort, such as a change in vital signs, restlessness, inability to relax or sleep, facial grimaces, and a guarding posture.

Rest and sleep patterns

Fatigue is common during the first week after delivery. The tiring last few weeks of pregnancy, the exhausting work of labor and delivery, and dramatic hormonal changes contribute to postpartal fatigue. Assess the client's rest and sleep patterns continually, keeping in mind that individual requirements for rest and sleep vary.

Reproductive system

Assess the uterus, lochia, and perineum every 15 minutes for the first hour after delivery, every 30 minutes for the second hour, then hourly for at least 4 hours. Thereafter, assess every 8 hours until discharge. Also, inspect the breasts during the first few days after delivery.

Uterus. Immediately after the placenta is delivered, uterine involution should begin. A gradual process that restores the uterus to a nonpregnant state, involution involves contractions of the myometrium (uterine muscle) and self-disintegration of cells or tissue.

Assessment of the uterus helps in evaluating the progress of involution. Uterine muscle tone should be sufficient for muscles to compress vessels, thereby controlling bleeding.

To ensure accurate assessment of the uterus, ask the client to void beforehand. Then locate the fundus—the rounded portion of the uterus above the level of the fallopian tube attachments. Just after delivery, the fundus should be located at or slightly above the midline at the level of the umbilicus. Each day thereafter, it should descend approximately 1 cm (about one fingerbreadth) toward the symphysis pubis (the slightly movable interpubic joint of the pelvis), until about the tenth postpartal day, when it is no longer palpable as an abdominal organ. (For assessment details, see Psychomotor Skills: *Postpartal assessment techniques*, page 530.)

Next, assess the consistency of the uterus. It should feel firm. A soft, pliable (boggy) uterus indicates uterine atony (poor muscle tone). This condition, which may lead to hemorrhage, most commonly results from bladder distention or uterine enlargement (such as in the client with hydramnios or one who gives birth to a very large neonate or more than one neonate). Uterine enlargement causes overstretching of muscle fibers, which then cannot contract effectively to compress vessels. Other risk factors for uterine atony include a prolonged or accelerated labor (both of which exhaust uterine muscles), general anesthesia, or administration of magnesium sulfate (for example, to stop premature labor or to prevent or control seizures in a client with PIH).

POSTPARTAL ASSESSMENT TECHNIQUES

Through careful assessment, the nurse can help ensure a normal postpartal recovery and may prevent complications. The nurse may use the techniques below to assess fundal position, evaluate the condition of the perineum, and detect thrombophlebitis.

Assessing fundal position

To assess the position of the fundus, place the right hand at the symphysis pubis to support the uterus while palpating the fundus with the left hand.

Document fundal height in centimeters from the umbilicus. For instance, if the fundus is located 1 cm below the umbilicus, record this as *U-1*. Also note the consistency of the uterus (for instance, firm or boggy).

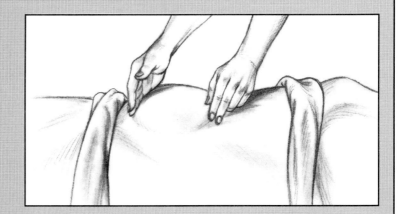

Inspecting the perineum

To evaluate for healing of an episiotomy or perineal lacerations, inspect the perineum regularly, using the following technique.

Verify adequate lighting, put on disposable gloves, and position the client appropriately. For example, if she has a right mediolateral episiotomy, position her on the right side. If she has a midline episiotomy, position her supine with knees flexed.

For optimal visualization in a side-lying client, flex the top leg upward at the knee. Standing behind her, gently lift the upper buttock to expose the perineum and anus.

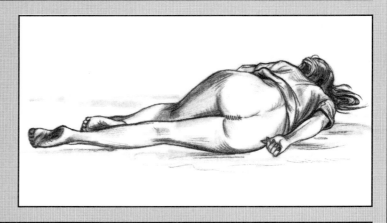

Eliciting Homans' sign

Coagulatory stimulation increases the risk of thromboembolism during the postpartal period. To assess for superficial thromboembolism, attempt to elicit Homans' sign.

Position the client supine. With one hand supporting her knee, lift the leg and dorsiflex the foot toward the ankle. If this maneuver causes pain, suspect superficial thromboembolism.

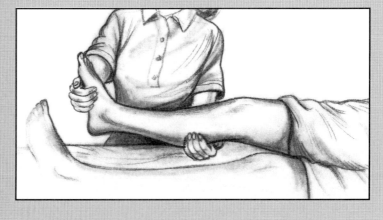

If the client has a boggy uterus, determine if it is caused by bladder distention. After delivery, the bladder may fill rapidly from postpartal diuresis, which eliminates the excess tissue fluid that accumulated during pregnancy as well as any I.V. fluids administered during labor. If bladder distention is responsible for the boggy uterus, expect the uterus to be displaced upward and to the right (above the symphysis); also expect an increased lochial flow. Be sure to review the client's labor and delivery history to check the time and amount of the last voiding or catheterization.

If the client had a cesarean delivery, take great care when assessing the uterus. With a slow, gentle motion, press on the abdomen toward the uterus, avoiding sutures or staples. Inspect the incision site every 15 minutes for the first hour, once an hour for the next 4 hours, then at least once every 8 hours. Evaluate the site for color, warmth, edema, discharge, degree of approximation (distance between the edges of the incision), and the condition of sutures, staples, dressing, or supportive abdominal binder.

Lochia. After the client has delivered, lochia should begin to flow from the vagina. Normally, lochia progresses through stages marked by changes in its appearance. During the first stage, lochia rubra, the discharge is bright red; this stage lasts for approximately 4 days. On about the fifth postpartal day, lochia serosa, the second stage, should begin. This pinkish, serous discharge typically extends through the seventh day. During the second and third postpartal weeks, the creamy white, brown, or colorless discharge known as lochia alba should be present.

Assess the type and amount of lochia. Lochia should progress through the stages described above without relapsing to an earlier stage. Evaluate the consistency of the discharge. Lochia should never contain large clots, tissue fragments, or membranes. If such material is passed, save all specimens for further evaluation. Also note the odor; normally, lochia has a fleshy, not foul, odor. A foul odor may signal infection (as may absence of lochia).

Jacobson (1985) suggests the following classifications to describe the amount of lochia:
• scant—blood appears on a tissue only when the vaginal area is wiped or the stain on the perineal pad is less than 1″ long
• light—the stain on the perineal pad measures 1″ to 4″ long
• moderate—the stain on the perineal pad is 4″ to 6″ long
• heavy—the pad becomes saturated within 1 hour.

If the client has a heavy lochial flow, begin a pad count to determine the amount of discharge more precisely. Record the number of pads used and the degree of saturation of each pad. To make lochial assessment more accurate, obtain the client's cooperation by teaching her about the lochial stages, including how to monitor them and how to describe consistency and amount.

Expect a relatively light lochial flow in the postcesarean client because the uterine contents are evacuated thoroughly during this procedure. In contrast, lochial flow may be slightly heavier during and after breast-feeding sessions from the effects of oxytocin, a hormone released during breast-feeding; the uterine contractions stimulated by oxytocin lead to expulsion of excess lochia. Also, lochial flow increases when the client rises from a lying to a standing position; lochia may escape down the legs as accumulated discharge and small clots are released. Tell the client to expect this so she will not become alarmed when it happens. To prevent her clothing from becoming stained, provide a hospital gown and disposable slippers.

Perineum. For accurate assessment of the perineum, arrange for adequate lighting and position the client properly; elevate the head of the bed no more than 30 degrees.

An episiotomy or perineal laceration should appear to be healing with no exudate; the site should be clean and not excessively tender. Assess the approximation of the incision or wound and check for such abnormalities as redness, warmth, tenderness, edema, ecchymosis, discharge, and hemorrhoids. If the perineum is ecchymotic, exquisitely painful, and grossly discolored, with a collection of blood under the skin surface, suspect a hematoma and report this to the physician.

Breasts. With the client supine and her bra removed, inspect the breasts for symmetry of size and shape. Then palpate in a circular direction as during a standard breast examination. Start by palpating the outer breast tissue, then move the fingers 1 cm toward the center of the breast and repeat. Continue with this pattern until all breast regions have been examined, noting any masses (which may indicate infection or a blocked milk duct). If the breasts are tense, warm, boardlike, and painful, suspect breast engorgement, which results from transient lymphatic and venous stasis. To help determine appropriate interventions, assess the extent of engorgement. Also inspect the nipples for erectility, cracking, and soreness.

If the client has chosen to breast-feed her neonate, colostrum should be secreted from the breasts and the client should be able to breast-feed comfortably every 2 to 4 hours on the first and second days after delivery. Also, she should be drinking an extra quart of fluids, increasing her food intake by 500 calories over her basic daily caloric needs, and wearing a support bra; the nipples should be free of cracks and reddened areas.

By the second or third postpartal day, the breast-feeding client should begin to feel tingling and throbbing in her breasts and notice some release of mature milk when her breasts are stimulated or when she hears her neonate cry. Mature milk is bluish, whereas colostrum is yellow.

Urinary system

Assessment of urinary elimination patterns is a key component of postpartal nursing assessment. Despite rapid urine production and bladder filling after delivery, many clients have difficulty voiding. For example, the client with severe perineal and urethral discomfort may not be able to relax the perineal muscles sufficiently to void; in the postcesarean client or a client who received regional anesthesia, the bladder may lack sensitivity to pressure, impairing the urge to void.

Failure to void within 6 to 8 hours after delivery may cause excessive uterine bleeding because bladder distention prevents uterine contractions and subsequent vessel compression. When voiding finally does occur after a delay, it may be incomplete, with substantial urine remaining in the bladder. This condition, called urinary stasis, may contribute to urinary tract infection.

To evaluate the client's bladder, palpate the suprapubic area. A full bladder is distended above the symphysis and can be palpated readily as a soft, movable mass. A uterus that is boggy, elevated, and deviated to one side supports the suspicion of a full bladder.

Once the client is ambulatory and can perform satisfactory self-care, determine her urine output pattern. Note the time of each voiding and the amount voided, and ask if her bladder feels empty afterward. Also find out if she is experiencing urinary frequency, burning, or urgency.

Cardiovascular system

The hypervolemia of pregnancy protects the postpartal client to some extent from the detrimental effects of blood loss during delivery. However, if the client has lost more than 500 ml of blood, suspect uterine hemorrhage. Commonly, hemorrhage has a sudden onset. To ensure early detection and avert serious consequences, be sure to monitor vital signs and assess her lochia carefully. (See Emergency Alert: *Postpartal hemorrhage*.)

Respiratory system

Assess the client's respiratory rate, rhythm, and depth. Respiratory assessment is especially important if the client had a prolonged labor or a complicated or surgical delivery or if she received an anesthesia that causes decreased sensation and motor activity. Because these circumstances increase the risk of respiratory complications, check for altered breathing patterns and poor gas exchange by auscultating the lungs every 4 hours for adven-

---

EMERGENCY ALERT

POSTPARTAL HEMORRHAGE

A leading cause of maternal mortality, postpartal hemorrhage demands prompt recognition and intervention to avert grave consequences. Normal blood loss at delivery is less than 500 ml; the nurse should suspect hemorrhage if the client's estimated blood loss exceeds 500 ml. Keep in mind that hemorrhage is not always obvious; sometimes it manifests as a slow but steady trickle of blood.

Postpartal hemorrhage commonly stems from uterine atony (poor muscle tone), lacerations of the cervix or vagina, or disseminated intravascular coagulation. Several weeks after delivery, the most common cause of hemorrhage is retention of placental fragments (secundines).

The nurse who suspects hemorrhage should notify the physician immediately, then continually monitor the client's vital signs, assess the condition of the uterus, and evaluate the amount and character of lochia. Refer to the chart below to help identify signs of postpartal hemorrhage and prepare for appropriate interventions.

Signs
- Boggy (soft, pliable) uterus
- Excessively large uterus located above the umbilicus at the midline (must be differentiated from a uterus displaced to the right, which results from bladder distention)
- Excessive lochia, possibly containing large blood clots with or without tissue fragments
- Lochia that flows in a steady trickle
- Increased pulse and respiratory rate with decreased blood pressure (may not arise until later, when shock occurs)

Nursing considerations
- Gently massage the uterus to stimulate contractions.
- Rapidly infuse oxytocin I.V. or administer carboprost, ergonovine, or methylergonovine by I.M. injection, as prescribed and necessary.
- Assess lochial flow to estimate the type and amount of blood loss and to detect any clots or tissue fragments. If lochia is bright red and flows in a slow trickle and the fundus is firm and located at the midline, suspect cervical or vaginal laceration as the cause of hemorrhage.
- Inspect for accumulated blood posterior to the perineum by turning the client from side to side and checking for blood on bed sheets and the perineal pad.
- Position the client flat on her back to facilitate circulation to vital organs.
- Make sure the blood bank has typed and cross-matched the client for possible blood replacement.
- As necessary, prepare the client for surgery.

---

titious sounds, such as crackles (rales) and rhonchi. Evaluate the breathing pattern regularly until the respiratory rate normalizes and the lungs are free of adventitious sounds.

Hematologic system

Usually, a complete blood count is performed 24 to 48 hours after delivery. Typically, the white blood cell (WBC) count is elevated, sometimes reaching 25,000/mm³ – especially if the client had a prolonged labor. Although the exact cause of this increase is unknown, Cunningham, McDonald, and Gant (1989) suggest it may result from the pronounced energy expenditure and stress of labor and delivery. Consequently, an elevated WBC count is not a reliable marker of postpartal infection. However, when accompanied by other potential infection signs, it may help to confirm an infection.

Compare the postpartal hemoglobin level and hematocrit to the corresponding predelivery levels. If the postpartal hemoglobin level is more than 3 g/dl below the predelivery level, the client is at risk for anemia; if it is 5 g/dl or more below the predelivery level, suspect heavy blood loss.

If the delivery was uncomplicated, measurement of coagulation factors usually is not necessary. Nonetheless, hypercoagulability – a result of decreased plasma volume – predisposes the postpartal client to thromboembolic disease. To check for this condition, which most often affects the lower extremities as thrombophlebitis, have the client lie supine with both legs extended. Inspect the legs for symmetry of shape and size, and palpate the thighs and calves to detect areas of warmth, edema, tenderness, redness, or hardness. Then attempt to elicit Homans' sign (pain in the calf when the foot is dorsiflexed).

Gastrointestinal system

Assess the client's progress toward reestablishing normal bowel function, documenting this progress daily. Bowel sounds should resume gradually on the first postpartal day. To determine the presence and quality of bowel sounds, assess the abdomen carefully in all four quadrants. Keep in mind that the postcesarean client may have diminished bowel sounds accompanied by abdominal distention and lack of peristalsis (from immobility, surgical manipulation, and anesthesia).

Inspect the rectal area for hemorrhoids, which may cause redness, discomfort, and itching. Hemorrhoids may arise during pregnancy or from the expulsive effort of labor and delivery. Usually, they disappear in the first few postpartal weeks. Document the presence of hemorrhoids and any associated signs and symptoms.

Neurologic system

If the client complains of headache, check for other signs and symptoms associated with PIH – edema, proteinuria, blurred vision, decreased blood pressure, and hyperactive reflexes. Try to determine the onset, intensity, duration, and location of the headache and find out if any specific factors seem to trigger or relieve it. Keep in mind that in a client who received some types of regional anesthesia, such as a spinal block, headache may result from loss of cerebrospinal fluid through the dural puncture site – a condition called postspinal headache.

During the first 4 hours after delivery, the client who received regional anesthesia should regain full sensory and motor function. Occasionally, however, residual neurologic effects may occur. To assess for the return of sensation and movement, ask the client to move her lower extremities and to report the level of feeling present. (As sensation and motor function return, the client may report a heightened awareness of discomfort and may need further evaluation to determine the need for pain relief.)

Musculoskeletal system

Assess breast and abdominal muscle tone, which commonly is diminished from overstretching and the effects of increased hormone levels during pregnancy. In some cases, the abdomen has become so stretched that the rectus abdominis muscles, which lie side-by-side, separate at the midline. This condition, called diastasis recti abdominis, rarely warrants treatment.

Many postpartal clients are concerned about poor muscle tone and eager to regain their prepregnancy figure. When conducting the assessment, provide an opening for the client to express such concerns and recommend appropriate exercises.

Immune system

Detection of postpartal infection is a primary nursing concern. In most cases, such infection involves the reproductive system. Besides regularly assessing the client's temperature, observe closely for subtle signs and symptoms of infection, such as chills, malaise, and pallor. Also review the client's chart for risk factors for puerperal infection, such as prolonged labor, prolonged time since rupture of the membranes, vaginal or cervical lacerations, and retention of placental fragments.

The client who received regional anesthesia has an increased risk of infection because of the invasive administration route used. Carefully and regularly inspect the spinal or epidural site for redness, warmth, edema, pain, and tenderness; promptly report any of these signs to the physician.

Also review the client's chart to assess her Rh status and rubella status.

Psychosocial status

The postpartal nurse has a unique opportunity to assess the client's and her partner's response to childbirth and to evaluate their interaction with the neonate. Typically, they focus initially on the neonate's sex, size, and facial similarities to their older children or to other relatives. Many facilities provide a place on the nursing record to describe parent-neonate interaction. If so, be sure to document this regularly.

Initial psychosocial assessment focuses on the client. Eventually, however, the nurse should broaden the assessment to include the father and other family members, such as siblings and grandparents.

Evaluating maternal emotional status. The client's emotional status can affect her interaction with the neonate and her adaptation to her role. To assess emotional status, evaluate the client's mood, attitude, energy level, feelings about the childbirth experience, level of confidence in caregiving, and sense of satisfaction with her neonate. Immediately after delivery, most clients have a positive mood and attitude from the joy and excitement they feel over the birth of the child. However, fatigue may set in quickly, and the client may seem disinterested in her neonate. To distinguish fatigue from disinterest, assess mother-neonate interaction just after the client awakens from a nap and has more energy for interaction.

A client who feels overwhelmed by becoming a mother may seem withdrawn. With such a client, check for other signs that indicate a potential for maladaptive parenting, such as depression, low self-esteem, lack of support, and a seeming preoccupation with physical discomfort.

Continue to assess the client's emotional status throughout her stay. Be sure to check for signs and symptoms of postpartal "blues," such as crying spells, irritability, insomnia, and poor appetite. When these problems persist for more than 2 weeks and impair the client's ability to cope with daily activities, she may have postpartal depression, a more serious disorder. In rare cases, postpartal psychosis develops; signs and symptoms of this disorder may include severe depression and suicidal impulses. The neonate may be at risk for neglect or abuse from the client's gross distortion of reality, delusions, confusion, agitation, and flight of ideas (Hamilton, 1982).

Although early discharge makes unlikely the nurse's detecting of postpartal depression or psychosis, the nurse who detects postpartal emotional problems should expect the client to be referred to a counselor, psychiatric nurse clinician, or a psychiatrist for early treatment. (For more information on postpartal depression and psychosis, see Chapter 26, Maternal Care at Home.)

Assessing mother-infant interaction. Observe the client and neonate together, and assess their interaction. If possible, observe during a feeding session because this is when the mother and neonate are most likely to interact. To ensure accuracy, assess interaction on at least two occasions; if the client is fatigued or in discomfort during one assessment, her behavior may give a false impression.

Note the amount of eye contact between the client and neonate. Does the client pay more attention to the observer or the neonate? Also note whether she holds the neonate close or at a distance, and assess the quality of her touch. Does she stroke, kiss, and fondle the neonate, or is her touch rough, quick, and unaffectionate? Does she talk to, smile at, or sing to the neonate when changing the diaper? These behaviors show that the client acknowledges the neonate's presence and seeks a response.

Listen to the client talk to her neonate. Does she speak directly in a soothing or playful way? If her tone is demanding or rejecting, assess this again on a subsequent occasion; if it continues, try to identify the cause.

Find out if the client worries about the neonate when the two are apart and if she believes the neonate knows her voice and notices her presence. Also pay close attention to the client's comments about the neonate. Does she express pleasure and satisfaction with the way her child is feeding? Note whether and how she talks about the neonate's characteristics. Does she use "claiming" expressions, such as, "He's got his daddy's eyes"? The client who claims her child has reconciled the real child with the "fantasy" child and has placed the child within the family context; this shows that interaction has begun. Other indications of claiming include referring to the neonate as "my baby" or "our baby" and calling the neonate by name rather than "it."

Also listen for attribution of negative personality traits to the neonate—for example, such statements as, "This baby is so stubborn; she just won't breast-feed." Lack of interaction also may be signaled by such comments as, "He's mad at me today" or, "She doesn't like me." In some cases, the client may state that the neonate prefers to be held by someone other than herself. Expression of continued disappointment with the neonate's gender or physical appearance also warns of a relationship at risk.

To help evaluate the client's feelings about her neonate, ask the client questions. (For examples of relevant assessment questions, see *Assessing psychosocial adaptation.*)

If the assessment uncovers a lack of interaction, suspect parental maladaptation and refer the client and neonate for consultation with a qualified counselor.

ASSESSING PSYCHOSOCIAL ADAPTATION

Depending on the client's and family's circumstances, the nurse may use questions similar to those shown below to determine how the client feels about her neonate and how she perceives her family's responses to the birth of the neonate. Rationales are given to explain the purpose of asking each question.

How do you feel about being a parent to this infant?
Rationale: This question gives the client a chance to express her concerns about parenting. The answer may reveal problems in bonding or in adaptation to the parental role. The remaining questions may help pinpoint some of her concerns.

How do you feel about your infant's behavior?
Rationale: If the client perceives the neonate as troublesome or abnormal, mother-infant interaction may be in jeopardy and the neonate may be at risk for abuse.

Does your infant look the way you expected?
Rationale: If the client perceives the neonate as unattractive or as having the "wrong" features, interaction may be compromised.

How do you feel about having a boy (or girl)?
Rationale: If the client was anticipating a child of the opposite sex, she will need to grieve over the loss of the fantasy child before she can bond with the real child.

Is the infant's father pleased with the infant?
Rationale: The client who receives support from the neonate's father has a better chance for a healthy adaptation to the parenting role.

Does the infant's father plan on helping you at home?
Rationale: The father who participates in child care or household tasks shows positive adaptation to his new role and tasks; this in turn may promote the client's adaptation.

How do you feel about having someone help you at home?
Rationale: Rejection of help or other indications of possessiveness toward the neonate may signify a problem in adaptation.

How do your other children feel about this infant?
Rationale: This question gives the client a chance to express any concerns she may have about the neonate's siblings. If the siblings are having problems adjusting to a new brother or sister, the client may need help coping.

What have the baby's grandparents said about this infant?
Rationale: Failure of the grandparents to accept the neonate or to offer emotional support to the client may create problems for the client adapting to the parental role.

Evaluating maternal sensitivity and response to neonatal communication cues. Observing how the client responds to the neonate's communication cues yields further information about the developing mother-infant relationship. Note how long the client takes to respond to the neonate's cues; ignoring the neonate may indicate a problem. Also evaluate the appropriateness of the client's responses. Some mothers cannot differentiate among communication cues that signal hunger, fatigue, the need to be held, the need for eye contact, and the need for a soothing or stimulating voice. If she misinterprets cues or overstimulates or understimulates the neonate, the interaction may be asynchronous. Aim to detect asynchrony early and intervene promptly before such behaviors become entrenched.

Signs that the client is responding inappropriately to communication cues include forcing or refusing eye contact with the neonate or stimulating a tired neonate. For example, she may talk to the neonate too much, too little, or at the wrong time. Also, she may overfeed or underfeed the neonate, hold the neonate too much or too little, or tickle or bounce a fatigued neonate. Ignoring the neonate also shows lack of sensitivity to neonatal communication cues and needs.

Assessing maternal adaptation. Assess whether the client is progressing normally through the stages of adaptation—taking in, taking hold, and letting go. Also determine whether she uses a consistent, intelligent approach toward her neonate, such as by asking questions about neonatal care and evaluating the effectiveness of her caregiving attempts.

Ask the client how her family feels about the neonate; the feelings of other family members can affect how the client perceives herself. For instance, the new mother tends to view others' acceptance of the neonate as acceptance of herself as a woman and mother. Such acceptance helps her adapt to the maternal role. On the other hand, if the neonate has an abnormal or unusual appearance that upsets family members, the client may interpret their response as a rejection of her.

Assessing paternal adaptation. To provide family-centered care, assess the adaptation of all family members, not just the client. The father's emotional status and adaptation to parenthood are particularly important. Because he usually serves as the client's main support person, his responses and behavior can play a key role in the client's adaptation to parenthood.

Many fathers have a great need to talk about the childbirth experience and their feelings but have no chance to do so except with the client. Thus, stay alert for signs that the father wants to unburden himself. If he had planned to participate actively in the birth but could not do so because of labor or delivery complications, assess for signs that he feels angry or disappointed.

Also determine the father's level of knowledge about neonatal behavior and care. Even if he will not be the primary caregiver, inadequate information about the neonate or lack of confidence in providing care can limit his interactions with the neonate.

Evaluate the father's expectations about the client's postpartal recovery and his understanding of the time and energy involved in caring for a neonate. Unrealistic expectations may lead to resentment, poor father-child interaction, and problems in the couple's relationship. For instance, if he is anticipating a rapid resumption of the client's normal energy level and desire for sexual activity, he may become resentful if her postpartal recovery takes longer than expected.

Also check for signs that the father is disappointed with the neonate's sex or is upset over a minor physical aberration. These feelings may jeopardize father-child interaction and cause the client to feel that he does not accept her as a woman or mother.

Assessing sibling adaptation. Observe the siblings as they interact with the neonate, checking for hostility, aggression, and jealousy. Also assess how the client and her partner deal with these problems.

Identifying support systems. Determine how much emotional and practical support is available to the client both inside and outside the family. The client with adequate practical and emotional support is more likely to adapt well to the maternal role. Evidence of such support includes visits, phone calls, gifts, and flowers. Also find out who will be available to help with child care or household tasks after discharge. In some cases, new parents fail to anticipate the need for help and then feel overwhelmed when the demands of child care become obvious.

Determining parental caregiving skills. To determine how much teaching the parents will need to gain competence in caring for the neonate, find out about their previous child-care experience and observe them as they provide care. With new parents, inexperience may be obvious. If the parents are experienced, however, do not automatically assume they are adept at giving care. Instead, ask them if they would like a refresher course, and give them the chance to ask questions.

NURSING DIAGNOSIS

After gathering assessment data, the nurse must review it carefully to identify pertinent nursing diagnoses for the client. (For a partial list of applicable diagnoses, see Nursing Diagnoses: *Postpartal client and family.*)

PLANNING AND IMPLEMENTATION

After assessing the client and formulating nursing diagnoses, the nurse develops and implements a plan of care.

When the client arrives on the postpartal unit, identify her by checking her identification band carefully. Provide a brief orientation to the unit, including such information as where the bathroom, telephone, and personal supplies are located and what time meals are served. Review visiting hours and rooming-in policy. If visiting hours are limited, promote client compliance by explaining that such limits are imposed for the client's and neonate's well-being. Also make sure the client understands why visitors must comply with infection-prevention measures, such as washing hands and putting on cover gowns before handling the neonate.

Ensuring safety

Various factors may contribute to weakness and light-headedness for the first few hours after delivery, leading to a nursing diagnosis of *high risk for injury related to blood loss, fatigue, limited food intake, or medication effects.* Consequently, advise the client to call for help when getting out of bed for the first time. Also show her how to raise or lower the bed rails. To prevent injury to the neonate, caution her against falling asleep in bed with the neonate.

If the client received regional anesthesia, she may have impaired motor or sensory function in the lower extremities. To guarantee safety, make sure all functions have returned to a satisfactory level before helping her out of bed.

Providing for adequate sleep and rest

For an hour or so after delivery, the client may be too excited to sleep or rest, despite her fatigue. Within a few hours, however, she may fall into a deep, although short, sleep. This sleep is especially crucial for the client who is recovering from a cesarean delivery or a prolonged, difficult labor and delivery. For the client with a nursing diagnosis of *fatigue related to pregnancy, labor, and delivery,* help determine rest and sleep requirements and encourage her to limit visitors and telephone calls. If necessary,

NURSING DIAGNOSES

POSTPARTAL CLIENT AND FAMILY

The following are potential nursing diagnoses for problems and etiologies that the nurse may encounter when caring for a client and her family during the postpartal period. Specific nursing interventions for many of these diagnoses are provided in the "Planning and implementation" section of this chapter.

Postpartal client
- Altered urinary elimination related to perineal and urethral edema and ecchymosis
- Anxiety related to new role development
- Constipation related to poor intestinal tone, diminished food intake, and immobility
- Fatigue related to pregnancy, labor, and delivery
- High risk for caregiver role strain related to demands of caring for a neonate
- High risk for injury related to blood loss, fatigue, limited food intake, or medication effects
- Impaired physical mobility related to bed rest, anesthesia, or inability to ambulate
- Impaired skin integrity related to the perineal wound
- Ineffective breathing pattern related to immobility following cesarean delivery
- Knowledge deficit related to self-care or parenting skills
- Pain related to the perineal wound
- Pain related to uterine contractions
- Sleep pattern disturbance related to hospitalization and caring for the neonate around the clock
- Social isolation related to sensory deprivation or separation from home, family, and friends

Postpartal family
- Altered family processes related to the neonate's birth
- Anxiety related to the stress of the changing family structure and the transition to parenthood
- Dysfunctional grieving related to loss of the fantasy child
- Family coping: potential for growth, related to the birth of a new family member
- Ineffective individual coping related to parenting tasks and responsibilities
- Knowledge deficit related to parenting tasks, infant care, and community resources
- Parental role conflict related to the birth of a new family member
- Potential altered parenting related to disappointment over the neonate's sex or appearance
- Social isolation related to the demands of caring for a neonate or an infant

ask visitors to leave the client's room when she feels tired to allow her to sleep.

The client may choose to have the neonate room-in with her. If she is undecided about rooming-in, inform her that this arrangement does not necessarily disrupt sleep. Keefe (1988) found that clients whose neonates spent the night in the nursery slept no longer or better than those whose neonates roomed-in.

Promoting uterine involution and preventing hemorrhage

The uterus should have sufficient tone after delivery to contract effectively so that vessels are compressed and involution proceeds normally. If the client has a boggy, or atonic, uterus, monitor her vital signs closely because hemorrhage can have a sudden onset. Interventions for uterine atony may vary with the underlying cause.

Facilitating voiding. If uterine atony stems from bladder distention (as indicated by a boggy uterus that is displaced upward and to the right), make every effort to keep the client's bladder empty. Within the first 4 hours after delivery, encourage her to walk to the bathroom; if she is confined to bed, offer a bedpan. Other nursing interventions that promote spontaneous voiding include turning on the faucet in the client's bathroom, irrigating the perineum, placing the client's hands in water, and providing plenty of fluids.

Failure to void within 8 hours of delivery necessitates urinary catheterization, as does bladder distention. Fortunately, many clients regain normal urinary elimination patterns after just a single catheterization.

If the client requires catheterization, be sure to use sterile technique to minimize the risk of infection. Also, conduct this procedure with extreme gentleness, offering appropriate explanations. Catheterization during the early postpartal period causes more discomfort than usual because of the edematous, bruised condition of the bladder, urethra, urinary meatus, labia, and perineum.

Massaging the uterus. When uterine atony does not stem from bladder distention, gentle massage of the uterus may be sufficient to stimulate uterine contractions, restoring firm tone. The nurse also may teach the client how to massage her own uterus. However, emphasize that she must do this gently to avoid overstimulation, which could prevent contractions.

Administering oxytocin. If massage fails to induce contractions, expect to administer an I.V. oxytocin preparation or I.M. carboprost. (For more information about these drugs and other drugs administered to postpartal clients, see Selected Major Drugs: *Drugs used during the postpartal period,* pages 538 and 539.) If hemorrhage occurs despite drug therapy, expect the client to undergo surgical exploration and evacuation of the uterus.

(Text continues on page 540.)

DRUGS USED DURING THE POSTPARTAL PERIOD

This chart summarizes the major drugs currently used during the postpartal period.

MAJOR INDICATIONS	USUAL ADULT DOSAGES	NURSING IMPLICATIONS
bromocriptine (Parlodel)		
Prevention of postpartal lactation	2.5 mg P.O. twice daily with meals for 14 to 21 days	• Monitor blood pressure. Transient hypotension may occur during the first 3 days of therapy. • Check for seizure activity. • Advise the client to use contraceptive methods other than oral contraceptives during treatment. • Warn the client to use caution when ambulating. • Do not initiate therapy sooner than 4 hours after delivery and not until signs have stablized.
carboprost (Prostin/M15)		
Postpartal hemorrhage from uterine atony that does not respond to conventional management	250 mcg deep I.M.; may repeat dose at 15- to 90-minute intervals; maximum total dosage should not exceed 2 mg	• Obtain vital signs; assess the amount and character of lochia and the condition of the fundus. • Administer cautiously to client with cervical lacerations. • Watch for adverse gastrointestinal (GI) effects. • Do not administer I.V.
codeine		
Mild to moderate postpartal pain	15 to 60 mg P.O. every 3 to 4 hours as needed (usually given with 325 to 650 mg of acetaminophen)	• Monitor respiratory and circulatory status and bowel function. • Observe the client for drowsiness; make sure she is alert when caring for her neonate.
diphenhydramine (Benadryl)		
Nighttime sedation	25 to 50 mg P.O. at bedtime	• Observe the client for drowsiness; make sure she is alert when caring for her neonate. • Assess the client for nausea and dry mouth.
docusate sodium (Colace)		
Stool softener	50 to 300 mg P.O. daily or until bowel movements are normal	• Assess the client for bowel activity, mild abdominal cramping, and diarrhea.
ergonovine maleate (Ergotrate Maleate)		
Prevention or treatment of postpartal hemorrhage from uterine atony or subinvolution	0.2 mg I.M. every 2 to 4 hours to a maximum of five doses; after initial I.M. dose, may give 0.2 to 0.4 mg P.O. every 5 to 12 hours for 2 to 7 days	• Monitor blood pressure, pulse rate, and uterine response. Report sudden changes in vital signs, frequent periods of uterine relaxation, and any change in the character or amount of lochia. • If ordered for severe uterine bleeding, dilute I.V. preparation to 5 ml with normal saline solution; administer over at least 1 minute while blood pressure and uterine contractions are monitored. • Contractions begin 5 to 15 minutes after P.O., 2 to 5 minutes after I.M., and immediately after I.V. administration and may continue 3 hours or more after P.O. or I.M. and 45 minutes after I.V. administration.

SELECTED MAJOR DRUGS

DRUGS USED DURING THE POSTPARTAL PERIOD (continued)

MAJOR INDICATIONS	USUAL ADULT DOSAGES	NURSING IMPLICATIONS
ibuprofen (Motrin)		
Mild to moderate postpartal pain	400 mg P.O. every 4 to 6 hours	• Assess the client for signs and symptoms of GI irritation, such as nausea, vomiting, diarrhea, and gastric discomfort. • Warn the client not to take more than 1.2 g/day without consulting her physician.
meperidine (Demerol)		
Moderate to severe postpartal pain (such as after cesarean delivery)	50 to 100 mg P.O., I.M., or S.C. every 3 to 4 hours; or by continuous I.V. infusion, 15 to 35 mg/hour as needed or around the clock	• Monitor the client's pulse rate. • Check for signs of central nervous system (CNS) depression, such as drowsiness or lethargy. Make sure the client is alert when caring for her neonate. • Assess the client's pain level. • To avoid toxic metabolites, give the smallest effective dosage.
methylergonovine (Methergine)		
Prevention and treatment of postpartal hemorrhage from uterine atony or subinvolution	0.2 mg I.M. every 2 to 4 hours for a maximum of 5 doses; after the initial I.M. dose, may give 0.2 to 0.4 mg P.O. every 6 to 12 hours for 2 to 7 days	• Monitor and record blood pressure, pulse rate, and uterine response. Report any sudden change in vital signs, frequent periods of uterine relaxation, and any change in lochia. • Decrease the dosage if severe cramping occurs. • Contractions begin 5 to 15 minutes after P.O. administration, 2 to 5 minutes after I.M. injection. They continue 3 hours or more.
morphine		
Severe pain (such as after cesarean delivery)	4 to 15 mg S.C. or I.M.; may be injected by slow I.V. infusion (over 4 to 5 minutes) diluted in 4 to 5 ml of water for injection	• Monitor for respiratory depression and hypotension. • Check for signs of CNS depression. Make sure the client is alert when caring for her neonate. • Drug may be injected into the epidural space for prolonged pain relief. Monitor the client for delayed respiratory depression. • If the client has pruritus after I.V. or epidural administration, expect to give antihistamines.
oxytocin (Pitocin)		
Reduction of postpartal bleeding after expulsion of the placenta	1 to 4 ml (10 to 40 units) in 1,000 ml of dextrose 5% in water or normal saline solution I.V., infused at a rate necessary to control bleeding (usually 20 to 40 milliunits/minute); or 10 units I.M.	• Administer by I.V. infusion, not I.V. bolus injection. • Record uterine contractions, heart rate, and blood pressure every 15 minutes. • Assess the amount and character of lochia and the condition of the fundus. • Check for increased pulse rate in response to pain from contractions.
simethicone (Mylicon)		
Flatulence, functional gastric bloating (such as after cesarean delivery)	40 to 80 mg after each meal and at bedtime	• Make sure the client chews tablets thoroughly. • Assess the client for bowel activity and abdominal distention.

Relieving discomfort from uterine contractions

The severity of uterine contractions, or afterpains, typically varies with parity. In the primiparous client, afterpains may not be noticeable; in the multiparous client, they may cause severe discomfort. Because breast-feeding promotes the release of oxytocin (which stimulates contractions), the breast-feeding client typically has more severe afterpains during and after feeding sessions. For the client with a nursing diagnosis of *pain related to uterine contractions,* expect to administer a mild analgesic (such as acetaminophen with codeine) or a nonsteroidal anti-inflammatory drug (such as ibuprofen).

Reducing perineal discomfort

Perineal lacerations or an episiotomy may cause considerable pain, possibly leading to a nursing diagnosis of *pain related to the perineal wound.* An ice pack applied to the perineum in the first few hours after delivery helps soothe the area by constricting vessels and reducing the vascular response of inflammation.

Warmth may be applied to the perineum 12 to 24 hours after delivery. Warmth causes vasodilation, which relieves discomfort and edema and promotes the local inflammatory response by hastening the arrival of leukocytes and antibodies at the site. A warm sitz bath can provide the necessary warmth. Typically, the client takes this treatment three or four times daily, with each bath lasting 15 to 20 minutes, until the discomfort has diminished or the perineum has healed. To ensure that the client can self-administer the bath correctly, provide complete instructions.

A topical spray or ointment also may be applied to relieve perineal discomfort. A topical spray may be an anesthetic, which provides local pain relief, or a steroid, which reduces edema and promotes healing.

Occasionally, the physician or nurse-midwife may order perineal heat lamp treatments, which promote perineal comfort and healing through a drying effect. Place the heat lamp between the client's legs, at least 18″ from the perineum. For client safety, limit treatments to the prescribed length, use a bulb no brighter than 40 watts, and make sure the bedclothes remain clear of the lamp. Also, make sure the lamp is positioned securely and cannot fall onto the client.

Other measures that may be used to reduce perineal discomfort include mild analgesia (such as oxycodone, propoxyphene, or codeine with acetaminophen), witch hazel compresses, and a commercial water and disinfectant spray (such as the Surgigator or Hygenique).

To keep the perineal region clean, show the client how to use a perineal irrigation, or squirt, bottle after each voiding. The client fills the bottle with warm water, then aims it at the perineum to rinse off any urine or lochia remaining on the surface.

Ensuring lactation suppression

For the client who chooses to bottle-feed her neonate, lactation is suppressed through drug therapy or a natural method. With either method, lactation ceases within 1 week.

Drug therapy typically involves bromocriptine. A synthetic ergot alkaloid derivative, bromocriptine inhibits secretion of prolactin, a hormone that stimulates milk production. If the client is receiving this drug, monitor for such adverse reactions as fatigue, dizziness, hypertension, hypotension, and seizures; contact the physician immediately if these problems arise. Advise her to finish all the medication in her prescription if no adverse reactions occur.

In the natural method of lactation suppression, the client must avoid any stimulation of the breasts and nipples and wear a tight support bra or breast binder. The client who has just delivered may prefer this method over taking a drug; for the client who wishes to discontinue breast-feeding after several weeks or months, this method is the only available option.

Promoting respiratory stability

Monitor the client's respiratory rate and effort. For the postcesarean client, who may have a nursing diagnosis of *ineffective breathing pattern related to immobility following cesarean delivery,* carry out measures that promote effective breathing patterns, thereby reducing the risk of pneumonia or atelectasis. For instance, have her cough and deep-breathe hourly; remind her to turn every 1 to 2 hours to promote oxygenation and prevent skin breakdown. Also, within a few hours after delivery, teach her how to use an incentive spirometer. This device maintains lung expansion and mobilizes secretions.

Preventing hematologic complications

If the client has a subnormal hemoglobin level and hematocrit, she may be in danger of anemia from blood loss. For a severely anemic client, expect the physician to order a blood transfusion. In less serious circumstances, provide a diet rich in iron to help prevent anemia, and teach the client about dietary iron sources.

Because the postpartal client—especially the multiparous client—is at risk for thrombophlebitis, stress the importance of early, moderate exercise (such as walking in the hallway). Unless the client received high doses of analgesics or anesthetics during labor and delivery, she should be able to walk around within a few hours of delivery. Also, instruct her to wear foot coverings that do not constrict the knee, to elevate her legs on a stool from time to time when sitting (to prevent blood stasis in the calves), and to avoid crossing her legs at the knee.

Promoting bowel elimination

Although bowel function usually returns to normal rapidly after delivery, various factors may hinder bowel elimination. To help avoid a nursing diagnosis of *constipation related to poor intestinal tone, diminished food intake, and immobility*, encourage early ambulation, plenty of fluids, and a well-balanced, high-fiber diet. Also advise her to act on any urge to defecate, taking adequate time to sit on the toilet at the time when her bowel movements normally occur. If she is reluctant to attempt a bowel movement out of fear that it will tear open her episiotomy suture line, reassure her that she will not damage the repaired wound by bearing down gently. The physician may order a stool softener, such as docusate, or a stimulant laxative, such as a bisacodyl suppository.

After the first few postpartal hours, the client may be hungry and thirsty. Provide cool liquids and a light meal, regardless of the time of day, and encourage the client to drink 1 or 2 quarts (four to eight 8-oz glasses) of fluid daily to replace fluids lost during labor and delivery.

Relieving abdominal distention and flatus accumulation

The postcesarean client may complain of abdominal distention accompanied by flatus accumulation. Interventions for this problem include insertion of a rectal tube to help expel flatus in the distal colon or suppositories to promote bowel activity and subsequent flatus expulsion. Also, the physician may order simethicone, which reduces flatus formation.

Encourage early ambulation and slow resumption of oral intake, beginning with ice chips and progressing to a liquid, then regular, diet. Advise the client to avoid carbonated beverages and gas-forming foods (such as cabbage, asparagus, and brussels sprouts).

Relieving hemorrhoidal discomfort

If the client has hemorrhoids, assure her that the acute discomfort should last only 2 to 3 days. In the meantime, apply soothing witch hazel compresses soaked in ice chips, use an anesthetic or steroid-based cream, or administer anti-hemorrhoidal suppositories. Other measures that help relieve hemorrhoidal discomfort include mild analgesics, sitz baths, and a side-lying position. Sometimes the hemorrhoid discomfort can be reduced by pushing the inflamed tissues back into the rectum with a finger

cot or a gloved, lubricated finger; if appropriate, teach the client how to do this herself.

Avoiding neurologic complications

The client who received spinal anesthesia may develop postspinal headache. If so, position her flat; or, if she is permitted to lie on her side, make sure her head is elevated no more than 30 degrees. Make sure she remains supine for 8 to 10 hours after anesthesia administration. Monitor her response to positioning; if she reports that the headache has worsened, lower the head of the bed. Because fluid replacement helps prevent postspinal headache, monitor fluid intake in a client at risk for this problem.

When headache results from PIH, interventions may include bed rest and administration of magnesium sulfate or sedatives.

Correcting musculoskeletal deficits

Beginning immediately after delivery, suggest mild exercises to improve muscle tone, such as arm, head, and shoulder raises or deep abdominal breathing with contraction of the abdominal muscles. Within a few days of delivery, the client may begin abdominal exercises, alternately contracting and relaxing the abdominal muscles. Advise her to reduce or stop exercising if lochial flow increases or if she becomes uncomfortable or fatigued.

Ensuring adequate immunologic status

If the client has signs and symptoms of postpartal infection, expect to administer antibiotics and to carry out measures to minimize or reverse any precipitating factors, such as anemia.

To prevent isoimmunization (development of antibodies against $Rh_o(D)$ antigens), most Rh-negative pregnant clients now receive Rh immune globulin (RhoGAM) during or near the twenty-eighth week of pregnancy. Cord blood is sampled after delivery to determine the neonate's Rh status. If the neonate is Rh-positive, make sure the client receives an additional RhoGAM injection within 72 hours of delivery, even if she received a prenatal injection.

If the client's antenatal rubella titer test revealed that she lacks immunity (indicated by a titer less than 1:10), she should be immunized before discharge. If she will receive the live vaccine (Meruvax II), warn her to avoid becoming pregnant for 3 months after immunization.

Promoting psychosocial adaptation

Postpartal hospitalization provides the client and her partner with an opportunity to adjust to their new role as parents and to review and receive information and feedback about the childbirth experience. The nurse should encourage the client to express her feelings—both positive and negative—about the experience. This helps prepare her for motherhood and future pregnancies (Konrad, 1987) and may avoid a nursing diagnosis of *anxiety related to new role development.* (If the client does not have a partner, identify a support person with whom she can share her feelings.) If appropriate, suggest that the client's partner participate in a fathers' support group to help him learn child care skills and coping strategies and to provide a forum where he can express his feelings (Taubenheim and Silbernagel, 1988).

Provide the client with positive feedback about her behavior during labor and delivery and her ongoing acquisition of parenting skills. If she has a negative perspective about the childbirth experience based on a misperception, provide a brief explanation to clarify the situation and promote positive feelings.

If the client is an adolescent, she poses a special challenge. To promote psychosocial adaptation, the nurse must understand adolescent behavior—especially the drive for independence, which plays a major role in adolescent judgment and decision making. A nonjudgmental approach—essential to developing a positive relationship with this client—may necessitate self-exploration of the nurse's own feelings and attitudes toward adolescent sexuality, pregnancy, and motherhood.

Promoting family adaptation. Make sure to include the father or significant other in nursing interventions, such as by inviting him to child-care demonstrations and giving him the opportunity to express his feelings and concerns. If he has questions about the events of childbirth or the mother's or neonate's condition, offer clarification. Also stay alert for signs that he feels inadequate as a labor partner, husband, or father. If such signs arise, reassure him that many new fathers have these doubts.

Offer anticipatory counseling so that the father knows what to expect in the months ahead. Topics that may be appropriate to include are resumption of sexual activity, the expected course of the mother's postpartal recovery, and the need to provide practical and emotional support at home.

Many siblings feel uncertain or jealous when a brother or sister is born. To help siblings adjust and thus avoid a nursing diagnosis of *altered family processes related to the neonate's birth,* urge the parents to let siblings visit the neonate in the health care facility (if facility policy allows). Be aware that studies have failed to support the notion that sibling visits increase the risk of neonatal infection (Solheim and Spellacy, 1988).

Encourage the client to call siblings on the telephone frequently and to spend uninterrupted time with them when they visit. Also, instruct her to watch for overt and subtle signs of sibling jealousy. Overt signs include hitting or throwing objects at the neonate; subtle signs include attempting to take the neonate out of the crib or covering the neonate with toys.

Encourage the parents to include the grandparents in their new family life because grandparents can serve as key support persons. However, keep in mind that changes in maternity and infant care practices over the past few decades may create conflicts between parents and grandparents. If such conflicts arise, help resolve them by providing teaching to grandparents and incorporating extended family issues in parenting classes. Also recommend that grandparents attend grandparent classes offered by the health care facility or community. Topics typically included in such classes include modern childbirth practices, parenting techniques, and the grandparent role.

Although many grandparents enjoy participating in caregiving, the nurse should not assume that all grandparents want to participate. Follow their lead in this matter, offering caregiving instruction only if they express a desire for it.

Grandparents also can help siblings adjust to the birth of the neonate. Encourage them to give siblings extra attention and a chance to express their feelings about the birth of a new family member. To help perpetuate a sense of family continuity, suggest that they relate family history to the siblings, including telling siblings about their parents' births.

Promoting psychosocial adaptation in special-needs clients. Special-needs clients include adolescent and older clients and those with sensory, mental, or physical disabilities.

Expect the adolescent client to have a greater need for teaching about neonatal and infant care. Ask how she plans to care for her child after discharge; if her arrangements seem inadequate, refer her to the appropriate resources.

The first-time mother over age 30 may feel anxious about her caregiving skills and her changing role. Particularly if she gave up a career to have a child, she may have a nursing diagnosis of *parental role conflict related to the birth of a new family member.* Urge this client to express her feelings about becoming a mother; if appropriate, refer her for counseling.

The disabled client will need individualized nursing care to ease the transition to parenthood. (For appropriate

HELPING THE DISABLED CLIENT ADAPT TO PARENTHOOD

Most disabled clients can develop a full, rewarding parenting role. Nursing care for these clients and their families necessitates extra creativity, empathy, and emotional support, with emphasis on communication and individualized interventions.

Vision-impaired client
Although a vision-impaired client cannot make eye contact with her neonate, she can use other senses to develop a bond. Give her the opportunity to touch, hear, and smell the neonate. Be sure to provide a thorough orientation to the surroundings, because the health care facility is an unfamiliar environment.

To help the client feel comfortable and confident when performing physical caregiving tasks, describe the motions involved. For example, when teaching her how to wrap the neonate in a blanket, describe this process step by step. Have her feel the position of the blanket and neonate at each stage, then guide her as she performs the actions, giving her ample time to become familiar with each step through touch.

Hearing-impaired client
When working with a hearing-impaired client, first determine if she can read lips or use sign language. The nurse who does not know sign language should seek help from a knowledgeable resource person. In some cases, a magic slate or tablet and pen can be used to communicate. (Be aware that federal law stipulates that facilities receiving federal funds must provide alternative ways of communicating with hearing-impaired clients.)

Although the client cannot hear her neonate, she may be able to feel sound vibrations. If she can vocalize, encourage her to do so with the neonate. Also consider recommending that she obtain a device that converts sound waves into a flashing light signal; this device can be placed on the nursery door at home to alert the client when the child is crying.

Mentally impaired client
A multidisciplinary team approach incorporating family and community support is required to address the needs of this client and her child. Unless severely impaired, the mentally impaired client can learn caregiving skills. If her social, communication, daily living, and independent living skills have not been assessed, refer her to the appropriate professional for evaluation.

If the client functions well enough to care for her neonate, implement a thorough plan for teaching child care tasks, taking into account her best learning method. Keep the teaching environment free from distractions, and ask the client to give return demonstrations of skills taught. Use an appropriate teaching pace, and if necessary, repeat teaching points.

Be sure to identify support resources and incorporate them into discharge planning. If the client lacks adequate support, help her make contact with a local support group, such as a parenting group. Refer her to a community health nurse or visiting nurse for follow-up assessment of her daily living skills.

Physically disabled client
Many parents with physical disabilities are quite creative in performing caregiving tasks. Base interventions on the client's particular strengths and weaknesses. For example, a client with psychomotor dysfunction may require referral to an occupational therapist, adaptation of the home environment, and an assistant caregiver until a comfortable and safe caregiving routine has been established.

---

nursing interventions, see *Helping the disabled client adapt to parenthood.*)

Implementing client teaching
The trend toward early discharge (within 24 to 48 hours of delivery) has made postpartal client teaching increasingly important—yet difficult to complete. Client teaching may be carried out by the postpartal nurse or a nurse who provides follow-up care at home after early discharge.

Teaching should focus on self-care and neonatal care. The former include such topics as postpartal danger signs, rest, nutrition, and exercises. (For more information, see Client Teaching: *Self-care after discharge,* page 544.)

Especially for the client with a nursing diagnosis of *knowledge deficit related to self-care or parenting skills,* consider using both individual and group teaching. During individual teaching, summarize important points in writing, perhaps listing them in a pamphlet that the client can take home to review. Also, keep in mind that creative teaching strategies make learning more enjoyable.

For the multiparous client, provide opportunities for teaching and discussion of topics of specific interest. Hiser (1987) found that most concerns of multiparous clients after discharge are affective rather than psychomotor. Appropriate affective topics might include how the client can meet the needs of other children, find time for herself, and regain a positive body image while caring for her neonate.

Postpartal examination. Make sure the client knows that she must visit the nurse-midwife or physician for the postpartal examination—usually 4 to 6 weeks after delivery, but as soon as 2 weeks if the client was discharged early. To reinforce this information, provide a written reminder. Also review danger signs the client should watch for after discharge. Advise her to call the nurse-midwife or physician if any of these signs arise.

SELF-CARE AFTER DISCHARGE

As you recover from delivery and welcome a new child into your life, you may experience dramatic physical and emotional changes. The guidelines below will help ensure your well-being during this challenging period.

Postpartal warning signs
If you have any of the following problems after discharge, notify your doctor promptly:
- heavy vaginal bleeding or passage of clots or tissue fragments
- a fever of 100.2° F or higher for 24 hours or longer
- a red, warm, painful area in either breast
- excessive breast tenderness not relieved by a support bra, pain pills, or warm or cool compresses
- pain on urination or voiding of only small amounts of urine
- a warm, red, tender area on either leg, especially the calf.

Hygiene, rest, and nutrition
- When using a sanitary belt and perineal pad, attach the front tab on the pad first and wear the pad with the blue line away from your body. To prevent contamination from fecal organisms, apply and remove the pad from front to back. Change the pad every 4 hours.
- Before emptying your bladder or moving your bowels, remove the perineal pad, using a front-to-back motion. Afterward, use a perineal squirt or spray bottle to cleanse the perineum. Wipe or pat the area gently with toilet tissue, again moving from front to back, then apply a fresh pad.
- After voiding or moving your bowels, wipe from front to back, then wash your hands thoroughly.
- Take a shower daily. Once the perineum has healed, you may take tub baths.
- Avoid sexual intercourse and do not place anything in your vagina (including tampons and douches) until after the postpartal examination (if your doctor advises).
- Rest frequently during the day, especially if you must awaken during the night to care for your infant.
- Consume a nourishing diet—at least 2,200 calories daily (2,500 calories if you are breast-feeding). Include foods from all four food groups. If you have trouble moving your bowels, add high-fiber foods (such as fresh fruits and vegetables, bran, and prunes) to your diet.

Breast care. Regardless of the infant feeding method the client is using, teach her to inspect her breasts daily, using a circular palpation pattern. This also is a good time to stress the importance of the monthly breast self-examination.

With the bottle-feeding client, who must suppress lactation, inform her that she may notice an occasional release of milk and may experience some breast fullness and discomfort until milk production ceases. Instruct her to drink adequate, but not excessive, amounts of fluids. For severe breast discomfort, recommend a mild analgesic or application of ice packs. Also instruct her to wear a snug bra day and night for the first few weeks after discharge and to wash her breasts daily with mild soap and water when she showers or bathes. Warn her not to let the shower stream run directly onto her breasts because this could stimulate them, causing lactation.

Rest and sleep requirements. Advise the client to anticipate increased sleep and rest requirements after discharge. Also counsel her to have realistic expectations of herself, her neonate, and her family. Some clients assume that they will be able to resume their usual schedule immediately, preparing all meals or returning to full-time work at home or at the office. Such expectations may prevent satisfactory adjustment to the new role. Consequently, recommend that the client limit her activities to caring for herself and the neonate for the first week after discharge, then increase other activities gradually over the following weeks.

If the client has limited support and must be self-sufficient after discharge, help her set priorities and reasonable goals so that she can get adequate rest. Also urge her to ask a friend or relative to help during the first week or two at home if possible. Such a person could assist with laundry, shopping, and care of older children.

Resumption of sexual activity. If the client does not ask when she can resume sexual intercourse, provide an opening—for instance, by saying, "Many clients are not sure when they can safely resume sexual intercourse and have questions about birth control." Inform her that she should avoid sexual intercourse until the nurse-midwife or physician has conducted the postpartal examination and evaluated her condition. If her postpartal recovery is satisfactory, the nurse-midwife or physician probably will inform her that she may resume sexual intercourse at that time. However, advise her that intercourse must be gentle at first because the vaginal and perineal areas may remain tender. Also, she may need to use a lubricant because postpartal hormonal changes may cause vaginal dryness.

Caution the client that she can become pregnant during the postpartal period—whether or not she is breast-feeding. Identify her need for family planning information by determining how she and her partner would feel about another pregnancy occurring so soon after this one.

Based on her teaching needs, review family planning methods and refer the client to appropriate follow-up resources.

Postpartal exercises. Provide the client with teaching materials on exercises. Also, inform her that after the postpartal examination the nurse-midwife or physician may approve more vigorous exercise, such as paced walking, swimming, and low-impact aerobics. If appropriate, recommend a community exercise program supervised by an experienced teacher.

For the client with especially poor abdominal tone, institute a teaching plan focusing on improving body tone before discharge or refer her to a postpartal exercise program.

Community resources. Despite the advantages of early discharge—lower health care facility costs, reduced exposure to pathogens, and enhanced parent-infant bonding (Jansson, 1985)—the practice has some drawbacks. Home visits to clients who were discharged early have uncovered breast-feeding problems, transitory depression, fatigue, neonatal icterus, and poor parent-infant bonding. To help prevent or minimize such problems, inform the client about community resources that can help her and her partner make a more satisfactory adjustment to parenthood. In many regions, for example, community health nurses make home visits to provide guidance, support, and counseling as well as assess the health of the client and neonate. The nurse also may offer information and support through follow-up telephone calls.

Preparing the client for discharge

When the client is ready for discharge, make sure she has sufficient supplies, such as perineal pads, a 24-hour supply of infant formula (if necessary), and satisfactory clothing for the neonate. If the family is having financial problems, refer them to a social worker, who may be able to provide some of these items.

If the family plans to go home by automobile, make sure an infant car seat or restraint is available; in many states, such a seat is required by law. Inform the parents that studies show that an adult's lap is not a safe place for the neonate to ride (Kidwell-Udin, Jacobson, and Jensen, 1987). In fact, a neonate held on the lap may suffer fatal injury in an accident.

EVALUATION

The following examples illustrate appropriate evaluation statements for the postpartal client and her family:

- The client maintained vital signs within a normal range.
- The client's uterus remained firm and the fundus descended 1 cm toward the symphysis each day.
- The client had a normal lochial flow with no large clots, tissue fragments, or membranes.
- The client demonstrated adequate healing of the episiotomy, with no exudate.
- The client ambulated within 2 hours of vaginal delivery.
- The client showed positive interaction with the neonate.
- The client knows how to care for her perineum.
- The client can determine whether her lochial flow is normal.
- The client can state danger signs to stay alert for after discharge.
- The client can state when to return to her nurse-midwife or physician for the postpartal examination.
- The client had early contact with the neonate and showed positive bonding behaviors, such as fondling, kissing, and cuddling.
- The client expressed an understanding of the best times to interact with the neonate.
- The client has responded appropriately to neonatal communication cues.
- The client showed increasing proficiency and confidence in caregiving skills.
- The client allowed the neonate's siblings to visit the neonate and called them on the telephone several times during her stay.
- The client's partner expressed realistic expectations for the client's postpartal recovery.
- The neonate's grandparents gave support and encouragement to the parents and siblings.

DOCUMENTATION

Thorough documentation not only allows the nurse to evaluate the effectiveness of the care plan, but it also makes this information available to other members of the health care team, helping to ensure consistency of care.

Documentation for the postpartal client should include:

- location and condition of the fundus
- amount, color, and consistency of lochia
- appearance of the perineum, episiotomy, or surgical incision
- physical findings from the examination of the breasts and extremities
- bowel and bladder elimination status
- client's comfort level and any necessary interventions to improve it
- client's activity level and rest and sleep patterns

- nature of the client's interaction with the neonate
- client teaching provided and the client's understanding of this teaching
- client's ability to use sitz baths and other perineal comfort measures
- client's use of a support bra.

Documentation of nursing care for the postpartal family should include:

- signs of positive bonding, or lack of such signs
- the quality of parent-neonate interaction
- client's ability to interpret and respond appropriately to neonatal communication cues
- evidence of reciprocity and synchrony in parent-neonate communication
- client's progression through the stages of maternal adaptation
- client's emotional status, including any signs of postpartal depression
- father's emotional status and adaptation to parenthood
- client's caregiving skills
- availability of practical and emotional support after discharge
- adaptation of siblings and grandparents to the neonate's birth.

CHAPTER SUMMARY

Chapter 24 described nursing care during the normal postpartal period. Here are the chapter highlights.

Parenting is a complex process with emotional and physical components. The birth of a neonate necessitates changes in family interrelationships and in tasks, responsibilities, and life-styles of individual family members.

The quality of parent-infant interaction has important implications for the future of the parent-child relationship and the child's psychological development.

Maternal adaptation to the parental role occurs in three phases: taking in (dependent phase), taking hold (dependent-independent phase), and letting go (interdependent phase).

Although father-neonate interactions and adaptation to the paternal role have not been studied thoroughly, research suggests that fathers have intense feelings toward their neonates and that early father-neonate contact eases the adjustment to parenthood.

In the first 24 hours after delivery, the client normally may have a slight temperature elevation. After this time, however, a persistent elevation may indicate an infection, which the nurse must report and investigate immediately.

Approximately 2 to 4 hours after delivery, the client's pulse typically decreases as the result of normal physiologic phenomena.

Decreased blood pressure may reflect excessive blood loss, as from uterine hemorrhage; increased blood pressure may indicate PIH.

The uterus should follow a predictable course of movement during involution. At all times, the fundus should feel firm and be located at the midline. A soft, or boggy, fundus suggests uterine atony; this in turn could lead to hemorrhage. To stimulate uterine contractions, the nurse may massage the uterus gently.

The nurse should monitor lochial discharge, noting its consistency and any deviation from the normal progression through the lochial stages—lochia rubra, lochia serosa, and lochia alba.

The nurse should make every attempt to keep the client's bladder empty. If the client cannot void because of pain, edema, or the effects of anesthesia, catheterization may be necessary.

Excitement, excessive blood loss, or medications used during labor and delivery may compromise respiratory status during the postpartal period. The postcesarean client is at increased risk for respiratory problems because of immobility and the effects of anesthesia.

Hypercoagulability resulting from decreased plasma volume places the postpartal client at increased risk for thromboembolism. To minimize this risk, the nurse should encourage early ambulation.

The nurse can help promote spontaneous bowel movements by providing a high-fiber, well-balanced diet; encouraging increased fluid intake and early exercise; and advising the client to heed the urge to defecate.

The nurse may suggest mild exercise shortly after delivery to improve muscle tone and improve lung expansion. Later, the physician may recommend a more comprehensive postpartal exercise program.

Although nursing assessment and interventions focus on the mother because she is the primary client, the nurse should incorporate other family members into the nursing process.

The nurse should assess the client's and family's interaction with the neonate and, if appropriate, document this information in the client's chart.

Sibling jealousy is a normal reaction to the birth of a new family member and usually diminishes over time.

Grandparents can help the postpartal family adapt to childbirth by giving emotional support and helping with child care. However, nursing interventions may be necessary to resolve conflicts between parents and grandparents over child-care practices.

With the increasing incidence of early discharge, the nurse must assess the client's learning needs quickly and effectively and implement an appropriate teaching plan. Postpartal teaching topics include postdischarge danger signs, breast care, rest and sleep requirements, resumption of sexual activity, postpartal exercises, and community resources.

STUDY QUESTIONS

1. What are the optimal conditions for parent-neonate interaction?

2. At 4 hours postpartum, Mrs. Segal, a 38-year-old multiparous client, has a boggy uterus that is displaced above and to the right of the umbilicus. After assessing Mrs. Segal, the nurse determines that her bladder is distended. Which interventions should the nurse carry out?

3. Mrs. Debra Reed, age 23, is a primiparous client. At 3 hours postpartum, she has a slight temperature elevation (99.9° F); however, her blood pressure has remained stable. What is the likely cause of the temperature elevation, and how should the nurse follow the client's condition?

4. Sandra Stelle, age 15, will be discharged in 18 hours. What should the nurse include in a teaching plan to prepare her to care for herself upon returning home?

5. Mrs. Dugan, age 24, and Mr. Dugan, age 25, have just had their first child. Which factors should the nurse assess to determine how well they are adapting to the birth of their child?

6. Which nursing interventions should the nurse carry out to enhance Mrs. Dugan's interaction with her neonate and promote effective maternal-infant communication?

7. On a visit to the nursery, Jimmy Gains, age 5, pinches his new baby brother. Which interventions should the nurse use to help his parents deal with his feelings of jealousy over the addition of a new family member?

BIBLIOGRAPHY

Blauvelt, H., and McKenna, J. (1961). Mother-neonate interaction capacity of the human newborn for orientation. In B.M. Forss (Ed.), *Determinates of infant behavior,* Vol. 1. New York: Wiley.

Condon, W.S., and Sander, L.W. (1974). Synchrony demonstrated between movements of the neonate and adult speech. *Child Development,* 45(2), 456-462.

de Chateau, P. (1976). Neonatal care routines: Influences on maternal and infant behavior and on breastfeeding. Thesis. Umea, Sweden.

Lang, R. (1972). *Birth book.* Ben Lomond, CA: Genesis Press.

Mead, G.H. (1934). *Mind, self and society.* Chicago: University of Chicago Press.

Mechanic, D. (1978). *Medical sociology* (2nd ed.) New York: Free Press.

Piaget, J. (1976). *Psychology of intelligence.* Lanham, MD: Littlefield.

Scott, L. (1988). *Time out for motherhood.* Los Angeles: Jeremy P. Tarcher.

Assessment

Clark, A. (1978). *Culture, childbearing, health professionals.* Philadelphia: F.A. Davis.

Cunningham, F., MacDonald, P., and Gant, N. (1989). *Williams obstetrics* (18th ed.). East Norwalk, CT: Appleton & Lange.

Gibbs, R.S., and Weinstein, A.J. (1976). Puerperal infection in the antibiotics era. *American Journal of Obstetrics and Gynecology,* 124(7), 769-787.

Jacobson, H. (1985). A standard for assessing lochia volume. *MCN,* 10(3), 174-175.

Rutledge, D.L., and Pridham, K.F. (1987). Postpartum mothers' perceptions of competence for infant care. *JOGNN,* 16(3), 185-194.

Intervention

Avant, K.C. (1988). Stressors on the childbearing family. *JOGNN,* 17(3), 179-185.

Fullar, S.A. (1986). Care of postpartum adolescents. *MCN,* 11(6), 398-403.

Gay, J.T., Edgil, A.E., and Douglas, A.B. (1988). Reva Rubin revisited. *JOGNN,* 17(6), 394-399.

Hampson, S. (1989). Nursing interventions for the first three postpartum months. *JOGNN,* 18(2), 116-122.

Jansson, P. (1985). Early postpartum discharge. *AJN,* 85(5), 547-550.

Kidwell-Udin, P., Jacobson, D., and Jensen, R. (1987). It's never too soon to teach car safety. *MCN,* 12(5), 344-345.

Konrad, C.J. (1987). Helping mothers integrate the birth experience. *MCN,* 12(4), 268-269.

Nice, F.J. (1989). Can a breastfeeding mother take medication without harming her infant? *MCN,* 14(1), 27-31.

Phillips, C.R. (1988). Rehumanizing maternal-child nursing. *MCN,* 13(5), 313-318.

Rubin, R. (1975). Maternal tasks in pregnancy. *MCN,* 4, 143-153.

Rubin, R. (1984). *Maternal identity and the maternal experience.* New York: Springer.

Taubenheim, A.M., and Silbernagel, T. (1988). Meeting the needs of expectant fathers. *MCN,* (13)2, 110-113.

Vezeau, T.M., and Hallsten, D.A. (1987). Making the transition to mother-baby care. *MCN,* 12(3), 193-198.

Parent-infant bonding

American Medical Association (1977, December 4-7). *Statement on parent and newborn interaction.* Presented at the meeting of the House of Delegates, Chicago.

Avant, P.K. (1980). Maternal attachment and anxiety: An exploratory study. *Dissertation Abstracts International,* 40, 165 B. University Microfilms No. 79-15863.

Avant, P.K. (1982). Anxiety as a potential factor affecting maternal attachment. *JOGNN,* 6, 416.

Bills, B.J. (1980). Enhancement of parental-newborn affectional bonds. *Journal of Nurse-Midwifery, 25*(5), 21-26.

Bowlby, J. (1969). *Attachment.* New York: Basic Books.

Brazelton, T.B. (1973). *Neonatal behavioral assessment scale.* Philadelphia: Lippincott.

Brazelton, T.B. (1974). Does the neonate shape his environment? In D. Bergsman (Ed.), *The infant at risk.* White Plains, NY: National Foundation of the March of Dimes.

Brazelton, T.B. (1978, Winter). The remarkable talents of the newborn. *Birth Family Journal, 5,* 187-191.

Brazelton, T.B., et al. (1974). The origin of reciprocity: The early mother-infant interaction. In M. Lewis and L.A. Rosenblum, (Eds.), *The origins of behavior,* Vol. 1: The effect of the infant on its caregiver. New York: Wiley.

Broussard, E.R. (1978). Psychosocial disorders in children: Early assessment of infants at risk. *Continuing Education for the Family Physician, 8*(2), 44-57.

Broussard, E.R., and Hartner, M.S.S. (1970). Maternal perception of the neonate as related to development. *Child Psychiatry and Human Development, 1*(1), 16-25.

Broussard, E.R., and Hartner, M.S.S. (1971). Further considerations regarding maternal perception of the newborn. In J. Hellmuth (Ed.), *Exceptional infant, Vol. 2, Studies in abnormalities.* New York: Brunner/Mazel.

Censullo, M., Lester, B., and Hoffmann, J. (1985). Rhythmic patterning in mother-newborn interaction. *Nursing Research, 34*(6), 342-346.

Cohler, B.J., Grunebaum, H.U., Weiss, J.L., Hartman, C.R., and Gallant, D.S. (1976). Child care attitudes and adaptation to the maternal role among mentally ill and well mothers. *American Journal of Orthopsychiatry, 46*(1), 123-134.

de Chateau, P. (1976a). The influence of early contact on maternal and infant behavior in primiparae. *Birth and the Family Journal, 3*(4), 149-155.

de Chateau, P. (1976b). Neonatal care routines: Influences on maternal and infant behavior and on breastfeeding. Thesis. Umea, Sweden.

de Chateau, P., and Wiberg, B. (1977a). Long-term effect on mother-infant behavior of extra contact during the first hour postpartum, I. First observation at 36 hours. *Acta Paediatrica Scandinavica, 66*(2), 137-143.

de Chateau, P., and Wiberg, B. (1977b). Long-term effect on mother-infant behavior of extra contact during the first hour postpartum, II. Follow-up at three months. *Acta Paediatrica Scandinavica, 66*(2), 145-151.

Field, T. (1978). Interaction behaviors of primary verus secondary caretaker fathers. *Developmental Psychology, 14*(2), 183-184.

Frommer, F.A., and O'Shea, G. (1973). Antenatal identification of women liable to have problems in managing their infants. *British Journal of Psychiatry, 123*(573), 149-156.

Giefer, M.A., and Nelson, C. (1981). Principles and practice: A method to help new fathers develop parenting skills. *JOGNN, 10*(6), 455-457.

Greenberg, M., and Morris, N. (1974). Engrossment: The newborn's impact upon the father. *American Journal of Orthopsychiatry, 44*(4), 520-531.

Hiser, P.L. (1987). Concerns of multiparas during the second postpartum week. *JOGNN, 16*(3), 195-203.

Humenick, S., and Bugen, L.A. (1987). Parenting roles: Expectation versus reality. *MCN, 12*(1), 36-39.

Jones, C. (1981). Father to infant attachment: Effects of early contact and characteristics of the infant. *Research in Nursing and Health, 4,* 183-192.

Keefe, M.R. (1988). The impact of infant rooming-in on maternal sleep at night. *JOGNN, 17*(2), 122-126.

Klaus, M.H, Jerauld, R., Kreger, N.C., McAlpine, W., Steffa, M., and Kennell, J.H. (1972). Maternal attachment: Importance of the first postpartum days. *New England Journal of Medicine, 286*(9), 460-463.

Klaus, M.H., and Kennell, J.H. (1976). Human maternal and parental behaviors. In M.H. Klaus and J.H. Kennell (Eds.), *Maternal-infant bonding.* St. Louis: Mosby.

Klaus, M.H., and Kennell, J.H. (1982). *Parent-infant bonding* (2nd ed.). St. Louis: Mosby.

Klaus, M.H., and Kennell, J.H. (1983). *Bonding: The beginnings of parent-infant attachment.* St. Louis: Mosby.

Klaus, M.H., Kennell, J.H., Plumb, N., and Zuehlke, S. (1970). Human maternal behavior at the first contact with her young. *Pediatrics, 46*(2), 187-192.

Korner, A.F. (1967). Individual differences at birth: Implications for early experience and later development. *Journal of the American Academy of Child Psychiatry, 6,* 676-690.

Lamb, M.E. (1982). Early contact and maternal-infant bonding: One decade later. *Pediatrics, 70*(5), 763-768.

Mercer, R.T. (1983). Parent-infant attachment. In L.J. Sonstegard (Ed.), *Women's Health, Vol. 2, Childbearing.* New York: Grune & Stratton.

Park, R.D. (1979). Perspectives on father-infant interaction. In J.D. Osofsky (Ed.), *The handbook of infant development.* New York: Wiley.

Porter, R.H., Cernoch, J.M., and McLaughlin, F.J. (1983). Maternal recognition of neonates through olfactory cues. *Physiology and Behavior, 1*(30), 151-154.

Porter, R.H., Cernoch, J.M., and Perry, S. (1983). The importance of odors in maternal-infant interactions. *MCN, 12*(3), 147-154.

Rodholm, M., and Larsson, K. (1979). Father-infant interaction at the first contact after delivery. *Early Human Development, 3*(1), 21-27.

Rubin, R. (1961). Maternal behavior. *Nursing Outlook, 9,* 682.

Rubin, R. (1963). Maternal touch. *Nursing Outlook, 11*(11), 828-831.

Stevenson-Hinde, J. and Parkers, C.M. (1982). *The place of attachment in human behavior.* New York: Basic Books.

Parental adjustment

Bell, R.Q., and Harper, L.V. (Eds.) (1980). *Child effects on adults.* Lincoln, NE: University of Nebraska Press.

Brim, O.G. (1960). Personality development as role learning. In I. Iscoe and H. Stevenson (Eds.), *Personality development in children.* Austin: University of Texas Press.

Brim, O.G. (1966). Socialization through the life cycle. In O.G. Brim and S. Wheeler (Eds.), *Socialization after childhood: Two essays.* New York: MacMillan.

Brim, O.G. (1977). Adult socialization. In D.L. Sills (Ed.), *International encyclopedia of the social sciences* (pp. 555-562). New York: Free Press.

Desmond, M.M., Rudolph, A., and Phitaksphraiwan, P. (1966). The transitional care nursery: A mechanism for preventive medicine in the newborn. *Pediatric Clinics of North America,* 13(3), 651-668.

Erikson, E.H. (1959). Identity and the life cycle: Selected papers. In *Psychological issues,* Vol. 1, No. 1. New York: International Universities Press.

Friedman, M.M. (1981). *Family nursing: Theory and assessment.* East Norwalk, CT: Appleton & Lange.

Garland, K.R. (1978, July-September). Factors in neonatal attachment, Part 1: Keeping abreast. Newborns are people, too! *Journal of Human Nurturing,* 206-213.

Haley, J. (1963). *Strategies of psychotherapy.* Philadelphia: Saunders.

Hamilton, G.H. (1982). Psychosis of pregnancy. *American Journal of Orthopsychiatry,* 49, 330.

Ventura, J.N. (1986). Parent coping, a replication. *Nursing Research,* 35(2), 77-80.

Family adaptation

Horn, M. and Manion, J. (1984). Creative grandparenting: Bonding the generations. *JOGGN,* 14(3), 233-236.

Maloni, J., McIndoe, J.E., and Rubenstein, G. (1987). Expectant grandparents class. *JOGGN,* 16(1), 26-29.

Marecki, M., et al. (1985). Early sibling attachment. *JOGNN,* 14(5), 418-423.

Olson, M.L. (1981). Fitting grandparents into new families. *MCN,* 6(6), 419-421.

Solheim, K., and Spellacy, C. (1988). Sibling visitation: Effects on newborn infection rates. *JOGNN,* 17(1), 43-48.

CHAPTER 25

POSTPARTAL COMPLICATIONS

OBJECTIVES

After reading and studying this chapter, the student should be able to:

1. Identify the major causes of puerperal infection.
2. Describe common causes of and treatments for postpartal hemorrhage.
3. Discuss postpartal nursing management of a client with pregnancy-induced hypertension.
4. Identify the assessment data that suggest thrombophlebitis.
5. Describe nursing considerations for a diabetic client during the postpartal period.
6. Identify a client at risk for a postpartal psychiatric disorder.
7. Discuss the postpartal care needs of a substance-abusing client.

INTRODUCTION

The postpartal period—the 6-week period following delivery—is a time of significant physiologic and psychological stress. Fatigue caused by labor, blood loss during delivery, and other conditions brought on by childbirth can cause complications—some of them critical—in the postpartal client. Prevention of such complications is a major focus of nursing care. Once a complication occurs, of course, the nurse must work to promote the client's recovery and ensure that the problem does not jeopardize the developing mother-neonate relationship.

This chapter focuses on common postpartal complications and related nursing care. It begins by discussing the physiology and etiology of postpartal complications, then shows how to apply the nursing process when providing care for the client with a complication.

PUERPERAL INFECTION

Puerperal infection—an infection of the reproductive tract occurring during the postpartal period—is a leading cause of childbearing-associated death throughout the world (Cunningham, MacDonald, and Gant, 1989). Labor and delivery reduce resistance to infection by bacteria normally found in or on the body. Most puerperal infections result from such bacteria as beta-hemolytic streptococci, staphylococci, and coliform. However, various other organisms may play a role.

Because the duration of labor and the incidence of infection are directly proportional, prolonged labor increases the risk of puerperal infection (Eschenbach and Wager, 1980). Also, rupture of the amniotic sac may allow bacterial entry; the intact amniotic sac normally acts as a barrier, preventing bacteria from ascending into the uterine cavity. Intrauterine manipulation during delivery of the fetus and placenta also can result in infection (Cunningham, MacDonald, and Gant, 1989), as can contamination by health care personnel during vaginal examination in the second stage of labor.

Types of puerperal infection

A puerperal infection develops from a local lesion or its extension. With a local lesion, the infection remains within the original infection site. The vagina, the cervix, a hematoma, an episiotomy, and any laceration of the vulva, vagina, or perineum are potential entry points for pathogenic organisms. An operation incision (such as from a cesarean delivery) also may be the source of infection; the morbidity rate from puerperal infection is two to four times higher after cesarean than after vaginal delivery (Petetti, 1985).

Extension of the original lesion occurs when a localized infection spreads to other areas via the blood or lymphatic vessels, leading to such infections as salpingitis, parametritis, peritonitis, or thrombophlebitis.

Localized wound infections. A localized infection may arise from a repaired external or internal wound. With infection of an external wound, such as an episiotomy, the apposing wound edges become edematous and separate; the wound then exudes pus and possibly sanguineous matter. An internal wound, such as a vaginal laceration, may become infected directly or by extension from the perineum. In this case, the vaginal mucosa becomes edematous and red; necrosis and sloughing follow. Cervical infection, which typically develops from a cervical laceration, may serve as the origin for a more distant infection.

Endometritis. After placental delivery, the placental attachment site is less than 2 mm thick, contains many small openings, and is infiltrated with blood, making it highly vulnerable to bacterial penetration; the remaining decidua also is susceptible to bacteria. Endometritis, the resulting infection, may involve the entire mucosa and sometimes impedes uterine involution (gradual return of the uterus to a nonpregnant size and condition).

Salpingitis. Commonly caused by gonorrheal organisms, this infection develops from bacterial spread into the lumen of the fallopian tubes. It usually manifests during the second week postpartum.

Parametritis. This infection, also called pelvic cellulitis, involves the retroperitoneal fibroareolar pelvic connective tissue; severe cases may involve connective tissue of all pelvic structures. Transmission may occur via lymphatic vessels from an infected cervical laceration or from a uterine incision or laceration. In some cases, however, parametritis represents ascent of an infection that began in a cervical laceration.

Peritonitis. This infection of the peritoneum arises in the same manner as parametritis. Generalized peritonitis poses a grave threat; bowel loops may become bound together by purulent exudate, and abscesses may develop in various pelvic sites.

Thrombophlebitis. This venous inflammation occurs when a puerperal infection spreads through veins – usually the ovarian veins, which drain the upper part of the uterus. In thrombophlebitis, a thrombus, or clot, forms and attaches to the vessel wall. The condition is known as pelvic thrombophlebitis when it involves the uterine and ovarian veins and as femoral thrombophlebitis when it involves the femoral, popliteal, or saphenous veins. (For more information on thrombophlebitis, see "Venous thrombosis" later in this chapter.)

Bacteremic (septic) shock. Parametritis, peritonitis, or thrombophlebitis may lead to systemic infection of the bloodstream, resulting in bacteremic shock. In this condition, vascular resistance decreases, causing a severe blood pressure decline and the threat of imminent death. Bacteremic shock most frequently stems from gram-negative organisms.

In toxic shock syndrome (TSS), a form of bacteremic shock, *Staphylococcus aureus* enters the bloodstream through micro-ulcerations, or small abrasions, in the vaginal or cervical mucosa. Because vaginal and cervical lacerations are common during vaginal delivery, the postpartal client is at increased risk for developing TSS.

ASSESSMENT

Review the client's history for risk factors. (For more information, see *Risk factors for puerperal infection,* page 552.) Because puerperal infection is associated with temperature elevation, obtain vital signs regularly. Suspect an infection if the client has a morbid temperature, defined by the Joint Committee on Maternal Welfare as one that exceeds 100.4° F (38° C) for 2 successive days after delivery, excluding the first 24 hours (Gibbs and Weinstein, 1976). However, be aware that a low-grade fever is common postpartally; during the first 24 hours after delivery, it most likely represents spontaneous sloughing of necrotic decidua and blood from the uterine cavity, not infection.

Be sure to note any complaints of chills, malaise, or generalized pain or discomfort because these signs and symptoms commonly accompany infection. Assess uterine tone and fundal height, and evaluate lochial discharge, noting the amount, color, consistency, and odor. Also obtain information about the client's sleep and rest patterns and hydration and nutritional status.

Laboratory analysis typically reveals an elevated white blood cell count and an increased erythrocyte sedimentation rate if infection is present. Blood and vaginal cultures may be analyzed to isolate the causative organism; however, isolation typically proves difficult because a blood or vaginal culture may become contaminated by various

RISK FACTORS FOR PUERPERAL INFECTION

The nurse should stay alert for signs and symptoms of infection in a postpartal client with any of the risk factors presented below.

Prenatal risk factors
• Anemia
• History of venous thrombosis
• Lack of prenatal care
• Poor nutrition

Intrapartal risk factors
• Cesarean delivery
• Chorioamnionitis (fetal membrane inflammation)
• Episiotomy
• Forceps delivery
• Numerous vaginal examinations during labor, especially after rupture of the membranes
• Intrauterine fetal monitoring
• Lacerations of the vaginal wall or perineum
• Prolonged rupture of membranes

Postpartal risk factors
• Inadequate infection control
• Postpartal hemorrhage
• Retained placental fragments

microorganisms, and a vaginal culture may become contaminated by blood.

For a localized wound infection, inspect for localized areas of edema, erythema, and tenderness; purulent drainage; gaping of wound edges; and dysuria. Stay alert for complaints of pain in a specific area. Lochial evaluation can be important; in a localized episiotomy infection, for instance, lochia may have a foul odor and appear yellow.

If endometritis is suspected, check for a fever (which may range from low-grade to 103° F [39.4° C]), malaise, lethargy, anorexia, chills, a rapid pulse, lower abdominal pain or uterine tenderness, and severe afterpains. Lochia may range from normal to foul-smelling, scant to profuse, and bloody to serosanguineous and brown.

Besides the signs and symptoms seen in endometritis, parametritis may cause a prolonged, sustained fever and tenderness on one or both sides of the abdomen.

The clinical picture presented by peritonitis also resembles that of endometritis. Other possible findings include vomiting, diarrhea, anxiety, tachycardia, shallow respirations, and bowel distention. Also check for abdominal guarding, rigidity, and rebound tenderness.

When thrombophlebitis is suspected, assess for tenderness, warmth, and redness in a portion of the vein; low-

grade fever; and a possible slight increase in the pulse. Try to elicit Homans' sign by dorsiflexing the foot; pain in the calf with this maneuver may signify thrombophlebitis. (For more information on assessing for thrombophlebitis, see "Venous thrombosis" later in this chapter.)

To assess for bacteremic shock in the client who has a suspected or diagnosed infection, stay alert for fever, confusion, nausea, chills, vomiting, and hyperventilation. In early shock, arterial blood gas (ABG) measurements typically reflect respiratory alkalosis. Later, the client becomes apprehensive, restless, irritable, and thirsty; flushing, tachycardia, tachypnea, hypothermia, and anuria are typical. ABG findings may show a progression to metabolic acidosis with hypoxemia.

Besides ABG analysis, the physician will order various studies to verify the diagnosis and guide intervention—hematologic tests, leukocyte analysis, creatinine and blood urea nitrogen tests, central venous pressure, pulmonary artery and wedge pressures, and hemodynamic values.

NURSING DIAGNOSIS

After gathering all of the assessment data, the nurse must review it carefully to identify pertinent nursing diagnoses for the client. (For a partial list of applicable diagnoses, see Nursing Diagnoses: *Postpartal complications*.)

PLANNING AND IMPLEMENTATION

For the client with a nursing diagnosis of *high risk for infection related to broken skin or traumatized tissue*, prevention is the best intervention. Careful aseptic technique, especially thorough hand washing, is crucial. To prevent cross-contamination among clients, make sure each client has her own sanitary supplies and that nondisposable items are cleaned after each use.

Also teach the client techniques that help prevent infection. (Client teaching is important even if an infection already is diagnosed.) To prevent contamination of the vagina with rectal bacteria, instruct her to use a front-to-back motion when applying perineal pads and cleansing the vulvar and perineal area.

For the client with a diagnosed infection, expect to administer antimicrobial and antipyretic therapy. The physician will choose an antibiotic based on the location and severity of the infection, the causative organism, and the client's physiologic status. Usually, the physician takes an aggressive treatment approach, choosing a broad-spectrum antibiotic because blood and vaginal cultures rarely identify specific causative organisms in puerperal

POSTPARTAL COMPLICATIONS

The following nursing diagnoses address problems and etiologies that the nurse may encounter when caring for a client with a postpartal complication. Specific nursing interventions for many of these diagnoses are provided in the "Planning and implementation" sections of this chapter.

- Altered health maintenance related to decreased capacity for deliberative and thoughtful judgment
- Altered peripheral tissue perfusion related to hypovolemia
- Anxiety related to perceived health status
- Body image disturbance related to birth canal injury
- Fluid volume deficit related to active postpartal hemorrhage
- High risk for infection related to broken skin, traumatized tissue, and altered blood glucose level
- High risk for infection related to a fistula, uterine prolapse, or venous stasis
- High risk for injury related to dislodgement of a blood clot
- High risk for injury related to seizure secondary to eclampsia
- High risk for violence: self-directed or directed at others, related to postpartal psychiatric disorder
- Ineffective breast-feeding related to an inability to initiate breast-feeding
- Ineffective individual coping related to a deficit in problem-solving skills
- Interrupted breast-feeding related to postpartal complication
- Knowledge deficit related to aseptic technique and perineal hygiene
- Knowledge deficit related to dietary and insulin requirements
- Knowledge deficit related to the etiology and treatment of the postpartal complication
- Pain related to birth canal injury
- Potential altered parenting related to interrupted mother-infant bonding
- Sexual dysfunction related to altered body structure secondary to a birth canal injury
- Sleep pattern disturbance related to the need for frequent monitoring

infection. Many clients require a combination of oral and I.V. antibiotics.

The physician also may order analgesics to help relieve general malaise, headache, and backache. For a localized wound infection, the physician may incise the infected area or remove sutures to promote drainage.

Independent nursing actions for the client with a puerperal infection focus on alleviating signs and symptoms and helping to meet the client's psychosocial needs. Thus,

be prepared to carry out comfort measures, ensure adequate rest, and provide a relaxed, quiet environment to counter malaise. To promote healing, provide sitz baths or a perineal heat lamp, if prescribed. Teach the client how to clean and change the dressing over the infected area and how to remove and apply perineal pads properly, using a front-to-back motion. Also, ensure a fluid intake of 2,000 ml/day.

Allow the client and neonate to spend as much time together as possible. If she has a nursing diagnosis of *knowledge deficit related to the etiology and treatment of the postpartal complication,* teach her and her family about her condition and treatment, and provide emotional support and encouragement. To help them work through anxiety and discouragement, encourage them to express their feelings.

EVALUATION

During this step of the nursing process, the nurse evaluates the effectiveness of the care plan by ongoing evaluation of subjective and objective criteria. Evaluation findings should be stated in terms of actions performed or outcomes achieved for each goal. The following examples illustrate appropriate evaluation statements for the client with a postpartal complication:

- The client's verbal and nonverbal behavior reflected an increased comfort level.
- The client's vital signs improved or remained within normal limits.
- The client demonstrated adequate wound healing.
- The client was able to interact with her neonate.
- The client demonstrated how to perform perineal hygiene.

For the client with a puerperal infection, these additional evaluation statements may be appropriate:

- The client's temperature is normal and drainage is no longer purulent.
- The client expressed an understanding of infection control measures.

DOCUMENTATION

All steps of the nursing process should be documented as thoroughly and objectively as possible. Thorough documentation not only allows the nurse to evaluate the effectiveness of the care plan, but it also makes this information available to other members of the health care team, helping to ensure consistency of care.

Documentation for the client with a postpartal complication should include the following:

- the client's vital signs
- the client's comfort level
- changes in status
- color, amount, consistency, and odor of lochia
- percentage of perineal pad saturation and time required for saturation
- laboratory results
- the client's feelings about her condition
- the client's ability to care for and interact with the neonate
- effect of the client's condition on her family.

For the client with a puerperal infection, also document:
- appearance of the affected area
- the client's understanding of the treatment course.

POSTPARTAL HEMORRHAGE

Postpartal hemorrhage occurs when a client loses more than 500 ml of blood during or after the third stage of labor. Postpartal blood loss is particularly dangerous because it is hard to quantify or, in some cases, collects in the uterus, remaining occult. Blood loss commonly is underestimated at the time of delivery because precise measurement is difficult; actual loss usually is twice that of estimated loss (Cunningham, MacDonald, and Gant, 1989).

Postpartal hemorrhage may occur early or late. Early (or immediate) postpartal hemorrhage arises within 24 hours after delivery; it occurs in approximately 5% of postpartal clients (Cunningham, MacDonald, and Gant, 1989). Late (or delayed) hemorrhage develops 2 days to 6 weeks postpartum and occurs in approximately 0.1% of postpartal clients (Danforth and Scott, 1986).

Causes

Any condition that results in trauma during childbirth can lead to postpartal hemorrhage. The most common causes are uterine atony (poor muscle tone); lacerations of the vagina, cervix, perineum, or labia; and retained placental fragments.

Uterine atony. This condition may stem from uterine enlargement, such as with hydramnios (excessive amniotic fluid), multiple gestation (more than one fetus), or delivery of a very large neonate. As the uterus enlarges, its muscle fibers become overstretched and cannot contract effectively to compress vessels; thus the uterus continues to bleed, setting the stage for hemorrhage.

Other causes of uterine atony include a prolonged or accelerated labor (both of which exhaust uterine muscles), general anesthesia (which relaxes muscles), or administration of magnesium sulfate (for instance, to stop premature labor). Also, the client with a history of postpartal hemorrhage has an increased risk for uterine atony.

Lacerations. Laceration of the vagina, cervix, perineum, or labia provides a potential hemorrhage site. A cervical laceration is particularly likely to hemorrhage because of increased cervical vascularity during pregnancy and immediately after delivery. Perineal and vaginal lacerations also may contribute to postpartal blood loss. However, these wounds are more likely to cause long-term damage by weakening the perineal muscles, which may necessitate later surgery.

Retained placental fragments. Retained placental fragments, which sometimes adhere to the uterus, can cause hemorrhage by impeding uterine contraction. In some cases, the entire placenta remains in the uterus at least 30 minutes after the second stage of labor (a condition known as retained placenta). Retained placental fragments are the major cause of late postpartal hemorrhage.

Hematoma. This collection of extravasated blood forms when blood escapes into the connective tissue beneath the skin of the external genitalia (vulvar hematoma) or beneath the vaginal mucosa (vaginal hematoma).

Episiotomy dehiscence. An episiotomy may dehisce (split open) in response to such factors as pressure caused by a vaginal hematoma. Also, a client who is obese or who has diabetes mellitus is more susceptible to episiotomy dehiscence because these conditions impair healing.

Uterine inversion. Hemorrhage immediately follows this condition, in which the uterus is turned inside out.

Uterine subinvolution. Uterine atony, retained placental fragments, or postpartal endometritis may cause this condition, in which the uterus fails to return to a nonpregnant size and condition after delivery.

Sequelae

A few clients who recover from severe postpartal hemorrhage suffer anterior pituitary gland necrosis, or Sheehan's syndrome. Other potential sequelae of postpartal hemorrhage include transfusion reactions, hepatitis, and renal failure from prolonged hypotension.

ANTICIPATING POSTPARTAL HEMORRHAGE

To ensure early detection of hemorrhage, the nurse should review the client's chart carefully for the following predisposing factors:

- Cesarean delivery
- Delivery of a large neonate
- Forceps or mid forceps rotation at delivery
- Hydramnios
- Intrauterine manipulation
- Lacerations of the birth canal
- Magnesium sulfate use during labor
- Manual removal of the placenta
- Multiparity
- More than one fetus
- Premature placental separation
- Previous history of uterine subinvolution
- Previous postpartal hemorrhage
- Prolonged labor
- Retained placental fragments
- Uterine atony
- Uterine inversion

ASSESSMENT

This condition can progress to shock, so be sure to assess the client carefully and thoroughly. Because hemorrhage usually can be predicted, review the client's history for such predisposing conditions as a prolonged labor or prenatal anemia. (For other predisposing conditions, see *Anticipating postpartal hemorrhage.*) If possible, quantify blood loss, keeping in mind that a loss exceeding 500 ml is ominous.

Early postpartal hemorrhage may manifest either as a large gush or as a slow, steady trickle of blood from the vagina. Even a seemingly innocuous trickle may lead to significant blood loss, which becomes increasingly life-threatening.

Late postpartal hemorrhage usually has a sudden onset; shock may ensue rapidly. When this occurs, immediate intervention is crucial to prevent cardiac arrest and death. Because late postpartal hemorrhage typically occurs after discharge (up to 1 month postpartum) and without warning, it can be especially dangerous to the unsuspecting client.

To detect trends that may reveal deteriorating status in a client with significant blood loss, measure vital signs regularly and assess skin turgor and color. A serious hemorrhage may cause the skin to turn pale and clammy. It also may trigger chills, visual disturbances, and a rapid, thready pulse. However, keep in mind that pulse and blood pressure may not change significantly until the client loses more than 10% of her blood volume. At this point, compensatory mechanisms triggered by hemorrhage fail and shock ensues; signs and symptoms then vary according to the stage of shock (as described earlier under "Bacteremic shock").

In a client with excessive vaginal bleeding, try to determine the cause to help guide intervention. For instance, assess uterine tone; a firmly contracted fundus rules out uterine atony and suggests an unrepaired cervical laceration as the cause of bleeding.

If the client has severe perineal pain with sensitive ecchymosis, suspect vulvar hematoma as the cause of hemorrhage. A vaginal hematoma, on the other hand, manifests as severe rectal pain and pressure and inability to void. Be aware that a vaginal hematoma is more difficult to visualize than a vulvar hematoma.

To assess for episiotomy dehiscence, another possible cause of hemorrhage, carefully inspect the area surrounding the episiotomy sutures and assess general perineal healing at least three times daily. Pain, a gaping suture line, and a reddened, edematous episiotomy suggest dehiscence.

Signs and symptoms of uterine subinvolution, which also may lead to hemorrhage, include a large, noncontracted uterus positioned above the umbilicus, prolonged lochial discharge, backache, and a heavy sensation in the pelvis.

NURSING DIAGNOSIS

For a partial list of applicable diagnoses, see Nursing Diagnoses: *Postpartal complications,* page 553.

PLANNING AND IMPLEMENTATION

Early identification and prompt, aggressive intervention are necessary to avert grave consequences of hemorrhage. As with puerperal infection, prevention is the optimal defense.

Prevention hinges on averting or treating underlying causes of hemorrhage. To detect retained placental fragments, the nurse-midwife or physician will inspect the delivered placenta for completeness; missing pieces warrant uterine exploration.

After placental separation, the physician may order an oxytocic drug to prevent uterine atony, another potential cause of hemorrhage. When administering an oxytocic drug, monitor vital signs and uterine contractions every 15 minutes. Gentle uterine massage also helps to stimulate uterine contractions. If oxytocic therapy and uterine massage fail to stimulate contractions, expect surgical exploration and evacuation of the uterus.

To prevent hemorrhage from a deep cervical laceration, immediate suturing is necessary. However, perfect repair is difficult, and suturing sometimes causes further complications (such as cervical eversion and exposure of the endocervical glands).

Blood loss from a hematoma commonly is underestimated, so be prepared for the possibility of hemorrhage in the client with a vulvar or vaginal hematoma. (Small hematomas, however, usually reabsorb naturally.) To prevent serious blood loss from a hematoma, the physician may incise and evacuate, or drain, the hematoma. Because incision and evacuation may cause infection, be sure to practice aseptic technique and teach the client how to perform perineal hygiene, especially if she has a nursing diagnosis of *knowledge deficit related to aseptic technique and perineal hygiene.*

To prevent serious hemorrhage from episiotomy dehiscence, the physician will incise and drain the area. If dehiscence results from an infection, the physician will order antibiotic therapy. Aseptic technique, frequent perineal pad changes, and careful hygiene are critical in the treatment of dehiscence.

If the client has suffered uterine inversion, blood replacement and surgical reinversion are needed to save the client's life.

To avert hemorrhage from uterine subinvolution, the physician may prescribe oxytocic agents to stimulate uterine contraction or increase uterine tone. Curettage may be performed to remove retained placental tissue. Because breast-feeding stimulates uterine contractions, thereby aiding involution, encourage the client to begin or continue breast-feeding (if she has chosen this feeding method).

When caring for the client with postpartal hemorrhage, be sure to conduct frequent, careful observations to detect status changes early. Closely monitor the following:
• vital signs
• fundal status, the amount and frequency of uterine massage administered, and any blood clots expressed
• number of perineal pads used, the percentage of pad saturation, and the time required to saturate the pad (weigh pads to assess blood loss)
• amount, color, consistency, and odor of lochia
• fluid intake and urine output (output should measure at least 30 ml/hour).

Check the client's level of consciousness frequently and report any changes to the physician. Be sure to maintain fluid replacement carefully because the client will have a nursing diagnosis of *fluid volume deficit related to active postpartal hemorrhage.*

When administering oxytocic therapy, check I.V. lines for patency, and document the effectiveness of therapy. Also document central venous pressure (CVP) recordings and perform CVP maintenance. As prescribed, type and crossmatch blood in anticipation of transfusion or surgery.

Because this client has a nursing diagnosis of *altered peripheral tissue perfusion related to hypovolemia,* be prepared to carry out the following measures:
• Increase the existing I.V. infusion rate or start an I.V. drip to boost circulating blood volume, as prescribed.
• Assist with insertion of a CVP line (if one was not inserted earlier).
• Administer an I.V. oxytocic agent, such as oxytocin (Pitocin) or methylergonovine (Methergine), as prescribed.
• Give supplemental oxygen at 6 liters/minute, as prescribed.
• Insert a urinary catheter, as prescribed.
• Lower the head of the bed, and position the client supine.
• Monitor the client's vital signs, urine output, blood loss, and general condition.
• Massage the fundus gently but firmly.
• Draw blood for a complete blood count; type and crossmatch for possible transfusion, as prescribed.
• Monitor vital signs every 5 to 15 minutes.
• Provide simple, appropriate explanations to the client to allay her anxiety.
• Keep a count of perineal pads applied, and document the percentage of saturation and saturation time.

EVALUATION

For the client with postpartal hemorrhage, appropriate evaluation statements may include general ones for any postpartal complication (see "Puerperal infection") as well as the following:
• The client's uterine tone improved.
• The client's lochial flow decreased to within normal limits.

DOCUMENTATION

Documentation for the client with postpartal hemorrhage should include the general documentation for any postpartal complication (see "Puerperal infection") as well as:
• fluid status, including intake and output, every 8 hours for at least 24 hours postpartum
• uterine tone and bladder status
• effectiveness of oxytocic therapy
• CVP measurements.

BIRTH CANAL INJURIES

Many clients suffer lacerations of the vagina and cervix during childbirth; also, labor and delivery normally cause changes in the position of pelvic structures.

Vaginal and perineal lacerations. Lacerations of the anterior vagina near the urethra are relatively common intrapartal events (Cunningham, MacDonald, and Gant, 1989). Typically, these injuries are accompanied by perineal lacerations; a deep perineal laceration may involve the anal sphincter and extend through the vaginal walls. Lacerations of the middle and upper thirds of the vagina, less common than anterior lacerations, usually result from forceps delivery; these wounds may lead to copious blood loss.

Cervical lacerations. Cervical lacerations up to 2 cm long are common during childbirth (Cunningham, MacDonald, and Gant, 1989). Normally, they heal uneventfully within 6 to 12 weeks and cause no further problems; however, the external os remains elongated permanently.

Deep cervical lacerations, an occasional result of precipitous labor, may lead to serious hemorrhage because of increased vascularity of the cervix and fragility of surrounding tissues. The tear may involve one or both sides of the cervix, possibly reaching up to or beyond the vaginal junction. Primiparous clients typically suffer more cervical lacerations than multiparous clients (Monheit, Cousins, and Resnik, 1980).

Levator ani injuries. The levator ani is one of a pair of muscles that lies across the pubic arch and pelvic diaphragm, supporting the perineal floor. Injury to this muscle results from overdistention of the birth canal; this in turn may cause muscle fibers to separate or decrease in tone. When this happens, the pelvis becomes relaxed; urinary incontinence may develop if the pubococcygeal muscle is involved (Cunningham, MacDonald, and Gant, 1989).

Pelvic joint injury. Pelvic immobility and subsequent joint injury may occur if the client's legs are positioned improperly during delivery or if she remains in stirrups for a prolonged period.

Pelvic relaxation. Exaggeration of the normal relaxation of pelvic support structures during childbirth may cause displacement of the uterus and other pelvic structures. Uterine prolapse (downward displacement) occurs in varying degrees. In mild prolapse, the cervix descends below its normal position in the vaginal canal; in moderate prolapse, the cervix reaches the introitus; in severe prolapse, the entire uterus protrudes from the vagina.

Enterocele (prolapse of the intestine into the posterior vaginal wall), cystocele (prolapse of the bladder into the anterior vaginal wall), and urethrocele (prolapse of the urethra into the anterior vaginal wall) sometimes accompany uterine prolapse. The combination of marked cystocele and uterine prolapse may cause obstruction of the lower ureter, with resulting hydronephrosis and renal dysfunction.

Fistula. An abnormal passage, a fistula may follow a traumatic delivery, such as a difficult forceps delivery or a delivery in which pressure is exerted during slow fetal descent. The fistula may be vesicovaginal or rectovaginal. A vesicovaginal fistula is an opening between the vagina and the urinary tract (urethra, bladder, or ureter); urine passes into and discharges from the vagina. A rectovaginal fistula is an opening between the rectum and vagina in which flatus and stool may be discharged through the vagina. This type of fistula usually forms after unsuccessful repair of an episiotomy or laceration; although a portion of the anal sphincter heals after repair, the area above the sphincter may break down.

ASSESSMENT

Injury to the birth canal may cause a wide range of signs and symptoms. To prevent further complications, these problems must be detected promptly. Review the client's history, especially the intrapartal records, for risk factors, which include:
- prolonged labor with protracted descent
- delivery of a large neonate
- abnormal fetal presentation
- cesarean, forceps, version, or vacuum extraction delivery
- previous history of cesarean delivery, traumatic delivery, uterine surgery, or postpartal hemorrhage
- uterine retroversion or anomaly.

Other key factors to assess for include the amount and color of vaginal bleeding, level of consciousness, subjective expressions of well-being, vital sign measurements and patterns, and fundal height and tone. Stay alert for signs of impending shock.

An extensive perineal laceration usually is apparent; this wound may bleed and interfere with normal voiding. The Redness, Edema, Ecchymosis, Discharge, Approximation (REEDA) scale may be used to assess the condition of the perineum. This scale, which provides a means for objective assessment, evaluates the five components of healing (as its name suggests). Daily documentation allows tracking of the healing. The total score may range from 1 to 15; the higher the total, the worse the condition of the perineum. A vaginal laceration may bleed and is visible on pelvic examination.

Signs and symptoms of a deep cervical laceration include bright red (arterial) vaginal bleeding with a firmly contracted uterus. The cervix appears lacerated, edematous, bruised, and ulcerated.

If a levator ani injury is present, the client may report a reduction in pleasure when she resumes sexual intercourse. Urinary incontinence may occur if the pubococcygeal muscle also was involved. If the injury caused weakening of the perineal floor, intercourse may be painful (a condition called dyspareunia).

With pelvic relaxation, uterine prolapse is visible on vaginal examination. To help determine the degree of prolapse, the examiner may ask the client to bear down during the examination. Also, the client may report a sensation of a lump in the vagina during prolonged standing or straining. If the cervix is irritated or eroded from its descent, vaginal discharge may occur (although this may be masked by lochial discharge). With cystocele and urethrocele, the client may retain urine, which may lead to frequency and urgency on urination and other signs and symptoms of urinary tract infection.

Pelvic relaxation may cause stress incontinence (involuntary discharge of urine on coughing, laughing, sneezing, or straining). Diagnosis of stress incontinence can be made on pelvic examination by manually restoring and maintaining the normal posterior urethrovesical angle to check for deformity (reflected by an increased angle).

Vesicovaginal fistula causes involuntary discharge of urine from the vagina. Rectovaginal fistula causes involuntary discharge of flatus and stool from the vagina.

NURSING DIAGNOSIS

For a partial list of applicable diagnoses, see Nursing Diagnoses: *Postpartal complications,* page 553.

PLANNING AND IMPLEMENTATION

Any birth canal injury may cause fatigue. Thus, group nursing procedures together to promote sleep and rest. Also, help the client participate in her recovery to the extent that she can. To help avoid a nursing diagnosis of *sexual dysfunction related to altered body structure secondary to a birth canal injury,* teach her how to perform Kegel exercises to strengthen pelvic floor muscles.

Depending on their size and location, some perineal and vaginal lacerations heal on their own. For the client with a nursing diagnosis of *pain related to birth canal injury,* provide pain relief measures and teach the client how to manage pain through the use of sitz baths, topical or oral medications, and distraction. If the client has difficulty voiding, insert an indwelling catheter, as prescribed, until healing begins.

An extensive perineal or vaginal laceration that bleeds profusely requires suturing, as does a deep cervical laceration. Because of their location, labial lacerations are difficult to repair and cause much discomfort during healing.

For a levator ani injury, medical and nursing management vary depending on the severity of the injury as well as the emotional impact on the client and family. In some cases, surgery is necessary; in others, the injury heals spontaneously.

For uterine prolapse, the physician manually repositions the uterus in the pelvis and may insert a pessary to elevate it and support the ligaments. Usually, the physician inserts the pessary initially, then the client removes it before going to bed and reinserts it each morning. Teach her how to insert the pessary correctly; instruct her to wash it with a mild antiseptic solution and to rinse it thoroughly before each insertion.

For a vesicovaginal fistula, the physician will attempt surgical repair. After surgery, the bladder must be drained for 10 days via an indwelling catheter. If surgical repair is not possible, the physician will order continuous bladder drainage because spontaneous closure of the fistula sometimes occurs. For a rectovaginal fistula, management involves surgical repair and antibiotic therapy. Because this client may have a nursing diagnosis of *body image disturbance related to birth canal injury,* be sure to provide emotional support. Passage of urine or stool through a fistula can make this injury particularly stressful for the client.

EVALUATION

For the client with birth canal injuries, appropriate evaluation statements may include general ones for any postpartal complication (see "Puerperal infection") as well as the following:

• The client demonstrated knowledge of pelvic floor exercises.

DOCUMENTATION

Documentation for the client with a birth canal injury should include the general documentation for any postpartal complication (see "Puerperal infection") as well as:
• fundal height
• uterine tone
• bowel status, including the presence or absence of bowel sounds and bowel movements.

PREGNANCY-INDUCED HYPERTENSION

Pregnancy-induced hypertension (PIH) refers to hypertensive disorders that develop between the twentieth week of pregnancy and the end of the first postpartal week. Preeclampsia refers to hypertension with albuminuria or edema. Eclampsia occurs in a client who has preeclampsia and involves seizures, possibly with coma; untreated, eclampsia usually is fatal.

Although the cause of PIH is unknown, inadequate prenatal care may be a contributing factor. Other possible predisposing factors include primigravidity, multiple gestation, preexisting diabetes mellitus or hypertension, and hydramnios. (For a detailed discussion of PIH, see Chapter 9, Antepartal Complications.)

ASSESSMENT

Evaluate the client for evidence of PIH. Usually, signs and symptoms of PIH subside rapidly after delivery. However, in the high-risk client, monitor blood pressure closely during the first 24 hours postpartum. Suspect PIH if systolic pressure rises at least 30 mm Hg and diastolic pressure increases at least 15 mm Hg above the baseline value. Be aware that an increase in blood pressure may signify an impending seizure.

With mild preeclampsia, expect generalized edema and proteinuria in addition to hypertension. With severe preeclampsia, blood pressure increases more sharply and the client typically complains of a severe, persistent headache and visual disturbances, such as blurring. She also may have epigastric pain, hyperreflexia (exaggerated reflexes), vomiting, apprehensiveness, photophobia, and sensitivity to noise.

Inspect the client's hands and feet for edema, which may make visualization of the joints impossible. Be sure to assess fluid intake and urine output; the latter may drop below 30 ml/hour even if the client is receiving I.V. fluids. Weigh the client daily to assess postpartal diuresis.

Promptly report urine output below 30 ml/hour, proteinuria, and other suggestive findings to the physician. In the preeclamptic client, blood volume may increase without an accompanying increase in hemoglobin; thus, an accurate hemoglobin measurement is important. The physician usually orders clotting studies to rule out disseminated intravascular coagulation (DIC), a grave bleeding disorder resulting from damage to the vessel wall. Such damage is a characteristic feature of preeclampsia (Cunningham, MacDonald, and Gant, 1989) and may predispose the client to DIC. (For a more detailed discussion of clinical findings in PIH, see Chapter 9, Antepartal Complications.)

NURSING DIAGNOSIS

For a partial list of applicable diagnoses, see Nursing Diagnoses: *Postpartal complications*, page 553.

PLANNING AND IMPLEMENTATION

Nursing management for preeclampsia and eclampsia focuses on preventing seizures and monitoring signs and symptoms of these disorders. The ultimate goal is to stabilize the client's status by intervening appropriately, providing optimal environmental conditions, and promoting psychosocial adjustment.

If the client was diagnosed as preeclamptic during pregnancy, the physician may order I.V. magnesium sulfate postpartally to decrease the seizure threshold, provide sedation, and dilate blood vessels. (See Chapter 9, Antepartal Complications, for a detailed discussion of nursing care for the client receiving magnesium sulfate.) A narcotic also may be prescribed. Immediately report any change in the client's condition.

Usually, the preeclamptic client will not receive oxytocic agents postpartally because of their hypertensive qualities; therefore, make sure to massage the uterus frequently to promote uterine contractions. Also encourage frequent voiding to keep the bladder empty and thus help avoid uterine atony.

The eclamptic client has a nursing diagnosis of *high risk for injury related to seizure secondary to eclampsia.* To help ensure client safety in case of a seizure, make sure bed rails are padded, an airway is at the bedside, and emergency equipment (including oxygen and suction apparatus) is readily available. During a seizure, do not attempt to force open the client's mouth. Strong muscle contractions prevent the jaws from opening without injury; also, the client may bite off a portion of any object in her mouth and aspirate it during the seizure. After the seizure is over, move the tongue aside with a tongue depressor and insert an oral airway.

Maintaining an optimal environment is crucial for the client with PIH. Minimize external stimulation by keeping the room dark and removing the telephone and television; the ring of a telephone or a flickering image on the TV screen may cause a seizure. Keep visitors to a minimum and visits short. Once the client shows signs of improvement, external stimuli can be reintroduced gradually.

When providing care, be thorough and efficient so as to disturb the client as little as possible. For instance, group together vital sign checks, hanging of I.V. solutions, dressing changes, pain assessments, and other routine nursing procedures. As soon as the client's condition improves, extend the time between vital sign checks.

The client who is not critically ill probably will express concern about her own and the neonate's physical safety, leading to a nursing diagnosis of *anxiety related to perceived health status*. Assure her that her condition is not permanent and probably will reverse. If the neonate is in the neonatal intensive care unit (NICU), encourage her to keep in touch with the NICU staff by telephone. Urge family members to visit the nursery so that they can tell the client about the neonate. If possible, place a photograph of the neonate at the client's bedside.

On the other hand, if the client is too ill or too sedated to inquire about the neonate or even to remember the delivery, suggest that the nurse who attended during labor and delivery talk to her to help her understand the circumstances.

EVALUATION

For the client with PIH, appropriate evaluation statements may include general ones for any postpartal complication (see "Puerperal infection") as well as the following:
• The client's blood pressure declined to within normal limits.
• The client remained free of seizures.
• The client maintained normal reflexes (2 +).
• The client's edema decreased.
• The client maintained a urine output greater than 30 ml/hour.

DOCUMENTATION

Documentation for the client with PIH should include the general documentation for any postpartal complication (see "Puerperal infection") as well as:
• daily weight
• fluid intake and urine output

• presence of urinary protein
• signs of edema
• status of deep tendon reflexes
• consciousness level.

VENOUS THROMBOSIS

Venous thrombosis (thrombus formation in a vein) affects less than 1% of postpartal clients (Easterling and Herbert, 1986). Various conditions predispose the postpartal client to this disorder: increased levels of certain blood-clotting factors; greater platelet number and adhesiveness; release of thromboplastin substances from deciduous tissues, placenta, and fetal membranes; and increased fibrinolysis inhibition. Hydramnios, preeclampsia, cesarean delivery, and immobility are additional risk factors. Since early ambulation has become the norm, the frequency of venous thrombosis has decreased dramatically.

When venous thrombosis occurs in response to inflammation of the vein wall, it is known as thrombophlebitis. When no inflammation is present, it is termed phlebothrombosis. In thrombophlebitis, the thrombus is attached firmly to the vein wall; it is less likely to break away and form a life-threatening pulmonary embolus than in phlebothrombosis, in which the thrombus is attached more loosely.

Typically, thrombophlebitis lasts 4 to 6 weeks, with symptoms subsiding gradually. In severe cases, potentially fatal abscesses develop. Thrombophlebitis is most common in a superficial vein (superficial thrombophlebitis) but may develop in a deep leg vein (deep-vein thrombophlebitis, or DVT). Typically, superficial thrombophlebitis manifests on the third or fourth postpartal day.

ASSESSMENT

Check the client's history for the following risk factors for venous thrombosis:
• obesity
• age over 40
• parity greater than three
• previous history of venous thrombosis
• anemia
• heart disease
• venous stasis from prolonged inactivity, such as after anesthesia and surgery.

With superficial thrombophlebitis, the affected vessel feels hard and thready or cordlike and is extremely sensitive to pressure. The surrounding area may be erythematous and feel warm; the entire limb may be pale, cold, and swollen. The client may have a low-grade fever.

In a client with suspected DVT or one who is at risk for DVT, perform a general assessment, including temperature measurement. Stay alert for complaints of cramping or aching pain in a specific region, especially if that region appears stiff, swollen, and red. Attempt to elicit Homans' sign; however, be aware that a negative Homans' sign does not rule out DVT. Other manifestations of DVT include malaise; edema of the ankle and leg with taut, shiny skin over the edematous area; fever; and chills. Measure leg, calf, and thigh circumferences to document any edema.

When the popliteal vein is involved, expect pain in the popliteal and lateral tibial areas; with anterior and posterior tibial vein involvement, the entire lower leg and foot are painful. Inguinal pain suggests femoral vein involvement; lower abdominal pain, iliofemoral vein involvement.

Pulmonary embolism, a potential complication of venous thrombosis, may manifest as sudden onset of dyspnea accompanied by diaphoresis, pallor, confusion, and a blood pressure decrease. The client may complain of chest pain accompanied by anxiety, tachycardia, and weakness. If these signs and symptoms occur, notify the physician immediately. Prompt initiation of therapy improves the chance for recovery.

NURSING DIAGNOSIS

For a partial list of applicable diagnoses, see Nursing Diagnoses: *Postpartal complications*, page 553.

PLANNING AND IMPLEMENTATION

Preventing and detecting pulmonary embolism are the highest priorities when caring for the postpartal client with venous thrombosis who has a nursing diagnosis of *high risk for injury related to dislodgement of a blood clot.* Monitor the client for dyspnea, a low-grade fever, tachycardia, chest pain, a productive cough, pleural friction rub, and signs of circulatory collapse. As prescribed, administer an anticoagulant, and monitor for therapeutic efficacy and adverse effects of the drug. Observe closely for signs of bleeding, and teach the client about the drug's purpose, adverse effects, and interactions with any other medications she is receiving. For thrombophlebitis, also expect to administer antibiotics.

Do not massage or rub the affected extremity and caution the client never to do this, especially if she has phlebothrombosis. Because the thrombus is loosely attached to the vessel wall, rubbing can dislodge it, increasing the risk of embolism.

Management of the client with superficial thrombophlebitis typically involves local heat application, elevation of the affected limb, bed rest, analgesics, and use of elastic stockings to help prevent blood from pooling in the legs. If these interventions are ineffective, the physician may prescribe an anticoagulant. For DVT, treatment typically includes I.V. heparin therapy, bed rest, analgesics, elevation of the affected limb, and elastic stockings.

Once symptoms subside, the client can resume ambulation gradually. Instruct her to wear elastic support stockings and to perform prescribed leg exercises. Caution her not to stand or sit for long periods and to avoid crossing her legs because this reduces circulation. Make sure she knows how to identify signs and symptoms of thrombus formation, and advise her to call the physician when they occur. Also teach her how to manage symptoms and relieve pain. For instance, warm, moist soaks increase circulation to the affected area, and analgesics provide pain relief. Throughout her stay in the health care facility, encourage her to visit with the neonate frequently to promote bonding.

EVALUATION

For the client with venous thrombosis, appropriate evaluation statements may include general ones for any postpartal complication (see "Puerperal infection") as well as the following:
• The client's condition remained stable, with no signs of pulmonary embolism.
• The client walked increasing distances without pain.
• The client's leg circumference decreased.
• The client expressed an understanding of the purpose, dosage, and adverse effects of anticoagulant medication and the necessity for continued medical supervision.

DOCUMENTATION

Documentation for the client with venous thrombosis should include the general documentation for any postpartal complication (see "Puerperal infection") as well as:
• clotting times and other laboratory values, such as prothrombin time and partial thromboplastin time.

MASTITIS

This inflammation of the breast, which occurs in 2% to 3% of breast-feeding clients, involves the tissue around the nipple and sometimes the periglandular connective tissue as well (Cunningham, MacDonald, and Gant, 1989). The most common cause is infection by *Staphylococcus aureus* bacteria; other causative organisms include beta-hemolytic streptococci, *Haemophilus influenzae, H. para-influenzae, Escherichia coli,* and *Klebsiella pneumoniae.* The pathogenic organism usually enters through a crack or abrasion in the nipple (however, mastitis can occur even in clients with intact nipples). Frequent breast-feeding helps prevent mastitis.

ASSESSMENT

Signs and symptoms of mastitis typically do not arise until 2 to 3 weeks after delivery. A portion of the breast is firm, tender, reddened, and warm; axillary lymph nodes may become enlarged. The client reports chills, malaise, headache, nausea, and aching joints. Typically, the body temperature measures 102° to 104° F (38.8° to 40° C). A culture of breast milk or the neonate's throat will identify the causative organism; elevated leukocyte and bacterial counts indicate infectious mastitis (Niebyl, 1985).

NURSING DIAGNOSIS

For a partial list of applicable diagnoses, see Nursing Diagnoses: *Postpartal complications,* page 553.

PLANNING AND IMPLEMENTATION

Because this infection usually manifests itself after discharge, teach the client how to prevent and detect mastitis when preparing her for discharge. The first line of defense against mastitis is prevention of cracked nipples. Advise the client not to use soap or alcohol to clean the nipples because these substances have a drying effect. Instead, instruct her to use plain water, allow the nipples to air dry, then apply a breast cream that does not contain lanolin. To avoid undue tension on the tissues, instruct her to remove the neonate from her breast carefully at the end of a feeding session. Because mastitis also may result from milk duct blockage and resulting milk stasis, advise the client to breast-feed frequently and to call the physician if her breasts become severely engorged.

Treatment for mastitis includes a full course of organism-specific antibiotic (usually lasting 10 days), bed rest

SELF-CARE FOR MASTITIS

To help ensure a complete recovery from mastitis, follow the guidelines below.

- Breast-feed your infant at least every 2 or 3 hours.
- Begin breast-feeding with the affected breast and continue with this breast until it feels completely soft.
- To allow your breast to empty completely, do not wear a brassiere or other restrictive clothing when breast-feeding.
- Breast-feed in different positions during each feeding session to promote full drainage of all milk ducts.
- Immediately before each feeding, apply a warm, wet washcloth to the affected area. Repeat this as often as desired.
- Gently massage the affected area while you breast-feed.
- Express by hand or pump any milk your infant does not remove from your breast.
- Increase your daily fluid intake by several glasses.
- Rest as much as possible, and ask your family and friends for help with other children and household chores.
- Contact the physician if your infant develops diarrhea (which may mean that your mastitis medication should be changed) or if you do not feel better after 48 hours of antibiotics and breast-feeding.

for at least 48 hours, close monitoring, and client teaching. (See Client Teaching: *Self-care for mastitis.*)

An untreated breast infection may result in an abscess, necessitating surgery. Even after surgery, however, the client usually can continue breast-feeding with no ill effects (Niebyl, 1985; Tully and Overfield, 1989). However, teach or remind her how to place the neonate's mouth carefully on the nipple. If postoperative breast-feeding is contraindicated, advise her to pump her breasts for several days until breast-feeding can resume. This may avert a nursing diagnosis of *ineffective breast-feeding related to an inability to initiate breast-feeding.*

EVALUATION

For the client with mastitis, appropriate evaluation statements may include general ones for any postpartal complication (see "Puerperal infection") as well as the following:

- The client expressed an understanding of breast care.

DOCUMENTATION

Documentation for the client with mastitis should include the general documentation for any postpartal complication (see "Puerperal infection") as well as:
• appearance of the affected area
• the client's understanding of the treatment course.

URINARY TRACT DISORDERS

Because of normal postpartal diuresis, urine production increases markedly in the first 48 hours after delivery; urine output typically measures 500 to 1,000 ml/voiding (Eschenbach and Wager, 1980). This increase in urine production heightens the risk of urinary tract infection. Other conditions that are common during the postpartal period, such as increased bladder filling and reduced sensitivity to the voiding urge, also may lead to urinary tract problems.

Cystitis. This inflammatory condition of the bladder and ureters may result from retention of stagnant urine in the bladder, catheterization, or bladder trauma during delivery. Usually, the infecting organisms ascend from the urethra to the bladder, then spread to the kidneys.

Pyelonephritis. This diffuse pyogenic inflammation of the pelvis and parenchyma of the kidney occurs when a bladder infection spreads to the ureters and kidneys; it begins in the interstitium and rapidly extends to the tubules, glomeruli, and blood vessels.

Bladder distention. This condition may follow urine retention, which results from increased bladder capacity and decreased sensitivity to the voiding urge (such as from bladder edema or anesthetics used during delivery). Also, the client with a distended bladder may void incompletely, leading to urine stasis—a condition that fosters bacterial growth and subsequent urinary tract infection. Bladder distention, in turn, may prevent uterine contractions and subsequent vessel compression, causing hemorrhage.

Urinary incontinence. Urinary incontinence may result from bladder distention with overflow or from relaxation of the pelvic floor muscles.

ASSESSMENT

With cystitis, expect urinary urgency and frequency, dysuria, discomfort over the bladder area, hematuria, and a low-grade fever. With pyelonephritis, expect urinary urgency, dysuria, nocturia, cloudy urine, chills, and flank pain accompanied by a temperature of 102° F or higher.

Bladder distention causes a boggy (soft) uterus that is displaced upward and to the right. Bladder distention with overflow is characterized by frequent voiding of small amounts (less than 75 ml).

NURSING DIAGNOSIS

For a partial list of applicable diagnoses, see Nursing Diagnoses: *Postpartal complications,* page 553.

PLANNING AND IMPLEMENTATION

Expect to administer antimicrobial therapy, provide comfort measures (such as sitz baths), and apply topical antiseptics. Catheterization may be necessary to prevent stagnant urine from accumulating in the bladder. Ensure a fluid intake of more than 3,000 ml/day, and record fluid intake and output. As prescribed, collect urine specimens for culturing.

EVALUATION

For the client with a urinary tract disorder, appropriate evaluation statements may include general ones for any postpartal complication (see "Puerperal infection") as well as the following:
• The client expressed an understanding of perineal care.
• The client's voiding patterns have returned to preinfection status.

DOCUMENTATION

Documentation for the client with a urinary tract disorder should include the general documentation for any postpartal complication (see "Puerperal infection") as well as:
• voiding patterns, including urinary frequency and amount.

DIABETES MELLITUS

Diabetes mellitus refers to a group of endocrine disorders characterized by impaired carbohydrate metabolism secondary to insufficient insulin secretion or resistance to insulin by target tissue. Because pregnancy alters carbohydrate metabolism and increases the need for insulin, the blood glucose level may be difficult to control during pregnancy. Thus, a pregnant client with previously stable diabetes may suffer complications. (For a detailed discussion of diabetes in pregnant clients, see Chapter 9, Antepartal Complications.)

In the early postpartal period, the diabetic client may need little or no exogenous insulin because the rapid postpartal decline in placental hormones and cortisol reduces opposition to insulin. However, as hormone levels begin to stabilize, the need for exogenous insulin increases. Throughout the postpartal period, the insulin dosage must be readjusted to achieve diabetic control in clients with insulin-dependent and noninsulin-dependent diabetes. Clients diagnosed with gestational diabetes usually resume a normal glucose status postpartally.

ASSESSMENT

If the client's history indicates that she has diabetes, be aware that she is at increased risk for developing other postpartal complications, including infection, hemorrhage, hypoglycemia, and hyperglycemia. Also, because of cardiovascular degeneration, the risk of preeclampsia is four times greater in diabetic clients than in the general population (Gilbert and Harmon, 1986).

Infection in the diabetic client typically involves the urinary tract; the vagina also is vulnerable because of altered pH and glycosuria, conditions conducive to bacterial growth (Gilbert and Harmon, 1986). If the client had a cesarean delivery, monitor her closely for infection at the incision site and the indwelling catheter site. If she delivered vaginally, assess episiotomy healing and evaluate lochia for signs of infection (such as foul odor or a yellow or greenish color).

Also assess for signs of hemorrhage; its risk in the diabetic client stems from her predisposition to hydramnios and fetal macrosomia (large fetal size). These conditions cause uterine overdistention, which in turn may lead to uterine atony and subsequent postpartal hemorrhage.

Hyperglycemia or hypoglycemia may develop as plunging levels of placental hormones alter postpartal glucose metabolism. Psychological stressors, such as strong postpartal emotions, and the physical work of labor contribute to glucose alterations. To detect hyperglycemia, assess for thirst, hunger, weight loss, and polyuria. Left untreated, hyperglycemia may lead to diabetic ketoacidosis. Also check for indications of hypoglycemia—tremulousness, cold sweats, piloerection, hypothermia, and headache. Confusion, hallucinations, bizarre behavior, and, ultimately, seizures and coma may occur in late hypoglycemia.

NURSING DIAGNOSIS

For a partial list of applicable diagnoses, see Nursing Diagnoses: *Postpartal complications,* page 553.

PLANNING AND IMPLEMENTATION

Caring for the postpartal diabetic client can be challenging because her blood glucose level may fluctuate widely, causing rapid changes in her exogenous insulin requirement. Medical management focuses on returning the client gradually to her prepregnancy insulin dosage. (The postpartal insulin dosage typically is half, or even less, of the prepregnancy dosage.) The client may return to her prepregnancy dosage within 48 hours to 1 month postpartum, although this varies with the intrapartal course of the disease (Robertson, 1987).

Nursing care centers on monitoring serial blood glucose measurements and observing for signs of hypoglycemia and hyperglycemia, preventing or controlling complications of diabetes, and teaching the client about her insulin needs. Also, ensure proper nutrition and promote mother-infant bonding.

Monitor the client's blood glucose level every 4 hours or more frequently, as needed. Instruct her to call for help immediately if she notices signs or symptoms of hypoglycemia or hyperglycemia. If hyperglycemia occurs, monitor urine for ketones every 4 hours.

This client has a nursing diagnosis of *high risk for infection related to broken skin, traumatized tissue, or altered blood glucose level.* To help detect infection, monitor the client's temperature at least every 4 hours for the first 24 hours postpartum, and notify the physician if it reaches 100.4° F (38° C) or more. To prevent hemorrhage, assess uterine tone and fundal height; evaluate lochia amount, color, and odor; check perineal pad saturation; and monitor bladder status. Good perineal hygiene and frequent hand-washing are imperative infection control practices.

Make sure the client understands the expected postpartal changes in her dietary and insulin requirements, especially if she has a nursing diagnosis of *knowledge deficit related to dietary and insulin requirements.* Emphasize that she should remain flexible and patient because postpartal diabetes control may be difficult to achieve, causing frustration and anger. Also, stress that she should not consider herself "cured" of diabetes if she is able to go a day or two without insulin and eat a regular diet during the postpartal period.

Because insulin does not enter breast milk, the client can breast-feed if she wishes (Gilbert and Harmon, 1986).

However, caution her that the additional 300 to 500 calories/day required to maintain breast-feeding will necessitate insulin adjustments, as may altered postpartal sleeping and eating patterns. Also inform her that the glucose content of breast milk rises along with the maternal blood glucose level.

If the client had gestational diabetes, advise her to have a follow-up oral glucose tolerance test 6 to 8 weeks postpartum. Inform her that she may develop gestational diabetes in future pregnancies, and advise her to seek prenatal care early if she becomes pregnant again.

EVALUATION

For the client with diabetes mellitus, appropriate evaluation statements may include general ones for any postpartal complication (see "Puerperal infection") as well as the following:

- The client's blood glucose level remained within normal limits.
- The client showed no signs or symptoms of hypoglycemia or hyperglycemia.
- The client remained free of infection.
- The client expressed an understanding of the effects of nutrition, rest, and breast-feeding on her insulin requirements.

DOCUMENTATION

Documentation for the client with diabetes mellitus should include the general documentation for any postpartal complication (see "Puerperal infection") as well as:

- serial blood glucose levels
- insulin administered
- signs or symptoms of hypoglycemia or hyperglycemia
- signs or symptoms of preeclampsia, infection, or hemorrhage
- client teaching about diet, exercise, insulin dosage and schedule, blood glucose monitoring schedule, signs and symptoms to report to the physician, and the need for regular follow-up medical care.

SUBSTANCE ABUSE

In some clients, substance abuse is not detected until the postpartal period, when the neonate shows neurobehavioral abnormalities or other effects of maternal substance abuse. The reason is twofold: Many pregnant substance abusers do not seek prenatal care, and even if signs of substance abuse manifest earlier, the client may deny her problem because of fear of possible legal and social ramifications.

ASSESSMENT

Because postpartal hospital stays are shorter than ever, remain alert for and report possible signs of substance abuse. These signs fall into three categories: physical, psychosocial, and obstetric.

Physical signs of substance abuse include chronic nasal congestion, dilated pupils, anorexia nervosa, tachycardia, irregular pulse, and needle marks on the skin. Physical signs in the neonate also may suggest substance abuse.

Psychosocial signs include memory loss, frequent mood swings, hostile or violent behavior, low self-esteem, and a drastic change in financial or social status.

Suggestive obstetric findings include a previous preterm delivery, history of abruptio placentae, hypertension, precipitous delivery, and previous delivery of a low-birthweight neonate.

The substance-dependent client may develop cardiovascular and central nervous system complications. Cocaine and certain other vasoconstrictive drugs may cause a transient increase in blood pressure, which may be mistaken for preeclampsia.

Abusing multiple substances is common and may complicate assessment, hindering anticipation of maternal and neonatal needs. To help detect any drugs ingested in the previous few hours or days, the physician may order toxicologic urine and blood screening. When assessing a client suspected of abusing drugs, try to establish a rapport and convey a caring, nonjudgmental attitude. If she admits to abusing substances, attempt to elicit the following information:

- extent and type of substance abused
- any substance abused by the client's partner
- previous participation in a substance-abuse treatment program
- degree of a commitment to stop substance abuse.

NURSING DIAGNOSIS

For a partial list of applicable diagnoses, see Nursing Diagnoses: *Postpartal complications,* page 553.

PLANNING AND IMPLEMENTATION

The substance-abusing postpartal client requires a multidisciplinary treatment approach. Besides the nurse and physician, a social worker, child protection worker, and community health worker may be involved in her care. Treatment depends on her willingness to admit her problem and comply with a drug treatment program, such as Alcoholics Anonymous or Narcotics Anonymous.

The client may be difficult to care for—irritable, manipulative, angry, defensive, and fearful. If necessary, set limits on acceptable behavior. However, remain nonjudgmental and avoid exacerbating any guilt the client may feel about her substance abuse, especially if her neonate is congenitally malformed or suffering other effects of maternal substance abuse.

Substance abuse may complicate accurate pain assessment and relief. To be effective, any analgesic administered must be equianalgesic to that of the substance (or substances) the client is accustomed to taking. Furthermore, creative nonpharmacologic pain relief methods, such as distraction, music therapy, and biofeedback, may prove challenging. However, having the client rate her pain on a scale of one to ten may aid efforts to evaluate the effectiveness of pain medication. Also, when possible, group together nursing procedures to decrease stimulation and increase rest for the client. Be aware, too, that care is more likely to be effective when provided consistently by a familiar staff.

Keep in mind that a substance-dependent client will not recover from her addiction during her short postpartal stay, even if she wants to. Treatment takes time, and its success depends greatly on the client's commitment and the treatment approach. (The client who received methadone before delivery should remain on the drug during the postpartal period. To establish trust and prevent drug withdrawal, make sure she receives the correct methadone dosage at the right time.)

For information about community substance abuse treatment programs, call the national drug treatment referral hotline (1-800-662-HELP), or urge the client to call this number. Provide the client with the telephone number of a crisis intervention or parent support hotline and arrange for follow-up medical care for both the client and neonate. This is especially important if the client has a nursing diagnosis of *ineffective individual coping related to a deficit in problem-solving skills* or *altered health maintenance related to decreased capacity for deliberative and thoughtful judgment*.

If the client expresses a desire to breast-feed, explain to her that the substance or substances she has been using may appear in her breast milk. If she seems likely to continue her substance abuse after discharge, explain the dangers to the neonate of breast-feeding under these conditions.

The increasing problem of maternal substance abuse has sparked debate on such issues as the rights of substance-abusing clients and their neonates and the responsibilities of all parties involved in their care.

Most states allow a substance-abusing client to be discharged from the health care facility with her neonate unless she has previously abused a child or health care professionals have sufficient reason to believe the neonate is at high risk for neglect or abuse. Early consultation with a social worker can initiate child welfare visits if the neonate is determined to be at high risk for abuse or neglect; a history of substance abuse usually is sufficient documentation to initiate such visits.

EVALUATION

For the substance-abusing client, appropriate evaluation statements may include general ones for any postpartal complication (see "Puerperal infection") as well as the following:
- The client acknowledges that she has been abusing substances.
- The client expressed readiness to enter an appropriate treatment program.

DOCUMENTATION

Documentation for the substance-abusing client should include the general documentation for any postpartal complication (see "Puerperal infection") as well as:
- signs and symptoms of drug withdrawal or continued drug use during hospitalization
- response to prescribed analgesics
- extent of the client's interaction with the neonate, her partner, and the health care team
- absence or presence of signs of mother-infant bonding
- expressions of willingness to be treated for substance abuse.

POSTPARTAL PSYCHIATRIC DISORDER

Childbirth can sometimes precipitate a major depressive episode. In many cases, the client with a major depressive episode must be admitted to a psychiatric hospital for treatment.

ASSESSMENT

This disorder usually arises after discharge. However, a review of the client's history may help anticipate a problem.

Signs and symptoms of postpartal major depressive episode, the most serious postpartal psychiatric disorder, include depressed mood, markedly diminished interest or pleasure in activities, significant weight loss or gain, insomnia or hypersomnia, psychomotor agitation, fatigue, feelings of worthlessness or excessive or inappropriate guilt, diminished ability to think, and recurrent thoughts of death. At least five of these symptoms must be present and at least one of them must be either depressed mood or loss of interest (American Psychiatric Association, 1987). The client may demonstrate a lack of bonding with the neonate, or she may express overt hostility and a desire to harm herself. She may feel unable to love her neonate and may lose her ability to cope with family life and its everyday tasks.

NURSING DIAGNOSIS

For a partial list of applicable diagnoses, see Nursing Diagnoses: *Postpartal complications,* page 553.

PLANNING AND IMPLEMENTATION

Supportive therapy, such as psychiatric consultation, should begin as early as possible. Many clients require hospitalization and psychotropic drugs. Electroconvulsant therapy may be used as a last resort (Theesen, Alderson, and Hill, 1989).

Allow the client to express her feelings freely, and respond in a supportive, empathetic manner. To give her a sense of control, encourage her to participate in her care and the neonate's care as much as possible. Recognize and reinforce all positive parenting behaviors.

If the client's behavior warrants a nursing diagnosis of *high risk for violence: self-directed or directed at others, related to postpartal psychiatric disorder,* notify the physician at once and, if necessary, initiate appropriate emergency procedures, as specified by facility policy. Make sure she remains under observation at all times.

EVALUATION

For the client with a postpartal psychiatric disorder, appropriate evaluation statements may include general ones for any postpartal complication (see "Puerperal infection") as well as the following:
• The client acknowledges that she has a problem
• The client did not harm herself (or others).
• The client expressed an understanding of her parenting abilities.

DOCUMENTATION

Documentation for the client with postpartal psychiatric disorder should include general documentation for any postpartal complication (see "Puerperal infection") as well as:
• the client's verbal and nonverbal behavior toward the neonate
• the client's perception of her parenting ability
• referral to or contact with other health practitioners, such as a psychiatrist
• treatment plans
• conferences with the client's support persons.

CHAPTER SUMMARY

Chapter 25 discussed nursing care of clients with postpartal complications. Here are the chapter highlights.

Puerperal infection is potentially life-threatening, but prompt recognition and intervention may prevent grave consequences. The infection may remain localized to a specific part of the reproductive tract or may spread to more distant sites. A morbid temperature is the hallmark of puerperal infection.

Postpartal hemorrhage can occur early or late in the postpartal period. Difficulty in quantifying blood loss sometimes delays recognition of hemorrhage. However, in many cases, hemorrhage can be predicted from such risk factors as uterine atony (and its underlying causes), lacerations, retained placental fragments, and uterine inversion. Identifying the cause of hemorrhage is essential to treatment.

Changes in pelvic support structures resulting from injury to the birth canal may be permanent. Such trauma is possible during any delivery but may be compounded by a prolonged labor and the use of instruments. For the client with pelvic relaxation, Kegel exercises are a key intervention to strengthen the pelvic floor.

Stasis, increased levels of certain blood-clotting factors, and other postpartal conditions may cause venous thrombosis and the attendant risk of pulmonary embolism. Common treatments include anticoagulant medication, bed rest, analgesics, use of antiembolism stockings, local heat, and elevation of the affected limb.

In the postpartal client with diabetes mellitus, fluctuating blood glucose levels can pose a management challenge. Diabetes also increases the risk of other postpartal complications, such as infection, hemorrhage, and PIH. Thus, prevention of these complications is an important part of nursing care.

The postpartal client who abuses substances is more readily identified now than previously. The nurse should stay alert for cardiovascular and central nervous system complications in this client; if she is addicted, she may experience withdrawal symptoms. A multidisciplinary health care approach can best meet the client's varied needs.

A postpartal psychiatric disorder rarely manifests before discharge. Treatment typically involves psychiatric evaluation, hospitalization, and medication; in rare cases, electroconvulsant therapy is needed.

Other complications that may arise during the postpartal period include mastitis and such urinary tract disorders as cystitis, pyelonephritis, bladder distention, and urinary incontinence.

STUDY QUESTIONS

1. How does a puerperal infection develop?
2. How much blood must the postpartal client lose to be diagnosed with postpartal hemorrhage?
3. What information should the nurse include in a discharge teaching plan for a client with thromboembolic disease?
4. When assessing a client for substance abuse, which physical signs might the nurse observe?
5. Mrs. Sarah Jennings, a primigravid client who is breast-feeding, is going to be discharged soon. What client teaching information should the nurse include in her discharge plan to prevent mastitis?

BIBLIOGRAPHY

Cunningham, F., MacDonald, P., and Gant, N. (1989). *Williams obstetrics* (18th ed.). East Norwalk, CT: Appleton & Lange.

Danforth, D.N., and Scott, J.R. (Eds.) (1986). *Obstetrics and gynecology* (5th ed.) Philadelphia: Lippincott.

Easterling, W., and Herbert, W. (1986). The puerperium. In D.N. Danforth and J.R. Scott (Eds.), *Obstetrics and gynecology* (5th ed.). Philadelphia: Lippincott.

Gilbert, E.S., and Harmon, J.S. (1986). *High-risk pregnancy and delivery: Nursing perspectives.* St. Louis: Mosby.

Gordon, M. (1989). *Manual of nursing diagnosis 1988-1989.* St. Louis: Mosby.

Monheit, A.G., Cousins, L., and Resnik, R. (1980). The puerperium: Anatomic and physiologic readjustments. *Clinical Obstetrics and Gynecology, 23*(4), 973-984.

Oxorn, H. (1986). *Oxorn-Foote human labor and birth* (5th ed.). East Norwalk, CT: Appleton & Lange.

Birth canal injuries

Davidson, N. (1974). REEDA: Evaluating postpartum healing. *Journal of Nurse-Midwifery, 19*(2), 6-9.

Postpartal hemorrhage

Bastin, J.P. (1989). Action STAT! Postpartum hemorrhage. *Nursing89, 19*(2), 33.

Rigby, P.G. (1987). Bleeding: Symposium on bleeding disorders in pregnancy. *American Journal of Obstetrics and Gynecology, 156*(6), 1422-1425.

Wahl, S.C. (1989). Septic shock: How to detect it early. *Nursing89, 19*(1), 52-59.

Puerperal infection

Eschenbach, D.A., and Wager, G.P. (1980). Puerperal infections. *Clinical Obstetrics and Gynecology, 23*(4), 1003-1037.

Gibbs, R.S., and Weinstein, A.J. (1976). Puerperal infection in the antibiotics era. *American Journal of Obstetrics and Gynecology, 124*(7), 769-787.

Gilstrap, L.C., and Cunningham, F.G. (1979). The bacterial pathogenesis of infection following cesarean section. *Obstetrics and Gynecology, 53*(5), 545-549.

Petetti, D.B. (1985). Maternal mortality and morbidity with cesarean delivery. *Clinical Obstetrics and Gynecology, 28*(12), 763.

Wager, G.P. (1983). Toxic shock syndrome. *American Journal of Obstetrics and Gynecology, 146*(1), 93-102.

Wolf, P.H., Perlman, J., and Fortney, J. (1987). Toxic shock syndrome. *JAMA, 258*(7), 908.

PIH

Chesley, L. (1978). Eclampsia: The remote prognosis. *Seminar on Perinatology, 2*(1), 99-111.

Mastitis

Niebyl, J. (1985). When the nursing mother has mastitis. *Contemporary OB/GYN, 29*(2), 31-32.

Tully, M., and Overfield, M. (1989). *Breastfeeding: A handbook for hospitals.* Indiana: Mead Johnson Nutritionals.

Diabetes mellitus

Hollander, P., and Maeder, E.C. (1985). Diabetes in pregnancy no longer a barrier to successful outcome. *Postgraduate Medicine, 77*(2), 137-146.

Leveno, K.J., and Whalley, P.J. (1980). Dilemmas in the management of pregnancy complicated by diabetes (symposium on diabetes mellitus). *Medical Clinics of North America, 66*(6), 1325-1346.

Robertson, C. (1987). When your pregnant patient has diabetes. *RN, 50*(11), 18-22.

White, P. (1980). Classification of diabetes, 1978. In K. Niswander (Ed.), *Manual of obstetrics.* Boston: Little, Brown.

Substance abuse

MacGregor, S.N., Keith, L., and Chasnoff, T. (1987). Cocaine use during pregnancy: Adverse perinatal outcome. *American Journal of Obstetrics and Gynecology, 157*(3), 686-690.

Madden, J.D., Payne, T.F., and Miller, S. (1986). Maternal cocaine abuse and effect on the newborn. *Pediatrics, 77*(2), 209-211.

Postpartal psychiatric disorder

American Psychiatric Association (1987). *DSM-III-R: Diagnostic and statistical manual of mental disorders* (3rd ed., rev.). Washington, DC: Author.

Mercer, R.T., and Ferketich, S.L. (1988). Stress and social support as predictors of anxiety and depression during pregnancy. *Advances in Nursing Science,* 10(2), 26-39.

O'Hara, M.W., Neunaber, D.J., and Zekoski, E.M. (1984). Prospective study of postpartum depression: Prevalence, course, and predictive factors. *Journal of Abnormal Psychology,* 93(2), 158-161.

Theesen, K., Alderson, M., and Hill, W. (1989). Caring for the depressed obstetric patient. *Contemporary OB/GYN,* 33(2), 123-129.

Watson, J.P., Elliott, S.A., Rugg, A.J., and Brough, D. (1984). Psychiatric disorder in pregnancy and the first postnatal year. *British Journal of Psychiatry,* 453-462.

CHAPTER 26

MATERNAL CARE AT HOME

OBJECTIVES

After reading and studying this chapter, the student should be able to:

1. Identify the advantages of caring for postpartal clients at home.

2. Discuss the factors involved in planning for a postpartal home nursing visit.

3. Describe how the nurse can help the postpartal client and her partner improve their parenting skills.

4. Discuss nursing interventions appropriate for a client with postpartal depression.

INTRODUCTION

Increasingly, clients are leaving the health care facility within 24 hours of delivery, with no further contact with health care professionals for 2 to 6 weeks.

More health care professionals now recognize that a neonate's birth necessitates adaptation by the entire family over an extended period. Also, consumers are demanding more personalized care than health care facilities traditionally have provided. Moreover, escalating health care costs and changing reimbursement policies have made early discharge more common; early discharge may increase the need for comprehensive follow-up care at home. Thus, postpartal follow-up has increasingly become a nursing intervention.

Today, a client may be discharged as early as 2 hours postpartum. In most cases, however, early discharge takes place 24 to 48 hours after delivery. Early discharge does not increase the risk of life-threatening complications. Norr and Nacion (1987) found no differences in the types and amount of morbidity between clients discharged early and those discharged later.

Thus, nurses now offer continued support for childbearing families in the home. The challenge for the home care nurse is to ensure continuity of care and maintain a high quality of care while taking advantage of the benefits of the home setting. By allowing a broader perspective for understanding the postpartal family, nursing care in the home enhances family-centered care. Also, because most clients are more relaxed in their own surroundings than in an institutional setting, mutual trust can be established quickly.

At home, the nurse can incorporate the realities of the client's home situation into all aspects of care, making that care holistic and more relevant. For the client, home care means that daily routines and schedules are dictated not by health care facility policy but by the family's normal activities and requirements. Most clients sleep better at home than in the health care facility and benefit from the freedom to choose their own food and visiting hours.

This chapter shows how the nurse can provide support in the home to help ensure a full postpartal recovery and help parents adapt to their new roles. The chapter begins by describing strategies that make home nursing care more effective. Then it describes how the nurse uses the nursing process when providing care at home, including ways of adapting standard nursing assessment methods and interventions to the home setting. The chapter concludes with a brief discussion of documentation.

NURSING STRATEGIES

The key to the success of home health care is close cooperation between health professionals within the health care facility and those providing care at home. The home care nurse should obtain a copy of the discharge plan and review it carefully before the first home visit.

Although most assessment methods and interventions used in the home are similar to those used in the health care facility, home care calls for thorough planning coupled with a flexible, innovative approach. Also, because the nurse is a guest in the client's home, establishing rapport and showing a regard for family customs and routines take on paramount importance.

Planning ahead

Unavoidable disruptions and distractions add an element of uncertainty to the home visit. Telephone calls and unplanned visits by relatives and friends may cause interruptions; noise made by children, televisions, and stereos may break the concentration needed in a teaching session. However, careful timing of visits can minimize this problem.

Setting specific appointment times and verifying them the day before helps ensure that the client will be at home when the nurse arrives. To reduce travel time, arrange to visit several clients living in the same area on the same day; get clear directions to the home and keep a road map in the car.

Establishing rapport

To provide family-centered care, establish a rapport based on mutual trust. Unlike the health care facility, the home is the family's territory; the family's unwritten rules, not health care facility policy, dictate acceptable behavior. Recognize and respect family beliefs, customs, and routines.

Keep in mind that some people are uncomfortable when a stranger comes into the home. To put the client at ease, begin the first visit by making introductions, then clarify the purpose of the visit and describe the services the nurse can provide. Determine whether the client requested the visit herself or was referred by a third party. If she was referred, find out if she understands the reason for the referral; a client who does not know why the nurse is there may refuse to share information freely or even to become involved in the process.

Maintain a friendly but professional manner and convey a caring attitude; also offer an accurate, complete description of the purpose and nature of home nursing visits.

The informality of a home visit can lead to role confusion, particularly in the less experienced nurse who confuses friendship with the professional helping relationship. To avoid this problem, keep in mind that the nursing role, unlike friendship, is goal directed; together with the client, the nurse continually evaluates progress toward goal achievement.

Be sure to consider how the client's cultural background may be affecting her postpartal recovery and her general life-style. Explore the client's culturally related beliefs about childbirth, postpartal recovery, and child rearing. Keep in mind that for some cultures, routine Western postpartal practices—early ambulation, exercise, showering, and warm sitz baths—may seem incomprehensible or even dangerous. In certain non-Western cultures, women may remain in seclusion, follow dietary restrictions, carefully time their exposure to heat and cold, and limit their activity. In a few cultures, women are considered impure during the postpartal period and must follow certain rituals to avoid spreading the impurities (Greener, 1989).

ASSESSMENT

For the postpartal client at home, a complete assessment includes a history, physical examination, psychosocial assessment, evaluation of mother-neonate interaction, and home assessment. However, not all clients may wish to be examined or to answer questions about their personal relationships; thus, the nurse must be sensitive to the client's right to refuse. (For specific questions on psychosocial assessment, see *Postpartal psychosocial assessment*, page 572.)

Assessment in the home has important advantages. If the client was discharged early, thorough assessment is particularly important to detect postpartal complications. Also, assessment in the home yields in-depth data about the client's family, life-style, beliefs, values, customs, and interests and information available only indirectly in an institutional setting.

If other family members are home during the assessment, the nurse can observe family interactions. The effects of relatives, friends, neighbors, and even household pets also can be incorporated into the assessment. By observing the family over time through serial home visits, the nurse gains greater insight into the client and her family, the safety and cleanliness of the home, and the degree to which the parents are providing a stimulating environment for child development.

Despite these advantages, assessment at home poses special problems. For instance, outside the institutional setting, which legitimizes and formalizes the caregiver's role, the client might find some assessment procedures embarrassing or an invasion of privacy. Also, the nurse cannot simply close the curtain for privacy when examining the client, as in the health care facility.

POSTPARTAL PSYCHOSOCIAL ASSESSMENT

To assess the postpartal client's psychosocial status and adaptation to the maternal role, explore her feelings by asking such questions as those shown here. Remember to keep all questions open-ended. If a client hesitates to answer any question, clarify and reword it; if she still seems resistant, go to the next question.

Daily activities
- How well are you managing your daily activities?
- How do you feel about your appetite and the amount of sleep you are getting?
- How would you rate your effectiveness in managing your responsibilities?

Impact of childbirth events
- What thoughts and feelings do you have when you look back at your childbirth experience?
- How do you think you handled the experience?
- What aspects of the experience stand out in your mind and why?

Mother-infant interaction
- How do you feel about yourself as a mother?
- How do you think your infant feels about you as a mother?
- What thoughts and feelings do you have when you are with your infant?
- What concerns do you have about your infant's health and safety? How do you handle these concerns?

Social activities and support
- In what stage are you in resuming your social activities and responsibilities with other adults?
- How is your relationship with your infant's father?
- Since delivery, which social activities have you engaged in that were pleasurable? Which were not pleasurable?

Self-esteem
- How would you rate yourself right now in terms of goodness?
- How well do you feel you are adjusting?
- What thoughts and feelings have you had about your physical attractiveness since the delivery?
- What is your predominant mood these days?
- How do you view your future?

Adapted with permission from Affonso, D.D. (1987). Assessment of maternal postpartum adaptation. *Public Health Nursing*, 4(1), 12. Reprinted by permission of Blackwell Scientific Publications, Inc.

To avoid infringing on the client's or family's privacy or personal space, use sensitivity, tact, and creativity. Let the client choose the best time and location for personal discussions and potentially embarrassing assessment pro-cedures, and obtain her verbal permission before beginning the assessment. If other members of the household are within hearing range, maintain confidentiality by conducting the assessment in another part of the home or tactfully asking others to move to another room for a few minutes.

History

The nurse who has had no previous contact with the client should review the antepartal and intrapartal records carefully.

When reviewing the immediate past pregnancy and delivery, note:
- whether it was a planned or unplanned pregnancy
- the extent of the client's prenatal care
- exposures during pregnancy (such as smoking, alcohol, drugs, X-rays, communicable diseases, and occupational hazards)
- hospital admissions or problems during pregnancy, such as bleeding or infection.

Assess the client's breast-feeding experience, if relevant, and ask about family planning and contraceptive use. Also question her about her sleeping and eating patterns and comfort level.

Physical examination

To assess the client's postpartal recovery and help detect or prevent complications, conduct a brief physical examination that focuses on evaluating postpartal recovery. During the examination, teach the client about postpartal physiologic changes and show her how to assess her progress toward recovery.

In the first few days after delivery, obtain vital signs, staying alert for a temperature above 100.4° F (38° C), which may signify infection. Note any increase in the pulse or respiratory rate or any decrease in blood pressure, which may indicate uterine hemorrhage.

Conduct a review of body systems to check for expected reversal of the changes that took place during pregnancy. To assess uterine involution, palpate the fundus; by the tenth day postpartum, it should no longer be palpable as an abdominal organ. Determine whether lochia is progressing through the normal stages; examine the perineum to determine if an episiotomy or laceration is healing properly. Check the breasts for engorgement, lactation stage, and nipple condition.

Psychosocial status

Ideally, obtain a psychosocial history, keying in on such topics as psychological problems after previous deliveries, the client's social support systems, and any recent or cur-

EVALUATING THE CLIENT'S HOME

To assess the safety, adequacy, and psychosocial environment of the client's home, the nurse should determine the answers to such questions as those shown below.

- How many rooms do the client and her family occupy? Has the addition of the neonate caused crowding?
- Does the family own or rent the home or apartment? Is the cost of housing burdensome to the family?
- Does the home have adequate heat, lighting, and ventilation to care for the neonate and client safely?
- Are the floors and stairs in safe condition?
- Does the neonate have a crib that meets safety standards? Does the client have a comfortable chair and a quiet place in which to breast-feed?
- Are safety hazards present that might impose a danger to the client or neonate, such as missing stair railings or uncovered electrical outlets?
- Does the home have running water and refrigeration? Can the client safely prepare and store formula for the neonate?
- Is the bathroom sanitary? Does it have a toilet, towels, and soap so that the client can carry out perineal care?
- How many bedrooms does the home have? Does the neonate sleep in the same room as the parents, in the parent's bed, or in another room?
- How do family members feel about their home? Do they consider it adequate for the needs of their growing family?

rent family stress. Also assess the client's economic status, review her work history, and ask about her child care plans.

Most postpartal clients express satisfaction and positive feelings; some, though, have ambivalent feelings, which may indicate conflicts that could compromise postpartal adaptation. Assess for other potential signs of poor adaptation, such as disinterest in the neonate, adults, or adult activities; lack of social participation; and social isolation.

The postpartal client may experience mood swings and emotional lability. To check for these problems, ask the client to describe her moods and feelings; be alert to extremes, such as elation and depression.

Postpartal mood swings may manifest as maternity blues, as a more severe alteration in mood swings, or as a major depressive episode.

Maternity blues ("baby blues"), a transient mood alteration, is characterized by sadness, crying episodes, fatigue, and low self-esteem. Usually arising within the first 3 weeks postpartum, it is experienced by 50% to 80% of postpartal clients (Hopkins, Marcus, and Campbell,

1984). Typically, it is self-limiting, lasting from 1 to 10 days (Condon and Watson, 1987).

A more severe alteration in mood swings occurs in approximately 20% of postpartal clients and manifests as tearfulness, despondency, feelings of guilt and inadequacy, and inability to cope with neonatal care. Generalized fatigue and complaints of ill health also are common. Signs and symptoms typically arise within a few weeks of delivery and may last from a few weeks to a year or more (Hopkins, Marcus, and Campbell, 1984).

Major depressive episode, a severe form of depression, occurs in approximately 0.1% of postpartal women and in many cases requires hospitalization (Hopkins, Marcus, and Campbell, 1984). A client with a major depressive episode will have at least five of the following symptoms: depressed mood, markedly diminished interest or pleasure in activities, significant weight loss or weight gain, insomnia or hypersomnia, psychomotor agitation, fatigue or loss of energy, feelings of worthlessness, diminished ability to think, and recurrent thoughts of death. At least one of the symptoms of this psychiatric disorder is depressed mood or loss of interest or pleasure (American Psychiatric Association, 1987).

Mother-infant interaction

In the home, the nurse can observe mother-infant interaction over time and within the natural setting, taking into account the effects of other family members and the home surroundings. An optimal time to observe is during a feeding session, when the client and infant are most likely to interact closely.

Home environment

Determine if the home is conducive to safe, adequate care of the client and neonate and whether it promotes positive psychosocial adaptation. For example, check for safety hazards and availability of basic necessities, such as water, electricity, and heat, and assess whether the client can obtain privacy in the home. (For more information about a home assessment, see *Evaluating the client's home*.)

NURSING DIAGNOSIS

After gathering all of the assessment data, the nurse must review it carefully to identify pertinent nursing diagnoses for the client. (For a partial list of applicable diagnoses, see Nursing Diagnoses: *Postpartal client receiving care at home,* page 574.)

POSTPARTAL CLIENT RECEIVING CARE AT HOME

For the postpartal client who is receiving nursing care at home, the nurse may find the following nursing diagnoses appropriate. Specific nursing interventions for many of these diagnoses are provided in the "Planning and implementation" section of this chapter.

- Altered family processes related to the birth of a neonate
- Altered role performance related to postpartal mood swings
- Altered sexuality patterns related to a painful episiotomy or fear of conception
- Fatigue related to the need to care for the neonate throughout the night
- High risk for caregiver role strain related to postpartal mood swings
- Impaired home maintenance management related to the demands of caring for the neonate
- Ineffective individual coping related to adaptation to the maternal role
- Knowledge deficit related to neonatal care
- Pain related to the perineal wound
- Potential altered parenting related to postpartal mood swings
- Situational low self-esteem related to loss of the prepregnancy figure
- Sleep pattern disturbance related to frequent demands of the neonate or infant
- Social isolation related to the neonate's constant care demands

PLANNING AND IMPLEMENTATION

After assessing the client and formulating nursing diagnoses, the nurse develops and implements a care plan. Nursing goals for the postpartal client receiving care at home include promoting postpartal recovery, helping the client adapt to the maternal role, promoting parenting skills, enhancing the couple's relationship, and helping siblings adapt to the birth of a new family member. Depending on the number of visits the nurse will make, meeting all of these goals may be a challenge.

To deal with newly emerging needs, the nurse also should be prepared to change goals at the last minute to address a sudden crisis. Suppose, for instance, that the nurse plans to teach neonatal care skills to a client with a nursing diagnosis of *knowledge deficit related to neonatal care*. On arrival, however, the nurse finds the client in tears because the neonate kept her up all night. In this case, the nurse should postpone interventions for the long-

term goal (correcting the knowledge deficit) and set new, short-term goals to deal with the client's immediate need for rest.

The nurse should plan each visit carefully in relation to the tentative goal set for the visit. If physical examination is planned, arrive with any equipment that will be needed. Forgetting a stethoscope, for instance, could mean that the goal for that visit remains unmet; scheduling another visit could be costly and time-consuming.

As appropriate, refer the client to community resources, such as self-help groups or parenting classes. Some prenatal instruction classes, for instance, include a fourth trimester class to discuss parenting.

Promoting postpartal recovery
If assessment reveals postpartal complications or delayed postpartal recovery, intervene as appropriate, referring the client to a physician if necessary. For example, after inspecting the episiotomy site, the nurse may determine that the client has a nursing diagnosis of *pain related to the perineal wound.* In this case, recommend a sitz bath three or four times daily, with each bath lasting 15 to 20 minutes. If the client does not know how to administer this treatment, provide teaching.

Helping the client adapt to the maternal role
To help avoid a nursing diagnosis of *ineffective individual coping related to adaptation to the maternal role,* use interventions that help the client regain control of her life. Encourage her to talk about the events of childbirth and her feelings about the experience. Be aware that many postpartal clients are afraid to admit that they feel confused and upset.

Offer praise and reassurance for her efforts to fulfill her responsibilities. If she feels overwhelmed by the tasks of her new role as parent, help her break down large tasks into smaller, more manageable parts. Keep in mind that a new mother needs some mothering herself, so encourage her to nurture and pamper herself, paying attention to her own needs as well as the neonate's.

Teach the client who is having trouble adapting to her new role because of a nursing diagnosis of *situational low self-esteem related to loss of prepregnancy figure* about proper diet and exercise. To help avoid a nursing diagnosis of *sleep pattern disturbance related to frequent demands of neonate,* advise her to sleep when the neonate sleeps.

If other family members are home during visits and are open to participating in teaching sessions, they may be included. For example, discuss with them the client's need for rest, and urge them to offer her physical and emotional support. This may necessitate an exploration of the

NURSING INTERVENTIONS FOR POSTPARTAL MOOD SWINGS

Chalmers and Chalmers (1986) have delineated four areas of concern for the client with postpartal mood swings, sometimes described as postpartal depression—the overwhelming nature of neonatal care, the meaning of motherhood, self-concept, and the relationship with her partner. The chart below shows nursing interventions to help the client deal with each concern.

CLIENT CONCERN	INTERVENTION
Overwhelming nature of neonatal care The time involved in caring for a neonate may seem overwhelming to the new mother. Her concept of herself as a mother may hinge on her ability to feed the neonate and cope with the neonate's crying; when feeding does not go well or the neonate is fretful, she feels she has failed.	• Mobilize the client's support system. • "Mother" the client. • Explore child care options. • Refer the client to a support group. • Teach the client various approaches to coping with a crying neonate. • Solicit the partner's support. • Advise the client to sleep when the neonate sleeps. • Instruct the client to break down large tasks into small, manageable parts. • Give positive reinforcement for a job well done.
Meaning of motherhood For the client with postpartal mood swings, the romanticized view of motherhood that she may have developed during pregnancy is replaced by feelings of confinement, isolation, and lack of time to herself. She feels overwhelmed by the responsibilities of being a mother 24 hours a day and may feel guilty about neglecting her partner and other children.	• Help the client grieve over the loss of her fantasies about motherhood. • Encourage the client to express her anger. • Help the client make social contacts so that she can share her concerns with other mothers. • Help the client find time to spend with her other children.
Self-concept After delivery, a client's self-concept may undergo dramatic changes. Disappointment related to the childbirth experience—for instance, an unexpected cesarean delivery—may lead to feelings of failure and guilt. Weight gain and poor muscle tone may cause the client to feel overweight and unattractive. In some clients, role conflicts lead to resentment and depression. For instance, the client may resent the neonate for interrupting her career; or if the client is compelled by economic circumstances or peer pressure to return to her job, she may feel guilty about leaving the child with someone else.	• Review the events of childbirth with the client and help her accept, understand, and integrate the experience. • Provide diet counseling. • Teach the client how to perform postpartal exercises, such as leg rolls, abdominal breathing, and arm raises, to help her regain her prepregnancy figure and thereby enhance her self-esteem. • Encourage the client to find time for herself.
Relationship with her partner The birth of a new family member triggers many changes in the couple's relationship. The neonate's constant care demands may restrict the couple's freedom, impose on their privacy, alter their sexual relationship, and result in general life-style changes. Also, the client may have role expectations that her partner cannot—or will not—fulfill.	• Reinforce the strengths of the relationship. • Provide counseling about resumption of sexual intercourse and family planning. • Explore the division of household labor and suggest changes, if necessary. • Encourage the partners to communicate openly.

division of household labor to determine which partner takes care of the neonate, looks after other children, buys groceries, prepares and cleans up after meals, cleans the house, and does the laundry. If the client now does most of these chores, suggest that other family members help relieve her of some of them.

If the client has a nursing diagnosis of *potential altered parenting related to postpartal mood swings,* refer her for

counseling or therapy. Also, because sleep deprivation may contribute to postpartal mood swings, help her plan ways to get adequate rest—for instance, by finding a babysitter. (For more information, see *Nursing interventions for postpartal mood swings.*)

For the client with a nursing diagnosis of *social isolation related to the neonate's constant care demands,* help her develop contacts within the community and refer her to appropriate community resources, such as counseling services, self-help groups, and babysitting services (sponsored by many churches).

If the client plans to return to work outside the home, give her an opportunity to discuss her feelings about this. Many parents seek approval for their decisions from health care professionals; provide emotional support to help the client feel better about her decision. As necessary, refer her to community resources, such as day care centers, and offer guidelines for selecting a day care provider. Advise her to consider the provider's personality, age, experience with infants, and fee and the availability of references and transportation. If the parents decide to use a babysitter, suggest that they hire one on a trial basis and invite the person to the home to meet them and to care for the child in their presence (Rothenberg, Hitchcock, Harrison, and Graham, 1983).

If the client is apprehensive about leaving her child with a day care provider, point out the benefits of this. For example, the child may gain independence and trust in others; the day care provider may help the client see the child from a different perspective and may suggest alternative ways of dealing with behaviors that are unfamiliar to the inexperienced mother.

Promoting parenting skills

With more women working outside the home and one-parent families increasing, many parents lack parenting skills and may have a nursing diagnosis of *knowledge deficit related to neonatal care.*

To increase their competence and confidence in caring for the neonate, reinforce discharge teaching of neonatal caregiving skills and provide information about infant growth and development. As appropriate, recommend fourth trimester classes, which offer anticipatory guidance and provide a forum for parents to share their concerns. Also teach the parents about their neonate's capacities and behavioral traits.

Most new parents also benefit from discussing their concerns with other parents, as in a parent support group. Besides offering first-hand knowledge and advice from experienced parents, a parent support group helps new parents feel that they are not alone in their concerns and that their child is not the first to behave in unexpected ways (Rothenberg, Hitchcock, Harrison, and Graham, 1983). Help the parents contact parent support groups by providing information and telephone numbers.

Enhancing the couple's relationship

The birth of a neonate leads to wide-ranging changes in family dynamics and interrelationships. The nurse who makes home visits can help the family adapt to these changes.

Ask the couple what they each enjoy most about their new role as parents, what they find most difficult about being parents, and how they expected the neonate's birth to affect their roles and relationships. Also ask how their relationship has changed and how they would like it to be. Point out that changes in a relationship affect both partners; the neonate's father may feel driven to work harder out of a sense of increased responsibility, whereas his partner may want him to help with child care. Each may feel that the other has the easier job. Discussing the division of household labor, as described earlier, may help clarify or resolve inequities in household responsibilities.

The birth of a child usually alters the couple's sexual relationship. Fischman, Rankin, Soeken, and Lenz (1986) found that the frequency of and desire for sex declines during the postpartal period. However, be aware that the couple may be embarrassed to ask questions about sex. Consequently, approach the topic gently by asking them to describe the changes that have taken place in their relationship, then asking, "And what about sex?" Urge them to share their feelings about sex with each other, emphasizing that many postpartal couples have concerns about sex.

Some clients are reluctant to resume sex out of fear of discomfort, leading to a nursing diagnosis of *altered sexuality patterns related to a painful episiotomy or fear of conception.* If this is the case, point out that intercourse usually can resume once the perineum has healed, bleeding has stopped, and the partners feel ready. However, caution the client that the first intercourse after childbirth may be somewhat painful because of perineal tenderness or vaginal dryness induced by hormonal changes. Recommend the use of lubricating jelly and positions that do not put pressure on the episiotomy site (if one is present), especially for the first postpartal intercourse.

If the client is afraid to resume sex out of fear of conception, provide teaching about family planning. Keep in mind that because oral contraceptives are contraindicated during breast-feeding, the breast-feeding client who used this contraceptive method before pregnancy may have special teaching needs in the early postpartal weeks.

Helping siblings adapt

Siblings may react to the birth of a neonate with jealousy, anger, and other negative behaviors, which may lead to a nursing diagnosis of *altered family processes related to the birth of a neonate.* Help the parents deal with this problem by advising them to spend time alone with each sibling and to let siblings participate in neonatal care.

EVALUATION

For postpartal home visits, the nurse makes two types of evaluations. Formative, or ongoing, evaluation takes place at the end of each visit as the nurse reviews mutually set goals and determines whether the client met the goals. Later, when the nurse and client decide to discontinue home visits, the nurse conducts summative evaluation.

The following examples illustrate appropriate evaluation statements for the client receiving nursing care at home:
• The client's postpartal recovery is progressing normally, without complications.
• The client and her partner show competence and confidence in neonatal caregiving skills.
• The client shows a positive adaptation to the maternal role.
• Other family members demonstrate a healthy adjustment to the birth of the neonate.

DOCUMENTATION

Documentation is particularly important for the client who receives nursing care at home; if care continues over an extended period, other health care professionals are likely to be involved. When nursing visits are terminated, the nurse should prepare a discharge summary.

Documentation of care should include the following points:
• progress of the client's postpartal recovery
• client's adaptation to her new role
• client's neonatal caregiving skills
• adaptation of other family members to the neonate's birth.

CHAPTER SUMMARY

Chapter 26 discussed maternal care at home. Here are the chapter highlights.

Providing nursing care for postpartal clients at home is both challenging and rewarding. As postpartal health care facility stays become shorter, the nurse can fill the gap in support that the client may experience when assuming the parental role.

Home visits call for planning and a flexible, innovative approach. The nurse may have to deal with such problems as distractions, client resistance, and nursing role confusion.

Assessment in the home can provide the nurse with important information about the client's needs, including life-style, beliefs, values, and interests. However, the nurse must respect family customs and practices and may have to find creative ways to ensure client privacy.

The home setting can enhance sharing and interaction between the nurse and client.

Nursing interventions focus on helping the client and her partner adapt to their new roles as parents, teaching them parenting and caregiving skills, and helping the family maintain or resume positive interrelationships.

Postpartal mood swings commonly are encountered by the home care nurse; mild forms usually respond well to nursing interventions.

STUDY QUESTIONS

1. Which strategies should the nurse use to help ensure the success of home nursing care?
2. The nurse makes the first home visit with Mrs. Cain and her neonate 2 days after delivery. Which features about the home environment should the nurse assess?
3. Mrs. Thomas greets the nurse with downcast eyes and a flat affect. Which other signs should the nurse look for to determine if the client is experiencing postpartal mood swings?
4. Ten weeks after delivery, Mrs. Short, age 25, reports that she is concerned because she and her husband have not resumed sex. How should the nurse intervene to help them?

BIBLIOGRAPHY

Balzer, J.W. (1988). The nursing process applied to family health promotion. In M. Stanhope and J. Lancaster (Eds.), *Community health nursing: Process and practice for promoting health* (2nd ed.; pp. 371-386). St. Louis: Mosby.

Fischman, S.H., Rankin, E.A., Soeken, K.L., and Lenz, E.R. (1986). Changes in sexual relationships in postpartum couples. *JOGNN,* 15(1), 58-63.

Flagler, S. (1988). Maternal role competence. *Western Journal of Nursing Research,* 10(3), 274-285.

Gorrie, T.M. (1986). Postpartal nursing diagnosis. *JOGNN,* 15(1), 52-56.

Greener, D.L. (1989). Transcultural nursing care of the childbearing woman and her family. In J.S. Boyle and M.M. Andrews (Eds.), *Transcultural concepts in nursing care.* Glenview, IL: Scott Foresman.

Hampson, S.J. (1989). Nursing interventions for the first three postpartum months. *JOGNN,* 18(2), 116-122.

Harrison, M.J., and Hicks, S.A. (1983). Postpartum concerns of mothers and their sources of help. *Canadian Journal of Public Health,* 74(5), 325-328.

Hiser, P.L. (1987). Concerns of multiparas during the second postpartum week. *JOGNN,* 16(3), 195-203.

Loveland-Cherry, C. (1988). Issues in family health promotion. In M. Stanhope and J. Lancaster (Eds.), *Community health nursing: Process and practice for promoting health* (2nd ed.; pp. 387-398). St. Louis: Mosby.

Rothenberg, B.A., Hitchcock, S., Harrison, M.L., and Graham, M. (1983). *Parentmaking: A practical handbook for teaching parent classes about babies and toddlers.* Menlo Park, CA: Banster.

Stevens, K.A. (1988). Nursing diagnoses in wellness childbearing settings. *JOGNN,* 17(5), 329-336.

Stolte, K.M. (1986). Nursing diagnosis and the childbearing woman. *MCN,* 11(1), 13-15.

Tegtmeier, D., and Elsea, S. (1984). Wellness throughout the maternity cycle. *Nursing Clinics of North America,* 19(2), 219-227.

Early discharge

Lemmer, C.M. (1987). Early discharge: Outcomes of primiparas and their infants. *JOGNN,* 16(4), 230-236.

Norr, K.F., and Nacion, K. (1987). Outcomes of postpartum early discharge, 1960-1986: A comparative review. *Birth,* 14(3), 135-141.

Postpartal assessment

Affonso, D.D. (1987). Assessment of maternal postpartum adaptation. *Public Health Nursing,* 4(1), 9-16.

Blackburn, S., Lyons, N., Stein, M., Tribotti, S., and Withers, J. (1988). Patients' and nurses' perceptions of patient problems during the immediate postpartum period. *Applied Nursing Research,* 1(3), 141-142.

Cropley, C. (1986). Assessment of mothering behaviors. In S.H. Johnson (Ed.), *Nursing assessment and strategies for the family at risk* (2nd ed.; pp. 15-40). Philadelphia: Lippincott.

Hans, A. (1986). Postpartum assessment: The psychological component. *JOGNN,* 15(1), 49-51.

Postpartal mood swings

Affonso, D.D. (1977). Missing pieces: A study of postpartum feelings. *Birth and the Family Journal,* 4(4), 159-164.

Affonso, D.D., and Domino, G. (1984). Postpartum depression: A review. *Birth,* 11(4), 231-245.

American Psychiatric Association (1987). *DSM-III-R: Diagnostic and statistical manual of mental disorders* (3rd ed., rev.). Washington, DC: Author.

Chalmers, D.E., and Chalmers, B.M. (1986). Postpartum depression: A revised perspective. *Journal of Psychosomatic Obstetrics and Gynecology,* 5, 93-105.

Condon, J.T., and Watson, T.L. (1987). The maternity blues: Exploration of a psychological hypothesis. *Acta Psychiatrica Scandinavia,* 76(2), 164-171.

Errante, J. (1985). Sleep deprivation or postpartum blues? *Topics in clinical nursing,* 6(4), 9-18.

Gennaro, S. (1988). Postpartal anxiety and depression in mothers of term and preterm infants. *Nursing Research,* 37(2), 82-85.

Hopkins, J., Marcus, M., and Campbell, S.B. (1984). Postpartum depression: A critical review. *Psychological Bulletin,* 5(3), 498-515.

Kraus, M.A., and Redman, E.S. (1986). Postpartum depression: An interactional view. *Journal of Marital and Family Therapy,* 12, 63-74.

Kruckman, L., and Asmann-Finch, C. (1986). *Postpartum depression: A research guide and international bibliography.* New York: Garland.

Petrick, J.M. (1984). Postpartum depression: Identification of high-risk mothers. *JOGNN,* 13(1), 37-40.

APPENDICES, MASTER GLOSSARY, AND INDEX

N.A.N.D.A. TAXONOMY OF NURSING DIAGNOSES

A taxonomy for classifying nursing diagnoses has evolved over several years. The following list is grouped around nine human response patterns endorsed by the North American Nursing Diagnosis Association, as of summer 1992.

PATTERN 1. Exchanging: A human response pattern involving mutual giving and receiving

1.1.2.1.	Altered nutrition: more than body requirements
1.1.2.2.	Altered nutrition: less than body requirements
1.1.2.3.	Altered nutrition: high risk for more than body requirements
1.2.1.1.	High risk for infection
1.2.2.1.	High risk for altered body temperature
1.2.2.2.	Hypothermia
1.2.2.3.	Hyperthermia
1.2.2.4.	Ineffective thermoregulation
1.2.3.1.	Dysreflexia
1.3.1.1.	Constipation
1.3.1.1.1.	Perceived constipation
1.3.1.1.2.	Colonic constipation
1.3.1.2.	Diarrhea
1.3.1.3.	Bowel incontinence
1.3.2.	Altered urinary elimination
1.3.2.1.1.	Stress incontinence
1.3.2.1.2.	Reflex incontinence
1.3.2.1.3.	Urge incontinence
1.3.2.1.4.	Functional incontinence
1.3.2.1.5.	Total incontinence
1.3.2.2.	Urinary retention
1.4.1.1.	Altered (specify type) tissue perfusion (renal, cerebral, cardiopulmonary, gastrointestinal, peripheral)
1.4.1.2.1.	Fluid volume excess
1.4.1.2.2.1.	Fluid volume deficit
1.4.1.2.2.2.	Potential fluid volume deficit
1.4.2.1.	Decreased cardiac output
1.5.1.1.	Impaired gas exchange
1.5.1.2.	Ineffective airway clearance
1.5.1.3.	Ineffective breathing pattern
1.5.1.3.1.	Inability to sustain spontaneous ventilation
1.5.1.3.2.	Dysfunctional ventilatory weaning response
1.6.1.	High risk for injury
1.6.1.1.	High risk for suffocation
1.6.1.2.	High risk for poisoning
1.6.1.3.	High risk for trauma
1.6.1.4.	High risk for aspiration
1.6.1.5.	High risk for disuse syndrome
1.6.2.	Altered protection
1.6.2.1.	Impaired tissue integrity
1.6.2.1.1.	Altered oral mucous membrane
1.6.2.1.2.1.	Impaired skin integrity
1.6.2.1.2.2.	Potential impaired skin integrity

PATTERN 2. Communicating: A human response pattern involving sending messages

2.1.1.1.	Impaired verbal communication

PATTERN 3. Relating: A human response pattern involving establishing bonds

3.1.1.	Impaired social interaction
3.1.2.	Social isolation
3.2.1.	Altered role performance
3.2.1.1.1.	Altered parenting
3.2.1.1.2.	Potential altered parenting
3.2.1.2.1.	Sexual dysfunction
3.2.2.	Altered family processes
3.2.3.1.	Parental role conflict
3.3.	Altered sexuality patterns

PATTERN 4. Valuing: A human response pattern involving the assigning of relative worth

4.1.1.	Spiritual distress (distress of the human spirit)

PATTERN 5. Choosing: A human response pattern involving the selection of alternatives

5.1.1.1.	Ineffective individual coping
5.1.1.1.1.	Impaired adjustment
5.1.1.1.2.	Defensive coping
5.1.1.1.3.	Ineffective denial
5.1.2.1.1.	Ineffective family coping: disabling
5.1.2.1.2.	Ineffective family coping: compromised
5.1.2.2.	Family coping: potential for growth
5.2.1.	Ineffective management of therapeutic regimen (individual)
5.2.1.1.	Noncompliance (specify)
5.3.1.1.	Decisional conflict (specify)
5.4.	Health-seeking behaviors (specify)

APPENDIX 1

N.A.N.D.A. TAXONOMY OF NURSING DIAGNOSES *(continued)*

PATTERN 6. Moving: A human response pattern involving activity

6.1.1.1.	Impaired physical mobility
6.1.1.1.1.	High risk for peripheral neurovascular dysfunction
6.1.1.2.	Activity intolerance
6.1.1.2.1.	Fatigue
6.1.1.3.	Potential activity intolerance
6.2.1.	Sleep pattern disturbance
6.3.1.1.	Diversional activity deficit
6.4.1.1.	Impaired home maintenance management
6.4.2.	Altered health maintenance
6.5.1.	Feeding self-care deficit
6.5.1.1.	Impaired swallowing
6.5.1.2.	Ineffective breast-feeding
6.5.1.2.1.	Interrupted breast-feeding
6.5.1.3.	Effective breast-feeding
6.5.1.4.	Ineffective infant feeding pattern
6.5.2.	Bathing or hygiene self-care deficit
6.5.3.	Dressing or grooming self-care deficit
6.5.4.	Toileting self-care deficit
6.6.	Altered growth and development
6.7.	Relocation stress syndrome

PATTERN 7. Perceiving: A human response pattern involving the reception of information

7.1.1.	Body image disturbance
7.1.2.	Self-esteem disturbance
7.1.2.1.	Chronic low self-esteem
7.1.2.2.	Situational low self-esteem
7.1.3.	Personal identity disturbance
7.2.	Sensory or perceptual alterations (specify—visual, auditory, kinesthetic, gustatory, tactile, olfactory)
7.2.1.1.	Unilateral neglect
7.3.1.	Hopelessness
7.3.2.	Powerlessness

PATTERN 8. Knowing: A human response pattern involving the meaning associated with information

8.1.1.	Knowledge deficit (specify)
8.3.	Altered thought processes

PATTERN 9. Feeling: A human response pattern involving the subjective awareness of information

9.1.1.	Pain
9.1.1.1.	Chronic pain
9.2.1.1.	Dysfunctional grieving
9.2.1.2.	Anticipatory grieving
9.2.2.	High risk for violence: self-directed or directed at others
9.2.2.1.	High risk for self-mutilation
9.2.3.	Post-trauma response
9.2.3.1.	Rape-trauma syndrome
9.2.3.1.1.	Rape-trauma syndrome: compound reaction
9.2.3.1.2.	Rape-trauma syndrome: silent reaction
9.3.1.	Anxiety
9.3.2.	Fear
9.4.1.	Caregiver role strain
9.4.2.	High risk for caregiver role strain

N.A.A.C.O.G. STANDARDS FOR THE NURSING CARE OF WOMEN AND NEWBORNS

The eight universal standards together encompass the field of nursing care of women and newborns. The first three are the universal standards of nursing practice; health education and counseling; and policies, procedures, and protocols. The remaining five are generic standards that relate to all aspects of nursing. They include professional responsibility and accountability, utilization of nursing personnel, ethics, research, and quality assurance.

Standard I: Nursing practice

Comprehensive nursing care for women and newborns focuses on helping individuals, families, and communities achieve their optimum health potential. This is best achieved within the framework of the nursing process.

Standard II: Health education and counseling

Health education for the individual, family, and community is an integral part of comprehensive nursing care. Such education encourages participation in, and shared responsibility for, health promotion, maintenance, and restoration.

Standard III: Policies, procedures, and protocols

Written policies, procedures, and protocols clarify the scope of nursing practice and delineate the qualifications of personnel authorized to provide care to women and newborns within the health care setting.

Standard IV: Professional responsibility and accountability

Comprehensive nursing care for women and newborns is provided by nurses who are clinically competent and accountable for professional actions and legal responsibilities inherent in the nursing role.

Standard V: Utilization of nursing personnel

Nursing care for women and newborns is conducted in practice settings that have qualified nursing staff in sufficient numbers to meet patient care needs.

Standard VI: Ethics

Ethical principles guide the process of decision making for nurses caring for women and newborns at all times and especially when personal or professional values conflict with those of the patient, family, colleagues, or practice setting.

Standard VII: Research

Nurses caring for women and newborns utilize research findings, conduct nursing research, and evaluate nursing practice to improve the outcomes of patient care.

Standard VIII: Quality assurance

Quality and appropriateness of patient care are evaluated through a planned assessment program using specific, identified clinical indicators.

Adapted with permission from NAACOG, the Organization for Obstetric, Gynecologic, and Neonatal Nurses (1991). *NAACOG Standards for the Nursing Care of Women and Newborns*, 4th ed. Washington, DC: NAACOG.

NEONATAL WEIGHT CONVERSION TABLE

The nurse can use the table below to convert a neonate's weight from customary units (pounds and ounces) to metric units (grams), or from metric to customary. The left column shows pounds; the top row shows ounces. The remaining numbers indicate grams.

Converting from customary to metric units
For a neonate weighing 4 pounds, 8 ounces, determine the weight in grams by finding *4 pounds* in the left column. Next, find *8 ounces* in the top row. The intersecting number (2041) is the neonate's weight in grams.

Converting from metric to customary units
For a neonate weighing 4224 grams, find *4224* in the gram section. Read across to the left column (*9 pounds*), then read upward to the top row (*5 ounces*) to determine the neonate's weight in customary units (9 pounds, 5 ounces).

Ounces	0	1	2	3	4	5	6	7	8	9	10	11	12	13	14	15
Pounds	**Grams**															
0	—	28	57	85	113	142	170	198	227	255	283	312	340	369	397	425
1	454	482	510	539	567	595	624	652	680	709	737	765	794	822	850	879
2	907	936	964	992	1021	1049	1077	1106	1134	1162	1191	1219	1247	1276	1304	1332
3	1361	1389	1417	1446	1474	1502	1531	1559	1588	1616	1644	1673	1701	1729	1758	1786
4	1814	1843	1871	1899	1928	1956	1984	2013	2041	2070	2098	2126	2155	2183	2211	2240
5	2268	2296	2325	2353	2381	2410	2438	2466	2495	2523	2551	2580	2608	2637	2665	2693
6	2722	2750	2778	2807	2835	2863	2892	2920	2948	2977	3005	3033	3062	3090	3118	3147
7	3175	3203	3232	3260	3289	3317	3345	3374	3402	3430	3459	3487	3515	3544	3572	3600
8	3629	3657	3685	3714	3742	3770	3799	3827	3856	3884	3912	3941	3969	3997	4026	4054
9	4082	4111	4139	4167	4196	4224	4252	4281	4309	4337	4366	4394	4423	4451	4479	4508
10	4536	4564	4593	4621	4649	4678	4706	4734	4763	4791	4819	4848	4876	4904	4933	4961
11	4990	5018	5046	5075	5103	5131	5160	5188	5216	5245	5273	5301	5330	5358	5386	5415
12	5443	5471	5500	5528	5557	5585	5613	5642	5670	5698	5727	5755	5783	5812	5840	5868
13	5897	5925	5953	5982	6010	6038	6067	6095	6123	6152	6180	6209	6237	6265	6294	6322
14	6350	6379	6407	6435	6464	6492	6520	6549	6577	6605	6634	6662	6690	6719	6747	6776
15	6804	6832	6860	6889	6917	6945	6973	7002	7030	7059	7087	7115	7144	7172	7201	7228

APPENDIX 4

TEMPERATURE CONVERSION TABLE

The nurse can use this table to determine Fahrenheit (°F) and Celsius (°C) temperature equivalents. Alternatively, temperatures can be converted with the following formulas.

To convert °C to °F:
$$°F = (°C \times 1.8) + 32$$

To convert °F to °C:
$$°C = (°F - 32) \div 1.8$$

DEGREES FAHRENHEIT	DEGREES CELSIUS	DEGREES FAHRENHEIT	DEGREES CELSIUS
93.2	34.0	101.5	38.6
93.6	34.2	101.8	38.8
93.9	34.4	102.2	39.0
94.3	34.6	102.6	39.2
94.6	34.8	102.9	39.4
95.0	35.0	103.3	39.6
95.4	35.2	103.6	39.8
95.7	35.4	104.0	40.0
96.1	35.6	104.4	40.2
96.4	35.8	104.7	40.4
96.8	36.0	105.2	40.6
97.2	36.2	105.4	40.8
97.5	36.4	105.9	41.0
97.9	36.6	106.1	41.2
98.2	36.8	106.5	41.4
98.6	37.0	106.8	41.6
99.0	37.2	107.2	41.8
99.3	37.4	107.6	42.0
99.7	37.6	108.0	42.2
100.0	37.8	108.3	42.4
100.4	38.0	108.7	42.6
100.8	38.2	109.0	42.8
101.1	38.4	109.4	43.0

1990 NUTRITIONAL GUIDELINES

The U.S. government has revised five of its seven dietary guidelines for Americans. The revisions reflect the use of a health-based definition for desirable weight, a focus on the total diet, and a focus on specific foods in the diet.

GUIDELINES

Modifications in the dietary guidelines address the intake of calories, fat, cholesterol, sodium, complex carbohydrates, and fiber. Excess intake of the first four and insufficient intake of the last two have been linked with obesity, heart disease, high blood pressure, stroke, diabetes, and some forms of carcinomas. Summaries of the specific recommendations follow.

Eat a variety of foods.
Because no single food can supply all nutrients in the amounts needed, a nutritious diet must contain a variety of foods. More than 40 nutrients are required to maintain health, including vitamins, minerals, amino acids, certain fatty acids, and sources of calories. To ensure variety, select foods daily from the five major food groups:
• vegetables
• fruits
• breads, cereals, rice, and pasta
• milk, yogurt, and cheese
• meats, poultry, fish, dry beans and peas, eggs, and nuts.

   Many pregnant women, women of childbearing age, teenage girls, and young children need an iron supplement. Also, some pregnant or breast-feeding women may need supplements to meet their increased requirements for other nutrients.

Maintain healthful weight.
Excess or inadequate weight increases the risk of developing health problems. Excess weight has been linked with hypertension, heart disease, stroke, diabetes mellitus, certain carcinomas, and other problems. Inadequate weight is associated with osteoporosis in women and an increased risk of early death in both sexes.

   A healthful weight depends on how much of the weight is fat, where the fat is located, and whether the person has weight-related problems or a family history of such problems. Healthful weight cannot be determined exactly; researchers are trying to develop more precise ways to describe it. However, the following guidelines can help the nurse judge whether a client's weight is healthy.
• *A weight within the range in the table for the client's age and height.* The table (see page 586) allows higher weights for people ages 35 and older compared to younger adults because research suggests that slightly increased weight among older people is not associated with health risks. The weight ranges given here are likely to change based on ongoing research. Also, the table shows weights in ranges because people of the same height with equal amounts of body fat may differ in amount of muscle and bone. The higher weights in each range are suggested for people with more muscle and bone. Weights above the range are unhealthful for most people; weights below the range may be healthful for some small-boned people but have been linked to health problems.
• *Body shape.* For adults, health depends on body shape as well as height. Research suggests that excess abdominal fat poses a greater health risk than excess fat in the hips and thighs.

   To assess body shape, find the waist-to-hip ratio. First, measure around the waist near the navel as the client stands relaxed. Then measure around the hips, over the buttocks where they are largest. Divide the waist measurement by the hip measurement to find the ratio. A ratio above 1 suggests a greater risk for several diseases.

Choose a diet low in unsaturated fat, saturated fat, and cholesterol.
Most health experts recommend that Americans eat less fat—both unsaturated and saturated fat—and cholesterol. Populations with high-fat diets have more obesity and certain types of carcinomas; high amounts of saturated fat and cholesterol increase the risk of cardiac disease. Also, with a low-fat diet, the variety of foods needed for nutrients can be consumed without exceeding caloric needs because fat contains more than twice the calories of an equal amount of carbohydrates or protein. A diet low in saturated fat and cholesterol can help maintain a desirable blood cholesterol level. (A blood cholesterol level above 200 mg/dl increases the risk of heart disease.)

   For adults, dietary fat should account for 30% or less of the total calories needed for healthy weight; saturated fat should provide less than 10% of calories. Because animal products are the source of all dietary cholesterol, eating less fat from animal sources will help lower both saturated fats and cholesterol.

Choose a diet with plenty of vegetables, fruits, and grain products.
Americans and other populations with diets low in dietary fiber and complex carbohydrates (such as starch) and high in fat tend to have more heart disease, obesity, and some carcinomas. To help ensure a varied diet, increase dietary fiber and carbohydrate intake, and decrease dietary fat intake, adults should eat at least three servings of vegetables, two servings of fruits, and six servings of grain products daily. Preferably, most dietary fiber should come from foods rather than supplements.

Use sugar in moderation.
Sugar and most foods containing large amounts of sugar are high in calories and low in essential nutrients. Therefore, most healthy people should eat these foods in moderation; people with low caloric needs should eat them sparingly. Sugar also contributes to tooth decay.

(continued)

APPENDIX 5

1990 NUTRITIONAL GUIDELINES *(continued)*

Use salt and sodium in moderation.
Most Americans consume more salt and sodium than they need. In populations with diets low in sodium, hypertension is less common than in the United States. Restriction of dietary salt and sodium may help reduce the risk of hypertension and usually helps decrease blood pressure in people with hypertension.

Drink alcoholic beverages in moderation, if at all.
Alcoholic beverages provide calories but little or no nutrients; they are linked with many health problems and accidents and can be addictive. Therefore, they should be consumed in moderation, if at all. The following individuals should not consume any alcoholic beverages:
• pregnant women or women trying to conceive
• people who plan to drive or engage in other activities requiring attention or skill
• people taking medications
• people who cannot limit their alcohol intake.

Weight table
The following table reflects ongoing research, which presently suggests that people can carry somewhat more weight as they age without added health risk. Because people of the same height may differ in muscle and bone makeup, weights are shown across a range for each height.

HEIGHT*	WEIGHT IN POUNDS†	
	Ages 19 to 34	Ages 35 and over
5'0"	97-128	108-138
5'1"	101-132	111-143
5'2"	104-137	115-148
5'3"	107-141	119-152
5'4"	111-146	122-157
5'5"	114-150	126-162
5'6"	118-155	130-167
5'7"	121-160	134-172
5'8"	125-164	138-178
5'9"	129-169	142-183
5'10"	132-174	146-188
5'11"	136-179	151-194
6'0"	140-184	155-199
6'1"	144-189	159-205
6'2"	148-195	164-210
6'3"	152-200	168-216
6'4"	156-205	173-222
6'5"	160-211	177-228
6'6"	164-216	182-234

*without shoes   †without clothes

Source: U.S. Department of Agriculture, U.S. Department of Health and Human Services (1990). *Nutrition and Your Health: Dietary Guidelines for Americans* (3rd ed.). Washington, DC.

GUIDELINES TO PREVENT H.I.V. TRANSMISSION

Human immunodeficiency virus (HIV), which causes acquired immunodeficiency syndrome (AIDS), is transmitted through sexual contact, exposure to blood and blood components, and perinatally from mother to neonate. The rising incidence of HIV infection increases the nurse's risk of exposure to blood of clients infected with HIV. To prevent exposure to blood and avoid infection, the nurse should follow universal and environmental precautions.

Universal precautions

Because medical history and examination cannot identify all clients infected with HIV, the nurse must take steps to prevent possible transmission. Use the following universal blood and body-fluid precautions when caring for all clients, especially during emergency care situations in which the client's infection status is unknown and the risk of blood exposure is increased.

1. When contact with a client's blood or body fluid is likely, use appropriate barrier precautions to prevent skin and mucous membrane exposure. Don gloves before touching a client's blood or body fluids, mucous membranes, or nonintact skin; before touching items or surfaces soiled with blood or body fluids; and before performing vascular access procedures. Change gloves after contact with each client. Wear a mask and protective eyewear or a face shield during procedures likely to generate droplets of blood or body fluids; wear a gown or apron during procedures likely to generate splashes of these fluids. If a glove is torn or a needlestick or other injury occurs, don a new glove as soon as the client's safety permits; remove the needle or item involved in the accident from the sterile field.

2. Wash hands and other skin surfaces immediately and thoroughly after any contact with blood or body fluids. Always wash hands immediately after removing gloves.

3. Take precautions to prevent injuries from needles and other sharp objects during and after procedures, when cleaning used instruments, and when disposing of used needles. To prevent needlesticks, do not recap used needles or manipulate them by hand in any manner. Place used disposable needles, scalpel blades, and other sharp objects in puncture-resistant containers (which should be located as close as possible to the work area). Place large-bore reusable needles in a puncture-resistant container to be transported for reprocessing.

4. To minimize the need for emergency mouth-to-mouth resuscitation, ensure that mouthpieces, resuscitation bags, or other ventilation devices are available wherever resuscitation procedures are likely.

5. A nurse with exfoliative dermatitis or exudative lesions should refrain from direct client care and from handling client care equipment.

6. A pregnant nurse should strictly follow all precautions to minimize the risk of HIV transmission; because HIV can be transmitted perinatally, the fetus also is at risk for infection.

These precautions apply to blood and any body fluid containing visible blood. Occupational transmission of HIV to health care workers by blood has been documented; infection control therefore focuses on preventing exposure to blood.

Universal precautions also apply to semen and vaginal secretions, which have been implicated in the sexual transmission of

HIV. The risk of occupational transmission is not known because exposure to semen is limited and gloves are worn routinely during vaginal examinations.

Universal precautions also apply to tissues, cerebrospinal fluid, synovial fluid, pleural fluid, peritoneal fluid, pericardial fluid, and amniotic fluid. HIV has been isolated in some of these substances, but HIV transmission by them is undocumented.

These precautions do not apply to feces, nasal secretions, sputum, sweat, tears, urine, and vomitus (unless they contain visible blood). Although HIV has been isolated in some, the transmission rate of HIV through them is very low or nonexistent. Human breast milk has been implicated in perinatal transmission of HIV, but universal precautions need not be taken because the neonate is infected after breast-feeding, not from the type of incidental exposure the nurse can expect. (However, wear gloves if exposure to breast milk is frequent.) Universal precautions do not apply to saliva because of the extremely low risk of infection, but follow general infection control practices — such as wearing gloves when examining mucous membranes — to minimize the risk further.

Environmental precautions

No environmental mode of HIV transmission has been documented. HIV survival outside the human body is brief, particularly in the concentrations typically found in a client's blood. Therefore, no changes in the recommended sterilization, disinfection, or housekeeping procedures are required. Take the following precautions during the care of all clients.

1. Follow the currently recommended sterilization and disinfection procedures for all client care equipment; these procedures are adequate to sterilize or disinfect instruments and other items contaminated by blood or other body fluids.

Before reusing them, sterilize instruments or devices that enter a client's sterile tissue or vascular system or that transport blood. Sterilize or disinfect items that touch intact mucous membranes. Use germicides registered with the U.S. Environmental Protection Agency as sterilants for sterilization or high-level disinfection, depending on contact time.

Thoroughly clean medical instruments and devices requiring sterilization or disinfection before exposing them to the germicide. Follow the manufacturer's specifications for compatibility of the device with the germicide.

HIV is inactivated rapidly when exposed to common commercially available germicides, even at low concentrations. In addition, a solution of sodium hypochlorite (household bleach) prepared daily makes an effective and inexpensive germicide, although it may not be compatible with certain medical devices. Concentrations between 1% and 10% are effective, depending

(continued)

GUIDELINES TO PREVENT H.I.V. TRANSMISSION

(continued)

on the amount of organic material on the surface to be cleaned.

2. Because walls, floors, and other environmental surfaces are not associated with HIV infection, extra measures to disinfect or sterilize them are not necessary. However, routine cleaning and removal of soil is recommended. Schedules and methods vary according to area, type of surface to be cleaned, and amount and type of soil present. Horizontal surfaces in client care areas usually are cleaned regularly when soiling or spills occur and when a client is discharged; vertical surfaces should be cleaned only if visibly soiled.

3. Use chemical germicides approved for use as hospital disinfectants to decontaminate spills of blood and other body fluids. In client care areas, remove visible material first and then decontaminate the area; in laboratories, flood the contaminated area with a liquid germicide before cleaning, then decontaminate with fresh germicide. Wear gloves when cleaning and decontaminating.

4. Hygienic storing and processing of linen is sufficient to prevent HIV infection from soiled linen. Handle soiled linen as little as possible and bag it at the location it was used; do not agitate it unnecessarily or sort or rinse it in client care areas. Place linen soiled with blood or body fluids in leak-proof bags. Linen should by washed with detergent in hot water (at least 160° F) or with suitable chemicals in cooler water.

5. Hospital waste has not been shown to be more infective than residential waste. To reduce any possibility of waste causing disease in the outside community, identify potentially infective wastes that should receive special precautions or disposal methods. These include microbiology laboratory waste, pathology waste, and blood or blood components. Such wastes should be incinerated or autoclaved before disposal in a sanitary landfill. Pour large amounts of blood, secretions, or excretions down a drain leading to a sanitary sewer; other infectious wastes can be ground and flushed into the sewer. Although potentially infective, items that have contacted blood, secretions, or exudates usually do not require the disposal methods listed above.

Strict adherence to these precautions will reduce exposure to blood and other substances possibly infected with HIV, thereby reducing the risk of transmission. Remember that these precautions do not eliminate the need for other disease-specific isolation precautions, such as isolation for pulmonary tuberculosis or enteric precautions for infectious diarrhea.

Source: U.S. Department of Health and Human Services (1989).
Guidelines for prevention of transmission of human immunodeficiency virus and hepatitis B virus to health-care and public safety workers.
Washington, DC: U.S. Government Printing Office.

APPENDIX 7

SELECTED RESOURCES FOR THE DISABLED PREGNANT CLIENT

A disability is defined as an impairment that limits major activities, such as hearing, seeing, or walking. Millions of women of childbearing age in the United States alone are disabled. Until recently, a disabled woman was discouraged from having a child; her family and friends worried that the neonate would inherit the disability and that the woman might be unable to care for the child. Health care professionals knew little about the effects of pregnancy, labor, and childbirth on the disabled woman's body.

Despite such discouragement, growing numbers of disabled women have chosen to become parents. To help provide a safe delivery and postpartal period for the disabled client and her neonate and to ensure the psychosocial well-being of the client and her partner, the nurse must be familiar with management techniques to use with the disabled client. These techniques involve client teaching, treatment planning, nursing care, and related subjects. The following resources can provide details.

AUDIOVISUALS

Arthritis Patient Services
1945 Randolph Road
Charlotte, NC 28207
704-331-4878

Eric Miller Company
Professional Video Programs
P.O. Box 443
114 Forrest Avenue
Narberth, PA 19072
215-667-3360

Multi-Focus, Inc.
1525 Franklin Street
San Francisco, CA 94109-4592
1-800-821-0514
415-673-5100

ORGANIZATIONS

American Association of Spinal Cord Injury Nurses
75-20 Astoria Boulevard
Jackson Heights, NY 11370
718-803-3782

American Foundation for the Blind
15 West 16th Street
New York, NY 10011
212-620-2000

American Occupational Therapy Association, Inc.
1383 Picard Drive
Rockville, MD 20850
301-948-9626

Arthritis Foundation
P.O. Box 19000
Atlanta, GA 30326
404-872-7100

Canadian Paraplegic Association
520 Sutherland Drive
Toronto, Ontario
Canada M4G 3V9
416-422-5644

International Childbirth Education Association
P.O. Box 20048
Minneapolis, MN 55420
612-854-8660

La Leche League International
9616 Minneapolis Avenue
Franklin Park, IL 60131
708-455-7730

Muscular Dystrophy Association
810 7th Avenue
New York, NY 10019
1-800-223-6333

National Head Injury Foundation
333 Turnpike Road
Southboro, MA 01772
1-800-444-6443

National Information Center on Deafness
Gallaudet University
800 Florida Avenue, NE
Washington, DC 20002
202-651-5051

National Multiple Sclerosis Society
205 E. 42nd Street, 3rd Floor
New York, NY 10017
212-986-3240

National Rehabilitation Information Center
8455 Colesville Road, Suite 935
Silver Spring, MD 20910-3319
301-588-9284

National Spinal Cord Injury Association
600 W. Cummings Park
Suite 2000
Woburn, MA 01801
1-800-962-9629
617-935-2722

Courtesy of Wilma Asrael, OTR, MHDL, ACCE.

APPENDIX 8

SUPPORT RESOURCES FOR FAMILIES WITH SPECIAL-NEEDS NEONATES

The nurse may wish to refer families with special-needs neonates to some of the following organizations for specific advice and coping techniques.

BIRTH DEFECTS

Association of Birth Defect Children, Inc.
Orlando Executive Park
5400 Diplomat Circle
Suite 270
Orlando, FL 32810
407-629-1466

March of Dimes Birth Defects Foundation
1275 Mamaroneck Avenue
White Plains, NY 10605
914-428-7100

CEREBRAL PALSY

United Cerebral Palsy Associations, Inc.
1522 K Street, Suite 1112
Washington, DC 20005
800-USA-5UCP

Canadian Cerebral Palsy Association
880 Wellington Street,
Suite 612
City Centre
Ottawa, Ontario
Canada K1R 6K7
613-235-2144

CRANIOFACIAL ABNORMALITIES

American Cleft Palate–Craniofacial Association
1218 Grandview Avenue
Pittsburgh, PA 15211
412-481-1376

Cleft Lip and Palate Program
Hospital for Sick Children
555 University Avenue
Toronto, Ontario
Canada M5G 1X8
416-598-6019

CYSTIC FIBROSIS

Cystic Fibrosis Foundation
6931 Arlington Road,
#200
Bethesda, MD 20814
301-951-4422

Canadian Cystic Fibrosis Foundation
2221 Yonge Street, Suite 601
Toronto, Ontario
Canada M4S 2B4
416-485-9149

DOWN'S SYNDROME

National Down Syndrome Society
666 Broadway
New York, NY 10012
212-460-9330

Down Syndrome Association of Metropolitan Toronto
P.O. Box 490
Don Mills, Ontario
Canada M3C 2T2
416-690-2503

HYDROCEPHALUS

National Hydrocephalus Foundation
22427 South River Road
Joliet, IL 60436
815-467-6548

(For a Canadian organization, see the Spina Bifida and Hydrocephalus Association of Ontario, below.)

INTRAVENTRICULAR HEMORRHAGE (IVH)

IVH Parents
P.O. Box 56-1111
Miami, FL 33256-1111
305-232-0381

MENTAL RETARDATION AND DELAYED DEVELOPMENT

Association for Retarded Citizens of the United States
2501 Avenue J
Arlington, TX 76006
817-640-0204

Canadian Association for Community Living
York University Kinsmen Building
4700 Keele Street
Downsview, Ontario
Canada M3J 1P3
416-661-9611

PHYSICAL DISABILITIES

National Easter Seal Society, Inc.
70 East Lake Street
Chicago, IL 60601
312-726-6200

Easter Seals Canada
45 Sheppard Avenue, East
Suite 801
Toronto, Ontario
Canada M2N 5W9
416-250-7490

RARE DISORDERS

National Organization for Rare Disorders
P.O. Box 8923
New Fairfield, CT 06812
800-999-NORD
203-746-6518

Lethbridge Society for Rare Disorders
100-542-7 Street, South
Lethbridge, Alberta
Canada T1J 2H1
403-329-0665

PARENTS OF PREMATURE AND HIGH-RISK INFANTS

Parent Care, Inc.
101½ South Union Street
Alexandria, VA 22314
703-836-4678

APPENDIX 8

SUPPORT RESOURCES FOR FAMILIES WITH SPECIAL-NEEDS NEONATES (continued)

PHENYLKETONURIA (PKU)

PKU Parents
c/o Dale Hilliard
8 Myrtle Lane
San Anselmo, CA 94960
415-457-4632

SEVERE HANDICAPS

**(TASH) The Association
for Persons with Severe
Handicaps**
7010 Roosevelt Way NE
Seattle, WA 98115
206-523-8446

SIBLING SUPPORT

**A.J. Pappanikou Center on
Special Education and
Rehabilitation**
991 Main Street, Suite 3A
East Hartford, CT 06108
203-282-7050

SICKLE CELL DISEASE

National Association for Sickle Cell Disease	**Canadian Sickle Cell Society**
4221 Wilshire Boulevard Suite 360 Los Angeles, CA 90010 800-421-8453 213-936-7205	1076 Bathurst Toronto, Ontario Canada M5R 3G8 416-537-3475

SPINA BIFIDA (MENINGOMYELOCELE)

Spina Bifida Association of America	**Spina Bifida and Hydrocephalus Association of Ontario**
1700 Rockville Pike Suite 250 Rockville, MD 20852 301-770-SBAA	55 Queen Street East Suite 300 Toronto, Ontario Canada M5C 1R6 416-364-1871

TECHNOLOGY-DEPENDENT CHILDREN

**SKIP: Sick Kids Need
Involved People**
990 Second Avenue
New York, NY 10022
212-421-9160

TURNER'S SYNDROME

**Turner's Syndrome
Society**
York University
Administrative Studies
Building, Room 006
Downsview, Ontario
Canada M3J 1P3
416-736-5023

VISUAL AND AUDITORY DEFICITS

American Society for Deaf Children	**Helen Keller National Center for Deaf-Blind Youths and Adults**
814 Thayer Avenue Silver Spring, MD 20910 301-585-5400 (international office)	111 Middle Neck Road Sands Point, NY 11050-1299 516-944-8900

MASTER GLOSSARY

ABO blood group incompatibility: isoimmune hemolytic anemia in which a maternal antigen-antibody reaction causes premature destruction of fetal red blood cells.

ABO incompatibility: condition in which the mother's blood type is O and the neonate's blood type is either A, B, or AB.

Abortion: spontaneous or induced termination of pregnancy before the fetus reaches the age of viability.

Abruptio placentae: premature separation of part or all of the placenta from the uterine wall after the twentieth week of pregnancy and before delivery; hemorrhage and shock are common complications.

Abuse: physical violence directed against one person by another who lives in that household, typically resulting in serious physical and psychological damage to the person; also called battering or domestic or family violence.

Acceleration: increase in the fetal heart rate from the baseline that lasts less than 15 minutes.

Accommodator: person who learns best from personal experience and hands-on demonstration.

Acquaintance: knowledge about another person that results from interaction; a prerequisite to parent-infant bonding.

Acquired immunodeficiency syndrome (AIDS): life-threatening disease that disables the immune system, rendering the body susceptible to opportunistic infection; present when an individual with human immunodeficiency virus (HIV) infection develops Kaposi's sarcoma, extrapulmonary cryptococcosis, *Pneumocystis carinii* pneumonia, or other designated diseases.

Acrocyanosis: bluish discoloration of the hands and feet caused by vasomotor instability, capillary stasis, and high hemoglobin levels.

Acrosome: membranelike covering on the head portion of a spermatozoon.

Active phase of labor: second phase of the first stage of labor, when the cervix dilates from 4 to 10 cm; includes three phases: acceleration, maximum slope, and deceleration (transition).

Acupressure: pressure on specific body points to promote energy flow and relieve pain.

Acupuncture: insertion of needles at specific body points to promote energy flow and relieve pain.

Adjuvant therapy: treatment in addition to the primary treatment.

Affirmation: technique used to reinforce a client's abilities, efforts, and self-esteem.

Age-related concerns: health concerns for an adolescent client (under age 19) or a mature client (over age 34) related to maternal, fetal, or neonatal risks during labor and delivery.

Agonist: substance that stimulates physiologic activity at cell receptors that are normally stimulated by naturally occurring substances.

Alcoholism: pathologic pattern of alcohol use marked by cognitive, behavioral, and physiologic symptoms that indicate inability to reduce intake, continued use despite adverse consequences, tolerance, and specific withdrawal symptoms; also called alcohol dependence.

Algesia: hypersensitivity to pain; hyperesthesia.

Allantois: diverticulum in the caudal end of the embryo; allantoic blood vessels help form those of the umbilical cord.

Alleles: pair of genes that may be different from each other but occupy corresponding sites (loci) on homologous chromosomes.

Alveolus: secretory unit of the mammary gland in which milk production takes place.

Ambivalence: conflicting feelings.

Amenorrhea: absence of menses.

Amino acids: building blocks of protein; divided into 9 essential amino acids (which the human body cannot make and must be provided in the diet) and 11 nonessential amino acids (which the body can make from the essentials in the diet).

Amniocentesis: prenatal needle aspiration procedure for obtaining amniotic fluid for analysis.

Amnionitis: inflammation of the inner layer of the fetal membranes, or amnion; most commonly a complication of early rupture of membranes.

Amniotic fluid: fluid within the amniotic sac that allows the fetus to move and cushions the fetus's head and umbilical cord during delivery.

Amniotic sac: membrane that surrounds the fetus, contains amniotic fluid, and eventually lines the chorion.

Amniotomy: artificial rupture of the amniotic membranes, performed by a physician or nurse-midwife to enhance or induce labor.

Amphetamine: drug that stimulates the sympathetic nervous system.

Analgesia: reduction of pain without loss of consciousness.

Androgen: class of hormone that stimulates the development of male secondary sex characteristics, such as facial hair and increased musculature.

Anemia: blood disorder characterized by a change in red blood cells or decreased hemoglobin, which may be related to a deficiency of iron, vitamin B_{12}, or folic acid.

Anencephaly: congenital absence of the cerebral hemispheres in which the cephalic end of the spinal cord fails to close during gestation.

MASTER GLOSSARY (continued)

Anesthesia: loss of sensation (total or partial) with or without loss of consciousness.

Anovulation: failure of the ovaries to produce, mature, or release ova.

Antagonist: substance that blocks the action of another, such as a drug, by binding to a cell receptor without causing a physiologic response.

Antepartal period: period during pregnancy and before labor and delivery.

Anteverted uterus: normal position in which the uterine corpus flexes forward at a less acute angle than an anteflexed uterus.

Anthropometry: science that deals with measurement of the size, weight, and proportions of the human body.

Antibody: protein produced in the body in response to invasion by a foreign agent (antigen); reacts specifically with the antigen.

Anticipatory grief: sadness in anticipation of loss.

Antigen: foreign substance that stimulates the immunologic system to formulate mechanisms with which to fight against it (antibody).

Apgar score: method of evaluating neonatal vigor at 1- and 5-minute intervals after delivery; ranging from 0 to 10, the score is based on assessment of heart rate, respirations, muscle tone, reflex irritability, and skin color.

Apnea: absence of spontaneous respirations.

Apnea monitor: device that sounds an alarm when breathing stops or drops below a preset level.

Appraisal support: type of support that includes affirmation and feedback.

Appropriate for gestational age: term used to describe a neonate whose birth weight falls between the tenth and ninetieth percentile for gestational age on the Colorado intrauterine growth chart.

AROM: artificial rupture of membranes (amniotic sac).

Asphyxia: condition caused by sustained oxygen deprivation and characterized by hypoxemia, hypercapnia, and acidosis.

Assessment: systematic collection of subjective and objective data about a client's health status; a step in the nursing process.

Asynclitism: lateral flexion of the fetus's head toward either the symphysis pubis (anterior asynclitism) or sacrum (posterior asynclitism) during labor.

Atony: lack of normal tone; uterine atony produces a boggy (soft, poorly contracted) organ and may lead to postpartal hemorrhage.

Attachment: process in which parent and child form an enduring relationship; sometimes differentiated from bonding.

Attitude: relationship of the parts of the fetus to one another.

Augmentation of labor: enhancement of uterine contractions from ineffectual to effectual during labor.

Autolysis: self-disintegration or self-digestion of tissue or cells.

Autosome: general term for any chromosome except a sex chromosome.

Azoospermia: absence of sperm in semen.

Back labor: labor that occurs when a fetus in the occiput posterior position presses on the sacral nerves during contractions.

Bacteremic shock: type of shock that occurs in septicemia (systemic infection of the bloodstream) when endotoxins are released from certain bacteria; also called septic shock.

Ballard gestational-age assessment tool: tool that examines seven physical (external) and six neuromuscular characteristics to determine a neonate's gestational age.

Ballottement: passive movement of the fetus elicited during pelvic examination in the fourth and fifth months of pregnancy.

Barbiturate: nonnarcotic, sedative drug that can cause physical and psychological dependence.

Basal body temperature (BBT) method: natural contraceptive method that predicts a client's fertile period by monitoring her daily BBT (the lowest body temperature of a healthy individual while awake).

Basal metabolic rate: rate at which cells use oxygen; lowest metabolic rate that preserves physiologic function.

Baseline fetal bradycardia: baseline fetal heart rate below 120 beats/minute.

Baseline fetal heart rate: resting pulse of the fetus assessed between contractions and without fetal movement; normal baseline fetal heart rate is 120 to 160 beats/minute.

Baseline fetal tachycardia: baseline fetal heart rate exceeding 160 beats/minute.

Battledore placenta: benign condition in which the umbilical cord implants at the edge of the placenta.

Bilirubin: yellow bile pigment; a product of red blood cell hemolysis.

Biparietal diameter: greatest transverse distance between the two parietal bones.

Biphasic pattern: sharp midcycle rise in basal body temperature followed by a return to the baseline.

Birth culture: beliefs, values, and norms held by a cultural or ethnic group about conception, conditions for procreation and childbearing, the mechanism of pregnancy and labor, and the rules of pre- and postnatal behavior.

MASTER GLOSSARY *(continued)*

Birthing chair: specialized chair that allows a client to give birth in an upright position.

Blastocyst: embryo precursor just after the morula stage.

Blastomere: daughter cell formed by mitosis just after fertilization of an ovum.

Blood-brain barrier: membrane that prevents harmful substances in the blood, such as anesthetic agents, from penetrating brain tissue.

Bloody show: blood-tinged vaginal discharge that occurs at the onset of labor when the cervical mucus plug is dislodged and small cervical capillaries break.

Body image: mental image of one's physical appearance, posture, gestures, personality, attitudes, and self-concept, and one's perception of others' reactions to that image.

Body language: nonverbal signals, such as facial expression, gestures, and body position.

Bonding: process through which an emotional attachment forms, which binds one person to another in an enduring relationship, as between parents and infant; sometimes called attachment.

Braxton Hicks contractions: painless uterine contractions that occur at irregular intervals throughout pregnancy but become more noticeable as term approaches; also called false labor contractions.

Brazelton neonatal behavioral assessment scale (BNBAS): tool that determines a neonate's interactive and behavioral capacities.

Breast engorgement: excessive fullness of the breasts resulting from temporary lymphatic and venous stasis; occurs during the early part of the lactation cycle.

Breast self-examination (BSE): procedure by which a woman assesses her breasts and accessory structures for signs of abnormality.

Breast shield: device worn late in pregnancy to draw out inverted nipples in preparation for breast-feeding.

Breech presentation: fetal position in which the buttocks or feet present first.

Bronchopulmonary dysplasia (BPD): lung disease characterized by bronchiolar metaplasia and interstitial fibrosis; associated with oxygen therapy and mechanical ventilation in preterm neonates.

Calorie: measurement of heat (energy); also called kilocalorie or kcal.

Caput succedaneum: generalized edema of the fetal scalp, usually caused by pressure on the fetal occiput during labor or vacuum extraction.

Carbohydrate: energy source providing 4 calories/g; found in the diet in the form of starches, sugars, and fiber (which provides no calories).

Cardiac decompensation: inability of the reserve power of the heart to compensate for impaired valvular functioning.

Cardiac disease: any heart disorder, especially one that places the client at high risk during the intrapartal period.

Cardinal movements of labor: series of positional changes that occur as the fetus passes through the pelvis; progression includes descent, flexion, internal rotation, extension, external rotation (restitution and shoulder rotation), and expulsion.

Carrier: person who has one normal and one abnormal gene at corresponding loci, when the abnormal gene is not expressed phenotypically; expression may occur in offspring if male and female carriers each transmit the abnormal gene.

Central venous pressure: pressure within the superior vena cava; represents the pressure under which blood returns to the right atrium.

Cephalocaudal: pertaining to the long axis of the body in a head-to-tail direction.

Cephalopelvic disproportion: condition in which the fetus's head is too large or the birth canal too small to permit normal vaginal delivery.

Cervical canal: structure extending from the external cervical os to the interior of the uterus.

Cervical cap: cup-shaped, flexible rubber device that fits over the cervix, is used with a spermicide, and acts as a barrier to spermatozoa.

Cervical mucus test: examination of cervical mucus for color, consistency, stretchiness, and quantity—all of which normally change throughout the menstrual cycle in response to hormonal stimulation; can predict a client's fertile period.

Cesarean delivery: surgical incision through the abdominal wall and uterus to deliver the fetus.

Childbirth exercises: activities designed specifically to tone and strengthen muscles stressed during pregnancy, labor, and childbirth.

Child life therapist: professional who uses play activities to help ill children cope with their illness and environment.

Chlamydia: sexually transmitted disease (STD) caused by *Chlamydia trachomatis,* which is typically asymptomatic; the most common STD in the United States.

Chloasma: pigment changes that typically appear on cheeks, temples, and forehead during pregnancy; also called melasma.

Chorioamnionitis: inflammation of the fetal membranes, typically caused by infection and producing maternal and fetal tachycardia, fever, uterine and other abdominal tenderness, and purulent vaginal secretions.

Chorionic villus sampling (CVS): prenatal diagnostic procedure for obtaining fetal tissue from the villous area of the chorion.

MASTER GLOSSARY *(continued)*

Chromosome: microscopic, threadlike structure in the cell nucleus that contains genetic information arranged in a linear sequence.

Chronic hypertension: persistently elevated arterial blood pressure that is present and observable before pregnancy, diagnosed by 20 weeks' gestation, or that extends past 42 days postpartum.

Chronic hypertension with superimposed preeclampsia: hypertension that is present and observable before pregnancy and that is complicated by the hypertensive syndrome associated with preeclampsia.

Circumcision: surgical removal of the prepuce (foreskin) covering the glans penis.

Cleansing breath: deep, relaxed breath before and after any patterned breathing during labor.

Cleft lip: congenital defect in which one or more clefts appear in the upper lip; caused by failure of the maxillary and median nasal processes to close during embryonic development.

Cleft palate: congenital defect in which a fissure appears in the palatal midline; caused by failure of the sides of the palate to close during embryonic development.

Climacteric: period of physiologic and psychological changes that occur toward the end of a female's reproductive years and includes a premenopausal, menopausal, and postmenopausal phase that may last up to 20 years; a male also may experience a climacteric stage as sexual activity decreases with age.

Clubfoot: congenital foot deformity characterized by unilateral or bilateral deviation of the metatarsal bones, causing the foot to appear clublike.

Clustering: process of grouping related assessment data to identify broad client needs; the nurse may then consult the NANDA taxonomy to choose an appropriate diagnostic category that addresses those needs.

Coagulopathy: abnormal clotting disorder characterized by hypothrombinemia, hypofibrinogenemia, and subnormal platelet count; caused by a major insult, such as abruptio placentae.

Cocaine: central nervous system stimulant derived from coca leaves that produces euphoria and anesthetizes nerve endings.

Cognitive-affective skills: skills that link mental processes with emotions.

Cognitive-motor skills: skills that link mental processes with physical activity.

Coitus interruptus: natural contraceptive method in which the male withdraws his penis from the vagina immediately before ejaculation; also called the withdrawal method.

Colostrum: thin, yellow, serous fluid secreted by the breasts during pregnancy and the first postpartal days before lactation be-gins; consists of water, protein, fat, carbohydrates, white blood cells, and immunoglobulins.

Conception: onset of pregnancy, starting with fertilization of an ovum and ending with its implantation in the uterine wall.

Conceptus: products of conception, including fetal membranes, placenta, and pre-embryo, embryo, or fetus.

Conditioned response: reaction acquired through training and repetition, as employed in the psychoprophylactic method of childbirth education.

Condom: sheath made of thin rubber, collagenous tissue, or animal tissue that is worn over the penis during intercourse to prevent sperm from entering the uterus.

Conduction: transfer of heat to a substance in contact with the body; a mechanism of heat loss or gain.

Congenital anomaly: abnormality present at birth; particularly, a structural abnormality that may be genetically inherited, acquired during gestation, or caused during delivery.

Congenital heart defect: one of five common defects: atrial septal defect or ventricular septal defect, tetralogy of Fallot, patent ductus arteriosus, valvular abnormality, or coarctation of the aorta.

Congenital hydrocephalus: condition characterized by accumulation of excessive cerebrospinal fluid within the cranial vault.

Congenital hypothyroidism: deficiency of thyroid hormone secretion during fetal development or early infancy; also called cretinism.

Consanguinity: kinship; blood relationship.

Consent: voluntary act in which one person agrees to an action by another person; not all consent given is informed consent.

Contraceptive sponge: doughnut-shaped device made of soft, synthetic material that contains spermicide.

Contraction: involuntary and intermittent tightening or shortening of uterine muscle fibers that leads to cervical dilation, effacement, and fetal descent.

Convection: transfer of heat away by movement of air currents; a mechanism of heat loss or gain.

Coping: process by which an individual deals with stress, solves problems, and makes decisions.

Coping mechanism: conscious response to stress that allows an individual to confront a problem directly and solve it.

Corona radiata: layer of granulosa cells that adheres to the zona pellucida before fertilization of an ovum.

Corpus luteum: spherical yellowish tissue that grows within a ruptured ovarian follicle after ovulation and secretes progesterone.

Couvade symptoms: pregnancy symptoms in an expectant father.

MASTER GLOSSARY *(continued)*

Crisis: period of instability or disorganization that follows failure of normal coping skills; risk is highest when a stressful event coincides with a crucial stage in family development.

Crossing-over: exchange of corresponding segments between homologous chromosomes while the chromosomes are paired during the first meiotic division.

Crowning: appearance of the fetus's head at the perineum.

Culdocentesis: use of a needle puncture or incision to remove intraperitoneal fluid (blood and purulent drainage) through the vagina.

Culture: integrated system of learned beliefs, values, and behaviors characteristic of a society's members.

Cyanosis: bluish skin discoloration caused by an excess of deoxygenated hemoglobin in the blood.

Cystitis: inflammatory condition of the urinary bladder and ureters characterized by dysuria, urinary frequency and urgency, hematuria, and other symptoms; may be caused by bacterial infection, calculus, or neoplasm.

Cystocele: herniation of the urinary bladder through the anterior vaginal wall.

Decidua: epithelial tissue of the endometrium during pregnancy.

Decidua basalis: portion of the decidua directly beneath the implanted ovum, attached to the myometrium.

Defense mechanism: unconscious response to stress that distorts reality and allows an individual to avoid, rather than directly cope with, an anxiety-producing situation.

Dehiscence: spontaneous opening of a surgical wound (such as an episiotomy).

Delirium tremens (DTs): acute, sometimes fatal psychotic reaction to alcohol withdrawal that occurs in about 5% of withdrawing alcoholics and usually lasts 2 to 4 days; characterized by fever, tachycardia, hypertension or hypotension, vivid hallucinations, seizures, and combativeness.

Denial: defense mechanism that involves refusal to acknowledge thoughts, feelings, desires, impulses, or facts that are consciously intolerable.

Dependent edema: interstitial accumulation of excess fluid in the lowest portions of the body.

Diabetes mellitus: endocrine syndrome in which heterogeneous chronic disorders are characterized by altered carbohydrate metabolism caused by inadequate insulin secretion by the beta cells of the islets of Langerhans in the pancreas or by ineffective use of insulin at the cellular level.

Diabetic ketoacidosis: emergency condition characterized by acidosis and accumulation of ketones in the blood, which results from faulty carbohydrate metabolism; occurs primarily as a complication of diabetes.

Diagnosis-related group (DRG): one of 470 groups of related diagnoses, each of which has an estimated length of hospital stay and cost; in the prospective payment system, DRGs are the basis for reimbursement by many private insurance companies and federal insurance programs.

Diaphragm: dome-shaped, flexible rubber device with a thick rim that contains a spring; it fits over the cervix, is used with a spermicide, and prevents pregnancy by blocking sperm passage into the uterus.

Dilatation: dilation; sometimes used to describe dilation of the cervical os during labor or to refer to an external means of dilation, such as drugs or instruments.

Dilatation and curettage (D & C): surgical method of pregnancy interruption that requires cervical dilation and uterine scraping with a metal curette to remove the products of conception; may be used as part of the treatment for endometriosis or as follow-up to an incomplete abortion.

Dilatation and evacuation (D & E): surgical method of pregnancy interruption that requires extreme cervical dilation and evacuation of uterine contents by large-bore suction equipment and crushing instruments.

Dilation: progressive widening of the external cervical os; also called dilatation.

Dimpling: breast skin puckering or depression, possibly caused by an underlying growth; also called retraction.

Diploid: having a full set of homologous chromosomes (46), as normally found in somatic cells.

Discharge planning: formulation of a program by the health care team, client, family, and appropriate outside agencies to ensure that the client's physical and psychosocial needs are met after discharge.

Displacement: defense mechanism that transfers emotions from an anxiety-producing object to a less threatening object.

Disseminated intravascular coagulation (DIC): abnormal clotting disorder characterized by hypoprothrombinemia, hypofibrinogenemia, and a subnormal platelet count; caused by a major insult to the body, such as abruptio placentae.

DNA: deoxyribonucleic acid; the chemical that carries genetic information.

Dominant: capable of genetic expression when a gene is present on only one of a pair of homologous chromosomes.

Down's syndrome: disorder in which birth defects are caused by an extra number 21 chromosome; also called trisomy 21.

Dubowitz gestational-age assessment tool: tool that examines 11 physical (external) and 10 neuromuscular characteristics to determine a neonate's gestational age.

Ductus arteriosus: tubular connection that shunts blood away from the pulmonary circulation during fetal development.

MASTER GLOSSARY (continued)

Ductus venosus: circulatory pathway that allows blood to bypass the liver during fetal development.

Dyad: pair of individuals in a close relationship.

Dysmaturity: undernourished fetus or neonate that is abnormally small for gestational age.

Dysmenorrhea: painful menstruation; a possible contraindication to intrauterine device (IUD) use.

Dyspareunia: painful or difficult intercourse; may result from vaginal dryness associated with menopause.

Dystocia: difficult delivery caused by fetal factors, such as malpresentation, malposition, macrosomia, and intrauterine fetal death; the client's pelvis; or uterine expulsive powers.

Dysuria: painful or difficult urination.

Early deceleration: innocuous waveform deceleration of the fetal heart rate that mirrors uterine contractions and typically occurs when the cervix is dilated 4 to 7 cm.

Early phase of labor: first phase of the first stage of labor, characterized by the onset of regular contractions and cervical dilation of up to 3 cm; also called the latent phase of labor.

Early postpartal discharge: discharge from the health care facility 2 to 72 hours after delivery.

Eclampsia: gravest, convulsive form of pregnancy-induced hypertension, affecting one of every 200 clients with preeclampsia, characterized by generalized tonic-clonic seizures and coma; occurs between the twentieth week of pregnancy and the end of the first postpartal week.

Ectoderm: outermost of the three primary germ cell layers of the embryo.

Ectopic pregnancy: implantation of the fertilized ovum outside the uterine cavity.

EDD: expected date of delivery.

Effacement: progressive thinning and shortening of the cervix during labor.

Effleurage: relaxation technique that uses light, rhythmic fingertip massage over the abdomen during labor; can help distract the client and decrease her pain.

Ejaculation: forceful expulsion of semen through the penile urethra.

Elective abortion: termination of pregnancy by choice before the age of viability.

Elective induction: initiation of labor for convenience in a term pregnancy.

Electronic fetal monitoring (EFM): direct (scalp electrode, intrauterine catheter) and indirect (ultrasound, tocodynamometer) devices that assess the relationship between the fetal heart rate and uterine contractions.

Embryo: developing organism after the pre-embryonic stage and before the fetal stage, usually occurring during weeks 4 through 8.

Emotional support: type of support that includes affection, trust, concern, and listening.

Empty nest syndrome: pattern of emotions that characterize a family whose children have recently left home.

Encephalocele: congenital neural tube defect in which the meninges and portions of brain tissue protrude through the cranium, typically in the occipital area.

Endocervix: inner portion of the cervix.

Endoderm: innermost of the three primary germ cell layers of the embryo.

Endogenous opiate theory: hypothesis that natural pain inhibitors found in the central nervous system bind at pain receptor sites and block transmission of pain impulses.

Endometriosis: abnormal condition in which endometrial tissue grows and functions outside the uterine cavity.

Endometrium: mucous membrane lining of the uterus, a portion of which forms the decidua during pregnancy.

En face position: position in which the neonate is held approximately 8″ (20 cm) in front of the parent or other observer; allows direct eye contact.

Engagement: descent of the fetal presenting part into the maternal pelvis; the widest diameter of the fetal presenting part is at or below the level of the ischial spines.

Engrossment: close face-to-face observation between parent and neonate; sometimes used to describe father-infant interaction.

Enterocele: herniation of the intestine into the posterior portion of the vagina.

Entrainment: phenomenon in which a neonate or an infant moves in rhythm to adult speech.

Epidural block: most common regional anesthesia technique, in which an anesthetic agent is injected into the epidural space between the dura mater and ligamentum flavum.

Episiotomy: surgical incision in the perineum to enlarge the vaginal opening for delivery; performed to prevent perineal tears, speed or facilitate delivery, or prevent excess stretching of perineal muscles and connective tissue.

Erythroblastosis fetalis: serious hemolytic disease of the fetus and neonate that produces anemia; jaundice; liver, spleen, and heart enlargement; and severe generalized edema; also called hydrops fetalis or hemolytic disease of the newborn.

Erythropoietin: hormone produced in the kidneys that regulates red blood cell production.

Ethics: discipline that attempts to identify, organize, analyze, and justify human acts by applying certain moral principles to a given situation.

MASTER GLOSSARY *(continued)*

Ethnicity: affiliation with a group of people classified according to a common racial, national, linguistic, or cultural origin or background.

Etiology: causal or contributing factor or factors.

Evaluation: determination of how successfully care plan goals have been met; a step in the nursing process.

Evaporation: conversion of fluid to vapor; a mechanism of heat loss.

Everted nipple: nipple that is turned outward and becomes more graspable with stimulation.

Exchange transfusion: procedure in which the neonate's blood is removed and replaced with fresh whole donor blood to remove unconjugated bilirubin in serum; used to treat hyperbilirubinemia and hemolytic anemia.

Expressivity: extent to which signs of a gene reveal themselves.

Extracorporeal membrane oxygenation (ECMO): technique that maintains gas exchange and perfusion by oxygenating blood outside the body through an arterial shunt; used mainly to treat refractory respiratory failure or meconium aspiration syndrome.

False labor: Braxton Hicks contractions.

Family-centered care: philosophical approach to health care that proposes that childbirth affects the entire family; incorporates such practices as paternal and sibling participation in childbirth and alternative birth settings.

Family functions: purposes for which the family exists and tasks necessary to attain those purposes; includes physical survival, sustenance, personal nurturing, education, and the passing on of values and beliefs.

Family pattern: overall organization of family relationships regardless of roles adopted by each member.

Family theory: set of assumptions and hypotheses that provides a reference point for studying and understanding the family.

Fat: energy source providing 9 calories/g; found in the diet in meat, dairy products, vegetable oils, and miscellaneous foods.

Father image: each man's concept of himself as a father, shaped from childhood memories of his own father, other role models, revision of his father image through other children, literature, and his imagination.

Female circumcision: religious or cultural procedure that removes a portion of the clitoris and labia.

Ferning: microscopic, fern-shaped pattern found in a smear of dried amniotic fluid, indicating rupture of the amniotic membranes.

Fertilization: penetration of a female gamete by a male gamete.

Fetal alcohol syndrome: syndrome caused by maternal alcohol consumption; characterized by altered intrauterine growth and development that results in mental and growth retardation, facial abnormalities, and behavioral deviations.

Fetal lie: relationship of the long axis of the fetus to the long axis of the mother.

Fetal-placental unit: umbilical cord, placental layers, and chorionic villus—through which placental transfer occurs.

Fetal position: relationship of the landmark on the fetal presenting part to the front, back, and sides of the maternal pelvis.

Fetal presentation: manner in which the fetus enters the pelvic passageway; for example, cephalic, shoulder, or breech.

Fetal scalp blood sampling: test that uses a fetal scalp blood sample to evaluate the fetus's acid-base status during labor; used as an adjunct to electronic fetal monitoring.

Fetal scalp stimulation: test that provides a reassuring sign of fetal well-being during labor by accelerating the fetal heart rate with pressure from the examiner's fingers or with application of an Allis clamp to the fetus's head.

Fetal station: relationship of the fetal presenting part to the maternal ischial spines.

Fetus: developing organism that forms after the embryonic stage from around week 9 through delivery.

Fibrin: insoluble protein formed from fibrinogen that is essential for blood clotting.

Fibrinogen: protein clotting factor in blood plasma that is converted to fibrin by the action of thrombin.

Fibroid: benign, slow-growing uterine neoplasm.

First stage of labor: stage of labor that begins with the onset of regular, rhythmic uterine contractions and ends with complete cervical dilation of 10 cm.

Fistula: abnormal passage between two internal organs or from an internal organ to the body surface.

Fixation: defense mechanism that stops development because of inability to resolve an issue.

Flashback phenomenon: auditory and visual hallucinations related to a previous frightening or pleasurable experience; may result from use of a psychoactive drug.

Flat nipple: nipple that is hard to distinguish from the areola; changes shape only slightly with stimulation.

Folic acid deficiency anemia: blood disorder in which immature red blood cells fail to divide, become enlarged, and decrease in number.

Follicle-stimulating hormone (FSH): anterior pituitary hormone; in women, it stimulates follicular growth; in men, it promotes spermatogenesis.

MASTER GLOSSARY *(continued)*

Fontanel: nonossified area of connective tissue between the skull bones where the sutures intersect; allows molding of the fetal skull for passage through the pelvis during delivery.

Foramen ovale: opening in the interatrial septum that directs blood from the right to left atrium during fetal development.

Forceps: two curved blades used to extract the fetus from the birth canal.

Foremilk: thin, watery breast milk secreted at the beginning of a feeding.

Formative evaluation: process in which the nurse and client judge progress toward goals during home care visits.

Fourchette: area of the female perineum between the posterior junction of the labia minora and labia majora.

Fourth stage of labor: period after delivery of the placenta, lasting about 1 hour.

Functional residual capacity (FRC): volume of air remaining in the lungs after a normal expiration.

Fundus: rounded portion of the uterus above the level of the fallopian tube attachments.

Funic souffle: blowing sound heard as fetal blood courses through the umbilical cord.

Galactorrhea: flow of breast milk unrelated to breast-feeding.

Galactosemia: hereditary autosomal recessive disorder in which deficiency of the enzyme galactose-1-phosphate uridyltransferase leads to galactose accumulation in the blood.

Gamete: male or female reproductive cell (spermatozoon or ovum).

Gamete intrafallopian transfer (GIFT): procedure in which oocytes (incompletely developed ova) are taken from the ovary, mixed with spermatozoa, and then instilled into the distal end of the fallopian tube; with GIFT, fertilization takes place in vivo (in the woman's own body).

Gametogenesis: developmental process by which spermatozoa and ova are formed.

Gastroschisis: congenital condition characterized by incomplete abdominal wall closure not involving the site of umbilical cord insertion; typically, the small intestine and part of the large intestine protrude.

Gate control theory: hypothesis that stimulation of larger-diameter, faster-traveling nerve fibers can block pain impulses carried on smaller-diameter, slower-traveling fibers, thus closing a gate that stops or modifies pain transmission.

Gene: self-reproducing biological unit of heredity; located at a specific locus (site) on a particular chromosome.

Genotype: individual's genetic constitution; may refer to the total genetic constitution or to specific alleles at a locus.

Gestational age: estimated age in weeks following conception.

Gestational-age assessment: evaluation of a neonate's physical and neurologic characteristics to determine approximate weeks of fetal development.

Gestational diabetes: type of diabetes first diagnosed during pregnancy, which may be asymptomatic except for impaired glucose tolerance test values; also called gestational diabetes mellitus.

Gestational edema: generalized interstitial accumulation of excess fluid (face, hands, sacrum, abdomen, ankles, tibia) after 12 hours of bed rest or a weight gain in excess of 2 kg (4 to 4½ lb) per week; the edema may be less significant than the weight gain.

Gestational hypertension: elevated blood pressures present on two occasions at least 6 hours apart characterized by systolic and diastolic pressure equal to or exceeding 140/90 mm Hg or a rise of 30 mm Hg systolic or 15 mm Hg diastolic above the client's baseline values.

Gestational proteinuria: protein in the urine just after labor recorded on two or more occasions at least 6 hours apart in a clean-catch or catheter-obtained specimen; protein must be 300 mg/liter or greater in a 24-hour specimen, or greater than 1 g/liter in a random daytime sample.

Glomerular filtration rate (GFR): volume of glomerular filtrate (a protein-free plasmalike substance) formed over a specific period.

Glucuronyl transferase: liver enzyme necessary for bilirubin conjugation.

Goal: desired outcome of nursing care that guides formation and implementation of nursing interventions.

Golgi body: complex membranous intracellular structure whose elements consist of flattened sacs; also called Golgi complex or Golgi apparatus.

Gonorrhea: sexually transmitted disease, caused by *Neisseria gonorrhoeae*, that may be asymptomatic or may produce vaginal discharge, urinary symptoms, dyspareunia, and menstrual irregularities.

Graafian follicle: mature ovarian vesicle located near the ovarian surface that contains an ovum; in response to hormonal stimulation during the menstrual cycle, the ovum matures and the vesicle ruptures.

Grand multiparity: having had more than five children.

Grief: intense sadness experienced after the loss of a valued person or object.

Grief process: cycle that follows a loss; the Kübler-Ross model progresses from denial through anger, bargaining, and depression to acceptance; stages may overlap or regress and may be repeated many times before acceptance is complete.

Habituation: gradual adaptation to a stimulus through repeated exposure.

MASTER GLOSSARY *(continued)*

Hallucinogen: psychotomimetic drug that alters consciousness and causes hallucinations.

Haploid: having only one-half of a set of homologous chromosomes (23), as normally found in gametes.

Health care facility: organization that provides health care services based on societal and client demands.

Health care provider: health care facility, agency, or professional that delivers services to clients.

Health maintenance organization (HMO): group practice that charges a flat fee for each insured client, regardless of the extent or type of services the group provides; emphasizes provision of government-mandated services that help maintain health and reduce inpatient hospital stays.

Hematocrit: volume percentage of red blood cells in whole blood.

Hematoma: collection of extravasated blood trapped in the tissues of the skin or in an organ, resulting from trauma or incomplete hemostasis, as after surgery.

Hemoglobin: protein in red blood cells that transports oxygen.

Hemoglobin F: hemoglobin produced by fetal erythrocytes; has a higher affinity for oxygen than does adult hemoglobin (hemoglobin A), helping to ensure adequate fetal tissue oxygenation.

Herpes genitalis: sexually transmitted disease caused by the herpes simplex virus; characterized by recurrent outbreaks of genital blisters that progress to shallow, painful ulcers.

Heterozygote: individual with two different alleles at corresponding loci on homologous chromosomes.

Hindmilk: high-fat breast milk secreted at the end of a feeding.

Hirsutism: excessive body hair; in women, its distribution follows a masculine pattern.

Hoffman's exercises: areola-stretching technique designed to facilitate breast-feeding by breaking adhesions and allowing inverted nipples to become more protractile.

Homans' sign: pain in the calf on dorsiflexion of the foot, indicating superficial thrombosis or thrombophlebitis.

Home health aide: person trained to provide personal care, such as bathing, dressing, and feeding, to the client at home.

Home health care: services, supplies, and equipment provided to a client in the home to maintain or promote physical, mental, and emotional health.

Home nursing visit: provision of nursing care in a client's home.

Homologous chromosomes: matching pair of chromosomes.

Homozygote: individual with identical alleles (normal or abnormal) at corresponding loci on homologous chromosomes.

Human immunodeficiency virus (HIV): retrovirus that can lead to acquired immunodeficiency syndrome (AIDS), which compromises the body's immune system and renders it susceptible to opportunistic infections.

Hydramnios: excessive amniotic fluid associated with congenital neonatal disorders and such maternal disorders as diabetes mellitus; also called polyhydramnios.

Hymen: fold of membranous tissue that occludes or partially blocks the vaginal orifice.

Hyperbilirubinemia: elevated serum level of unconjugated bilirubin.

Hyperemesis gravidarum: abnormal prenatal condition characterized by excessive nausea or vomiting leading to dehydration and starvation.

Hyperemia: increased amount of blood.

Hyperesthesia: increased sensitivity, usually of the skin, which may occur late in labor.

Hyperglycemia: abnormally high serum glucose level.

Hyperplasia: increase in cell number.

Hypertonia: condition in which the uterus resists stretching.

Hypertrophy: increase in cell size.

Hypocalcemia: decreased serum calcium level.

Hypofibrinogenemia: abnormally low fibrinogen (a coagulation agent) in the blood.

Hypoglycemia: abnormally low serum glucose level.

Hypotonic: having reduced muscle tension; describes a muscle that is relaxed, not well contracted.

Hypovolemia: abnormally diminished volume of circulating fluid.

Hysteroscopy: visual examination of the uterus through a hysteroscope (illuminated tube) that has been passed through the vagina; during this procedure, the client can be sterilized by passing silicone through the hysteroscope and using it to occlude the fallopian tubes.

Imagery: relaxation technique in which the client focuses on a mental representation of a real or imagined place; also called visualization.

Imperforate anus: congenital defect characterized by abnormal closure of the anus.

Implantation: attachment of the blastocyst to the uterine wall; occurs 6 to 7 days after fertilization of the ovum.

Implementation: nursing actions that carry out interventions described in the nursing care plan to achieve established goals; a step in the nursing process.

Inborn error of metabolism: abnormal metabolic condition caused by an inherited defect of a single enzyme or other protein.

Incompetent cervix: condition in which the cervix will not maintain a pregnancy to term.

MASTER GLOSSARY *(continued)*

Incontinence: inability to control urination or defecation.

Incubator: fully enclosed, single-walled or double-walled bed containing a heating source and a humidification chamber.

Indicated or nonelective induction: initiation of labor for medical or obstetric reasons that threaten the health of the fetus or client.

Induction of labor: attempts to speed labor by starting or augmenting uterine contractions.

Infertility: inability to conceive after 1 year of regular intercourse without contraception or inability to carry a pregnancy to birth.

Informational support: type of support that includes advice, suggestions, directives, and other information.

Informed consent: legal rule in which a client is entitled to receive certain information about a proposed course of treatment or surgery; usual required information includes risks, benefits, and alternatives.

Inhalation analgesia: anesthetic agent inhaled in small concentrations to produce analgesia without loss of consciousness.

Instrumental support: type of support that includes money, time, and other such resources.

Intervention: action performed by the nurse to implement the nursing care plan.

Intrapartal period: period during labor and delivery.

Intrauterine device (IUD): plastic contraceptive device that contains copper or progesterone and is inserted in the uterine cavity; may prevent pregnancy by altering endometrial physiology and inhibiting implantation of the fertilized ovum.

Intrauterine growth retardation (IUGR): abnormal process in which fetal development and maturation are impeded or delayed by maternal disease, genetic factors, or fetal malnutrition caused by placental insufficiency; seen in the small-for-gestational-age neonate.

Intrauterine pressure catheter: pliable, water-filled tube inserted into the uterus to assess uterine tone and the frequency, duration, and intensity of uterine contractions.

Intraventricular hemorrhage: bleeding into the ventricles.

Inverted nipple: nipple that turns inward; occurs in three types: pseudoinverted (becomes erect with stimulation), semi-inverted (retracts with stimulation), and truly inverted (inverted both at rest and when stimulated).

In vitro fertilization: procedure during which oocytes are taken from the ovary, mixed with spermatozoa, and fertilized and incubated in a glass petri dish; up to four viable embryos then are placed in the woman's uterus.

Involution: retrogressive changes in vital processes or in organs after fulfilling their functions; return of the reproductive organs to a nonpregnant state.

Iron deficiency anemia: blood disorder in which a lack of iron leads to production of smaller (microcytic) red blood cells, reducing oxygen transport throughout the body.

Isoimmune hemolytic anemia: disorder in which an antigen-antibody reaction leads to premature destruction of red blood cells.

Isoimmunization: development of antibodies in response to isoantigens (blood group antigens).

Jaundice: yellow skin discoloration caused by bilirubin accumulation in the blood and tissues.

Karyotype: chromosome complement arranged by relative size, centromere position, and staining pattern and depicted by photomicrograph.

Kegel exercises: isometric exercises in which the muscles of the pelvic diaphragm and perineum are contracted voluntarily (also called pubococcygeus exercises); helps increase contractility of the vaginal introitus and improve urine retention.

Ketosis: condition characterized by an abnormally high concentration of ketone bodies in body tissues and fluids; also called ketoacidosis.

Klinefelter's syndrome: disorder caused by an extra X chromosome in the male (XXY).

Labor: process that occurs from the onset of cervical effacement and dilation to delivery of the placenta.

Lactation: synthesis and secretion of milk from the breasts.

Lactogenesis: initiation of breast milk production.

Lactose intolerance: condition in which an individual lacks sufficient lactase (the enzyme necessary to break down lactose, or milk sugar); symptoms include diarrhea, abdominal cramps, and flatulence after ingesting milk or milk products.

Laminaria tents: dried hygroscopic seaweed cones used to dilate the cervix.

Lanugo: fine hair covering the face, shoulders, and back of the fetus or neonate before 28 weeks' gestation.

Laparoscopy: visual examination of the internal abdomen through a laparoscope (illuminated tube) inserted into the abdomen via a 1″ (2.5-cm) incision; during this procedure, a woman's reproductive organs can be assessed for causes of infertility, or sterilization can be performed by ligating the fallopian tubes through the laparoscope.

Laparotomy: 4″ to 5″ (10- to 13-cm) abdominal incision below the umbilicus; during this procedure, female sterilization can be performed by crushing, ligating, banding, or electrocoagulating the fallopian tubes.

Large for gestational age (LGA): term used to describe a neonate whose birth weight exceeds the ninetieth percentile for gestational age on the Colorado intrauterine growth chart.

MASTER GLOSSARY *(continued)*

Late deceleration: nonreassuring waveform of the fetal heart rate indicating placental insufficiency; occurs after a uterine contraction begins but does not return to baseline until the contraction is over.

Leopold's maneuvers: four abdominal palpation procedures used to determine the fetal lie, position, and presentation.

Let-down reflex: milk ejection from the breast triggered by nipple stimulation or an emotional response to the neonate.

Levator ani: one of a pair of muscles of the pelvic diaphragm that stretches across the bottom of the pelvic cavity, supporting the pelvic organs; separates into the pubococcygeus and the iliococcygeus.

Libido: psychic energy or instinctual drive associated with sexual desire, pleasure, or creativity.

Lie: relationship of the fetal long axis to the maternal long axis; may be longitudinal, oblique, or transverse.

Lightening: subjective sensation the client may feel as the fetus descends into the pelvic inlet and changes the shape and position of the uterus near term.

Linea nigra: dark line extending from the umbilicus or above to the mons pubis.

Linkage: association of genes located on the same chromosome, resulting in a tendency for some nonallelic genes to be associated in inheritance.

Lipolysis: decomposition of fat.

LMP: first day of the last menstrual period.

Lochia: vaginal discharge after delivery occurring in three distinct stages; composed of blood, tissue, leukocytes, and mucus.

Locus: the specific site of a particular gene in a chromosome (plural, loci).

Long-term variability: rhythmic fluctuations of 5 to 20 beats/minute above and below the baseline fetal heart rate, normally occurring 3 to 5 times per minute.

Low birth weight: birth weight of 1,500 to 2,500 g.

Lumpectomy: breast cancer surgery that removes only the lump; usually followed by radiation therapy.

Luteal phase: second half of the menstrual cycle from ovulation to menstruation.

Luteinizing hormone (LH): anterior pituitary hormone that stimulates ovulation and corpus luteum development.

Lymphedema: excess fluid collected in tissues of the hand and arm when lymph nodes or vessels are removed or blocked.

Macrosomia: excessively large fetus, typically weighing over 4,000 g.

Major depressive episode: disorder of emotional origin that sometimes is precipitated by childbirth; characterized by depressed mood, markedly diminished interest or pleasure in activities, significant weight loss or gain, insomnia or hypersomnia, psychomotor agitation, fatigue, feelings of worthlessness or excessive or inappropriate guilt, diminished ability to think, or recurrent thoughts of death; at least five of these symptoms must be present and at least one of the five must be either depressed mood or loss of interest.

Malformation: developmental defect.

Malpresentation: abnormal fetal presentation, such as transverse lie or breech presentation.

Marijuana: commonly abused drug obtained from the flowering tops, stems, and leaves of the hemp plant; also called cannabis sativa, weed, grass, pot, or tea.

Mastectomy: surgical removal of the breast.

Mastitis: inflammmation of breast tissue.

Maternity blues: postpartal disorder characterized by transient mood alteration involving crying episodes and sadness (also called "baby blues"); usually lasts 1 to 10 days.

Maturational crisis: intensification of problems or symptoms linked to the developmental level of an individual or family.

Mature neonate: neonate of 38 to 42 weeks' gestation; also called term neonate.

Meconium: thick, sticky, green-to-black material that collects in the fetal intestines and forms the first neonatal stool; when present in amniotic fluid, may indicate fetal distress.

Meconium aspiration syndrome (MAS): lung inflammation resulting from inhaling meconium-stained amniotic fluid in utero or when the neonate takes the first few breaths.

Meditation: relaxation technique that achieves an altered state of consciousness by slow deep-breathing and focusing on a single mental stimulus.

Megaloblastic anemia: blood condition in which immature blood cells become abnormally large, possibly because of nutrient deficiencies.

Meiosis: specialized form of cell division that produces gametes.

Menarche: onset of menses, usually occurring between ages 12 and 13.

Meningomyelocele: congenital neural tube defect in which part of the meninges and spinal cord protrudes through the vertebral column.

Menopause: cessation of menses with the decline of cyclic hormonal production and function, usually between ages 40 and 60; may begin at an earlier age—for example, after surgical removal of the uterus, ovaries, or both.

MASTER GLOSSARY (continued)

Menorrhagia: abnormally heavy or long menstrual flow; also called hypermenorrhea.

Menstruation: cyclic discharge of blood and mucosal tissue from the uterus between menarche and menopause, except during pregnancy or lactation.

Mesoderm: middle layer of the three primary germ layers of the embryo.

Methadone: synthetic narcotic used in detoxification programs to replace heroin.

Metrorrhagia: bleeding or spotting between menstrual periods.

Microcephaly: congenital anomaly characterized by abnormal smallness of the head relative to the rest of the body and by underdevelopment of the brain, with resulting mental retardation.

Minerals: nonorganic substances necessary for normal body functioning; those needed in large amounts, such as calcium, phosphorus, sodium, and magnesium, are called macrominerals; those needed in small amounts, such as iron, iodine, zinc, and fluoride, are called microminerals, trace minerals, or trace elements.

Minilaparotomy: ¾″ to 1¼″ (2- to 3-cm) abdominal incision above the pubis; during this procedure, female sterilization can be performed by crushing, ligating, banding, or electrocoagulating the fallopian tubes.

Mitosis: cell division characteristic of all cell types except gametes.

Mitral valve prolapse: cardiac disease in which the mitral valve leaflets protrude into the atrium during ventricular systole.

Mittelschmerz: abdominal pain near the ovaries during ovulation; a symptom that may help predict fertile periods in the sympto-thermal contraceptive method.

Molding: shaping of the fetal head by overlapping of the sutures, which helps the head conform to the birth canal.

Monophasic pattern: relatively flat basal body temperature that does not vary more than 0.05 degree F each day.

Monosomy: absence of one chromosome of a homologous pair.

Morbid temperature: oral temperature exceeding 100.4° F (38° C) that persists for 2 successive days after delivery, excluding the first 24 hours.

Morning-after contraceptive: oral medication given 24 to 72 hours after sexual intercourse to prevent conception; typically used in emergencies, such as rape, condom breakage, or expulsion of an intrauterine device.

Moro reflex: normal neonatal reflex elicited by dropping the neonate's head backward in a sudden motion, resulting in extension and abduction of all extremities, formation of a "C" with the fingers, and adduction, then flexion, of all extremities (as in an embrace).

Morula: small mass of cells formed after a zygote undergoes several mitotic divisions.

Mother image: each woman's concept of herself as a mother, shaped from childhood memories of her own mother, other role models, revision of her mother image through other children, literature, and her imagination.

Motivation: incentive or reason to act.

Motor maturity: full development of muscle tone and posture, including muscle coordination, muscle movements, and reflexes.

Mourning: actions or expression of grief.

Mucus plug: protective mucus barrier that blocks the cervical canal during pregnancy; caused by estrogen stimulation.

Multiparous: having given birth to one or more children.

Music therapy: relaxation technique that uses musical sounds to alter physiologic responses to stress.

Mutation: any permanent inheritable change in DNA.

Myoepithelial cells: smooth-muscle cells surrounding breast alveoli and ducts; with the let-down reflex, these cells contract and eject milk into breast ductules and sinuses.

Myometrial contractions: postpartal uterine contractions that reduce uterine size; also called afterpains.

Myometrium: uterine muscle.

Myotonia: increased muscle tension that causes voluntary and involuntary muscle contractions; a physiologic response to sexual stimulation.

Nagele's rule: method of calculating the expected date of delivery using a client's first day of the last menstrual period.

Necrotizing enterocolitis: acute inflammatory bowel disorder occurring mainly in preterm neonates.

Negligence: failure to act as a reasonable person would given similar training, experience, and circumstances.

Neonatal adaptation: physiologic and behavioral changes during the first 24 hours after delivery through which the neonate makes the transition from the intrauterine to the extrauterine environment.

Neonatal intensive care unit (NICU): nursery that provides the highest level of life-support management, including ventilatory support; heart rate, blood pressure, cardiorespiratory, and blood gas monitoring; I.V. fluid therapy; and experienced round-the-clock medical and nursing care.

Neonatal mortality: number of deaths per 1,000 live births within the first 28 days after birth.

Neonatal social behaviors: neonatal responses to actions by caregivers and others, such as smiling, gazing, cuddling, and following voices with the eyes.

MASTER GLOSSARY (continued)

Neuromuscular dissociation: relaxation technique that uses tension and relaxation of specific muscle groups to develop awareness of muscle tension.

Neutral thermal environment: narrow range of environmental temperatures at which the least amount of energy is required to maintain a stable core temperature.

Nicotine: addictive alkaloid found in tobacco.

Nipple confusion: condition in which the infant does not know how to suck properly from a nipple; caused by frequent nipple changes (such as from use of supplemental bottles during breast-feeding).

Nipple inversion: inturning or depression of the nipple.

Noncompliance: failure to act in accordance with requests, instructions, demands, or requirements.

Nondisjunction: failure of homologous chromosomes or chromatids to separate during mitosis or meiosis, resulting in daughter cells that contain unequal numbers of chromosomes.

Nonpitting edema: condition in which pressure does not leave a depression despite interstitial accumulation of excess fluid.

Nonshivering thermogenesis: heat production by lipolysis of brown fat; primary method through which the neonate produces heat.

Notochord: rod-shaped structure that defines the primitive axis of the body and forms the central developmental point of the axial skeleton.

Nuclear family: traditional family structure that includes father, mother, and their biological children.

Nulliparous: never having given birth to a child.

Nursing care plan: written guide to a client's care encompassing the assessments, nursing diagnoses, planning, goals, and interventions throughout the course of care; the plan is revised and updated as needed.

Nursing diagnosis: descriptive statement identifying actual or potential client health problems that can be resolved or diminished by nursing care; a step in the nursing process.

Nursing process: systematic problem-solving method that forms the framework for nursing practice; consists of five steps: assessment, nursing diagnosis, planning, implementation, and evaluation.

Objective data: information about a client's health status obtained through physical assessment and diagnostic study results.

Occiput posterior position: variation of the normal fetal position, in which the head enters the pelvic inlet with the occiput facing posteriorly in the oblique diameter, causing back labor.

Oligohydramnios: presence of less than 300 ml of amniotic fluid at term.

Oligospermia: abnormally low number of spermatozoa in semen.

Omphalocele: congenital anomaly in which a portion of the intestine protrudes through a defect in the abdominal wall at the umbilicus.

Oogenesis: process by which ova develop.

Opiate: narcotic drug derived from opium (such as codeine, morphine, and heroin) that may relieve pain or induce sleep.

Oral contraceptive: hormonal compound (estrogen, progestin, or both) that is taken by mouth and inhibits ovulation.

Orientation: neonate's ability to respond to visual and auditory stimuli.

Osteoporosis: decreased bone mass, occurring most commonly in menopausal women.

Out-of-phase endometrium: discrepancy of 2 or more days between the ovulatory date, cycle date, and histologic date of the endometrium.

Ovaries: female gonads; glands located on each side of the pelvis that contain ova and secrete the hormones estrogen and progesterone.

Ovulation: maturation and discharge of an ovum from the ovary in response to hormonal stimulation during the menstrual cycle.

Ovum: female gamete (plural, ova).

Oxytocin: hormone secreted by the posterior pituitary gland that stimulates uterine smooth-muscle contractions and breast milk ejection; also, a synthetic hormone (Pitocin) that simulates the actions of the natural hormone.

Oxytocin receptors: cellular structures in the breast that are sensitive to the effects of oxytocin.

Paced breathing: learned breathing technique that aids relaxation and helps the client maintain control during labor contractions; may be slow, modified, or patterned.

Papanicolaou (Pap) test: cytologic study of stained exfoliated cells to detect and diagnose certain conditions in the female reproductive tract, particularly premalignant and malignant conditions, such as cancer of the vagina, cervix, and endometrium.

Paracervical block: regional anesthesia technique that blocks nerve conduction on both sides of the cervix, relieving uterine pain during the first stage of active labor.

Parity: obstetric classification of a woman by the number of births and stillbirths that occur after 28 weeks of gestation.

Patent ductus arteriosus: abnormal opening between the pulmonary artery and the aorta; results from failure of the fetal ductus arteriosus to close after birth (seen mainly in the preterm neonate).

MASTER GLOSSARY *(continued)*

Pathologic jaundice: condition marked by yellow skin discoloration and an increase in the serum bilirubin level (above 13 mg/dl); arising within 24 hours after birth, it results from blood type or blood group incompatibility, infection, or biliary, hepatic, or metabolic abnormalities.

Pathologic mourning: mourning that does not lead to resolution of grief.

Peau d'orange: orange-peel-like appearance of breast skin caused by edema.

Pedigree: diagram of a family tree depicting occurrence of one or more traits in the various family members.

Pelvic examination: assessment of the external and internal genitalia by inspection and palpation.

Pelvic inflammatory disease (PID): infection of the oviducts, ovaries, and adjacent tissue; may result from intrauterine device use or a sexually transmitted disease.

Pelvis: bony structure made up of the sacrum, coccyx, and innominate bones; passageway through which the fetus travels during labor.

Penetrance: frequency with which a gene manifests itself in phenotypes of individuals with that gene.

Perceived support: belief that help is available if needed.

Perimenopausal: occurring during the climacteric stage.

Perinatal period: period extending from the twenty-eighth week of gestation to the end of the fourth week after birth.

Perineum: region between the vulva and anus; bounded in front by the pubic arch and the arcuate ligaments, in back by the tip of the coccyx, and laterally by the inferior rami of the pubis and ischium and the sacrotuberus ligaments.

Periods of neonatal reactivity: predictable, identifiable series of behavioral and physiologic characteristics occurring during the first hours after birth; characterized by distinctive changes in vital signs, state of alertness, and responsiveness to external stimuli.

Peripartum cardiomyopathy: cardiac disease in which the left ventricle functions abnormally during the last month of pregnancy or first 6 postpartal months.

Pessary: device inserted into the vagina to treat uterine prolapse, uterine retroversion, or cervical incompetence.

Phenotype: observable expression of a genetically determined trait.

Phenylketonuria: autosomal recessive disorder characterized by the abnormal presence of metabolites of phenylalanine (such as phenylketone) in the urine.

Physiologic jaundice: common condition of the full-term neonate marked by yellow skin discoloration and an increase in the serum bilirubin level (4 to 12 mg/dl); arising 48 to 72 hours after birth and peaking by the third to fifth day, it results from neonatal hepatic immaturity.

Pica: consumption of nonfood items.

Pitting edema: condition in which pressed tissues leave a small depression or pit; caused by interstitial accumulation of excess fluid.

Placenta accreta: condition in which part or all of the placenta adheres firmly to the uterine wall.

Placenta increta: condition in which placental villi invade the uterine myometrium.

Placenta percreta: condition in which placental villi penetrate the myometrium to the peritoneal covering of the uterus.

Placenta previa: abnormally low implantation of the placenta so that it encroaches onto the internal cervical os.

Placental insufficiency: inadequate or improper functioning of the placenta leading to a compromised intrauterine environment that jeopardizes the fetus.

Planning: one step in the nursing process that includes setting and prioritizing goals for each nursing diagnosis, formulating interventions to help the client achieve these goals, and developing the nursing care plan.

Pleiotropy: multiple signs and symptoms caused by one or two genes.

Poikilotherm: neonate who takes on the temperature of the environment.

Polar body: small, nonfunctional cell produced along with a functioning ovum during oogenesis.

Polycystic kidney disease: condition characterized by formation of multiple cysts within the kidney, leading to kidney enlargement and destruction of adjacent tissue.

Polycythemia: abnormal increase in the number of red blood cells; in the neonate, it results from maternal-fetal transfusion, delayed umbilical cord clamping, or placental insufficiency.

Polydipsia: excessive thirst; a characteristic symptom of diabetes mellitus.

Polymenorrhea: increased frequency of menstrual bleeding.

Polyphagia: excessive hunger; a characteristic symptom of diabetes mellitus.

Polypharmacy: practice of taking different drugs simultaneously in varying dosages.

Polyuria: excessive urine excretion; a characteristic sign of diabetes mellitus.

MASTER GLOSSARY (continued)

Position: relationship of the leading fetal presenting part to a point on the maternal pelvis.

Posterior urethral valves: congenital anomaly characterized by urinary tract obstruction, hydronephrosis, and impaired urine flow.

Postpartal hemorrhage: abnormally large amount (more than 500 ml) of bleeding after delivery, which may be caused by uterine atony, rupture, lacerations, inversion, or hematoma.

Postpartal period: approximately 6-week period following delivery during which the anatomic and physiologic changes resulting from pregnancy resolve; also called puerperium.

Postterm neonate: neonate born after completion of week 42 of gestation; also called postmature neonate.

Pre-embryo: developing organism from implantation through week 3, when—according to most authorities—the organism becomes an embryo.

Precipitate labor: labor that proceeds very rapidly, usually lasting less than 3 hours.

Precipitous delivery: unusually rapid delivery.

Preeclampsia: nonconvulsive form of pregnancy-induced hypertension characterized by the onset of acute hypertension, proteinuria, and edema after the twenty-fourth week of gestation; called eclampsia when it includes seizures and coma.

Pregnancy-induced hypertension (PIH): group of potentially life-threatening hypertensive disorders that may develop in the second or third trimester; includes preeclampsia and eclampsia.

Premenstrual syndrome (PMS): cyclic cluster of signs and symptoms, such as breast tenderness, fluid retention, and mood swings, that usually occurs after ovulation and before or during menses.

Presentation: fetal part that enters the maternal pelvis first and can be touched through the cervix; may be cephalic, breech, or shoulder.

Presenting part: portion of the fetus that first enters the pelvic passageway.

Preterm neonate: neonate born before completion of week 37 of gestation; also called premature neonate.

Primary infertility: failure to conceive by a couple in which the woman has never been pregnant.

Primiparous: giving birth for the first time.

Primitive streak: small aggregation of cells at the caudal end of the embryo that offers early evidence of the embryonic axis.

Progressive muscle relaxation: systematic muscle contraction and relaxation to reduce tension.

Projection: defense mechanism that involves attributing to someone else traits that are unacceptable in oneself.

Prolactin: hormone causing breast milk production; secreted by the anterior pituitary gland in response to tactile stimulation of the breast.

Prolonged deceleration: decrease in the fetal heart rate from the baseline lasting several minutes or longer in response to a sudden stimulus of the vagal system, such as uterine tachysystole, anesthetics, or maternal hypotension.

Prostaglandin: naturally occurring hydroxy fatty acid that stimulates uterine contractions.

Protein: energy source, essential in various body functions, that provides 4 calories/g; can be complete (providing all 9 essential amino acids in the proportion needed for growth) or incomplete.

Proteinuria: presence in the urine of abnormally large amounts of protein, usually albumin.

Protractility: state of nipple protrusion rather than inversion.

Psychoprophylactic method: childbirth preparation technique developed by Ferdinand Lamaze that emphasizes concentration, relaxation, and education.

Psychosis: major mental disorder of organic or emotional origin characterized by extreme personality derangement or disorganization; commonly accompanied by severe depression, agitation, regressive behavior, illusions, delusions, and hallucinations so severe that the individual loses touch with reality, cannot function normally, and usually requires hospitalization.

Puberty: developmental stage early in adolescence when reproductive ability begins and secondary sex characteristics develop.

Pudendal block: regional anesthesia technique used during the second stage of labor to numb the perineum and vagina, primarily for episiotomy repair.

Puerperal infection: invasion by microorganisms of the reproductive tract during the postpartal period.

Puerperium: 6-week period after childbirth.

Pyelonephritis: acute inflammation of the ureters and kidneys, commonly caused by *Escherichia coli*; produces the effects of cystitis plus fever, chills, flank pain, and other signs and symptoms.

Quickening: first awareness of fetal movement, typically felt after 16 to 20 weeks.

Radiant warmer: open bed with an overhead radiant heat source.

Radiation: transfer of heat from one surface to another without contact between the surfaces; a mechanism of heat loss or gain.

Rationalization: defense mechanism that involves creation of reasons to justify painful or unacceptable situations or actions.

Reaction formation: defense mechanism that involves behaving in a way exactly opposite to an unconscious wish.

MASTER GLOSSARY *(continued)*

Received support: activities performed to assist a person.

Recessive: incapable of genetic expression unless the responsible allele is carried on both members of a pair of homologous chromosomes.

Reciprocity: process in which a neonate gives cues and the parent or other caregiver interprets, then responds to, the cues.

Recommended dietary allowances (RDAs): specific quantities of essential nutrients for different ages, sexes, and conditions judged adequate to maintain nutritional status of nearly all healthy people by the Food and Nutrition Board of the National Academy of Sciences.

Rectocele: herniation of the rectum into the vagina.

Reflex: involuntary function or movement of any organ or body part in response to a stimulus.

Refractory period: time after an orgasm when restimulation and orgasm are not possible for a man.

Regional anesthesia: direct nerve block following injection of a local anesthetic agent.

Regionalization of care: system that avoids costly duplication of services and ensures availability of essential services in a geographical area; hospitals and special facilities, such as neonatal intensive care units and trauma units, are classified as primary, secondary, and tertiary health centers, depending on the facilities and personnel available, the population served, the number of beds in the facility, and other criteria.

Regression: defense mechanism of retreat to an earlier developmental phase to reduce the demands of maturity.

Renal agenesis: congenital absence of one kidney (unilateral renal agenesis) or both kidneys (bilateral renal agenesis).

Repression: defense mechanism of unconscious exclusion from the conscious mind of painful impulses, desires, or fears.

Respiratory distress syndrome: acute, potentially fatal neonatal lung disorder (most common in preterm neonates), resulting from surfactant deficiency; characterized by a respiratory rate greater than 60 breaths/minute, lung inelasticity, nasal flaring, expiratory grunts, chest retractions, and peripheral edema.

Respite care: care provided by a secondary caregiver to relieve the primary caregiver; may be required for hours or weeks.

Retained placenta: condition in which the placenta remains in the uterus 30 minutes after the second stage of labor.

Retinopathy of prematurity (ROP): disease of the retinal vasculature associated with oxygen therapy in the preterm neonate; formerly called retrolental fibroplasia.

Retroflexed uterus: position in which the uterine corpus flexes toward the rectum and the cervix lies in the normal position.

Retroverted uterus: position in which the uterine corpus flexes toward the rectum at a less acute angle than a retroflexed uterus.

Rheumatic heart disease: cardiac disease in which an untreated streptococcal infection leads to bacterial invasion and alteration of the mitral or tricuspid valve.

Rh incompatibility: isoimmune hemolytic anemia in which maternal antibodies cause destruction of fetal red blood cells, leading to severe anemia and jaundice in the neonate.

Rh isoimmunization: sensitization of maternal blood antibodies against fetal blood antigens, which can create a serious blood incompatibility during pregnancy and can lead to erythroblastosis fetalis.

Rhythm method: natural contraceptive method that predicts a fertile period by analyzing the length of eight previous menstrual cycles; also called calendar method.

Ripe cervix: soft, effaced, dilated cervix.

Role: set of repetitive behaviors adopted consciously or unconsciously that provides consistency in family relationships and accomplishment of tasks.

Rooting reflex: normal neonatal response elicited by stroking the cheek or corner of the mouth with a finger or nipple, resulting in turning of the head toward the stimulus.

Rugae: transverse folds in the vaginal mucosa.

Rupture of the membranes: rupture of the amniotic sac, followed within 24 hours by labor in about 80% of women.

Salpingitis: inflammation or infection of the fallopian tube.

Scalp electrode: small spiral electrode attached to the fetal scalp to provide direct monitoring with a fetal electrocardiogram.

Scanning: technique for relieving stress by identifying and then relaxing tense muscles.

Scarf sign: term describing the distance that the neonate's elbow can be extended across the chest toward the opposite side; an index of gestational age.

Secondary infertility: failure to conceive by a couple in which the woman has been pregnant before but now cannot conceive or carry a pregnancy to term.

Second stage of labor: period that begins with complete cervical dilation and ends with delivery of the neonate.

Secretory phase: first half of the menstrual cycle from menstruation to ovulation.

Secundines: placenta and membranes expelled after delivery; the afterbirth.

Self-care: active and assertive participation in attaining one's health care goals.

MASTER GLOSSARY *(continued)*

Self-differentiation: personal growth characterized by identification of one's abilities, actions, and relationships with others.

Self-esteem: degree to which one values oneself.

Self-quieting behaviors: actions the neonate uses to quiet the self when crying, including hand-to-mouth movements, fist sucking, and attending to external stimuli (evaluated during the behavioral assessment).

Semen: white, viscous secretion of male reproductive organs consisting of spermatozoa and nutrient fluids ejaculated through the penile urethra.

Sexuality: ongoing process of recognizing, accepting, and expressing oneself as a sexual being.

Sexually transmitted disease (STD): disorder acquired through vaginal, anal, or oral intercourse.

Short-term variability: Beat-to-beat changes in the fetal heart rate (FHR); normal short-term variability is 2 to 3 beats/minute from the baseline FHR.

Sibling rivalry: competition between siblings for parental love and approval.

Sickle cell anemia: autosomal recessive blood disorder in which hemoglobin molecules become sickle- or crescent-shaped, which affects their oxygen-carrying capacity and causes vessel obstruction.

Situational crisis: intensification of problems or symptoms linked to a traumatic event.

Small for gestational age (SGA): term used to describe a neonate who experienced intrauterine growth retardation and whose birth weight falls below the tenth percentile for gestational age on the Colorado intrauterine growth chart.

Smegma: sebaceous secretion that accumulates under the foreskin of the penis and at the base of the labia minora.

Smith's minor abnormalities: neonatal physiologic variations, such as abnormal dermal ridges, that may indicate major anomalies (for example, Down's syndrome).

Somatic complaints: physical symptoms caused by psychological concerns.

Spermatogenesis: process by which spermatozoa develop.

Spermatozoon: male gamete (plural, spermatozoa).

Spermicide: chemical substance that kills spermatozoa; the active ingredient in contraceptive foams, creams, suppositories, and jellies.

Spinnbarkeit: stretchiness of cervical mucus at ovulation; caused by estrogen.

Spontaneous abortion: abrupt termination of pregnancy from natural causes before the age of viability.

Square window sign: term describing the degree to which the neonate's wrist can be flexed against the forearm; an index of gestational age.

Standardized nursing care plan: care plan developed for a group of clients with similar physical, emotional, or learning needs that reflects common standards of care.

Standards of care: acts that a reasonable person would have performed or omitted under specific circumstances; conduct against which the defendant's actions are judged in a malpractice case.

Station: relationship of the fetal presenting part to the maternal ischial spine.

Sterilization: process that terminates fertility, rendering an individual unable to reproduce.

Striae gravidarum: pink streaks in the skin caused by separated connective tissue; typically appear on the breasts, abdomen, buttocks, or thighs and turn silvery after childbirth; also called stretch marks.

Subjective data: assessment information obtained from the client and others with intimate knowledge of the client, typically through interviews.

Substance abuse: maladaptive pattern of continued substance use despite knowledge of impaired social, occupational, psychological, or physical functioning caused or exacerbated by the substance; abused substances can include nicotine (in tobacco), alcohol, and legal and illegal drugs.

Substance dependence: cluster of cognitive, behavioral, and physiologic symptoms that indicate impaired control of substance use as evidenced by tolerance and withdrawal symptoms.

Sucking reflex: normal neonatal reflex elicited by inserting a finger or nipple in the neonate's mouth, resulting in forceful, rhythmic sucking.

Summative evaluation: process in which the nurse and client judge progress toward goals after home visits are discontinued.

Support: feelings of affection, trust, affirmation, and the sharing of advice, information, and time between people.

Support person: partner, friend, or family member who provides continuous support during labor and delivery.

Surfactant: phospholipid produced by Type II alveolar cells in the alveolar lining of the lungs; decreases alveolar inflation pressures, improves lung compliance, and provides alveolar stability, thereby decreasing effort in breathing.

Sympto-thermal method: natural contraceptive method that predicts fertile periods based on basal body temperature, cervical mucus changes, and such symptoms as mittelschmerz and changes in libido.

MASTER GLOSSARY (continued)

Synactive theory of development: Als's theory proposing that the neonate continuously interacts with the environment and that the neonate's physiologic status depends on the environmental stimuli received and processed.

Synchrony: interaction in which each party acts and reacts in a manner appropriate to the cues given.

Synclitism: state in which the fetal biparietal diameter is parallel to the plane of the maternal pelvic inlet.

Syphilis: sexually transmitted disease caused by *Treponema pallidum*, which produces painless, papular lesions (chancres) and may progress through various stages to heart damage, seizures, and death.

T$_4$ lymphocyte: type of lymph cell that is vital to the body's immune response.

Tachysystole: contractions occurring more frequently than every 2 minutes.

Tenesmus: persistent, ineffectual spasms of the rectum or bladder accompanied by the desire to empty the bowel or bladder.

Teratoma: congenital neoplasm consisting of various cell types, none of which normally occur together.

Term neonate: neonate of 38 to 42 weeks' gestation; also called mature neonate.

Testes: male gonads; reproductive glands contained in the scrotum that produce spermatozoa and the androgenic hormone testosterone.

Tetanic uterine contraction: sustained uterine contraction lasting 70 seconds or longer, occurring more than once every 3 minutes, and increasing intrauterine pressure to 75 mm Hg or more.

Therapeutic abortion: termination of a pregnancy for medical reasons (physiologic or psychological) before the age of viability.

Therapeutic communication: interaction that focuses on attaining client goals rather than on the mutual pleasure received from social communication.

Therapeutic empathy: ability to view experiences, emotions, and thoughts from a client's perspective and to use that knowledge to build the client's awareness and help set goals.

Thermoregulation: maintenance of body temperature by complex interaction between environmental temperature and body heat loss and production.

Third stage of labor: period that begins with complete delivery of the neonate and ends with delivery of the placenta.

Thrombophlebitis: formation of a thrombus (clot) in response to inflammation of the vein wall.

Tocodynamometer: externally applied pressure-sensitive device that records the frequency and duration of uterine contractions.

TORCH infections: acronym for a group of infections, including toxoplasmosis, other infections (chlamydia, group B beta hemolytic streptococcus, syphilis, and varicella zoster), rubella, cytomegalovirus, and herpesvirus type 2.

Touch therapy: relaxation technique that uses tactile stimulation to alter perceptions of discomfort during labor.

Toxic shock syndrome (TSS): rare, potentially fatal, multisystem disorder caused by a toxin secreted by *Staphylococcus aureus;* has been associated with improper tampon use and typically causes sudden high fever, vomiting, diarrhea, myalgia, vaginal redness or discharge, skin rash, and sore throat.

Toxicity: quality or quantity of a substance that makes it poisonous.

Transcutaneous electric nerve stimulation (TENS): use of electric current to counterstimulate nerve fibers and thus block pain transmission.

Transient tachypnea: neonatal disorder characterized by rapid, shallow breathing (possibly accompanied by cyanosis) that lasts a few hours or days; caused by the retention of fetal lung fluid that follows cesarean delivery.

Transitional period: time during which the neonate experiences biological and behavioral adaptations to extrauterine life; normally lasts about 24 hours.

Transverse lie: presentation in which the long axis of the fetus is perpendicular to that of the mother.

Trichomoniasis: sexually transmitted disease caused by *Trichomonas vaginalis*, which is characterized by vaginal discharge, urinary symptoms, and vulvar edema, pruritus, and tenderness.

Trisomy: presence of an extra chromosome in a diploid cell.

Trophoblast: layer of ectoderm on the outside of the blastocyst that implants the embryo in the uterine wall and forms the chorion, amnion, and chorionic villi.

True labor: characterized by regular contractions that increase in intensity and duration as the intervals between them decrease, along with progressive effacement and cervical dilation.

Ultrasound: method of external electronic fetal monitoring that sends low-energy, high-frequency sound waves through the abdominal wall in the direction of the fetal heart; waves are translated into audible fetal heart tones and fetal heart rate waveforms.

Universal precautions: infection control measures that treat all blood and body fluids as potentially infectious.

Urethritis: urethral inflammation caused by a lower urinary tract infection, which produces the same effects as cystitis.

Urinary tract infection (UTI): invasion by microorganisms of one or more structures of the urinary tract; most commonly caused by gram-negative bacteria.

MASTER GLOSSARY *(continued)*

Uterine atony: poor uterine muscle tone.

Uterine inversion: abnormal condition in which the uterus is turned inside out so that the internal surface protrudes into or beyond the vagina; usually caused by excessive traction on the umbilical cord.

Uterine involution: gradual return of the uterus to a nonpregnant size and condition after labor and delivery.

Uterine prolapse: downward displacement of the uterus from its normal position in the pelvis.

Uterine souffle: blowing sound heard with a stethoscope as blood flows through the uterine arteries to the placenta.

Uterine subinvolution: failure of the uterus to return to a nonpregnant size and condition after labor and delivery.

Vacuum curettage: surgical method of pregnancy interruption that requires cervical dilatation and suction equipment to evacuate the uterine contents.

Vacuum extraction: procedure using a cup-shaped suction device applied to the fetus's scalp to provide traction for delivery.

Vaginal introitus: entrance to the vagina.

Vaginitis: vaginal inflammation that may be caused by fungi, protozoa, or bacteria.

Variability: beat-to-beat changes in the fetal heart rate that reflect the degree of tonic balance between the sympathetic and parasympathetic nervous systems.

Variable deceleration: nonuniform deceleration pattern indicating cord compression of variable significance; the most common deceleration pattern in labor, usually well tolerated by the fetus.

Varicosity: enlarged, tortuous area of a vessel; in pregnancy, typically venous varicosities of the legs, rectum, or vulva.

Vasectomy: male sterilization procedure that requires cutting and tying or cauterizing of part of the vas deferens.

Vasocongestion: blood vessel engorgement and increased blood flow to tissues; a physiologic response to sexual stimulation.

VBAC: vaginal birth after cesarean delivery.

Vegetarian: individual who avoids all animal products (vegan), all but eggs and milk (lacto-ovo vegetarian), all but poultry (pollo-vegetarian), or all but fish (pesco-vegetarian).

Ventouse: suction cup used in vacuum extraction.

Ventral suspension: term describing the degree to which the neonate extends the back, flexes the arms and legs, and holds the head upright when an examiner positions the neonate prone and places a hand under the chest; an index of gestational age.

Vernix caseosa: grayish white, cheeselike substance composed of sebaceous gland secretions and desquamated epithelial cells that covers the near-term fetus and neonate.

Version: procedure for turning the fetus in utero to a position favorable for delivery.

Very low birth weight: birth weight of 500 to 1,500 g.

Viability: age and weight at which the fetus is capable of surviving outside the uterus (usually 24 weeks and 50l g).

Vitamins: compounds needed in small amounts for normal body functioning; may be fat-soluble (stored in fat) or water-soluble (incapable of being stored by the body).

Vulvitis: vulvar inflammation, which may be caused by fungi, protozoa, bacteria, other organisms, chemical irritation, or allergic reaction.

Womb name: nickname by which expectant parents refer to the fetus during pregnancy.

Zona pellucida: noncellular layer covering the surface of a mature ovarian follicle.

Zygote: diploid cell formed by the union of a haploid ovum and spermatozoon; develops into an embryo.

INDEX

i refers to an illustration; t, to a table.

i refers to an illustration; t, to a table.

i refers to an illustration; t, to a table.

i refers to an illustration; t, to a table.

i refers to an illustration; t, to a table.

i refers to an illustration; t, to a table.

i refers to an illustration; t, to a table.

i refers to an illustration; t, to a table.

i refers to an illustration; t, to a table.